Second Edition

PHYSICAL ACTIVITY EPIDEMIOLOGY

Rod K. Dishman, PhD

University of Georgia, Athens

Gregory W. Heath, DHSc, MPH

University of Tennessee, Chattanooga

I-Min Lee, MBBS, MPH, ScD

Harvard Medical School, Boston

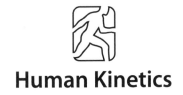

Human Kinetics

Library of Congress Cataloging-in-Publication Data

Dishman, Rod K.
  Physical activity epidemiology / Rod K. Dishman, Gregory W. Heath, I-Min Lee. -- 2nd ed.
      p. ; cm.
  Includes bibliographical references and index.
  ISBN 978-0-7360-8286-0 (hardcover) -- ISBN 0-7360-8286-7 (hardcover)
  I. Heath, Gregory. II. Lee, I-Min. III. Title.
  [DNLM: 1. Exercise. 2. Epidemiologic Methods. 3. Health Promotion. QT 255]

  613.7'1--dc23

                              2012009493

ISBN-10: 0-7360-8286-7 (print)
ISBN-13: 978-0-7360-8286-0 (print)

The web addresses cited in this text were current as of March 2012, unless otherwise noted.

Acquisitions Editor: Myles Schrag; **Managing Editor:** Katherine Maurer; **Assistant Editors:** Steven Calderwood, Brendan Shea, and Kali Cox; **Copyeditor:** Joyce Sexton; **Indexer:** Nancy Ball; **Permissions Manager:** Dalene Reeder; **Graphic Designer:** Fred Starbird; **Graphic Artist:** Yvonne Griffith; **Cover Designer:** Keith Blomberg; **Photographer (cover):** Ken Straiton/ First Light/age fotostock; **Visual Production Assistant:** Joyce Brumfield; **Photo Production Manager:** Jason Allen; **Art Manager:** Kelly Hendren; **Associate Art Manager:** Alan L. Wilborn; **Art Style Development:** Joanne Brummett; **Illustrations:** © Human Kinetics unless otherwise indicated; **Printer:** Edwards Brothers Malloy

Printed in the United States of America   10 9 8 7 6 5 4 3 2 1

The paper in this book is certified under a sustainable forestry program.

Human Kinetics
Website: www.HumanKinetics.com

United States: Human Kinetics
P.O. Box 5076
Champaign, IL 61825-5076
800-747-4457
e-mail: humank@hkusa.com

Canada: Human Kinetics
475 Devonshire Road Unit 100
Windsor, ON N8Y 2L5
800-465-7301 (in Canada only)
e-mail: info@hkcanada.com

Europe: Human Kinetics
107 Bradford Road
Stanningley
Leeds LS28 6AT, United Kingdom
+44 (0) 113 255 5665
e-mail: hk@hkeurope.com

Australia: Human Kinetics
57A Price Avenue
Lower Mitcham, South Australia 5062
08 8372 0999
e-mail: info@hkaustralia.com

New Zealand: Human Kinetics
P.O. Box 80
Torrens Park, South Australia 5062
0800 222 062
e-mail: info@hknewzealand.com

E4800

To serious students.

To Henry J. Montoye and Ralph S. Paffenbarger Jr. To Sharon and our scholar-athletes, Jessica, Corinne, Adrienne, Ben, Jackson, Emme, and Paris. To my mother, Virginia, and the memory of my father, Willard, a hardworking farmer who knew about quality of life and outlived his birth cohort.

> Knowing is not enough; we must apply.
> Willing is not enough; we must do.
> —*Johann Wolfgang von Goethe*
>
> Rod K. Dishman

To my mother, Lovell, and the memory of my father, Ernest, who as a physician taught me that good science has hands and a heart. To John Holloszy and Ken Powell, who did their best to equip me as an applied physiologist and epidemiologist.

> A student is not above his teacher,
> but everyone who is fully trained will be like his teacher.
> —*Saint Luke 6:40*
>
> Gregory W. Heath

To the memory of three people who were physically active before science deemed it healthful: my grandmother, Ng Phoy Lan; my mentor and friend, Ralph S. Paffenbarger Jr.; and my esteemed colleague and friend, Jerry Morris.

To my parents, Keng Yew and Nguk Huong, and my husband, Geoff.

> I-Min Lee

CONTENTS

PART THREE

Physical Activity and Risk Factors

· 143 ·

PART SIX

Physical Activity and Special Concerns

· 377 ·

Physical activity has endured as an important part of hygiene in many cultures since antiquity. This book is about how the methods of epidemiology are being used to confirm scientifically that physical inactivity is a burden on public health and what can be done about it. Epidemiology is the study of the distribution of disease and other health events in a population. Behavioral epidemiology is the observation and study of behaviors that lead to disease or premature death and of the distribution of these behaviors. In this way, behavioral epidemiology goes beyond the traditional focus of epidemiology on infectious diseases, the containment of bacterial and viral contagion. Though traditional epidemiology is concerned with preventive measures, the emphasis is on environmental intervention (e.g., sewage disposal, water purification, or inoculation programs for viruses). In behavioral epidemiology, the focus shifts to understanding behaviors that decrease or increase the risk of people's developing diseases (e.g., hand washing, medical screening for tumors, sharing of hypodermic needles by drug abusers). Behavioral epidemiology is especially important for understanding and preventing chronic diseases, which develop over periods of years largely as a result of people's habits, such as physical inactivity.

Physical activity epidemiology is a specific branch of behavioral epidemiology. Thus, physical activity epidemiology is composed of two main features. The first is the study of relationships between physical activity, and conversely physical inactivity, and disease using the traditional methods of epidemiology. The second feature is the study of the distribution and putative determinants of physical activity in a population. Once it is established by convincing epidemiologic evidence that physical activity appears causally linked with disease, injury, or early death, the next goal of physical activity epidemiology is to determine how physical activity can be altered in order to reduce the frequency of disease, injury, or early death.

Physical activity epidemiology is a new field, about 60 years old, but it has evolved from old ideas dating to the use of structured exercise for health promotion in China around 2500 BC; the ancient Indian Ayurveda system of medicine of the ninth century BC; and the use of vigorous exercise (gymnastics) by ancient Greek physicians Herodicus, Hippocrates, Asclepiades, and Galen. Even during the Middle Ages in Europe, when the influence of Greek writings was obscured until the Renaissance, the Greek medical tradition of using exercise was preserved by the Arabs and later translated from Arabic into Latin medical manuals, the *Tacuinum Sanitatis*. The work *Sirr al-asrar,* reportedly written by Aristotle, is believed to be the basis of the famous poem of medicine, *Regimen Sanitatis Salernitanum,* which was published at the medical school at Salerno, Italy, in the 12th century and which mentioned the healthful benefits of physical activity. Rabbi Moses ben Maimum, the Jewish philosopher of the 12th century and physician to Saladin, the sultan of Egypt, advocated healthful exercise in the *Mishnah Torah.* During the Renaissance, scholars in Italy renewed interest in classical Greek gymnastics and recommended it as a fundamental part of education. The 14th-century Italian poet laureate, Francesco Petrarca, encouraged exercise as a natural remedy to replace medicines that "poison the body" in his 1354 work, *Invective Contra Medicum (Protest Against the Doctor).* In 1772, Benjamin Rush, Philadelphia physician and father of American psychiatry, delivered a "Sermon on Exercise" in which he recommended sports and exercises for people of all ages. His plan of a Federal University included exercise, laying the foundation for exercise and fitness in preventive medicine, which was perpetuated during the mid-to-late 19th century by early American physician educators at Harvard and Yale universities.

The modern history of physical activity epidemiology is short, however. Though many researchers have contributed, modern physical activity epidemiology has its roots in the studies by Dr. Jeremy Morris, professor emeritus of public health at the London School of Hygiene and Tropical Medicine of the University of London, who found in the early 1950s that the highly active conductors on London's double-decker buses were at lower risk of coronary heart disease than the drivers, who sat through their shifts at the steering wheel. That work was shortly followed, in the 1960s and 1970s, by the first of many studies by Dr. Ralph Paffenbarger, professor emeritus of medicine at Stanford University, who found that the risk of heart disease was inversely related to the amount of work done by San Francisco longshoremen and the amount of leisure-time physical activity among Harvard alumni. During that time, Henry Montoye began his pioneering development of measures of physical activity and fitness for use in epidemiologic studies. The impact of these men's work was especially noteworthy at the time because physical activity was not yet considered by epidemiologists to be an important influence on public health worthy of study.

Despite traditional epidemiologists' lack of acceptance that physical activity had a proven benefit to health, in 1980 the U.S. Public Health Service identified physical fitness and exercise as one of 15 areas of focus of the national objectives for improving people's health. Recognizing, however, that the scientific basis of physical activity as a national health objective was not yet solid, the Centers for Disease Control and Prevention (CDC) created the Behavioral Epidemiology and Evaluation Branch (BEEB) within the Center for Health Promotion and Education of the Division of Health

Education. Under the direction of Dr. Kenneth Powell, its main purpose was monitoring progress of the nation's 1990 goals for physical activity and fitness. To help with this purpose, the Behavioral Risk Factor Surveillance System (BRFSS) was begun to monitor activity in most of the United States, and the Workshop on Epidemiologic and Public Health Aspects of Physical Activity and Exercise was held in Atlanta on September 24 and 25, 1984, which culminated in the publication of summaries of current knowledge and directions for future research in physical activity epidemiology.

Another historical focal point in the modern history of physical activity epidemiology was the first International Conference on Exercise, Fitness, and Health, organized by Professor Claude Bouchard under the auspices of the Canadian Association of Sport Sciences and the Ontario Ministry of Tourism and Recreation. Held in Toronto in the spring of 1988, the conference resulted in scientific consensus statements summarizing the world's knowledge about exercise, fitness, and health. The widespread impact of that conference and the resulting book, as well as a rapidly growing knowledge base, led to the Second International Consensus Symposium on Physical Activity, Fitness, and Health, held in Toronto in May 1992, which updated the knowledge summarized in the first conference.

Key documents published in the United States include a position statement by the American Heart Association in 1992 recognizing physical inactivity as an independent risk factor for coronary heart disease and recommendations on physical activity and public health, prepared jointly by the Centers for Disease Control and Prevention and the American College of Sports Medicine and published in the *Journal of the American Medical Association* in 1995. In the historical benchmark *Physical Activity and Health: A Report of the Surgeon General,* published in 1996, nearly 100 experts, led by Steven Blair, then director of epidemiology and clinical applications at the Cooper Institute for Aerobics Research in Dallas, outlined the consensus in the scientific community about the beneficial effects of physical activity. That capstone publication signaled the maturation of the field of physical activity epidemiology by providing a scientific footing for the development of public health guidelines and policy about physical activity and by outlining a host of questions for future study. That scientific basis grew exponentially, and in 2008 the first-ever federal *Physical Activity Guidelines for Americans* was published. In that same year, the International Society for Physical Activity and Health was incorporated as a professional society for the advancement of the science and practice of physical activity and health worldwide. The society's incorporation was another sign of the maturity of the field of physical activity epidemiology.

The purpose of this book is to summarize this still growing body of knowledge, the methods used to obtain it, its implications for public health, and the important questions that remain. A unique feature of the book is the application of the cardinal principles used by epidemiologists to infer cause-and-effect relationships about physical activity and health risk. Other novel features of the book are chapters that specifically address the measurement and surveillance of physical activity and fitness in a population and the problem of motivating large numbers of youth and adults to become more physically active in their leisure time. In this second edition of *Physical Activity Epidemiology*, we kept the original topics of the first edition but updated the content extensively to be contemporary with the rapidly expanding body of evidence. For example, separate chapters are now dedicated to all-cause mortality and cardiovascular disease mortality. A large section on studies of patients with inflammatory diseases has been added to the chapter on immunology to give it a more clinical perspective. More information on people from special populations and health disparities has been added to the chapter on disability, and a new section on the built environment and social interventions to promote physical activity participation has been added to the chapter on adoption and maintenance of physical activity. In addition, this new edition includes expanded coverage of pathophysiology and biological plausibility and of the effects of physical activity on cognitive function, dementia, and HIV/AIDS.

The social significance of exercise and other forms of physical activity in developed and developing nations has never been greater. In the United States, physical inactivity is a burden on the public's health, accounting for an estimated 200,000 deaths annually from coronary heart disease, type 2 diabetes mellitus, and colon cancer. The combined effect of physical inactivity and excess caloric intake accounts for an estimated 300,000 deaths each year and is a key contributor to the 50% increase in the prevalence of obesity, as well as a similar increase in the risk of type 2 diabetes, among U.S. adults and youth during the past decade. For the first time, obesity is a bigger world health problem than malnutrition. Growing evidence also supports that physical inactivity is a risk factor for poor mental health, especially depression, which the World Health Organization has projected will be second only to cardiovascular disease as the world's leading cause of death and disability by the year 2020 and will be first by 2030.

The promotion of leisure-time physical activity has emerged as an important initiative for public health and quality of living in many economically developed nations. *Healthy People 2020,* the national health goals of the U.S. Department of Health and Human Services, includes several objectives that collectively call for increasing physical activity in all segments of the U.S. population and also provide new developmental objectives for public policy to promote physical activity. Similar policy statements about the health importance of physical activity have been issued during the decade in Australia, Canada, and Europe. It is especially noteworthy that the theme for World Health Day in 2002 was "Move for Health." Nonetheless, leisure-time physical activity levels have remained below recommendations in nations that keep population statistics about physical activity. In the

United States, insufficient levels of leisure-time physical activity have not changed appreciably during the past decade. Despite widespread attempts to increase physical activity in the general population, 25% to 40% of U.S. adults aged 18 years or older do not participate in leisure-time physical activity, a rate largely unchanged since the first edition of the book was published. Objective measurements show that less than 10% of U.S. adults participate at a recommended level for health. Less than one half of American youth participate in vigorous physical activity at the recommended level of one hour each day. A recent study showed that by age 16 or 17, nearly a third of white American girls and more than half of African American girls said they did not participate in any regular leisure physical activity. To organize efforts to promote physical activity in the United States, the *National Plan for Physical Activity* was launched in 2010 to complement similar efforts already underway in several other nations worldwide.

This book is dedicated to understanding how leisure-time physical activity can be effectively promoted to enhance people's longevity and quality of life. The book is intended for use as the first textbook for upper-level undergraduates and master's degree students who are being introduced to physical activity epidemiology for the first time or as a companion text for broader-based courses in public health or health promotion and education that include physical activity among other health-related behaviors.

A textbook's worth is judged by how well it serves teaching. A good introductory textbook should raise a lot of questions but answer most of them. It should also teach beginning students that knowledge is an ever-growing and changing thing. We think that ingredients key to effective teaching are common to an effective text: namely, up-to-date, logically sequenced content illustrated by clear examples. Keeping those ingredients in mind, we have strived to avoid merely presenting superficial summaries of trendy topics and reviews of research literatures rendered uninformative after being watered down to be easily read by a lay audience. We have selected classical and contemporary topics that we feel have a sufficiently large body of knowledge to justify inclusion in a textbook and that we felt capable of presenting with at least a modest degree of competence. Certainly, other topics have public health importance and would be of interest to many people. Examples include osteoarthritis, chronic obstructive lung disease, chronic fatigue, chronic pain, and quality of life and independent living among older adults. Our undergirding purpose has been to provide a text that has fidelity to the science but translates that science in ways that will engage, inform, and challenge serious students. We hope to dispel the myth that researchers don't write textbooks and can't teach.

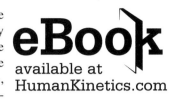

Instructor Resource

New to *Physical Activity Epidemiology, Second Edition,* is an image bank. This resource is free to course adopters and provides instructors with all of the figures and tables from the text to use in custom presentations and course materials.

ACKNOWLEDGMENTS

We will accept the blame when the book falls short of its goals. When it succeeds, we must share the credit with the many people who offered material for the book, ideas about what that material should be or how it would be best presented, and an environment that permitted the book to become a reality. Those people include the pioneers of physical activity epidemiology who served as mentors and exemplars; students who imparted to us questions and tactics for attacking them; colleagues who motivate us to constantly raise the standard of excellence; and our families, who nurture us and sustain our pursuit of that excellence.

We also gratefully acknowledge the contributions by Rik Washburn to the book's first edition and the people of Human Kinetics: Mike Bahrke and Myles Schrag, acquisitions editors; Kate Maurer, developmental editor; Dalene Reeder, permissions manager; as well as Joyce Sexton, the copyeditor who superbly forced us to be clear and accurate.

INTRODUCTION

When meditating over a disease, I never think of finding a remedy for it,
but instead, a means of preventing it.

• Louis Pasteur •

I propose that the theme for World Health Day 2002 be "Move for Health."
This will give particular visibility to ways in which individuals and
communities can influence their own health and well being.

• Gro Harlem Brundtland •
Director-General, World Health Organization

If we can now develop and implement effective policies and programs to encourage and
enable more people be more active more of the time, this will truly be a "Triumph of Epidemiology."

• Steven N. Blair and Jeremy N. Morris (2009, p. 256) •

The essence of epidemiology is captured by the opening words of the French chemist Louis Pasteur. This book is about the role played by physical activity in public health, namely, preventing chronic diseases and premature death. It is about population medicine more than clinical medicine, which focuses on the care of individuals, usually people who are already sick. The main goals of clinical medicine are diagnosis and treatment of disease. Treatment can take the form of secondary prevention, which is reducing the odds that a disease will recur, or tertiary prevention, which is minimizing the negative impact of a disease on a person's quality of daily life. Epidemiology is more aligned with population medicine, which focuses on a community of individuals and includes those who are not sick. The main goals of population medicine are the control and primary prevention of disease within a large group of people. People who are at risk for developing a disease are identified, and measures are then taken to reduce those odds by identifying and altering factors that cause disease.

▷ **THIS BOOK** is about why physical inactivity is a burden on public health and what can be done about it.

The role of physical activity in promoting the longevity and health of the public has become increasingly important for most developed, and many developing, nations around the world (Danaei et al. 2009), as evidenced by the theme of World Health Day 2002, "Move for Health," sponsored by the World Health Organization in São Paulo, Brazil, on April 7, 2002. In addition to the cost of human suffering resulting from poor health, the financial burden of poor health is great, as illustrated in figure 0.1.

Percentage of gross domestic product has increased steadily during the past 50 years, from about 4% in the 1940s to a projection of 18% in 2010. This means that 18 cents of every dollar spent in the United States is spent on some aspect of health care. The cost for each person in the United States was about $8,000 in 2007 and is approaching $9,000 a year, which is higher than in other leading economies worldwide including Canada, France, Germany, Japan, and the United Kingdom, which all have longer life expectancies (figure 0.2). The rate of increase in health expenditures in the United States is expected to be 6.2% each year through 2018. The distribution of U.S. health care costs is illustrated in figure 0.3.

Containment of health care costs in the United States is a national priority. The burden of cardiovascular disease illustrates this clearly. Not only are cardiovascular diseases (CVD) the most common (affecting more than 80 million Americans each year) and the most deadly (accounting for about 864,000 deaths each year, or 35% of all deaths), they are the most expensive, costing an estimated $475 billion each year. Coronary heart disease (CHD) alone accounts for 20% of deaths in the United States each year. Other

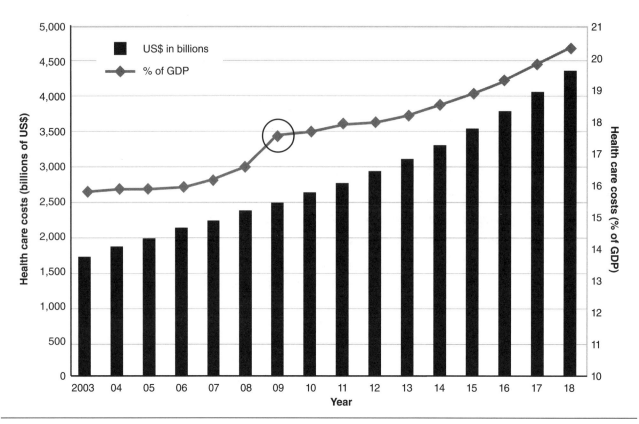

Figure 0.1 The trend in U.S. health costs, expressed in billions of dollars and as a percentage of gross domestic product (GDP).

Data from Centers for Medicare and Medicaid Services, Office of Actuary National Health Expenditures, 2009.

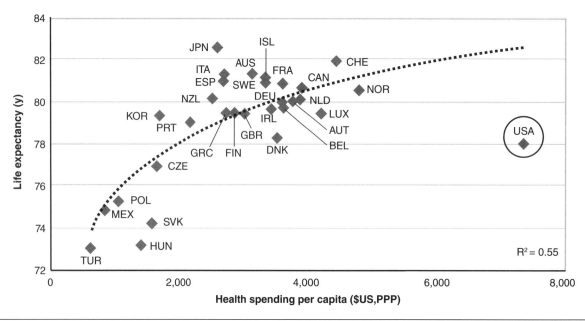

Figure 0.2 Health care expenditures and life expectancy in the United States and other nations.

Data from OECD Health Data 2009. Available: http://www.oecd.org/health/healthdata

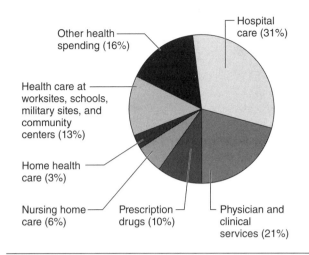

Figure 0.3 Where the U.S. health dollar was spent, 2007.

diseases and conditions that are common, deadly, and costly in the United States and that can be helped by physical activity are listed in table 0.1. The statistics in this table illustrate the three main ways by which the health impact of diseases, and the health-promoting potential of physical activity, are traditionally judged in the field of epidemiology. CHD is a prime concern for public health not only because of its frequency of occurrence (ranking near the top), but also because it ranks second only to all cancers in annual mortality. In contrast, diabetes is more common and costly than CHD, but it accounts for far fewer deaths. These three diseases cause two of every three deaths in the United States (Eyre et al. 2004).

Osteoporosis and depression each have comparably high prevalence rates, but they are less costly and do not have

directly attributable death rates as high as those of CHD and diabetes. Hence, the number of people affected, odds of death, and overall financial burden make a strong case that the highest priority for public health is determining whether and to what extent physical activity protects against CHD.

Certainly, other criteria can be used to render such judgments (such as lost function and lowered quality of life), but this example provides one way to reach decisions about allocating resources for research and policy regarding physical activity in public health. It also partly explains, as will become apparent in chapters dealing with specific chronic diseases, why more is currently known about the association between physical activity and risk for CHD than for other chronic diseases. Heart disease has received more research attention. For these reasons, the evidence that physical activity and physical fitness reduce the risk of CHD mortality is presented in chapter 5 as the model of how behavioral epidemiologists study the association between physical activity and disease and make decisions about whether the scientific evidence permits cause-and-effect conclusions. We will see that indeed the association between physical activity and health is sufficiently strong to justify the inclusion of physical activity and fitness as key indicators of health promotion in the United States.

Figure 0.4 shows how many deaths from leading diseases in the United States might be attributable to exposure to 12 risk factors. Death rates are U.S. National Center for Health Statistics estimates for 2005. Relative risks and prevalence rates of the risk factors were taken from major U.S. national health surveys. Of the 2.5 million U.S. deaths in 2005, nearly half a million were associated with tobacco smoking, and about 400,000 were associated with high blood pressure;

Table 0.1   Disease Statistics for U.S. Adults, 2007

Disease	Annual prevalence	Annual deaths	Costs in U.S. dollars (direct medical costs)
CVD	80-83.4 million	864,000	475 billion (187 billion)
CHD	13.7-16.8 million	425,000-446,000	165 billion
Stroke	5.4-6.5 million	144,000	69 billion
Cancer	16.4 million	560,000-595,000	228 billion (93 billion)
Diabetes	17 million (plus 6.4 million undiagnosed)	75,000-190,000	174 billion
Obesity	55.4-74.1 million	112,000	147 billion (61 billion)
Osteoporosis	10 million (plus 34 million with low bone mass)	60,000-87,000 (after hip fractures alone)	30 billion from hip, vertebral, and wrist fractures (14 billion)
Depression	14 million	29,000 (suicide)	83 billion (26 billion)
Sedentariness	84.8 million	191,000 (CVD, cancer, diabetes)	76 billion (24 billion from CVD)

Adapted from CDC 2009; American Heart Association 2009; Kessler et al. 2003; Finkelstein et al. 2009; Greenberg et al. 2003; Danaei et al. 2009. Based on National Health and Nutrition Examination Survey 2005-2006; Behavioral Risk Factor Surveillance Survey 2005; American Cancer Society, Cancer Facts & Figures, 2009; National Institute of Arthritis and Musculoskeletal and Skin Diseases 2009.

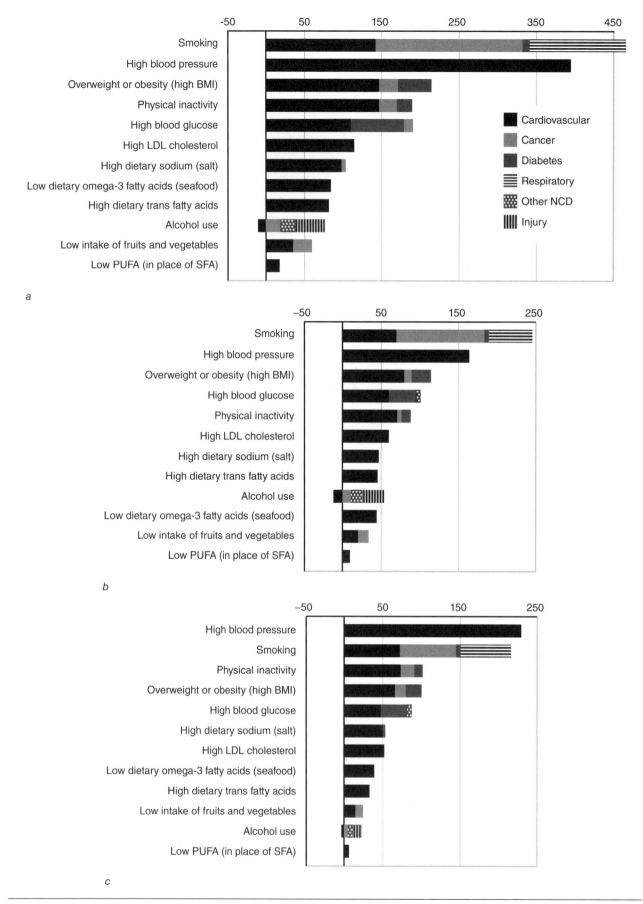

Figure 0.4 Deaths in 2005 attributed to physical inactivity and other health risk factors in U.S. adults younger than 70 years of age, shown for (a) both sexes, (b) men, and (c) women.

Reprinted, by permission, from G. Danaei et al., 2009, "The preventable causes of death in the United States: comparative risk assessment of dietary, lifestyle, and metabolic risk factors," *Plops Medicine* 6(4), e1000058. Licensed under Creative Commons License 2.5.

each accounted for about 1 in 5 deaths in U.S. adults. Physical inactivity accounted for nearly 1 in 12 deaths.

A summary of 10 studies from six countries (three from the United States; two each from Canada and the Netherlands; and one each from Australia, Switzerland, and the United Kingdom), using population estimates of physical inactivity with relative risks of inactivity for specific diseases, estimated that the annual excess cost in 2003 U.S. dollars (direct, indirect, or both) per inactive person per year ranged from $109 to $1305 (median $172) (Andrews et al. 2004). Similarly, estimated annual direct medical costs of physical inactivity per inactive person for five U.S. states (Georgia, Minnesota, New York, South Carolina, and Washington) ranged from a low of $20 in Washington to $80 in Georgia (Garrett et al. 2004). The yearly cost directly attributable to inactivity in the United States is an estimated $23 to $76 billion, or 1.5% to 5.0% of national health care expenditures (Finkelstein et al. 2004; Oldridge 2008). The total economic costs of physical inactivity were estimated as 2.6% of the total health care costs in Canada in 2001 (Katzmarzyk and Janssen 2004).

Disease is medically defined as reduced, abnormal, or lost structure or function of cells, organs, or systems of the body. The main adverse effects of disease include impairment of bodily functions, disfigurement, and death. Diseases usually have distinctive signs (i.e., objective measures), symptoms (i.e., what people feel and can report), causes, and courses of treatment, though the cause may not be known and the treatment may be only partly effective. However, many chronic diseases, such as CHD or acquired immunodeficiency syndrome (AIDS), that lead to dysfunction of organs or systems are progressions from cellular diseases that initially have no outward signs or symptoms. Hence, a person can appear healthy yet have diseased coronary vessels without heart dysfunction or can be infected with the human immunodeficiency virus (HIV) that causes AIDS without impairment of the immune system sufficient to result in the overt signs and symptoms that characterize AIDS. In either case, the person has a disease but is not yet overtly ill or infirm.

▷ **THE MAIN** goals of population medicine are the control and primary prevention of disease within a large group of people.

Conversely, health is not simply defined as the opposite of disease. In 1946, the World Health Organization (WHO) defined **health** as a "state of complete physical, mental, and social well-being and not merely the absence of disease or infirmity" (WHO 1946). That idealistic definition expanded the concept of health beyond the confines of medicine and biology, but it didn't define health using measurable benchmarks that are necessary for setting public health goals and evaluating progress toward them. At the 54th World Health Assembly in 2001, all 191 WHO Member States adopted the International Classification of Functioning, Disability and Health, the ICF, as a way to classify health and health-

related domains according to features of the body, the whole person, and society. Each of those features is further described through lists of (1) body functions and structure, (2) personal activities, and (3) participation in society (WHO 2000). Because a person's level of functioning or disability occurs in a context, the ICF also includes a list of environmental factors that can affect people's functioning. Several nations are developing population norms for some ICF domains, including physical activity.

Hence, health is relative rather than absolute. Lost function results from illness, but it can also occur in the absence of disease. For example, lost strength and mobility can result from wasting of muscle and reduced joint flexibility after insufficient use regardless of whether or not someone is free of disease. Much of this book is about aging, because the odds that people will develop a chronic disease increase directly as they age. Though people of the same age can certainly differ in risk for disease, exposure—the primary risk factor for disease and death—naturally increases with age. Expressed cynically, the longer you live, the closer you are to dying. Though longevity has been a longstanding benchmark in the field of epidemiology, WHO recently adopted the concept of healthy life expectancy as a better index of health around the world (figure 0.5). This concept is based on disability-adjusted life expectancy, which subtracts years according to the prevalence and severity of diseases that impair human functioning and quality of living (Murray and Lopez 1997a, 1997b; Mathers et al. 2001). This is not a new idea, though. Plutarch, the Greek essayist of the first century AD, wrote in *Consolation to Apollonius*, "The measure of a man's life is the well spending of it, and not the length." Based on analysis of 1990 disease and injury rates worldwide by the United Nations Global Program on Evidence for Health Policy, the United States ranked 24th of 191 countries, with a per capita healthy life expectancy of 70 years, compared with the highest-ranked countries, Japan, Australia, France, Sweden, Spain, and Italy, which had healthy life expectancies ranging from 73 years to around 74.5 years. By 2007, the United States ranked 38th. Figure 0.5 illustrates that men

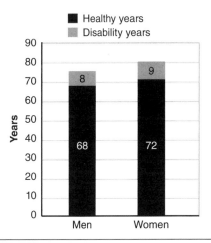

Figure 0.5 Healthy life expectancy for U.S. men and women.

Table 0.2   Top 12 Leading Causes of Disability-Adjusted Life Years Among Men and Women in the United States

Men	Women
Coronary heart disease	Coronary heart disease
Motor vehicle accidents	Major depression
Lung or throat cancer	Cerebrovascular disease
HIV/AIDS	COPD
Alcohol use	Lung or throat cancer
Cerebrovascular disease	Breast cancer
COPD	Osteoarthritis
Homicide	Dementia and other neurological disorders
Self-inflicted	Diabetes
Major depression	Motor vehicle accidents
Diabetes	Alcohol use
Osteoarthritis	Asthma

Reprinted, by permission, from C.M. Michaud et al., 2006, "The burden of disease and injury in the United States 1996," *Population Health Metrics* 4: 1-49.

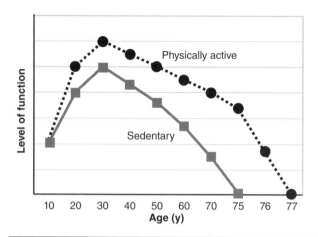

Figure 0.6   Physical functioning across age for active compared to sedentary people.

and women in the United States can now expect to live their last eight to nine years with some type of disability; leading causes are described in table 0.2.

It has been estimated that interventions to increase physical activity recommended by the U.S. Task Force on Community Preventive Services would cost between $14,000 and $69,000 per person for each year of increased healthy life expectancy population-wide (Roux et al. 2008). Similar estimates from Australia are $3,000 to $79,000 (Australian dollars) (Cobiac, Vos, and Barendregt 2009).

The focus of the chapters that follow is on the evidence that physical activity can help reduce the risks of major chronic diseases that negatively affect healthy life expectancy. Most of those diseases increase in prevalence as people age, so the importance of physical activity to public health will surely continue to increase as the population ages during the coming years. The World Health Organization and the United Nations have predicted that the proportion of U.S. adults older than 60 years will nearly double from the current figure, 16%, to 27% by the year 2050.

▷ **THE WORLD** Health Organization has defined healthy life expectancy as disability-adjusted life expectancy; the United States ranks 38th worldwide, with a per capita healthy life expectancy of 78.2 years.

Loss of function, which contributes to disability, increases with increasing age but usually geometrically; the loss is proportionally greatest in the later years rather than in the middle years of life. The ultimate goals of community medicine and epidemiology are to find and implement ways to lessen the slope of the decline of the aging curve (figure 0.6), to square off the rapidly accelerating

loss in the later years of life, and add a few healthy years as well. Put simply, the goals are for people to get sick later, lose function more slowly, live longer, and then die quickly when it's time. Thus, this book is about the quality of years lived, as well as the number of years lived. As the English author and moralist Samuel Johnson was quoted in 1769, "It matters not how a man dies, but how he lives. The act of dying is not of importance, it lasts so short a time" (Boswell 1769).

Research confirms that both men and women who are physically active and have normal body mass index (a measure of fatness) maintain higher cardiorespiratory fitness throughout adulthood when compared with people who are inactive and obese (see figure 0.7). Other evidence supports that people with low physical activity are twice as likely to die early and 50% less likely to report excellent health prior to death compared to people who stay physically active as they age (Kaplan, Baltrus, and Raghunathan 2007).

This book presents the theory and the evidence that a habit of physical activity contributes in a meaningful way to both quantity and quality of life. It also teaches you how to think like an epidemiologist and critically evaluate cause and effect from research studies conducted in the field of epidemiology. The book is organized into six parts: part I, "Introduction to Physical Activity Epidemiology"; part II, "Physical Activity and Disease Mortality"; part III, "Physical Activity and Risk Factors"; part IV, "Physical Activity and Chronic Diseases"; part V, "Physical Activity, Cancer, and Immunity"; and part VI, "Physical Activity and Special Concerns." The first chapter in part I, "Origins of Physical Activity Epidemiology," presents an abridged history of physical activity and health, which provides the background for appreciating the modern field of physical activity epidemiology. Chapter 2, "Concepts and Methods in Physical Activity Epidemiology," and chapter 3, "Measurement and Surveillance of Physical Activity and Fitness," introduce the traditions and techniques used by

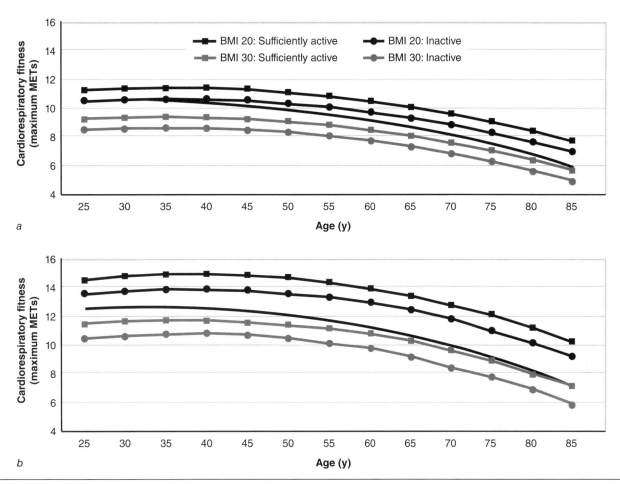

Figure 0.7 Age-related change in cardiorespiratory fitness (metabolic equivalents, METs) in (*a*) women and (*b*) men according to physical activity level and body mass index (BMI). Solid linear lines indicate decline with age adjusted for physical activity level and percent body fat and estimated from cross-sectional age groups. Broken curvilinear lines show decline in fitness according to normal weight or overweight status and sufficient physical activity or inactivity estimated from longitudinal analysis.

Data from Jackson et al. 2009; Jackson et al. 1995; and Jackson et al. 1996.

behavioral epidemiologists to study the distribution and causes of chronic diseases, including the measurement and surveillance of physical activity and physical fitness in segments of a population. Part II deals with all-cause mortality (chapter 4), coronary heart disease mortality (chapter 5), and mortality from cerebrovascular disease and stroke (chapter 6). Chapters 7, 8, and 9 in part III address the impact of physical activity on reducing hypertension, dyslipidemia, and obesity, respectively. Each of these conditions is a disease in its own right but also is a major risk factor for the development of cardiovascular diseases. Parts IV and V comprise chapters that describe the effects and **etiology** of major chronic diseases and the evidence that physical activity offers protection against these diseases: chapter 10 (diabetes), chapter 11 (osteoporosis), chapter 12 (colon, breast, and other cancers), and chapter 13 (the immune system). Part VI covers special concerns, including mental health (chapter 14); concerns of special populations, including those with disabilities (chapter 15); hazards that people face when they are physically active (chapter 16);

and the challenge of promoting an active lifestyle (chapter 17). A glossary of terms is also provided.

A special feature of all the chapters is discussion of the cardinal principles used by epidemiologists to judge the strength of evidence that physical activity or physical fitness reduces the risk of chronic disease in a direct, causal way that can be explained biologically. Finally, a unique feature of the book is the discussion in chapter 17 of the features of people, environments, and even physical activity itself that are associated with physical inactivity during leisure time. The chapter addresses the crucial problem of motivating the large numbers of people who are sedentary to begin and sustain a regular habit of physical activity in their leisure time. Though a good argument can be made that moderate-to-vigorous physical activity is one of the most important behaviors for improving the health of people who live in developed nations, it is possibly the least commonly practiced of all health behaviors. In sum, this book is designed to show why physical inactivity is a burden on public health and what can be done about it.

BIBLIOGRAPHY

Andrews, R., M. Pratt, B. Lankenau, G. Wang, and A. Neiman. 2004. The economic impact of physical activity. In *Proceedings of the International Conference on Health Benefits of Physical Activity,* Beijing, China, October 26-27, pp. 153-163.

Blair, S.N., and J.N. Morris. 2009. Healthy hearts and the universal benefits of being physically active: Physical activity and health. *Annals of Epidemiology.* 19: 253–256.

Boswell, J. 1769. *Boswell's life of Johnson.* London: Oxford University Press, 1946.

Centers for Medicare and Medicaid Services, Office of the Actuary, National Health Statistics Group. www.cms.hhs.gov/NationalHealthExpendData/.

Cobiac, L.J., T. Vos, and J.J. Barendregt. 2009. Cost-effectiveness of interventions to promote physical activity: a modelling study. *PLoS Medicine* 6 (7): e1000110. [Epub, July 14]

Danaei, G., E.L. Ding, D. Mozaffarian, B. Taylor, J. Rehm, C.J. Murray, and M. Ezzati. 2009. The preventable causes of death in the United States: Comparative risk assessment of dietary, lifestyle, and metabolic risk factors. *PLoS Medicine* 6 (4): e1000058.

Eyre, H., R. Kahn, R.M. Robertson, et al. 2004. Preventing cancer, cardiovascular disease, and diabetes: A common agenda for the American Cancer Society, the American Diabetes Association, and the American Heart Association. *Circulation* 109: 3244-3255.

Finkelstein, E.A., G. Wang, I.M. Lee, et al. 2004. *National and state-specific inactivity attributable medical expenditures for six diseases.* Final report prepared for the Centers for Disease Control and Prevention by the Research Triangle Institute. Research Triangle Park, NC: CDC and Research Triangle Institute.

Garrett, N.A., M. Brasure, K.H. Schmitz, M.M. Schultz, and M.R. Huber. 2004. Physical inactivity: Direct cost to a health plan. *American Journal of Preventive Medicine* 27: 304-309.

Jackson, A.S., E.F. Beard, L.T. Wier, R.M. Ross, J.E. Stuteville, and S.N. Blair. 1995. Changes in aerobic power of men, ages 25-70 yr. *Medicine and Science in Sports and Exercise* 27: 113-120.

Jackson, A.S., L.T. Wier, G.W. Ayers, E.F. Beard, J.E. Stuteville, and S.N. Blair. 1996. Changes in aerobic power of women, ages 20-64 yr. *Medicine and Science in Sports and Exercise* 28 (7):886-894.

Jackson, A.S., X. Sui, J.R. Hébert, T.S. Church, and S.N. Blair. 2009. Role of lifestyle and aging on the longitudinal change in cardiorespiratory fitness. *Archives of Internal Medicine* 169 (19): 1781-1787.

Kaplan, G.A., P.T. Baltrus, and T.E. Raghunathan. 2007. The shape of health to come: Prospective study of the determinants of 30-year health trajectories in the Alameda County Study. *International Journal of Epidemiology* 36: 542.

Katzmarzyk, P.T., and I. Janssen. 2004. The economic costs associated with physical inactivity and obesity in Canada: An update. *Canadian Journal of Applied Physiology* 29 (1): 90-115.

Mathers, C.D., R. Sadana, J.A. Salomon, C.J. Murray, and A.D. Lopez. 2001. Healthy life expectancy in 191 countries, 1999. *Lancet* 357: 1685-1691.

Michaud, C.M., M.T. McKenna, S. Begg, N. Tomijima, M. Majmudar, M.T. Bulzacchelli, S. Ebrahim, M. Ezzati, J.A. Salomon, J.G. Kreiser, M. Hogan, and C.J. Murray. 2006. The burden of disease and injury in the United States 1996. *Population Health Metrics* 4: 1-49.

Murray, C.J., and A.D. Lopez. 1997a. Alternative projections of mortality and disability by cause 1990–2020: Global Burden of Disease Study. *Lancet* 349: 1498-1504.

Murray, C.J., and A.D. Lopez. 1997b. Global mortality, disability, and the contribution of risk factors: Global Burden of Disease Study. *Lancet* 349: 1436-1442.

Oldridge, N.B. 2008. Economic burden of physical inactivity: Healthcare costs associated with cardiovascular disease. *European Journal of Cardiovascular Prevention and Rehabilitation* 15 (2): 130-139.

Roux, L., M. Pratt, T.O. Tengs, M.M. Yore, T.L. Yanagawa, J. Van Den Bos, C. Rutt, R.C. Brownson, K.E. Powell, G. Heath, H.W. Kohl 3rd, S. Teutsch, J. Cawley, I.M. Lee, L. West, and D.M. Buchner. 2008. Cost effectiveness of community-based physical activity interventions. *American Journal of Preventive Medicine* 35 (6): 578-588.

United Nations, Department of Economic and Social Affairs, Population Division. 2007. World population prospects: The 2006 revision, highlights. Working Paper No. ESA/P/WP.202 New York: United Nations.

World Health Organization. 1946. Constitution of the World Health Organization. Geneva.

World Health Organization. 2000. *International Classification of Functioning, Disability and Health (ICIDH-2).* Geneva: World Health Organization.

World Health Organization. Burden of Disease database. www.who.int/whosis/indicators/2007HALE0/en/.

PART ONE

Introduction to Physical Activity Epidemiology

This book is dedicated to understanding how leisure-time physical activity can enhance people's quantity and quality of life. The promotion of leisure-time physical activity has emerged as an important initiative to improve public health and quality of living in many economically developed and developing nations. The U.S. Surgeon General's report on physical activity and health, published in 1996, provided the scientific consensus on the benefits of physical activity for chronic diseases and mental well-being; and the subsequent Surgeon General's report on mental health, published in 1999, acknowledged a role for physical activity as part of mental hygiene. *Healthy People 2020,* the national health goals of the U.S. Department of Health and Human Services, includes several objectives that collectively call for increasing physical activity in all segments of the U.S. population. Similar policy statements about the importance of physical activity

to health were issued during the 1990s in Australia, Canada, and Europe. It was especially significant that World Health Day 2002, sponsored by the World Health Organization (WHO), was dedicated to physical activity and fitness. The WHO subsequently adopted the "Global Strategy on Diet, Physical Activity and Health" in May 2004. In 2008, the U.S. Department of Health and Human Services published *Physical Activity Guidelines for Americans*, the first-ever physical activity guidelines issued by the federal government to recommend the types and amounts of physical activity that promote health. The National Physical Activity Plan in the United States was launched in 2010. The chapters in this section provide historical and contemporary views of the field of physical activity epidemiology and explain how it is applied to determine whether physical activity appears causally linked with health and longevity.

CHAPTER 1

Origins of Physical Activity Epidemiology

Health is the vital principle of bliss,
And exercise, of health.

• James Thomson, 1748 •
The Castle of Indolence

The cure for this ill is not to sit still,
Or frowst with a book by the fire;
But to take a large hoe and a shovel also,
And dig till you gently perspire.

• Rudyard Kipling, 1890 •
The Cameelious Hump

CHAPTER OBJECTIVES

▸ Describe key people and events in antiquity that set the historical foundation for the role of physical activity in health

▸ Identify key people and events in modern times that shaped the use of epidemiological methods to study physical activity and health risks

▸ Briefly discuss the landmark population studies that exemplify physical activity epidemiology

▸ Provide examples of international consensus about physical activity in health and its place in the 2008 Physical Activity Guidelines for Americans and in the Healthy People 2020 goals for the United States

▸ Identify and briefly discuss national plans for promoting physical activity worldwide

Physical activity epidemiology emerged as a new field of study about 60 years ago and has expanded to include intervention during the past 25 years as its scientific undergirding has grown. However, the ideas that underlie the field are not new but are based in antiquity, dating to the use of structured exercise for health promotion in China around 2500 BC (Lyons and Petrucelli 1978). The main purpose of this chapter is to recount key events in the ancient and modern history of physical activity and health to provide perspective on the present and future of physical activity epidemiology through an understanding of its past.

Ancient History of Physical Activity and Health

The Code of Hammurabi, king of Babylon, had laws about health practices and physicians as early as 2080 BC. However, modern-day preventive medicine and public health can be traced mainly to ancient cultures in India and subsequently Greece. In Homer's *Iliad,* Asclepius, the son of Apollo and god of medicine, was killed by a thunderbolt from Zeus because he had saved the lives of mortals and cheated Hades, god of the dead. His legacy continued, though, because his daughters inherited his powers. Panacea, goddess of healing, gave medicines to the sick, while Hygeia, goddess of health, taught people to protect their bodies by prudent living. Even today, we use the word "panacea" to refer to a healing agent and "hygiene" to refer to healthy practices.

Hippocrates (460-377 BC), known as the "father of medicine," was trained in the tradition of Asclepius, but he has also been described as the first epidemiologist. He kept records of associations between diseases and climate, living conditions, and habits such as diet and exercise. He distinguished endemic diseases that differ in prevalence between places from epidemic diseases that vary in prevalence across time (Duncan 1988). In his *Regimen in Health,* Hippocrates wrote this about exercise:

> Eating alone will not keep a man well; he must also take exercise. For food and exercise, while possessing opposite qualities, yet work together to produce health. . . . And it is necessary . . . to discern the power of various exercises, both natural exercises and artificial, to know which of them tends to increase flesh and which to lessen it; and not only this, but also to proportion exercise to bulk of food, to the constitution of the patient, to the age of the individual. . . . Exercise should be many and of all kinds, running on the double track increased gradually, . . . sharp walks after exercises, short walks in the sun after dinner, many walks in the early morning, quiet to begin with, increasing till they are violent and then gently finishing.

Allen J. Ryan, MD, founding editor of the primary care journal *The Physician and Sportsmedicine* and a pioneer in the field of sports medicine at the University of Wisconsin during the 1960s and 1970s, wrote one of the first modern accounts of the history of physical activity and health. In it he concluded that "the concept of health is older than knowledge about the causes of disease" (Ryan 1984).

In his book *De Sanitate Tuenda (On Hygiene),* the second-century Greco-Roman physician Claudius Galenus, a.k.a. Galen (1951), extolled the virtues of exercise:

> The uses of exercise, I think, are twofold, one for the evacuation of the excrements, the other for the production of good condition of the firm parts of the body. For since vigorous motion is exercise, it must needs be that only these three things result from it in the exercising body, hardness of the organs from mutual attrition, increase of the intrinsic warmth, and accelerated movement of respiration.

Exercise as Medicine

The written history about the use of physical activity and exercise for the protection and rehabilitation of health can be traced back to the ancient Indian system of medicine of the ninth century BC, the **Ayurveda** (Sanskrit for "the knowledge of living"), which recommended exercise and massage for the treatment of rheumatism (Guthrie 1945). The Indian physician Sushruta prescribed moderate daily exercise as early as 600 BC for the treatment of diabetes. Sushruta also recognized physical activity as preventive medicine, viewing sedentary living as a cause of obesity, diabetes, and early death (Tipton 2008).

Around 480 BC, the Greek physician Herodicus specialized in therapeutic **gymnastics** (one of three classes of medical practice at that time). He based his therapies mainly on vigorous exercise. Herophilus and Eristratus of Alexandria, Egypt, in the fourth century BC recommended moderate exercise, and Asclepiades of Bithynia, a Greek reformer of Hippocratic therapy in the first century BC, recommended walking and running for his patients (Vallance 1995). Later, Aristotle, the Greek philosopher and tutor of Alexander the Great in the court of Macedonia, extended those views, stating, "The following are examples of the results of action: bodily health is the result of a fondness for gymnastics; a man falls into ill health as a result of not caring for exercise" (Aristotle 1908).

Even during the Middle Ages in Europe, when the influence of Greek writings was obscured awaiting their rediscovery in the Renaissance, the Greek medical tradition of using exercise was preserved by the Arabs and later translated from Arabic into Latin medical manuals, the *Tacuinum Sanitatis* (Arano 1976). The *Canon of Medicine,* written by the Persian physician Ibn Sine (a.k.a. Avicenna) in 1025, was the most influential medical text in Europe during the 15th and 16th centuries. Walking was recommended in its chapter, "Regimen of Old Age," which is regarded as the forerunner of geriatric medicine (Howell 1987). The work *Sirr al-asrar,* reportedly written by Aristotle, is believed to be the basis of the famous poem of medicine, *Regimen Sanitatis Salernitanum,* which was published at the medical school at Salerno, Italy, in the 12th century and which mentioned the healthful benefits of walking after a meal and the use of exercise as a purgative (Cummins 1976). Rabbi Moses ben Maimum (also known as Maimonides), the Jewish philosopher-physician of the 12th century who was chief rabbi in Cairo and physician to Saladin, the sultan of Egypt, wrote in the Mishnah Torah: "Anyone who lives a sedentary life and does not exercise . . . even if he eats good foods and takes care of himself according to proper medical principles—all his days will be painful ones and his strength shall wane. . . . The most beneficial of all types of exercise is physical gymnastics to the point that the soul rejoices" (Maimonides 1990).

Exercise and Health Education

During the Renaissance, scholars in Italy renewed interest in classical Greek gymnastics and recommended it as a fundamental part of education. The 14th-century Italian poet laureate, Francesco Petrarca, encouraged exercise as a natural remedy to replace medicines that "poison the body" in his 1354 work, *Invective Contra Medicum (Protest Against the Doctor)* (Struever 1993). In the mid-1400s, Leon Battista Alberti recommended physical exercise beginning in early infancy for strengthening the muscles, stimulating the circulation, and adapting the nervous system. He also stated that exercise for those purposes became even more important with increasing age. Maffeus Vegius, in his 15th-century *Education of Children and Their Good Habits,* distinguished between light recreational exercises and heavy exercise designed to strengthen the body, advising moderation in all physical activity.

Although the great educators of the 15th century recommended exercise as a lifelong habit, contemporary physicians did not embrace exercise. This was changed during the Renaissance by the Italian physician Hieronymus Mercurialis, who urged all people who led sedentary lives to exercise. His *Six Books on the Art of Gymnastics,* printed in 1569, laid the foundation for modern rehabilitative medicine by recommending that convalescents and weakened older people do special exercises, based on specific diagnoses, that should not worsen their infirmities.

For the purpose of health, Mercurialis replaced passive exercises, which had been recommended by early Renaissance experts, with vigorous exercise involving heavy breathing and physical effort, including mountain climbing among three types of walking. He considered running, jumping, rope climbing, and wrestling healthy forms of exercise and suggested ball games to strengthen the upper body.

One of the first physicians since the classical Greeks to attempt to explain the benefits of exercise was the French-born Swiss pharmacologist Joseph Duchesne, who in 1648 wrote in *Ars Medica Hermetica,* "The essential purpose of gymnastics for the body is its deliverance from superfluous humors, the regulation of digestion, the strengthening of the heart and joints, the opening of the pores of the skin, and the stronger circulation of blood in the lungs by strenuous breathing."

In 1772, Benjamin Rush, Philadelphia physician and father of American psychiatry, delivered a "Sermon on Exercise," in which he recommended sports and exercises for young and old alike. His "Plan of a Federal University" included exercises to improve the body's strength and health (Runes 1947). Soon afterward, in 1802, the British physician William Heberden reported a case history of heart disease in which he concluded, "I know one who set himself a task of sawing wood half an hour every day, and was nearly cured" (Heberden 1802). But it was not until the years between the U.S. Civil War and World War I that physicians became the main proponents of exercise to promote good health. Their influence was the basis for our present-day acceptance of the relationship between exercise and a more rewarding and healthier life, as well as for our contemporary knowledge about the developing science of exercise as a form of preventive medicine.

After Edward Hitchcock Jr. (1828-1911) graduated from Harvard Medical School in 1853, he and his father published a discussion of the relationship between exercise and health for boys and girls, which argued that gymnastics was as important to schools and colleges as were academic libraries (Hitchcock and Hitchcock 1860). Hitchcock was appointed director of the Department of Physical Education and Hygiene at Amherst College in 1861 and kept the position for 50 years, lecturing on anatomy, physiology, physical culture, and **hygiene.** In 1885 he was elected the first president of the Association for the Advancement of Physical Education.

The role of physical fitness in preventive medicine was advocated further by Dudley Sargent, an 1878 graduate of Yale Medical School who was the first director of the Hemenway Gymnasium at Harvard in 1880. One of the first men he tested for fitness at Harvard was Theodore Roosevelt. Sargent also established a private gymnasium in Cambridge, Massachusetts, known as the Sanatory Gymnasium, where he directed an exercise program for the female Harvard students who studied in the Harvard Annex, which later became Radcliffe College. Sargent published *Health, Strength, and Power* in 1904, in which he argued for the importance of regular vigorous exercise for health and presented exercises for children and men of all ages designed to increase fitness.

R. Tait McKenzie (1867-1938), a Canadian who completed his undergraduate and medical degrees at McGill University, sustained Hitchcock's impetus. After graduation and a short medical practice, McKenzie returned to McGill as a lecturer in anatomy and became medical director of physical education. He moved to the University of Pennsylvania in 1904, where he was professor and director of physical education. McKenzie published *Exercise in Education and Medicine* in 1909, which discussed the physiology of exercise and systems used for physical conditioning. He also described physical education for people with disabilities. The second half of the book discussed the use of exercise to treat diseases, providing the foundation of modern physical medicine and rehabilitation.

The impetus provided by those early physician-educators continued in the United States and Europe during the first half of the 20th century and culminated in the founding of the American College of Sports Medicine in 1954. Though

many contributors to the application of physiological methods and principles to the study of physical activity and fitness are noteworthy and have been chronicled elsewhere (e.g., Buskirk 1992; Costill 1994; Tipton 1998), much of their work focused on performance or secondary prevention of disease and rehabilitation. The pioneering efforts of Thomas K. Cureton are especially noteworthy as they relate to the role of fitness in the primary prevention of chronic diseases and the maintenance of physical function with aging. After his appointment as director of the Physical Fitness Research Laboratory at the University of Illinois in 1944, Dr. Cureton's seminal studies on the physiology of fitness formed the cornerstone for today's recognition that multiple components of fitness are each related to the public's health. He led by example, too, holding 14 World and National Masters Swimming records, beginning at age 72 when he won five gold medals at the first National Masters Swimming Championships in Chicago in 1973 (Berryman 1996). Moreover, the subsequent contributions of his many doctoral students, including Henry Montoye (recipient in 1949 of the first PhD awarded in physical education in the United States) and five presidents of the American College of Sports Medicine (Montoye, Charles Tipton, James Skinner, Michael L. Pollock, and William Haskell), to the study of physical activity, fitness, and health provided, and continue to provide, much of the experimental evidence that supports the modern epidemiological study of physical activity. In Europe, the now-burgeoning contributions of physiologists and physicians to the epidemiology of physical activity can be traced in part to early work by Marti J. Karvonen, former Surgeon General of Finland, who led the Finnish Cohort of the famous Seven Countries Study of diet and health practices, started in 1959 by renowned University of Minnesota nutrition researcher Ancil Keys. Keys founded the Laboratory of Physiological Hygiene at the University of Minnesota in 1948, which has since produced five Citation and Honor award winners from the American College of Sports Medicine and has been a key influence on physical activity epidemiology. The legacy of exercise physiologists to understanding of mechanisms whereby physical activity contributes to health has grown exponentially since the impetus provided by these pioneers, extending to the molecular biology of exercise and disease (Booth et al. 2002).

Modern History of Physical Activity and Health

The modern history of physical activity epidemiology is short; its beginnings can be traced to the late 1940s and a growth spurt in the mid-1980s that has continued exponentially up to the present time (Blair and Morris 2009; Paffenbarger, Blair, and Lee 2001). Though many researchers have contributed, modern physical activity epidemiology has its roots in the work of Dr. Jeremy Morris, professor emeritus of public health at the London School of Hygiene and Tropical Medicine of the University of London, and Dr. Ralph Paffenbarger, professor emeritus of medicine at Stanford University and adjunct professor emeritus at Harvard University. Their impact was heightened because they were respected epidemiologists at a time when physical activity was not considered by their peers an important influence on public health worthy of study.

Dr. Morris served for many years as professor of social medicine and director of the Medical Research Council's Social Medicine Unit at the London Hospital Medical College, where he authored *Uses of Epidemiology* (1957), the first text to apply classical epidemiology to emerging health problems of chronic, noncommunicable disease. Dr. Morris and his coworkers helped establish the epidemiologic method for the collection, analysis, and interpretation of data on the causes of chronic diseases (Morris 2009).

Dr. Paffenbarger also made important scientific contributions to epidemiology prior to his studies of physical activity. Early in his career, Dr. Paffenbarger worked with Dr. David Bodian at Johns Hopkins University on the mechanisms of transmission and the pathogenesis of poliomyelitis, one of the most disabling and fatal childhood diseases of the first half of the 20th century. Dr. Paffenbarger also did some of the earliest research on postpartum depression and other mental illnesses more than 40 years ago. His work on potential causes of reproductive cancers included some of the first studies of leisure physical activity and cancer risk. Dr. Paffenbarger also led by example. A distinguished masters athlete, he ran more than 150 races of marathon distance (42.2 km) or longer, including completion of the Western States 100-mile (161 km) run five times and the Boston Marathon more than 20 times.

Landmark Research

The association of physical activity and physical fitness with reduced risk of chronic diseases was not understood scientifically until Dr. Morris and his colleagues began to study **coronary heart disease (CHD)** in the late 1940s. In the early 1950s, Morris formulated the hypothesis that "men in physically active jobs suffer less coronary—ischaemic—heart disease than comparable men in sedentary jobs, such disease as the active do develop is less severe and strikes at later ages" (Morris et al. 1953).

The hypothesis evolved when Morris observed what appeared to be a protective effect of occupational physical activity against CHD, observations that were viewed skeptically by the scientific community at the time. The first study by Morris and colleagues (1953) showed that the highly active conductors on London's double-decker buses were at lower risk of CHD than the drivers, who sat through their shifts at the steering wheel. If conductors developed the disease, it was less severe and occurred at later ages. The London bus study sparked the modern era of physical activity epidemiol-

ogy. Morris later reported a similar observation, that postmen delivering the mail on foot had lower rates of CHD than sedentary office clerks and telephone operators.

Several important studies of occupational and leisure-time physical activity and disease began around the world after Dr. Morris published his work, including studies of Finnish lumberjacks (Karvonen 1962), U.S. railroad workers (Taylor et al. 1969), and CHD in men in the Seven Countries Study (Keys 1967). Studies of entire communities—such as the Framingham (Massachusetts) Heart Study, begun in 1948 (Dawber, Meadors, and Moore 1951; Kannel 1967), and the Tecumseh (Michigan) Community Health Study, begun in 1957 (Montoye 1975)—soon added measures of fitness and physical activity.

Framingham Heart Study

This ongoing community study began in 1948, when a random sample of 5209 men and women aged 30 to 62 years who lived in Framingham, Massachusetts, located 20 miles west of Boston, agreed to participate in a long-term study funded by the National Heart Institute (now the National Heart, Lung, and Blood Institute) of the National Institutes of Health. The original participants underwent physical examinations every two years, including a resting electrocardiogram, chest X ray, and urine and blood tests. In 1971 the Offspring Study of 5135 adult children of the original participants and their spouses began; and in 1995, 500 of Framingham's minority residents were added to begin the Omni Study. Thus, although 75% of the original participants have died, mainly from cardiovascular disease, these new recruits will ensure that the Framingham Study will continue to provide important information about health risks. Notably, data from the Framingham study linked physical activity with reduced risk of heart disease (Kannel 1967), soon after it had been discovered in 1960 and 1961 that cigarette smoking, cholesterol, and high blood pressure were risk factors for heart disease.

Tecumseh Community Health Study

In the 1940s, Dr. Thomas Francis Jr., an epidemiologist at the University of Michigan, had the idea that a study of an entire community, including the biological, physical, and social environment, might reveal how some people maintain good health while others are more susceptible to disease (Francis 1961; cf. Montoye 1975). With funding from the state of Michigan and later from the National Institutes of Health, such a community study was started in 1957 in Tecumseh, Michigan, a mixed rural–urban community with a population of about 9500 located 55 miles southwest of Detroit. There were three cycles of health examinations. From 1959 to 1960, over 8600 people (88% of those eligible for the study) aged 20 years or older underwent physical examinations, including resting electrocardiograms, lung function tests, chest X rays, anthropometric tests, and blood and urine tests. A second cycle of testing from 1961 to 1965 reexamined most of the original participants and added 2500 new residents. In addition to adding hand and cervical X rays to the examination, the researchers assessed physical activity of men aged 16 to 69 via a questionnaire and interview and used a simple submaximal step test to estimate fitness from heart rate response and recovery after exercise. A treadmill exercise test was later added for some participants during a third testing cycle, conducted from 1967 to 1969. Montoye (1975) published a comprehensive summary of the relationships among physical activity, fitness, and health risk factors discovered in this study.

Longshoremen and College Alumni Studies

The most sustained and compelling studies of physical activity and health were conducted in the United States by Dr. Paffenbarger, who is most recognized for his seminal reports from the San Francisco Longshoremen Study and the ongoing College Health Study (at Harvard College and the University of Pennsylvania) begun in the 1960s and 1970s (Paffenbarger et al. 1966, 1970, 1978). Those large studies helped fuel scientific and public interest in physical activity as an important component of health promotion and focused the broader fields of preventive medicine and public health on physical inactivity as a significant public health problem.

Aerobics Center Longitudinal Study

The Aerobics Center Longitudinal Study (ACLS) is an ongoing examination of the impact that diet, physical activity, and other lifestyle factors have on mortality and chronic disease risk. The ACLS is the largest prospective study of its kind, based on objective measures of fitness for more than 80,000 patients seen since 1970 at the Cooper Clinic, a preventive medicine practice in Dallas, Texas. Unique features of the ACLS are clinical examinations and fitness tests including strength testing and treadmill tests of aerobic power. The cohort comprises about 90% non-Hispanic whites, and nearly 80% have graduated from college. More than 5000 deaths occurred in the cohort through 2004. Periodic mailback surveys from the patients during the 1980s and 1990s and in 2004 have been used to identify cases of disease and provide surveillance of health habits, including physical activity. For 26 years, the study was managed through the Cooper Institute—the nonprofit research arm of the Cooper Clinic—by Dr. Steven Blair, who is currently a professor in the departments of Exercise Science and Epidemiology and Biostatistics in the Arnold School of Public Health at the University of South Carolina. More than 100 studies of fitness and lowered risks of mortality, cardiovascular disease, cancer, obesity, diabetes, hypertension, depression, and metabolic syndrome have been published from the ACLS. The first ACLS paper on fitness-reduced mortality risk among men and women (Blair et al. 1989) is one of the most highly cited papers in physical activity epidemiology. It has been cited by other scientists more than 1500 times.

The U.S. Nurses' Health and Health Professionals Studies

The Nurses' Health Study is considered the "grandmother" of women's health studies and is the longest-running cohort study of women. It was established in 1976 by Dr. Frank Speizer at Harvard Medical School and Brigham and Women's Hospital to study the association between the use of oral contraceptives and cigarette smoking and the risk of chronic diseases in more than 120,000 married registered nurses between the ages of 30 and 55. The study included questions about exercise in 1980 through 1982 and has included more detailed questions approximately every other year since 1986. Nearly 240,000 female nurses have participated. Participants receive detailed questionnaires every two years about their medical histories and every four years about their physical activity habits during the past 24 to 48 months.

The Health Professionals Follow-Up Study was started in 1986 by Drs. Walter Willett and Meir Stampfer at the Harvard School of Public Health as a complement to the Nurses' Health Study for the purpose of evaluating nutrition and health risks of cancer and cardiovascular diseases among men. At the outset of the study, more than 51,000 male health professionals were recruited. That group comprised approximately 30,000 dentists, 4000 pharmacists, 3750 optometrists, 2200 osteopathic physicians, 1600 podiatrists, and 10,000 veterinarians. There was small representation by about 500 African Americans and 900 Asian Americans in the cohort. Participants fill out questionnaires about diseases and health behaviors including physical activity every two years. The web-based Health Professionals Follow-Up Study 2 began in spring 2009, recruiting male health professionals aged 30 to 60 years nationwide.

Contemporary Physical Activity Epidemiology

Despite the growing evidence that physical activity is linked with lowered risk for heart disease, in 1975 Milton Terris, former president of the American Public Health Association, concluded in a keynote address at the Sixth Annual Meeting of the Society for Epidemiologic Research that "physical fitness and physical education have no respected place in the American public health movement." He stated,

> On the subject of physical fitness I speak with no authority. Having spent a large portion of my life seated at a desk, I have no personal acquaintance with the concept. On a more intellectual level, I have been far too bound by the philosophical rigidities of the American public health movement to become knowledgeable in the literature of this field, and

am therefore in no position to judge the relation of physical exercise and physical fitness to performance of activities of daily living and to "physical, mental and social well-being," that is, to "positive health," vitality, and joy of life. These are issues which are eminently worth studying.

—Terris 1975, p. 1039

Despite traditional epidemiologists' lack of acceptance that physical activity was a proven benefit to health, in 1980 the U.S. Public Health Service identified physical fitness and exercise as one of 15 areas of focus of the national objectives for improving people's health (U.S. Department of Health and Human Services 1980). Recognizing, however, that the scientific basis of physical activity as a national health objective was not yet solid, the Centers for Disease Control (CDC) created the Behavioral Epidemiology and Evaluation Branch (BEEB) within the Center for Health Promotion and Education of the Division of Health Education. Under the direction of Dr. Kenneth Powell, its main purpose was monitoring progress of the nation's 1990 goals for physical activity and fitness. To help fulfill this purpose, the Behavioral Risk Factor Surveillance System (BRFSS) was begun to monitor activity in most of the United States. This system is still operating today. The BEEB staff organized and conducted the Workshop on Epidemiologic and Public Health Aspects of Physical Activity and Exercise in Atlanta on September 24 and 25, 1984, which culminated in the publication of summaries of current knowledge and directions for future research in 10 areas (Powell and Paffenbarger 1985).

In contrast to the low status of physical activity in public health prior to the mid-1980s, a testament to the modern acceptance of physical activity epidemiology was given in 1996, when Drs. Morris and Paffenbarger jointly received the first Olympic Prize in Sports Science, awarded biannually by the Medical Commission of the International Olympic Committee through 2004. The Olympic Prize was the "Nobel Prize" of sport and exercise science.

International Consensus

Another historical focal point in the modern history of physical activity epidemiology was the first International Conference on Exercise, Fitness, and Health, organized by Professor Claude Bouchard under the auspices of the Canadian Association of Sport Sciences and the Ontario Ministry of Tourism and Recreation and held in Toronto in the spring of 1988. Sixty-two papers from that conference, together with scientific consensus statements summarizing the world's knowledge about exercise, fitness, and health, were published (Bouchard et al. 1990). The widespread impact of that conference and the resulting book, as well as a rapidly growing knowledge base, led to the Second International Consensus

Symposium on Physical Activity, Fitness, and Health, held in Toronto in May 1992 as part of Canada's celebration of 125 years of confederation.

A sequel book, titled *Physical Activity, Fitness, and Health: International Proceedings and Consensus Statement,* contained 70 chapters that updated the knowledge summarized in the first conference and book (Bouchard, Shephard, and Stephens 1994). This book was an important prelude to *Physical Activity and Health: A Report of the Surgeon General* (U.S. Department of Health and Human Services 1996).

U.S. Government Reports

Key documents published in the United States include a position statement by the American Heart Association in 1992, which recognized physical inactivity as an independent risk factor for coronary heart disease (Fletcher et al. 1992), and recommendations on physical activity and public health prepared jointly by the Centers for Disease Control and Prevention and the American College of Sports Medicine (Pate et al. 1995).

In the historical benchmark *Physical Activity and Health: A Report of the Surgeon General* (U.S. Department of Health and Human Services 1996), nearly 100 experts, led by Steven Blair, director of epidemiology and clinical applications at the Cooper Institute for Aerobics Research in Dallas, outlined the consensus in the scientific community about the beneficial effects of physical activity on overall mortality, cardiovascular diseases, cancer, type 2 diabetes, osteoarthritis, osteoporosis, obesity, mental health, health-related quality of life, risk of musculoskeletal injury, and risk of sudden death.

A recent benchmark for physical activity and public health in the United States was the inaugural publication in 2008 of *Physical Activity Guidelines for Americans* by the U.S. Department of Health and Human Services. These are the first-ever physical activity guidelines for Americans issued by the federal government, similar in purpose to the long-standing Dietary Guidelines for Americans. They describe the types and amounts of physical activity that offer substantial health benefits to participants (see table 1.1). The guidelines were based on a report submitted by the Physical Activity Guidelines Advisory Committee, a group of 13 leading experts in the field of exercise science and public health. The committee conducted an extensive review of the scientific data relating physical activity to health published since the release of the 1996 Surgeon General's report on physical activity and health. The guidelines provide sufficient depth and flexibility to target specific population subgroups, such as seniors, children, and persons with disabilities. They represent an extension of the HealthierUS Initiative, launched by President George Bush in June 2002, which identified four pillars for healthier living—being physically active every day, eating a diet consistent with the Dietary Guidelines for Americans, getting prevention screenings, and avoiding risky behaviors.

Table 1.1 Physical Activity Guidelines in the United States: Classification of Total Weekly Amounts of Aerobic Physical Activity Into Four Categories

Levels of physical activity	Range of moderate-intensity minutes a week	Summary of overall health benefits	Comment
Inactive	No activity beyond baseline (i.e., light-intensity activities of daily life, such as standing, walking slowly, and lifting lightweight objects)	None	Being inactive is unhealthy.
Low	Activity beyond baseline but fewer than 150 min of moderate-intensity activity or 75 min of vigorous-intensity exercise each week	Some	Low levels of activity are clearly preferable to an inactive lifestyle.
Medium	150 min to 300 min of moderate-intensity activity or 75 min of vigorous-intensity exercise (or their combination equivalent to 500 to 1000 MET-minutes) each week	Substantial	Activity at the high end of this range has additional and more extensive health benefits than activity at the low end.
High	More than 300 min a week	Additional	Current science does not allow researchers to identify an upper limit of activity above which there are no additional health benefits.

Adapted from U.S. Department of Health and Human Services 2008.

Physical Activity for Health Promotion in the United States and the World

In 1995 the CDC and the Prevention Research Center at the University of South Carolina started offering widely renowned postgraduate training courses for physical activity and public health researchers and practitioners, which continue today. Largely as an outgrowth of those courses, the U.S. National Society of Physical Activity Practitioners in Public Health was formed in 2006. In 1998, the CDC WHO Collaborating Center for Physical Activity and Health Promotion was founded as part of CDC's Division of Nutrition and Physical Activity for the purpose of fostering global health policy about physical activity, guiding evidence-based interventions and surveillance, and spreading training courses worldwide (Pratt, Epping, and Dietz 2009).

At the May 2002 World Health Assembly, member nations mandated that the World Health Organization (WHO) create a Global Strategy on Diet, Physical Activity and Health. In 2003, the WHO and the Food and Agriculture Organization of the United Nations published the technical report "Diet, Nutrition, and the Prevention of Chronic Diseases," which summarized evidence for the role of physical activity in reducing risks of some chronic diseases related to diet (e.g., cardiovascular disease, colon and breast cancer, and unhealthy weight gain) and presented policy statements about the importance of surveillance and promotion of physical

activity for public health. In May 2004, the WHO adopted the Global Strategy on Diet, Physical Activity and Health, which has four main objectives:

- **Reduce risk factors for chronic diseases** that stem from unhealthy diets and physical inactivity through public health actions.
- **Increase awareness and understanding** of the influences of diet and physical activity on health and the positive impact of preventive interventions.
- **Develop, strengthen, and implement global, regional, national policies and action plans** to improve diets and increase physical activity that are sustainable and comprehensive and that actively engage all sectors.
- **Monitor science and promote research** on diet and physical activity.

Consistent with those goals, the International Congress on Physical Activity and Public Health met first in Atlanta in 2006 and then in Amsterdam in 2008 and Toronto in 2010. The International Society for Physical Activity and Health was founded by Harold (Bill) Kohl III in 2008.

Global and National Physical Activity Plans

The United States was, until 2010, one of the few industrialized countries in the world without a national physical activity plan. Canada, England, Finland, Northern Ireland, Pakistan,

Scotland, Switzerland, the Netherlands, and Western Australia, among others, have had such a plan for several years. The European network for the promotion of health-enhancing physical activity (HEPA Europe) is a collaborative project for better health through the promotion of physical activity in the WHO European Region.

However, on July 1, 2009, the Centers for Disease Control and Prevention and the Prevention Research Center at the University of South Carolina launched the inaugural organizing conference in Washington, D.C., for the National Physical Activity Plan (which was officially launched in May 2010). Dr. Russ Pate and the Arnold School of Public Health at the University of South Carolina are providing the organizational infrastructure for the developing plan, which is a growing network of organizations and individuals dedicated to supporting a broad and comprehensive national effort to increase physical activity throughout the U.S. population.

Health Goals for the Nation

Behavioral epidemiologists are helping shape public health policy for the purpose of promoting participation in physical activity by the public. In each decade since 1980, the U.S. Department of Health and Human Services has published a set of health objectives for the nation, policy goals for improving the nation's health. Objectives for increasing physical activity and physical fitness have figured prominently among these objectives. For realistic national objectives to be set, surveillance systems are necessary for monitoring progress. Such systems have been available only since the mid-1980s. The midcourse status of the objectives for physical activity and fitness established in 2000 for the year 2010 was evaluated in 2005 by the Centers for Disease Control and Prevention (2010). The final report was released in Fall 2011 and is summarized alongside the mid-course progress report in figure 1.1.

None of the objectives were met, perhaps in part because there was no national plan in place to help reach them. However, figure 1.1 shows that modest progress was made toward meeting targets in five areas for adults and two areas for adolescents in grades 9 through 12. For example, in 1997, 40% of adults said they engaged in no leisure-time physical activity. That rate was 37% in 2003 and 36% in 2008, although other national surveys have estimated the rate at 25%. The decrease of 4% by 2008 represents just a 10% reduction in sedentariness, but it represents 20% progress toward the targeted objective of cutting the rate of inactivity by half to 20% (i.e., 10% / 50% = 20%). However, there was no sustained increase in moderate or vigorous

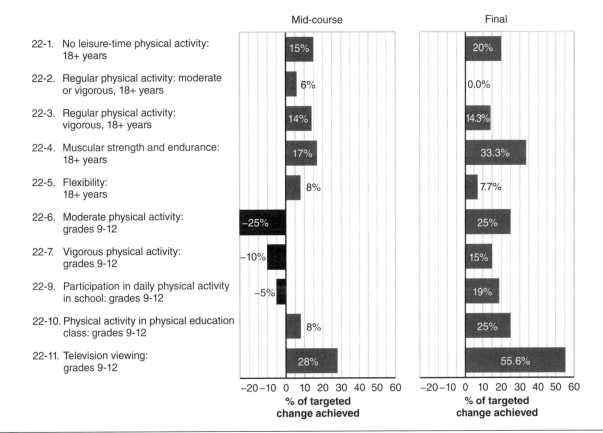

Figure 1.1 Mid-course and final reviews of progress toward Healthy People 2010 objectives for physical activity and fitness.

Adapted from CDC 2010 and Healthy People. Available: http://www.cdc.gov/nchs/data/hpdata2010/hp2010_final_review.pdf.

Health Disparities in Meeting the Objectives of Healthy People 2010

Nearly all of the objectives had significant health disparities of 10% or more among select population groups (Sondik et al. 2010). For example:

- White non-Hispanics had the best rate for objectives 22-1, 22-2, 22-3, 22-4, 22-6, 22-7, and 22-11; the Hispanic or Latino population had the best rate for objectives 22-9 and 22-10
- Males had better rates than females for objectives 22-1, 22-4, 22-7, and 22-10

- People with some or more college education had the best rates for objectives 22-1 through 22-4 and 22-5
- Residents of urban or metropolitan areas had better rates than residents of rural areas for objective 22-1
- People without disabilities had better rates than people with disabilities for objectives 22-1 through 22-4

For more on physical activity and diverse populations, see chapter 15.

physical activity among adults, despite 6% progress in 2003, and participation in regular vigorous physical activity stayed at about 24% of adults between 1997 and 2008, just 14% of the way to its target of 30%. In contrast, one-third of the targeted change was achieved for muscular strength and endurance among adults, showing a positive linear trend during the decade. Among high school students, there was 19% progress toward students taking daily physical education and 25% progress toward the objective of increased physical activity during physical education classes. Also, mid-course drops in vigorous and moderate physical activity seen in 2003 were reversed by 2009, resulting in overall gains of 15-25% toward the 2010 targets. The importance of the progress made toward less TV watching is hard to judge, because current evidence does not show a strong, direct association between time spent watching TV and overall physical inactivity in children and adolescents

(Gorely et al. 2004; Nilsson et al. 2009). Other changes not shown included a 24% increase in adults walking for the purpose of transportation, but 33-38% drops in adults and children bicycling for transportation (e.g., to work or school) and a 64% drop in physical education requirements in high schools.

Partly based on that midcourse evaluation, physical activity objectives (usually a 10% gain above current estimates) were recently established for the year 2020 and are provided in table 1.2. Objective 8, limiting screen time (watching television or videos and playing computer video games), is not listed here. Also not presented are new developmental objectives for which no baseline data were available to set targets. These include muscle strengthening for adolescents, adult participation in employer-based exercise programs, and legislative policies for the built environment that enhance physical activity opportunities.

Table 1.2   Select Physical Activity Objectives in the United States for 2020

Objective	2008 baseline	2020 target
1. Reduce the proportion of adults who engage in no leisure-time physical activity.	36.2%	32.6%
2. Increase the proportion of adults who meet current federal physical activity guidelines for aerobic physical activity and for muscle-strengthening activity.		
2.1 Increase the proportion of adults who engage in aerobic physical activity of at least moderate intensity for at least 150 min/week, or 75 min/week of vigorous intensity, or an equivalent combination.	43.5%	47.9%
2.2 Increase the proportion of adults who engage in aerobic physical activity of at least moderate intensity for more than 300 min/week, or more than 150 min/week of vigorous intensity, or an equivalent combination.	28.4%	31.3%
2.3 Increase the proportion of adults who perform muscle-strengthening activities on two or more days of the week.	21.9%	24.1%
2.4 Increase the proportion of adults who meet the objectives for aerobic physical activity and for muscle-strengthening activity.	18.2%	20.1%

Objective	2008 baseline	2020 target
3. Increase the proportion of adolescents who meet current federal physical activity guidelines for aerobic physical activity and for muscle-strengthening activity.		
3.1 Aerobic physical activity	18.4%	20.2%
4. Increase the proportion of the nation's public and private schools that require daily physical education for all students.		
4.1 Elementary schools	3.8%	4.2%
4.2 Middle and junior high schools	7.9%	8.6%
4.3 Senior high schools	2.1%	2.3%
5. Increase the proportion of adolescents who participate in daily school physical education.	33.3%	36.6%
6. Increase regularly scheduled elementary school recess in the United States.		
6.1 Increase the number of states that require regularly scheduled elementary school recess.	7 states	17 states
6.2 Increase the proportion of school districts that require regularly scheduled elementary school recess.	57.1%	62.8%
7. Increase the proportion of school districts that require or recommend elementary school recess for an appropriate period of time.	61.5%	67.7%
9. Increase the number of states with licensing regulations for physical activity provided in child care.		
9.1 Require activity programs providing large muscle or gross motor activity, development, and/or equipment.	25 states	35 states
9.2 Require children to engage in vigorous or moderate physical activity.	3 states	13 states
9.3 Require number of minutes of physical activity per day or by length of time in care.	1 state	11 states
10. Increase the proportion of the nation's public and private schools that provide access to their physical activity spaces and facilities for all persons outside of normal school hours.	28.8%	31.7%
11. Increase the proportion of physician office visits that include counseling or education related to physical activity.		
11.1 Increase the proportion of office visits made by patients with a diagnosis of cardiovascular disease, diabetes, or hyperlipidemia that include counseling or education related to exercise.	13%	14.3%
11.2 Increase the proportion of physician visits made by all child and adult patients that include counseling about exercise.	7.9%	8.7%

Adapted from U.S. Department of Health and Human Services 2010.

Summary

Acknowledgment of the potential health benefits of physical activity is as old as recorded history. Since the inclusion of physical activity in the practice of ancient medicine in China, India, and Greece, its recognition in the Bible and the Mishnah Torah, its preservation in medical practice by the Arabs, and its reintroduction to Western medicine of the 16th through 18th centuries (by physicians such as the Italian physician-educator Mercurialis, the French pharmacologist Duchesne, the British cardiologist Heberden, and the American physician Rush), physical activity has endured as an important part of hygiene in many cultures. However, physical activity epidemiology as a formal field of research has a short history of about 25 years. British epidemiologist Jeremy Morris is credited with the seminal research that spawned modern physical activity epidemiology in the late 1940s, and his work was expanded by Ralph Paffenbarger and other investigators in the United States and Europe during the late 1960s and 1970s. Systematic inquiry into physical activity epidemiology did not gather full steam until landmark scientific consensus meetings in Atlanta in 1984, organized by Ken Powell of the Centers for Disease Control, and in Toronto in 1988, organized by Claude Bouchard and the Canadian government.

The capstone publication of the report of the U.S. Surgeon General, *Physical Activity and Health*, spearheaded by Steven Blair, signaled the maturation of the field by summarizing current knowledge pertinent to public health guidelines and policy and by outlining a host of questions for future study. The Physical Activity Guidelines Advisory Committee updated that knowledge base in 2008. The purpose of the chapters that follow is to summarize this knowledge, the methods used to obtain it, its implications for public health, and the important questions that remain.

· BIBLIOGRAPHY ·

American Heart Association. 2009. Heart Disease and Stroke Statistics – 2009 Update. *Circulation* 119: e21-e181.

Arano, L.C. 1976. *Tacuinum sanitatis.* Milan: Electa Edifice.

Aristotle. 1908. *The works of Aristotle.* Translated by W.D. Ross. Oxford: Clarendon Press, 1908-1952.

Berryman, J.W. 1996. Thomas K. Cureton, Jr.: Pioneer researcher, proselytizer, and proponent for physical fitness. *Research Quarterly for Exercise and Sport* 67: 1-12.

Blair, S.N., H.W. Kohl III, R.S. Paffenbarger Jr., D.G. Clark, K.H. Cooper, and L.W. Gibbons. 1989. Physical fitness and all-cause mortality: A prospective study of healthy men and women. *Journal of the American Medical Association* 262: 2395-2401.

Blair, S.N., and J.N. Morris. 2009. Healthy hearts—and the universal benefits of being physically active: Physical activity and health. *Annals of Epidemiology* 19 (4): 253-256.

Booth, F.W., M.V. Chakravarthy, S.E. Gordon, and E.E. Spangenburg. 2002. Waging war on physical inactivity: Using modern molecular ammunition against an ancient enemy. *Journal of Applied Physiology* 93: 3-30.

Bouchard, C., R.J. Shephard, and T. Stephens, eds. 1994. *Physical activity, fitness, and health: International proceedings and consensus statement.* Champaign, IL: Human Kinetics.

Bouchard, C., R.J. Shephard, T. Stephens, J.R. Sutton, and B.D. McPherson, eds. 1990. *Exercise, fitness, and health: A consensus of current knowledge.* Champaign, IL: Human Kinetics.

Burton, R. 1632. *The anatomy of melancholy.* Printed by Ion Lichfield for Henry Cripps.

Buskirk, E.R. 1992. From Harvard to Minnesota: Keys to our history. *Exercise and Sport Sciences Reviews* 20: 1-26.

Centers for Disease Control and Prevention, National Center for Health Statistics. 2000. *Healthy people 2000 review, 1998-99.* Washington, DC: U.S. Government Printing Office.

Centers for Disease Control and Prevention, National Center for Health Statistics. 2009. Series 10, Number 240. Washington, DC: U.S. Government Printing Office.

Centers for Disease Control and Prevention, National Center for Health Statistics. 2010. *Healthy people 2010 final review.* Washington, DC: U.S. Government Printing Office. Available at www.cdc.gov/nchs/data/hpdata2010/hp2010_final_review. pdf. Accessed March 8, 2012.

Costill, D.L. 1994. Applied exercise physiology. In *40th anniversary lectures,* pp. 69-80. Indianapolis: American College of Sports Medicine.

Cummins, P.W. 1976. *A critical edition of le regime tresutile et tresproufitable pour conserver et garder la santé du corps humain.* Chapel Hill, NC: North Carolina Studies in the Romance Languages and Literatures.

Danei, G., E.L. Ding, D. Mozaffarian, B. Taylor, J. Rehm, C.J.L. Murray, and M. Ezzati. 2009. The preventable causes of death in the United States: Comparative risk assessment of dietary, lifestyle, and metabolic risk factors. *PLoS Medicine* 6 (4): e1000058.

Dawber, T.R., G.F. Meadors, and F.E.J. Moore. 1951. Epidemiological approaches to heart disease: The Framingham Study. *American Journal of Public Health* 41: 279-286.

Duncan, D. 1988. Epidemiology: Basis for disease prevention and health promotion. New York: Macmillan.

Fletcher, G.F., S.N. Blair, J. Blumenthal, C. Caspersen, B. Chaitman, S. Epstein, H. Falls, E.S. Froelicher, V.F. Froelicher, and I.L. Pina. 1992. Statement on exercise: Benefits and recommendations for physical activity programs for all Americans. A statement for health professionals by the Committee on Exercise and Cardiac Rehabilitation of the Council on Clinical Cardiology, American Heart Association. *Circulation* 86: 340-344.

Francis, T. Jr. 1961. Aspects of the Tecumseh Study. *Public Health Reports* 76: 963-966.

Galen, C. 1951. *De sanitate tuenda.* Translated by R.M. Green. Springfield, IL: Charles C Thomas.

Gorely, T., S.J. Marshall, S.J. Biddle, N. Cameron, and I. Murdey. 2004. Couch kids: Correlates of television viewing among youth. *International Journal of Behavioral Medicine* 11 (3): 152-163.

Greenberg, P.E., R.C. Kessler, H.G. Birnbaum, S.A. Leong, S.W. Lowe, P.A. Berglund, and P.K. Corey-Lisle. 2003. The Economic Burden of Depression in the United States: How Did It Change Between 1990 and 2000? *Journal of Clinical Psychiatry* 64: 1465-1475.

Guthrie, D. 1945. *A history of medicine.* London: Thomas Nelson.

Heberden, W. 1802. *Commentaries on the history and cure of diseases.* London: T. Payne, News-gate.

Hitchcock, E., and E. Hitchcock Jr. 1860. *Elementary anatomy and physiology for colleges, academies, and other schools.* New York: Ivison, Phinney & Co.

Howell, T.H. 1987. Avicenna and his regimen of old age. *Age and Ageing* 16: 58-59.

Joseph, L.H. 1949. Gymnastics from the middle ages to the 18th century. *Ciba Symposia* 10 (March-April): 5.

Kannel, W.B. 1967. Habitual level of physical activity and risk of coronary heart disease: The Framingham Study. *Canadian Medical Association Journal* 96: 811-812.

Karvonen, M.J. 1962. Arteriosclerosis: Clinical surveys in Finland. *Proceedings of the Royal Society of Medicine* 55: 271-274.

Kessler, R.C., P. Berglund, O. Demler, R. Jin, D. Koretz, K.R. Merikangas, J. Rush, E.E. Walters, and P.S. Wang. 2003. The epidemiology of major depressive disorder: Results from the National Comorbidity Survey Replication (NCS-R). *Journal of the American Medical Association* 289 (23): 3095-3105.

Keys, A. 1967. Epidemiological studies related to coronary heart disease: Characteristics of men aged 40-59 in seven countries. *Acta Medica Scandinavica* 460 (Suppl.): 1-392.

Lyons, A.S., and R.J. Petrucelli. 1978. *Medicine: An illustrated history,* p. 130. New York: Harry N. Abrams.

Maimonides, M. 1199. *Three treatises on health.* Translated by F. Rosner with bibliographies by J.I. Dienstege. Haifa, Israel: Maimonides Research Institute, 1990.

McGinnis, J.M. 1992. The public health burden of a sedentary lifestyle. *Medicine and Science in Sports and Exercise* 24 (Suppl. 6): S196-S200.

McKenzie, R. 1909. *Exercise in education and medicine.* Philadelphia: Saunders.

Montoye, H.J. 1975. *Physical activity and health: An epidemiologic study of an entire community.* Englewood Cliffs, NJ: Prentice Hall.

Morris, J.N. 1957. *Uses of epidemiology.* London: Churchill Livingstone.

Morris, J.N. 2009. Physical activity versus heart attack: A modern epidemic - personal observations. In *Epidemiologic methods in physical activity studies,* edited by I-M. Lee, pp. 3-12. New York: Oxford University Press.

Morris, J.N., J.A. Heady, R.A.B. Raffle, C.G. Roberts, and S.W. Parks. 1953. Coronary heart disease and physical activity of work. *Lancet* 2: 111-120, 1053-1057.

Nilsson, A., L.B. Andersen, Y. Ommundsen, K. Froberg, L.B. Sardinha, K. Piehl-Aulin, and U. Ekelund. 2009. Correlates of objectively assessed physical activity and sedentary time in children: A cross-sectional study (The European Youth Heart Study). *BMC Public Health* 9 (September 7): 322.

Paffenbarger, R.S. Jr., S.N. Blair, and I.M. Lee. 2001. A history of physical activity, cardiovascular health and longevity: The scientific contributions of Jeremy N Morris, DSc, DPH, FRCP. *International Journal of Epidemiology* 30: 1184-1192.

Paffenbarger, R.S. Jr., M.E. Lauglin, A.S. Gima, and R.A. Black. 1970. Work activity of longshoremen as related to death from coronary heart disease and stroke. *New England Journal of Medicine* 282: 1109-1114.

Paffenbarger, R.S. Jr., A.L. Wing, and R.T. Hyde. 1978. Chronic disease in former college students: XVI. Physical activity as an index of heart attack risk in college alumni. *American Journal of Epidemiology* 108: 161-175.

Paffenbarger, R.S. Jr., P.A. Wolf, J. Notkin, and M.C. Thorne. 1966. Chronic disease in former college students: I. Early precursors of fatal coronary heart disease. *American Journal of Epidemiology* 83: 314-328.

Pate, R.R., M. Pratt, S.N. Blair, W.L. Haskell, C.A. Macera, C. Bouchard, D. Buchner, W. Ettinger, G.W. Heath, A.C. King, et al. 1995. Physical activity and public health: A recommendation from the Centers for Disease Control and Prevention and the American College of Sports Medicine. *Journal of the American Medical Association* 273: 402-407.

Physical Activity Guidelines Advisory Committee. 2008. *Physical Activity Guidelines Advisory Committee report.* Washington, DC: U.S. Department of Health and Human Services.

Powell, K.E., and R.S. Paffenbarger Jr. 1985. Workshop on epidemiologic and public health aspects of physical activity and exercise: A summary. *Public Health Reports* 100: 118-126.

Pratt, M., J.N. Epping, and W.H. Dietz. 2009. Putting physical activity into public health: A historical perspective from the CDC. *Preventive Medicine,* June 23. [Epub ahead of print]

Runes, D. 1947. *Selected writings of Benjamin Rush.* New York: Philosophical Library.

Ryan, A.J. 1984. Exercise and health: Lessons from the past. In *Exercise and health: The academy papers,* edited by H.M. Eckert and H.J. Montoye, Vol. 17, pp. 3-13. American Academy of Physical Education. Champaign, IL: Human Kinetics.

Sargent, D.A. 1904. *Health, strength, and power.* New York: Dodge.

Sondik, E.J., D.T. Huang, R.J. Klein, and D. Satcher. 2010. Progress toward the Healthy People 2010 goals and objectives. *Annu Rev of Public Health* 31(1): 271–81.

Struever, N. 1993. Petrarch's invective contra medicum: An early confrontation of rhetoric and medicine. *Modern Language Notes* 108: 659-679.

Taylor, H.L., H. Blackburn, V. Puchner, R.W. Parlin, and A. Keys. 1969. Coronary heart disease in selected occupations of American railroads in relation to physical activity. *Circulation* 40 (Suppl. 3): 202.

Terris, M. 1975. Approaches to an epidemiology of health. *American Journal of Public Health* 65: 1037-1045.

Tipton, C.M. 1998. Contemporary exercise physiology: Fifty years after the closure of Harvard Fatigue Laboratory. *Exercise and Sport Sciences Reviews* 26: 315-339.

Tipton, C.M. 2008. Susruta of India, an unrecognized contributor to the history of exercise physiology. *Journal of Applied Physiology* 104: 1553-1556.

U.S. Department of Health and Human Services. 1980. *Promoting health/preventing disease: Objectives for the nation.* Washington, DC: U.S. Government Printing Office.

U.S. Department of Health and Human Services. 1991. *Healthy people 2000: National health promotion and disease prevention objectives.* DHHS Publication No. [PHS] 91-50212. Washington, DC: U.S. Government Printing Office.

U.S. Department of Health and Human Services. 1996. *Physical activity and health: A report of the Surgeon General.* Atlanta: U.S. Department of Health and Human Services, Centers for Disease Control and Prevention, National Center for Chronic Disease Prevention and Health Promotion.

U.S. Department of Health and Human Services. 2000. *Healthy people 2010: Understanding and improving health.* 2nd edition. With *Understanding and improving health* and *Objectives for improving health.* 2 vols. Washington, DC: U.S. Government Printing Office.

U.S. Department of Health and Human Services. 2008. *Physical activity guidelines for Americans.* ODPHP Publication No. U0036. Washington, DC: U.S. Government Printing Office.

U.S. Department of Health and Human Services. 2010. *Healthy people 2020: Improving the health of Americans.* Washington, DC: U.S. Government Printing Office.

Vallance, J.T. 1995. *The lost theory of Asclepiades of Bithynia.* Oxford: Clarendon Press.

CHAPTER 2

Concepts and Methods in Physical Activity Epidemiology

Nothing has such power to broaden the mind as the ability to investigate systematically and truly all that come under thy observation in life.

• Marcus Aurelius (AD 121-180) •
Meditations

When you have excluded the impossible, whatever remains, however improbable, must be the truth.

• Sir Arthur Conan Doyle, 1892 •
"The Adventure of the Beryl Coronet," *The Adventures of Sherlock Holmes*

CHAPTER OBJECTIVES

▸ Introduce and explain the basic measures and statistics used in epidemiology to estimate health risks

▸ Describe and give examples of common study designs used in epidemiologic research

▸ Provide examples of tools for decision making about health outcomes in clinical trials

▸ Introduce and explain the use of standard criteria used to evaluate the strength of evidence that physical activity and physical fitness have causal associations with health risks and outcomes

The term **epidemiology** is derived from the Latin roots *epi* (upon) and *demo* (the people). In simple terms, epidemiology is the study of the distribution and determinants of disease in a population. More specifically, the term is defined as the application of the scientific method to the study of the distribution and dynamics of disease in a population for the purposes of identifying factors that affect the distribution and then modifying these risk factors to reduce the frequency of **morbidity** and mortality from the disease. A **risk factor** is a characteristic that, if present, increases the probability of disease in a group of individuals who have the characteristic compared with a group of individuals who do not have the characteristic.

Hippocrates described environments and behaviors that he associated with disease in *On Airs, Waters, Places.* But British physician John Snow (1813-1858) is usually regarded as the first modern epidemiologist because of his careful compilation and logical analysis of facts and figures to deduce the source of contagion during an 1854 cholera outbreak in the Soho region of London. Cholera first appeared in England in 1831, and health officials thought it was spread by "bad air"; this was the prevailing view before Pasteur popularized the germ theory of infectious disease. In contrast, in a widely dismissed book, *On the Mode of Communication of Cholera,* published in 1849, Snow speculated that cholera was spread by contaminated water. The 1854 outbreak let him test his idea in what he termed "the grand experiment," described in a second edition of the book published the next year. Within three days of the Soho outbreak, 89 people living near Broad Street died. When Snow plotted the location of the cases on a map of Soho (figure 2.1), he observed an association between the density of cholera cases and a single well located on Broad Street. In the 1855 edition of his book, Snow wrote,

On proceeding to the spot, I found that nearly all the deaths had taken place within a short distance of the [Broad Street] pump. There were only ten deaths in houses situated decidedly nearer to another street-pump. In five of these cases the families of the deceased persons informed me that they always went to the pump in Broad Street, as they preferred the water. . . . In three other cases, the deceased were children who went to school near the pump in Broad Street . . . there were 61 instances in which I was informed that the deceased persons used to drink the pump water from Broad Street, either constantly or occasionally. . . .

Snow also noted only five cases among 535 inmates of the Poland Street workhouse (a debtor's prison), located near the pump. However, the workhouse had its own well. If the mortality rate in the workhouse had equaled the rate among residents in the three surrounding streets, more than a hundred inmates would have died. There were no cases among 70 workers at a Broad Street brewery, where the men were given free beer every day and never drank from the pump.

Removing the pump handle of the Broad Street well ended the epidemic. It was discovered later that the well was only 3 ft (about 1 m) from an old cesspit that had begun to leak fecal bacteria reportedly rinsed from the diapers of an infected child. Snow was unaware that Fillipo Pacini, the famous Italian anatomist, had in the same year identified the bacterium that causes cholera.

Snow's investigation exemplified that epidemiology has three distinct goals: (1) to describe the distribution of disease, for example, who gets the disease and when and where the

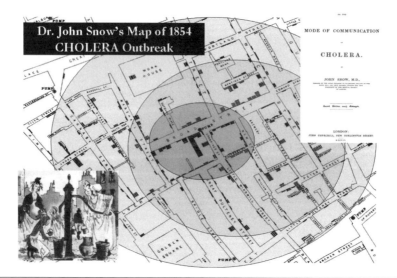

Figure 2.1   John Snow's map showing cholera deaths in London in 1854, with the cover of his 1855 text *On the Mode of Communication of Cholera.*

Adapted from J. Snow, 1855, *On the mode of communication of cholera, London* (England: John Churchill). Image courtesy of Ralph Frerichs, Department of Epidemiology, School of Public Health, UCLA.

disease occurs; (2) to analyze this descriptive information to identify risk factors that are associated with an increased probability of disease occurrence; and (3) to prevent disease occurrence by modifying the identified risk factors.

Physical activity epidemiology studies factors associated with participation in a specific behavior—that is, physical activity—and how this behavior relates to the probability of disease or injury. Examples of this type of study include description of the level of physical activity in a population, comparison of levels of physical activity among populations, determination of factors associated with participation in physical activity, and investigation of the association between physical activity and the risk for chronic diseases such as coronary heart disease (CHD), stroke, diabetes, osteoporosis, and cancer.

▷ **EPIDEMIOLOGY IS** the use of the scientific method to study the distribution of disease in a population, to identify risk factors that likely cause the disease, and then to change the risk factors in order to reduce sickness and death from the disease.

Epidemiologic Measures

A fundamental measurement in epidemiology is the frequency with which an event under study occurs, usually an injury, disease, or cause of death in a population. **Incident cases** are the new occurrences of these events in the study population during the time period of interest. In other words, incident cases are those cases in which health status changes—that is, from alive to dead, from not injured to injured, or from not sick to sick—during the period of observation. In contrast, **prevalent cases** represent the number of persons in the population who have a particular disease or condition at some specific point in time. Prevalence of a disease is a function of both incidence and duration. The prevalence of a disease can increase as a result of an increase in either the number of new cases (incidence) or the length of time during which individuals have the disease before they die or recover.

If the incidence or prevalence of a condition is known, the incidence rates and prevalence rates can be calculated. The rate is simply the frequency or number of events that occur over some defined time period divided by the average size

of the population at risk. The usual estimate of the average number of people at risk is the population at the midpoint of the time interval under study. The general formula for calculating a rate is

Rate = Number of cases / Average population size.

Because incidence and prevalence rates are usually less than 1, they are generally expressed per some power of 10 (e.g., per 100 [percent], per 1000, or per 10,000) for ease of discussion. Therefore, if the death rate in the United States was calculated to be 0.009 deaths per year, 0.009 could be multiplied by 1000 and expressed as 9 deaths per 1000 individuals in the population per year.

Cumulative incidence rates are the number of incident cases over a defined time period divided by the population at risk over that time period. Actual incidence rates are cases divided by person-years of risk. Incidence rates provide a measure of the rate at which people without disease develop disease over a specified time interval. Likewise, prevalence rates are calculated as the number of prevalent cases divided by the size of the population at a particular time. Prevalence rates indicate only how many people have a particular disease or engage in a behavior, such as physical activity or smoking, at a particular time. Prevalence rates are useful for planning purposes. For example, a survey of a city might show that the prevalence of people with CHD is particularly high. Therefore it may be economically feasible for a local hospital to consider opening a cardiac rehabilitation program. However, prevalence data are not useful when the purpose is to try to determine factors that may be related to an increased probability of disease because high prevalence does not necessarily indicate high risk; it could reflect increased survival. For example, the high prevalence of CHD in a city survey might not necessarily indicate that people in that city are at increased risk of getting CHD but could reflect high-quality emergency services and medical care that increase the rate of survival. In contrast, low prevalence might simply reflect rapid death or rapid cure, not low incidence. The problem of using prevalence data alone is that you don't know which of the possible interpretations is true.

It is particularly important to be sure that the information you use to make comparisons among groups is based on actual rates. This may seem obvious, but this fact has been overlooked in a number of real-world examples. For example, a sports medicine physician reports that he has seen 100 cases of ruptured patellar tendons in runners over the past year. Does this indicate that running is the cause of this problem and that indeed it is a large problem that needs to be dealt with? The answer is that, with information only on the number of cases (numerator) and no information regarding the number of people at risk (denominator), it is impossible to tell. To make these assessments, you need to know how many runners visited the clinic over the course of the year. If 100 runners were seen and 100 cases of ruptured patellar tendons were diagnosed, then the incidence would be 100%, a potentially serious problem! On the other hand, if 1000 runners were seen, the rate would be only 10%, requiring a completely different interpretation. The use of numerator data, the number of cases, without consideration of the size of the population at risk should be avoided. However, numerator data like these can often be found in the sports medicine literature.

Crude, Specific, and Standardized Rates

Three general categories of rates are commonly used in epidemiology: crude, specific, and standardized. Rates that are based on a total population without consideration of any of the population characteristics, such as the distribution of age, sex, and ethnicity, are referred to as *crude rates*. When rates are calculated separately for population subgroups (typically age, sex, and ethnicity), they are called *specific rates* (e.g., age-specific rates, sex-specific rates). Standardized rates are crude rates that have been standardized (adjusted) for some population characteristic, such as age or sex, to allow valid comparisons of rates among populations where the distribution of the given characteristic may be quite different.

Crude rates, because they depend on the characteristics of the population from which they are calculated, can be misleading. For example, the crude prevalence of participation in vigorous physical activity in Boulder, Colorado, would be expected to be higher than that in a community such as Sun City, Arizona, simply because of the difference in the age distribution of residents in those communities. Likewise a comparison of breast cancer rates in two populations where the sex distribution varies greatly could be misleading. There are two solutions to this problem. First, valid comparisons among populations can be made if specific rates are used. In the preceding examples, it would be reasonable to compare the rates of participation in vigorous physical activity between Boulder and Sun City by five-year age groups, or the rates of breast cancer for men and women separately. Although the use of specific rates provides a valid comparison, the procedure can become cumbersome, particularly when numerous categories, such as five-year age groups over a large age range, need to be compared. Therefore, to make comparisons of rates between two populations with unequal distributions of risk factors, standardized rates should be used.

Standardized rates, which are also referred to as adjusted rates, are simply crude rates that have been adjusted to control for the effect of some population characteristic, such as age or sex. The most common method for the adjustment is called direct standardization. In practice, the standardization process is performed by readily available computer software packages. The following example shows how the direct standardization process actually works. The data in table 2.1 represent the death rates from two different populations. The crude death rate in population A is 4.51% and in population B is 3.08%. This is curious, and misleading, when you consider that the age-specific death rate in population B is twice that

Table 2.1   Illustration of the Principle of Direct Standardization of Crude Rates From Two Hypothetical Populations

Age group	Number	Population A, age-specific death rate	Expected	Number	Population B, age-specific death rate	Expected
Calculation of crude rate						
20-49	2,000	0.001	2	8,000	0.002	16
50-79	10,000	0.01	100	10,000	0.02	200
80 and over	8,000	0.1	800	2,000	0.2	400
Total	20,000		902	20,000		616
Crude death rate	902/20,000 = 4.51%			616/20,000 = 3.08%		
Calculation of standardized rates using the combined population to form the standard population						
20-49	10,000	0.001	10	10,000	0.002	20
50-79	20,000	0.01	200	20,000	0.02	400
80 and over	10,000	0.1	1,000	10,000	0.2	2,000
Total	40,000		1,210	40,000		2,420
Standardized death rate	1210/40,000 = 3.03%			2420/40,000 = 6.05%		

of population A. An inspection of the age distributions in these populations suggests the problem. Population A has a higher proportion of individuals in the older age group, where the age-specific death rate is highest, than population B does. To make a valid comparison of the death rates in these two populations, it is necessary to adjust death rates to account for the difference in age distribution. The direct standardization method involves applying the age-specific rates of the populations to be compared to that for a single standardized population. The standard population can be any reasonable or realistic population. In this example, the standard population is simply the combination of populations A and B. In practice, the population of a particular state or the entire United States is often used. Because the age distribution in the standard population is the same for all the age-specific death rates that are applied to it, the effect of the different age distribution in the two actual populations being compared is eliminated. This procedure allows the overall death rates in the two populations to be compared without the **bias** introduced by differences in the age distribution.

As illustrated in table 2.1, after adjustment for age, the overall death rate in population B (2420/40,000 = 6.05%) is twice that of population A (1210/40,000 = 3.03%), accurately reflecting the fact that the age-specific death rates in population B are twice as high as those in population A. The same principles of direct standardization can be used to compare incidence rates of disease or injury in populations that differ in their distributions of sex, health status, **cholesterol** or blood pressure level, or any other characteristic that might bias the rate comparison. Though standardized rates are useful for making valid comparisons across populations, it must be remembered that they are fictional rates. The adjusted rates can vary, depending on the standard population that is used in the adjustment process. Therefore, the adjusted rate can be misleading and should be used only for comparison purposes.

Research Design in Epidemiologic Studies

A **research design** is the way that participants are grouped and compared according to behavior or attributes (e.g., physical activity or fitness), the health-related events being studied, time, and factors other than physical activity or fitness that

could explain the occurrence of health-related events. The goal of a design in physical activity epidemiologic research is to make sure that comparisons of groups based on differences in physical activity or fitness are not biased by other factors. In other words, the research design used determines whether it is reasonable to infer that physical inactivity was a direct, or the only, explanation for the occurrence of an injury, disease, or death.

▷ **THE RESEARCH** design used is an important consideration in evaluation of the likelihood of a cause-and-effect association between physical activity and the occurrence of death or disease.

In a strong research design, passage of time is needed between the change in the **independent variable** (i.e., the manipulated or fluctuating variable, such as physical activity, thought to be associated with the outcome) and the subsequent change in the **dependent variable** (i.e., the outcome variable, such as heart disease). When the change occurs as the result of **natural history** (i.e., is self-initiated by the people being studied), the design is observational. When change in the independent variable is manipulated by the investigator, the design is experimental. When the independent and dependent variables are observed or manipulated across a period of time, the design is longitudinal or prospective. When the study looks back in time after the occurrence of injury, disease, or death in an attempt to reconstruct an influencing factor, such as physical activity habits, the design is retrospective.

Several types of research designs are commonly used in epidemiologic research: cross-sectional surveys, case–control studies, cohort studies, and randomized controlled trials (table 2.2). The design employed in any particular study depends on the questions to be answered, the time and financial resources available, and the availability of data. The major advantages and disadvantages of the commonly used epidemiologic study designs are summarized in table 2.3.

Cross-Sectional Surveys

Cross-sectional surveys, sometimes called prevalence studies, measure both risk factors and the presence or absence of disease at the same point in time. Although this approach

Table 2.2 Study Designs

Type of study	Time		
	Past	Present	Future
Cross sectional		Assess risk factors and disease outcome	
Case-control	Inquire about exposure to risk factors	Assess outcome, that is, case or control	
Prospective cohort		Assemble cohort Assess risk factors	Assess outcomes
Randomized trial		Randomly assign to experimental groups	Assess outcomes

Table 2.3   Study Designs in Epidemiologic Research: Advantages and Disadvantages

Design	Advantages	Disadvantages
Cross-sectional survey	Is quick and easy to conduct. Is appropriate for hypothesis generation.	No temporal relationship between risk factors and disease. Is not appropriate for hypothesis testing.
Case–control study	Is appropriate for the study of rare events. Can study multiple risk factors. Is inexpensive and quick to perform.	Cannot determine absolute risk. Subject to recall bias. Can study only one disease at a time. Temporal relationships may be uncertain.
Cohort study	Provides an absolute measure of risk. Allows the study of multiple disease outcomes.	Is expensive and time-consuming to conduct. Is not appropriate for studying rare outcomes. Results can be affected by loss to follow-up. Can assess the effect only of risk factors obtained at baseline.
Randomized controlled trial	Investigator has control over the research process. Is the gold standard for evaluation of interventions.	Is expensive and time-consuming to conduct. Generalizability is often limited. Lack of compliance and dropouts can cause problems.

Definitions of Study Designs

- **Cross-sectional study.** Both risk factors and the presence or absence of disease are measured at the same point in time.
- **Case–control study.** Participants are selected based on the presence (i.e., cases) or absence (i.e., **controls**) of a disease of interest. Cases and controls are matched on several possible causes of disease; then a comparison of the frequency of past exposure to other potential risk factors for the disease is made between the two groups.
- **Prospective cohort study.** A group of individuals is selected at random from a defined population.

After the **cohort** is selected, baseline information on potential risk factors is collected, and individuals are followed over time to track the incidence of disease between those people subsequently exposed or not exposed to the risk factors of interest.

- **Randomized controlled trial.** Participants are selected and randomly assigned to receive an experimental manipulation or a control condition. Baseline and outcome measurements are obtained to determine the size of changes after the experimental manipulation compared with the control condition.

is expedient and relatively inexpensive, it does not allow determination of the temporal relationship between a potential cause and effect. For example, in a cross-sectional survey of 556 female participants in the Health and Religion Project, Eaton and colleagues (1995) reported significant negative correlations between physical activity and body mass index, systolic and diastolic blood pressure, and total cholesterol.

While those results indicate that the women with lower levels of physical activity had higher levels of important cardiovascular disease risk factors, it is not possible to determine whether low activity or high risk factors came first. The use of a cross-sectional study design precludes

our knowing whether the women were less active because they had high body mass, blood pressure, or cholesterol, or whether they had high levels of these risk factors because they were less active. Cross-sectional surveys can be useful for generating hypotheses regarding potential associations between risk factors and diseases and also for assessment of the prevalence of risk factors or behaviors in a defined population. For example, the U.S. Centers for Disease Control and Prevention, in cooperation with state health departments, conducts the Behavioral Risk Factor Surveillance Survey each year to determine the prevalence of several disease risk factors, including smoking and sedentary behavior. An **ecological study** is a specific type of cross-sectional survey in which the frequency of some risk factor of interest, for instance sedentary behavior, is compared with an outcome measure, such as obesity, in a particular geographic region, for example a city, county, or state. For example, surveys conducted in a particular state might find high rates of sedentary behavior as well as high rates of obesity. Though this type of information may suggest the hypothesis that sedentary behavior results in obesity, drawing this conclusion is unjustified. Data from this type of survey should never be used to make any conclusion regarding cause and effect because these data are not associated with individual persons. There is no way to know whether the individuals who are sedentary are the same individuals who are obese. This problem is referred to as the **ecological fallacy,** that is, erroneously concluding that an association between variables exists based on an ecological study.

Case–Control Studies

In a case–control study, subjects are selected based on the presence of a disease of interest and matched with controls without the disease. After cases and controls are selected, the frequency of past exposure to potential risk factors for the disease and the odds of having the risk factors between the case and control groups are compared. Risk factor information is typically obtained by personal interview or a review of medical records. A number of case–control studies are available in the physical activity epidemiology literature, particularly in the area of physical activity and cancer. The case–control methodology is ideal for the study of diseases like cancer that occur rather infrequently and have a long latent period between exposure to a risk factor and actual manifestation of the disease. Prospective study designs are not practical if the period between the exposure to a risk factor and the development of a disease is long, as the investigator would have to wait up to 20 years in many situations before having any cases of disease to study.

For example, a group of investigators in the Netherlands reported on a case–control study of physical activity as a risk for breast cancer in women ages 20 to 54 years. A sample of 918 women who had been diagnosed with invasive breast cancer between 1986 and 1989 were selected from a cancer registry. Each patient was matched by age and region of residence with a control subject. Both cases and controls were interviewed in their homes to collect information about lifetime physical activity and other risk factors, including reproductive and contraceptive history, family history of breast cancer, smoking, alcohol use, and premenstrual and menstrual complaints. To ensure recall of past behavior over the same time interval in cases and controls, control subjects were assigned a date of pseudo-diagnosis, that is, a date that corresponded with the date on which the controls were the same age as their matched case subject at actual diagnosis. The analysis was restricted to risk events that occurred prior to actual diagnosis or pseudo-diagnosis to ensure the correct temporal association between the risk factor and disease. Results indicated that women who had been more active than their peers at ages 10 to 12 years were at significantly reduced risk of breast cancer. Also, women who had ever engaged in recreational physical activity at any point prior to diagnosis were also at significantly reduced risk for breast cancer. These data support the hypothesis that recreational physical activity decreases the risk of breast cancer in women, but the results must be interpreted in the light of potential problems associated with the case–control study design, including recall bias and nonrepresentativeness of the control group.

There are several disadvantages to the case–control study design. As discussed later in this chapter in the section on evaluating associations, the case–control design does not allow a direct determination of the **absolute risk** of the disease because the incidence rates are not available; a group of individuals is not followed over time. However, an estimate of the risk of disease in those exposed to the risk factor compared with those not exposed can be calculated. An additional disadvantage of the case–control design is difficulty in obtaining a truly representative control group. To obtain a representative group of controls that are generally matched with cases by age, sex, and race, controls are often obtained from the same setting as the cases (e.g., the hospital where the cases were diagnosed or the same neighborhood where the cases reside). Investigators often use multiple control groups to increase the probability of obtaining a representative comparison group. Another limitation of case–control studies is recall bias, which may result in a spurious association between a risk factor and disease. Recall bias is the phenomenon in which individuals who have experienced an adverse event (e.g., cancer, heart attack) may think more about why they had this problem than healthy individuals and thus might be more likely to recall exposure to potential risk factors. Case–control studies of mortality are also vulnerable to recall bias because information must be obtained from a witness to past behavior, such as a spouse. The spouse or other close relatives of the deceased might be more likely to recall previous risk behaviors than individuals who have not lost a loved one. Another disadvantage of case–control studies is the inability to study more than one disease outcome at a time, although sometimes cases of two cancers (e.g., colon and rectal) are compared to the same control group to make the study more economical.

Case–control studies offer several advantages over other epidemiologic study designs. They are relatively quick and inexpensive to conduct, are useful for studying rare disease outcomes, require a relatively small number of subjects, and allow the study of multiple risk factors. These advantages make this design particularly useful for the initial development and testing of hypotheses to determine whether conducting a more time-consuming and expensive cohort study or randomized trial is warranted.

Prospective Cohort Studies

The term *cohort* comes from the Latin word for a division of a Roman army consisting of 300 to 600 soldiers. In epidemiology, a cohort is a clearly identified group to be studied. Prospective cohort studies, sometimes referred to as *incidence* or *longitudinal follow-up studies,* involve the selection of a group of individuals at random from some defined population or the selection of groups exposed or not exposed to a risk factor of interest.

After the cohort is selected, baseline information on potential risk factors is collected, and individuals are followed over time to track the incidence of disease. A number of prospective cohort studies—for example, the Nurses' Health Study, the Framingham Heart Study, the Harvard Alumni Study, the Honolulu Heart Study, the Physicians' Health Study, and the Aerobics Center Longitudinal Study—have generated valuable information regarding the association of physical activity, physical fitness, and health outcomes. For example, the Aerobics Center Longitudinal Study to date has measured physical fitness, defined as endurance time on a treadmill test, in over 10,000 men and 3000 women when they visited the Cooper Clinic in Dallas, Texas, for preventive medical examination. In one analysis, total mortality in the cohort was assessed for about eight years of follow-up. During the period of observation, 240 deaths among men and 43 deaths among women occurred after about 110,000 **person-years** of exposure (one person followed for one year equals one person-year). Age-adjusted death rates (per 10,000 person-years of exposure) from all causes were lower with each successive level of fitness, from the least fit (64 deaths among men and 40 deaths among women) to the most fit (19 deaths among men and 9 deaths among women). The effects of higher fitness were independent of age, smoking, cholesterol level, systolic blood pressure, blood sugar, and parental history of CHD. Much of the decrease in the total mortality rate in the fitter subjects was explainable by reduced rates of cardiovascular disease and cancer.

The prospective approach is more costly and time-consuming than either a cross-sectional survey or a case–control study, it cannot be used to study diseases that occur infrequently, and it can assess the effects only of risk factors that were measured at baseline (i.e., the beginning of the study). The major advantage of the prospective study is that the risk profile is established before the outcome is assessed. Therefore, any information obtained at baseline cannot be biased by the knowledge of results. However, results can still be biased when many cases are lost to follow-up. Prospective studies also allow the investigator to control the data collection as the study proceeds, to assess changes in risk factors over time, to classify the disease end points (e.g., CHD, diabetes, osteoporosis) correctly, and to study multiple disease outcomes, some of which may not have been planned at the outset of the study. Perhaps most importantly, a prospective design allows the estimation of the true absolute risk of developing a disease. Definition and measurement of risk are discussed later in this chapter.

Randomized Controlled Trial

The randomized controlled trial is the gold standard of research designs for testing a research hypothesis. This design gives the researcher more control than with any of the other epidemiologic research designs. In a randomized controlled trial, participants are selected for study and randomly assigned to receive an experimental manipulation or a control condition. Measurements are made before and after the intervention period in both groups to assess the difference in the outcomes of interest between the intervention and control conditions. The key to this approach is randomization, which ensures that the experimental and control groups are comparable with respect to all factors, known or unknown, except for the factor addressed by the experimental intervention.

Although the randomized controlled trial is the optimal research design, actually conducting these trials poses a number of challenging problems. For example, potential participants in a randomized trial must agree to participate without knowing whether they will be assigned to the intervention or control group. This can be particularly problematic in an exercise intervention trial in which the motivation to participate is to receive the intervention, not to be assigned to a control condition. If possible, it is best to conduct a randomized trial in a double-blind manner; that is, neither the participants nor the observers who collect the data are aware of group assignments. The double-blind approach is obviously not possible in exercise intervention research, for which only single-blind trials (with only the data collection personnel unaware of group assignments) are feasible. Biases can be introduced by poor compliance with the intervention (i.e., some experimental participants fail to fully participate in the intervention) and by dropouts in either the intervention or control group (i.e., groups are no longer equivalent by the end of the study). Because of the difficulty in recruiting participants for large randomized trials, these trials are often conducted using highly select samples. This reduces external validity, the ability to generalize the study results to other populations, especially when loss to follow-up is high. For example, the Physicians' Health Study, which was conducted to determine the **effectiveness** of aspirin on cardiovascular disease and of beta-carotene on cancer and which included a measurement of physical activity, had as subjects mostly white, healthy, middle-aged, male physicians. The generalizability of these results to other groups, such as young men, women, minorities, or nonphysicians, is questionable.

Although the randomized controlled trial is the research design of choice for hypothesis testing, many important questions in physical activity epidemiology cannot be answered with this approach. For example, researchers may be interested in knowing what type, frequency, intensity, and duration of exercise are most beneficial for reducing the incidence of CHD. In theory, an experiment could be conducted in which individuals are randomly assigned to a specific exercise regimen or a control condition and followed for incidence of heart disease. This approach is not practical for several reasons. First, the risk of a first **myocardial infarction** in healthy middle-aged men is about 7 per 1000 per year. Hence, the study would need to involve about 20,000 men, randomly assigned to an exercise intervention group and a control group and followed over a one-year period, to obtain 140 potential cases of myocardial infarction for study! All 20,000 men would need to undergo extensive evaluation prior to randomization to ensure that they are free of heart disease. Steps would have to be taken to ensure that the exercise group adheres to the exercise frequency, intensity, and duration stipulated in the program and that the control group does not start an exercise program during the intervention year. Given the large numbers of subjects needed, a study of this type would have to be conducted at multiple sites across the country, adding additional complexity to maintaining quality control over both the intervention program and other measures of interest (e.g., risk factors). It is obvious that such a study would be exceedingly expensive and a logistical nightmare. Needless to say, a trial of this type has never been and most likely will never be undertaken. The randomized trial has a place in physical activity studies, where smaller, more manageable trials can be conducted on the effects of different levels of physical activity or exercise training on muscle performance, balance, gait, CHD risk factors (such as lipid levels, obesity, blood pressure, insulin levels), and where it is expected that disease rates will be very high, for example in the secondary prevention of cardiovascular diseases in cardiac rehabilitation trials.

Summary

The ultimate goal of a research design is to assess the degree to which change in an independent variable (e.g., physical activity or fitness) is causally associated with change in a dependent variable (e.g., injury, disease, or death). It is important to remember the inherent strengths and weaknesses of the various study design options as we discuss the evidence for physical activity in reducing the risk of chronic disease.

Evaluating Associations in Epidemiologic Studies

Conceptually, epidemiologic research is simply a comparison of groups formed based on the presence or absence of a risk factor under study, the independent variable (e.g., physical activity, smoking, obesity), and the presence or absence of a disease or condition of interest, the dependent variable (e.g., CHD, diabetes, osteoporosis). The goal is generally to identify the risk factors for a particular disease and to determine how much of an impact those factors have on the probability of disease. In practice, the situation can easily become much more complex in that it is often desirable to study several independent variables at the same time and to determine how those variables interact to affect disease risk. For example, epidemiologists are interested in studying the association of physical activity and the incidence of type 2 diabetes while considering the influence of age, sex, body fat, family history of diabetes, diet, smoking, and so on. They may also be interested in assessing the effect of different levels of exercise (i.e., low, moderate, or high intensity) and durations of exposure to a risk factor on disease outcome.

Regardless of how complex the issues under study become, most epidemiologic research can be conceptually framed in a standard 2 × 2 table (see table 2.4). There are slight differences in the interpretation of the 2 × 2 table, depending on whether data were obtained from a prospective cohort or a case–control study. Both study designs are discussed in further detail in the following sections.

Table 2.4 The 2 × 2 Table for Assessing the Association Between Risk Factors and Disease

Risk factor status	Disease status		
	Present	Absent	Total
Present	a	b	a + b
Absent	c	d	c + d
Total	a + c	b + d	a + b + c + d

a = Subjects with both risk factor and disease
b = Subjects with risk factor but no disease
c = Subjects with no risk factor and disease
d = Subjects with no risk factor and no disease

a + b = All subjects with risk factor
a + c = All subjects with disease
b + d = All subjects with no disease
c + d = All subjects with no risk factor
a + b + c + d = All subjects

Prospective Cohort Study

The interpretation of the 2 × 2 table for a prospective cohort study is presented in table 2.5. Recall that in a prospective cohort study, a population is selected, baseline measurements are obtained, and the population is followed over time to document the development of disease. Table 2.6 provides data from a hypothetical prospective cohort study on the association between physical activity at baseline and the incidence of CHD to illustrate the process of assessing the strength of the association between a risk factor and disease.

In the example, 500 men in the total sample of 10,000 developed CHD. The overall incidence rate is then 500 cases per 10,000 population, or 0.05 (5%). The question of interest is, What impact does risk factor status (i.e., level of physical activity) have on the incidence of disease? To answer this question, we need to calculate the incidence of disease in both the active and sedentary groups. The incidence rate, or risk, for CHD in the sedentary group is $a/(a + b) = 400/(400 + 5600) = 400/6000 = 0.067$, or 6.7%. The incidence rate, or risk, of disease in the active group is $c/(c + d) = 100/(100 + 3900) = 100/4000 = 0.025$, or 2.5%. With this information, the effect of sedentary behavior on CHD risk can be evaluated. The **risk difference** is simply the risk of disease in the group exposed to the risk factor minus the risk of disease in the unexposed group. In the example, the risk in the exposed (sedentary) group is 6.7%, and the risk in the unexposed (active) group is 2.5%, so the risk difference is 6.7% − 2.5% = 4.2%. Obviously, if the levels of risk in

the exposed and unexposed groups are the same, the risk difference is zero.

If exposure to the risk factor is harmful, as is the case for sedentary behavior in the example, then the risk difference is greater than zero. If exposure is protective (e.g., exposure to a drug that lowers cholesterol level), then the risk difference is less than zero. The risk difference is also called the **attributable risk;** it is an estimate of the amount of risk attributed to the risk factor. In the example, 4.2% of the risk of CHD in this population is attributed to exposure to the risk factor of sedentary behavior. The **relative risk (RR),** or **risk ratio,** is the ratio of the risk in the exposed group to the risk in the unexposed group. In the example, the relative risk of CHD between the exposed (sedentary) group and the unexposed (active) group is

$$RR = [a/(a + b)]/[c/(c + d)]$$

$$= [400/(400 + 5600)]/[100/(100 + 3900)]$$

$$= 0.067/0.025 = 2.68.$$

If the risk of disease in the exposed and unexposed groups is the same, the relative risk is 1.0. If the risks in the two groups are not the same, calculation of the relative risk provides an easily interpretable method of demonstrating, in relative terms, how much greater or smaller the risks are. In the example, the risk of CHD in the sedentary group is 2.68 times higher than in the active group. When considering risk assessments, it is important to remember the difference between absolute and relative risk. In the example, the absolute risk for developing CHD—that is, the true risk in the exposed (sedentary) group—is 6.7%, but that level of risk is 2.68 times higher than the absolute risk in the active group (2.5%). In some cases the relative risk can be extremely high even while the absolute risk in both groups is rather low. For example, the relative risk of a myocardial infarction after heavy physical exertion in a group of men and women who do not exercise regularly has been shown to be approximately 100 times the risk of myocardial infarction in men and women who are regular exercisers. This is an extremely high relative risk; however, the absolute risk of myocardial infarction following heavy exertion, even for sedentary individuals, is actually quite low. Considering that the absolute risk of a myocardial infarction during any given hour in a healthy, middle-aged adult man is approximately one per million, even with a hundredfold increase the absolute risk is still quite small ($0.000001 \times 100 = 0.0001$, or an absolute risk of 1 per 10,000).

Relative risks can also be used to judge the efficacy of clinical outcomes in randomized controlled trials. If, for example, 20% of heart patients in a control group who get usual care or no treatment die from a second heart attack, but the rate is only 10% in an exercise group, the absolute risk difference between the groups is 10%. Inverting that difference (i.e., $1.0/0.10 = 10$) yields what is known as the **number**

Table 2.5   The 2 × 2 Table for a Prospective Cohort Study

Risk factor status	Follow-up			Incidence rate of disease
	Develop disease	Do not develop disease	Total	
Present	a	b	$a + b$	$a/(a + b)$
Absent	c	d	$c + d$	$c/(c + d)$

Table 2.6   Hypothetical Cohort Study on Physical Activity and Coronary Heart Disease

Risk factor status	Follow-up		Incidence rate of disease
	Develop disease	Do not develop disease	
Present (sedentary)	$a = 400$	$b = 5600$	6.7%
Absent (active)	$c = 100$	$d = 3900$	2.5%
Total	500	9500	

needed to treat (NNT). In this example, an additional life would be saved for every 10 patients treated with exercise.

The Cox Proportional Hazards Ratio is a common rate ratio used in survival analysis (i.e., death rates) in both observational studies and clinical trials. It is an estimate of the ratio of incidence rates of disease between an exposed or untreated group and an unexposed or treated group. The hazard rate is the probability that an event will occur during a future period of time divided by the length of that time period. In this book, we will refer to hazards ratios as relative risks for simplicity. Like the relative risk, the **odds ratio (OR)** compares the likelihood of an event between two groups. For a prospective study, it is calculated by dividing cases by noncases in each of the exposed and unexposed groups and computing the ratio of those rates.

$$OR = (a/b)/(c/d)$$

$$= ad/bc.$$

In the standard 2×2 table (see table 2.4), the risk of disease in the exposed group, as discussed previously, is $a/(a + b)$, whereas the odds of disease in the exposed group (i.e., the chance of having vs. not having the disease) in the exposed group is simply a/b. Based strictly on the mathematics, if a is small compared with b, which it often is, then the odds and the risk are quite similar. We can illustrate this by calculating the OR for the hypothetical data in table 2.6. Here the OR is $(400/5600)/(100/3900) = 2.79$ or $(400 \times 3900)/(100 \times 5600) = 1,560,000/560,000 = 2.79$, which is quite similar to the relative risk of 2.68. Therefore, an OR will approximate a relative risk when the prevalence of a disease is low and the number of cases is therefore a small portion of the population. However, an OR is best used in a case–control design.

Case–Control Study

A case–control study doesn't permit computation of a relative risk directly since the people studied are selected because they already have a disease rather because they have been exposed to a risk factor. In a case–control study, participants are selected based on disease status (i.e., whether the disease is present or absent). Table 2.7 is a 2×2 table illustrating the organization of data from a case–control study. The analysis in a case–control study is a comparison of the proportion of cases exposed to a suspected risk factor, $a/(a + c)$, with

the proportion of controls exposed to the same risk factor, $b/(b + d)$. If exposure to the risk factor is positively related to the disease, then the proportion of cases exposed to the risk factor should be greater than the proportion of controls exposed to the risk factor. In a case–control study, the only measure of the strength of the association between the risk factor and disease is the OR (ad/bc). Conceptually, the OR is an estimate of the risk of disease given the presence of a particular risk factor compared with the risk of disease if the risk factor is not present. Although the odds of having the risk factor are estimated in the diseased group, there is no way to accurately estimate probability of disease (i.e., risk) in people who have the risk factor. When disease cases are selected first and then matched with controls without disease, the overall prevalence of the disease in the two groups combined can be much higher than in a population.

Nonetheless, in most instances the ORs from well-conducted case–control studies are reasonable estimates of the relative risk that would have been derived from a prospective cohort study, provided that the overall risk of disease (i.e., prevalence or incidence rates) in the population is low (i.e., less than 5%).

Interpreting Relative Risks and Odds Ratios

If the risk of disease is the same in the groups exposed and not exposed to the risk factor, the relative risk and OR will be 1.0. Typically, when relative risk is calculated, the incidence of disease in the exposed group is placed in the numerator and the incidence of disease in the unexposed group in the denominator, as was done with the data from the hypothetical prospective cohort study in table 2.6, where the calculated relative risk was 2.68. This makes sense because as the impact of the risk factor increases (in this case the impact of sedentary behavior on CHD incidence), the relative risk increases. However, it is also acceptable to reverse the fraction and place the incidence of disease in the exposed group in the denominator. Then the relative risk would be $0.025/0.067 = 0.37$, indicating that the risk in the active group is about one-third that of the sedentary group.

Although the formula for calculating the OR is different from that for calculating relative risk, the interpretation of magnitude of the actual value is virtually the same. Usually the OR is expressed with the group exposed to the risk factor in the numerator. However, the interpretation of the strength of the observed OR is not changed if the exposed group is placed in the denominator. The 95% **confidence interval** is a measure of the degree of confidence that the observed relative risk or OR is meaningful. The 95% confidence interval gives an estimate of the lowest and highest values that might be expected 95 times if the study were to be repeated 100 times using other samples of the same number of people. The confidence interval can be used to determine whether

Table 2.7   The 2 × 2 Table for a Case–Control Study

		Cases (disease)	Controls (no disease)
Risk factor status	Present	a	b
	Absent	c	d
Proportion exposed		$a/(a + c)$	$b/(b + d)$

the observed relative risk or OR differs statistically from 1.0. A relative risk or OR of 1.0 indicates that there is no difference in the risk of disease between those exposed and not exposed to the risk factor. If the relative risk of CHD in sedentary individuals (2.68 in our hypothetical study) had a 95% confidence interval ranging from 0.72 to 3.15, the relative risk would not be statistically significant because the confidence interval includes a value of 1.0. However, if the same relative risk had a 95% confidence interval ranging from 1.5 to 3.5, the relative risk would be significantly different from 1.0 because 1.0 does not fall within the calculated confidence interval.

Attributable Risk

An important function of epidemiologic research is to estimate the amount of disease burden in a population that results from a potentially modifiable risk factor. For example, researchers might ask this question: In the U.S. population, how much CHD mortality is the result of sedentary behavior, high blood pressure, obesity, and other modifiable risk factors? This type of information is extremely important for making decisions about which risk factors intervention efforts should target to maximize the benefits to public health. Also, the public may be more interested in and likely to comply with intervention efforts if the importance of such efforts to their individual health can be demonstrated.

The concept of attributable risk is credited to Morton Levin (Levin 1953), who also was among the first to link smoking with cancer risk. Several epidemiologic measures are used to assess the impact of exposure on disease risk factors. These include the attributable risk percentage in the exposed group, **population attributable risk,** and population attributable risk fraction (i.e., percentage). The following paragraphs describe these measures using the hypothetical data in table 2.6 as an illustration.

Attributable Risk (AR) Fraction in the Exposed

The AR percentage estimates the total risk of disease that results from a risk factor among those who are exposed to that risk factor. Either of two formulas can be used to calculate the AR fraction:

$$(1)\ AR\% = (Risk_{exposed} - Risk_{unexposed})/Risk_{exposed}$$

$$(2)\ AR\% = (RR - 1)/RR$$

Using the data from table 2.6 with formula 1 to calculate the AR percentage of CHD among the sedentary,

$$AR\% = (0.067 - 0.025)/0.067$$

$$= 0.042/0.067$$

$$= 0.6268$$

$$= 62.7\%.$$

Using formula 2,

$$AR\% = (2.68 - 1)/2.68$$

$$= 1.68/2.68$$

$$= 0.6268$$

$$= 62.7\%.$$

Therefore, among those who are sedentary, 62.7% of the risk for CHD is attributable to sedentary behavior. The AR percentage in the exposed can also be calculated for a case–control study by substituting the OR for the relative risk in formula 2.

Population Attributable Risk (PAR)

Population attributable risk is the risk of disease in the total population minus the risk in the unexposed group. In the CHD example of table 2.6, the calculation of the PAR allows a determination of how much of the total risk of CHD is attributable to sedentary behavior. In this example, the risk of CHD in the total population is 500/10,000 = 0.05, or 5 per 100 per year. The risk of disease in the active group is 100/4000 = 0.025, 2.5 per 100 per year. Therefore, PAR = 5 − 2.5 = 2.5; in other words, 2.5 cases per 100 population per year are attributable to sedentary behavior.

Population Attributable Risk (PAR) Fraction

PAR percentage is the percentage of the risk of a disease that is attributable to a particular risk factor. It is PAR expressed as a percentage rather than an absolute value.

$$PAR\% = (Risk_{total} - Risk_{unexposed})/Risk_{total}$$

Using the data from table 2.6,

$$PAR\% = (5 - 2.5)/5$$

$$= 0.5$$

$$= 50\%.$$

Therefore, 50% of the total risk for CHD in this population is attributable to sedentary behavior. Hypothetically, half the CHD cases would be prevented in this population if sedentary people became physically active.

From a public health perspective, this formula is a more useful approach to the calculation of PAR fraction:

$$PAR\% = (P_{exposed})(RR - 1)/[1 + (P_{exposed})(RR - 1)],$$

where $P_{exposed}$ is the proportion of the population exposed to the risk factor and RR is the relative risk of disease associated with the risk factor.

This formula allows a comparison of the impact of different risk factors on disease risk in a population. For example, the proportion of CHD risk due to sedentary behavior could be compared with that due to cigarette smoking. Let us assume that the relative risk for CHD associated with sedentary behavior is 2.0 and that 50% of the U.S. population is sedentary ($P_{exposed}$). Let us also assume that the relative risk of CHD associated with cigarette smoking is 5.0 and that 20% of the U.S. population smokes. With this information, the PAR percentage for both sedentary behavior and cigarette smoking can be calculated as follows:

$$PAR\% \text{ (sedentary behavior)} = 0.5(2.0 - 1)/$$
$$[1 + (0.5)(2.0 - 1)]$$
$$= 0.5/1.5$$
$$= 0.333$$
$$= 33.3\%$$

$$PAR\% \text{ (smoking)} = 0.2(5.0 - 1)/[1 + (0.2)(5.0 - 1)]$$
$$= 0.2(4)/[1 + (0.2)(4)]$$
$$= 0.8/(1 + 0.8)$$
$$= 0.444$$
$$= 44.4\%$$

Thus, in this example, approximately 33% of the CHD in the population is attributable to sedentary behavior and 44% to cigarette smoking. In theory, if all sedentary individuals become active, there would be 33% fewer cases of CHD in the population. Similarly, if all the cigarette smokers quit, there would be 44% fewer CHD cases.

PAR percentage thus allows comparison of the impact of risk factors that vary in relative risk and prevalence in the population. A risk factor might have a very high relative risk but a low prevalence in the population; modification of that risk factor thus would have limited impact on public health. The PAR percentage of sedentary behavior as it relates to several disease outcomes, including CHD and cancer, is evaluated in subsequent chapters.

Diagnostic Tests

Diagnostic tests make use of the same information used in computing RR and OR, but for the purpose of predicting the odds that a person has a disease based on the results of a laboratory test. This is more common in preventive medicine than in epidemiology. However, some risk factors that physical activity modifies rely on laboratory tests (e.g., cholesterol and triglycerides for CHD and insulin or glucose levels for diabetes), so a basic understanding of diagnostic tests and how they are judged for usefulness is important in epidemiology too. Standard diagnostic terms are defined in table 2.8, and their uses are shown in table 2.9.

A useful test first should be sensitive, which means it can detect a disease that is present. A sensitive test has a high proportion of true positives and few false negatives. A test should also be specific, which means it doesn't falsely detect a disease that isn't present. A specific test has a high proportion of true negatives and few false positives. Usually, **sensitivity** and **specificity** rates of 80% or more are considered to be potentially useful. However, sensitivity and specificity don't alone determine the predictive value

Table 2.8 Terms Used in Diagnostic Tests

Term	What it means
True positive (TP)	Patients with the disease who have a positive test
True negative (TN)	Patients with the disease who have a negative test
False positive (FP)	Patients without the disease who have a positive test
False negative (FN)	Patients with the disease who have a negative test
Bayes' theorem	The odds of having or not having the disease based on the test result and the prevalence of the disease
Likelihood ratio of a positive test result (LR+)	The increase in the odds of having the disease after a positive test result
Likelihood ratio of a negative test result (LR−)	The decrease in the odds of having the disease after a negative test result

Table 2.9 Diagnostic Statistics

Sensitivity (Sen)	Probability of positive test if diagnosis is positive	$Sen = TP/(TP + FN)$
Specificity (Spc)	Probability of negative test if diagnosis is negative	$Spc = TN/(TN + FP)$
Positive predictive value (Ppv)	Probability of positive diagnosis if test is positive	$Ppv = TP/(TP + FP)$
Negative predictive value (Npv)	Probability of negative diagnosis if test is negative	$Npv = TN/(TN + FN)$

of a test. The prevalence of the outcome in a population must also be considered. Thus, a test's predictive value depends on the frequency of the trait that underlies the test and the prevalence of the disease, relative to the decision point on the diagnostic test. For example, when a disease is highly prevalent (e.g., in more than 50% of a population), a poor test can have high sensitivity. If prevalence were 60%, just guessing that a disease is present would be better than tossing a coin. This illustrates **Bayes' theorem,** which roughly states that the odds of event A (e.g., disease) being dependent upon event B (positive test result) are an inverse function of the prior probability of A and B before the test is administered. In practice, the odds that a positive test result will give an accurate prediction of disease is given by a **positive likelihood ratio** (PLR) = sensitivity/(1 − specificity) multiplied by the prior odds of the disease (prevalence/[1 − prevalence]). Likewise, the odds that a negative test result will give an accurate prediction of the absence of disease is given by the prior odds multiplied by a **negative likelihood ratio** (NLR) = ([1 − sensitivity]/specificity). A more easily computed positive predictive value is given by the number of true positives divided by true positives + false positives. Negative predictive value is given by the number of true negatives divided by true negatives + false negatives.

Table 2.10 uses the same data given in tables 2.5 and 2.6 to compute these diagnostic statistics. They show that physical inactivity has good sensitivity (i.e., 80%) as a "test" of CHD (it detected 400 of the 500 cases), but it has poor specificity (i.e., 41%) and very low positive predictive value (i.e., 6.67%). This is because of the high number of false positives (i.e., 5600), which exceeds the number of true negatives (i.e., 3900). In contrast, a negative test result (in this case, being physically active) has very good negative predictive value (i.e., 97.5%) because only 100 of 4000 active people (i.e., 2.5%) had CHD. Note that the ratio PLR/NLR = 2.79, which is the same value as the OR computed from these data in the example of table 2.4. Thus, the OR for a prospective cohort design is equivalent to the ratio of the positive and negative likelihood ratios, which depend on the sensitivity and specificity of the risk factor and the prevalence of the disease. It is the application of these statistics that differs in purpose between the OR and evaluation of a diagnostic test.

Models in Physical Activity Epidemiology

To understand the role of physical activity and fitness in health, it is necessary to view these factors in the context of the models used by epidemiologists to understand the independent and interactive causes of disease, injury, or death.

The three most commonly used models for this purpose are presented in figure 2.2. The first and most common model is the epidemiologic triangle, consisting of the host (i.e., the person), the environment (e.g., physical, social), and the agent (e.g., physical activity or fitness). This model evolved from the early days of infectious disease epidemiology and has been superseded by more recent models that are more applicable to chronic disease epidemiology, in which the cause of disease is generally multifactorial. The web of causation holds that a disease has no single, isolated cause. Hence, a study of physical activity and fitness as risk factors for a disease must consider how they interact with other potential causes of the disease. The strength of the web—namely, its acknowledgment that the causes of disease interact with each other—is also its weakness, because its complexity leads to difficulty with regard to understanding the etiology of disease and predicting health outcomes. The wheel is probably the most valid model of epidemiologic inquiry because it views the development of the host as intertwined with the environment, and it recognizes that the host develops from a genetic core that is modifiable to varying degrees by the biological, physical, and social environments to which the host is exposed.

Exercise scientists Claude Bouchard and Roy Shephard have integrated the traditional epidemiologic models to illustrate how the independent and interactive effects on health of heredity, habits other than physical activity, the physical environment, the social environment, and personal attributes might be conceptualized (Bouchard and Shephard 1994). Their model is presented in figure 2.3 and simplified in figure 2.4.

As shown in figures 2.3 and 2.4, heredity, or genetic factors, is directly associated with all other parts of the model. Although we cannot alter genetic factors, at least at this point in time, it is important to be aware of the role that genetic factors might play in the association of physical activity

Table 2.10 Computing Diagnostic Statistics

Test groups	Cases (CHD)	Noncases (No CHD)	
Positive test Inactive (exposed)	400 True positive test	5600 False positive test	Ppv 400/6000 = 6.67%
Negative test Active (unexposed)	100 False negative test	3900 True negative test	Npv 3900/4000 = 97.5%
	Sensitivity 400/500 = 80%	Specificity 3900/9500 = 41%	

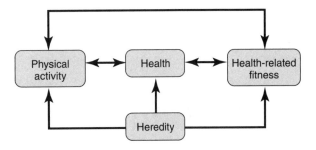

Figure 2.4 An integration of the traditional epidemiological models illustrates how the independent and interactive effects on health of heredity, habits other than physical activity, the physical environment, the social environment, and personal attributes might be conceptualized.

(1) The epidemiologic triangle

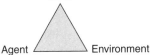

(2) The web of causation

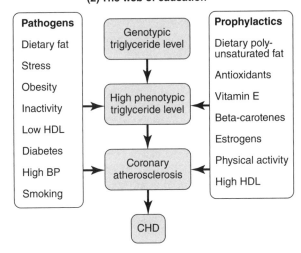

(3) The wheel

Figure 2.2 The three traditional epidemiological models.

Adapted from Mausner and Kramer 1985.

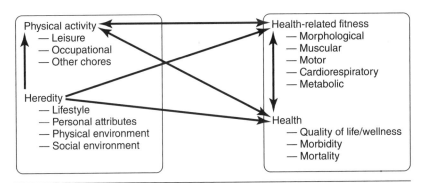

Figure 2.3 Plausible causal paths for physical activity, fitness, and health.

and health. Humans differ widely in genetic makeup. For example, there appears to be as much variation in DNA sequence within each race as there is among the races. Given these circumstances, an equal state of health and of physical and mental well-being is unlikely to be achieved for all. Individuals of a particular genetic makeup are less susceptible to disease and disability than others. Genetic predisposition explains, at least in part, why we are not equally prone to hypertension, atherosclerosis, diabetes, osteoporosis, cancer, or heart attacks. Genetic factors also may play a significant role in determining an individual's level of physical activity and physical fitness (muscular strength, aerobic capacity, etc.) and explain a major part of the difference in people's physiological response (e.g., body fat, cholesterol, blood pressure, aerobic capacity) to identical diets or exercise training programs.

There is equally wide variation in the physical and social environments to which people are exposed among and within societies. Those differences can be in climate, population density, natural resources, economy, educational level, and cultural values. All these factors can singly and collectively affect exposure to disease risk factors (including behaviors) and disease vulnerability. These influences are evidenced by the fact that only about 20% to 50% of the variation in people's physical activity and about 40% of the variation in their cardiorespiratory fitness are explainable by variation in **genotypes** (i.e., genetic inheritance). Moreover, even among monozygotic (i.e., identical) twins, biological adaptations to vigorous physical activity, including fitness changes, can vary by as much as 50% (Bouchard et al. 1994). Hence, even gene expression in response to physical activity is apparently influenced by the environment during the life span. On the other hand, although age, sex, and ethnicity are not strong influences on adaptations to physical activity, people's initial phenotypes (i.e., their observable **traits**) are major predictors of responses to exercise training for some variables (e.g., submaximal heart rate and blood pressure) but not others (e.g., maximal oxygen uptake and high-density lipoprotein cholesterol; Bouchard and Rankinen 2001).

Inferring Cause in Epidemiologic Studies

The epidemiologic models previously described provide a framework for considering the association among variables in an attempt to determine cause and effect. In the context of epidemiology, causal association can be defined as an association between categories of events or characteristics in which an alteration in the frequency or quality of one category is followed by a change in the other category. To determine whether an observed association between a risk factor and disease is likely causal, it is first necessary to demonstrate a statistical association between the risk factor and disease outcome. Next, it is necessary to rule out that the association is explained by bias (i.e., that the people studied don't represent the population of interest). Even when a strong, statistically significant, and unbiased association between a risk factor and disease is demonstrated, there is always the possibility that the observed association is noncausal. Two issues, confounding and effect modification, can result in noncausal associations.

Confounding

Confounding is the confusion of the effect of the presumably causal variable under study with the effects of other extraneous variables so that all or part of the supposed causal effect of the "causal" variable on the dependent variable is actually explainable by the extraneous variables. For example, in men, baldness is associated with the risk of myocardial infarction; however, this is most likely not a causal association. Age increases both the likelihood of baldness and the risk of myocardial infarction; thus, age confounds the association between baldness and myocardial infarction. Confounding takes place when two or more potential risk factors co-occur in a group so that it is not possible to determine the independent effect of either risk factor. A confounder must be associated with both the exposure variable (e.g., physical inactivity) and the health outcome (e.g., disease, injury, or death) and also with the health outcome independently of the exposure variable. Said another way, if a physically active group of people were observed to have a lower rate of disease than a sedentary group but also were younger and smoked less tobacco, it would not be possible to conclude that physical activity protected against disease independently of age and smoking. Rather, the higher rate of disease in the sedentary group might be explainable by older age and smoking, not by the group's low physical activity. Figure 2.5 illustrates age as a confounder.

Of the 500 active people, 250 have disease and 250 do not. So, the rate is 50%. Of 500 inactive people, 400 have disease. So, their rate is 80%, 1.6 times the rate among the

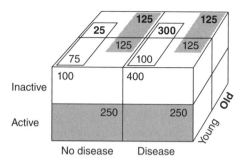

Figure 2.5 Age as a confounder of lower coronary heart disease risk in physically active adults.

active. However, this difference in rates is confounded by age differences between the active and inactive. Both the diseased and not diseased active people are equally split between young and old. However, 75% of inactive people are old (25 of 100 without disease and 300 of 400 with disease). Hence, the higher rate of disease among the inactive might be explained by their higher age.

The possibility of confounding is higher in observational studies, which are common in physical activity epidemiology, than in randomized controlled trials. This is so because the random assignment of participants to groups in randomized trials reduces the likelihood that the comparison groups (e.g., exposed vs. not exposed) differ with regard to a potential confounding variable.

For example, many observational studies have shown greater physical activity at baseline to be associated with lower risk of all-cause mortality. Does increased physical activity cause the lower mortality risk, or are more-active people generally in better health and therefore at lower risk of dying? Does overall health status confound the observed association between more physical activity and decreased mortality? Most well-conducted observational studies use statistical techniques to adjust, or attempt to adjust, for indicators of health status such as blood pressure, lipid levels, obesity, and cigarette smoking to determine whether the association of physical activity with morbidity or mortality risk has **independence** from confounders. A simple way to determine this is to divide the number of cases by the suspected confounder. For example, if higher age is positively associated with a higher rate of disease and negatively associated with physical activity, dividing the number of cases of each of the exposed and unexposed groups by their cumulative ages would standardize the rates according to age (i.e., the denominator for the rate becomes person-years of exposure) and remove most of the confounding influence of age.

Case–control studies can minimize the effects of confounding by matching each diseased case with one or more nondiseased persons who have the same scores on risk factors that are possible **confounders.** Nevertheless, many studies report that the association of physical activity and all-cause mortality persists after adjustment for the measured confounders. The association may still be the result of **residual confounding**, though as most studies do not measure all potential confounders or do not measure these confounders perfectly or do not determine whether they change across time. For example, other diseases that may affect both physical activity and mortality, such as diabetes or depression, are often not taken into consideration. This points to the difficulty for any single observational study to account for all potential confounders and therefore to provide definitive evidence that the apparent effect of physical activity in reducing risk is wholly independent of other possible explanations for the reduced risk.

The accumulation of results of numerous investigations using different samples and measuring different confounding variables adds weight to a causal association between physical activity and chronic disease risk.

Effect Modification

In addition to confounding, effect modification, also called *interaction,* needs to be considered in any evaluation of the possibility of causal associations. Effect modification in epidemiology refers to a situation in which two or more risk factors modify one another's effects on an outcome. For dichotomous variables (variables with only two levels or categories, e.g., yes or no, sedentary or active), effect modification means that the effect of the exposure on the outcome depends on the presence of another variable. For example, the effect of the physical activity categories sedentary or active on the presence or absence of CHD might differ depending on some third factor, such as sex; physical activity might reduce the risk of disease among men but not in women. In such a case, sex would be termed an **effect modifier.** We can evaluate the effect modification of continuous variables by determining the extent to which the effect of exposure on outcome depends on the level of some other variable.

For example, the effect of physical activity assessed by questionnaire on the risk for CHD may depend on the body mass index (BMI, body weight in kilograms divided by the square of height in meters). The risk of disease among the least-active people might be greatest among those having the highest BMI. If so, BMI would be considered an effect modifier in the association between activity and CHD. Figure 2.6 illustrates age as an effect modifier. Mortality decreases linearly with higher levels of physical activity. However, the slope of the decrease is much steeper among older people. The least-active older person has a much higher mortality rate than does the least-active young person. But the mortality rates for older people become increasingly similar to those of young people at higher levels of physical activity. Said another way, low activity is a bigger problem for older people, but high activity protects against mortality regardless of age. Hence, age modifies the effect of physical activity for reducing mortality risk.

Determining the degree to which certain factors act as effect modifiers can provide important information for the development of preventive strategies. For example, if it were

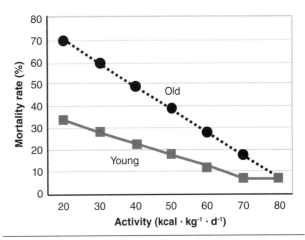

Figure 2.6 Age as an effect modifier of lower coronary heart disease risk in physically active adults.

demonstrated that individuals with high BMIs are at higher risk of CHD only if they also are relatively inactive compared with those who have normal or low BMIs, the evidence for effect modification might be sufficient to prompt interventions designed specifically to increase physical activity among individuals with high BMIs. The potential for confounding and effect modification increases the difficulty of interpreting epidemiologic studies of the direct effects of physical activity on health. Age can be a confounder because of a direct association between age and increased risk for death and most chronic diseases. Therefore, to examine the association between physical activity and health outcomes, the effect of age needs to be removed. Age can also change the magnitude of risk associated with other variables. Thus, age is also considered an effect modifier. For example, the risk of CHD increases with age, increased blood pressure, and decreased levels of physical activity. But age is also associated with decreased physical activity and increased blood pressure. Therefore, to determine whether there is an association between physical activity and CHD risk, the effect of both age and blood pressure must be controlled. In epidemiologic studies, this type of control is typically done by statistical analysis.

When you read and interpret information about the association of physical activity and health outcomes, it is important to be aware of the potential consequences of confounding (i.e., the confusion of two supposedly causal variables) and effect modification (i.e., the influence of a third variable on the strength or direction of the association between two other variables) and to determine whether these issues have been satisfactorily addressed.

Criteria for Causation

Epidemiologists are like detectives, building a circumstantial case for likely causes of disease, injury, or early death. When a strong enough case is built, the conduct of experiments (e.g., randomized controlled trials) is justified to provide more confirming evidence that the suspected culprit is guilty. However, population experiments can be impractical and too costly to carry out, and they are often not ethical. That is why there has never been a population-wide experiment with humans to show that smoking causes CHD or lung cancer. It would not be ethical to have people start smoking since the odds are so strong that they would die because of smoking. Doing so would be similar to having people jump from airplanes without a parachute in order to prove that parachutes can save lives (Smith and Pell 2003). When a statistical association between a risk factor and a disease outcome can be demonstrated and the results of confounding and effect modification have been accounted for, there are several criteria that, if satisfied, increase the probability that the association is real and causal. The general approach taken to judge the strength of scientific evidence about whether a risk factor is a likely cause of chronic disease or early mortality has a long history. Its contemporary roots are mainly found in the process used to produce the U.S. Surgeon General's 1964 report, *Smoking and Health,* and in similar ideas later popularized by the British epidemiologist Austin Bradford Hill in his seminal paper—"The Environment and Disease: Association or Causation?"—presented in 1965 to the Royal Society of Medicine in London. Although Hill stated, "None of my nine viewpoints can bring indisputable evidence for or against the cause-and-effect hypothesis" (Hill 1965, p. 299),

they are often cited as the "Bradford Hill criteria," or **Hill's criteria** (see table 2.11).

However, the classical rules of inquiry used in contemporary epidemiology have a long evolution. They have common threads in logic and medicine that span centuries, stemming from the logic of deduction used by Greek philosophers such as Plato and Aristotle; their application to medicine by the Greco-Roman physician Galen and the Persian philosopher physician Ibn Sīnā; refinement of the scientific method by the English empiricist Francis Bacon; universal application by the Scottish philosopher David Hume; and finally, extension to groups and populations by the British philosopher John Stuart Mill.

Ibn Sīnā (a.k.a. Avicenna) (980-1037) was a translator of Aristotle and Galen and is most famous for writing the *Canon of Medicine,* a standard medical text in Europe through the Renaissance. He extended Aristotelian syllogistic logic to principles for testing the clinical efficacy of drugs and medicines. In *Novum Organum (New Instrument),* published in 1620, Francis Bacon revised Aristotle's logic into methods of agreement, difference, and concomitant variation and formalized the scientific method. Those ideas were further elaborated as eight "rules by which to judge of causes and effects" by David Hume in his 1739 *A Treatise of Human Nature.* Hume's rules were intended for universal application, but they parallel Hill's ideas of strength of association, con-

Table 2.11   Austin Bradford Hill's Viewpoints on Inferring Cause

Hill's criteria, 1965	Hume's rules, 1739
Strength of association: Rate of disease is higher in the exposed group.	"There must be a constant union betwixt the cause and effects." (Rule 3)
Consistency: Association is repeatedly observed by different persons and in different places, circumstances, and times.	"Multiplicity of resembling instances constitutes the very essence of power or connexion." (not a rule but a premise)
Specificity: Association is limited to one disease and a single group or location with no other likely explanation. However, diseases can have more than one cause.	"The same cause always produces the same effect, and the same effect never arises but from the same cause." (Rule 4)
Temporality: The effect must occur after the exposure, especially for diseases that develop slowly.	"The cause must be prior to the effect." (Rule 2)
Biological gradient: A dose–response gradient. More exposure should be associated with a higher rate of disease. A linear gradient is the best evidence, but other patterns of association may be causal.	"When any object increases or diminishes with the increase or diminution of its cause." (Rule 7)
Plausibility: Findings are explainable by existing biological knowledge and can be altered.	Biology did not evolve as part of scientific inquiry until the 19th century.
Coherence: A causal interpretation should not conflict with knowledge about the natural history of the disease and its known pathophysiology.	In the 18th century, it was thought that infectious diseases were spread among people by breathing bad air (miasma theory). Germ theory of disease did not take hold until Robert Koch's proofs in the late 19th century.
Experiment: Manipulation of the presumed cause should result in a lower rate of disease.	Although Bacon had popularized the scientific method a century earlier, Hume's rules were being applied to universal logic, not scientific inquiry.
Analogy: Weaker evidence may be accepted as causal, if similar factors have already been accepted as a cause of the disease.	"Like effects imply like causes." (Rule 5)

Adapted from Hill 1965; Morabia 1991.

sistency, specificity, temporality, dose response, and analogy applied to epidemiology more than 200 years later (Morabia 1991). Hume's eighth rule, "that an object, which exists for any time in its full perfection without any effect, is not the sole cause of that effect, but requires to be assisted by some other principle," implies the idea of effect modification. In 1843, John Stuart Mill described five canons or methods of inquiry in *A System of Logic: Ratiocinative and Inductive* (Mill 1843) that provided a logical basis for research designs and principles used in classical epidemiology (Susser 1973). For example, the method of agreement provides a basis of consistency; the method of concomitant variation illustrates dose response; the method of difference is illustrated by a randomized controlled trial (Susser 1973). These canons were elaborations of the ideas of Bacon and Hume except for Mill's method of residues, which specified that the effects of a cause must be isolated from other competing causes. This forms the basis of controlling for confounders in case–control designs and cohort designs to ensure that a risk factor has an independent association with disease. Hence, judging the strength of inferences about cause from observational studies can't be traced to a single source.

Causal inference about chronic diseases developed gradually in textbooks of epidemiology during the 1960s and '70s; it wasn't mentioned in Austin Bradford Hill's 1961 text on medical statistics (Zhang et al. 2004). And, application of biological science to the study of chronic disease wasn't central to epidemiologic inquiry until its use in the 1964 report of the U.S. Surgeon General on the hazards of cigarette smoking. Because Mill applied these ideas to the social sciences, he extended causal logic to thinking about groups, providing the historical linchpin for the methods of inquiry used by classical epidemiology (MacMahon and Pugh 1970; Susser 1973). Thus, we use the term **Mill's canons** to describe the modern-day principles for inferring causality from observations in a population. If they are met, an observed association is more likely to be causal. Nonetheless, Mill emphasized the necessity of experiments. "Suppose that, by a comparison of cases of the effect, we have found an antecedent which appears to be, and perhaps is, invariably connected with it:

we have not yet proved that antecedent to be the cause until we have reversed the process, and produced the effect by means of that antecedent. . . .Observation, in short, without experiment (supposing no aid from deduction) can ascertain sequences and co-existences, but cannot prove causation" (Mill 1892, p. 277).

The determination of a causal relationship when direct experimental evidence is absent, as is often the case for the association of physical activity and health outcomes, is not easy, nor is it entirely objective. Individuals often have different interpretations of the available evidence. In this text we summarize and present, to the best of our ability, the evidence that physical activity and fitness have a causal association with major chronic diseases and injury.

Summary

This chapter on methods and concepts presents the rudimentary principles and skills of logical inquiry that epidemiologists use to study physical activity. Odds ratios, relative risks, and attributable risks help determine whether physical activity can reduce the rate of disease, injury, or death among people at risk. The research design used in an epidemiologic study—whether a cross-sectional, case–control, or cohort observational design or an experimental, randomized controlled trial—determines the strength of the inference that lower risk is explainable solely by physical activity or fitness and not by other confounding or effect-modifying factors. Ultimately, the strength of the evidence for concluding the existence of a cause and an effect is judged by Mill's canons: temporal sequence, strength of association, consistency, dose–response relationship, and biological plausibility.

This chapter provides the foundation for understanding how epidemiologists determine whether people's attributes or behavior influences their risk of disease, injury, and death. The next chapter on behavioral epidemiology discusses the definition and measurement of physical fitness and physical activity, the attributes and behavior central to physical activity epidemiology.

Mill's Canons

1. **Temporal sequence:** Exposure to the risk factor must precede development of the disease with sufficient time to account for disease progression.

2. **Strength of association:** There is a large and clinically meaningful difference in disease risk between those exposed and those not exposed to the risk factor.

3. **Consistency:** The observed association is always observed if the risk factor is present

(e.g., regardless of sex, race, age, or methods of measurement).

4. **Dose response:** The risk of disease associated with the risk factor is greater with stronger exposure to the risk factor.

5. **Biological plausibility:** The observed association is explainable by existing knowledge about possible biological mechanisms of the disease, which may be alterable (e.g., by physical activity).

· BIBLIOGRAPHY ·

Altman, F. 1994. *Practical statistics for medical research,* 2nd edition, pp. 409-417. London: Chapman Hall.

Bhopal, R.S. 2008. Cause and effect: The epidemiological approach. In *Concepts of Epidemiology: Integrating the ideas, theories, principles and methods of epidemiology,* 2nd edition, chapter 5. New York: Oxford University Press.

Bouchard, C., and T. Rankinen. 2001. Individual differences in response to regular physical activity. *Medicine and Science in Sports and Exercise* 33 (Suppl. 6): S446-S451.

Bouchard, C., and R.J. Shephard. 1994. *Physical activity, fitness, and health: International proceedings and consensus statement.* Champaign, IL: Human Kinetics.

Bouchard, C., A. Tremblay, J.P. Despres, G. Theriault, A. Nadeau, P.J. Lupien, S. Moorjani, D. Prudhomme, and G. Fournier. 1994. The response to exercise with constant energy intake in identical twins. *Obesity Research* 2: 400-410.

Brenner, H., and O. Gefeller. 1997. Variation of sensitivity, specificity, likelihood ratios and predictive values with disease prevalence. *Statistics in Medicine* 16: 981-991.

Caspersen, C.J. 1989. Physical activity epidemiology: Concepts, methods, and applications to exercise science. *Exercise and Sport Sciences Reviews* 17: 423-474.

Dean, A.G. 1999. Epi Info and Epi Map: Current status and plans for Epi Info 2000. *Journal of Public Health Management and Practice* 5 (4): 54-57.

Dean, A.G., J.A. Dean, D. Coulombier, K.A. Brendel, D.C. Smith, A.H. Burton, R.C. Dicker, K. Sullivan, R.F. Fagan, and T.B. Arner. 1996. *Epi Info, version 6.04a, a word-processing, database, and statistics program for public health on IBM-compatible microcomputers.* Atlanta: Centers for Disease Control and Prevention.

Eaton, C.B., K.L. Lapane, C.E. Graber, A.R. Assaf, T.M. Lasater, and R.A. Carleton. 1995. Physical activity, physical fitness, and coronary heart disease risk factors. *Medicine and Science in Sports and Exercise* 27: 340-346.

Hill, A.B. 1961. *Principles of medical statistics.* New York: Oxford University Press.

Hill, A.B. 1965. The environment and disease: Association or causation. *Proceedings of the Royal Society of Medicine* 58: 295-300.

Jekel, J.F., J.G. Elmore, and D.L. Katz. 1996. *Epidemiology, biostatistics and preventive medicine.* Philadelphia: Saunders.

Laupacis, A., D.L. Sackett, and R.S. Roberts. 1988. An assessment of clinically useful measures of the consequences of treatment. *New England Journal of Medicine* 318: 1728-1733.

Levin, M.L. 1953. The occurrence of lung cancer in man. *Acta Unio Internationalis Contra Cancrum* 9 (3): 531-541.

MacMahon, B., and T.F. Pugh. 1970. *Epidemiology: Principles and methods.* Boston: Little, Brown.

MacMahon, B., and D. Trichopoulos. 1996. *Epidemiology: Principles and methods.* 2nd edition. Boston: Little, Brown.

Mausner, J., and S. Kramer. 1985. *Mausner and Bahn epidemiology: An introductory text.* 2nd edition. Philadelphia: Saunders.

Mill, J.S. 1843. *A system of logic, ratiocinative and inductive, being a connected view of the principles of evidence and the methods of scientific investigation.* Vol. 1, pp. 1-580. London: John W. Parker, West Strand.

Mill, J.S. 1892. *A system of logic, ratiocinative and inductive, being a connected view of the principles of evidence and the methods of scientific investigation.* 8th edition. New York: Harper & Brothers, Publishers, Franklin Square.

Mittleman, M.A., M. Maclure, G.H. Tofler, J.B. Sherwood, R.J. Goldberg, and J.E. Mullen. 1993. Triggering of acute myocardial infarction by heavy exertion: Protection against triggering by regular exertion. *New England Journal of Medicine* 329: 1677-1683.

Morabia, A. 1991. On the origin of Hill's causal criteria. *Epidemiology* 2 (5, September): 367-369.

Morabia, A., ed. 2004. *History of epidemiologic methods and concepts.* Basel, Switzerland: Birkhäuser Verlag.

Paffenbarger, R.S. Jr. 1988. Contributions of epidemiology to exercise science and cardiovascular health. *Medicine and Science in Sports and Exercise* 20: 426-438.

Smith, G.C., and J.P. Pell. 2003. Parachute use to prevent death and major trauma related to gravitational challenge: Systematic review of randomised controlled trials. *British Medical Journal* 327: 1459-1461.

Stebbing, W. 1875. *Analysis of Mr. Mill's system of logic.* New edition. London: Longmans, Green, and Co.

Susser, M. 1973. *Causal thinking in the health sciences: Concepts and strategies of epidemiology.* New York: Oxford University Press.

Szklo, M., F.J. Nieto, and F. Javier. 2000. *Epidemiology: Beyond the basics.* Gaithersburg, MD: Aspen.

U.S. Department of Health, Education, and Welfare. 1964. *Smoking and health. Report of the Advisory Committee to the Surgeon General.* Public Health Service Publication No. 1103. Washington, DC.

Zhang, F.F., D.C. Michaels, B. Mathema, S. Kauchali, A. Chatterjee, D.C. Ferris, et al. 2004. Evolution of epidemiologic methods and concepts in selected textbooks of the 20th century. *Sozial- und Praventivmedizen* 49: 97-104.

CHAPTER 3

Measurement and Surveillance of Physical Activity and Fitness

*The office of the scholar is to . . . guide men by showing them facts
amidst appearances. He plies the slow, unhonored, and unpaid task of observation. . . .
He is the world's eye.*

• Ralph Waldo Emerson, 1837 •

CHAPTER OBJECTIVES

▸ Introduce and define how physical activity and fitness are part of the field of behavioral epidemiology

▸ Discuss the definition and measurement of physical activity and fitness as the central behaviors and attributes that define physical activity epidemiology

▸ Describe the concept of dose–response relations between exposure to physical activity and health outcomes

▸ Present federal guidelines for healthful participation in physical activity

▸ Describe national and international surveillance systems that estimate prevalence and trends in physical activity participation

Behavioral epidemiology is the observation and study of behaviors, including physical inactivity or sedentariness, that lead to disease or premature death and of the distribution of these behaviors. Thus, behavioral epidemiology encompasses two main features. The first is the study of relationships between behavior and disease, the traditional approach introduced in chapters 1 and 2. The second feature is the study of the behavior, its distribution in a population, and its determinants (Mason and Powell 1985). Once it is established, using epidemiologic methods, that a behavior appears causally linked with disease, injury, or early death, the next critical step is to determine how the behavior can be altered. In this way, behavioral epidemiology goes beyond traditional infectious disease epidemiology, which is concerned mainly with the containment of bacterial and viral contagion. Removal of the handle from the Broad Street pump after John Snow linked the 1848 cholera outbreak in London with contaminated well water is an early example of behavioral epidemiology.

However, even though that example had to do with preventive measures, the emphasis of traditional epidemiology has been on environmental intervention (e.g., sewage disposal, inoculation programs for schoolchildren). In modern behavioral epidemiology, the focus shifts to understanding behaviors that increase or decrease the risk of people developing the disease (e.g., hand washing or sharing hypodermic needles by drug abusers, which can spread diseases). Behavioral epidemiology is especially important for understanding and preventing chronic diseases that develop over periods of years largely as a result of people's habits. The discussion of behavioral epidemiology in this book focuses on who is physically active or inactive and why, as well as on how health professionals and public policy makers can help the physically inactive to become active in ways that reduce chronic diseases and premature death and promote health. This chapter introduces a fundamental step in the application of behavioral epidemiology to physical activity, namely the measurement and **surveillance** of physical activity and fitness. Chapter 17 concludes this book by describing environmental and personal factors that are associated with physical activity and interventions designed to increase it.

▷ **BEHAVIORAL EPIDEMIOLOGY** is the study of behaviors, including physical inactivity or sedentariness, that lead to disease or premature death and of the distribution of these behaviors.

Why Is Behavioral Epidemiology Important?

Until the middle of the 20th century, the major threat from disease was infectious contagion. For example, the great flu **epidemic** of 1918 killed 40,000,000 people worldwide, including 675,000 Americans, in just 11 months. Fears over such **pandemic** catastrophes (a pandemic is an epidemic that spreads widely across a region or the world) spurred growth in the field of epidemiology. Indeed, in 1927, the physician Wade Hampton Frost defined epidemiology as the science of the mass phenomena of infectious diseases. Similar concerns exist today about AIDS and deadly hemorrhagic diseases caused by viruses, such as the Ebola virus, which had case fatality rates of 50% to 90% between 1976 and 2003 in Zaire (now the Democratic Republic of the Congo). A new strain of Ebola discovered in Uganda in late 2007 killed 37 of 149 cases. Ebola is classified as a biosafety level 4 threat, the highest biocontainment level reserved for infectious agents that cause severe to fatal disease in humans and do not as yet have approved vaccines available. By comparison, flu viruses are usually considered a level 2 threat. Infectious diseases remain a serious threat to public health, ranking as the third leading cause of death worldwide. Failure to maintain public sanitation and vaccination can lead to an exponential growth of death from infectious disease in a short period of time.

Despite the importance to public health of sustaining efforts to observe and control infectious and contagious diseases, the early definition of epidemiology no longer suffices. Noninfectious diseases are now the top causes of illness, disability, and death. Though early epidemiologists were concerned mainly about infectious contagions resulting directly from physical and chemical **pathogens** (e.g., bacteria and viruses causing diseases that can spread to humans) arising from environmental conditions or contaminants, most infectious diseases are now controllable. Modern-day epidemiologists are equally concerned about chronic diseases. Chronic diseases may be partly caused by pathogens such as bacteria or viruses, but they are diseases that typically require many years to fully develop; their signs and symptoms manifest themselves usually in middle age or later. Their gradual adult, rather than congenital or adolescent, onset suggests that environmental factors other than direct exposure to pathogens are very important in determining their age of onset and severity. For example, non-insulin-dependent diabetes (i.e., type 2 diabetes) has traditionally been also called adult-onset diabetes. However, the increasing rate of type 2 diabetes has nearly reached epidemic status, especially in American Indian youths. Among all U.S. youths 10 to 19 years of age, the incidence rate of type 1 diabetes (15,000 new cases or 1.9%) is nearly four times higher than that for type 2 diabetes (3700 new cases or 5.3%). In American Indian youth, those rates are reversed. This is most likely because of increasing obesity linked to overeating and physical inactivity. One of every six U.S. youth who are overweight has prediabetes (i.e., higher than normal blood glucose).

It is now known that about half the mortality from the top 10 leading causes of death in the United States can be traced directly or indirectly to behavior. Hence, it is understood that certain behaviors, such as insufficient physical activity, can be pathogenic. Today, epidemiologists are as concerned

· WEB RESOURCES ·

www.cdc.gov. The home page of the federal Centers for Disease Control and Prevention (CDC) in Atlanta, Georgia. Provides quick access to many health databases pertinent to physical activity epidemiology and to the *Morbidity and Mortality Weekly Report.*

www.cdc.gov/mmwr/. *Morbidity and Mortality Weekly Report,* which compiles national health data and reports from state health departments.

www.cdc.gov/brfss/. The site for the Behavioral Risk Factor Surveillance System (BRFSS), the world's largest telephone survey, which tracks health risks, including physical inactivity, in the United States.

www.cdc.gov/nccdphp/dnpa/surveill.htm. The site of the National Center for Chronic Disease Prevention and Health Promotion of the CDC, Division of Nutrition, Physical Activity, and Obesity. Provides access to information about the major survey and surveillance systems for measuring and tracking physical activity in the United States.

www.cdc.gov/nchs/nhis.htm. The site for the National Health Interview Survey, which tracks health behaviors in the United States.

www.cdc.gov/nccdphp/dash/yrbs/. The site of the Youth Risk Behavior Survey, which tracks health risks, including physical inactivity, among youth in the United States.

www.fedstats.gov/agencies/. Provides links to statistics from several U.S. federal health agencies, including the National Center for Health Statistics.

https://sites.google.com/site/theipaq/. Describes the development and validation of the International Physical Activity Questionnaire.

www.who.int. Site of the World Health Organization in Geneva, Switzerland. Provides information on world diseases and lifestyles.

www.cdc.gov/nccdphp/dnpa/physical/health_professionals/data/physical_surveys.htm. Site maintained by the CDC. Provides a summary of physical activity surveillance systems used in the United States.

https://sites.google.com/site/compendiumofphysicalactivities/. Provides the updated 2011 Compendium of Physical Activities, a list of updated MET codes for activities where evidence has been published to support the new MET values.

with the prevention of behaviors that cause disease as with containing diseases once they occur. This is evidenced by the 1992 name change of the federal Centers for Disease Control, established in 1946, to the Centers for Disease Control and Prevention.

What Is Physical Activity?

Physical activity is defined as "any bodily movement produced by skeletal muscle that results in energy expenditure" (Caspersen, Powell, and Christenson 1985); it includes occupational work, domestic chores, leisure activity, playing sports, and **exercise** that is planned for fitness or health purposes. It also includes fidgeting and maintaining upright posture (Levine 2007). Physical activity is the most variable component of an individual's total daily energy expenditure, which consists of basal metabolic rate (i.e., the energy needed to maintain the body at rest) and the thermic effect of food (i.e., the energy required to digest food) in addition to physical activity. The high degree of both intra- and interindividual variability in daily physical activity makes the assessment of this behavior in free-living populations a very difficult task. Without a valid and reliable measure of daily or weekly physical activity, epidemiologists would be unable to evaluate the association between physical activity and the risk for chronic disease. In addition, measures of physical activity are needed for the **descriptive epidemiology** of physical activity (i.e., the assessment of variation in physical activity by age, sex, race, ethnicity, health status, and geographic location), for surveillance systems that

track population trends in physical activity over time, and for assessing mediators of physical activity, as well as the effectiveness of interventions designed to increase the level of physical activity.

Measures of Physical Activity

Several methods are available for physical activity assessment, including occupational classification, behavioral observation, physiological markers (heart rate, doubly labeled water), dietary intake, motion sensors, and self-report questionnaires. Prior to 1970, 20 of the 24 epidemiologic studies of the association between physical activity and coronary heart disease (CHD) used occupational classification as the measure of physical activity. Although these studies provided interesting information on the potential association between physical activity and heart disease, they ignored the influence of leisure-time physical activity. It was not until the mid-1960s that Dr. Henry J. Montoye quantified both the occupational and leisure-time physical activity habits recalled by participants using a questionnaire interview in the Tecumseh (Michigan) Community Health Study (Montoye 1975). Since that time, about 50 physical activity questionnaires have been developed.

Before discussing the specifics of physical activity questionnaires, it is important to consider the problem of establishing the validity of these instruments. Using physical activity questionnaires, epidemiologists can obtain data on the physical activity habits of a large number of people in a very cost- and time-efficient manner. But how do we know that the questionnaire provides a valid assessment of physical activity? The problem in answering this question is that there is no acceptable criterion measure or gold standard with which to compare questionnaire results. Though direct observation of behavior might provide such a criterion, it has been impractical, and socially unacceptable, to implement objective round-the-clock surveillance of people. Therefore, epidemiologists must be satisfied with assessing questionnaire validity using imperfect measures of physical activity, such as dietary intake, physiological variables like doubly labeled water and heart rate monitoring, motion sensors, direct or indirect **calorimetry,** or using other variables influenced by physical activity such as body fat, blood pressure, blood lipids, muscular strength and endurance, or aerobic power.

The goal of most physical activity questionnaires is to estimate the energy expenditure attributable to participation in specific types of physical activity, such as household, occupational, or leisure activity. Energy expenditure in kilocalories or kilojoules (1 kcal is the amount of heat required to increase the temperature of 1 kg of water 1 °C; 1 kcal = 4.2 kJ) can be accurately measured using direct or indirect calorimetry. An average daily energy expenditure of about 4.3 kcal/min or greater is frequently used to classify individuals as physically active in epidemiologic studies. Direct calorimetry involves the measurement of heat production of an individual in a sealed, insulated chamber. This technique is highly accurate (<1% error); however, the engineering problems associated with developing and maintaining a direct calorimeter are substantial, and the size of the chamber limits the potential for physical activity. Therefore, this technique is infrequently used in the development or validation of physical activity questionnaires. **Indirect calorimetry** involves estimating energy expenditure from oxygen consumption and carbon dioxide production by applying the caloric equivalent of oxygen: 5 kcal per liter of oxygen consumed. Laboratory systems to measure energy expenditure by indirect calorimetry have been in use for decades; however, in the recent past, light, portable systems such as the Cosmed K4b2, capable of measuring oxygen during unrestricted physical activity outside the laboratory, have become available. These devices are particularly useful for assessing the energy costs of specific activities that can be used to develop scoring algorithms for physical activity questionnaires and for assessing the validity of a variety of motion-sensing devices as measures of physical activity.

Currently, three methods of physical activity assessment—doubly labeled water, heart rate monitoring, and motion sensors—are commonly used both as measures of physical activity in small-scale studies and as criterion measures for validation of physical activity questionnaires. Heart rate monitors and motion sensors are the most popular because they are accurate and feasible to use. Doubly labeled water is expensive and not very feasible for most applications, but it is the most accurate and unobtrusive measure of energy expenditure that can be used in natural settings. The following sections provide a detailed description of these methods. Table 3.1 rates methods by cost; interference with normal activity; acceptability; and ability to measure specific features of physical activity, including type, **intensity,** duration, frequency, and timing.

▷ **A GOOD MEASURE** of physical activity provides reliable and valid information on specific features of physical activity, including type, intensity, duration, frequency, and timing.

Table 3.1 Characteristics of Physical Activity Assessment Procedures

Activity assessment procedure	Group size	Age	Study costs[1]		Subject costs[1]		Probability of interfering[1]	Acceptability		Activity specifics
			Money	Time	Time	Effort		Personal	Social	
Calorimetry										
Direct	Single	Infant-elderly	VH	VH	VH	H-VH	H-VH	No	No	Yes
Indirect	Single-small	Young adult-elderly	H-VH	VH	VH	M-VH	H-VH	No	No	Yes
Surveys										
Indirect calorimetry diary	Single-small	Young adult-elderly	M-H	M-H	M-H	M-H	VH	No	No	Yes
Task-specific diary	Small-large	Adolescent-elderly	L-M	L-M	H-VH		VH	?	Yes	Yes
Recall questionnaire	Small-large	Adolescent-elderly	L-M	L-M	M-H		L	Yes	Yes	Yes
Quantitative history	Small-large	Adolescent-elderly	L-M	L-M	L-M		L	Yes	Yes	Yes

Activity assessment procedure	Group size	Age	Study costs[1]		Subject costs[1]		Probability of interfering[1]	Acceptability		Activity specifics
			Money	Time	Time	Effort		Personal	Social	
Physiological markers										
Cardiorespiratory fitness	Small-large	Child-elderly	M-VH	M-H	M-H	M-VHM	L	?	?	No
Doubly labeled water	Single-small	Infant-elderly	H-VH	M-VH	M		L-H	Yes	Yes	No
Mechanical and electronic monitors										
Heart rate monitor	Single-small	Infant-elderly	H-VH	M-VH	M-H	M-H	L-M	Yes	Yes	No
Stabilometer	Single-small	Infant	M-H	M	H-VH	L	L	Yes	Yes	No
Horizontal time monitor	Single-small	Child-elderly	M-H	M	H-VH	L-M	L-M	?	Yes	No
Pedometer	Single-small	Child	L-M	L	L	L	L-M	Yes	Yes	No
Gait assessment	Single-large	Child-elderly	H-VH	M-VH	L-M	M-H	L-M	Yes	Yes	
Electronic motion sensor	Single-large	Child-elderly	M-H	L	L	L	L-M	?	Yes	No
Accelerometer	Single-large	Infant-elderly	L-M	L-M	L	L	L-M	Yes	Yes	No
Other										
Dietary measures	Large	Adolescent-elderly	M-H	M	M-H	M-H	L	Yes	Yes	No
Job classification	Large	Employed only	L-M	L-M	L	L	L	Yes	Yes	?
Behavioral observation	Single-small	Infant-elderly	H-VH	H-VH	H-VH	L-H	L-VH	?	?	Yes

[1]L = low; M = moderate; H = high; VH = very high; ? = unclear whether the approach has personal or social acceptability.

Reprinted from LaPorte, Montoye, and Caspersen 1985.

Doubly Labeled Water

At the present time, the **doubly labeled water (DLW)** technique is the best overall field measure of total daily energy expenditure (Schoeller 1999). This technique was developed by Lifson and colleagues at the University of Minnesota based on their observation that the oxygen atoms exhaled in carbon dioxide and those in body water were in isotopic equilibrium (Lifson, Gordon, and McClintock 1955). Thus, it was assumed that the kinetics of water elimination and respiration were linked. With use of this method, the participant drinks a measured amount of water that has been labeled with stable isotopes of hydrogen and oxygen ($^2H^1H^{18}O$). These isotopes are tracers that transform the body's water into a virtual metabolic recorder that integrates H_2O output and CO_2 production. Urine samples are obtained during a seven- to 14-day period, and the overall energy expenditure over the evaluation period can be estimated from CO_2 production without the need to collect respiratory gases. When the labeled water is drunk, the two isotopes are rapidly distributed in body water and

begin to be eliminated from the body. The ^2H is eliminated as ^2HHO and is a measure of water flux. The ^{18}O is eliminated from the body as both $H_2^{18}O$ and $C^{18}O_2$ and is thus a measure of water and carbon dioxide flux.

The difference between these elimination rates is, thus, an estimate of carbon dioxide flux, as shown in figure 3.1. Using the equations of indirect calorimetry and assuming a value for the respiratory quotient (RQ), energy expenditure can be estimated by the known oxidative cost, and hence caloric expenditure, of burning fat, carbohydrate, and protein. This is explained later in this chapter in the section on lipid metabolism as a component of physical fitness. In addition, assumptions regarding the amount of total body water and the amount of body water lost in the evaporation of sweat and through the respiratory tract must be made.

The DLW method was validated first under laboratory conditions in mice (McClintock and Lifson 1957) and was later shown to be feasible for use with humans (Lifson et al. 1975; Schoeller and van Santen 1982). Theoretically, the coefficient of variation of the DLW method is between

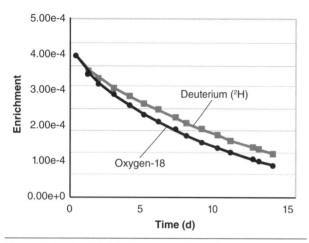

Figure 3.1 Doubly labeled water. The Δ between slopes of ^2H and $^{18}O = CO_2$ production, an indirect measure of metabolic rate, which can be converted to calories or joules based on the chemical composition of food being oxidized (which affects the energy equivalence of each liter of CO_2 produced).

Adapted, by permission, from A.M. Prentice, 1990, *International atomic energy agency NAHRES-4, IAEA, Vienna* (Lausanne, Switzerland: I/D/E/C/G International Dietary Energy Consultancy).

4% and 8%; however, the error is exaggerated when normal metabolism is disrupted, which can easily occur in individuals in uncontrolled field settings.

The DLW technique has the advantage of using nonradioactive isotopes, and it allows the assessment of energy expenditure over a relatively long time period (one to two weeks) in an unobtrusive manner. The major disadvantages are cost (several hundreds of dollars per person); the need for expensive equipment (ratio mass spectrometer) for analysis of urine samples; and the lack of direct information on energy expenditure from physical activity, its specific components, or the pattern of energy expenditure over time. Although the DLW technique is often considered the most accurate measure of daily energy expenditure in free-living humans, a number of sources of error with this technique must be considered (Prentice 1990). For example, a change in body water, which can be estimated from changes in body weight, increases the error in estimated total energy expenditure. Approximately 4% of the ^2H molecules and 1% of the ^{18}O molecules are incorporated into nonaqueous tissue, which results in an overestimation of their dilution space in body water. Deuterium isotopes are lost as vapor at a slower rate than ^1H molecules, which can result in approximately a 2.5% error in estimated energy expenditure. Approximately 2% of the isotopes are lost in feces rather than in urine. Each variation in RQ of 0.01 from an assumed value of 0.85 results in a 1% error in estimates. This can be especially problematic in individuals who consume large amounts of alcohol, because hydrogen used in the metabolism of ethanol reduces the difference in the elimination rates of ^2H and ^{18}O, which results in an underestimation of energy expenditure.

Since the mid-1980s, use of the DLW technique has become more common in studies of human energy expenditure (Westerterp et al. 1984, 1988; Westerterp 1998); however, its primary value is as a validation measure against which to compare other physical activity assessment methods. The DLW method provides the best measure of total energy expenditure that can be obtained while people live naturally outside a laboratory. However, the high cost of the ^{18}O tracer isotope, as well as the need for a ratio mass spectrometer to determine its rate of elimination in the urine, makes the method infeasible in epidemiologic studies with large numbers of participants.

Heart Rate Monitors

A variety of heart rate monitors are currently available commercially. The most useful heart rate monitors measure the electrical activity of the heart, typically by attaching a transmitter with chest electrodes to a chest strap that transmits the electrocardiographic signal to a digital wristwatch receiver. A computer chip in the wristwatch uses the R–R interval (the period of the heartbeat measured as the time difference in milliseconds between successive R-waves of the electrocardiogram) to calculate the minute-by-minute heart rate and stores this information in a memory cell, which can be downloaded to a personal computer for analysis. Studies have indicated that this type of heart rate monitor provides a highly accurate measure of heart rate when compared with the heart rate determined from the conventional hard-wired electrocardiogram.

However, the conversion of heart rate to a measure of energy expenditure, which is based on a linear association between heart rate and oxygen consumption, is problematic. Typically, a linear regression is calculated between heart rate and oxygen consumption measured during exercise on a treadmill or cycle ergometer, sometimes along with heart rate and oxygen consumption measured during sitting, standing, or other typical daily physical activities. The mean heart rate during daily activities is then used with the laboratory-developed regression equation to estimate oxygen consumption and thus energy expenditure. Considerable error in energy expenditure estimates can occur because the average daily heart rate is typically at the low end of the heart rate–oxygen consumption calibration, where the association between those variables is not linear. The need to develop calibrations for each participant makes the use of heart rate to estimate energy expenditure both time-consuming and expensive and thus impractical for large-scale studies. In addition, the heart rate–oxygen consumption relationship varies with posture, environmental temperature, emotional state, type of muscular contraction (static or dynamic, small or large muscle mass), level of cardiovascular fitness, and fatigue, all of which are potential sources of error.

It has been suggested that the difference between an individual's resting heart rate and mean daily heart rate may provide a useful index of physical activity. The utility of heart rate monitors may be in assessing the pattern of physical activity over the course of a day to assess the intensity of physical activity.

Motion Sensors

The pedometer, a device for counting steps, was first conceived by Leonardo da Vinci over 500 years ago. Research using older, gear-driven, mechanical pedometers indicated that these devices showed poor validity and **reliability** as a step counter, even under highly controlled laboratory conditions (Gayle, Montoye, and Philpot 1977; Washburn, Chin, and Montoye 1980). However, research on the reliability and validity of newer electronic pedometers that use a coiled spring-suspended lever, such as the Digi-Walker SW-200 (manufactured by Yamax, Inc., Tokyo, and now distributed by New-Lifestyles, Lees Summit, Missouri; ~$20), is more encouraging. For example, Bassett and colleagues (1996) reported that the Digi-Walker recorded the number of both left and right steps during outdoor walking in 20 adults with only a trivial 1% overestimate of actual steps taken. Similarly, Welk and colleagues (2000) showed that the mean step counts from the Digi-Walker during walking and running both on a treadmill and on a track by 31 adult volunteers were within 3% to 5% of the actual values. However, in the same sample, Welk and coauthors reported a rather low correlation ($r = 0.34$) between the average daily step count over a one-week period and average daily energy expenditure assessed by the Stanford Seven-Day Physical Activity Recall Questionnaire. When participants removed the Digi-Walker during all structured vigorous and moderate physical activity, the correlation

between the step counts and energy expenditure estimated by the recall questionnaire was near zero ($r = -0.07$).

In general, there are some concerns about the interunit reliability of these devices. Also, the most widely validated pedometers (e.g., the Digi-Walker SW-200) do not have a time stamp or data storage capacity; thus, participants must record numbers from the devices at the beginning and end of the day. Most spring-levered pedometers have 95% accuracy for counting steps at walking speeds above 3 mph (4.8 km/h), but they vary between 50% and 90% at slower speeds, especially among older people who can develop a shuffling gait (Melanson et al. 2004). Newer, more expensive pedometers have a digital clock, use a piezoelectric mechanism that is more accurate than spring-levered pedometers for slow walking, and have a computer-downloadable memory (up to 40 days) (e.g., Omron model HJ-720ITC). It has been suggested that pedometers may serve as a useful criterion measure for validating self-report estimates of walking and as motivational devices for interventions designed to increase walking (Bravata et al. 2007; Lubans, Morgan, and Tudor-Locke 2009).

Although pedometers can't capture all physical activities accurately, they are being used worldwide to describe physical activity levels in both adults and children (see figure 3.2). Typical pedometer counts of steps vary according to group, but a common public health goal has been 10,000 steps a day.

The development of portable **accelerometers** as physical activity assessment devices was prompted by laboratory studies conducted in the late 1950s that suggested an association between the integral of vertical acceleration with respect to time and energy expenditure (Brouha and Smith 1958; Montoye, Servais, and Webster 1986). Montoye and colleagues

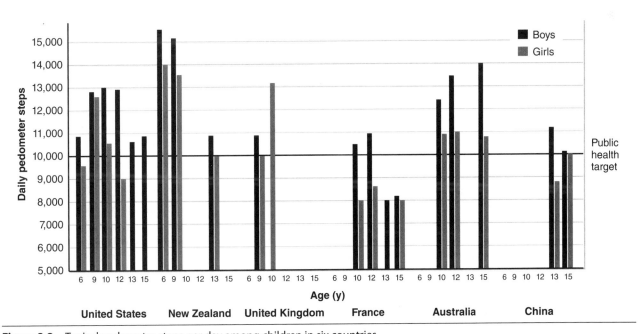

Figure 3.2 Typical pedometer steps per day among children in six countries.

Data from Beets et al. 2010.

at the University of Wisconsin–Madison were the first to use this principle to develop the prototype for a portable accelerometer later marketed under the name Caltrac. The Caltrac, like most portable accelerometers, uses a transducer, made of two layers of piezoceramic material with a brass center layer. When the body accelerates, the transducer, mounted on a cantilever beam, bends, producing an electric charge proportional to the force exerted. An internal computer chip integrates the area under the acceleration–deceleration curve over a defined time interval, stores that value in computer memory, and resets the integrator.

Though pedometers are simply event counters, portable accelerometers, designed to be worn on a belt at the waist, provide a measure of both frequency and intensity of movement. Currently available portable accelerometers have the advantage of collecting and storing data sequentially over time so that the pattern of physical activity over a day or a number of days can be assessed. The disadvantages of these devices include their cost (approximately \$300 to \$500 per unit), their unsuitability for aquatic activities, and their unresponsiveness to static activity or activities that involve minimal movement of the body's center of gravity, such as rowing, cycling, or most types of resistance exercise (e.g., weightlifting). Despite these limitations, portable accelerometers are a useful addition to the methodology of physical activity assessment.

The Caltrac, unlike the newer generation of portable accelerometers, does not store data in a time sequence but provides only an estimate of total physical activity in a given time period. A number of studies, in both laboratory and field settings, have shown Caltrac readings to be significantly associated with energy expenditure measured by indirect calorimetry during walking and running on level surfaces ($r = 0.68$ to 0.94) and with energy expenditure during daily activities measured by doubly labeled water over a seven-day period. The lack of data storage capability, the rather large size, and poor quality control in manufacturing have led researchers away from using the Caltrac to using more sophisticated portable accelerometers, such as the one made by Computer Science and Applications, Inc. (CSA, in Shalimar, Florida), the Biotrainer, and the Tritrac.

The CSA Model 7164 portable accelerometer (now marketed as the Actigraph by Manufacturer's Technology, Inc., in Pensacola, Florida) is a small ($5.1 \times 3.8 \times 1.5$ cm; 43 g), single-plane portable accelerometer that uses a piezoelectric transducer. Data can be downloaded via an optical interface to the serial port of a personal computer for analysis. The investigator can set the start time and data collection interval. The Actigraph accelerometer can store minute-by-minute data for up to 22 days. Studies have indicated moderate associations between the Actigraph accelerometer's counts per minute and energy expenditure measured by indirect calorimetry during both treadmill and overground walking and running at increasing speeds ($r = 0.66$ to 0.82; Hendelman et al. 2000; Melanson and Freedson 1995). As with all

portable accelerometers, however, the Actigraph accelerometer's counts per minute do not well reflect increases in energy cost due to increased grade. The association between Actigraph accelerometer readings and energy expenditure during other types of physical activity, such as housecleaning, golf, and yard work, are lower ($r = 0.59$; Hendelman et al. 2000; Welk et al. 2000).

The Biotrainer (manufactured by IM Systems, Baltimore, Maryland) is a single-plane accelerometer similar in size to the Actigraph accelerometer, while the Tritrac (made by Reining International, Madison, Wisconsin) is a three-plane accelerometer that is considerably larger than the others (170 g). Welk and colleagues (2000) compared Actigraph accelerometer, Biotrainer, and Tritrac output with energy expenditure measured by indirect calorimetry from 52 adults who completed two 30-min activity scenarios, including treadmill walking or jogging and simulated lifestyle activities. The correlation between accelerometer readings and energy expenditure was higher for treadmill activity (mean $r = 0.86$) than for lifestyle activities (mean $r = 0.55$). Correlations among the Actigraph accelerometer, Biotrainer, and Tritrac were high for both treadmill ($r = 0.86$) and lifestyle activity ($r = 0.70$), suggesting that similar information is obtained from all three accelerometers.

In theory, a multiplane accelerometer should provide a better estimate of body movement and thus energy expenditure; however, studies (e.g., Welk et al. 2000; Hendelman et al. 2000) have shown little advantage to using the larger and more complex three-plane Tritrac accelerometer over smaller and less complex single-plane accelerometers (such as the Actigraph and the Biotrainer).

In the future, the use of motion sensors in epidemiologic research will continue to increase. The GT3X three-plane Actigraph became available in 2009. It is pricey (\$335, plus software), but there will surely be increasing growth in its application to physical activity surveillance and in research that compares the performance of single-plane and multiplane scoring of the device's counts. Accelerometer counts have also been combined with speed-of-movement estimates from satellite global positioning devices to classify some types of physical activity (Troped et al. 2008). Additionally, researchers at the University of Massachusetts are exploring the use of artificial intelligence scoring algorithms to "train" accelerometers to detect the most likely type of physical activity people engage in through computer modeling of variations in the frequency patterns of oscillations in counts that may be unique to different types of movement (e.g., locomotion, vigorous sports, and household activities) (Staudenmayer et al. 2009). Researchers have also used accelerometers to detect fidgeting and changes in posture that can contribute to energy expenditure accumulated during the day (Allen et al. 2006; Luinge and Veltink 2004; Mathie et al. 2004). As the price of this technology declines, the feasibility of monitoring a large number of individuals over several days will increase. In the meantime, portable accelerometers will continue to be a useful criterion measure for the validation of self-reported physical activity instruments.

To provide a better understanding of the dose–response relationship between physical activity intensity and chronic disease risk, better self-report measures of physical activity intensity must be developed. Heart rate monitoring and portable accelerometers have been suggested as criterion measures for assessing the intensity of daily physical activity. Several investigators have attempted to define cut points for Actigraph accelerometer counts per minute that correspond to various levels of activity measured in metabolic equivalents, or **METs;** however, the results of these studies have not been encouraging. For example, activity intensity of 3 METs or greater varied from 191 to 1952 Actigraph accelerometer counts per minute, a 10-fold difference between reports!

Figure 3.3 shows how accelerometer counts can be used to estimate METs of increasing intensities of physical activity and define count thresholds for moderate or vigorous physical activity. Healthy 8th-grade girls wore Actigraph accelerometers on the hip and a Cosmed portable metabolic unit to allow estimation of METs through measurement of oxygen consumption during 10 activities ranging from sedentary TV watching and computer games to jogging at a pace of about 5 mph (8 km/h) (Treuth et al. 2004). Sedentary activities required less than 2 METs of energy expenditure and registered fewer than 50 counts during 30-s periods of recording. Although there was an overall pattern whereby METs and accelerometer counts both increased between sedentary activities and physical activities, the scatter between METs and accelerometer counts shown in the figure illustrates large differences among girls within each type of activity. Bicycle riding shows this most clearly. The horizontal range in counts is narrower than the vertical range in METs. This means that several girls who registered similar accelerometer scores varied widely in their energy expenditure. So, there was a poor correlation between counts and METs for bicycling. That's not surprising, because the up-and-down movement of the hips during leg cycling is small despite the work being done by the legs. With bicycling excluded, counts predicted 84% of the variation in METs across all other physical activities, but the standard error of that prediction was 1.4 METs. This means that roughly 68% of the scatter of counts ranged 1.4 METs above or below a true prediction.

What is the practical impact of that much error? Simply put, it shows that the accelerometer wasn't accurate for ranking girls or specific types of activities according to energy expenditure (Schmitz et al. 2005), but it might be useful for distinguishing between categories of sedentary, moderate, and vigorous levels of intensity that differ from each other by more than 1.4 METs. Indeed, the purpose of the study was to use the counts to classify girls' participation in activities that were at least moderately intense (about 4.6 METs in the study). Using a threshold of 1500 counts led to the fewest classification errors, about 6%. Some girls had that many counts while doing sedentary or low-intensity activities (i.e., watching TV, playing a computer game, sweeping the floor, or walking slowly), and some girls had less than 1500 counts while they were actually doing moderately intense activities (e.g., fast walking, stair climbing, or jogging). The 1500-count threshold was most accurate for detecting whether girls were walking slowly (2.5 mph, or 4 km/h) or walking briskly (3.5 mph, or 5.6 km/h).

An advantage of an accelerometer is that it can provide real-time assessments of the patterning of physical activity.

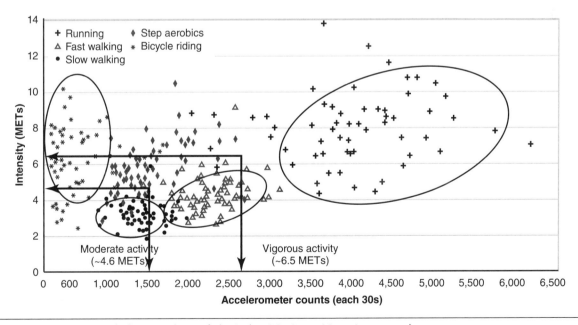

Figure 3.3 Estimating metabolic equivalents of physical activity intensities using an accelerometer.

Data from Treuth et al. 2004. Courtesy of Diane Cattelier, University of North Carolina-Chapel Hill.

It estimates both total physical activity accumulated while it is worn and individual epochs of physical activity and sedentary activity that contribute to the total accumulation. Thus, an accelerometer permits profiling of the variability of physical activity, which is likely an important part of a person's exposure to physical activity (Elsiger and Tremblay 2007). To date, only a diary could provide such a measure of variability, but a diary is intrusive and is a burden to keep, requiring verification by an objective measure. Nonetheless, present-day applications of accelerometers have not been the answer to the problem of accurately assessing the intensity of activities of daily living. In a recent study of adults aged 20 to 60 years, correlations between accelerometer counts and estimated energy expenditure were moderately strong during treadmill walking or jogging ($r \sim .80$), but were weak during activities of daily living ($r \sim .35$) (Howe, Staudenmayer, and Freedson 2009). The accelerometer overestimated energy expenditure for level treadmill walking or jogging by 20% and underestimated energy expenditure for activities that use the arms (e.g., basketball, cleaning, painting, and tennis) by $\sim$25% to 65% and for climbing by nearly 75%. The accelerometer accurately gauged energy expenditure only for gardening, raking, mowing, and treadmill walking or jogging uphill, and only when averaged across people. Errors for individuals could be much larger. When only counts in the vertical plane were used, errors were similar to those when counts from side-to-side and front-to-back movements were also registered.

An unresolved question is whether using accelerometers to rank people on their physical activity gives a better estimate of usual participation in health-promoting physical activity than using self-reports of physical activity (Corder et al. 2009). Self-reports of physical activity commonly overestimate physical activity levels when compared to objective monitoring by accelerometers. So, it is likely that self-reports of physical activity will provide inflated estimates of whether people meet recommended levels of sufficient physical activity compared with estimates derived by objective methods. Nonetheless, some recent evidence argues against this. A recent cross-sectional study of 90 British men aged 45 to 64 years described 24-h surveillance of all physical activity using accelerometers and heart rate monitors (Thompson et al. 2009). A high point prevalence of sufficient physical activity (about 73%) was observed during a week in that study, similar to the rate reported in the International Physical Activity Prevalence Study using the International Physical Activity Questionnaire (IPAQ) (Bauman et al. 2009). This occurred in both studies when sufficient activity included all forms of physical activity and was defined in a way that is similar to recent U.S. recommendations for levels sufficient to promote health (i.e., at least 450-500 METs $\cdot$ min^{-1} $\cdot$ week^{-1} of physical activities at intensities $\geq$3 METs accumulated in bouts of 10 or more minutes) (Haskell et al. 2007; U.S. Department of Health and Human Services 2008). Similarly, 70% of men and 62% of women in the NHANES 2005-2006 survey of U.S. adults said they had been active enough during the past 30 days to meet the current federal guideline of 500 METs $\cdot$ min^{-1} $\cdot$ week^{-1} or more of moderate or vigorous physical activities. However, in contrast to the aforementioned 24-hr surveillance of British men, only 58% of men and 33% of women met that guideline when accelerometer counts during the past seven days were used as the gauge (Tucker, Welk, and Beyler 2011). When federal guidelines are defined as 150 min of moderate physical activities or 75 min of vigorous activity each week, or an equivalent combination, just 10% to 11% of men and 7% to 9% of women meet them when accelerometer counts are used to define sufficient levels of physical activity (Tucker, Welk, and Beyler 2011).

Further work is needed to more clearly define these cut points for activity intensity and to clearly delineate the physical activity characteristics for which the cut points are valid. Technologies such as global positioning systems and body-mounted cameras are also beginning to be used for physical activity assessment. New technologies will give researchers additional options for future work on the validation of self-report instruments to assess physical activity.

Physical Activity Questionnaires

The most practical and most often used method of assessing physical activity in epidemiologic studies is self-report physical activity questionnaires or interviews. This method allows researchers to obtain physical activity information from a large number of individuals in a time- and cost-efficient manner. Since the early 1970s, over 30 survey instruments have been developed for physical activity assessment. Pereira and colleagues (1997), Montoye and colleagues (1996), and Washburn and Montoye (1986) published descriptions of survey instruments, as well as information on their reliability and validity.

These questionnaires differ on several important factors, such as the time period over which activity is assessed (from the past week to the respondent's lifetime), type of activity assessed (leisure, household, transportation, occupation), length of the questionnaire, administration mode (interviewer- or self-administered), and outcome measurement (e.g., kilocalories, MET-hours, unitless score). Physical activity questions used in U.S. surveillance systems were designed mainly to detect prevalence of meeting federal guidelines for participation in moderate or vigorous physical activity. Because most questions in those systems have remained the same during the past decade, they can be used to estimate population trends across successive years. However, only a few studies have been conducted to confirm their reliability and validity, which appear only fair to moderate in strength (Brownson et al. 1999; Nelson et al. 2001; Rosenbaum 2009; Yore et al. 2007).

Three validated questionnaires have been commonly used in epidemiology research and have special historical significance: the Minnesota Leisure Time Physical Activity Questionnaire (MLTPAQ), the Harvard Alumni/Paffenbarger Physical Activity Survey, and the Stanford Seven-Day Physical Activity Recall Interview. Others are noteworthy because they were designed to measure physical activity worldwide in nations with differing languages and cultures (International Physical Activity Questionnaire and the Global Physical Activity Questionnaire) or in special groups such as youths (3-day Physical Activity Recall) or older adults (CHAMPS).

Minnesota Leisure Time Physical Activity Questionnaire

The MLTPAQ is an interview-administered instrument that asks respondents to recall their participation in a list of leisure-time physical activities over the past year. Respondents are asked to provide the number of months, average number of times per month, and the average amount of time spent on each occasion of each activity reported. The outcome is scored as an activity metabolic index per week based on MET values associated with each reported activity. A number of studies have indicated reasonable validity and reliability for this instrument. Physical activity assessed by the MLTPAQ has been associated with reduced risk of CHD in two reports from the Multiple Risk Factor Intervention Trial (Leon et al. 1987; Leon and Connett 1991).

Harvard Alumni/Paffenbarger Physical Activity Survey

This instrument was designed for a study of the association of physical activity habits and chronic disease risk in a population of Harvard University alumni (Paffenbarger, Wing, and Hyde 1978). The time frame can range from the past week to several past years. The survey is brief and contains the following items: "How many city blocks do you normally walk each day? How many flights of stairs do you climb up each day? List any sports or recreation you have actively participated in during the past year." Values in kilocalories are assigned to walking, stair climbing, and recreational activity and summed to obtain a score in kilocalories per week. Physical activity assessed with this survey has been associated with reduced risk for chronic disease in the Harvard alumni population (Paffenbarger et al. 1993b; Lee, Hsieh, and Paffenbarger 1995; Lee and Paffenbarger 2000; Lee, Sesso, and Paffenbarger 2000; Sesso, Paffenbarger, and Lee 2000).

Stanford Seven-Day Physical Activity Recall Interview

This instrument was designed for use in the Stanford Five-City Project (Sallis et al. 1985; Blair et al. 1985). It is an interviewer-administered survey that requests information on sleep and physical activity, such as aerobic exercise, work-related activity, gardening, walking, and leisure-time

physical activity of moderate intensity or greater, over the past seven days. Respondents are shown a list of possible activities in each category. The amount of time remaining each day after activities of moderate intensity or greater have been accounted for is assumed to have been spent performing light-intensity activity. The outcome is expressed in kilocalories per kilogram (or simply kilocalories if the respondent's body weight is known) per week or per day.

International Physical Activity Questionnaire (IPAQ)

The IPAQ records physical activity as hours and additional minutes of participation during the past seven days in activities rated according to multiples of METs expressed as MET-minutes per week. It assesses frequency and duration of moderate (4 METs) and vigorous (8 METs) physical activity and walking (3.3 METs) appropriate for categorization of individuals as meeting public health guidelines for sufficient regular physical activity. Time spent in activities is aggregated across leisure, work, domestic chores, and transportation. The IPAQ has acceptable measurement properties for monitoring population levels of physical activity among 18- to 65-year-old adults in diverse settings. Studies conducted in 12 countries on six continents using standardized methods indicate that IPAQ questionnaires yield repeatable data (Spearman's rho ~0.80) (Craig et al. 2003). Criterion validity judged against accelerometry is comparable to that for other self-report measures (a median validity coefficient of rho ~0.30). The "usual week" and "last 7 d" reference periods perform similarly, and the reliability of the self-administered form is similar to that of the telephone interview.

Global Physical Activity Questionnaire (GPAQ)

The GPAQ was developed as part of the World Health Organization's STEPWISE Approach to Chronic Disease Risk Factor Surveillance (STEPS), a feasible approach to monitoring trends in eight major health risk factors including physical inactivity, especially in developing nations (Armstrong and Bull 2006). It has 16 questions administered by interview or self-report questionnaire that are designed to assess time (typical day or week) spent in physical activities done in separate contexts, including paid jobs or unpaid work (including household chores, harvesting, hunting or fishing for food), transport, and leisure or recreation. Both moderate and vigorous activities are assessed for work and leisure. Walking or cycling for transport is summed. One question is about time spent in sedentary activities. Reliabilities across three to seven days are approximately 0.70 to 0.80. GPAQ scores and IPAQ scores were moderately correlated with each other (0.45 to 0.65) but were weakly correlated with pedometer or accelerometer counts in studies from nine countries (Bull, Maslin, and Armstrong 2009).

3-Day Physical Activity Recall (3-D PAR)

This instrument has been validated against accelerometry in 8th- and 9th-grade girls (Pate et al. 2003). Vigorous physical activity (VPA) as measured by the 3-D PAR was correlated ($r = 0.41$) with VPA estimated by accelerometry. The 3-D PAR uses a script and graphic figures to explain the intensity level of common activities. Light activities are described as requiring little or no movement with slow breathing, moderate activities as some movement and normal breathing, hard activities as moderate movement and increased breathing, and very hard activities as quick movements and hard breathing. The instrument is administered by a trained research assistant. Participants are asked to recall their activities on the previous three days (e.g., Tuesday, then Monday, then Sunday). For each day recalled, participants complete a grid, which is divided into 30-min time blocks, beginning at 7 a.m. and ending at midnight. Participants report the predominant activity in each 30-min block. A list of 58 common physical activities and sedentary behaviors is provided. The list includes an option to add an "other" activity performed; participants enter the number of an activity and indicate whether the activity was performed at a light, moderate, hard, or very hard intensity. The average number of 30-min blocks of vigorous physical activity (VPA, ≥ 6 METs) is calculated, and whether or not participants accumulated one or more 30-min blocks of VPA per day and two or more blocks of moderate-to-vigorous physical activity (MVPA, ≥ 3 METs) is determined. MET values are obtained from the Compendium of Physical Activities (Ainsworth et al. 2000).

CHAMPS Physical Activity Questionnaire

This self-report measure was developed initially to evaluate outcomes of the Community Healthy Activities Model Program for Seniors (CHAMPS), an intervention to increase physical activity (Stewart et al. 2001). The questionnaire assesses weekly frequency and duration of various leisure-time and domestic physical activities typically undertaken by older adults over the past four weeks. Scoring yields an estimate of weekly calories expended during physical activity and summaries of weekly frequency of moderate-intensity activities (≥ 3 METs) or all physical activities. Six-month stability reliability has ranged from 0.58 to 0.67. Correlations between scores from the CHAMPS measure with scores from other validated measures of physical activity designed for older adults (i.e., the Physical Activity Scale for the Elderly [PASE] and the Yale Physical Activity Scale [YPAS]) are moderately large (0.58 to 0.68) (Harada et al. 2001). Also, correlations of CHAMPS scores with performance-based measures of physical function and physical activity measured by accelerometer counts and pedometer steps are moderately large (~0.40 to 0.70) but slightly smaller than those observed for the PASE and YPAS (Stewart et al. 2001; Giles and Marshall 2009), which each have been partially validated against doubly labeled water (Bonnefoy et al. 2001).

An important issue to consider when evaluating the epidemiologic literature on the association between physical activity and health outcomes is the physical activity assessment method that was used. Did the investigators use an instrument with established validity and reliability for the type of sample under study? If not, do the authors provide any evidence for the validity and reliability of the instrument that was used?

Many large epidemiologic studies that provide physical activity and health information were designed to evaluate other health risk factors; physical activity was of only secondary interest in many such studies, and thus the physical activity assessment methods were often less than optimal and sometimes of poorly established validity and reliability. For example, the Physicians' Health Study was a randomized, double-blind, placebo-controlled trial designed to determine whether aspirin in low doses decreases the risk of CHD and whether beta-carotene decreases the risk of both CHD and cancer. Physical activity in this study was assessed by the question, "How often do you exercise vigorously enough to work up a sweat?" Response categories were "daily," "5 to 6 times/week," "2 to 4 times/week," "once/week," "1 to 3 times/month," or "rarely/never." There is some evidence for the validity of this item as an indicator of physical activity level (Siconolfi et al. 1985; Washburn, Chin, and Montoye 1990), and activity assessed with "sweat" questions has been associated with health outcomes (Manson et al. 1992). However, this item assesses a very specific type of physical activity in which only a small and highly select segment of the population may engage.

The Nurses' Health Study is a prospective study, begun in 1976, of health and lifestyle factors in 121,700 female registered nurses. In addition to other types of leisure-time physical activity, respondents are asked to report the average amount of time spent in walking or hiking outdoors per week during the past year and to estimate their usual walking pace as easy or casual, average, brisk, or very brisk. The validity and reliability of self-reports of walking distance and speed have not been established.

▷ **SELF-REPORTS OF** physical activity are the most feasible method for measuring physical activity in national surveys and surveillance systems. Objective measures, such as motion sensors, heart rate monitors, and doubly labeled water, can estimate different components of physical activity and are commonly used to validate self-report measures.

There are currently a number of well-established **physical activity surveys** for individuals of all ages, from adolescents to adults over 65 years old. However, physical activity surveys specifically for women and ethnic minorities or surveys designed to assess specific aspects of physical activity that may be related to health outcomes, such as high-load weight-bearing activities or activities that increase muscular strength, have yet to be validated.

It is generally thought that individuals tend to overestimate participation in vigorous activities and underestimate participation in light- to moderate-intensity activities (Sallis and Saelens 2000). Further work needs to be done to enhance recall of physical activity intensity on self-report measures so that the amount and intensity of physical activity required to reduce chronic disease risk can be determined.

What Is Physical Fitness?

Physical fitness is an attribute that has a genetic basis but is also sensitive to changes in type and amount of physical activity, especially as people age. It is important to measure fitness both as an outcome of physical activity and as a moderator or mediator of physical activity's effect on disease morbidity and mortality and injury.

The measurement of fitness should become an important part of surveillance systems that track physical activity and risks for disease or injury. Defining physical fitness is a harder task than one might first think. The World Health Organization has defined fitness as "the ability to perform muscular work satisfactorily." That definition does not specify the ways in which physical, social, and psychological circumstances can vary to determine what is satisfactory, nor does it acknowledge that fitness comprises several abilities rather than a single overall ability. Physical fitness is better understood when the specific components that can be measured, and the circumstances under which those components relate to bodily function and health or reduced disease, are defined.

According to scientific consensus from the Second International Conference on Physical Activity, Fitness, and Health (Bouchard, Shephard, and Stephens 1994), the components of **health-related physical fitness,** listed in table 3.2, can be categorized as morphological, muscular, motor, cardiorespiratory, and metabolic.

Fitness can be classified as performance related when the ability to perform (e.g., competitive sports, military maneuvers, or occupational work) is considered. Tests of **performance-related fitness** are designed to measure psychomotor skills, maximal and submaximal cardiorespiratory power, muscular strength, power and endurance in the limbs and trunk for propulsion, body size, and body composition. High scores on these tests depend on genetic endowment as well as good nutrition and high motivation to train and to perform maximally during the testing. Measures of performance-related fitness show only a limited relationship to health, with the exceptions of cardiorespiratory capacity and body composition.

Health-related fitness components are more easily improved by regular physical activity and more directly relate to health. In addition to maximal cardiorespiratory power and body composition, which are important for both performance and health, health-related fitness components include body mass for height, subcutaneous fat distribution, abdominal visceral fat, bone density, strength and endurance of the

Table 3.2   The Components of Health-Related Fitness

Component	Measures
Morphological	Body mass for height Body composition Subcutaneous fat distribution Abdominal visceral fat Bone density Flexibility
Muscular	Power Strength Endurance
Motor	Agility Balance Coordination Speed of movement
Cardiorespiratory	Submaximal exercise capacity Maximal aerobic power Heart functions Lung functions Blood pressure
Metabolic	Glucose tolerance Insulin sensitivity Lipid and lipoprotein metabolism Substrate oxidation characteristics

Reprinted, by permission, from C. Bouchard, R.J. Shephard, and T. Stephens, 1994, *Physical activity, fitness, and health: International proceedings and consensus statement* (Champaign, IL: Human Kinetics), 81.

muscles in the abdomen and low back, heart and lung functions, blood pressure, glucose and insulin metabolism, blood lipoproteins, and the ratio of lipid to carbohydrate oxidation.

Morphological Component

Many population-based studies have shown associations between disease or death rates and measures of body size, shape, and composition. Understanding these associations is important for evaluating the biological plausibility that increased physical activity or physical fitness decreases rates of disease and death.

Fatness

The human body is governed by the first law of thermodynamics, that is, the principle of conservation of energy. Hence, changes in a person's body fat mass are determined by the balance between energy intake from food and energy expenditure, which results from basal or resting cell metabolism, the thermic effect of digestion, and physical activity. The amount of energy released by the body can be expressed in absolute terms (in kilojoules or kilocalories) or as a ratio relative to body mass and the estimated surface area of the body (e.g., per kilogram of body mass or fat-free mass). The relationship of body mass with fatness is most commonly expressed as Quetelet's body mass index (BMI; body mass in kilograms divided by height in meters squared).

A high BMI is a risk factor for all-cause mortality and increases risk for high blood pressure, high **triglycerides,** high cholesterol, impaired glucose tolerance, and high insulin levels. A BMI from 20 to 25 is considered normal or desirable for young to middle-aged adults. A very low BMI increases risk for all-cause death, but it is not clear that the risk is independent from smoking or wasting effects associated with disease. Most population studies have defined overweight as a BMI exceeding 27 for males and 28 for females, because those levels are associated with a doubling of risk for all-cause death. However, contemporary standards define overweight and obesity as a BMI exceeding 25 and 30, respectively, for both men and women. For children, overweight is defined as a BMI above the 95th percentile for age; the 85th percentile marks at-risk for overweight.

It is important to distinguish *overweight,* indicating high total mass, from *overfat,* indicating that a high percentage of total mass is fat. Proportions for constituents that compose fat-free body mass are about 73% water, 7% mineral, 19% to 20% protein, and less than 1% carbohydrate. These proportions vary little among people. In contrast, the rest of body mass, which is fat, varies widely and commonly composes 30% to 60% of total body mass in people who are obese. The association between increased risk for disease and death and BMI is assumed to exist because BMI estimates percent body fat accurately to within about ±5% in 7 of every 10 people in the population. Nonetheless, the use of BMI as an index of fatness is not appropriate among athletes or otherwise well-conditioned people who have a large fat-free body mass, or among frail elderly people or pregnant women.

Population-based studies that measure percent body fat and its association with disease or death have not been conducted, but clinical studies with small groups have shown that percent body fat and total fat mass are significantly correlated with high blood pressure and high blood levels of triglycerides, cholesterol, and insulin. The distribution of fat mass throughout the body is another risk factor for cardiovascular disease and death and for type 2 or non-insulin-dependent diabetes mellitus (NIDDM). A concentration of regional fat predominantly on the trunk is more common among men and is referred to as an android pattern, or apple shape. A concentration of regional fat predominantly on the hips is more common among women and is referred to as a gynoid pattern, or pear shape. Based on girth measurements, waist-to-hip ratios of 0.85 or lower for women and 0.95 or lower for men are regarded as normal in terms of health risk. In both men and women, waist-to-hip ratios exceeding those values are associated with high blood pressure, insulin resistance, elevated blood insulin levels, high blood triglycerides, and high cholesterol. The elevated risk for premature death posed by upper body fat can be partly explained by fat cells in the abdomen that drain into the portal circulation to the liver, thus affecting insulin levels and the metabolism of glucose, triglycerides, and cholesterol.

Bone Mass

Bone mass is typically measured by the density of mineral per area of bone (in grams per centimeter squared) using **dual X-ray absorptiometry (DXA),** a special X-ray scan. The potential maximal bone mineral density seems to be determined by young adulthood and peaks in women from ages 30 to 40 years and in men from ages 40 to 50. After those ages, new bone is formed more slowly than old bone is absorbed by the body, leading to bone involution, which is a risk factor for developing clinical osteoporosis. Aside from body deformities, the main health problem resulting from osteoporosis is increased risk of fractures associated with falls among the elderly.

Risk factors for osteoporosis include inherited susceptibility (80% of the cases are older women, especially white women), decreased estrogen levels (usually after menopause or in young women who have amenorrhea), low dietary intake of calcium, and a low level of physical activity. Bone mineral content is higher in people with a high fat-free body mass and is increased by weight-bearing and resistance exercises, most specifically in the body areas most used during those exercises. The effects of physical activity on bone mass are discussed in chapter 11.

Flexibility

Flexibility is generally defined as the range of motion at a specific joint or linked joints during both passive and dynamic movements. Flexibility is determined by the structure of bone and its surface, including cartilage, and the soft tissues around the articulating surfaces of the joint. As a measure of physical fitness, flexibility is usually distinguished from the laxity of a joint, which is a measure of joint instability governed largely by the tightness of ligaments. Flexibility for fitness is improved mainly by the stretching of muscles, their surrounding connective tissues, and tendons. The loss or gain of flexibility is very specific to each joint and its customary range of motion.

Muscular Component

Muscular strength, power, and endurance are the three main features of muscular fitness that are most related to physical performance and health. In sedentary men and women, a marked loss of fat-free body mass accompanies aging. This wasting is largely the result of lack of use of muscles and contributes to loss of mobility. In the frail elderly, important activities of daily living—such as lifting objects from the floor or over the head, carrying groceries, or rising out of a chair or bed—become impossible. Even a moderate amount of muscular fitness permits a person to engage in daily chores or leisure-time recreational activities with greater endurance, less subjective fatigue, and better circulation to exercising muscles. Maintaining muscular fitness in the trunk may also reduce the risk for low back pain, which is very common among adults in developed industrialized nations that have come to depend on technology for lifting and transporting objects, apparently causing a decline in normal trunk strength and endurance.

▶ **BY MAINTAINING** strength as they age, people can do daily chores and leisure physical activity with more endurance and less fatigue. Trunk strength can also reduce risk of low back pain, which is a prevalent health complaint in middle-aged and older adults.

Motor Component

Speed of movement, agility, balance, and coordination are the principal components of motor fitness, which is more accurately termed *psychomotor fitness* because those components are influenced by the senses. Motor fitness is especially important for children because it enhances exploring and challenging the physical environment during growth and maturation. Motor fitness is a limiting factor in the process of acquiring basic psychomotor skills. Children's performance on tests of other components of fitness is limited by their degree of motor fitness.

Low motor fitness in childhood may have a long-lasting impact, contributing indirectly to sedentary living among adults who did not develop the psychomotor skills needed for many leisure physical activities. Though motor fitness does not appear to explain differences in health among young adults, poor coordination and balance increase the risks of falls and fractures and the subsequent loss of independence or years of life among frail elderly men and women.

Cardiorespiratory Component

From the late 1950s to the early 1990s, most physicians and exercise scientists came to regard **cardiorespiratory fitness** as the most important component of fitness for health. This occurred mainly because cardiorespiratory fitness was most logically related to heart disease, the most prevalent killer of adults; because it could be defined and measured with greater precision than other components of fitness; and because, among single components of fitness, it provided the best explanation of why some people can sustain more work than others. For those reasons, and because it is the only component of fitness to have been

measured and associated with reduced death rates from all causes and from CHD specifically in population-based epidemiologic studies, cardiorespiratory fitness still holds the premier position among health-related components of fitness. However, epidemiologists now place more emphasis on measuring other components of fitness in studies of disease, injury, and death in order to obtain a more complete view of how physical fitness is related to health.

Cardiorespiratory fitness changes with age, increasing during adolescence (but declining in American girls in their late teens) (see figure 3.4) and then decreasing at an accelerated rate after age 45 (see figure 0.7 in the introduction). Because fitness is associated with better health, it is important to understand how it can be increased at all ages.

Maximal Aerobic Capacity

Population-based studies have defined cardiorespiratory fitness mainly as **maximal aerobic power,** or maximal oxygen uptake (i.e., $\dot{V}O_2$), during an exercise test consisting of gradual increments of intensity until a peak or plateau of oxygen uptake by skeletal muscles (or until voluntary fatigue) that appeared to the testers to be maximal. Today, a broader view of cardiorespiratory fitness and how it may relate to health is emerging.

Submaximal Exercise Capacity

Aerobic endurance performance is defined as the ability to sustain an intensity of power output ranging from moderate to high, but below maximal, for a prolonged period of time.

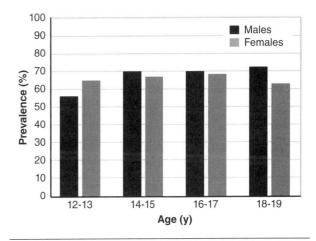

Figure 3.4 Prevalence of U.S. adolescents meeting health-related fitness standards, NHANES 1999-2002.

Data from R.R. Pate et al., 2006, "Cardiorespiratory fitness levels among US youth 12 to 19 years of age, *Archives of Pediatric and Adolescent Medicine,* 160: 1005-1012.

Cardiac Function

Heart function is usually assessed through measurement of cardiac muscle functions, including the heart rate for a given power output (adjusted for body mass), cardiac ejection fraction, myocardial shortening rate, stroke volume, and cardiac output, using exercise electrocardiography and imaging techniques.

Pulmonary Function

Lung function is clinically assessed by measuring static and dynamic lung volumes. These include tidal volume (amount of air inspired or expired during a normal breath), minute ventilation (volume of air expired in 1 min), vital capacity (the maximal volume of air that can be expired after a maximal inspiration), forced expiratory volume (FEV_1; volume of air expired during the first second of vital capacity), and peak flow (highest rate of expired air volume during vital capacity). Though maximal oxygen uptake depends in part on maximal minute ventilation, cardiorespiratory fitness in most healthy adults is limited by heart function, not by differences among people in lung function. Exceptions are cases of severe chronic obstructive lung diseases (COPD; diseases characterized by persistent slowing of airflow during forced expiration) such as cystic fibrosis, emphysema, and asthma.

Blood Pressure

Regular exercise lowers blood pressure at rest and during exercise at submaximal intensities. This is an important part of physical fitness for two reasons. (1) High resting blood pressure is associated with an increased risk of heart attack, stroke, ruptured arteries, kidney failure, death from CHD, and sudden cardiac death not necessarily resulting from coronary disease. (2) Lowered systolic blood pressure at a given heart rate during exercise provides a rough index that the oxygen consumption of the heart is lower, thus lowering the risk of arrhythmia and ischemia during exercise.

Metabolic Component

Metabolic fitness is the newest component of fitness recognized by exercise physiologists and epidemiologists who study health. It appears especially useful for understanding the potential health benefits of physical activity for preventing diabetes and atherosclerosis, the disease process leading to CHD and stroke.

Glucose Tolerance

People with impaired glucose tolerance are at risk for developing type 2 diabetes, a leading cause of cardiovascular disease and death and of circulatory diseases of the eyes, kidneys, and extremities. Regular physical activity affects glucose metabolism in ways that appear to protect against glucose intolerance. These include normalizing hormonal secretion of insulin and glucagon from the pancreas, increasing the sensitivity of

muscle cells to insulin, and an insulin-like action of muscle contraction that enhances glucose uptake from the blood.

Blood Lipid and Cholesterol Profiles

High blood levels of triglycerides, total cholesterol, and low-density lipoprotein cholesterol (LDL-C) and low blood levels of high-density lipoprotein cholesterol (HDL-C) are risk factors for CHD and stroke. Because regular physical activity affects lipid metabolism in ways that apparently lead to lowered triglycerides and elevated HDL-C, the concept of metabolic fitness can help explain how physical activity helps protect against atherosclerotic diseases that lead to CHD and stroke.

> ▶ **METABOLIC FITNESS** is the newest component of fitness recognized by exercise physiologists and epidemiologists who study health. It is especially useful for understanding the potential health benefits of physical activity for preventing diabetes and cardiovascular disease.

Lipid Oxidation

The ratio of carbon dioxide exhaled to oxygen consumed each minute is known as the respiratory exchange ratio (RER), which provides an index of the relative oxidation of lipids to carbohydrate in the cell, the respiratory quotient (RQ). At rest, RER is approximately 0.83 for a person whose diet has the usual mixture of calories from protein, carbohydrate, and fat. An RER of 0.70 would indicate that only fat was oxidized, while an RER of 1.0 would indicate that only carbohydrate was oxidized. A relatively low RER at rest or during prolonged submaximal exercise indicates that a person is burning more lipids than carbohydrates as fuel. A high rate of lipid oxidation also appears to alter cholesterol metabolism and reduce body fat so as to decrease risk of cardiovascular disease and premature death. Sustained muscular effort for prolonged periods of time depends on high initial levels of glucose stored in the liver and muscle as glycogen and on normal levels of glucose maintained in the blood during exercise. However, using fat as a fuel in cell respiration is also important for endurance performance by helping spare glucose.

Exercise Training

Exercise is a specific type of physical activity performed regularly, usually for the purpose of improving or maintaining physical fitness, physical skills, or health. Enough is known about the ways in which some biological systems (e.g., cardiorespiratory and neuromuscular) respond to differing amounts of exercise that professional guidelines have been adopted for optimal exercise prescription by exercise and health professionals.

The most established exercise training guidelines, which outline the recommended frequency, intensity, time, and type or mode of exercise for fitness (cleverly referred to as the F.I.T.T. principles), were pronounced by the American

College of Sports Medicine (ACSM) in 1978 and revised in 1990 and 1998 (table 3.3; Pollock et al. 1998). Those guidelines generally encompass recommendations for moderate physical activity endorsed by the ACSM and the American Heart Association and adopted in the 2008 Physical Activity Guidelines for Americans (U.S. Department of Health and Human Services 2008). The key difference between the ACSM guidelines and the federal guidelines is the emphasis in the ACSM guidelines on gradual progression to vigorous-intensity exercise for fitness and the emphasis in the Physical Activity Guidelines for Americans on moderate, as well as vigorous, physical activities for total energy expenditure.

▶ **EXERCISE TRAINING** guidelines for fitness endorsed by the ACSM focus on the F.I.T.T. principles: recommended frequency, intensity, time, and type or mode of exercise for fitness.

Frequency

The recommended frequency of exercise depends on a person's goals. A range of three to five days per week is recommended for increasing cardiorespiratory fitness or decreasing body fat, although a sedentary person can improve by exercising two days per week during the first few weeks of training. Gains are proportional to frequency within the range of three to five days. A frequency beyond five days each week increases risk for injury, even among people who are well conditioned.

Muscular strength and endurance, fat-free body mass, and flexibility can be increased and maintained through participation in resistance exercise (e.g., weightlifting) at least two or three days per week.

Intensity

Because people differ in their initial level of fitness, the recommended intensity of exercise is always relative to a person's maximal capacity. For cardiorespiratory fitness, the recommended intensity of training ranges from 50% to 85% of maximal oxygen uptake reserve, which is calculated by adding 50% to 85% of the difference between resting and maximal $\dot{V}O_2$ measured during exercise testing to a person's resting $\dot{V}O_2$. For very sedentary, older, or obese people, 40% may be a more appropriate and effective beginning intensity. Because heart rate (HR) reserve (a percentage, usually 50% to 85%, of the difference between maximal exercise HR and

Table 3.3   ACSM 1998 and 2008 Federal Physical Activity Guidelines for Americans

Category	ACSM Guidelines for Fitness 1998	Physical Activity Guidelines for Americans 2008	ACSM Recommendations 2011
Cardiorespiratory training	20 to 60 min (at least 10 min each session) 3 to 5 days/week 40/50% to 85% capacity	≥150 min/week moderate (3.0-5.9 METs), or ≥75 min/week vigorous (6.0+ METs), or equivalent combination (at least 10 min each session, spread throughout the week)	Moderate-intensity cardiorespiratory exercise training for ≥30 min/d on ≥5 d/wk for a total of ≥150 min/wk, vigorous-intensity cardiorespiratory exercise training for ≥20 min/d on ≥3 d/wk (≥75 min/wk), or a combination of moderate- and vigorous-intensity exercise to achieve a total energy expenditure of ≥500-1000 MET·min^{-1}·wk^{-1}.
		For added benefits: ≥300 min/week moderate or ≥150 min/week vigorous or equivalent combination	
Strength training	Strength activities (major muscle groups) 2 or 3 days/week	Strength activities (major muscle groups) ≥2 days/week	Resistance exercises for each of the major muscle groups 2 or 3 days/week Exercises involving balance, agility, and coordination; and flexibility exercises for each of the major muscle–tendon groups (a total of 60 s /exercise) on ≥2 days/week
Progression	Progression to vigorous intensities	Gradual increase in physical activity	
Population	Recommendations are for healthy adults	Includes guidelines for children, older adults, pregnant women, people with disabilities, and children and adolescents: ≥60 min daily of moderate or vigorous physical activities (≥3 days/week)	Recommendations are for healthy adults

Based on Pollock et al. 1998; DHHS 2008; and ACSM 2011.

resting HR, added to resting HR) is linearly related to $\dot{V}O_2$ reserve in the 50% to 85% range and is much more practical to use, an intensity of 50% to 85% of HR reserve can serve as a surrogate for percent $\dot{V}O_2$ reserve. A range of 65% to 90% of maximal heart rate is equivalent to 50% to 85% of HR reserve.

For increasing or maintaining muscular strength and endurance and fat-free body mass, the intensity of resistance exercise has traditionally been expressed relative to a person's 1-repetition maximum (1RM). Some experts recommend that the resistance fall within a range of percentages of 1RM, such as the range of 50% to 85% proposed for cardiorespiratory fitness. Another common approach is to use the highest resistance that can be repeated a certain number of times before fatigue (commonly 8RM-15RM). A lower RM value (i.e., a higher resistance) promotes strength more than it does endurance, while a higher RM (i.e., a lower resistance) promotes more endurance. The ACSM recommendations do not specify intensity; rather, they suggest a minimum of 8 to 10 different resistance exercises using the major muscle groups. People under 50 years of age are advised to complete 8 to 12 repetitions of each exercise, and people over 50 are advised to complete 10 to 15 repetitions.

For flexibility training, the ACSM recommends that the joints involved with the major muscle groups be stretched, using both static and dynamic methods, but does not mention intensity. In common practice, intensity is judged by the person based on the sensation of stretch without pain.

Time or Duration

The recommended daily time or duration for exercise for increasing or maintaining cardiorespiratory fitness or reducing body fat ranges from 20 to 60 min. While fitness improvements are proportional to exercise time within those ranges, the risk of injury, especially musculoskeletal injuries and heat injury in hot or humid environments, also increases with longer durations. The ACSM has not offered specific recommendations for the duration of resistance and stretching exercises, probably because the benefits of training for strength and flexibility depend more on the number of repetitions than on the rate at which the repetitions are completed; in contrast, in exercise training for cardiorespiratory fitness, improved fitness is proportional to the rate of energy expenditure. However, some recent research suggests that several intermittent bouts of aerobic exercise (e.g., three separate sessions of 10 min each) can increase cardiorespiratory fitness.

Type or Mode

The type or mode of exercise refers to the form of the activity, its rate or pace, and its continuity. Activities that involve large muscle groups (e.g., walking or hiking, run-

ning or jogging, cycling, cross-country skiing, aerobic dance or aerobic group exercise, rope skipping, rowing, stair climbing, swimming, skating, and endurance games), that are performed rhythmically, and that can be sustained continuously for 20 to 60 min at a time are recommended when the goal of exercise is cardiorespiratory fitness or fat loss. When the frequency, intensity, and time spent are similar, gains in cardiorespiratory fitness and fat loss are similar, regardless of the type of physical activity.

Resistance exercises (e.g., weightlifting) are used for muscular strength and endurance, and stretching exercises are used for flexibility training. Because body systems respond in very specific ways to the challenges imposed by different modes of exercise, a well-balanced exercise training program includes several modes. Certain types of physical activity that affect specific components of physical fitness might be especially effective in reducing the risk of specific diseases (table 3.4).

▶ **THE PERCENT** gains in fitness after exercise training are very similar for males and females of all ages. The effects of frequency, intensity, and duration on fitness are interrelated. For example, similar increases in fitness can occur at relatively lower intensities if the frequency and duration of the activity are increased. Similarly, if the intensity of the exercise is increased, the frequency and duration can be reduced. This algebraic relationship among intensity, duration, and frequency allows the exercise training program to be individualized based on initial fitness or readiness for exercise, age, and personal fitness goals.

Dose Response of Physical Activity and Health

Observe moderation.
> —Hesiod, eighth century BC

Keep the Golden Mean.
> —Cleobu'los, king of Rhodes (630-559 BC)

Not too strong, not too fast, not too often, not too long.
> —T.L. De Lorme, 1945

Establishing dose response is one of Mill's canons for determining the causality of a health risk factor and also has practical importance for public policy recommendations about the types and amounts of physical activity that are healthful. Subsequent chapters discuss the dose–response evidence for each aspect of health covered in this book. Here we provide an overview of the current evidence.

Table 3.4 Dimensions of Physical Activity With Proposed Mechanism of Effect, Diseases or Conditions Affected, and Potential Surveillance Definitions

Physical activity dimension	Possible mechanisms	Diseases or conditions affected	Potential operational definitions for surveillance purposes
Caloric expenditure	Energy use	CHD, type 2 diabetes, obesity, cancer	Kilocalorie score; total time spent in or pattern of regular, sustained activities
Aerobic intensity	Enhanced cardiac function	CHD, type 2 diabetes, cancer	Kilocalorie score; total time spent in or pattern of intense activities
Weight bearing	Gravitational force	Osteoporosis	Total time spent in or pattern of weight-bearing activities
Flexibility	Range of motion	Disability	Total time spent in or pattern of activities that promote or require flexibility
Muscular strength	Muscle force generation	Disability	Total time spent in or pattern of activities that promote or require muscular strength

Reprinted, by permission, from C.J. Caspersen, R.K. Merritt, and T. Stephens, 1994, International physical activity patterns: A methodological perspective. In *Advances in exercise adherence*, edited by R.K. Dishman (Champaign, IL: Human Kinetics), 90.

Since the Second International Consensus Symposium on Physical Activity, Fitness, and Health in Toronto in 1992 (Bouchard, Shephard, and Stephens 1994), worldwide attention has been paid to the question of whether, and in what forms, dose–response relationships exist between the frequency, intensity, and duration of different types of physical activity and reduced risks of disease, injury, and premature death. Hypothetical dose–response relationships between the amount of physical activity and several risk factors for CHD (Haskell 1994) and between intensity of physical activity and general health benefits and hazards (Dehn and Mullins 1977) are depicted in figures 3.5 and 3.6, respectively. As illustrated next, whether the apparent health-protective effects of physical activity are best described by a linear, dose-dependent relationship was controversial over the past decade and remains undecided today.

▷ **ESTABLISHING DOSE** response is one of Mill's canons for determining the causality of a health risk factor, but it is also important for public policy recommendations about the types and amounts of physical activity that are healthful.

National Runners' Health Study

Circumstantial evidence supportive of a linear dose–response relationship between activity and health outcomes was provided by the National Runners' Health Study conducted at the University of California at Berkeley. This cross-sectional study included about 2600 female (Williams 1996) and over 8200 male runners (Williams 1997). After runners with history of heart attack or medication that might affect CHD, smokers, and vegetarians were excluded, 1837 women and 7059 men remained in the study for data analysis. Participants completed a two-page questionnaire, which was distributed at races and sent to subscribers of *Runner's World* magazine. The questionnaire obtained information on demographic characteristics (age, race, and education); running history (age when the participant began running at least 12 miles per week, average weekly distance run and number of marathons run in the preceding five years, best marathon and 10 km times); weight history (highest and current weight; weight when the participant started running; lowest weight as a runner); circumferences of the chest, waist, and hips; diet (whether vegetarian; weekly intake of alcohol, red meat, fish, fruit, vitamin C, vitamin E, and aspirin); current and past cigarette use; history of heart attack and cancer; and medications taken to treat high blood pressure, thyroid conditions, high cholesterol levels, or diabetes. In addition to the questions asked of the men, women were asked about menstrual history (whether currently having periods and age at menarche) and hormone use (birth control pills, postmenopausal estrogen replacement, or progesterone). The questionnaire also requested permission to obtain the participants' height, weight, plasma cholesterol and triglyceride concentrations, blood pressure, and heart rate at rest from their physicians. Risk for CHD was estimated using the Framingham Heart Study equation for predicting CHD risk by combining runners' scores on blood levels of cholesterol, triglycerides, uric acid, and glucose.

Among men, results indicated a linear reduction in estimated overall risk for CHD with each successive 16 km increment (about 10 miles) in weekly running distance, from less than 16 km up to 80 km (about 50 miles) per week. Risk was 30% lower in male runners who averaged 64 km or more each week than in those running less than 15 km each week. Nonetheless, male runners covering 80 km or more per week had the same CHD risk as those running 64 to 79 km per week.

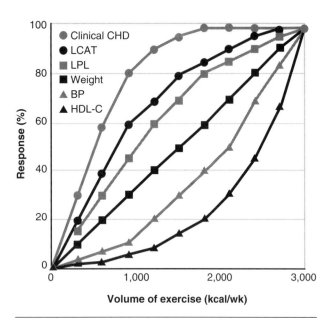

Figure 3.5 Hypothetical dose–response relationships between the amount of physical activity exposure and several health-related outcomes.

Reprinted, by permission, from W.L. Haskell, 1994, Dose-response issues from a biological perspective. In *Physical activity, fitness, and health: International proceedings and consensus statement,* edited by C. Bouchard, R.J. Shephard, and T. Stephens (Champaign, IL: Human Kinetics), 1037.

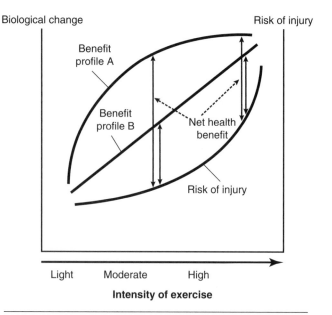

Figure 3.6 The relationship of exercise intensity to biological change (for two dose–response profiles) and risk of adverse events (e.g., injury) is shown. Net health benefit for moderate- and high-intensity exercise is also displayed.

Reprinted from M. Dehn and C. Mullins, 1977, "Physiologic effects and importance of exercise in patients with coronary heart disease," *Cardiovascular Medicine* 2: 365. By permission of Michael Dehn.

The results for women also suggested a dose–response relationship between reduction in CHD risk and physical activity as distance run each week increased. There was a 30% reduction in the overall risk of CHD and a 45% reduction in risk of CHD death among the women who ran the most. Those risk reductions were statistically independent of BMI, age, education, menstrual status, alcohol consumption, diet, estrogen, progesterone, and the use of birth control pills. The clearest findings were for increased HDL-C: The women who ran the most (more than 64 km each week) had HDL-C levels that were nearly 10 mg/dl (0.25 mmol/L) higher than those of the women who ran the least (16 km or less each week).

Whether there was a dose–response relationship for running intensity and health outcome was also examined, based on runners' reports of pace (in kilometers per hour) during their best recent 10 km race; this was used as a surrogate measure of their exercise intensity during training (Williams 1998b). After adjustments for weekly running distance, age, consumption of alcohol, and diet, both men and women who ran faster (i.e., at greater intensity) had lower blood pressures; triglyceride levels; ratios of total cholesterol to HDL-C; BMIs; and waist, hip, and chest girths. Relative to the effect of running distance, running velocity was associated with a 13.3 times greater effect on systolic blood pressure, a 2.8 times greater effect on diastolic blood pressure, and a 4.7 times greater calculated effect on

waist circumference. Among women, running velocity was associated with a 5.7 times greater effect on systolic blood pressure. In contrast, running distance had a more than sixfold greater calculated effect on HDL-C levels in both sexes than did running velocity.

Other findings from the National Runners' Health Study suggest that associations between running distance and reduced risk factors extended to older runners (Williams 1998a). Among 935 men in their 60s and 175 men in their 70s, the associations of weekly running distance with higher levels of plasma HDL-C and lower plasma triglycerides, lower ratio of total cholesterol to HDL-C, lower systolic and diastolic blood pressure, and lower BMI were similar to those seen in runners younger than age 60. In contrast, the inverse relationship between running distance and LDL-C was smaller than that observed among younger men.

An important question is whether these results are generalizable to the U.S. population at large. Because all subjects were runners, even the least-active subjects in the study were more active than the least-active subjects in other studies of physical activity and CHD risk that included sedentary subjects. Hence, the National Runners' Health Study suggested a dose–response reduction in CHD that is linear for most runners, but it did not permit a test of whether there is a proportionately greater reduction in risk in low-mileage runners compared with sedentary peers. Also, the study predicted risk based on 10 years of running experience at the time of the survey (the average subject had been running about 8.5 years), but the study did not actually observe the runners for 10 years, nor were actual CHD events measured; the likelihood of CHD events was computed using a prediction formula derived from men in the Framingham Heart Study. Moreover, the National Runners' Health Study showed a benefit plateau at about 50 miles run per week. That finding is pertinent for evaluating the public health benefits versus costs of exercise; we later consider the risk of injuries among runners, which appears to increase with increased running distance.

The results of the National Runners' Health Study and many other studies suggest that regular physical activity has great potential for reducing health risk factors associated with all-cause and coronary heart and vascular disease (CVD) mortality in a dose–response manner. However, this was a cross-sectional study, not a prospective cohort or controlled trial, and was limited to relatively high-distance runners who expended many more calories than the typical person, who might benefit from less physical activity.

Current Scientific Consensus

A consensus symposium on the dose–response relationship between physical activity and health was held in October 2000 at Hockley Valley Resort near Toronto (Bouchard 2001). Twenty-four invited experts from six countries reviewed the available research literature and evaluated the cumulative evidence in several areas of health according to four scientific categories that considered the quality of the research designs and the quantity and agreement of findings in each area.

Consensus was reached that an inverse, and generally linear, relationship exists between physical activity and rates of all-cause mortality, CVD mortality, and the incidence of type 2 diabetes. Consensus was not reached about dose response for the other health outcomes evaluated, mainly because (1) in some areas not enough studies examined the dose–response question, (2) measures of physical activity were imprecise, (3) some responses to physical activity were too small to allow examination of the dose influence, and (4) confounding influences such as genetic variability and body fatness were inadequately controlled.

Given the wide variability in people's adaptations to similar physical activity stimuli, it is not too surprising that as yet it has been difficult to define precisely a dose–response pattern for physical activity and many health outcomes. As figure 3.7 shows, changes in maximal oxygen uptake in response to exercise training vary widely. For example, in the HERITAGE Family Study of several hundred sedentary adults' responses were widely varied, despite subjects' exposure to the same exercise stimulus (i.e., 20 weeks of cycling exercise three days per week at an intensity of 65% of maximal oxygen uptake; Bouchard and Rankinen 2001).

Similarly, wide variations have been found for other outcomes of exercise training such as HDL-C, the good choles-

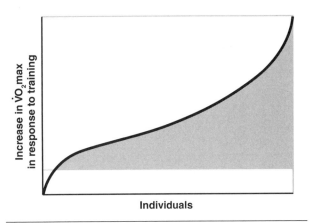

Figure 3.7 General pattern of heterogeneity in $\dot{V}O_2$max training response among individuals. A pattern similar to this one was found in the HERITAGE study.

terol. The HERITAGE Family Study found that responses to training are relatively the same for adults regardless of age, sex, and race. However, people's initial levels are a strong predictor of training response for some attributes, including submaximal exercise heart rate and blood pressure, but weakly influence changes in maximal oxygen uptake and HDL-C. Moreover, family inheritance (i.e., shared environment and genetics) is a significant influence on variation in people's response to regular physical activity (Bouchard and Rankinen 2001).

Current conclusions about people's average responses in specific health outcomes to various amounts of physical activity are categorized in table 3.5 according to the strength of the evidence: strong—agreement among numerous randomized controlled trials; substantial—agreement or mixed evidence among a limited number of randomized controlled trials or among nonrepresentative samples; moderate—agreement among uncontrolled trials or observational studies (Physical Activity Guidelines Advisory Committee 2008).

Surveys and Surveillance of Physical Activity

Before physical activity can be increased in a population, the prevalence rates of physical activity and its trends across time among geographic regions and subgroups within the population must be established. Surveys are used to determine the prevalence of physical activity by asking a sample of the population about their physical activity habits. Trends in physical activity prevalence are determined by surveillance systems, which repeatedly and regularly conduct the same survey in a population every year or every several years. Surveillance is necessary to measure **secular trends** (i.e., naturally occurring change in the population) and response to public health interventions. Surveys and surveillance systems

Table 3.5 Summary of Evidence for Dose–Response Effects of Physical Activity on Adult Health

Health outcome	Risk reduction	Strength of evidence	Dose response	Effective dose
All-cause mortality	30%	Strong	Clear inverse	2 to 2.5 h per week of moderate-to-vigorous physical activity (MVPA)
Cardiorespiratory health (CHD, CVD, stroke)	20% to 35%	Strong	Clear inverse	800 MET-minutes per week of MVPA
Metabolic health (type 2 diabetes and metabolic syndrome)	30% to 40%	Strong	Inverse	2 to 2.5 h per week of MVPA
Bone health (hip fracture)	36% to 41%	Moderate	Inverse	540 to 876 MET-minutes per week of MVPA
Functional health (disability or role limitations with aging)	30%	Moderate to strong	Inverse	Not clear
Cancer (breast or colon)	20% to 30%	Strong	Inverse (shape unclear)	210 to 420 min per week of MVPA
Mental health (depression or cognitive decline with aging)	20% to 30%	Strong	Inverse (depression)	Not clear

that measure and track changes in physical activity prevalence are necessary to determine population segments that need intervention and to judge the effectiveness of population-based intervention. In this section we consider some surveys and surveillance systems in developed nations worldwide and their estimates of physical activity prevalence. We then turn to key national surveys and surveillance systems in the United States and their results.

Though it is tempting to compare nations, varying definitions and methods used by many of the different surveys make it difficult to make direct comparisons. The International Consensus Group for Physical Activity Measurement met in Geneva, Switzerland, in 1998 to launch the development of a set of valid instruments that can be used internationally to obtain comparable estimates of physical activity worldwide (Booth 2000). Subsequently, the International Physical Activity Prevalence Study began, using translations of the same self-report measure of physical activity, the International Physical Activity Questionnaire, administered by mail-out questionnaire or by telephone or face-to-face interview. Preliminary data are available from that study, permitting comparisons of low, moderate, and high physical activity levels among many nations, based on the frequency and duration of participation in activities of differing intensities. Moderate and high levels are generally regarded as sufficient for promoting public health. See figures 3.8 and 3.9.

The Health Behavior in School-aged Children (HBSC) survey of physical activity, carried out in 31 European

nations, Israel, Canada, and the United States during 2001 and 2002, found that, averaged across nations, 34% of boys and girls reported being physically active for at least 60 min five or more days each week (Roberts, Tynjala, and Komkov 2004). There was wide variation among the countries, but none met the World Health Organization recommended level of 60 min of moderate-to-vigorous physical activity each day (Borraccino et al. 2009).

National Surveys in Developed Nations

The World Health Organization (WHO) MONICA Optional Study of Physical Activity (MOSPA) was developed and is managed by the Centers for Disease Control and Prevention (CDC) for the purpose of comparing estimates of physical activity among nations that participate in the WHO MONICA surveillance system, which monitors cardiovascular disease trends worldwide. Thirteen of the 40 WHO MONICA survey sites in Europe and Asia participated from 1988 to 1994. In addition, several countries, including the United States, include questions about leisure-time physical activity in periodic national surveys about health and behavior. Those surveys provide a basis for comparing prevalence of physical activity among population subgroups and changes in prevalence over time. Table 3.6 describes the features of the surveys in several nations.

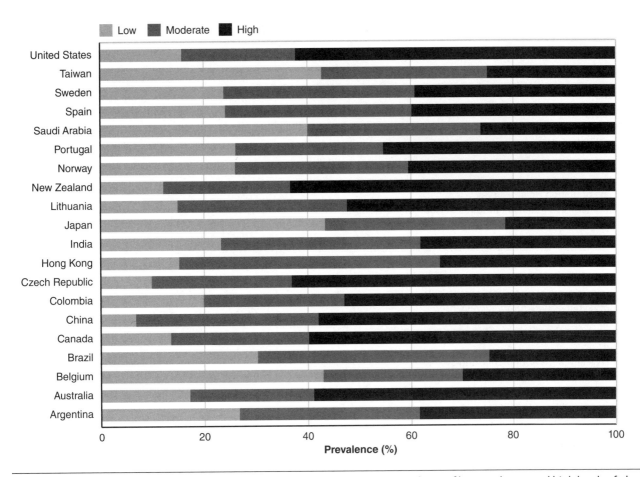

Figure 3.8 Results of the International Prevalence Study on Physical Activity. Prevalence of low, moderate, and high levels of physical activity in 20 nations.

Data from Bauman et al. 2009.

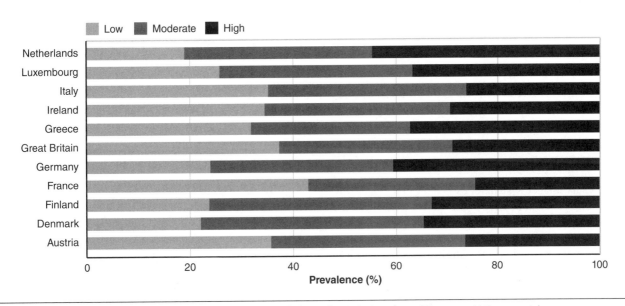

Figure 3.9 Prevalence of low, moderate, and high levels of physical activity in selected European Union countries.

Adapted from Sjöström et al. 2006.

Table 3.6   Features of Population Surveillance of Physical Activity in Selected Nations

Country, survey name, year(s) of survey	Mode of administration	Ages	Recall period
Australia National Nutrition and Physical Activity Survey Children 2007, adults 2009 www.health.gov.au/	Telephone interview, household	Children: pedometers for 6 days; 48-h recall ages 9+	Past week Average week in past 6 months
Canada National Population Health Survey Biennial since 1994-1995, longitudinal tracking of individuals since 2000/2001 www.statcan.gc.ca/	Telephone interview, household	12+	Past 3 months
England National Health Survey for England 1991-1994, every year since 1997 except 2001 www.surveynet.ac.uk/sqb/qb/surveys/hse/hseintro.htm	Computer-assisted household interview since 1999	16+	Past 4 weeks
Finland National Health Behaviour Monitoring System 1978-2008 www.ktl.fi/portal/english/ research__people___programs/ health_promotion_and_chronic_disease_prevention/ units/health_promotion_research_unit/ health_behaviour_monitoring_systems/	Postal survey	15-64	Past 4 weeks Past year Usual workday
New Zealand Active New Zealand Survey 2007/2008 www.activenzsurvey.org.nz/	Face-to-face interview	16+	Past 7 days
Scotland Scottish Health Survey 1995, 1998, 2003, annually since 2008 www.surveynet.ac.uk/sqb/qb/surveys/ShealthS/shealthsintro.htm	Computer-assisted household interview	Children 2-15 Adults 16+	Past 4 weeks
Wales Welsh Health Survey 2003-2004, 2005-2006, annually since 2007 http://wales.gov.uk/topics/statistics/theme/health/health-survey/?lang=en	Self-report questionnaire after face-to-face interview	Adults 16+	Past 7 days

The United States

The first surveillance system for estimating and monitoring leisure-time physical activity in the United States was the Behavioral Risk Factor Surveillance System (BRFSS), which was developed by the Behavioral Epidemiology and Evaluation Branch of the Division of Health Education of the CDC's Center for Health Promotion and Education (Bradstock et al. 1984). Five additional national surveillance surveys of physical activity in the United States are managed by the CDC in Atlanta. These are summarized in table 3.7 and described in more detail in the following sections.

Behavioral Risk Factor Surveillance System

The BRFSS uses a population-based telephone survey and has provided estimates of national and state trends in physical activity, as well as obesity and fruit and vegetable consumption, since 1984. Its creation was prompted mainly by the 1990 health objectives for the nation established in 1980 (U.S. Department of Health and Human Services 1980), which for the first time emphasized physical activity and fitness. Those objectives highlighted the need to estimate current and future prevalence rates of physical activity in order to judge whether the participation objectives were appropriate and could be met.

Table 3.7 Summary of U.S. Physical Activity Surveillance Data Sources

Survey	Mode of data collection	Target population	Frequency of data collection	Physical activity domain(s)
BRFSS	Telephone interview	Adults (>18 years of age) in U.S. states, territories, and the District of Columbia. Sample is about 225,000 people.	Ongoing—annual	Leisure time, domestic, transportation Leisure: Usual week, ≥10 min each time
NHIS	Personal interview	Adults and children in U.S. states and the District of Columbia. Sample is about 100,000 people from 40,000 households.	Ongoing—annual	Leisure time Usual leisure, at least ≥10 min each time
NHANES	Interview/examination	About 5000 to 10,000 children and adults in the United States.	Ongoing—annual	Leisure time, domestic, transportation Children: past 7 days, ≥60 min each day Adults: typical week, ≥10 min each time
YRBSS	School-based survey	Approximately 15,000 high school students in the United States.	Every 2 years	Leisure time, domestic, transportation
NHTS	Household survey	About 25,000 U.S. households.	Every 5-7 years	Transportation
SHPPS	Mail survey	U.S. school districts, state education organizations, and classrooms.	Periodic	Physical activity policies and curricula

Source: Division of Nutrition, Physical Activity and Obesity, National Center for Chronic Disease Prevention and Health Promotion. www.cdc.gov/nccdphp/dnpa/physical/health_professionals/data/physical_surveys.htm

National estimates of physical activity and other health risk behaviors among adults had been provided by surveys regularly conducted by the National Center for Health Statistics (NCHS), but those surveys had not emphasized physical activity and health behaviors and were not designed to provide estimates for individual states, which might differ from the national average. Initially, from 1981 to 1983, BRFSS conducted point-prevalence surveys in 28 states and the District of Columbia. Since 1994, all states, the District of Columbia, and three territories (Puerto Rico, the U.S. Virgin Islands, and Guam) have administered the BRFSS by telephone. They send their results to the National Center for Chronic Disease Prevention and Health Promotion (NCCDPHP) at the CDC for compilation. Beginning in 2001, new questions were designed to incorporate three physical activity domains into the overall score: leisure time, domestic, and transportation.

National Health Interview Survey

The National Health Interview Survey (NHIS) is a large household survey conducted since 1957 by the National Center for Health Statistics (NCHS) at the CDC that uses family interviews to provide the main source of information on the health of the civilian noninstitutionalized population of the United States. It provided the baseline estimates of physical activity prevalence in the Healthy People 2010 and Healthy People 2020 objectives of the U.S. Department of Health and Human Services (2000, 2010). NHIS questions

assess physical activities that are light to moderate in intensity, as well as vigorous, whereas other questionnaires focus only on moderate- and vigorous-intensity activities.

National Health and Nutrition Examination Survey (NHANES)

NHANES, managed by the NCHS, provides statistics about the health- and nutrition-related behaviors of Americans using personal interview and direct physical examination. It is smaller than the BRFSS or NHIS but provides more detailed information than can be collected in the other surveys. The current physical activity questions in NHANES were first used in 1999. The physical examination includes a cardiovascular fitness evaluation (submaximal treadmill test) and a musculoskeletal fitness test (strength testing), which provide the only national data available on physical fitness among adults.

Youth Risk Behavior Surveillance System

The Youth Risk Behavior Surveillance System (YRBSS) is a national school-based survey conducted by state, territorial, and local education and health agencies and tribal governments. Results are compiled by the NCCDPHP at the CDC. It was begun in 1990 to monitor physical activity, nutrition, and other health risk behaviors among youths in grades 9 to 12. More detailed questions about physical activity were asked in 2010 and will be asked every other year.

National Household Travel Survey

The U.S. Department of Transportation conducts the National Household Travel Survey (NHTS) (formerly the Nationwide Personal Transportation Survey) to provide estimates of daily trip frequency, trip distance, means of transportation, and trip time for persons 5 years of age and older. Trends in walking and bicycling have been provided since 1969 and are currently being used by the Active Community Environments Initiative to promote physical activity through environmental change.

School Health Policies and Programs Study (SHPPS)

SHPPS is a periodic national survey mailed to state education agencies, district-level representatives, and designated school staff classroom faculty. Results are compiled by the NCCDPHP at the CDC. The survey is designed to assess school health policies and programs at the state, district, and classroom level in elementary, middle, and high schools. Physical activity questions on the SHPPS assess physical education curriculum offerings, availability of recess and intramural sport programs, and state and district curricular requirements for physical education.

Physical Activity in the United States

Physical activity levels in the United States seem generally similar to those in other economically developed nations that have a surveillance system for estimating the prevalence of leisure physical activity. Based on NHIS estimates (which are used to judge progress toward national physical activity goals in the United States), only about 30% of U.S. adults have said they regularly participate in either moderate or vigorous leisure-time physical activity for roughly the past decade. This is well below the 2010 national target of 50% participation, as shown in figure 3.10.

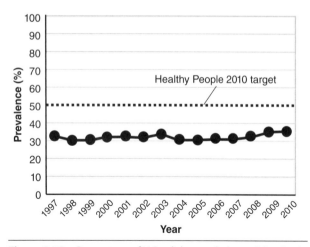

Figure 3.10 Percentage of U.S. adults regularly participating in moderate or vigorous leisure-time physical activity, 1997-2010.

Data from NHIS.

For 2005, age-adjusted prevalence estimates of regular participation and inactivity were similar for NHIS (30% and 41%) and NHANES (34% and 32%), but were 48% and 14% for BRFSS (Carlson et al. 2009). This suggests that the BRFSS overestimates regular physical activity and underestimates inactivity by wide margins. The YRBSS has estimated that a third of adolescents participate in less than 20 min of vigorous physical activity three days a week. In 2009, the YRBSS estimated that only 11% of girls and 25% of boys met the new guideline of an hour or more of moderate-to-vigorous physical activity every day. About 30% of girls and 17% of boys said they hadn't spent an hour exercising on any of the past seven days (CDC 2010). Those estimates have not changed since 2005.

Geographic Variation

There is wide variation across the United States in participation in regular physical activity, defined as either 20 or more minutes of vigorous physical activity (e.g., 6 METs or more) on three or more days each week or sustained physical activity of any intensity for about 30 min on five or more days each week.

Generally, western states are most active, and southern states are least active. Differences in the prevalence of regular moderate or vigorous physical activity in the United States according to region of the country are presented in figure 3.11. The two maps suggest improvements between 2005 and 2007 in the number of states and territories meeting the Healthy People 2010 target of 50% participation. In 2007, about half the states had met the target. However, estimates fluctuate based on how many people respond. Figure 3.12 shows that seven of the states that met the target might actually not have done so if other surveys had been conducted, and that 14 of the states that didn't meet the target were so close that they might have met it with other surveys.

Population Subgroups

Within the United States, physical activity differs by race or ethnic group, sex, age, and education level. Regions may differ in physical activity in part because they also differ in those demographic factors. Figure 3.13 shows that on average, physical activity levels are lower among women, older people, minority groups, and those who have less formal education. Note the big discrepancy between the estimates of overall participation at the recommended level.

The BRFSS and NHIS, which are the two main surveys of adult physical activity in the United States, differ widely in their estimates of sufficient physical activity defined as meeting the Healthy People 2010 recommendation for regular participation in either moderate or vigorous physical activity. The BRFSS estimate for 2007 was nearly 49% averaged across the nation, while the NHIS estimate was about 31%. The proportion of adults who said they got no leisure-time physical activity in 2007 was estimated as

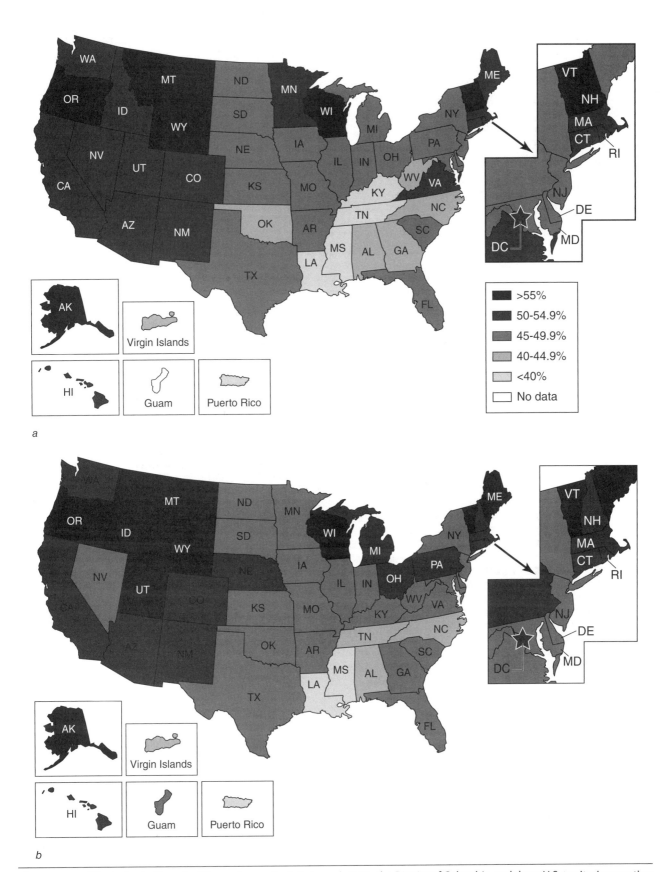

Figure 3.11 Who's physically active? Percentages of adults in each state, the District of Columbia, and three U.S. territories meeting the Healthy People 2010 recommendation for either regular vigorous physical activity (≥20 min per day on three or more days per week) or regular moderate activity (≥30 min per day on five or more days per week) in (a) 2005 and (b) 2007.

Based on BRFSS 2008.

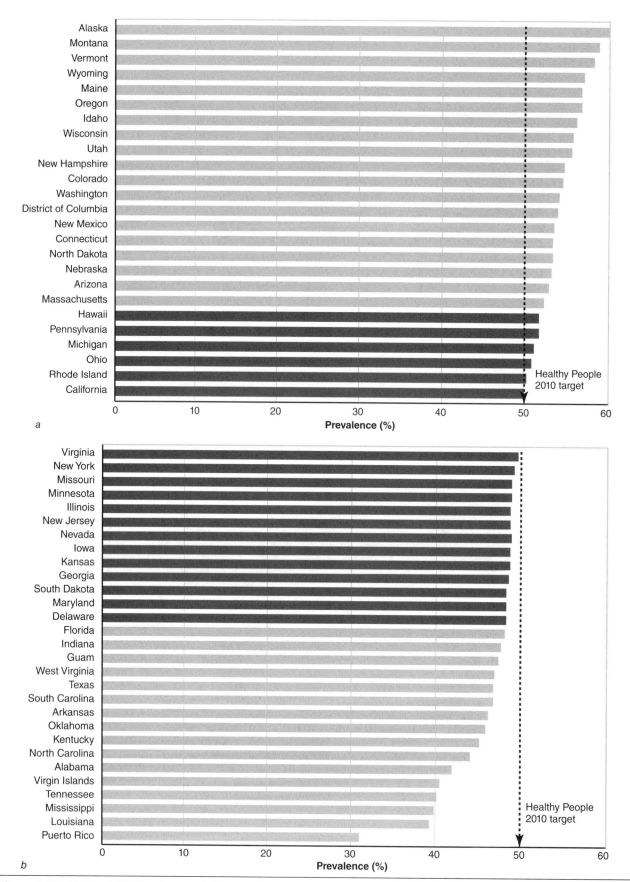

Figure 3.12 Regional BRFSS estimates of *(a)* states that were judged to meet the Healthy People 2010 goal of sufficient physical activity in 2007 and *(b)* states that were judged as not having met the goal. Dark bars indicate states that might have been falsely judged as meeting or not meeting the goal of 50%.

Data from Center for Disease Control 2008, *Prevalence of self-reported physically active adults U.S.,* 2007.

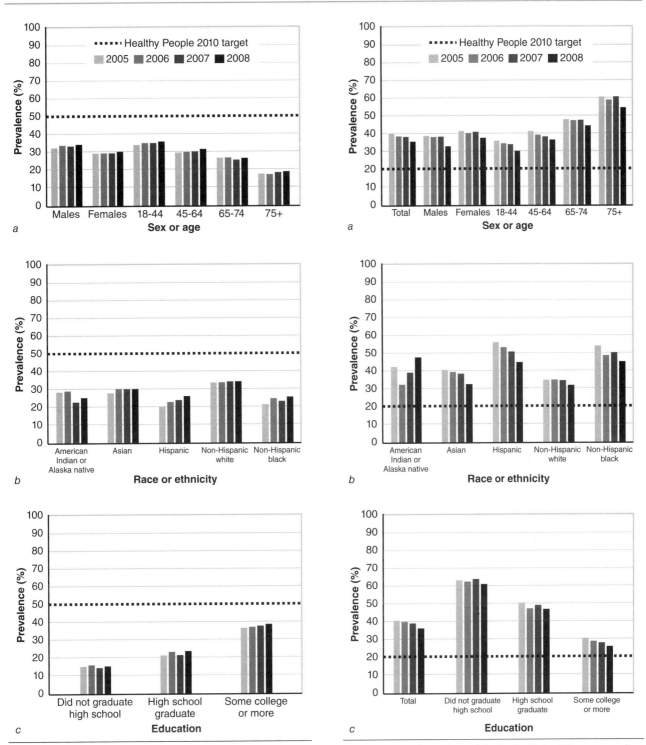

Figure 3.13 Regular physical activity in the United States according to (a) gender and age, (b) race/ethnicity, and (c) education level. The dashed line indicates the national goal of 50%.

Data from Centers for Disease Control and Prevention, Health, United States, 2008. Available: www.cdc.gov/nchs/hus/updatedtables.htm.

Figure 3.14 Physical inactivity in the United States according to (a) gender and age, (b) race/ethnicity, and (c) education level. The dashed line indicates the national goal of 20%.

Data from Centers for Disease Control and Prevention, Health, United States, 2008. Available: www.cdc.gov/nchs/hus/updatedtables.htm.

24% by BRFSS but as 39% by NHIS. Figure 3.14 shows that on average, physical inactivity levels are higher among women, older people, minority groups, and those who have less formal education. As for levels of sufficient physical activity, there is a big gap between the estimates of overall participation and the recommended level.

Figure 3.15 shows declining physical activity measured by daily pedometer steps across age groups in American Indians from 13 communities in Arizona, Oklahoma, and the Dakotas. Few adults approached the public health goal of 10,000 steps each day. In another sample of nearly 5000 adults living in Arizona and South Dakota, 48% said they got at least 150 min a week of moderate physical activity, mainly household chores (Duncan et al. 2009). Almost 20% said they engaged in no leisure-time physical activity; this percentage is similar to that for the U.S. population.

Approximately 27% of adults say they participate in strength activities (i.e., weightlifting or calisthenics) during their leisure time. Rates are higher in men in all age groups except those aged 65 to 74 years. Figure 3.16 shows that participation by both men and women drops by nearly two-thirds from the ages of 18 to 24 to age 75.

Because people tend to inflate how much time they are active and underestimate the time they spend in sedentary behaviors, even the NHIS figure is likely an overestimate of true physical activity. To get a more objective estimate of physical activity in the United States, the NHANES survey

recruited people to wear an accelerometer during the 2003-2004 sampling period. Figure 3.17 shows the prevalence rates of meeting public health recommendations for youths aged 6 to 15 years (≥60 min of MVPA each day) and adults ages 16+ (≥30 min of MVPA each day accumulated in sessions of ≥10 min each time) on five or more days during seven days of recording. The objectively measured rates are strikingly lower than those estimated from people's self-ratings of their physical activity. Likewise, figure 3.18 shows that Americans spend nearly half their waking hours in sedentary behaviors.

After entering adolescence, girls in the United States and several European countries show a bigger reduction in both school-based and leisure physical activity than do boys. Whether this is explainable by social factors is not yet

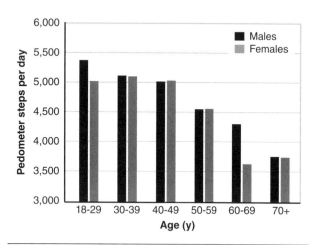

Figure 3.15   Daily pedometer steps in American Indians.

Data from Storti et al. 2009.

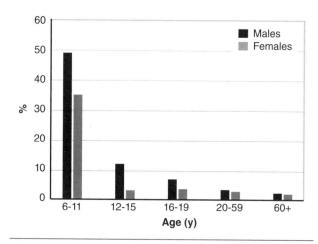

Figure 3.17   Percentages of various age groups meeting public health recommendations for sufficient physical activity, as measured by accelerometer.

Data from Troiano et al. 2008.

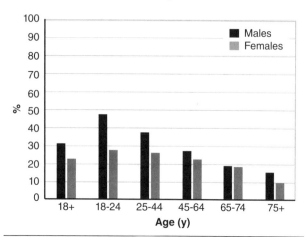

Figure 3.16   Percentage of adults aged ≥18 years who engaged in leisure-time strengthening activities, by age group and sex.

Data from Centers for Disease Control 2009.

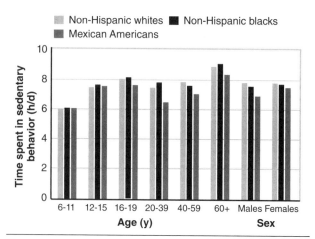

Figure 3.18   Time spent in sedentary behaviors in the United States during 2003-2004 sampling period, as measured by accelerometer.

Data from Matthews et al. 2008.

known, but there seems to be nothing biologically inherent about being female that would cause girls and women to be less active than males. Though girls become fatter than boys after puberty, cultural factors seem more likely than biology to explain most of the reduced activity.

▷ **SECULAR CHANGES** in culture can strongly influence the prevalence of physical activity. Examples are increased television viewing and computer use among youths and a decrease in daily physical education during the past decade.

Mixed positive and negative trends in physical activity among youths during the 1990s seem to support the hypothesis that long-term trends in the culture are strong influences on youth. The results from the YRBSS shown in figure 3.19 show the proportion of U.S. high school students who were sufficiently active and attended physical education classes daily in 2005 and 2007. The decline in both rates from the 9th through 12th grades is more steep in girls than boys. Both of these trends are plausibly explained by social factors.

Population-based studies using accelerometers also show that boys and girls are insufficiently active. A study of

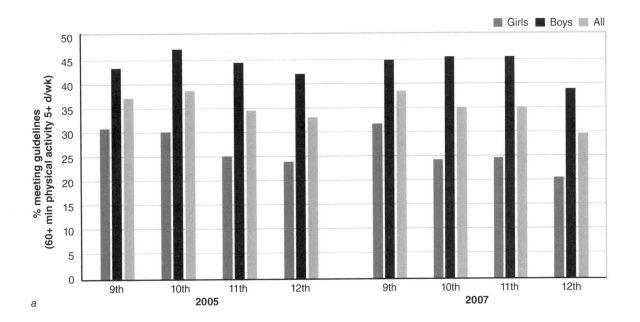

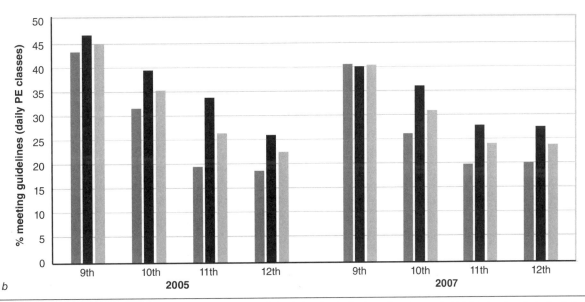

Figure 3.19 Prevalence of (a) sufficient physical activity and (b) daily physical education classes in U.S. high school students in 2005 and 2007.

Sources: CDC MMWR 55(SS-5), 2006; CDC MMWR 57(SS-4), 2008

6th-grade girls from six regions of the United States found that the girls averaged just 24 min each day of moderate-to-vigorous physical activity (Pate et al. 2006). A similarly large cohort study of English boys and girls showed that 12-year-old boys averaged 25 min a day and girls averaged just 16 min per day (Ness et al. 2007); only 5% of boys and 0.4% of girls in that cohort met the current public health recommendation of at least 1 h of moderate-to-vigorous physical activity each day (Riddoch et al. 2007).

Physical Activity, Fitness, and Aging

Though it seems reasonable that people will become less active as they age, perhaps as a result of lost mobility, it is probably incorrect to assume that age is an independent and unavoidable cause of reduced activity. Figure 3.20 illustrates this by comparing changes from 1962 to 1977 in the percentage of Harvard alumni who were judged to be active according to age cohort or birth cohort. Population studies that extend over many years often begin keeping records in different years on different waves of people. People are frequently placed into the same age cohort for analyses even though they were born in different years. A birth cohort contains only people born in the same year. Figure 3.20 shows the common observation that the percentage of each age group that is physically active steadily declines from the youngest age group (34-39 years) to the oldest age group (65-69 years). In contrast, however, the lines connecting birth cohorts as they aged show that in most instances, men born in the same year maintained their level of stair climbing and walking as they aged and in many instances increased the time they spent playing sports.

▶ **THOUGH SURVEYS** typically show that physical activity declines when groups of older people are compared with younger people, this can be an artifact of using **absolute intensity** rather than relative intensity, which adjusts for decreasing fitness with age. Harvard alumni who were tracked individually actually increased physical activity during the transition from middle age to old age.

Studies have overestimated the decline in physical activity at older ages because they have used the same absolute standards of the rate of energy expenditure for young and old people, despite the fact that a person's maximal rate of energy expenditure declines linearly with increasing age. Dr. Carl Caspersen, a physical activity epidemiologist with the CDC, elegantly showed the impact of inappropriately using such absolute standards for gauging trends in physical activity patterns among older people (Caspersen, Merritt, and Stephens 1994). In his analysis of data on U.S. men from the 1985 National Health Interview Study (NHIS), the trend of declining physical activity with age that appears when the common recommendation of 3 kcal per kilogram per day of

energy expenditure is used as the standard did not appear with use of another common recommendation based on frequency, duration, and rate of energy expenditure relative to capacity. The decline in the proportion of men participating in physical activity was less steep, and men older than 75 actually were more active, when the relative intensity standard was used to define the recommendation than when the absolute standard was used.

Likewise, the trend for declining participation by older men in physical activities requiring 6 METs or more was reversed among men aged 75 years or older when a relative standard of activities requiring 60% or more of maximum METs was used. The concept of METs was introduced in 1936 by exercise physiologist David Bruce Dill to express exercise intensity relative to metabolic rate and independently of body mass. Basal or resting metabolic rate represents 1 MET, which is the equivalent, on average, of 3.5 ml O_2 consumed per kilogram of body mass per minute or 1 kcal $\cdot$ kg^{-1} $\cdot$ h^{-1}. Exercise intensity is expressed as a multiple of a MET. For example, a woman with a maximal aerobic capacity of 35 ml $O_2 \cdot$ kg$^{-1} \cdot$ min^{-1} would, on average, raise her metabolism 10 times above its resting level while exercising at her peak capacity. Participation rates among older men in the aforementioned NHIS study were underestimated because they were based on standard activities that simply were too intense for the older men, who apparently were choosing activities that, though lower in absolute intensity, were appropriately intense relative to the men's declining fitness levels. Though the analysis was limited to men, the general idea should apply equally to older women. In fact, new studies have shown that standard MET values should be adjusted to account for differences in resting metabolic rate (i.e., lower or higher than 3.5 ml $O_2 \cdot$ kg$^{-1} \cdot$ min^{-1}) in males and females who vary in body mass, height, and age (Byrne et al. 2005; Kozey et al. 2010). Table 3.8 shows this adjustment for seven activities using the standard and MET values corrected for a middle-aged (35 yrs) normal weight male and female along with an older (55 yrs) overweight male and female. A summary value in MET-minutes (MET × minutes an activity is performed) is computed for each column using 30 min of participation per activity for comparison purposes.

Summary

This chapter introduces the commonly accepted definitions and measures of physical activity and physical fitness. The descriptive epidemiology of differences in physical activity by geographic region, race or ethnic group, sex, age, and education level is introduced. Surveillance of physical activity prevalence and trends among groups and regions is necessary to monitor progress toward public health objectives for increasing physical activity.

Because physical activity occurs in many forms, intensities, and amounts, it is possible that its relationship with the

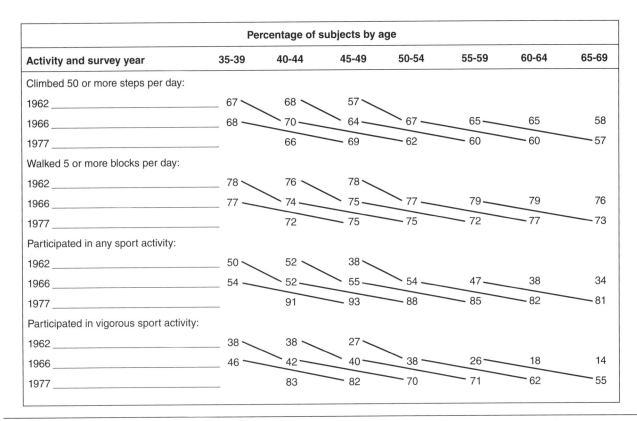

Activity and survey year	Percentage of subjects by age						
	35-39	40-44	45-49	50-54	55-59	60-64	65-69
Climbed 50 or more steps per day:							
1962	67	68	57				
1966	68	70	64	67	65	65	58
1977		66	69	62	60	60	57
Walked 5 or more blocks per day:							
1962	78	76	78				
1966	77	74	75	77	79	79	76
1977		72	75	75	72	77	73
Participated in any sport activity:							
1962	50	52	38				
1966	54	52	55	54	47	38	34
1977		91	93	88	85	82	81
Participated in vigorous sport activity:							
1962	38	38	27				
1966	46	42	40	38	26	18	14
1977		83	82	70	71	62	55

Figure 3.20 Birth- versus age-cohort effect on physical activity with aging. Changes over time in specific physical activities among Harvard alumni by cross-sectional age group and by cohort, 1962-1977.

Reprinted, by permission, from K.E. Powell and R.S. Paffenbarger, 1985, "Workshop on epidemiologic and public health aspects of physical activity and exercise: A summary," *Public Health Reports* 100(2): 118-126.

Table 3.8 Standard and Corrected MET Values for Selected Activities

Activity	2011 compendium METs	Female		Male	
		Normal weight, 35 yrs	Overweight, 55 yrs	Normal weight, 35 yrs	Overweight, 55 yrs
Rope jumping	12.3	13.5	16.5	12.9	15.4
Running, 6 mph	9.8	10.7	13.1	10.3	12.3
Bicycling, general	7.5	8.2	10.0	7.9	9.4
Pushing stroller	4.0	4.4	5.4	4.2	5.0
Calisthenics	3.5	3.8	4.7	3.7	4.4
Shopping	2.3	2.5	3.1	2.4	2.9
Watching TV	1.3	1.4	1.7	1.4	1.6
Total MET-minutes	1221	1335	1635	1294	1530

Total MET-minutes are based on 30 min of participation in each activity. Values are based on a normal weight woman 168 cm in height and weighing 60 kg, an overweight woman 168 cm in height and weighing 77 kg, a normal weight man 178 cm in height and weighing 70 kg, and an overweight man 178 cm in height and weighing 91 kg.

Reprinted, by permission, from B.E. Ainsworth et al., 2011, *The compendium of physical activities tracking guide* (Healthy Lifestyles Research Center, College of Nursing and Health Innovation, Arizona State University). Available: https://sites.google.com/site/compendiumofphysicalactivities/.

development of disease and with premature death differs according to those features. Determining whether this is so is fundamentally necessary to satisfy Mill's canon of dose response. It is also practically important for public policy about recommended types and amounts of physical activity and to determine which components of physical fitness are related to the risk of mortality or to the development of specific diseases. Determining whether physical fitness has specific effects on disease risk is also important for forming public policy and for satisfying Mill's canon of biological plausibility. That is, it is expected that many physiological adaptations to physical activity that favorably influence the pathophysiology of diseases would also be reflected in changes in some component of physical fitness. The following chapters address these issues, starting in chapter 4, "All-Cause Mortality."

· BIBLIOGRAPHY ·

Ainsworth, B.E., W.L. Haskell, M.C. Whitt, et al. 2000. Compendium of physical activities: An update of activity codes and MET intensities. *Medicine and Science in Sports and Exercise* 32: S498-S516.

Allen, F.R., E. Ambikairajah, N.H. Lovell, and B.B. Celler. 2006. Classification of a known sequence of motions and postures from accelerometry data using adapted Gaussian mixture models. Physiological Measurement 27 (10): 935-951.

American College of Sports Medicine. 2011. American College of Sports Medicine position stand. Quantity and quality of exercise for developing and maintaining cardiorespiratory, musculoskeletal, and neuromotor fitness in apparently healthy adults: Guidance for prescribing exercise. *Medicine and Science in Sports and Exercise* 43 (7): 1334-1359

Armstrong, T., A. Bauman, and J. Davies. 2000. *Physical activity patterns of Australian adults: Results of the 1999 National Physical Activity Survey.* Canberra, Australia: Australia Institute of Health and Welfare.

Armstrong, T., and F. Bull. 2006. Development of the World Health Organization Global Physical Activity Questionnaire (GPAQ). *Journal of Public Health* 14: 66-70.

Bassett, D.R., B.E. Ainsworth, S.R. Leggett, C.A. Mathien, J.A. Main, D.C. Hunter, and G.E. Duncan. 1996. Accuracy of five electronic pedometers for measuring distance walked. *Medicine and Science in Sports and Exercise* 28 (8): 1071-1077.

Bassett, D.R. Jr., B.E. Ainsworth, A.M. Swartz, S.J. Strath, W.L. O'Brien, and G.A. King. 2000. Validity of four motion sensors in measuring moderate intensity physical activity. *Medicine and Science in Sports and Exercise* 32 (Suppl. 9): S471-S480.

Bauman, A.E., F.C. Bull, T. Chey, et al. 2009. International physical activity prevalence estimates: Results from the International Prevalence Study in 20 countries. *International Journal of Behavioral Nutrition and Physical Activity* 6: 21. doi: 10.1186/1479-5868-6-21.

Beets, M.W., D. Bornstein, A. Beighle, B.J. Cardinal, and C.F. Morgan. 2010. A 13 country review of pedometer measured physical activity patterns of youth. *American Journal of Preventive Medicine* 38 (2): 208-216.

Blair, S.N., W.L. Haskell, P. Ho, R.A. Paffenbarger Jr., K.M. Vranizan, J.W. Farquhar, and P.D. Wood. 1985. Assessment of habitual physical activity by seven-day recall in a community survey and controlled experiments. *American Journal of Epidemiology* 122 (5): 794-804.

Bonnefoy, M., S. Normand, C. Pachiaudi, J.R. Lacour, M. Laville, and T. Kostka. 2001. Simultaneous validation of ten physical activity questionnaires in older men: A doubly labeled water study. *Journal of the American Geriatrics Society* 49: 28-35.

Booth, M.L. 2000. Assessment of physical activity: An international perspective. *Research Quarterly for Exercise and Sport* 71: 114-120.

Borraccino, A., P. Lemma, R.J. Iannottii, A. Zambon, P. Dalmasso, G. Lazzeri, M. Giacchi, and F. Cavallo. 2009. Socioeconomic effects on meeting physical activity guidelines: Comparisons among 32 countries. *Medicine and Science in Sports and Exercise* 41: 749-756.

Bouchard, C. 2001. Physical activity and health: Introduction to the dose–response symposium. *Medicine and Science in Sports and Exercise* 33 (Suppl. 6): S347-S350.

Bouchard, C., and T. Rankinen. 2001. Individual differences in response to regular physical activity. *Medicine and Science in Sports and Exercise* 33 (Suppl. 6): S446-S451.

Bouchard, C., and R.J. Shephard. 1994. Physical activity, fitness, and health: The model and key concepts. In *Physical activity, fitness, and health: International proceedings and consensus statement,* edited by C. Bouchard, R.J. Shephard, and T. Stephens, pp. 77-88. Champaign, IL: Human Kinetics.

Bouchard, C., R.J. Shephard, and T. Stephens, eds. 1994. *Physical activity, fitness, and health: International proceedings and consensus statement.* Champaign, IL: Human Kinetics.

Bradstock, M.K., J.S. Marks, M. Forman, E.M. Gentry, G.C. Hogelin, and F.L. Trowbridge. 1984. Behavioral risk factor surveillance, 1981-1983: CDC Surveillance Summaries. *Morbidity and Mortality Weekly Report* 33 (1): 1SS-4SS.

Bravata, D.M., C. Smith-Spangler, V. Sundaram, A.L. Gienger, N. Lin, R. Lewis, C.D. Stave, I. Olkin, and J.R. Sirard. 2007. Using pedometers to increase physical activity and improve health: A systematic review. *Journal of the American Medical Association* 298 (19): 2296-2304.

Brouha, L., and P.E. Smith Jr. 1958. Energy expenditure of motions [abstract]. *Federation Proceedings of the American Society for Experimental Biology* 17: 20.

Brownson, R.C., A.A. Eyler, A.C. King, Y.L. Shyu, D.R. Brown, and S.M. Homan. 1999. Reliability of information on physical activity and other chronic disease risk factors among US women aged 40 years or older. *American Journal of Epidemiology* 149 (4): 379-391.

Bull, F.C., T.S. Maslin, and T. Armstrong. 2009. Global physical activity questionnaire (GPAQ): Nine country reliability and validity study. *Journal of Physical Activity and Health* 6: 790-804.

Byrne, N.M., A.P. Hills, G.R. Hunter, R.L. Weinsier, Y. Schutz. 2005. Metabolic equivalent: one size does not fit all. *Journal of Applied Physiology* 99 (3): 1112-1119.

Carlson, S.A., D. Densmore, J.E. Fulton, M.M. Yore, and H.W. Kohl 3rd. 2009. Differences in physical activity prevalence and trends from 3 U.S. surveillance systems: NHIS, NHANES, and BRFSS. *Journal of Physical Activity and Health* 6 (Suppl. 1): S18-27.

Caspersen, C.J. 1989. Physical activity epidemiology: Concepts, methods, and applications to exercise science. *Exercise and Sport Sciences Reviews* 17: 423-475.

Caspersen, C.J., R.K. Merritt, and T. Stephens. 1994. International physical activity patterns: A methodological perspective. In *Advances in exercise adherence,* edited by R.K. Dishman. Champaign, IL: Human Kinetics.

Caspersen, C.J., K.E. Powell, and G.M. Christenson. 1985. Physical activity, exercise, and physical fitness: Definitions and distinctions for health-related research. *Public Health Reports* 100 (2): 126-130.

Centers for Disease Control and Prevention (CDC). 1996. State-specific prevalence of participation in physical activity—Behavioral Risk Factor Surveillance System, 1994. *Morbidity and Mortality Weekly Report* 45 (31): 673-675.

Centers for Disease Control and Prevention. 2007. Prevalence of regular physical activity among adults—U.S., 2001 and 2005. *Morbidity and Mortality Weekly Report* 56 (46): 1209-1212.

Centers for Disease Control and Prevention. 2008a. Health, United States, 2008. From www.cdc.gov/nchs/hus/updatedtables.htm.

Centers for Disease Control and Prevention. 2008b. Prevalence of self-reported physically active adults—U.S., 2007. *Morbidity and Mortality Weekly Report* 57 (48): 1297-1300.

Centers for Disease Control and Prevention. 2010. Youth Risk Behavior Surveillance—United States, 2009. Surveillance Summaries. *Morbidity and Mortality Weekly Report* 59 (SS-5): 117-126.

Corder, K., S. Brage, and U. Ekelund. 2007. Accelerometers and pedometers: Methodology and clinical application. *Current Opinion in Clinical Nutrition and Metabolic Care* 10 (5): 597-603.

Corder, K., U. Ekelund, R.M. Steele, N.J. Wareham, and S. Brage. 2008. Assessment of physical activity in youth. *Journal of Applied Physiology* 105 (3): 977-987.

Corder, K., E.M. van Sluijs, A. Wright, P. Whincup, N.J. Wareham, and U. Ekelund. 2009. Is it possible to assess free-living physical activity and energy expenditure in young people by self-report? *American Journal of Clinical Nutrition* 89 (3): 862-870.

Craig, C.L., A.L. Marshall, M. Sjöström, A.E. Bauman, M.L. Booth, B.E. Ainsworth, M. Pratt, U. Ekelund, A. Yngve, J.F. Sallis, P. Oja, and the IPAQ Consensus Group and the IPAQ Reliability and Validity Study Group. 2003. International Physical Activity Questionnaire (IPAQ): 12-country reliability and validity. *Medicine and Science in Sports and Exercise* 35: 1381-1395.

Dehn, M., and C. Mullins. 1977. Physiologic effects and importance of exercise in patients with coronary heart disease. *Cardiovascular Medicine* 2: 365.

De Lorme, T.L. 1945. Restoration of muscle power by heavy resistance exercise. *Journal of Bone and Joint Surgery* 27: 645-647.

Dipietro, L., C.J. Caspersen, A.M. Ostfeld, and E.R. Nadel. 1993. A survey for assessing physical activity among older adults. *Medicine and Science in Sports and Exercise* 25: 628-642.

Dishman, R.K., R.A. Washburn, and D.A. Schoeller. 2001. Measurement of physical activity. *Quest: American Academy of Kinesiology and Physical Education Papers* 53: 295-309.

Duncan, G.E., J. Goldberg, D. Buchwald, Y. Wen, and J.A. Henderson. 2009. Epidemiology of physical activity in American Indians in the Education and Research Towards Health cohort. *American Journal of Preventive Medicine* 37 (6): 488-494.

Esliger, D.W., and M.S. Tremblay. 2007. Physical activity and inactivity profiling: The next generation. *Canadian Journal of Public Health* 98 (Suppl. 2): S195-207.

European Commission. 1999. *A pan-EU survey on consumer attitudes to physical activity, body weight and health.* Luxembourg: Office for Official Publications of the European Communities.

Freedson, P.S., and K. Miller. 2000. Objective monitoring of physical activity using motion sensors and heart rate. *Research Quarterly for Exercise and Sport* 71: 21-29.

Gayle, R., H.J. Montoye, and J. Philpot. 1977. Accuracy of pedometers for measuring distance walked. *Research Quarterly* 48 (3): 632-636.

Giles, K., and A.L. Marshall. 2009. Repeatability and accuracy of CHAMPS as a measure of physical activity in a community sample of older Australian adults. *Journal of Physical Activity and Health* 6: 221-229.

Harada, N.D., V. Chiu, A.C. King, and A.L. Stewart. 2001. An evaluation of three self-report physical activity instruments for older adults. *Medicine and Science in Sports and Exercise* 33: 962-970.

Haskell, W. 1994. Dose–response issues from a biological perspective. In *Physical activity, fitness, and health: International proceedings and consensus statement,* edited by C. Bouchard, R.J. Shephard, and T. Stephens, pp. 1030-1039. Champaign, IL: Human Kinetics.

Haskell, W.L., I.M. Lee, R.R. Pate, K.E. Powell, S.N. Blair, B.A. Franklin, C.A. Macera, G.W. Heath, P.D. Thompson, and A. Bauman. 2007. Physical activity and public health: Updated recommendation for adults from the American College of Sports Medicine and the American Heart Association. *Circulation* 116: 1081-1093.

Health Canada. 1999. *Physical activity of Canadians. 2.1 Description of the survey and reports.* National Population Health Survey Highlights, No. 2. Ottawa, ON: Health Canada.

Helakorpi, S., A. Uutela, R. Prättälä, and P. Puska. 1999. *Health behaviour and health among Finnish adult population, spring 1999.* Helsinki: National Public Health Institute.

Hendelman, D., K. Miller, C. Baggett, E. Debold, and P. Freedson. 2000. Validity of accelerometry for the assessment of moderate intensity physical activity in the field. *Medicine and Science in Sports and Exercise* 32 (Suppl.): S442-S449.

Howe, C.A., J.W. Staudenmayer, and P.S. Freedson. 2009. Accelerometer prediction of energy expenditure: Vector magnitude versus vertical axis. *Medicine and Science in Sports and Exercise* 41 (12): 2199-2206.

Jackson, A.S., X. Sui, J.R. Hebert, T.S. Church, and S.N. Blair. 2009. Role of lifestyle and aging on the longitudinal change in cardiorespiratory fitness. *Archives of Internal Medicine* 169: 1781-1787.

Jacobs, D.R., B.E. Ainsworth, T.J. Hartman, and A.S. Leon. 1993. A simultaneous evaluation of 10 commonly used physical activity questionnaires. *Medicine and Science in Sports and Exercise* 25: 81-91.

Kearney, J.M., M.J. Kearney, S. McElhone, and M.J. Gibney. 1999. Methods used to conduct the pan–European Union survey on consumer attitudes to physical activity, body weight and health. *Public Health Nutrition* 2: 79-86.

Kesaniemi, Y.A., E. Danforth Jr., M.D. Jensen, P.G. Kopelman, P. Lefebvre, and B.A. Reeder. 2001. Dose–response issues concerning physical activity and health: An evidence-based symposium. *Medicine and Science in Sports and Exercise* 33 (Suppl. 6): S351-S358.

Kozey, S., K. Lyden, J. Staudenmayer, P. Freedson. 2010. Errors in MET estimates of physical activities using 3.5 ml $O_2 \cdot kg^{-1} \cdot min^{-1}$ as the baseline oxygen consumption. *Journal of Physical Activity and Health* 7 (4): 508-516

Kriska, A.M., and C.J. Caspersen. 1997. Introduction to a collection of physical activity questionnaires. *Medicine and Science in Sports and Exercise* 29 (Suppl. 6): S5-S9.

LaPorte, R.E., H.J. Montoye, and C.J. Caspersen. 1985. Assessment of physical activity in epidemiologic research: Problems and prospects. *Public Health Reports* 100: 131-146.

Lee, I.M., C.C. Hsieh, and R.S. Paffenbarger Jr. 1995. Exercise intensity and longevity in men: The Harvard Alumni Health Study. *Journal of the American Medical Association* 273 (15): 1179-1184.

Lee, I.M., and R.S. Paffenbarger Jr. 2000. Associations of light, moderate, and vigorous intensity physical activity with longevity: The Harvard Alumni Health Study. *American Journal of Epidemiology* 151 (3): 293-299.

Lee, I.M., H.D. Sesso, and R.S. Paffenbarger Jr. 2000. Physical activity and coronary heart disease risk in men: Does the duration of exercise episodes predict risk? *Circulation* 102: 981-986.

Leon, A.S., and J. Connett. 1991. Physical activity and 10.5 year mortality in the Multiple Risk Factor Intervention Trial. *International Journal of Epidemiology* 20: 690-697.

Leon, A.S., J. Connett, D.R. Jacobs Jr., and R. Rauramaa. 1987. Leisure-time physical activity levels and risk of coronary heart disease and death: The Multiple Risk Factor Intervention Trial. *Journal of the American Medical Association* 258 (17): 2388-2395.

Levine, J.A. 2007. Nonexercise activity thermogenesis—liberating the life-force. *Journal of Internal Medicine* 262 (3): 273-287.

Lifson, N., G.B. Gordon, and R. McClintock. 1955. Measurement of total carbon dioxide production by means of D2 18O. *Journal of Applied Physiology* 7: 704-710.

Lifson, N., W.S. Little, D.G. Levitt, and R.M. Henderson. 1975. D2 18O method for CO2 output in small animals and economic feasibility in man. *Journal of Applied Physiology* 39: 657-663.

Lubans, D.R., P.J. Morgan, and C. Tudor-Locke. 2009. A systematic review of studies using pedometers to promote physical activity among youth. *Preventive Medicine* 48 (4): 307-315.

Luinge, H.J., and P.H. Veltink. 2004. Inclination measurement of human movement using a 3-D accelerometer with autocalibration. *IEEE Transactions on Neural Systems and Rehabilitation Engineering* 12 (1): 112-121.

Manson, J.E., D.M. Nathan, A.S. Sroleswski, M.J. Stampfer, W.C. Willett, and C.H. Hennekens. 1992. A prospective study of exercise and incidence of diabetes in U.S. male physicians. *Journal of the American Medical Association* 268: 63-67.

Mason, J.O., and K.E. Powell. 1985. Physical activity, behavioral epidemiology, and public health. *Public Health Reports* 100: 113-115.

Mathie, M.J., A.C. Coster, N.H. Lovell, and B.G. Celler. 2004. Accelerometry: Providing an integrated, practical method for long-term, ambulatory monitoring of human movement. *Physiological Measurement* 25 (2): R1-20.

McClain, J.J., and C. Tudor-Locke. 2009. Objective monitoring of physical activity in children: Considerations for instrument selection. *Journal of Science and Medicine in Sport* 12 (5): 526-533.

McClintock, R., and N. Lifson. 1957. Applicability of the D2 18O method to the measurement of the total carbon dioxide output of obese mice. *Journal of Biological Chemistry* 226: 153-156.

Melanson, E.L. Jr., and P.S. Freedson. 1995. Validity of the Computer Science and Applications, Inc. (CSA) activity monitor. *Medicine and Science in Sports and Exercise* 27 (6): 934-940.

Melanson, E.L., J.R. Knoll, M.L. Bell, W.T. Donahoo, J.O. Hill, L.J. Nysse, L. Lanningham-Foster, J.C. Peters, and J.A. Levine. 2004. Commercially available pedometers: Considerations for accurate step counting. *Preventive Medicine* 39 (2): 361-368.

Montoye, H.J. 1975. *Physical activity and health: An epidemiologic study of an entire community.* Englewood Cliffs, NJ: Prentice Hall.

Montoye, H.J., H.C.G. Kemper, W.H.M. Saris, and R.A. Washburn. 1996. *Measuring physical activity and energy expenditure.* Champaign, IL: Human Kinetics.

Montoye, H.J., S.B. Servais, and J.G. Webster. 1986. Estimation of energy expenditure from a force platform and an accelerometer. In *Sport science,* edited by J. Watkins, T. Reilly, and L. Burwitz, pp. 375-380. London: Spon.

Nelson, D.E., D. Holtzman, J. Bolen, C.A. Stanwyck, and K.A. Mack. 2001. Reliability and validity of measures from the Behavioral Risk Factor Surveillance System (BRFSS). *Social and Preventive Medicine* 46 (Suppl. 1): S03-S42.

Ness, A.R., S.D. Leary, C. Maddocks, et al. 2007. Objectively measured physical activity and fat mass in a large cohort of children. *PLoS Medicine* 4: e97.

Paffenbarger, R.S. Jr., S.N. Blair, I.M. Lee, and R.T. Hyde. 1993a. Measurement of physical activity to assess health effects in free-living populations. *Medicine and Science in Sports and Exercise* 25: 60-70.

Paffenbarger, R.S. Jr., R.T. Hyde, A.W. Wing, I.M. Lee, D.L. Jung, and J.B. Kampert. 1993b. The association of changes in physical activity level and other lifestyle characteristics with mortality among men. *New England Journal of Medicine* 328 (February 23): 538-545.

Paffenbarger, R.S. Jr., A.L. Wing, and R.T. Hyde. 1978. Physical activity as an index of heart attack risk in college alumni. *American Journal of Epidemiology* 108: 165-175.

Pate, R.R., R. Ross, M. Dowda, S.G. Trost, and J. Sirard. 2003. Validation of a three-day physical activity recall instrument in female youth. *Pediatric Exercise Science* 15: 257-265.

Pate, R.R., J. Stevens, C. Pratt, et al. 2006. Objectively measured physical activity in sixth-grade girls. *Archives of Pediatric and Adolescent Medicine* 160: 1262-1268.

Pereira, M.A., S.J. Fitzgerald, E.W. Gregg, M.L. Joswiak, W.J. Ryan, R.R. Suminski, A.C. Utter, and J.M. Zmuda. 1997. A collection of physical questionnaires for health-related research. *Medicine and Science in Sports and Exercise* 29 (6): S3-S205.

Perusse, L., A. Tremblay, C. LeBlanc, and C. Bouchard. 1989. Genetic and familial environmental influences on level of habitual physical activity. *American Journal of Epidemiology* 129: 1012-1022.

Physical Activity Guidelines Advisory Committee. 2008. *Physical Activity Guidelines Advisory Committee report.* Washington, DC: U.S. Department of Health and Human Services.

Pollock, M.L., G.A. Gaesser, J.D. Butcher, J.P. Despres, R.K. Dishman, B.A. Franklin, and C.E. Garber. 1998. Recommended quantity and quality of exercise for developing and maintaining cardiorespiratory and muscular fitness, and flexibility in healthy adults. *Medicine and Science in Sports and Exercise* 30: 975-991.

Powell, K.E. 1988. Habitual exercise and public health: An epidemiological view. In *Exercise adherence: Its impact on public health,* edited by R.K. Dishman, pp. 15-40. Champaign, IL: Human Kinetics.

Powell, K.E., and R.S. Paffenbarger. 1985. Workshop on epidemiologic and public health aspects of physical activity and exercise: A summary. *Public Health Reports* 100 (2): 118-126.

Prentice, A.M., ed. 1990. *The doubly-labeled water method for measuring energy expenditure: A consensus report by the IDECG working group. Technical recommendations for use in humans.* International Atomic Energy Agency NAHRES-4. Vienna: International Dietary Energy Consultancy Group.

Prior, G. 1999. Physical activity. In *Health survey for England: Cardiovascular disease '98,* edited by B. Erens and P. Primatesta, pp. 181-219. London: Stationery Office.

Riddoch, C.J., C. Mattocks, K. Deere, J. Saunders, J. Kirby, K. Tilling, S.D. Leary, S.N. Blair, and A.R. Ness. 2007. Objective measurement of levels and patterns of physical activity. *Archives of Disease in Childhood* 92: 963-969.

Roberts, C., J. Tynjala, and T.J. Komkov. 2004. Physical activity. In *Young people's health in context: Health Behaviour in School-aged Children (HBSC) study: International report from the 2001/2002 survey,* edited by C. Currie, C. Roberts, A. Morgan, et al. *Health Policy for Children and Adolescents,* No. 4, pp. 90-97. Copenhagen: World Health Organization Regional Office for Europe.

Rosenbaum, J.E. 2009. Truth or consequences: The intertemporal consistency of adolescent self-report on the Youth Risk Behavior Survey. *American Journal of Epidemiology* 169 (11): 1388-1397.

Russell, D.G., and N.C. Wilson. 1991. *Life in New Zealand commission report.* Vol. 1, *Executive overview.* Dunedin, New Zealand: University of Otago.

Sallis, J.F., W.L. Haskell, P.D. Wood, S.P. Fortmann, T. Rogers, S.N. Blair, and R.S. Paffenbarger Jr. 1985. Physical activity assessment methodology in the five-city project. *American Journal of Epidemiology* 212 (1): 91-106.

Sallis, J.F., and B.E. Saelens. 2000. Assessment of physical activity by self-report: Status, limitations, and future directions. *Research Quarterly for Exercise and Sport* 71: 1-14.

Schmitz, K.H., M. Treuth, P. Hannan, R. McMurray, K.B. Ring, D. Catellier, and R. Pate. 2005. Predicting energy expenditure from accelerometry counts in adolescent girls. *Medicine and Science in Sports and Exercise* 37 (1): 155-161.

Schoeller, D.A. 1999. Recent advances from application of doubly labeled water to measurement of human energy expenditure. *Journal of Nutrition* 129 (10): 1765-1768.

Schoeller, D.A., and E. van Santen. 1982. Measurement of energy expenditure in humans by doubly-labeled water method. *Journal of Applied Physiology* 53: 955-959.

Schoenborn, C.A., and M.A. Barnes. 2002. Leisure-time physical activity among adults: United States, 1997-98. *Advance Data* 325 (April 7): 1-24.

Schuit, A.J., E.G. Schouten, K.R. Westerterp, and W.H. Saris. 1997. Validity of the Physical Activity Scale for the Elderly (PASE): According to energy expenditure assessed by the doubly labeled water method. *Journal of Clinical Epidemiology* 50: 541-546.

Servais, S.B., J.G. Webster, and H.J. Montoye. 1984. Estimating human energy expenditure using an accelerometer device. *Journal of Clinical Engineering* 9: 159-171.

Sesso, H.D., R.S. Paffenbarger Jr., and I.M. Lee. 2000. Physical activity and coronary heart disease in men: The Harvard Alumni Health Study. *Circulation* 102: 975-980.

Siconolfi, S.F., T.M. Lasater, R.C.K. Snow, and R.A. Carleton. 1985. Self-reported physical activity compared with maximal oxygen uptake. *American Journal of Epidemiology* 122: 101-105.

Sirard, J.R., and R.R. Pate. 2001. Physical activity assessment in children and adolescents. *Sports Medicine* 31: 439-454.

Sjöström, M., P. Oja, M. Hagströmer, B.J. Smith, and A. Bauman. 2006. Health-enhancing physical activity across European Union countries: The Eurobarometer study. *Journal of Public Health* 14: 291-300.

Stamatakis, E., U. Ekelund, and N.J. Wareham. 2007. Temporal trends in physical activity in England: The Health Survey for England 1991 to 2004. *Preventive Medicine* 45 (6): 416-423.

Staudenmayer, J., D. Pober, S. Crouter, D. Bassett, and P. Freedson. 2009. An artificial neural network to estimate physical activity energy expenditure and identify physical activity type from an accelerometer. Journal of Applied Physiology 107 (4): 1300-1307.

Stewart, A.L., K.M. Mill, A.C. King, W.L. Haskell, D. Gillis, and P.L. Ritter. 2001. CHAMPS physical activity questionnaire for older adults: Outcomes for interventions. *Medicine and Science in Sports and Exercise* 33 (7): 1126-1141.

Storti, K.L., V.C. Arena, M.M. Barmada, C.H. Bunker, R.L. Hanson, S.L. Laston, J.L. Yeh, J.M. Zmuda, B.V. Howard, and A.M. Kriska. 2009. Physical activity levels in American-Indian adults: The Strong Heart Family Study. American Journal of Preventive Medicine 37 (6): 481-487.

Strath, S.J., A.M. Swartz, D.R. Bassett Jr., W.L. O'Brien, G.A. King, and B.E. Ainsworth. 2000. Evaluation of heart rate as a method for assessing moderate intensity physical activity. *Medicine and Science in Sports and Exercise* 32 (Suppl. 9): S465-S470.

Thompson, D., A.M. Batterham, D. Markovitch, N.C. Dixon, A.J. Lund, and J.P. Walhin. 2009. Confusion and conflict in assessing the physical activity status of middle-aged men. *PLoS One* 4 (2): e4337.

Treuth, M.S., K. Schmitz, D.J. Catellier, R.G. McMurray, D.M. Murray, M.J. Almeida, S. Going, J.E. Norman, and R. Pate. 2004. Defining accelerometer thresholds for activity intensities in adolescent girls. *Medicine and Science in Sports and Exercise* 36 (7): 1259-1266.

Troped, P.J., M.S. Oliveira, C.E. Matthews, E.K. Cromley, S.J. Melly, and B.A. Craig. 2008. Prediction of activity mode with global positioning system and accelerometer data. *Medicine and Science in Sports and Exercise* 40: 972-978.

Tucker, J.M., G.J. Welk, and N.K. Beyler. 2011. Physical activity in U.S.: Adults compliance with the Physical Activity Guidelines for Americans. *American Journal of Preventive Medicine* 40 (4): 454-461.

Tudor-Locke, C., and D.R. Bassett Jr. 2004. How many steps/day are enough? Preliminary pedometer indices for public health. *Sports Medicine* 34 (1): 1-8.

Tudor-Locke, C., T.L. Hart, and T.L. Washington. 2009. Expected values for pedometer-determined physical activity in older populations. *International Journal of Behavioral Nutrition and Physical Activity* 6: 59.

Tudor-Locke, C., J.J. McClain, T.L. Hart, S.B. Sisson, and T.L. Washington. 2009. Expected values for pedometer-determined physical activity in youth. *Research Quarterly for Exercise and Sport* 80 (2): 164-174.

U.S. Department of Health and Human Services. 1980. *Promoting health/preventing disease: Objectives for the nation.* Washington, DC: U.S. Government Printing Office.

U.S. Department of Health and Human Services. 1996. *Physical activity and health: A report of the Surgeon General.* Atlanta: Centers for Disease Control and Prevention, National Center for Chronic Disease Prevention and Health Promotion.

U.S. Department of Health and Human Services. 2000. *Healthy people 2010: Understanding and improving health.* 2nd edition. Washington, DC: U.S. Government Printing Office.

U.S. Department of Health and Human Services. 2008. *2008 Physical activity guidelines for Americans.* ODPHP Publication No. U0036, pp. 1-61. Washington, DC: U.S. Government Printing Office.

U.S. Department of Health and Human Services. 2009. Summary Health Statistics for U.S. Adults: National Health Interview Survey, 2008. *Vital and Health Statistics.* Series 10, number 242. DHHS Publication No (PHS) 2010-1570 (pp. 42-43). From www.cdc.gov/nchs/data/series/sr_10/sr10_242.pdf.

U.S. Department of Health and Human Services. 2010. *Healthy people 2020: Understanding and improving health.* 2nd edition. Washington, DC: U.S. Government Printing Office.

Washburn, R., M.K. Chin, and H.J. Montoye. 1980. Accuracy of pedometers in walking and running. *Research Quarterly for Exercise and Sport* 51 (4): 695-702.

Washburn, R.A., S.R.W. Goldfield, K. Smith, and J.B. McKinlay. 1990. The validity of exercise induced sweating as a measure of physical activity. *American Journal of Epidemiology* 132: 107-113.

Washburn, R.A., and H.J. Montoye. 1986. The assessment of physical activity by questionnaire. *American Journal of Epidemiology* 123 (4): 563-576.

Washburn, R.A., K.W. Smith, A.M. Jette, and C.A. Janney. 1993. The Physical Activity Scale for the Elderly (PASE): Development and evaluation. *Journal of Clinical Epidemiology* 46: 153-162.

Welk, G.J., J.A. Differding, R.W. Thompson, S.N. Blair, J. Dziura, and T. Hart. 2000. The utility of the Digi-Walker step counter to assess daily physical activity patterns. *Medicine and Science in Sports and Exercise* 32 (Suppl.): S481-S488.

Westerterp, K.R. 1998. Alterations in energy balance with exercise. *American Journal of Clinical Nutrition* 68 (4): 970S-974S.

Westerterp, K.R. 1999. Physical activity assessment with accelerometers. *International Journal of Obesity and Related Metabolic Disorders* 23 (Suppl. 3): S45-S49.

Westerterp, K.R., F. Brouns, W.H.M. Saris, and F. Ten Hoor. 1988. Comparison of doubly labelled water with respirometry at low- and high-activity levels. *Journal of Applied Physiology* 65: 53-56.

Westerterp, K.R., J.O. de Boer, W.H.M. Saris, P.F.M. Schoffelen, and F. Ten Hoor. 1984. Measurement of energy expenditure using doubly-labeled water. *International Journal of Sports Medicine* 5 (Suppl.): 74-75.

Williams, P.T. 1996. High-density lipoprotein cholesterol and other risk factors for coronary heart disease in female runners. *New England Journal of Medicine* 334 (20): 1298-1303.

Williams, P.T. 1997. Relationship of distance run per week to coronary heart disease risk factors in 8283 male runners: The National Runners' Health Study. *Archives of Internal Medicine* 157: 191-198.

Williams, P.T. 1998a. Coronary heart disease risk factors of vigorously active sexagenarians and septuagenarians. *Journal of the American Geriatrics Society* 46 (2): 134-142.

Williams, P.T. 1998b. Relationships of heart disease risk factors to exercise quantity and intensity. *Archives of Internal Medicine* 158 (3): 237-245.

Yore, M.M., S.A. Ham, B.E. Ainsworth, J. Kruger, J.P. Reis, H.W. Kohl 3rd, and C.A. Macera. 2007. Reliability and validity of the instrument used in BRFSS to assess physical activity. *Medicine and Science in Sports and Exercise* 39 (8): 1267-1274.

PART TWO

Physical Activity and Disease Mortality

Today, the average life expectancy of a U.S. citizen, about 75 years for men and 80 years for women, ranks near the lowest among industrialized nations. Because many scientific studies show that people's behavior influences their health and risk of premature mortality, understanding the role of physical activity in reducing mortality risk has great public health importance in the United States, as it does in other developed and developing nations. Physical inactivity is a burden to the public health in the United States, accounting for an estimated 191,000 deaths each year from all causes. Two leading causes of death are (a) coronary heart disease and (b) stroke and other cerebrovascular diseases; these account for about 22% of all deaths worldwide and 26% of deaths in high-income countries. The chapters in this section focus on the evidence that physical activity protects against premature death from all causes, as well as the evidence that it protects against the development of coronary heart disease and stroke. (The term "cardiovascular disease" is used to refer to a category of diseases involving the heart or blood vessels; in the studies discussed in this section, cardiovascular disease comprises primarily coronary heart disease and stroke.)

All-Cause Mortality

CHAPTER 4

*It is not the rich nor the great, not those who depend on medicine,
who became old, but such as use much exercise.*

• James Easton, 1799 •

CHAPTER OBJECTIVES

▸ Introduce information on life expectancy and major causes of mortality

▸ Review epidemiologic evidence on the association of occupational and leisure-time physical activity and reduced all-cause mortality

▸ Review epidemiologic evidence on the association of physical fitness and reduced all-cause mortality

▸ Discuss and evaluate the strength of the evidence to critically examine whether the associations between physical activity and reduced all-cause mortality are real and likely to be causal in nature

The conclusion by the early English epidemiologist James Easton was drawn in his 1799 book, *Human Longevity*, in which he chronicled the lives of 1712 people who lived to 100 years of age or older between the years 66 AD and 1799 (Easton 1799). This chapter examines whether Easton's view was accurate based on modern epidemiologic evidence. Subsequent chapters of the book present evidence for the associations of physical inactivity with increased risks of developing specific diseases that are major contributors to all-cause mortality, such as coronary heart disease, stroke, type 2 diabetes, and cancer, as well as the associations of physical inactivity with increased risks of chronic medical conditions such as hypertension, hyperlipidemia, obesity, osteoporosis, and depression.

In this chapter, we review the evidence to support the hypothesis that physical inactivity (or low physical fitness) increases the risk of all-cause mortality (i.e., increases the risk of premature mortality). It is not our goal to provide an exhaustive review of this topic since the body of literature is large, but rather to present a sample of classic and contemporary studies, as well as to summarize current issues including dose response and optimal amount of physical activity to reduce the risk of premature mortality. For comprehensive reviews on the topic of physical activity or fitness and all-cause mortality, see Lee and Skerrett (2001), Kodama and colleagues (2009), Lollgen and colleagues (2009), and Woodcock and colleagues (2011).

Life Expectancy at Birth

Today, the average life expectancy of a person living in the United States is among the lowest in high-income countries. Overall, Japan has the highest life expectancy at birth (82.6 years), while the United States ranks only 38th (78.2 years) (United Nations 2007). As indicated in table 4.1, the highest average life expectancy at birth belongs to men in Iceland (80.2 years) and women in Japan (86.1 years), while in the United States, life expectancy is 75.6 years for men and 80.8 years for women.

Death rates are lower among women than men at all ages in the United States, starting at ages 35 years, as shown by male:female ratios of <100 men for every 100 women in the population of ages 35 and older (figure 4.1). Possible, though unproven, explanations include sex hormones: Testosterone has been linked with hazardous behavior and undesirable cholesterol levels, while estrogen is an antioxidant (which might protect against cell damage) and appears to regulate enzymes that favorably affect cholesterol metabolism. Evolutionary biologists argue that long life in women is linked with a genetic advantage for childbirth and care of the young (Perls and Fretts 1998). However, many other social and environmental influences might interact to explain the longer life expectancy of women. Paradoxically, females are less physically active than males. Nonetheless, living longer does not necessarily ensure more years of good health. Where data are available,

Table 4.1   Life Expectancy by Country, 2005-2010

Rank	Country	Life expectancy at birth (years)
Men		
1	Iceland	80.2
2	Hong Kong	79.4
3	Japan	79
3	Switzerland	79
5	Australia	78.9
6	Sweden	78.7
7	Israel	78.5
7	Macau	78.5
9	Canada	78.3
10	New Zealand	78.2
11	Singapore	78
12	Norway	77.8
13	Spain	77.7
14	Italy	77.5
14	Netherlands	77.5
16	Malta	77.3
17	United Kingdom	77.2
17	United Arab Emirates	77.2
19	France	77.1
19	Greece	77.1
	United States	75.6
Women		
1	Japan	86.1
2	Hong Kong	85.1
3	Switzerland	84.2
3	Spain	84.2
5	France	84.1
6	Australia	83.6
7	Italy	83.5
8	Iceland	83.3
8	U.S. Virgin Islands	83.3
10	Sweden	83
11	Canada	82.9
12	Israel	82.8
12	Macau	82.8
14	Puerto Rico	82.7
15	Austria	82.6
16	Norway	82.5
17	Finland	82.4
18	Martinique	82.3
18	Belgium	82.3
20	New Zealand	82.2
20	Guadeloupe (France)	82.2
20	South Korea	82.2
	United States	80.8

Data from United Nations, Department of Economic and Social Affairs, Population Division, 2007.

· WEB RESOURCES ·

www.health.gov/paguidelines/. This site provides access to the first-ever Physical Activity Guidelines for Americans issued by the federal government in 2008. The site also provides access to the 2008 Physical Activity Guidelines Advisory Committee report, which is a comprehensive documentation of the scientific background and rationale for the 2008 physical activity guidelines.

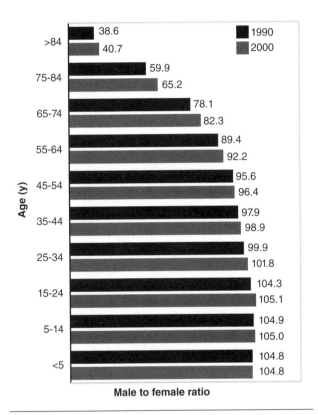

Figure 4.1   Male:female ratio (number of men per 100 women) by age group, United States, 1990 and 2000.

Reprinted from U.S. Census Bureau 2000.

Table 4.2   Leading Causes of Death Overall and in Selected Age Groups: United States, 2006

Age group	Cause	% of all deaths
All ages	Heart disease	26
	Cancer	23.1
	Cerebrovascular disease	5.7
5 to 14 years	Accidents	36.7
	Cancer	14.8
	Birth defects	5.6
25 to 44 years	Accidents	25.8
	Cancer	13.9
	Heart disease	12.4
65 years and older	Heart disease	29
	Cancer	22
	Cerebrovascular disease	6.7

Adapted from Heron 2010.

we will discuss how physical activity and fitness affect disease risk and health outcomes similarly and differently in women and men.

Major Causes of Mortality

In 2006, 2.4 million men and women in the United States died (Heron 2010). Table 4.2 shows that the three leading causes of death overall were heart disease, cancer, and cerebrovascular disease, accounting for more than half of all the deaths occurring. Heart disease and cancer also were the two leading causes of death in men and in women looked at separately. Among men, the third leading cause of death was accidents; in women, it was cerebrovascular disease.

In later chapters, we examine the associations of physical activity and physical fitness with each of the leading

causes of death separately: coronary heart disease, cancer, and cerebrovascular disease. You will see there is strong evidence showing that physical activity or fitness is inversely associated with the risk of developing each of these diseases. Thus, it is not surprising that physical activity or fitness also is inversely related to lower all-cause mortality rates (i.e., lower risk of premature mortality). In this chapter, we present the evidence showing an inverse association of physical activity or fitness with all-cause mortality rates.

Physical Activity and All-Cause Mortality

In a review by the 2008 Physical Activity Guidelines Advisory Committee (an expert panel appointed by the federal government) of the cumulative evidence from 73 studies published after 1996, the committee reported that 67 studies found a significant inverse relation between physical activity and all-cause mortality rates (Physical Activity Guidelines Advisory Committee 2008). The median relative risk (RR), comparing most active with least-active subjects, was 0.69 across all studies, indicating a 31% risk reduction with physical activity. This was similar for men (median RR = 0.71) and women (median RR = 0.67), and for studies in which both sexes were analyzed together (median RR = 0.68). Inverse associations were noted for persons aged <65 years and for those 65 years and older. While limited data were available for minority race–ethnic groups, the data suggested inverse associations for groups other than Caucasian populations. The committee also found strong evidence of an inverse dose–response relation, which will be discussed in more detail later in this chapter.

A subsequent meta-analysis of 38 studies published in 2009 reported essentially similar findings, observing that highly active men had a 22% (RR: 0.78; 95% confidence interval, CI: 0.72-0.84) lower risk of all-cause mortality compared with low-active men, while highly active women had a 31% lower risk (RR: 0.69; 95% CI: 0.53-0.90) (Lollgen, Bockenhoff, and Knapp 2009). Meanwhile, moderately active men and women had 19% and 24% lower risks, respectively, indicative of an inverse dose–response relation.

Occupational Physical Activity and All-Cause Mortality

The early studies of physical activity and risk of developing coronary heart disease conducted among London transport workers, described later in this textbook, stimulated other investigators to examine death rates among physically active and sedentary workers in various occupations. Here we consider two such studies. (As a note, many of the early studies of occupational physical activity examined heart disease mortality rates specifically, the main contributor to all-cause mortality rates in high-income countries. These studies are described in chapter 5.)

U.S. Railroad Workers

In an early study of occupational physical activity, 191,609 men who had worked in the U.S. railroad industry for at least 10 years by 1951, and who were employed in 1954, were classified by level of occupational activity as sedentary (clerks) or active (switchmen or section men, the most active) (Taylor et al. 1962). Men aged 40 to 64 years were then followed for all-cause mortality in 1955 and 1956. The age-adjusted death rates (per 1000) were 11.7 for clerks, 10.3 for switchmen, and 7.6 for section men. Although the mortality rate was significantly lower among the most active men, the results should be interpreted cautiously because data on potential confounding factors, such as smoking, body mass index (BMI), blood pressure, and cholesterol, were not available and thus the analysis did not adjust for them.

Men and Women in Eastern Finland

In a study published two decades later, Salonen, Puska, and Tuomilehto (1982) followed about 4000 men aged 30 to 59 years and 3700 women aged 35 to 59 years from two counties in eastern Finland for seven years. Occupational physi-

cal activity was assessed in 1972 using a single item on a questionnaire with four levels of responses. This information was then dichotomized into low or high physical activity at work. The relative risk of all-cause mortality associated with low, compared with high, occupational physical activity adjusted for age, BMI, cigarette smoking, diastolic blood pressure, and serum cholesterol was 1.9 (95% CI: 1.5-2.5) in men and 2.2 (95% CI: 1.5-3.3) in women. (Investigators also examined leisure-time physical activity, using a single item on a questionnaire, and observed findings similar to those for occupational activity.)

Leisure-Time Physical Activity and All-Cause Mortality

While early studies of physical activity and all-cause mortality tended to focus on occupational physical activity, later studies—in particular, those conducted in the 1980s and later—increasingly focused on leisure-time physical activity because physical activity in the workplace had declined in Western developed nations during the late 1950s to early 1960s as industry moved from manual to mechanized labor. In this section we consider several classic and contemporary prospective cohort studies of leisure-time physical activity and all-cause mortality rates. (This study design was chosen because the majority of studies on this topic have been prospective cohort studies; additionally, this study design is less susceptible to bias than case–control studies.)

Harvard Alumni Health Study

The Harvard Alumni Health Study, one of the most influential investigations of physical activity and chronic disease risk, is an ongoing cohort study of the predictors of chronic disease in men who entered Harvard University as undergraduates between 1916 and 1950 (no women were admitted during these years). The original prospective cohort was composed of 21,582 alumni who returned a mail questionnaire on medical history and health habits in 1962 or 1966.

In a classic study published in 1986, Paffenbarger and colleagues (1986) followed approximately 17,000 men, who were aged 35 to 74 years in 1962 or 1966 and who were free of heart disease, for 12 to 16 years until 1978 for mortality, during which 1413 men died. The investigators assessed physical activity on questionnaires by asking men about the number of flights of stairs climbed daily, the number of city blocks walked daily, and the types of sports and recreational activities they engaged in, as well as the duration (hours per week) spent on these activities. These self-reports were then used to estimate energy expenditure in kilocalories per week. There was a steady decline in all-cause death rates across weekly energy expenditure categories, from 94 per 10,000 person-years among men expending less than 500 kcal/week to 54 per 10,000 person-years among men expending ≥2000 kcal/week (figure 4.2).

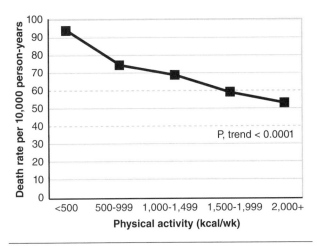

Figure 4.2 Age-adjusted death rates according to physical activity, Harvard Alumni Health Study, 1962-1978.

Investigators also estimated the number of years of life gained from being physically active. For these analyses, men were classified as active, expending 2000 kcal/week or more, or inactive, expending <500 kcal/week. Overall, after adjustment for differences in age, smoking, BMI, blood pressure, and age of parental death, active men could expect to live 2.15 years longer up to age 80, compared with inactive men. Obviously, younger men could expect to gain more years to age 80 than older men; for example, active men aged 35 to 39 years at the start of the study could expect to gain 2.51 years compared to inactive men; active men aged 70 to 74 years, 0.42 years.

These analyses were extended in a subsequent study by Lee, Hsieh, and Paffenbarger (1995), who wanted to investigate what intensity of physical activity was needed in order to decrease all-cause mortality rates. In this study, investigators additionally excluded men with stroke, cancer, and chronic obstructive pulmonary disease to minimize bias, since such men may decrease their activity levels and also have increased risk of dying. Men were then classified into categories of vigorous (activities requiring 6 metabolic equivalents [METs] or more) energy expenditure (<150, 150-399, 400-749, 750-1499, and ≥1500 kcal/week) and categories of nonvigorous energy expenditure (activities requiring <6 METs, also categorized as <150, 150-399, 400-749, 750-1499, and ≥1500 kcal/week). In addition to adjusting for age, smoking, BMI, hypertension, diabetes, and early parental mortality, analyses mutually adjusted for vigorous and nonvigorous activities. During a follow-up of up to 26 years (3728 deaths), there was a significant, inverse dose–response relation between vigorous energy expenditure assessed at baseline (1962 or 1966) and all-cause mortality rates (p, trend = 0.007), but not between nonvigorous energy expenditure and all-cause mortality rates (p = 0.36). When physical activity information was updated in 1977, similar patterns were observed.

Investigators thus concluded that the data showed that vigorous-intensity physical activity was needed in order to

reduce the risk of premature mortality. However, they also acknowledged that alternate explanations were possible for the findings. First, nonvigorous activities tend to be less precisely reported than vigorous activities; thus, the lack of significant findings with nonvigorous energy expenditure may merely reflect the imprecision with which these activities were reported by alumni. Additionally, investigators did not separate out light-intensity activities from those of moderate intensity. Thus, they were unable to make any conclusions specific to moderate-intensity activities.

To address moderate-intensity activities specifically, Lee and Paffenbarger (2000) conducted a subsequent study. In this study, Harvard alumni were categorized according to groups of energy expenditure from light- (<4 METs), moderate- (4-<6 METs), and vigorous-intensity physical activity, based on information provided in 1977 and using the same categories for each intensity as the groupings listed earlier. Men were then followed for mortality through 1992, during which period 2539 men died. Investigators observed that light-intensity activities were not associated with all-cause mortality rates (p, trend = 0.72); there was a trend of borderline significance for moderate-intensity activities (p, trend = 0.07) and a significant trend for vigorous-intensity activities (p, trend <0.001). When walking, a moderate-intensity physical activity, was examined separately, there was a significant trend across categories of walking <5, 5 to <10, 10 to <20, and ≥20 km/week; p, trend = 0.004. Investigators concluded that these data clearly indicated a benefit of vigorous-intensity activities while providing some support for moderate-intesity activities in lowering all-cause mortality rates.

Seventh Day Adventist Study

The associations of work and leisure-time physical activity with all-cause and disease-specific mortality rates were examined among nearly 9500 Seventh Day Adventist men aged 30 years or older in 1958 who were followed from 1960 through 1985; 4000 died during follow-up (Lindsted, Tonstad, and Kuzma 1991). Questionnaires assessed physical activity by asking men "How much exercise do you get (work or play)?" and offering four possible responses: none, slight, moderate, or heavy. In analyses, the bottom two categories were combined to form an inactive group. After adjustment for race, marital status, education, smoking, BMI, medical illness, and diet, all-cause death by age 50 was reduced among men with moderate activity, compared to inactive men (RR = 0.61; 95% CI: 0.50-0.74), and for men with heavy activity (RR = 0.66; 95% CI: 0.50-0.87). Moderate physical activity remained associated with reduced mortality rates up to age 80; but neither moderate nor heavy activity was significantly associated with lower mortality rates at age 90.

Iowa Women's Health Study

The studies described in the preceding sections included only men. In the Iowa Women's Health Study, investigators observed an inverse relation between physical activity and all-cause mortality rates in women also. Kushi and colleagues (1997) evaluated the association between physical activity and all-cause mortality in a cohort of 40,417 postmenopausal women living in Iowa. Women, aged 55 to 69 years, were sent a questionnaire at baseline in 1986 that asked about health habits and personal medical history. Physical activity was assessed through questions about whether the women participated in regular physical activity, as well as about their participation in moderate- and vigorous-intensity activities. In analyses, women were classified as having low, moderate, or high activity levels. A high activity level was defined as participating in vigorous-intensity activities more than two times a week or moderate-intensity activities more than four times a week; moderate activity level was defined as participating in vigorous-intensity activities once a week or moderate-intensity activities one to four times a week; low activity level was defined as all other patterns of physical activity. During a follow-up of seven years, 2260 women died.

After adjustment for age, age at menarche, age at menopause, age at first live birth, parity, alcohol intake, total energy intake, cigarette smoking, estrogen therapy, BMI (baseline and at age 18), waist-to-hip ratio, education, marital status, and history of hypertension or diabetes, the relative risks of all-cause mortality associated with moderate and high physical activity, compared with low, were 0.77 (95% CI: 0.69-0.86) and 0.68 (0.60-0.77) (p, trend <0.001), respectively. Similar results were obtained after excluding women with heart disease and cancer at baseline, and excluding the first three years of follow-up, to prevent a bias from illness leading to decreased physical activity. When investigators examined moderate- and vigorous-intensity activities separately, they found that both were related to lower risks of dying during follow-up. Compared with women who rarely or never participated in moderate-intensity physical activity, the relative risk was 0.71 (95% CI: 0.63-0.79) for those who participated in such activities once a week to a few times per month, 0.63 (0.56-0.71) for those who participated two to four times per week, and 0.59 (0.51-0.67) for those who participated more than four times per week; p, trend <0.001. For vigorous-intensity activity, the corresponding relative risks were 0.83 (0.69-0.99), 0.74 (0.59-0.93), and 0.62 (0.42-0.90), respectively; p, trend = 0.009.

Cardiovascular Health Study

The Cardiovascular Health Study is a prospective cohort study designed to determine the extent to which subclinical disease, functional health, and personal characteristics jointly predict mortality among older adults aged ≥65 years (Fried et al. 1998). A main cohort of 5201 men and women who were 95% white and a supplemental cohort of 685 African American men and women were recruited from four U.S. communities in California, Maryland, North Carolina, and Pennsylvania. Physical activity was assessed by interview in 1989 and 1990 using a modified Minnesota Leisure Time Activity Questionnaire, which evaluated the frequency and

duration of participation in 15 leisure-time activities. Using this information, the energy expended in kilocalories per week was estimated, and subjects were categorized into quintiles. The African American cohort, enrolled in 1992-1993, was not included in this physical activity analysis.

After five years of follow-up, there were 646 deaths (12%) in the main cohort. Twenty characteristics of the participants were independently associated with mortality, including older age, male sex, income less than $50,000 per year, low weight, smoking for more than 50 pack-years, high brachial systolic blood pressure (>169 mmHg), elevated fasting glucose level (>7.2 mmol/L, or >130 mg/dl), abnormal left ventricular ejection fraction, major electrocardiographic abnormality, and lack of physical activity. Neither high-density lipoprotein cholesterol (HDL-C) nor low-density lipoprotein cholesterol (LDL-C) was associated with mortality in this cohort. A prediction equation for mortality computed from the main cohort using the variables just mentioned also accurately predicted mortality in the African American cohort.

With regard to physical activity, men and women who expended >980 to 1890 kcal/week had about a 30% lower risk of mortality during follow-up (RR = 0.72; 95% CI: 0.55-0.93), and those expending >1890 kcal/week had about one half the risk (RR = 0.56; 95% CI: 0.43-0.75), compared to those expending <68 kcal/week, after adjustment for several potential confounding factors, including age, sex, smoking, BMI, alcohol use, blood pressure, serum cholesterol, and presence of various chronic diseases. There also was a significant inverse dose–response relation across quintiles of energy expenditure, p <0.005.

Honolulu Heart Program

The studies described so far included primarily Caucasian subjects. The Honolulu Heart Program included non-Caucasian participants; subjects were men of Japanese ancestry living in Hawaii. In a study of physical activity and all-cause mortality, about 700 nonsmoking older men, who were aged 61 to 81 years and who were physically capable, were followed over 12 years, during which 208 men died (Hakim et al. 1998). Between 1980 and 1982, men were asked to report the distance they walked per day. After adjustment for age, alcohol, diet, total and HDL cholesterol, hypertension, and diabetes, the relative risks for all-cause mortality associated with walking 1 to 2 miles and 2.1 to 8 miles per day were 0.7 (95% CI: 0.5-0.9) and 0.6 (0.4-0.8), respectively, compared with walking <1 mile/day.

Finnish Twin Study

In this research, investigators used data from the Finnish Twin Study to determine whether genetic factors or family health habits during childhood could explain part of the protective effects of physical activity against premature death (Kujala et al. 1998). A cohort of 7925 healthy men and 7977 healthy women aged 25 to 64 years, who were members of twin pairs, responded to a mailed questionnaire at baseline in 1975 asking about physical activity habits and other known risk factors for mortality. Leisure-time physical activity was assessed through questions about the frequency, duration, and intensity of exercise sessions. Those who reported exercising at least six times per month with an intensity equivalent to at least vigorous walking, for an average duration of 30 min each time, were classified as conditioning exercisers. Those who reported no leisure physical activity were classified as sedentary, and all other subjects were classified as occasional exercisers. There were 1253 deaths in the whole cohort and 434 discordant deaths among same-sex twin pairs (i.e., one twin died and the other was still alive) in the period 1977 through 1994.

In the whole cohort, after age, sex, smoking, occupation, and alcohol use were controlled for, the relative risk for all-cause mortality was 0.80 (95% CI: 0.69-0.91) among occasional exercisers and 0.76 (0.59-0.98) among conditioning exercisers, compared with sedentary subjects. Also, there was a dose–response reduction in risk of dying with increasing quintiles of estimated energy expended on exercise; p, trend = 0.002. In analyses restricted only to the 434 same-sex twin pairs discordant for death, the corresponding odds ratios for all-cause mortality were 0.73 (0.50-1.07) for occasional exercisers and 0.56 (0.29-1.11) for conditioning exercisers; p, trend = 0.06. While the results in the 434 pairs were not statistically significant, the magnitude of risk reduction was larger than that seen in the whole cohort. Thus, the lack of statistical significance was likely due to reduced statistical power because of the small sample size.

These results suggest that the inverse relation between physical activity and mortality rates is likely to be causal and is unlikely to be due to genetic factors. That is, it is unlikely that the genes that contribute toward making a person physically active or fit are the same genes that contribute to longevity. The results would have been more persuasive if only monozygotic twin pairs (identical twins) had been analyzed, since they share genetic information more completely than dizygotic twins (nonidentical twins). However, in only one of the 120 monozygotic Finnish twins who were discordant for mortality was one twin sedentary and the other a conditioning exerciser. The correlation between the estimated daily energy expenditure of twins was about 0.40 for both male and female monozygotic twins, about twice as large as that for dizygotic twins. In a study from the Swedish Twin Registry, described later, investigators were able to examine dizygotic and monozygotic twins separately and observed results that support those from the Finnish Twin Study.

Canada Fitness Survey Cohort

More than 6000 men and 8,000 women, aged 20 to 69 years, who participated in the Canada Fitness Survey between 1981 and 1988 and who were free of cardiovascular disease, were studied for the associations of physical activity and all-cause mortality (Villeneuve et al. 1998). Physical activity was assessed using a modified Minnesota Leisure Time Physical Activity Questionnaire, and subjects were categorized into five groups: 0 to <0.5, 0.5 to <1.5, 1.5 to <3.0, 3.0 to <0.5, and ≥0.5 kcal · kg^{-1} · day^{-1} of energy expended on leisure-time activities. During a follow-up of seven years, 614 men and 502 women died. After adjustment for age and smoking, men in the most active group had a relative risk for all-cause mortality of 0.82 (95% CI: 0.65-1.04), that is, an 18% risk reduction that was not statistically significant. For women, similar findings were observed (RR: 0.88; 95% CI: 0.68-1.04).

Particularly in women, investigators hypothesized that leisure-time physical activity alone might not adequately reflect total activity levels, since women tend to be less active during leisure time, compared with men, but carry out more household activities. Thus, they also analyzed total physical activity, captured using the same leisure-time physical activity questionnaire and self-reports of household chores. Women were categorized into quartiles of total energy expenditure; in age-adjusted analyses, higher levels of total physical activity were significantly related to lower mortality rates. The relative risks for all-cause mortality associated with total activity quartiles (lowest to highest) were 1.0 (referent), 0.66 (95% CI: 0.50-0.87), 0.68 (0.51-0.89), and 0.71 (0.50-0.87), respectively (Weller and Corey 1998).

Nurses' Health Study

The Nurses' Health Study began in 1976, when 121,700 female registered nurses 30 to 55 years of age residing in 11 large U.S. states completed a mailed questionnaire regarding their medical history and lifestyle, including physical activity. Since then, women have been followed every two years via questionnaires to update risk factor information and health status. Physical activity was first assessed in 1980, and information on physical activity was updated every two to four years. Initially, women were asked about the average number of hours of participation in vigorous activity (1980 and 1982) and in moderate activity (1980). In 1986, the physical activity questions were expanded so that they were now similar to those used in the Harvard Alumni Health Study. Women were asked to report their usual walking pace outdoors and the number of flights of stairs climbed daily. Additionally, they were asked about the average time per week spent on each of several specified leisure-time activities.

One report from this cohort (Rockhill et al. 2001) addressed physical activity in relation to all-cause mortality among 80,348 women free of cardiovascular disease and cancer in 1980. Women were classified as participating in <1.0, 1.0 to 1.9, 2.0 to 3.9, 4.0 to 6.9, and ≥7.0 h/week of physical activity. During follow-up from 1982 to 1996, 4746 women died. After adjustment for age, smoking, alcohol, height, BMI, and postmenopausal hormone use, the relative risks of dying during follow-up were 1.00 (referent), 0.82 (0.76-0.89), 0.75 (0.69-0.81), 0.74 (0.68-0.81), and 0.71 (0.61-0.82), respectively. Thus, there appeared to be a curvilinear dose–response relation, with a tapering of the reduction in risk occurring after about 2 h/week of physical activity.

In an updated analysis following women through 2000, investigators continued to observe lower mortality rates among women with higher physical activity levels (Hu et al. 2004). In particular, this inverse relation was observed among women with normal weight, those who were overweight, and those who were obese. Physical inactivity and obesity increased the risk of mortality, with women having no risk factors at lowest risk, those with either risk factor at intermediate risk, and those with both risk factors at highest risk. Using normal-weight (BMI <25.0 kg/m^2), active women (≥3.5 h/week of physical activity) as referent, obese women (BMI ≥30.0 kg/m^2) with the same level of physical activity had a significantly elevated relative risk of 1.91 (95% CI: 1.60-2.30) for all-cause mortality after adjustment for potential confounders. Normal-weight women who were inactive (<1 h/week) also had a higher relative risk, 1.55 (1.42-1.70), while obese inactive women experienced the highest relative risk, 2.42 (2.14-2.73).

Health, Aging, and Body Composition (Health ABC) Study

This represents the only study to date that has used an objective assessment of physical activity to examine its association with all-cause mortality. A total of 302 high-functioning adults, aged 70 to 82 years, residing in Pittsburgh, Pennsylvania, and Memphis, Tennessee, participated in an energy expenditure substudy in 1997 and 1998 (Manini et al. 2006). Total energy expenditure was assessed over a two-week period using doubly labeled water, an accurate method of measuring energy expenditure. The researchers then estimated energy expended on free-living activities by subtracting the thermic effect of food (estimated at 10% of total energy expenditure) and resting metabolic rate (measured using indirect calorimetry) from total energy expenditure. Subjects were divided into thirds of free-living energy expenditure: <521, 521 to 770, and >770 kcal/day.

During an average of 6.2 years of follow-up, 55 subjects died. Survival curves indicated that the most active participants survived at the highest rate, the least-active participants at the lowest rate. After adjustment for age, sex, study site, weight, height, percent body fat, sleep duration, and history of various chronic diseases, the relative risks for all-cause mortality in the three activity groups as defined earlier were 1.00 (referent), 0.65 (0.33-1.28), and 0.33 (0.15-0.74), respectively; *p,* trend 0.007.

Thus, this study, using an objective measure of physical activity, reported findings parallel to those from studies using self-reported physical activity assessed on questionnaires. While the magnitude of risk reduction seen here is larger than that generally observed in epidemiologic studies using self-reported measures, in which an average risk reduction of approximately 30% to 5% is noted when extreme groups are compared (Physical Activity Guidelines Advisory Committee 2008; Lollgen, Bockenhoff, and Knapp 2009), individual studies of self-reported physical activity have reported reductions as large as that seen in the Health ABC Study (e.g., 76% risk reduction, comparing extreme categories, in a study of about 2000 persons aged ≥65 years conducted in Taiwan [Lan, Chang, and Tai 2006]).

The Swedish Twin Registry Study

As with the Finnish Twin Study, the aim of the Swedish Twin Registry Study was to investigate whether genetic factors could explain the inverse relation between physical activity and all-cause mortality rates. Subjects were all same-sex twins, born from 1926 through 1958, who were alive and living in Sweden in 1970 (Carlsson et al. 2007). Included were 5240 monozygotic twin pairs and 7869 dizygotic twin pairs aged 14 to 46 years at baseline in 1972. Physical activity was assessed on questionnaires using a single question about average leisure-time physical activity over the past year, with seven possible responses ranging from "almost never" to "very much." In analyses, these were collapsed into three levels—low, moderate, and high physical activity.

During follow-up from 1973 through 2004, 1800 men and women died. In analyses of the whole cohort, after adjustment for age and smoking, the relative risks for all-cause mortality among men with moderate and high, compared with low, physical activity levels were 0.84 (95% CI: 0.72-0.98) and 0.64 (0.50-0.83), respectively. In women, they were 0.82 (0.70-0.96) and 0.75 (0.50-1.14), respectively. Investigators then analyzed twin pairs discordant for physical activity (i.e., accounting for genetic inheritance). Specifically, among 3112 monozygotic twins (1556 pairs), the odds ratio, adjusted for age and smoking, associated with a higher physical activity level was 0.80 (0.65-0.99); that is, even among persons sharing much genetic data in common, the more active twin was 20% less likely to die during follow-up, supporting a causal relation between physical activity and lower all-cause mortality rates.

Sedentary Behavior and All-Cause Mortality

As discussed in chapter 5, sedentary behavior, or sitting, may represent an independent risk factor for heart disease, separate from physical inactivity. Because heart disease is the leading cause of death in the United States and in most high-income countries, one might expect sedentary behavior also to be a risk factor for all-cause mortality. Epidemiologic data are emerging to support this hypothesis.

In the Canada Fitness Survey, more than 17,000 men and women, aged 18 to 90 years, were followed for 12 years for mortality (Katzmarzyk et al. 2009). At baseline in 1981, participants were asked to report the time spent sitting on most days of the week as almost none, approximately one-fourth, half, three-fourths, or almost all of the time. During follow-up, 1832 men and women died. After adjustment for age, sex, smoking, alcohol intake, and leisure-time physical activity, the relative risks of all-cause mortality associated with the five categories of sitting were 1.00 (referent), 1.00 (95% CI: 0.86-1.08), 1.11 (0.94-1.30), 1.36 (1.14-1.63), and 1.54 (1.25-1.91), respectively; *p,* trend <0.0001. Even among individuals active enough to meet physical activity recommendations, those spending more time sitting were at increased risk of all-cause mortality compared with those sitting less. The age-adjusted relative risks among such physically active men and women were 1.00, 0.92, 1.01, 1.31, and 1.40, respectively. The corresponding age-adjusted relative risks among those who did not meet physical activity recommendations were 1.00, 0.99, 1.21, 1.50, and 1.86, respectively.

The relation between sedentary behavior and all-cause mortality rates was also investigated in the American Cancer Society's Cancer Prevention Study II (Patel et al. 2010). A total of 53,440 healthy men and 69,776 healthy women, aged 50 to 74 years, reported on the average number of hours that they spent sitting per day, not counting time during work, in 1992. During follow-up through 2006, 11,307 men and 7923 women died. Compared with men sitting 0 to <3 h/day, the relative risks for mortality (adjusted for age; race; marital status; education; smoking; BMI; alcohol intake; total caloric intake; presence of high blood pressure, diabetes, and high cholesterol; and physical activity) among men sitting 3 to 5 h/day and ≥6 h/day were 1.07 (1.03-1.12) and 1.17 (1.11-1.24), respectively. In women, the relative risks were 1.13 (1.07-1.18) and 1.34 (1.25-1.44), respectively. As in the Canada Fitness Survey, more sitting time was associated with higher mortality rates, regardless of how much subjects exercised during their leisure time. Additionally, the association held among persons of normal-weight, overweight, or obese status.

Physical Fitness and All-Cause Mortality

Thus far, we have discussed studies of physical activity and all-cause mortality. Physical fitness is a concept different from but related to physical activity. Physical fitness represents a physiologic condition; physical activity represents a behavior. While physical fitness has a genetic component, regular physical activity can improve cardiorespiratory fitness in most individuals (Timmons et al. 2010). In the studies already discussed, physical activity was primarily assessed using self-reports, likely resulting in imprecise measures and possible underestimation of the true magnitude of the association between physical activity and all-cause mortality. Physical fitness, on the other hand, tends to be objectively measured in epidemiologic studies (e.g., with use of a maximal treadmill exercise test), which may potentially yield stronger associations with all-cause mortality.

In a meta-analysis of >100,000 subjects from 33 studies (Kodama et al. 2009), investigators estimated that a 1-MET higher level of maximal aerobic capacity was associated with a 13% reduction in risk of all-cause mortality (RR: 0.87; 95% CI: 0.84-0.90). When cardiovascular fitness was categorized into low (<7.9 METs), intermediate (7.9-10.8 METs), or high (≥10.9 METs), the relative risks for all-cause mortality were 1.00 (referent), 0.68 (0.52-0.66), and 0.64 (0.68-0.76), respectively.

Thus, while individual studies (see examples in the following sections) may show stronger associations between physical fitness and all-cause mortality than studies of physical activity and all-cause mortality, overall this meta-analysis indicates associations of similar magnitude in studies of physical activity and physical fitness. That is, on average, investigations indicate a 31% reduction in all-cause mortality rates among the most active compared with the least-active individuals (Physical Activity Guidelines Advisory Committee 2008) and a 36% risk reduction among most, compared with least-fit, persons (Kodama et al. 2009).

U.S. Railroad Workers

In an analysis of 2431 white men aged 22 to 79 years, who were employed in the U.S. railroad industry and were free from cardiovascular disease at the baseline exam, physical fitness was assessed based on heart rate response to a sub-maximal treadmill exercise test (Slattery and Jacobs 1988). The men were followed for mortality from the baseline exam, conducted from 1957 to 1960, until 1977, during which time there were 631 deaths. With men divided into approximate fourths, the risk for all-cause mortality in the least-fit group was 1.23 times (95% CI: 1.17-1.30) that of the fittest group after adjustment for age, blood pressure, cigarette smoking, and serum cholesterol.

Aerobics Center Longitudinal Study

The Aerobics Center Longitudinal Study is an observational cohort study of over 25,000 men and 7000 women who received preventive medical examinations at the Cooper Institute in Dallas, Texas, beginning in 1970. It is an open cohort; that is, subjects continue to be added to the cohort study over time.

In a 1989 study, Blair and colleagues reported on the relationship between maximal treadmill time (an estimate of cardiorespiratory fitness that predicts maximal oxygen uptake with about 80% accuracy) and mortality rates in 10,224 men and 3120 women from this cohort who were followed for an average of about eight years until 1985, during which 240 men and 43 women died (Blair et al. 1989). The age-adjusted all-cause mortality rate for the least-fit men (bottom quintile, i.e., the lowest 20% of the cohort) was more than three times greater (RR: 3.44; 95% CI: 2.05-5.77) than for the most fit (top quintile). Among women, in whom the number of deaths was very small, the mortality rate for the least-fit women was 4.65 times greater (95% CI: 2.22-9.75) than for the most fit women. In both sexes, it appeared that the largest risk reduction occurred between the bottom quintile and the next 20% of fitness, with only minor additional decrements in risk at higher quintiles of fitness. Thus, later analyses from this cohort often categorized subjects as belonging to low-fit (bottom 20%) or higher-fit groups (top 80%).

In an updated analysis with follow-up extended to an average of 10 years, with 1025 deaths in men, investigators confirmed these earlier observations (Wei et al. 1999). Further, they reported that low fitness was associated with higher all-cause mortality rates regardless of whether men were normal weight, overweight, or obese. Among normal-weight men, the relative risk for all-cause mortality adjusted for age and examination year among those in the bottom 20% of cardiorespiratory fitness, compared with the upper 80%, was 2.00 (1.8-2.8). For overweight and obese men, these rates were 2.5 (2.1-3.0) and 3.1 (2.5-3.8), respectively. Similar findings were observed in a study of women from this cohort, who were followed for an average of over 12 years, with 292 deaths occurring (Farrell et al. 2010). In another study of 2603 adults aged 60 and older, maximal exercise treadmill tests were conducted between 1979 and 2001, and subjects were followed for mortality through 2003, during which period 450 subjects died (Sui et al. 2007). The relative risks of all-cause mortality, associated with quintiles of fitness and adjusted for age, sex, examination year, smoking, abnormal exercise EKG response, history of chronic health conditions, BMI, waist circumference, and percent body fat and fat-free mass, were 1.00 (referent), 0.54 (0.41-0.72), 0.44 (0.33-0.59), 0.44 (0.33-0.59), and 0.31 (0.22-0.43), respectively. Regardless of the BMI of subjects, lower fitness (bottom 20% of distribution) was associated with higher all-cause mortality rates (figure 4.3).

These analyses, jointly examining the associations of physical activity, adiposity, and all-cause mortality rates, raised an issue sometimes referred to as the "fit versus fat"

hypothesis. That is, these data suggested that higher levels of cardiorespiratory fitness could remove the excess risk of mortality associated with being overweight or obese. For example, in the 2007 analyses conducted by Sui and colleagues, compared with older adults who were of normal BMI (18.5-24.9 kg/m²) and who were fit (top 80%), those with BMI ≥30.0 to 34.9 kg/m² but who were fit had a relative risk of all-cause mortality of 1.12 (0.76-1.66). Compared to the same group, those who were of normal BMI but who were unfit (bottom 20%) had a relative risk of 3.63 (2.47-5.32). These relative risks were adjusted for age, sex, examination year, smoking, abnormal exercise EKG response, and history of chronic health conditions. Thus, these data suggested that it was better to be "fit and fat" than "unfit and thin."

Not all studies have agreed with these conclusions. Other studies of physical activity and mortality, including the Harvard Alumni Health Study (Lee and Paffenbarger 2000) and the Nurses' Health Study (Hu et al. 2004), show that that either risk factor—being physically inactive or being overweight or obese—is associated with increased risk of premature mortality, of approximately equal magnitude, and that possessing both risk factors increases risk yet further. In these two studies, being active did not remove the excess risk associated with being overweight or obese. A review examining the "fit versus fat" hypothesis agreed that findings related to all-cause mortality were mixed (Fogelholm 2010). However, the data related to the risk of developing another outcome, type 2 diabetes, were more clear in showing that being overweight or obese greatly increased the risk of type 2 diabetes, and that being physically fit or active did not remove the excess risk associated with being overweight or obese.

Veterans Study

In another study of cardiorespiratory fitness and all-cause mortality in men, 6213 consecutive male veterans who were referred for treadmill exercise testing from 1987 onward, based on clinical reasons, were investigated (Myers et al. 2002). Of these, 2534 men had no history of cardiovascular disease (CVD) and had a normal exercise test result; the remainder had a history of CVD, an abnormal exercise test result, or both. The mean age of subjects was 59 years; during a mean follow-up of 6.2 years, 1256 men died. For each 1-MET higher peak exercise capacity, the age-adjusted relative risk of all-cause mortality was 0.84 (0.79-0.89). Cardiorespiratory fitness was inversely associated with mortality in men both without and with a history of CVD. When men were divided into quintiles of fitness, the least-fit quintile had more than four times the risk of dying during follow-up compared with the most fit quintile. The magnitude of increased risk of mortality for this risk factor, low fitness, was higher than the magnitudes associated with other traditional risk factors, such as smoking; obesity; high cholesterol level; or history of hypertension, diabetes, or chronic obstructive pulmonary disease.

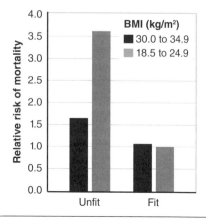

Figure 4.3 Cardiorespiratory fitness, body mass index, and all-cause mortality rates in men and women ≥60 years of age, Aerobics Center Longitudinal Study, 1979-2003.

St. James Women Take Heart Project and Economics of Noninvasive Diagnosis Study

The studies discussed so far have examined largely men (although the Aerobics Center Longitudinal Study did include a small group of women). A study by Gulati and colleagues (2005) investigated women exclusively, with the aim of examining whether the findings seen largely in men also extended to women. A total of 5721 asymptomatic women from the Chicago metropolitan area with mean age 52 years who were participating in the St. James Women Take Heart Project underwent a treadmill test in 1992 to assess cardiorespiratory fitness. Another 4471 women with cardiovascular symptoms and mean age 61 years who were participating in the Economics of Noninvasive Diagnosis Study underwent a treadmill test between 1990 and 1995.

During follow-up through 2000, 180 asymptomatic women and 537 symptomatic women died. Among women in the former group, as compared with those whose exercise capacity was ≥85% of age-predicted value, those whose exercise capacity was <85% of age-predicted value (i.e., the less fit women) had a relative risk of all-cause mortality of 2.03 (1.51-2.71). For symptomatic women, the corresponding relative risk was similar, 2.37 (1.90-2.37).

Veterans Affairs Health Care System Study

The aim of this study was to investigate the association between cardiorespiratory fitness and all-cause mortality specifically in blacks, since most of the subjects in previous studies, such as those discussed earlier here (except for the Economics of Non-invasive Diagnosis Study, in which 28% of the women were black), were white. A total of 6749 black men (mean age, 58 years) and 8911 white men (mean age, 60 years) who received medical care from the Veterans Health Care System in Washington, D.C., and Palo Alto, California, were studied (Kokkinos et al. 2008). These men received a symptom-limited exercise tolerance test, either for routine evaluation or for evaluation of exercise-induced ischemia. Fitness was assessed based on peak exercise time on a treadmill using the Bruce protocol and expressed in METs. During a mean follow-up of 7.5 years, 3912 men died.

In the whole cohort, for each 1-MET increase in peak exercise capacity, the relative risk of dying during follow-up decreased by 18% (RR: 0.82; 95% CI: 0.81-0.83). The findings were similar for black and white men, with relative risks of 0.79 (0.78-0.81) and 0.83 (0.82-0.84), respectively. When men were categorized into groups achieving <5, 5 to 7, 7.1 to 10, and >10 METs of peak exercise capacity, in black men the relative risks were 1.00, 0.81, 0.50, and 0.26, respectively; in white men they were 1.00, 0.79, 0.52, and

0.34, respectively. These analyses were adjusted for age, BMI, CVD medications, and CVD risk factors. When men without CVD were analyzed separately, similar findings were observed. Investigators concluded that the inverse relation between cardiorespiratory fitness and all-cause mortality, previously observed primarily in white subjects, also extended to African Americans.

Changes in Physical Activity or Fitness and All-Cause Mortality

As you can see from the preceding discussion, all of the studies relating physical activity or fitness to all-cause mortality have been observational epidemiologic studies. Studies of this design cannot prove cause and effect (for further discussion, refer to chapter 2). However, observational studies of changes in physical activity or fitness in relation to all-cause mortality can provide information that strengthens the premise of a causal link. Though not as convincing as evidence from a randomized controlled trial (in which physical activity or fitness is manipulated by investigators), evidence that a naturally occurring change in an independent variable such as physical activity or fitness results in a change in a dependent variable, such as all-cause mortality, can provide further evidence for a cause-and-effect association of those variables.

Several studies have now been published on the impact of changing physical activity habits or changing levels of physical fitness on the subsequent risk for all-cause mortality. Next we consider two exemplar studies of changes in physical activity and two of changes in physical fitness in relation to all-cause mortality. These consistently indicate that changing from low to high physical activity or fitness levels is associated with lower mortality rates compared with remaining at low levels. Conversely, changing from high to low levels is associated with mortality rates similar to those associated with remaining at low levels. Thus, these data are consistent with a causal relation between physical activity or fitness and decreased all-cause mortality rates.

Harvard Alumni Health Study

This was the first investigation of the association of changes in physical activity with all-cause mortality rates, as well as estimated years of life gained by changing from low to high levels of physical activity (Paffenbarger et al. 1993). A total of 10,269 healthy Harvard alumni, aged 45 to 84 years in 1977, were followed until 1985 for mortality. Changes in physical activity (assessment of physical activity in this study was described earlier) between 1962 or 1966 and 1977 were related to mortality rates during follow-up, when 476 men died.

In analyses, men were dichotomized into two groups at each time: not participating in moderate-intensity recreational activities (≥4.5 METs), deemed "inactive," or participating in such activities, deemed "active." Investigators reported that compared to men who were inactive both in 1962 or 1966 and in 1977, men who changed from being inactive to active between the 1960s and 1977 had a significant 23% lower all-cause mortality rate (RR = 0.77; 95% CI: 0.58-0.96), after adjustment for age, cigarette smoking, hypertension, and BMI. In fact, their risk reduction was comparable in magnitude to that of men who were active at both times (RR = 0.71 [0.55-0.96]). On the other hand, men who changed from being active to inactive were as badly off as those who had remained inactive, with a relative risk of 1.15 (0.73-1.15); that is, there was no significant difference in mortality rates between these two groups.

Overall, men who changed from being inactive to active gained 0.72 years of life, compared to those who remained inactive. This gain in life expectancy was similar to the gain associated with not increasing one's BMI (0.65 years) and remaining normotensive (0.91 years), though somewhat less than the gain associated with quitting smoking cigarettes (1.46 years).

Study of Osteoporotic Fractures

These findings among male Harvard alumni also extend to women. In the Study of Osteoporotic Fractures, women aged 65 years and older were enrolled from four research centers in Baltimore, Maryland; Portland, Oregon; Minneapolis, Minnesota; and Monongahela Valley, Pennsylvania. At their baseline visit, in 1986 to 1988, physical activity was assessed using a modified version of the Harvard Alumni Health Study questionnaire (Gregg et al. 2003). Physical activity was again assessed at a follow-up visit in 1992 to 1994. Of the 7553 women included in these analyses, 1029 died over a median of 6.7 years after the follow-up visit.

In analyses, women in the lowest 40% of distribution and expending <595 kcal/week were classified as sedentary, and the remaining 60% were classified as active. Women who were sedentary at both times or who changed from being active to sedentary were most likely to die during follow-up. Those who were active at both times or changed from being sedentary to active had the lowest mortality rates. With women who were sedentary at both times as referent, those who changed from being sedentary to active had a relative risk for all-cause mortality of 0.52 (95% CI: 0.40-0.69) after adjustment for age, smoking, BMI, self-rated health, various chronic medical conditions, and baseline physical activity. Meanwhile, those who changed from being active to sedentary had a relative risk of 0.92 (0.77-1.09), not significantly different from that of the women who had remained sedentary. The associations were similar in women without and with chronic diseases but tended to be weaker in women aged 75 years or more.

Aerobics Center Longitudinal Study

The Aerobics Center Longitudinal Study was the first study to examine the association of changes in physical fitness with all-cause mortality. These analyses included 9177 men (6219 healthy and 2958 with a history of myocardial infarction, stroke, diabetes, or hypertension), aged 20 to 82 years, who received two preventive medical exams between 1970 and 1987 (Blair et al. 1995). The mean interval between examinations was 4.9 years. Physical fitness was assessed by time on a treadmill in a maximal exercise protocol, and subjects were classified by investigators as unfit (lowest 20% of distribution of cardiorespiratory fitness for age) or fit (the remaining 80%). During an average follow-up of 5.1 years after the second examination, 223 men died.

Results indicated that the lowest age-adjusted mortality rates were in men who were fit at both examinations, while the highest mortality rates were in those unfit at both examinations. The age-adjusted relative risk for all-cause mortality among men who were fit at both examinations, compared to those who were unfit at both, was 0.33 (95% CI: 0.23-0.47). Men who changed fitness category from unfit to fit had a relative risk of 0.52 (0.38-0.72). This trend was observed among men of different age groups, ranging from those 20 to 39 years through those aged 60 years and older. In additional analyses treating physical fitness as a continuous variable, for each minute of increased treadmill time (equivalent to about 1-MET increase in fitness) between the first and second examination, mortality risk was reduced by 7.9%.

In comparing the association of favorable change in fitness with decreases in all-cause mortality rates against the associations of favorable changes in other cardiovascular risk factors (BMI, systolic blood pressure, cholesterol, and smoking), investigators reported that the magnitude was most favorable for fitness. Thus, these findings on changes in cardiorespiratory fitness in relation to all-cause mortality rates are parallel to those on changes in physical activity.

Norwegian Men

A cohort of 1428 healthy Norwegian men aged 50 to 70 years underwent a clinical examination during 1972 through 1975 that included an exercise test on a bicycle (Erikssen et al. 1998). A second identical examination was given in 1980 through 1982, after which men were followed for mortality through 1994. During follow-up, 238 men died. After adjustment for age, baseline fitness, physical activity, smoking, BMI, resting heart rate, blood pressure, vital capacity, total cholesterol, triglycerides, and abnormal exercise test result, there was a significant relation between increasing physical fitness from examination 1 to examination 2 and lower all-cause mortality rates (RR = 0.70; 95% CI: 0.62-0.79) per 1-unit standard deviation of increase.

Are the Associations Real?

In looking at data from studies on the association of physical activity or fitness with all-cause mortality, we see that all the data have been observational. As a first step toward determining that the observed association is causal, we have to ensure that the observed associations are valid and not the result of some other factor such as chance, bias, or confounding.

The role of chance can be assessed through examination of the statistical significance of the findings. By convention, we accept that chance is an unlikely explanation if we obtain a p-value of <0.05 for the findings. The p-value obtained depends on the size of the study (small numbers of subjects may lead to an underpowered study, such that a significant p-value is not obtained, even if there is a true association), as well as the magnitude of effect (large magnitudes of effect require a smaller sample size to allow observation of a significant result). Many of the studies discussed in the preceding sections did show statistically significant results, indicating that chance is an unlikely explanation. Moreover, meta-analyses that have combined many studies to examine the relation of physical activity or fitness with all-cause mortality, thus ensuring adequate sample size, consistently report significantly lower rates of mortality among more active (or fit) men and women compared with less active (or fit) persons (Lollgen, Bockenhoff, and Knapp 2009, Kodama et al. 2009).

Could bias explain the findings we see in the studies discussed here? Several biases need to be considered. Selection bias is a bias that occurs when the selection of participants into a study is related to both exposure and outcome. This is a bias that is more likely to occur in case–control and retrospective cohort studies because both exposure and outcome have occurred at the initiation of the study. For example, consider the hypothetical situation in which death certificates are more readily available for clerical workers in a shipping company because they are less likely to be injured in their job than other types of workers and stay on longer in the same position. They continue to receive benefits, including death benefits for heirs. When they die, their beneficiaries need to file a death certificate to obtain the benefits. Cargo workers in the same company are more likely to change jobs because of injury and so tend to lose benefits. When they die, the company may be unaware of the fact because their heirs do not file for benefits. Suppose we conduct a retrospective study of occupational physical activity and mortality in this company. Our findings may be biased by the selection of subjects into the study—we are more likely to see data for sedentary subjects (clerks) who die, less likely to see data for active subjects (cargo workers) who die. This will result in a bias of higher death rates among sedentary persons. Certainly, this bias is a possibility; however, this chapter has presented findings primarily from prospective cohort studies in which selection bias is less of a possibility since the outcome has not yet occurred at the start of the study. In these prospective studies, we observe documentation of lower mortality rates among more active or fit persons.

Loss to follow-up is a particular concern in prospective cohort studies. Subjects who are sick—and thus more likely to die—may tend to drop out of the study. If they also are persons who are less active, we would observe a dilution of the true effect of physical activity on mortality since we observe a falsely low death rate among inactive subjects. In the studies described thus far, loss to follow-up is not a major concern. While many studies did not report follow-up rates, many used national systems to ascertain deaths (e.g., National Death Index in the United States), which tend to be complete. Of the studies that did report follow-up rates, these tended to be very high (Physical Activity Guidelines Advisory Committee 2008).

Another bias to consider is what has sometimes been referred to as "reverse causation." This bias results when sick persons, who are more likely to die, decrease their activity levels because of their ill health. The observed association between low physical activity level and high mortality rates may not be due to the former causing the latter, but rather reflecting that sick persons, who are more likely to die, are less physically active. Reducing the potential for this bias has been addressed in different ways. Many studies include only ostensibly healthy subjects (primarily free of CVD and cancer, the most common diseases present among the populations of high-income countries, in which many of the studies discussed here are based) to prevent the bias. Additionally, several studies have excluded initial follow-up from analyses, when sick subjects—who may have decreased their activity levels because of ill-health—are likely to die, thus minimizing this potential bias. Also, with longer follow-up periods, the effect of this bias is diluted since sick persons die early in follow-up. The median length of follow-up in the studies of physical activity and all-cause mortality is about 12 years; thus, the effect of such a bias would be minimal (Physical Activity Guidelines Advisory Committee 2008).

Misclassification of physical activity can potentially lead to a bias. Many of the studies on this topic collected physical activity information using self-reports by subjects, and this is likely to be imprecise. However, in order for a bias to occur, the misclassification has to be systematically related to both exposure and outcome. In prospective cohort studies, physical activity is assessed at the beginning of the study, prior to the occurrence of any outcomes. Thus the misclassification cannot be systematically related to the outcome of all-cause mortality. Instead, any misclassification is likely to be random, which leads to dilution of results rather than a systematic bias. One study, the Health ABC Study, assessed physical activity using doubly labeled water, considered a gold standard for measuring energy expenditure (Manini et al. 2006). This study showed, as did the studies using self-reports, an inverse relation between physical activity and all-cause mortality rates.

With regard to confounding, physically active persons tend to have other healthy habits as well, which may explain the association of higher physical activity or fitness levels with lower all-cause mortality rates. However, this is unlikely to have explained the inverse relation observed because the association persisted after the investigators controlled for several potential confounders (including age, sex, race, education, smoking, BMI, alcohol, diet, personal and family medical history, and reproductive variables in women).

Thus, the observation of lower all-cause mortality rates among persons with higher levels of physical activity or fitness is likely to be a real association and unlikely to be due to alternate explanations of chance, bias, or confounding.

Strength of the Evidence

While we conclude that the association of physical activity with lower mortality rates is real, is the association one of cause and effect? Only well-designed and well-conducted randomized controlled trials can provide data supportive of a causal relationship. To date, there have been no data from randomized controlled trials of physical activity and mortality among persons at usual risk. Thus, the available observational data cannot prove that there is a causal relation between higher levels of physical activity (or fitness) and lower mortality rates. We previously discussed observational studies showing that persons who change from being inactive to active (or unfit to fit) have lower mortality rates than persons who have remained inactive (or unfit) all along, lending credence to the assumption of cause and effect. Further, while no randomized clinical trials have been conducted among persons at usual risk, such trials have been conducted among persons who have coronary heart disease. A meta-analysis of 48 randomized clinical trials involving 8940 patients with myocardial infarction or coronary artery revascularization procedures found an odds ratio for total mortality of 0.80 (95% CI: 0.68-0.93) among patients assigned to cardiac rehabilitation that included exercise as compared with usual care (Taylor et al. 2004).

Additionally, we can apply several criteria to observational epidemiologic data to judge whether the observed associations are likely to be causal (see chapter 2 for additional discussion): temporal sequence, strength of association, consistency of results, biological plausibility, and dose response. Each of these is discussed next in the context of observational epidemiologic studies of physical activity or fitness and all-cause mortality.

Temporal Sequence

If an association were causal, the exposure—in this case, physical activity or fitness—would have to precede the outcome, mortality. All of the studies discussed here were prospective cohort studies, in which the appropriate temporal sequence occurred. Prospective cohort studies have demonstrated consistent associations of higher activity or fitness levels with lower mortality rates (Lollgen, Bockenhoff, and Knapp 2009, Kodama et al. 2009).

Strength of Association

The magnitude of the inverse association between physical activity or fitness and all-cause mortality, based on observational epidemiologic studies, is moderate. In the meta-analysis by Lollgen and colleagues (2009), the most active subjects had a 31% risk reduction compared with the least active. For physical fitness, the meta-analysis by Kodama and colleagues (2009) showed a risk reduction of 36% for the most fit compared with the least-fit subjects. These meta-analyses indicate an average across all studies; individual studies have reported magnitudes of effect that are smaller or larger.

With regard to changes in physical activity or fitness, data from the Harvard Alumni Health Study (Paffenbarger et al. 1993) and the Aerobics Center Longitudinal Study (Blair et al. 1995) suggest that the strength of association related to beneficial changes in activity or fitness is comparable to that seen for beneficial changes in other cardiovascular risk factors such as BMI, blood pressure, cholesterol, and smoking.

Consistency of Results

Data on the association of physical activity or fitness with all-cause mortality have been consistently reported across many studies, and in men and women. The studies, conducted at different times using different methodologies and subjects from different countries, have yielded overall similar results, supporting a causal association.

Biological Plausibility

One of the most important criteria for helping to establish a causal relation is evidence for the biological plausibility of the observed association. Earlier in this chapter, we stated that the leading causes of death in the United States are heart disease, cancer, and cerebrovascular disease, accounting for more than half of all deaths. In chapters 5, 6, and 12, we discuss potential biological underpinnings for an inverse relation between physical activity or fitness and each of these major causes of mortality. It is clear that many plausible biological mechanisms exist to explain why physically active or fit men and women should have lower rates of these diseases, and thus all-cause mortality.

Dose Response

The presence of a dose–response relation between physical activity or fitness and all-cause mortality rates can help support the case for a cause-and-effect relationship. (It is worth noting that the absence of a dose–response relation does not necessarily mean that a causal relation does not exist.) The available data do support an inverse, curvilinear relationship. In the 2009 meta-analysis of leisure-time physical activity (for which the most data are available) and all-cause mortality previously discussed, the relative risks for low-active, moderately active, and highly active men were 1.00, 0.81, and 0.78, respectively (Lollgen, Bockenhoff, and Knapp 2009). Among women, they were 1.00, 0.76, and 0.69, respectively. In the 2009 meta-analysis of cardiorespiratory fitness and all-cause mortality by Kodama and colleagues, the relative risks for low, intermediate, and high fitness categories were 1.00, 0.68, and 0.64, respectively.

Thus, these data indicate a larger magnitude of risk reduction between low and intermediate categories, and a smaller magnitude of risk reduction between intermediate and high categories, indicating a curvilinear dose–response relation.

How Much Physical Activity Is Needed to Decrease Risk of Premature Mortality?

In order to provide clear public health recommendations for physical activity, it is important to specify how much physical activity is required. The question of "how much" can refer to the total volume of energy expended on physical activity, the intensity, the duration, or the frequency of physical activity. As can be seen from the exemplar studies described earlier, most studies have presented their findings in terms of the volume of energy expended. There are relatively few data to clarify requirements related to the other dimensions of physical activity.

Based on a comprehensive review of the literature, the 2008 Physical Activity Guidelines Advisory Committee concluded that the available data indicate that it is the overall volume of energy expended—regardless of whether this is from leisure-time physical activity (assessed in most studies), occupational activity, household activity, or commuting activity (such as walking and bicycling)—that is important for lowering the risk of premature mortality (Physical Activity Guidelines Advisory Committee 2008). The data are clear in showing that the equivalent of 2 to 2.5 h per week of moderate-intensity physical activity is sufficient to significantly decrease all-cause mortality rates. Several studies specifically on walking also show clearly that walking 2 or more hours per week is associated with a significantly lower risk of all-cause mortality. As discussed in the section on dose response, the existing data support an inverse dose–response relation. Thus, the 2 to 2.5 h per week of moderate-intensity physical activity or walking does not represent an "all or nothing" threshold level for risk reduction. It represents a useful target for public health recommendations, since benefit is clearly seen at this level. Additionally, the studies to date

consistently support an inverse dose–response relation for the total volume of energy expended, indicating that while the goal is 2 to 2.5 h per week of moderate-intensity physical activity, any amount of physical activity is useful, and more activity is associated with additional risk reductions in mortality rates. This supports a "some is good; more is better" approach toward the amount of physical activity required for lowering all-cause mortality rates (U.S. Department of Health and Human Services 2008; Wen et al. 2011).

With regard to the intensity of physical activity required, studies indicate that moderate- or vigorous-intensity physical activity is associated with lower all-cause mortality rates (Physical Activity Guidelines Advisory Committee 2008). However, it is unclear whether vigorous-intensity physical activity is associated with additional risk reduction in mortality rates, compared with lower-intensity activities, beyond its contribution to the total energy expended. That is, for the same volume of energy expended, does vigorous intensity activity confer additional benefits compared to moderate- or light-intensity activity? While several studies have investigated activities of different intensities in relation to all-cause mortality, few have tried to tease out confounding by the volume of energy expended (that is, accounting for the fact that, for example, 30 min of vigorous-intensity activity expends more energy than does 30 min of moderate-intensity activity). A few studies, providing limited data, suggest that higher intensities of physical activity are associated with additional risk reductions for all-cause mortality beyond their contribution to greater total volume of energy expended (U.S. Department of Health and Human Services 2008).

With regard to the duration and frequency of physical activity required, there are no data on these dimensions that are independent of their contributions to the total volume of energy expended. Various studies have indeed examined different durations of physical activity, or different frequencies of physical activity, in relation to all-cause mortality rates. But these studies did not adjust for confounding by volume of physical activity, so the findings related to duration (or frequency) may be reflecting the dose–response relation between the total volume of energy expended and risk of all-cause mortality. Stated in another way, it is unknown whether multiple short bouts of physical activity versus a single long bout that expends the same energy are differentially associated with all-cause mortality rates (Physical Activity Guidelines Advisory Committee 2008). Finally, one study examined the association of all-cause mortality with physical activity carried out one or two days a week that generated sufficient energy expenditure to meet current physical activity recommendations (i.e., the so-called "weekend warrior" pattern) (Lee et al. 2004). Overall, the relative risk for mortality among weekend warriors, compared with sedentary men, was 0.85 (95% CI: 0.65-1.11). This relation was significantly different among men at low and high CVD risk. Among men without major cardiovascular risk factors, weekend warriors had a significantly lower risk of dying compared with sedentary men (RR = 0.41 [0.21-0.81]). This was not seen among men with at least one major risk factor (RR = 1.02 [0.75-1.38]).

Summary

A large body of observational epidemiologic studies consistently shows that physically active or fit individuals have lower rates of premature mortality than inactive or unfit individuals. The findings from these studies are unlikely to be the result of chance, bias, or confounding. And, while observational studies cannot prove cause and effect, using the guidelines of temporal sequence, strength of association, consistency of results, biological plausibility, and dose response, the available data from the observational studies strongly support a causal relation. This association is present in both men and women and in persons of different ages. While data are more limited with regard to persons of different race–ethnic groups, the available data suggest that the association is present for persons of different race-ethnicities.

Current guidelines recommend 150 min/week of moderate-intensity aerobic activity or 75 min/week of vigorous-intensity physical activity, or the equivalent energy expenditure in moderate plus vigorous activities, for health, including lowering all-cause mortality rates (U.S. Department of Health and Human Services 2008). And, encouragingly for persons who are sedentary, the available data further suggest that any physical activity, even at levels lower than recommended, may be helpful. Because there is a dose–response relation, for persons able and willing to expend more total energy, to engage in activities of higher intensities, or to do both, additional risk reductions in mortality rates will occur.

· BIBLIOGRAPHY ·

Blair, S.N., H.W. Kohl III, C.E. Barlow, R.S. Paffenbarger Jr., L.W. Gibbons, and C.A. Macera. 1995. Changes in physical fitness and all-cause mortality: A prospective study of healthy and unhealthy men. *Journal of the American Medical Association* 273: 1093-1098.

Blair, S., H. Kohl, R. Paffenbarger, D. Clark, K. Cooper, and L. Gibbons. 1989. Physical fitness and all-cause mortality: A prospective study of healthy men and women. *Journal of the American Medical Association* 262: 2395-2401.

Blair, S.N., and M. Wei. 2000. Sedentary habits, health, and function in older women and men. *American Journal of Health Promotion* 15: 1-8.

Carlsson, S., T. Andersson, P. Lichtenstein, K. Michaelsson, and A. Ahlbom. 2007. Physical activity and mortality: Is the association explained by genetic selection? *American Journal of Epidemiology* 166: 255-259.

Easton, J. 1799. *Human longevity; recording the name, age, place of residence, and year of the decease, of 1712 persons who attained a century, & upwards, from A.D. 66 to 1799.* Salisbury, England: Author.

Erikssen, G., K. Liestol, J. Bjornholt, E. Thaulow, L. Sandvik, and J. Erikssen. 1998. Changes in physical fitness and changes in mortality. *Lancet* 352: 759-762.

Farrell, S.W., S.J. Fitzgerald, P.A. McAuley, and C.E. Barlow. 2010. Cardiorespiratory fitness, adiposity, and all-cause mortality in women. *Medicine and Science in Sports and Exercise* 42: 2006-2012.

Fogelholm, M. 2010. Physical activity, fitness and fatness: Relations to mortality, morbidity and disease risk factors. A systematic review. *Obesity Reviews* 11: 202-221.

Fried, L.P., R.A. Kronmal, A.B. Newman, D.E. Bild, M.B. Mittelmark, J.F. Polak, J.A. Robbins, and J.M. Gardin. 1998. Risk factors for 5-year mortality in older adults: The Cardiovascular Health Study. *Journal of the American Medical Association* 279: 585-592.

Gregg, E.W., J.A. Cauley, K. Stone, T.J. Thompson, D.C. Bauer, S.R. Cummings, and K.E. Ensrud. 2003. Relationship of changes in physical activity and mortality among older women. *Journal of the American Medical Association* 289: 2379-2386.

Gulati, M., H.R. Black, L.J. Shaw, M.F. Arnsdorf, C.N.B. Merz, et al. 2005. The prognostic value of a nomogram for exercise capacity in women. *New England Journal of Medicine* 353: 468-475.

Hakim, A.A., H. Petrovitch, C.M. Burchfiel, W. Ross, B.L. Rodriguez, et al. 1998. Effects of walking on mortality among nonsmoking retired men. *New England Journal of Medicine* 338: 94-99.

Heron, M. 2010. Deaths: Leading causes for 2006. *National Vital Statistics Reports,* Vol. 58, No. 14. Hyattsville, MD: National Center for Health Statistics.

Hu, F.B., W.C. Willett, T. Li, M.J. Stampfer, G.A. Colditz, and J.E. Manson. 2004. Adiposity as compared with physical activity in predicting mortality among women. *New England Journal of Medicine* 351: 2694-2703.

Katzmarzyk, P.T., T.S. Church, C.L. Craig, and C. Bouchard. 2009. Sitting time and mortality from all causes, cardiovascular disease, and cancer. *Medicine and Science in Sports and Exercise* 41: 998-1005.

Kodama, S., K. Saito, S. Tanaka, M. Maki, Y. Yachi, et al. 2009. Cardiorespiratory fitness as a quantitative predictor of all-cause mortality and cardiovascular events in healthy men and women: A meta-analysis. *Journal of the American Medical Association* 301: 2024-2035.

Kokkinos, P., J. Myers, J.P. Kokkinos, A. Pittaras, P. Narayan, et al. 2008. Exercise capacity and mortality in black and white men. *Circulation* 117: 614-622.

Kujala, U.M., J. Kaprio, S. Sarna, and M. Koskenvuo. 1998. Relationship of leisure-time physical activity and mortality: The Finnish twin cohort. *Journal of the American Medical Association* 279: 440-444.

Kushi, L.H., R.M. Fee, A.R. Folsom, P.J. Mink, K.E. Anderson, and T.A. Sellers. 1997. Physical activity and mortality in postmenopausal women. *Journal of the American Medical Association* 277: 1287-1292.

Lan, T.Y., H.Y. Chang, and T.Y. Tai. 2006. Relationship between components of leisure physical activity and mortality in Taiwanese older adults. *Preventive Medicine* 43: 36-41.

Lee, I.M., C.C. Hsieh, and R.S. Paffenbarger Jr. 1995. Exercise intensity and longevity in men. The Harvard Alumni Health Study. *Journal of the American Medical Association* 273: 1179-1184.

Lee, I.M., and R.S. Paffenbarger Jr. 2000. Associations of light, moderate, and vigorous intensity physical activity and longevity: The Harvard Alumni Health Study. *American Journal of Epidemiology* 151: 293-299.

Lee, I.M., H.D. Sesso, Y. Oguma, and R.S. Paffenbarger Jr. 2004. The "weekend warrior" and risk of mortality. *American Journal of Epidemiology* 160: 636-641.

Lee, I.M., and P.J. Skerrett. 2001. Physical activity and all-cause mortality: What is the dose–response relation? *Medicine and Science in Sports and Exercise* 33 (Suppl. 6): S459-S471.

Lindsted, K.D., S. Tonstad, and J.W. Kuzma. 1991. Self-report of physical activity and patterns of mortality in Seventh-Day Adventist men. *Journal of Clinical Epidemiology* 44: 355-364.

Lollgen, H., A. Bockenhoff, and G. Knapp. 2009. Physical activity and all-cause mortality: An updated meta-analysis with different intensity categories. *International Journal of Sports Medicine* 300: 213-224.

Manini, T.M., J.E. Everhart, K.V. Patel, D.A. Schoeller, L.H. Colbert, et al. 2006. Daily activity energy expenditure and mortality among older adults. *Journal of the American Medical Association* 296: 171-179.

Myers, J., M. Prakash, V. Froelicher, D. Do, S. Partington, and J.E. Atwood. 2002. Exercise capacity and mortality among men referred for exercise testing. *New England Journal of Medicine* 346: 793-801.

Paffenbarger, R.S. Jr., R.T. Hyde, A.L. Wing, and C.C. Hsieh. 1986. Physical activity, all-cause mortality, and longevity of college alumni. *New England Journal of Medicine* 314: 605-613.

Paffenbarger, R.S. Jr., R.T. Hyde, A.L. Wing, I-M. Lee, D.L. Jung, and J.B. Kampert. 1993. The association of changes in physical-activity level and other lifestyle characteristics with mortality among men. *New England Journal of Medicine* 328: 538-545.

Patel, A.V., L. Bernstein, A. Deka, H.S. Feigelson, P.T. Campbell, et al. 2010. Leisure time spent sitting in relation to total mortality in a prospective cohort of US adults. *American Journal of Epidemiology* 172: 419-429.

Perls, T.T., and R.C. Fretts. 1998. Why women live longer than men. *Scientific American,* June.

Physical Activity Guidelines Advisory Committee. 2008. *Physical Activity Guidelines Advisory Committee report.* www.health.gov/paguidelines/.

Rockhill, B., W.C. Willett, J.E. Manson, M.F. Leitzmann, M.J. Stampfer, D.J. Hunter, and G.A. Colditz. 2001. Physical activity and mortality: a prospective study among women. *American Journal of Public Health* 91: 578-83.

Salonen, J.T., P. Puska, and J. Tuomilehto. 1982. Physical activity and risk of myocardial infarction, cerebral stroke and death: A longitudinal study in Eastern Finland. *American Journal of Epidemiology* 115: 526-537.

Slattery, M.L., and D.R. Jacobs Jr. 1988. Physical fitness and cardiovascular disease mortality: The U.S. Railroad Study. *American Journal of Epidemiology* 127: 571-580.

Sui, X., M.J. LaMonte, J.N. Laditka, J.W. Hardin, N. Chase, S.P. Hooker, and S.N. Blair. 2007. Cardiorespiratory fitness and adiposity as mortality predictors in older adults. Journal of the American Medical Association 298: 2507-2516.

Taylor, H.L., E. Klepetar, A. Keys, R.W. Parlin, and H. Blackburn. 1962. Death rates among physically active and sedentary employees of the railroad industry. *American Journal of Public Health* 52: 1697–1707.

Taylor, R.S., A. Brown, S. Ebrahim, J. Jolliffe, H. Noorani, K. Rees, B. Skidmore, J.A. Stone, D.R. Thompson, and N. Oldridge. 2004. Exercise-based rehabilitation for patients with coronary heart disease: Systematic review and meta-analysis of randomized controlled trials. *American Journal of Medicine* 116: 682-692.

Timmons, J.A., S. Knudsen, T. Rankinen, L.G. Koch, M. Sarzynski, et al. 2010. Using molecular classification to predict gains in maximal aerobic capacity following endurance exercise training in humans. *Journal of Applied Physiology* 108: 1487-1496.

United Nations, Department of Economic and Social Affairs, Population Division. 2007. *World population prospects: The 2006 revision, highlights.* Working Paper No. ESA/P/WP.202. New York: United Nations.

U.S. Department of Health and Human Services. 2008. *2008 Physical activity guidelines for Americans.* www.health.gov/paguidelines/.

Villeneuve, P.J., H.I. Morrison, C.L. Craig, and D.E. Schaubel. 1998. Physical activity, physical fitness, and risk of dying. *Epidemiology* 9: 626-631.

Wei, M., J.B. Kampert, C.E. Barlow, M.Z. Nichaman, L.W. Gibbons, et al. 1999. Relationship between low cardiorespiratory fitness and mortality in normal-weight, overweight, and obese men. *Journal of the American Medical Association* 282: 1547-1553.

Weller, I., and P. Corey. 1998. The impact of excluding non-leisure energy expenditure on the relation between physical activity and mortality in women. *Epidemiology* 9: 632-635.

Wen, C.P., J.P.M. Wai, M.K. Tsai, Y.C. Yang, T.Y.D. Cheng, M.-C. Lee, T.C. Hui, K.T. Chwen, S.P. Tsai, and X. Wu. 2011. Minimum amount of physical activity for reduced mortality and extended life expectancy: a prospective cohort study. *Lancet* 378: 1244-1253.

Woodcock J., O.H. Franco, N. Orsini, and I. Roberts. 2011. Nonvigorous physical activity and all-cause mortality: systematic review and meta-analysis of cohort studies. *International Journal of Epidemiology* 40: 121-138.

CHAPTER 5

Coronary
Heart Disease

With respect to the treatment of this complaint (angina pectoris) . . .
I knew one who set himself a task of sawing wood for half an hour
every day, and was nearly cured.

• William Heberden, 1818 •

CHAPTER OBJECTIVES

▸ Describe the public health burden of coronary heart disease, including its prevalence, trends, and major risk factors

▸ Discuss the pathophysiology of coronary heart disease

▸ Review epidemiologic evidence that physical activity reduces the risk of developing coronary heart disease

▸ Summarize data from studies investigating how much physical activity is needed to reduce the risk of developing coronary heart disease

▸ Review epidemiologic evidence that physical fitness reduces the risk of developing coronary heart disease

▸ Discuss and evaluate the strength of the evidence to examine whether the observed associations between physical activity and coronary heart disease are real and likely to be causal in nature

While coronary heart disease (CHD) has traditionally been viewed as a disease of high-income countries, there is increasing realization today that chronic, noncommunicable diseases—of which CHD is a major component—are important health problems also in low- and middle-income countries (Strong et al. 2005). Indeed, because the population of the low- and middle-income countries is larger than that of the high-income countries, the absolute number of deaths due to CHD in low-income countries, where CHD is not the leading cause of death, exceeds that in high-income countries, where it is the leading cause of death. In this chapter, we examine the relation of CHD with physical inactivity, a major risk factor for the development of the disease.

History and Magnitude of the Problem

The recorded history of CHD dates to around AD 150, when Galen wrote about dyscrasias of the heart (an abnormal condition of the body attributed to materials affecting blood cells). In 1628, the British physician William Harvey explained that blood was pumped by the heart in a circuit. He was the first to describe a myocardial infarction (heart attack). A century later, in 1768, William Heberden coined the term **angina pectoris** to refer to the chest pain resulting from inadequate circulation of blood to the heart. Soon afterward, the English surgeon John Hunter discovered coronary artery disease (another term for CHD) while conducting an autopsy of a patient who had apparently died in an angry rage. Ironically, Hunter died about 20 years later of a heart attack, reportedly enraged after an acrimonious meeting. In 1912 an American physician, James Harrick, speculated that CHD resulted from a hardening of the arteries that supply blood to the heart.

Today CHD represents a major public health problem worldwide. According to the National Heart, Lung, and Blood Institute (1998), heart disease (i.e., CHD, hypertensive heart disease, and rheumatic heart disease) has been the number-one cause of death in the United States since the early 1920s. However, mortality from heart disease in the United States dropped by 59% from 1950 to 1999, and by 36% between 1996 and 2006 (Lloyd-Jones et al. 2010). Worldwide, the annual rates of heart attack and coronary death in middle to early old age (35 to 64 years) also have dropped in both men (a 2.7% decline) and women (a 2.1% decline) since the 1980s (Tunstall-Pedoe et al. 1999). These U.S. and worldwide trends probably occurred because of reduced cigarette smoking by adults, better medication for hypertension, greater public awareness about the importance of a healthy diet, and better medical treatment for heart attacks.

▷ **MORTALITY FROM** heart disease in the United States dropped by 59% from 1950 to 1999, and by 36% between 1996 and 2006. Nonetheless, CHD remains the number-one cause of death in the United States, costing an estimated $177 billion in 2010, more than one-third of the costs of all cardiovascular diseases.

Currently, an estimated 17.6 million persons aged 20 years and older in the United States have CHD (Lloyd-Jones et al. 2010). The annual incidence of acute myocardial infarction (MI; a major manifestation of CHD), both first and recurrent attacks, is about 935,000, and the annual number of CHD deaths is about 425,000. It is estimated that approximately every 25 s, an American will suffer a coronary event and that approximately every minute, one American will die from such an event. Coronary heart disease accounts for over 50% of cardiovascular deaths and 1 of 6 deaths each year in the United States. About half of American men and a third of American women will develop CHD. The average age at first MI for men is about 65 years; for women, it's 70 years. Compared with men, women are protected from CHD before menopause. The economic burden of CHD in the United States also has been high during the past several years, accounting for an estimated $177 billion in 2010, or more than one-third of the annual cost of all cardiovascular diseases. Coronary heart disease is a major contributor to disability and lost productivity.

▷ **THE ANNUAL** incidence of acute MI is about 935,000, and the average annual number of cardiac deaths is about 425,000. It is estimated that approximately every 25 s, an American will suffer a coronary event and that approximately every minute, one American will die from such an event.

Coronary Heart Disease Risk Factors

The major risk factors for CHD include genetic susceptibility, male sex, age, elevated serum cholesterol, low levels of high-density lipoprotein cholesterol, cigarette smoking, high blood pressure, obesity, diabetes mellitus, and physical inactivity. Major risk factors that are modifiable by physical activity (e.g., hypertension, dyslipidemia, obesity, and diabetes) are described in more detail in chapters 7 through 10 of this book.

In addition, inflammation, abnormalities in regulatory proteins of the hemostatic system (which control blood clotting mechanisms), and possibly elevated homocysteine (which is associated with vascular injury) appear to directly contribute to the pathogenesis of CHD. These are discussed in the following section, which describes the etiology of CHD.

· WEB RESOURCES ·

www.heart.org/HEARTORG/GettingHealthy/PhysicalActivity/Physical-Activity_ UCM_001080_SubHomePage.jsp. This website provides information on physical activity and heart health from the American Heart Association.

www.health.gov/paguidelines. This site provides access to the federal government's (U.S. Department of Health and Human Services) physical activity guidelines and the scientific basis for these guidelines.

Major Modifiable Risk Factors for Coronary Heart Disease

- Tobacco smoke
- High blood cholesterol
- High blood pressure
- Physical inactivity
- Diabetes mellitus
- Obesity
- Stress
- High triglycerides
- Alcohol abuse (moderate use, one to two drinks a day, reduces risk)

American Heart Association 2010 (Lloyd-Jones et al. 2010).

Coronary Heart Disease Etiology

The process that leads to CHD and ischemic stroke is **atherosclerosis,** which is a form of **arteriosclerosis** (i.e., hardening of an artery) characterized by fatty deposits called **atheromas** (from the Greek words *athere,* meaning "gruel," and *oma,* meaning "tumor"), which contribute to narrowing and obstruction of medium and large arteries.

Plaques (large, more solid atheromas) vary in size and shape. They may protrude into the lumen (interior diameter) of a coronary artery but often extend into the artery wall, making them difficult to detect by common clinical tests such as **angiography.** Though vessel occlusion (blockage) by large plaques is the main cause of angina pectoris, smaller plaques covered by scar tissue are more apt to rupture and release cholesterol into the blood, triggering **thrombosis** (clot formation) and increasing the risks of **ischemia,** heart attack, and injury to or death of myocardial cells downstream from the occluded region of the vessel.

The atherosclerotic process in coronary arteries begins in childhood. Its severity is related to the level of blood cholesterol and its **lipoprotein** constituents. Low-density lipoprotein (LDL) cholesterol accelerates atherosclerosis, while high-density lipoprotein (HDL) cholesterol retards it. Cigarette smoking, high blood pressure, and dietary intake of **saturated fat** and cholesterol also contribute to atherosclerosis. In contrast, physical activity retards the atherosclerotic process, in part through its beneficial effects on LDL and HDL levels and blood pressure.

Atherogenesis

The process of atherogenesis begins with a lesion of the **intima** (the innermost lining) of a coronary artery. The lesion results from tissue injury to cells of the **endothelium,** which can be physical damage from lipoprotein levels or chemical damage from tobacco smoke. The initial response to the injury (figure 5.1*a*) involves several interactions between circulating blood platelets and arterial endothelial cells. Platelets adhere to connective tissue at the site of injury, which activates fibrinogen (figure 5.1*b*); fibrinogen increases platelet aggregation and releases platelet-derived growth factor, which is **chemotactic** for smooth muscle, and **fibroblasts** (the most common cells of connective tissue); smooth muscle and fibroblasts proliferate into the arterial intima and lead to plaque formation (figure 5.1*c* and *d*).

Renegade Low-Density Lipoprotein

Contributing to the atheromas in response to endothelial injury are abnormal molecules of LDL that have become free radicals after **oxidation** (i.e., $LDL + O_2$). A **free radical** is an atom or group of atoms that transiently exists in an unstable state by carrying an unpaired electron until an electron can be stolen from another atom. When oxygen loses an electron from one of its four pairs during normal metabolism, it becomes a free radical. Hence, oxidation occurs when another element becomes a free radical by losing an electron as it combines with oxygen. Oxidation of LDL in the atheromas can lead to disintegration of a cell after damaging the cell membrane.

Oxidized LDL stimulates secretion of monocyte chemoattractant protein-1 (MCP-1), which results in a fatal attraction for immune cells known as **macrophages,** already drawn to the arterial lesion to ingest the debris of injured endothelial

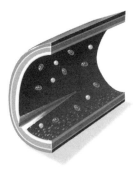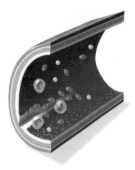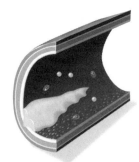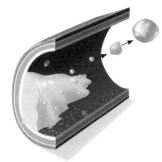

a A blood-borne irritant injures the arterial wall, disrupting the endothelial layer and exposing the underlying connective tissue.

b Blood platelets and circulating immune cells known as monocytes are then attracted to the site of the injury and adhere to the exposed connective tissue. The platelets release a substance referred to as platelet-derived growth factor (PDGF) that promotes migration of smooth muscle cells from the media to the intima.

c A plaque, which is basically composed of smooth muscle cells, connective tissue, and debris, forms at the site of injury.

d As the plaque grows, it narrows the arterial opening and impedes blood flow. Lipids in the blood, specifically low-density lipoprotein cholesterol (LDL-C), are deposited in the plaque.

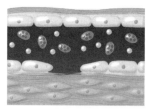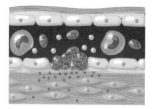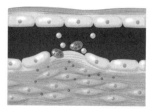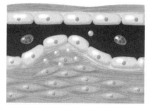

Figure 5.1   Process of atherogenesis.

Reprinted, by permission, from L. Kenney, J. Wilmore, and D. Costill, 2012, *Physiology of sport and exercise*, 5th ed. (Champaign, IL: Human Kinetics). 528.

cells. In this way, the renegade LDL leads to foam-filled macrophages on the endothelium, which contribute to the growing atheroma; this in turn can eventually block arteries or contribute to a coronary thrombosis. Oxidized LDL is also **cytotoxic** to endothelial cells and thus adds to cell injury. Smoking increases renegade LDL, but beta-carotene (vitamin A) and vitamin E are antioxidants. Observational epidemiologic studies have shown that diets rich in antioxidants are associated with lower rates of CHD, although randomized controlled trials of single antioxidant vitamins have not been shown to protect against the development of CHD. Antioxidants can give up electrons to free radicals without becoming free radicals themselves. Monounsaturated fats, such as olive oil, also prevent LDL from becoming a free radical.

Inflammation

An emerging body of evidence from laboratory, case–control, and prospective clinical studies during the past decade has shown that atherosclerotic disease involves inflammatory processes (Libby, Ridker, and Maseri 2002) as well as macrophages, as discussed earlier. Major risk factors for cardiovascular disease (CVD), including dyslipidemia, hypertension, diabetes, and obesity, all have pro-

inflammatory features, as do bacterial and viral infection. Inflammation also appears to play a role in acute coronary events, such as cardiac sudden death resulting from thrombosis (Rifai and Ridker 2002). Prospective epidemiologic studies in both men and women have reported that increased risk of CVD (CHD and stroke) is associated with elevated levels of cytokines involved with regulation of the acute-phase response to infection and acute-phase markers such as fibrinogen and **C-reactive protein** produced by the liver. Most evidence thus far has focused on C-reactive protein because it is easily measured, has a long half-life (making it stable in the blood over time), and influences several inflammatory responses that plausibly affect the progression of atherosclerosis, including uptake of LDL by macrophages, attraction of **monocytes** to the endothelium of arteries, and production of MCP-1 (Libby, Ridker, and Maseri 2002). Several prospective cohort studies have shown that men and women who have high levels of C-reactive protein, a marker of low-grade inflammation, have approximately 2.5 to 4.5 times the risk of developing CVD as people with low or normal levels (Albert et al. 2002; Libby, Ridker, and Maseri 2002). And, a recent randomized clinical trial testing a statin drug, rosuvastatin, in healthy men and women with normal LDL cholesterol levels but elevated C-reactive protein showed that the drug lowered both LDL cholesterol (by 50%) and C-reactive protein levels (by 37%), and resulted in a 44% reduction in the occurrence of a first cardiovascular event (Ridker et al. 2008). Other markers of inflammation, including white blood cell counts and fibrinogen, have also been associated with the development of CHD (Folsom et al. 2002). Finally, several treatment strategies currently used to prevent CHD, including diet, smoking cessation, aspirin, cholesterol-lowering statin drugs, and physical activity, also have anti-inflammatory effects that may explain part of their benefits. The anti-inflammatory effect of physical activity may be mediated through beneficial changes in body weight. The basic immunology of infection and inflammation and the acute inflammatory response to exercise are discussed in chapter 13.

> ▶ **AN EMERGING** body of evidence from laboratory, case–control, and prospective clinical studies during the past decade has shown that atherosclerotic disease involves inflammatory processes. The anti-inflammatory effect of physical activity may be mediated through beneficial changes in body weight.

Hemostasis

Studies have shown that hemostatic factors (i.e., factors that regulate blood clotting) are risk factors for CVD. Principal factors that affect **hemostasis** include blood **viscosity,** coagulation factors, platelet aggregability or stickiness, fibrinogenesis, and fibrinolysis. Coagulation or clotting of blood involves platelet aggregation and fibrinogenesis. Platelet stickiness is increased in the morning and by hormones such as adrenaline and noradrenaline, and is reduced by aspirin, ethanol, and flavonoids (chemicals such as resveratrol found in the skin of red grapes).

Platelet aggregation is catalyzed by **fibrinogenesis,** which involves the conversion of the blood protein fibrinogen to **fibrin** in the presence of calcium by the hydrolytic **protease** enzyme **thrombin.** Normally, that process is opposed by **fibrinolysis,** which is the hydrolysis of fibrin by the enzyme **plasmin.** Plasmin is formed in the blood from **plasminogen** by **tissue-type plasminogen activator (tPA),** which is released from endothelial cells in blood vessels or by drugs such as streptokinase and **trypsin.** A major contributor to impaired fibrinolysis is a high blood level of plasminogen activator inhibitor-1 (PAI-1), which also is released by blood vessel endothelial cells and inhibits tPA.

Results from the Framingham Heart Study have shown that blood **hematocrit,** the percentage of blood volume occupied by cells, is a risk factor for CVD. High hematocrit is associated with increased blood thickness and **coagulability;** these characteristics increase the contact between platelets and endothelial cells, which can promote aggregation.

The concentration of fibrinogen in the blood also is a risk factor for heart attack and stroke. The cumulative results from 13 prospective, five cross-sectional, and four case–control population-based studies done in several nations between 1984 and 1998 indicated that a high level of fibrinogen in blood plasma doubles the risk of developing CVD (when the upper tertile was compared with the lowest) and increases recurrent MI and ischemic stroke by 8%, independently of overall CVD risk status, smoking, and age (Maresca et al. 1999).

Low fibrinogen offers some protection against MI or sudden cardiac death in people who report angina even if they have high serum cholesterol. In contrast, studies have found that high PAI-1 is a risk factor for first heart attack or stroke, a recurrent heart attack among heart attack survivors, and cardiac death among people reporting angina. Beneficial effects of physical activity on hemostatic factors may be one of the pathways through which physical activity decreases the risk of developing CVD.

> ▶ **BLOOD CLOTTING** factors such as fibrinogen and plasminogen activator inhibitor-1 are associated with increased risk of ischemic heart attack and stroke. People who are physically active tend to have lower levels of such clotting factors.

Homocysteine

Elevated levels of **homocysteine** in the blood are associated with a higher risk of developing CVD, although whether this link is causal is unclear (Homocysteine Studies Collaboration 2002). Homocysteine, a natural intermediate amino acid, is formed during the metabolism of an essential amino acid, methionine. The homocysteine hypothesis of CVD is credited to physician Kilmer McCully (1969), who observed that children with the genetic condition **homocystinuria** (which leads to abnormally high levels of homocysteine because of deficiencies in metabolic enzymes) usually died from arteriosclerosis at an early age.

A high blood level of homocysteine is associated with buildups of collagen and calcium, degeneration of elastin, and endothelial cell damage in the lumen of coronary arteries, each of which contributes to the formation of atherosclerotic plaques. The leading hypothesis is that homocysteine damages endothelial cells by producing hydrogen peroxide, which then results in the atherosclerotic cascade of platelet aggregation and blood clotting, leading to arterial occlusion.

A meta-analysis examining the association of blood homocysteine levels with risk of CHD showed a weaker association in prospective cohort studies, where findings are less likely to be biased, than in case–control studies, where disease may have altered homocysteine levels. The cumulative results from 12 prospective cohort studies showed that the adjusted odds ratio for CHD associated with a 25% lower homocysteine was 0.83 (95% confidence interval, CI: 0.77-0.89); from 13 case–control studies using population controls, it was 0.67 (0.62-0.71) (Homocysteine Studies Collaboration 2002).

While these observational epidemiologic studies have suggested lower risks of CHD with lower homocysteine levels, a recent randomized clinical trial testing a combination pill containing folic acid, vitamin B_6, and vitamin B_{12}, which help break down homocysteine in the body, showed no effect of this pill on CVD among >5000 women at high risk of CVD (either because they had a history of CVD or because they had at least three CVD risk factors), despite significant lowering of blood homocysteine. After an average follow-up of more than seven years, the relative risk for CVD for women assigned to the combination pill versus placebo was 1.03 (0.90-1.19) (Albert et al. 2008). Thus, the American Heart Association does not recommend widespread use of folic acid and B vitamin supplements to reduce the risk of CVD; however, it does recommend getting a daily diet containing sufficient folic acid and vitamins B_6 and B_{12}.

Reducing dietary intake of protein and increasing intake of B vitamins are the frontline preventive treatments for moderate elevations in homocysteine. Other factors believed to increase the risk of high homocysteine levels include age, male sex, environmental toxins, high blood cholesterol, and lack of physical activity.

Physical Activity and Coronary Heart Disease

In 1802, Scottish physician William Heberden reported that a patient of his was nearly cured of his angina pectoris after "sawing wood for half an hour every day" (Heberden 1818). Physical inactivity is recognized by the American Heart Association (Fletcher et al. 1996), the U.S. federal government, the International Society and Federation of Cardiology, and the World Health Organization (Bijnen, Caspersen, and Mosterd 1994) as a major independent risk factor for CHD. The following sections describe early studies on the association between occupational activity and CHD risk, followed by discussion of early, as well as more recent, case–control and retrospective and prospective cohort studies on the association of leisure-time physical activity and CHD risk.

▷ **THE DATA** indicate that on average, physical activity during middle age cuts the risk of CHD by 30% to 40% for both men and women.

In a recent review by the 2008 Physical Activity Guidelines Advisory Committee (an expert panel appointed by the federal government) of the cumulative evidence from more than 60 studies published after 1996, the committee concluded that more active men and women have lower rates of CHD than less active persons (Physical Activity Guidelines Advisory Committee 2008). The data from prospective cohort studies indicate that on average, physical

activity during middle age cuts the risk of CHD by 30% to 40% for both men and women.

Occupational Activity and Coronary Heart Disease Risk

British epidemiologist Jeremy Morris began the modern study of exercise and heart disease with his hallmark hypothesis that physical activity protects against CHD, testing this hypothesis in pioneering research on London transport workers and other occupational groups in the 1950s (Morris et al. 1953).

▷ **IN THE** early 1950s, British physician and epidemiologist Jeremy Morris hypothesized that physical activity was protective against CHD.

London Bus Conductors

The first study by Morris showed that the physically active conductors on London's double-decker buses were at lower risk of CHD than the drivers, who sat through their shifts at a steering wheel. Among conductors who did develop CHD, the disease was also less severe and occurred at later ages. Morris later reported the similar observation that postmen delivering mail on foot had lower rates of CHD than sedentary office clerks and telephone operators. Subsequent studies were conducted to investigate other explanations for those initial observations. Blood pressure levels were lower in the conductors, but among men with the same blood pressure level, the conductors still had less heart disease than the drivers. Bus drivers also were more obese, but among men of similar body mass, the rate of sudden coronary death continued to be higher in the drivers than in the conductors.

San Francisco Longshoremen

In the United States, Ralph Paffenbarger Jr. and W.E. Hale (1975; Paffenbarger et al. 1977) tracked over 6300 San Francisco longshoremen (dock workers), aged 35 to 74 years, for 22 years or until death or age 75. Physical activity of the men was classified according to job title, and job switches were checked annually. Cargo handlers who loaded and unloaded ships were classified as more physically active than foremen and clerks. Union rules required all workers to serve at least their first five years as cargo handlers (the average was 13 years), which helped control for self-selection of unfit men into the easy jobs.

The death rate from CHD expressed per 10,000 person-years of work among men who expended at least 8500 kcal each week, estimated from occupational activity, was about half that of less active men. Their rate of sudden cardiac death was nearly two-thirds lower. After adjustments for cigarette smoking, systolic blood pressure, body weight, and glucose tolerance, those relative rate reductions were smaller but remained different (figure 5.2).

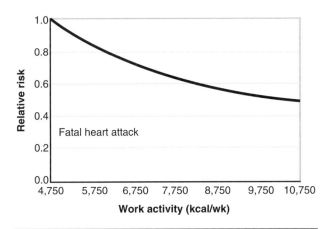

Figure 5.2 The San Francisco Longshoremen Study shows that the death rate from coronary heart disease, expressed per 10,000 man-years of work, among men who expended at least 8500 kcal each week was about half that of less active men.

Reprinted, by permission, from G. Thomas et al., 1981, *Exercise and health: The evidence and the implications* (Cambridge, MA: Oelgeschlager, Gunn, and Hain).

Other Studies of Occupational Activity

In addition to the classic studies just described, studies have compared incidence and prevalence rates of CHD among men performing jobs that required different levels of physical activity, including railroad workers, farmers, employees of utility companies, civil servants, police officers, and firefighters. Generally, these studies showed that physically active workers had one-third to three-fourths fewer total or fatal CHD events than the least-active workers.

However, studies of occupational physical activity, estimated based on job classifications, are difficult to interpret. This is so because the actual energy expenditure of people having the same job title can differ widely; also, it is hard to keep track of people who switch jobs after the study begins. Railroad switchmen had a lower rate of CHD than clerks and executives in one study (Taylor et al. 1962), but the apparently protective effect of physical activity might have been explained by job transfers by sicker workers from more active to inactive jobs. Studies of civil service employees in Los Angeles (Chapman and Massey 1964) and employees of several public utility companies (Hinkle et al. 1968; Mortensen, Stevensen, and Whitney 1959; Paul et al. 1963) showed no association between CHD events and physical activity on the job. The reason could have been that most of the jobs at the utility company required a similar, low level of energy expenditure. Further, the leisure-time physical activity of workers was not measured. People who have sedentary jobs might be very active in their leisure, just as laborers might choose to be sedentary during leisure time.

To add to the challenge of interpreting the findings of the early studies on occupational activity and CHD risk, many studies did not adjust for differences in other CHD risk factors, such as smoking and dietary habits, between workers with different occupational activity levels. For example, in Finland, vigorously active lumberjacks had a higher rate of mortality from CHD and greater frequency of abnormal electrocardiograms than did less active farmers from the same region (Punsar and Karvonen 1976). However, the lumberjacks smoked more, consumed more saturated fat, and had lower socioeconomic status than the farmers. The high prevalence of these other risk factors may have offset the potential protective effect of the high daily energy expenditure of lumberjack work. In another study of Iowa men 20 to 64 years of age, farmers had 10% less CHD and total mortality than nonfarmers (Pomrehn, Wallace, and Burmeister 1982). However, although the Iowa farmers were twice as physically active and more physically fit, they also used less tobacco and alcohol, which might have accounted for their better health. Farmers in studies conducted in Georgia (Cassell et al. 1971) and North Dakota (Zukel et al. 1959) also smoked less than nonfarmers, which precludes a definitive conclusion that their higher physical activity was an independent explanation for their lower rate of heart disease.

A retrospective cohort study of Israeli workers in kibbutzim (communal settlements) was better able to control for other risk factors that may have confounded the physical activity–heart disease association (Brunner et al. 1974). Individuals in this study were of similar ethnic origin, lived in the same environment, consumed a common diet, and had the same access to medical care. Nearly 5300 men and over 5200 women ages 40 to 64 years were classified as either sedentary or active based on the portion of the workday that they spent in manual labor or sitting. The active and sedentary groups had similar body weights and serum cholesterol and triglyceride levels. Thus, these factors cannot explain the observation of relative risks for nonfatal and fatal heart attacks over a 15-year period being 2.5 times higher among sedentary men and three times higher in sedentary women.

Leisure-Time Physical Activity and Coronary Heart Disease Risk

Nearly all of the studies published before 1978 measured only occupational physical activity based on job descriptions. Occupational physical activity decreased precipitously in Western developed nations during the late 1950s to early 1960s as industry moved from manual to mechanized labor. As a result, more attention was directed at understanding whether physical activity in leisure time could reduce CHD risk. In general, the findings from studies of leisure-time physical activity and CHD risk have been consistent in showing an inverse relation between physical activity and CHD risk. In the following sections, we briefly describe exemplar case–control and retrospective cohort studies, followed by more detailed discussions of the more methodologically sound prospective cohort studies.

Case–Control Studies

Though scientifically a weaker study design than prospective cohort studies, case–control and retrospective cohort studies typically cost less to conduct. Promising findings from such studies provided justification for the more costly prospective studies that followed. Case–control studies remain useful today for providing preliminary evidence about new hypotheses that can later be better examined by prospective cohort studies.

The Netherlands

In this case–control study, nearly 500 heart attack victims in Holland, or their immediate relatives, and 800 controls from the same communities were interviewed about their past physical activity habits (Magnus, Matroos, and Stracklee 1979). A significant inverse association was found between heart attack and habitual (defined as more than eight months per year) walking, cycling, and gardening, but not if those activities were performed only sporadically or seasonally (four to eight months per year). Vigorous exercise was not associated with any further risk reduction compared with moderate activities.

King County, Washington

For this study, leisure-time physical activity during the past year of 163 people who had suffered primary cardiac arrest and an equal number of matched controls ages 25 to 75 who lived in Seattle and suburban King County, Washington, was estimated by interviews with the spouses of cases and controls (Siscovick et al. 1982). The risk of cardiac arrest was 55% to 65% lower for men and women in the two upper quartiles of high-intensity physical activity compared with those who had not engaged in any high-intensity physical activity (figure 5.3).

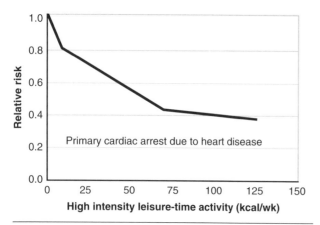

Figure 5.3 The King County, Washington, residents study shows the relative risk of primary cardiac arrest due to heart disease versus high-intensity leisure-time activity.

Reprinted, by permission, from K.E. Powell, 1988, Habitual exercise and public health: An epidemiological view. In *Exercise adherence: Its impact on public health,* edited by R.K. Dishman (Champaign, IL: Human Kinetics), 30.

Retrospective Cohort Study: Health Insurance Plan of New York.

One of the first population studies to assess both leisure-time and occupational physical activity was a retrospective study of 55,000 men ages 25 to 64 years enrolled in the Health Insurance Plan of New York (Shapiro et al. 1969). On-the-job and leisure-time physical activities were assessed by a questionnaire and interviews with the insured or his widow. Subjects' activity levels were classified as light, moderate, or heavy. Considerations were made for time spent walking and sitting at work, transportation to and from work, total working hours, and time spent lifting and carrying objects. The incidence of MI in both the heavy- and moderate-activity groups was about half that of the light-activity group; furthermore, the least-active men had a 4.5 times greater mortality rate following MI than the most active men. The reductions in risk for MI and death after MI were independent of body mass and smoking.

Prospective Cohort Studies

In the past 30 years, a number of prospective cohort studies conducted in Europe and the United States have evaluated the association between leisure-time physical activity and CHD risk. These studies were generally designed to follow representative samples of initially healthy people living in different geographic regions or samples from selected groups, such as Harvard alumni or British civil servants, for extended periods to determine what factors, including physical activity, were associated with the risk of developing CHD. While early studies tended to include primarily men, many studies published after 1996 also included women (Physical Activity Guidelines Advisory Committee 2008). While the results of most, but not all, of these studies show that leisure-time physical activity is inversely associated with CHD morbidity or mortality, the overall data clearly show higher levels of physical activity to be associated with lower CHD rates. A meta-analysis that included 26 studies, enrolling 513,472 subjects who experienced 20,666 CHD events, reported that the relative risk of CHD associated with a moderate, compared with a low, level of leisure-time physical activity was 0.88 (95% CI: 0.83-0.93) (Sofi et al. 2008). For high compared with low level of leisure-time physical activity, the relative risk was 0.73 (0.66-0.80). And, another meta-analysis that quantitatively analyzed the relation reported that individuals who engaged in the equivalent of 150 min/week of moderate-intensity leisure-time physical activity (i.e., meeting current U.S. guidelines) had a 14% lower risk (relative risk, 0.86 [0.77-0.96]) compared with those reporting no leisure-time physical activity, while those engaging in twice that amount (the equivalent of 300 min/week) had a 20% lower risk (relative risk, 0.80 [0.74-0.88]) (Sattelmair et al. 2011). In the next sections we provide details for several representative studies.

British Civil Servants

The prospective cohort studies of British civil servants represent some of the classic studies conducted on physical activity and CHD risk. In an initial investigation, Morris and colleagues studied about 18,000 middle-aged executive-level British civil servants who were apparently without CHD and had sedentary desk jobs (Morris et al. 1973, 1980). The men were asked to complete a detailed record of their physical activity during a Friday and Saturday. The activity records were used to classify the men as vigorous exercisers or nonvigorous exercisers.

Vigorous exercise was defined as exercise at an intensity of at least 7.5 kcal/min (a level common in heavy industrial work) and included sports, swimming, jogging, rapid walking, hiking, hill climbing, or heavy work around the home. About 20% of the men in the study were classified as vigorous exercisers. Vigorous exercisers reported participating in at least 5 min per day of sports or recreational activities at or above that intensity, or at least 30 min of heavy chores such as digging in the garden. The men were then observed for an average of 8.5 years, providing 150,000 person-years of exposure. During that period, 475 men died from CHD. The rate of CHD death was more than twice as high in the nonvigorous group (2.9%) as in the vigorous group (1.1%), a relative risk of about 2.6. Aerobic exercise (e.g., swimming, brisk walking, and cycling) was associated with lower incidence of CHD, but no association was observed with time spent in leisure gardening and household chores.

Adjustments between the active and less active men for differences in a wide range of risk factors did not eliminate the main finding that participation in vigorous exercise was inversely related to CHD death. Contrary to expectation, the prevalence of heart attack was not lower among people with higher overall leisure-time activity. However, Morris reported a smaller increase with age in both fatal and nonfatal first attacks in the men who reported more exercise, which was persistent across the period of observation, eliminating the possibility that the low physical activity resulted from illness.

Morris and colleagues (1980) also demonstrated that the incidence rates of CHD were low only among men who were active recently or currently. High rates of CHD were found among those who had stopped participating in moderate leisure activity from five to over 40 years before the study was conducted. Also, men who played vigorous sports at the time they were questioned had the same low incidence of CHD during follow-up whether or not they had been physically active during the years preceding the study.

In a further investigation, Morris and colleagues (1990) studied over 9000 male British civil servants, ages 45 to 64 years, who recalled their physical activity during the preceding month. After 87,500 person-years of observation over a nine-year period, 272 men had died from CHD. Another 202 men had had nonfatal heart attacks. The rate of CHD events was significantly lower among men who had been classified as vigorous aerobic exercisers. Other physical activities were not associated with either heart attack or CHD death. Lower-intensity aerobic activities were associated with lower CHD rates for the older men (55 to 64 years at the start of the study), suggesting that dose response varies with age.

Harvard Alumni Health Study

This represents another classic study of physical activity and CHD risk. In an early investigation of about 17,000 male alumni of Harvard University who were mainly employed in sedentary occupations or retired, alumni reported their physical activities on mailed questionnaires (Paffenbarger, Wing, and Hyde 1978). The age-adjusted incidence rate of CHD was inversely related to the energy expended on walking, stair climbing, and playing sports and to the composite energy expenditure on all these activities in kilocalories per week. Men expending fewer than 2000 kcal per week were at a 64% higher risk than their former classmates who were less active (figure 5.4). Coronary heart disease risk decreased about 10% more when the energy expenditure occurred in vigorous sports rather than in walking or climbing stairs. The inverse association between risk of CHD and level of physical activity remained strong when adjustments were made for other risk factors, including cigarette smoking, hypertension, diabetes mellitus, obesity, and parental history of heart attack. Another important finding from the study was that alumni who had been athletes during college but did not continue exercising were at greater risk for CHD than physically active alumni who had not been college athletes. That is, only contemporary physical activity, not prior athletic history in college, was associated with reduced CHD events—an observation similar to that made by Morris in the British civil servants. Hence, the protective effects of

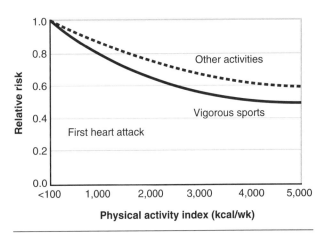

Figure 5.4 The Harvard Alumni Health Study shows the relative risk of first heart attack versus physical activity index.

Reprinted, by permission, from K.E. Powell, 1988, Habitual exercise and public health: An epidemiological view. In *Exercise adherence: Its impact on public health*, edited by R.K. Dishman (Champaign, IL: Human Kinetics), 30.

exercise appear to be independent of constitutional factors that would favor success in youth athletics and that might be expected to retard disease in later years.

> ▷ **MALE HARVARD** alumni who had been athletes during college and did not continue exercising were at greater risk for CHD than physically active alumni who had not been college athletes. Only contemporary physical activity, not prior athletic history in college, was associated with reduced CHD events.

Follow-up of these alumni (Lee, Sesso, and Paffenbarger 2000; Sesso, Paffenbarger, and Lee 2000) confirmed lower rates of CHD among men who were physically active in middle age, compared with less active men, even after accounting for differences in other health characteristics including smoking, alcohol intake, diet, use of vitamin/mineral supplements, hypertension, diabetes, and early parental death. For example, in an analysis that compared men expending <1000, 1000 to 1999, 2000 to 2999, 3000 to 3999, and ≥4000 kcal/week, the multivariate relative risks for CHD were 1.00 (referent), 0.80 (95% CI: 0.57-1.12), 0.80 (0.55-1.18), 0.74 (0.47-1.17), and 0.62 (0.41-0.96), respectively; p, trend = 0.046 (Lee, Sesso, and Paffenbarger 2000).

The Harvard cohort has provided some of the most well-controlled and long-term data for examining the association between leisure physical activity and risk of chronic diseases, including specific cancers, diabetes, depression, and CVD. Perhaps the most valuable of Dr. Paffenbarger's contributions was the observation of persistent dose–response relationships, indicating optimal reductions in CHD morbidity and mortality at around 2000 kcal of leisure physical activity per week.

> ▷ **THE WELL-CONTROLLED** Harvard Alumni Health Study has consistently shown a dose–response relationship between leisure physical activity and reduced risk of CHD morbidity and mortality, with an optimal weekly expenditure of about 2000 kcal in leisure physical activity.

Framingham Heart Study

In the Framingham Heart Study—a follow-up study of 1909 men and 2311 women who lived in Framingham, Massachusetts—a statistically significant inverse relationship was found between an index of overall job and leisure-time physical activity determined by a questionnaire and 14-year CHD mortality in men, but not women (Kannel and Sorlie 1979). The relative risk of developing CHD for the least-active men 45 to 64 years of age compared with the most active was small (1.3) but statistically significant (figure 5.5). One possible explanation for the lack of an association seen in women is that the physical activity questionnaire may not have captured physical activity well in women, since women of that era tended to do few leisure-time activities.

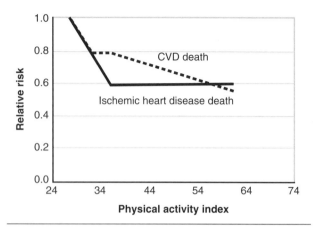

Figure 5.5 The Framingham Heart Study (men only) shows the relative risk of death due to cardiovascular disease versus physical activity index.

Reprinted, by permission, from K.E. Powell, 1988, Habitual exercise and public health: An epidemiological view. In *Exercise adherence: Its impact on public health*, edited by R.K. Dishman (Champaign, IL: Human Kinetics), 30.

Seven Countries Study

The Seven Countries Study involved 16 cohorts of men in seven countries who were 40 through 59 years old at the start of the study (Keys 1980). Differences between 10-year CHD incidence and mortality rates among populations were unrelated to the proportion of sedentary men in the population. Other risk factors, particularly serum cholesterol levels and dietary intake of saturated fat, appeared to better explain the differences in CHD rates among countries. In only three of the seven countries there was an inverse association between physical activity (mostly occupational) and CHD; and in the others, there was no association. For example, in Finland, the country with the highest CHD incidence and mortality, the 10-year follow-up revealed no difference in CHD mortality between men classified as sedentary and the most active men. However, relatively few men were classified as sedentary in the Finnish cohorts.

Finnish Cohorts

Karvonen (1982) followed the two Finnish cohorts in the Seven Countries Study for an additional five years and reassessed the original 10-year data after studying in greater detail the men's physical activity habits through use of an extensive structured interview. Reevaluation of the original 10-year data revealed that, for men ages 50 to 69 years, higher CHD incidence was clearly associated with sedentary habits. Subsequent five-year CHD mortality and combined fatal and nonfatal MI rates in this age group also were inversely related to physical activity status; however, the majority of men who died of CHD had already been diagnosed with CHD before the five-year follow-up (i.e., in the first 10 years). Thus it is unclear whether physical activity had a protective effect on CHD during the additional five-year follow-up or whether the high incidence of CHD among the least-active men was related to already-present CHD.

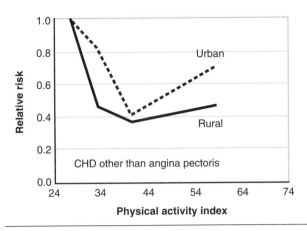

Figure 5.6   The Puerto Rico study of men shows the relative risk of CHD other than angina pectoris versus the physical activity index.

Reprinted, by permission, from K.E. Powell, 1988, Habitual exercise and public health: An epidemiological view. In *Exercise adherence: Its impact on public health*, edited by R.K. Dishman (Champaign, IL: Human Kinetics), 30

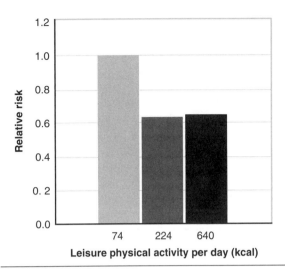

Figure 5.7   The MRFIT study shows the relative risk of CHD versus leisure physical activity.

Adapted from Leon et al. 1987.

Puerto Rico Heart Health Program

The Puerto Rico Heart Health Program (Garcia-Palmieri et al. 1982) used a physical activity rating index similar to the one used in the Framingham Heart Study to evaluate the activity levels of 8793 men, initially 45 to 65 years of age. Over an 8.5-year follow-up, there was an inverse association between physical activity and incidence of CHD events other than angina pectoris (figure 5.6); the highest risk was twice as large as the lowest.

Multivariate analysis to control for confounding by other CHD risk factors confirmed that reduced physical activity contributed independently to risk of CHD. The association also persisted after the data were reanalyzed to exclude CHD events in the first two and a half years in order to eliminate men whose low levels of physical activity might have been caused by subclinical disease.

Multiple Risk Factor Intervention Trial (MRFIT)

The MRFIT involved over 12,000 men, initially 35 to 57 years old, who were in the top 10% to 15% for risk of CHD based on cigarette smoking, blood pressure, and serum cholesterol. Men's exercise habits were estimated by a detailed interview (Minnesota Leisure Time Physical Activity Questionnaire [MLTPAQ]) in which they recalled participation in about 60 leisure-time physical activities during the preceding year (Leon et al. 1987). Frequency, duration, and intensity (in metabolic equivalents, METs) of the physical activities were used to calculate total energy expenditure spent in leisure-time physical activity. During six to eight years of follow-up, 488 men died. Mortality rates from all causes and from CHD among the two most active tertiles of men were about 67% of the rates in the least-active tertile, who averaged 74 kcal/day in leisure-time physical activity (figure 5.7). Mortality rates were very similar in the second and third tertiles, even though men in the most active tertile averaged 640 kcal a day while

the middle tertile had an average expenditure of about 220 kcal. This finding suggests a threshold of benefit somewhere between 75 and 220 daily kilocalories for these men rather than a linear dose response, for which we would expect a further decrease in CHD mortality rate with an increase in energy expenditure from 220 to 640 daily kilocalories. Results were unchanged after adjustment for age and other cardiovascular risk factors, so the reduced relative risk of CHD mortality seen in the more active men was independent of several confounding factors.

Subsequently, with longer follow-up and more deaths observed, investigators were able to analyze men according to deciles (instead of tertiles) of physical activity. In a study conducted 16 years later, the men in the least-active decile, who had averaged 5 min/day of leisure-time physical activity at the beginning of the study, had 22% higher CHD death rates than men in the second to fourth least-active deciles, who had averaged about 20 min/day of mainly light- and moderate-intensity physical activity (Leon, Myers, and Connett 1997). Exercising longer than 20 min a day was associated with no additional reduction in the risk of dying from CHD. Hence, even a modest amount of daily physical activity was better than being sedentary for middle-aged and older men at high risk for CHD.

British Regional Heart Study

In this prospective cohort study, investigators followed 7735 men ages 40 to 59 years from 24 general practice clinics across Britain for eight years (Shaper, Wannamethee, and Weatherall 1991). At the start of the study, men reported on questionnaires their regular walking or cycling, recreational activities, and sporting activities. A physical activity score was derived based on the frequency of these activities (i.e., an index of energy expended based on both the frequency and intensity of activities), and men were categorized into six groups: inactive, occasional, light, moderate, moderately vigorous, and vigorous. During follow-up, 488 men suffered at least one major heart attack. After adjustment for several potential confounders, the relative risks for heart attack for the six groups of physical activity were 1.00 (referent), 0.9 (95% CI: 0.5-1.3), 0.9 (0.6-1.4), 0.5 (0.2-0.8), 0.5 (0.3-0.9), and 0.9 (0.5-1.8), respectively. A similar relation was seen in men without, and with (about one-quarter of men), ischemic heart disease at the start of the study. It is unclear why physical activity was not related to lower risk among the most active men; this may have been due in part to the small number of men in the most active category.

Nurses' Health Study

The Nurses' Health Study is a prospective cohort study designed primarily to investigate the associations of diet with health. The relation between physical activity and CHD risk also has been studied in this cohort. In an eight-year follow-up begun in 1986 of 72,488 female nurses ages 40 to 65 years who were free of CVD or cancer, 645 nonfatal heart attacks or deaths from CHD were observed (Manson et al. 1999). Physical activity was assessed on questionnaires using questions similar to those for the Harvard Alumni Health Study, with women queried about their walking, stair climbing, and participation in leisure-time activities every four years. Based on these reports, total energy expenditure was estimated in MET-hours per week. There was a strong, graded, inverse association between total energy expenditure and CHD risk. After adjustments were made for risk factors in addition to age (smoking, body mass index [BMI], menopausal status, use of postmenopausal hormones, parental history of early-onset MI, use of vitamin supplements, alcohol use, hypertension, diabetes, hypercholesterolemia, and aspirin use), the relative risks of CHD for increasing quintiles of total energy expenditure were 1.00 (referent), 0.88 (95% CI: 0.71-1.10), 0.81 (0.64-1.02), 0.74 (0.58-0.95), and 0.66 (0.51-0.86) respectively. The women in the top two quintiles who had significantly lower relative risks for CHD were physically active at the equivalent of at least 3 h of brisk walking or 1.5 h of vigorous exercise each week. Walking was sufficient to lower CHD risk: Among women who did not report any vigorous activities, the corresponding relative risks for increasing quintiles of walking were 1.00 (referent), 0.78 (0.57-1.06), 0.88 (0.65-1.21), 0.70 (0.51-0.95), and 0.65 (0.47-0.91), respectively. Again, the women in the top two quintiles of walking had significantly lower relative risks for CHD; their walking was ≥3.9 MET-hours per week, or the equivalent of 1.3 h or more of brisk walking per week.

Women's Health Study

The Women's Health Study was a randomized controlled trial testing low-dose aspirin and vitamin E for the prevention of heart disease and cancer among approximately 40,000 women aged 45 years and older, conducted between 1992 and 2004. Following the completion of the trial, women continue to be followed for morbidity and mortality. In this study, physical activity was assessed at baseline and updated

every two or three years using a questionnaire very similar to that used in the Nurses' Health Study. In an analysis that included an average follow-up of five years, during which 244 women developed CHD, the relative risks of CHD associated with <200, 200 to 599, 600 to 1499, and ≥1500 kcal/week expended in leisure-time physical activities were 1.00 (referent), 0.79 (95% CI: 0.56-1.12), 0.55 (0.37-0.82), and 0.75 (0.50-1.12), respectively, after adjustment for differences in age, smoking, alcohol intake, diet, menopausal status, use of postmenopausal hormones, and parental history of early-onset MI (Lee et al. 2001). One contribution of this study has been to provide data on the relation between walking, a moderate-intensity activity, and the risk of developing CHD. Among women who did not participate in any vigorous activities, those who walked as little as 1 to 1.5 h per week had significantly lower risk of CHD: Compared with the risk for women who did not usually walk, the multivariate relative risks for CHD associated with walking <1, 1 to 1.5, and ≥2 h/week were 0.86 (0.57-1.29), 0.49 (0.28-0.86), and 0.48 (0.29-0.78), respectively.

Women's Health Initiative Observational Study

The Women's Health Initiative is a study of approximately 162,000 ethnically diverse, postmenopausal women ages 50 to 79 years in four major study components: three randomized clinical trials and a prospective cohort study, the Women's Health Initiative Observational Study, which comprises approximately 94,000 women. An analysis of women from the observational study examined the association of physical activity with the risk of developing CVD (Manson et al. 2002). Women reported the frequency and duration of walking and participation in "mild," "moderate," and "strenuous" activities at baseline between 1994 and 1998. During a mean follow-up of 3.2 years, 1551 CVD events occurred. In multivariate analyses that adjusted for several potential confounders, the relative risks for CVD with increasing quintiles of energy expenditure were 1.00 (referent), 0.89 (95% CI: 0.75-1.04), 0.81 (0.68-0.97), 0.78 (0.66-0.93), and 0.72 (0.59-0.87), respectively. The women in the top three quintiles who had significantly lower relative risks for CVD all expended at least 7.3 MET-hours per week, the equivalent of approximately 2.5 h per week of brisk walking. Investigators also examined walking and vigorous activities separately, in relation to CVD risk, and observed comparable risk reductions when comparing CVD rates between top and bottom quintiles for each kind of activity.

Health Professionals Follow-Up Study

In this prospective cohort study of over 44,000 U.S. men ages 40 to 75 years, designed primarily to examine diet and health, physical activity also was assessed via questionnaire every four years, using questions similar to those in the Nurses' Health Study and the Women's Health Study. In a follow-up of men observed between 1986 and 1998, investigators examined associations between CHD risk and the amount, type, and intensity of physical activity (Tanasescu et al. 2002). They found that total physical activity, running, weight training, and rowing were each inversely and linearly related to risk of CHD after adjustment for age, smoking, and several CHD risk factors. Running for an hour or more per week was associated with a 42% risk reduction (relative risk [RR] = 0.58; 95% CI: 0.44-0.77). Weight training for 30 min or more per week was associated with a 23% risk reduction (RR = 0.77; 95% CI: 0.61-0.98). Rowing for 1 h or more per week was associated with an 18% risk reduction (RR = 0.82; 95% CI: 0.68-0.99). A half hour per day or more of brisk walking was associated with an 18% risk reduction (RR = 0.82; 95% CI: 0.67-1.00). Walking pace was associated with reduced CHD risk independent of the number of walking hours. However, there were no significant associations of jogging, cycling, swimming, or racket sports with CHD risk. Average exercise intensity was associated with reduced CHD risk independent of the total amount of physical activity. The risk reductions (95% CIs) corresponding to moderate (4-5.9 METs) and high (≥6 METs) activity intensities were 0.94 (0.83-1.04) and 0.83 (0.72-0.97) compared with low-intensity (<4 METs) activities.

Other Kinds of Physical Activity and Coronary Heart Disease Risk

In recent years, because of low levels of physical activity during leisure time, there has been interest in other kinds of physical activity, particularly activity undertaken as part of transportation (e.g., walking or cycling during commuting). There appears to be a modest inverse association between commuting physical activity and risk of cardiovascular end points. In a meta-analysis, the pooled relative risk for a combination of various cardiovascular end points (CHD, stroke, hypertension, or diabetes) associated with commuting physical activity in men was 0.91 (95% CI: 0.80-1.04); in women, it was 0.87 (0.77-0.98). There are few data on household or domestic physical activity, and the data are mixed regarding their association with reduced CVD risk (Hamer and Chida 2008); this may be due in part to the reduced precision with which such activities are assessed.

Sedentary Behavior and Coronary Heart Disease Risk

Sedentary behavior may represent an independent risk factor for CHD, separate from physical activity. Even if an individual follows current recommendations for physical activity, such as by walking briskly, 30 min a day, on five days a week, there remain many hours in which one can be sedentary. For example, assuming 8 h of sleep and 30 min of brisk walking, there are still 15.5 h of the day in which one can be sedentary, sitting most of the time, or one can stand and make many brief, spontaneous movements (e.g., fidgeting, standing up and sitting down). Animal studies show that experimentally decreasing spontaneous standing and ambulatory time in rats had a deleterious effect on lipoprotein lipase regulation far greater in magnitude than the beneficial effect of adding exercise to rats' normal activity (Hamilton, Hamilton, and Zderic 2007). In humans, investigators who followed >17,000 men and women in the Canada Fitness Study, ages 18 to 90 years, for 12 years reported recently that increased sitting time was directly related, in a dose–response fashion, to CVD mortality (Katzmarzyk et al. 2009). The multivariate relative risks associated with sitting almost none, one-fourth, half, three-fourths, and almost all of the time were 1.00 (referent), 1.01 (95% CI: 0.77-1.31), 1.22 (0.94-1.60), 1.47 (1.09-1.96), and 1.54 (1.09-2.17), respectively, trend <0.0001. Of interest was the observation that even among individuals active enough to meet physical activity recommendations, those spending more time sitting were at increased risk of CVD mortality compared with those sitting less. The age-adjusted relative risks among such physically active men and women were 1.00, 0.92, 1.01, 1.31, and 1.40, respectively.

Physical Fitness and Coronary Heart Disease Risk

The imprecise methods used in most studies to assess regular physical activity (primarily self-reports) may result in an underestimation of the true magnitude of the association between all-cause and CHD mortality by misclassifying some inactive people as active and some active people as inactive. More objective measurement of fitness potentially yields a more accurate estimate of risk. While physical fitness has a genetic component, regular physical activity also contributes to higher levels of physical fitness. Low physical fitness is associated with increased risk of CHD and CVD. The reported relative risks are higher in some studies, although a meta-analysis of studies of physical fitness in relation to CHD or CVD risk reported a relative risk, adjusted for potential confounding factors, of similar magnitude to studies of physical activity, 0.64 (95% CI: 0.57-0.72), comparing high versus low levels of physical (specifically, cardiorespiratory) fitness (Kodama et al. 2009). Alternately, comparing low versus high levels instead, the relative risk was 1.56 (1.39-1.75). In this section we discuss the findings from several representative studies of physical fitness and CHD risk. There are several components of physical fitness, including muscular endurance (or cardio-respiratory fitness), muscular strength, body composition, and flexibility. Most studies of fitness and CHD risk have assessed cardiorespiratory fitness.

▷ **THE TRUE** size of the protective effect of physical activity against CHD risk is probably underestimated by the current methods used to measure physical activity, which undoubtedly misclassify some inactive people as active and some active people as inactive.

Los Angeles Public Safety Employees

Cardiorespiratory fitness was estimated by the heart rate response to submaximal cycling exercise among 2779 healthy male fire and law enforcement workers younger than 55 years in Los Angeles County, who were then followed for an average of about five years, during which 36 heart attacks occurred (Peters et al. 1983). The relative risk of heart attack after controlling for other conventional CHD risk factors was 2.2 (95% CI: 1.1-4.7) for the men who had below-average physical fitness, compared with men with above-average fitness, measured at the beginning of the study. The relative risk for men with below-average, compared with above-average, fitness was 6.6 (2.3-27.8) if they also had at least two of the following risk factors: high total cholesterol, elevated systolic blood pressure, or cigarette smoking.

Lipid Research Clinics Prevalence Study

Findings from the Lipid Research Clinics study indicated a strong association between cardiorespiratory fitness and lower CHD incidence and mortality. Ekelund and colleagues (1988) measured the fitness of over 3100 healthy white men ages 30 to 69 years old using a submaximal treadmill exercise test. After an average follow-up of 8.5 years, there were 45 CVD deaths. The relative risk of CHD death for men in the least-fit quartile, compared with those in the most fit quartile, was 6.5 (95% CI: 1.5-28.7); and for CVD death the relative risk was 8.5 (2.0-36.7). Although based on small numbers, as shown in figure 5.8, there was a striking dose–response gradient across fitness categories.

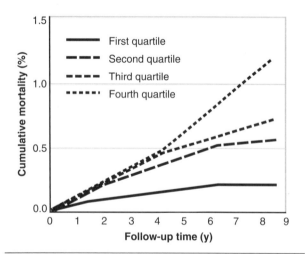

Figure 5.8 Cumulative rates of death from cardiovascular diseases in healthy men according to quartiles of exercise test heart rate. Men who were most active (first quartile) had the lowest CVD death rate. Divergence of mortality curves over follow-up indicates that the effect on cardiovascular mortality is unlikely to be due to bias.

Based on Ekelund et al. 1988.

Aerobics Center Longitudinal Study

The often-cited Aerobics Center Longitudinal Study, a follow-up of over 25,000 men and 7000 women conducted by the Cooper Institute for Aerobics Research in Dallas, Texas, found that mortality rates from CVD and from all causes were lower in fit men and women than in the unfit (Blair et al. 1989). Cardiorespiratory fitness in this study was estimated from time on a treadmill during a maximal test protocol. The greatest difference in mortality rates was seen between the low- and moderate-fitness categories for both sexes, but there was a further reduction between the moderate- and high-fitness categories. The CVD mortality rate for the highly fit men (top 40%) was about half that of the moderately fit (middle 40%), but the rate for the least-fit men (bottom 20%) was more than three times that of moderately fit men. Among women, based on only seven CVD deaths, similar observations were noted in that less fit women had higher rates of CVD mortality than more fit women.

Subsequent analyses that included longer follow-up with more CVD deaths continued to show that unfit men and women experienced higher CVD mortality rates compared with fit men and women, even after accounting for potential confounders (Blair et al. 1989; Sui et al. 2008). And the increased risk of CVD mortality associated with low fitness was observed to be similar in magnitude to, or even stronger than, that associated with other CVD risk factors such as smoking, hypertension, diabetes, or hypercholesterolemia.

St. James Women Take Heart Project

In another study of women, 5721 volunteers from the Chicago metropolitan area who were 35 years and older and who were healthy underwent a symptom-limited treadmill test to estimate cardiorespiratory fitness levels (Gulati et al. 2005). During follow-up that averaged over eight years, 180 women died, 58 from cardiac causes. In analyses that adjusted for age differences, the relative risks for cardiac death among high-, medium-, and low-fit women were 1.00 (referent), 2.02 (95% CI: 0.46-8.82), and 4.27 (1.03-17.6), respectively.

Summary

Although cardiorespiratory fitness is partly explainable by genetic inheritance, a high proportion of the variation in cardiovascular fitness is explained by physical activity habits. Hence, the agreement of findings among studies that measured either physical activity or fitness supports the hypothesis of a causal relationship between regular physical activity and reduced risk of CHD.

Individuals With Other Risk Factors or Existing Coronary Heart Disease

In the early investigations of leisure-time physical activity and CHD risk in British civil servants (Morris et al. 1973, 1980) and Harvard alumni (Paffenbarger, Wing, and Hyde 1978), investigators showed that even among men with other CVD risk factors (such as smoking; short stature; high BMI; history of hypertension, stroke, or diabetes; and parental history of early-onset CVD), higher levels of physical activity were associated with lower CHD risk. In the MRFIT study (Leon et al. 1987), physical activity also was shown to be significantly associated with reduced CVD risk in men who smoked cigarettes and had high blood pressure and high serum cholesterol. Other studies have also contributed support for this hypothesis, showing that the association of physical activity with reduced risk of CHD is present in men and women without and with CVD risk factors, and that the magnitude of the association is generally similar among those without and with CVD risk factors (e.g., Nurses' Health Study, Women's Health Study, Women's Health Initiative, Health Professionals Follow-Up Study).

For example, in the Aerobics Center Longitudinal Study (Blair et al. 1996), low physical fitness was shown to be an important predictor of CHD mortality in both smokers and nonsmokers, those with and without high cholesterol or blood pressure, and those who were considered healthy and unhealthy (as indicated by an abnormal electrocardiogram or history of CHD, stroke, hypertension, diabetes, or cancer).

▷ **PHYSICAL INACTIVITY** contributes substantially to the public health burden. Eliminating inactivity would have an impact on reducing excess mortality as great as, or greater than, eliminating other major CHD risk factors.

In an analysis published in 1999 from the Aerobics Center Longitudinal Study (Wei et al. 1999), results indicated that low (bottom 20%), compared with high (top 80%), cardiorespiratory fitness resulted in significant increases in the relative risk for CVD mortality in all weight categories (normal weight, BMI ≤24.9 kg/m^2: RR = 1.7, 95% CI: 1.1-2.5; overweight, BMI 25.0-29.0 kg/m^2: RR = 1.9, 95% CI: 1.4-2.5; obese, BMI ≥30.0 kg/m^2: RR = 2.0, 95% CI: 1.2-3.6). The strongest relative risk for CVD mortality, as expected, was associated with the presence of baseline CVD (normal weight: RR = 4.6, 95% CI: 3.1-6.8; overweight: RR = 3.5, 95% CI: 2.6-4.7; obese: RR = 5.8, 95% CI: 3.5-9.7). The other risk indicators (diabetes, high cholesterol, hypertension, and smoking) also generally showed comparable increases for CVD mortality in normal-weight, overweight, and obese men.

Higher levels of physical activity after a heart attack also appear to be associated with lower mortality among patients with CVD. Cumulative results of 48 randomized clinical trials involving 8940 patients with MI or coronary artery revascularization procedures, where the median intervention duration was three months and the median follow-up was 15 months, indicated that the odds ratios for total mortality (OR = 0.80; 95% CI: 0.68-0.93) and cardiac mortality (OR = 0.74 [0.61-0.96]) were lowered in groups that received cardiac rehabilitation, compared with usual care (Taylor et al. 2004).

Cardiac rehabilitation programs typically include components of not only exercise, but also education, behavior change, counseling, support, and strategies aimed at targeting cardiovascular risk factors. Thus, a benefit on mortality rates cannot be entirely attributed to physical activity. In the meta-analysis described above by Taylor et al. (2004), investigators also separately examined 12 randomized controlled trials that compared cardiac rehabilitation programs with only an exercise component versus usual care. Total mortality also was reduced for cardiac patients assigned to exercise-only cardiac rehabilitation (OR = 0.76 [0.59-0.98]). In another meta-analysis of randomized controlled trials examining secondary prevention for CHD patients, investigators reported that cardiac rehabilitation programs that did not include an exercise component were associated with a smaller reduction in all-cause mortality (OR = 0.87 [0.73-0.99]) than programs that included only an exercise component (OR = 0.72 [0.54-0.95]) (Clark et al. 2005).

A prospective cohort study reported findings congruent with the randomized clinical trials discussed above in the meta-analyses by Taylor et al. (2004) and Clark et al. (2005). Among 837 men and women with a history of CVD, sport activity or walking was associated with between 26% and 68% lower rates of all-cause and CVD mortality during follow-up (Hamer and Stamatakis 2009).

▷ **EXERCISE-ONLY CARDIAC** rehabilitation programs in patients with CHD reduce mortality rates by 24% on average, compared with usual care.

Physical Inactivity Compared With Other Risk Factors

In chapter 2, we introduced the concept of population attributable risk (PAR), which is an estimate of the reduction in disease rate that might occur if all individuals with a specific risk factor (e.g., smoking, hypertension, obesity, inactivity) eliminated that factor. Population attributable risk is a theoretical calculation that depends on accurate information regarding both the relative risk for the factor being investigated and the percentage of the population exposed to the risk factor; it assumes a cause–effect association, the persistence of the risk factor into the future, and an equal distribution of potential confounding factors in the groups being compared. While all these conditions might not be fulfilled, theoretical PAR calculations can still provide epidemiologists with a useful method to quantify and compare the public health burden of different disease risk factors.

A number of studies have estimated the PAR for physical inactivity and compared this with the PAR for other cardiovascular risk factors. On the basis of prevalence estimates of sedentary lifestyle in the United States, Powell and Blair (1994) estimated the PAR for sedentary lifestyle (defined as no leisure-time physical activity) on CHD mortality to be 16%.

Using data from the Harvard Alumni Health Study, Paffenbarger and colleagues (1993) estimated the PAR for CHD mortality associated with no participation in moderately vigorous sport activity (≥4.5 METs) at 14%. Thus, if all men in this sample had taken up moderately vigorous sport activity, the CHD mortality rate would have been reduced by 14%. In the Harvard alumni sample, the PAR for CHD mortality associated with low physical activity was comparable to those for cigarette smoking (13%), hypertension (20%), and overweight (BMI ≥26, 11%). Haapanen-Niemi, Vuori, and Pasanen (1999) used data from a number of population-based studies of Finnish men ages 30 to 63 to estimate PAR for low physical activity and other cardiovascular risk factors for CHD mortality. Population attributable risks for various risk factors were cigarette smoking, 10% to 33%; high serum cholesterol, 9% to 21%; hypertension, 6% to 15%; overweight, 3% to 6%; and low leisure-time physical activity, 22% to 39%. Wei and colleagues (1999) used data from the Aerobics Center Longitudinal Study to compare the effects of low cardiovascular fitness with other risk indicators, including type 2 diabetes, high cholesterol, high blood pressure, and cigarette smoking. Results indicated that low fitness had a PAR for CVD mortality that was similar to, if not larger than, those associated with the other measured risk factors. For example, in obese men (BMI ≥30 kg/m²), the PAR for CVD mortality associated with low fitness (bottom 20% of distribution) was 39%, which was comparable to, or higher than, the PAR for baseline CVD (51%), type 2 diabetes (15%), high cholesterol (26%), hypertension (15%), and cigarette smoking (6%).

As might be expected, PAR estimates vary across studies. However, it appears that physical inactivity contributes substantially to the public health burden and that eliminating this behavior would have an impact on reducing excess CHD or CVD mortality at least comparable to, if not greater than, elimination of other major cardiovascular risk factors.

Are the Associations Real?

The data presented in this chapter regarding the inverse association between physical activity or fitness and risk of CHD were obtained from observational studies. With this study design, individuals are not randomly assigned to groups based on activity level; therefore, it cannot be assumed that high levels of physical activity or fitness caused the low CHD rates. An initial step in establishing that the observed associa-tion is causal is to ensure that the observed associations are valid and not the result of some other factor, such as chance, bias, or confounding.

The role of chance can be assessed by examining the statistical significance of the findings. Since many of the results were statistically significant, and meta-analysis of data across many studies shows significant results, chance is an unlikely explanation for the findings. Bias in study results can arise from selection bias, loss to follow-up, or imprecision of measurement of physical activity or fitness. Selection bias is more likely to occur in case–control studies. This bias operates when participation in a study is differential depending on disease status; for example, if persons who are physically active are more likely to participate as controls in a study, this may result in an over-estimation of the benefit of physical activity. The possibility that individuals with undiagnosed disease might decrease their physical activity (hence be less fit), resulting in a biased observation of higher CHD incidence in those with low activity or fitness levels, needs to be carefully evaluated. Minimizing this type of bias in an observational study is achieved by careful initial screening of participants to try to eliminate those with diseases and by observing disease incidence or mortality over a long follow-up period. Individuals in the study cohort who have undiagnosed diseases at baseline are likely to develop disease or die early in the follow-up period, resulting in a cohort of healthy survivors as the length of follow-up increases.

The majority of studies on activity or fitness and CHD risk discussed earlier in this chapter used what would be considered a sufficiently long follow-up period of six to 26 years to reduce the likelihood that the results would be affected by undiagnosed disease at baseline. Moreover, many investigators conducted additional analyses that did not include cases occurring early in the follow-up period, thus minimizing the possibility of bias due to undiagnosed disease.

Additionally, studies that find changes in physical activity or fitness to be associated with changes in disease risk are also less likely to reflect bias due to disease causing lower activity levels. For example, the results of both Paffenbarger and colleagues (1993) and Blair and colleagues (1995) indicated that individuals who changed either physical activity or physical fitness levels had a change in mortality risk in the hypothesized direction; that is, a change from low to high activity or fitness was associated with a decrease in mortality risk, and a change from high to low was associated with an increase. Most of these deaths in men were caused by CVD.

▷ **A FINDING THAT** changes in physical activity or fitness are associated with changes in disease risk is less likely to reflect bias due to disease causing lower activity levels.

Other factors such as loss to follow-up, misclassification of individuals' physical activity or fitness, or differences in risk characteristics other than physical activity or fitness can also lead to invalid results in a prospective cohort study.

Loss to follow-up may be related to the level of physical activity or fitness; those lost to follow-up also may have discontinued participation in the study because of the development of illness, thus biasing the results. This is generally not thought to be a problem, considering that the follow-up rates reported in cohort studies on activity and fitness and mortality were 90% or higher. As discussed in chapter 3, measurement of physical activity in population studies presents a major challenge. Also, most prospective studies measure physical activity only at baseline and do not consider changes in activity over the follow-up period (although in several of the studies described earlier, such as the Nurses' Health Study, the Women's Health Study, and the Health Professionals Follow-Up Study, physical activity information was updated over time). It is generally thought that since physical activity is measured before the disease outcome is known, misclassification of physical activity levels would be random with respect to outcome. Random misclassification by activity level tends to reduce the magnitude of the true association between activity and CHD outcome, suggesting that the magnitude of decreased CHD risk associated with physical activity reported in the literature is most likely an underestimate.

▶ **BECAUSE INACTIVE** or unfit participants may be less likely to continue in a study, loss to follow-up may bias study findings.

It is also likely that individuals who are physically active or fit differ from sedentary or unfit individuals in other health habits or disease risk factors, such as cigarette smoking, alcohol intake, blood pressure, BMI, lipid profile, and dietary habits, which may influence the association of physical activity or fitness with reduced CHD risk. This phenomenon in epidemiologic studies is referred to as "confounding." Well-conducted cohort studies have statistically controlled for many potential risk factors, and the significant inverse association of activity and fitness with CHD risk persists. The adjustment of study results for CVD risk factors, particularly the major ones such as cholesterol, blood pressure, and obesity, is controversial. Some researchers have argued that a favorable change in a risk factor that is associated with a change in activity or fitness is part of the causal pathway through which physical activity and fitness affect CHD risk and therefore should not be controlled in the analysis. Thus, studies that have adjusted for these CVD risk factors may, indeed, be underestimating the true benefit of physical activity or fitness on CHD risk.

Strength of the Evidence

After consideration of the roles of chance, bias, and confounding in the preceding sections, we can reasonably conclude that a valid association of physical activity and fitness

with lower CHD risk does exist. The next question to ask is, Are the observed associations causal? As outlined in chapter 2, epidemiologists apply at least five main criteria that, if satisfied, help establish that the observed associations are likely to be causal. These criteria, Mill's canons, are temporal sequence, strength of association, consistency of results, biological plausibility, and dose response.

Temporal Sequence

In a prospective cohort design, the independent variable (activity or fitness) is measured before the outcome occurs, thus demonstrating the appropriate temporal sequence. Prospective cohort studies have demonstrated consistent associations of higher activity or fitness levels with lower CHD risk.

Strength of Association

In their review of the literature on physical activity and CHD mortality, Powell and coworkers (1987) reported that the relative risk associated with inactivity varied across studies but ranged from 1.5 to 2.4, with a median of about 1.9 for all 47 determinations of relative risk obtained from the studies considered. Therefore, the risk of CHD mortality was almost twice as high for sedentary individuals as for physically active individuals (or, conversely, active individuals had about half the risk that sedentary individuals did). In more recent reviews, such as the qualitative review conducted by the Physical Activity Guidelines Advisory Committee (2008) and recent meta-analyses (Sattelmair et al. 2011; Sofi et al. 2008), the magnitude of the association was somewhat smaller, with most active subjects observed to have approximately 20% to 40% reduction in CHD risk compared with least-active subjects.

Earlier we noted that the PAR of CHD mortality associated with low physical activity was comparable to, or larger than, that of other risk factors, such as cigarette smoking, high blood pressure, high serum cholesterol, and overweight.

Consistency of Results

The data on the association of activity and fitness with all-cause and CHD mortality are remarkably consistent for men and women. Most studies, even though they were conducted at different times using different methodologies and samples from different parts of the world, have yielded overall similar results.

Biological Plausibility

An important consideration in establishing causality is evidence for the biological plausibility of the observed association. The biological mechanisms that explain the protective effect of physical activity against CHD are not fully known but include factors mainly related to myocardial oxygen supply and demand and myocardial electrical stability. Increased levels of HDL cholesterol, decreased body weight and blood pressure, improved glucose tolerance, favorable changes in hemostatic variables, and decreased inflammation are among the mechanisms best supported by current scientific evidence. An investigation using data from the Women's Health Study indicated that 59% of the reduction in CVD risk associated with physical activity was explained by several traditional and novel CVD risk factors (Mora et al. 2007). The largest contribution was from inflammatory and hemostatic biomarkers, 32.6%, with lower contributions from blood pressure, 27.1%; traditional lipids (total, LDL, and HDL cholesterol), 19.1%; novel lipids (lipoprotein [a], apolipoprotein A1 and B100), 15.5%; BMI, 10.1%; and hemoglobin A1c/diabetes, 8.9%. The remaining proportion, 41%, of the reduction in risk of CVD with physical activity may be due to other mechanisms not assessed in the study, such as myocardial oxygen supply and demand and myocardial electrical stability.

▷ **REGULAR PHYSICAL** activity reduces CHD risk independently of other risk factors, but it can also favorably influence cardiovascular risk factors such as blood pressure, body weight, blood lipids, blood clotting factors, and inflammatory markers.

Myocardial Oxygen Supply and Demand

Normal adaptations to exercise training include lowered blood cholesterol and triglycerides, which should decrease the risk of atherosclerotic plaques and help maintain normal blood supply to the heart. Another common adaptation is a lowering of heart rate and blood pressure at rest and during submaximal exercise. Those factors combined (e.g., systolic blood pressure × heart rate) are an index of the metabolism (i.e., the oxygen demand) of the heart. In addition, a few postmortem necropsy studies have shown less coronary atherosclerosis or injury to the myocardium among men who had been regular exercisers. These studies include a widely publicized autopsy on famous lifelong marathon runner Clarence DeMar (Currens and White 1961) and studies in Westchester County, New York (Stamler et al. 1970); Great Britain (Morris and Crawford 1958); Israel (Mitrani, Karplus, and Bunner 1970); and Finland (Rissanen 1976). Even when the prevalence of severe coronary atherosclerosis was similar among men who had been sedentary, moderately active, or very active, physically active men had larger lumens in the coronary arteries. Moreover, physically active men were less likely to have complete occlusions of major coronary arteries and had less scarring from ischemic events and healed infarcts, even when they had advanced atherosclerosis. Experimental studies on rats and monkeys also have reported that the interior diameters of coronary arteries were larger after regular exercise (Leon 1972; Leon and Bloor 1977). In another study of monkeys, regular exercise reduced the severity of coronary atherosclerosis in animals fed a high-fat, high-cholesterol diet (Kramsch et al. 1981).

▷ **REGULAR EXERCISE** lowers the oxygen demands of the heart during physical activity of a fixed intensity, thus reducing the risk of ischemia during physical work.

Hemostatic and Inflammatory Biomarkers

Several lines of research suggest that physical activity might reduce the risk of coronary thrombosis via favorable changes in hemostatic and inflammatory biomarkers. Decreased hematocrit resulting from an expansion of plasma volume is a hallmark response to regular physical activity. Thus, exercise training should lead to reduced viscosity (thickness) of the blood, which might reduce coagulability and platelet stickiness. Regular physical activity also might decrease platelet aggregation through changes in the metabolism of **prostaglandins.**

Results from some cross-sectional, population-based studies are consistent with such views. For example, leisure-time physical activity, but not job activity, was inversely related to plasma viscosity among 3500 men and women ages 25 to 64 years (Koenig et al. 1997), even after adjustment for age, cholesterol, smoking, blood pressure, and body weight for height. Strenuous exercise also was associated with lower activity of clotting factor VII in a cross-sectional study of nearly 4000 men ages 45 to 69 years (Connelly, Cooper, and Meade 1992). Low leisure-time physical activity was associated with high levels of clotting factor VII, independently of total serum cholesterol, BMI, and insulin levels, each of which was associated with higher levels of clotting factor VII (Bladbjerg, Moller, and Jespersen 1998).

Several hemostatic factors also are markers of inflammation, and recent studies suggest that the protective effects of physical activity against the development of CHD may partly result from effects on inflammation as well as hemostasis. For example, the association between physical activity and markers of inflammation was examined in a healthy cohort of 5888 men and women 65 or more years old in the cross-sectional Cardiovascular Health Study (Geffken et al. 2001). Blood levels of C-reactive protein, fibrinogen, white blood cells, and albumin and clotting factor VIII activity were compared among the cross section, which was divided into quartiles by self-reported physical activity. After adjustment for age, sex, race, smoking, BMI, CVD, diabetes, and hypertension, people in the highest quartile of physical activity had 19% lower concentration of C-reactive protein, 6% lower white blood cell count, 4% lower concentration of fibrinogen, and 3% less clotting factor VIII activity than people in the lowest quartile. Further analysis suggested that the lower levels of inflammatory markers among the more active people might be largely explained by their lower BMI and blood glucose levels.

Another, larger cross-sectional study, the National Health and Nutrition Examination Survey III (NHANES III, 1988-1994), examined the association between C-reactive protein and physical activity among 13,748 adults 20 years of age or older (Ford 2002). After adjustment for age, sex, ethnicity, education, work status, smoking, hypertension, BMI, waist-to-hip ratio, HDL-C concentration, and aspirin use, the odds ratios for elevated C-reactive protein concentration (defined as the 85th percentile or higher for each sex) were 0.98 (95% CI: 0.78-1.23), 0.85 (0.70-1.02), and 0.53 (0.40-0.71) for participants who engaged in light, moderate, and vigorous physical activity, respectively, during the previous month compared with participants who did not engage in any leisure-time physical activity.

A companion analysis of the NHANES III study examined the relationship between physical activity and elevated inflammation as indicated by a high C-reactive protein level, white blood cell count, and fibrinogen level in 3638 apparently healthy men and women 40 years and older (Abramson and Vaccarino 2002). After adjustment for age, sex, race, education, blood pressure, HDL and LDL levels, blood glucose, BMI, waist-to-hip ratio, smoking, alcohol use, dietary fat, and vitamin C and E supplementation, the odds of having an elevated C-reactive protein level were reduced among people who were active 22 or more times per month (OR = 0.63; 95% CI: 0.43-0.93) when compared with those engaging in physical activity zero to three times per month. Similar associations were seen for white blood cell count and fibrinogen levels.

In addition to those studies of physical activity, cardio-respiratory fitness levels were inversely associated with C-reactive protein levels in a sample of 722 men from the Aerobics Center Longitudinal Study after adjustments for age, BMI, vitamin use, statin medication use, aspirin use, the presence of inflammatory disease, CVD, diabetes, and smoking habit (Church et al. 2002). In another cross-sectional study of 135 black, white, and Native American middle-aged overweight women, plasma C-reactive protein levels decreased linearly across tertiles of cardiorespiratory fitness and increased across tertiles of BMI (LaMonte et al. 2002). After adjustment for BMI, smoking, diabetes, and estrogen use, the differences in C-reactive protein levels among fitness tertiles remained except in the black women. Among all women, after adjustment for race and the confounders, the odds of high-risk C-reactive protein levels (>0.19 mg/dl) were 0.67 (95% CI: 0.19-2.4) among fit (>6.5 METs) versus unfit women. Though these cross-sectional studies suggest that regular physical activity might have protective effects against chronic, low-grade inflammation, they lack the proper temporal sequence needed to permit an inference of cause and effect. Prospective studies, though limited, have yielded similar findings of a favorable effect of physical activity on hemostasis and inflammation.

In the British Regional Heart Study, a cross-sectional analysis of 3810 men aged 60 to 79 years showed inverse dose–response relations between physical activity and several of the hemostatic factors just discussed, including blood viscosity, platelet count, coagulation factors VIII and IX, fibrinogen, and C-reactive protein (Wannamethee et al. 2002). Additionally, physical activity information was available on these men from 20 years previously. While statistical power was limited, analysis of change in physical activity from 20 years ago to the present, in relation to current hemostatic and inflammatory variables, generally showed associations similar to those in the cross-sectional analyses after adjustment for the possible confounders of age, BMI, smoking, and alcohol use. Men who increased their physical activity over the 20 years had levels of the biomarkers similar to those of the men who were physically active at both assessments, whereas the men who decreased their activity level over the 20 years had levels similar to those of the men who were inactive at both assessments.

In an experimental study of the effects of exercise training on some peripheral inflammatory markers associated with endothelial dysfunction, blood levels of granulocyte-macrophage **colony-stimulating factor** (GM-CSF), macrophage chemoattractant protein-1 (MCP-1), soluble intercellular adhesion molecule-1 (ICAM-1), and soluble vascular cell adhesion molecule-1 (VCAM-1) were measured before and after 12 weeks of exercise in 12 patients who had stable congestive heart disease (Adamopoulos et al. 2001). A crossover research design was used in which patients were randomly assigned first to either exercise or usual care, followed by the other condition, thus serving as their own controls. The exercise training increased the patients' maximal oxygen uptake by 13% and was accompanied by significant reductions in serum GM-CSF, MCP-1, ICAM-1, and VCAM-1. Thus, exercise training appears to favorably affect peripheral inflammatory markers of the interaction between macrophages and endothelial cells among patients with congestive heart failure.

In a recent randomized clinical trial, the Inflammation and Exercise (INFLAME) study examined the effect of aerobic exercise training, without dietary intervention, on C-reactive protein levels in individuals with elevated C-reactive protein (Church et al. 2007). Subjects were 162 sedentary men and women, mean age 49.7 years and mean BMI 31.8 kg/m², with elevated C-reactive protein levels defined as ≥2.0 mg/L. Participants were randomized into an exercise group that trained for four months or a nonexercise control group. The intervention consisted of supervised exercise at a dose of 16 kcal/kg body weight per week, or approximately 150 to 210 min/week of moderate-intensity physical activity. Following the exercise intervention, cardiorespiratory fitness levels increased by 12% in the exercise group. There was no significant difference in median change in C-reactive protein levels between the exercise and control groups ($p = 0.4$). However, change in C-reactive protein level was significantly correlated with changes in weight and fat mass (both $p < 0.01$). Thus, while data from the observational studies indicate an association between physical activity and decreased inflammation even after adjusting for BMI, the results from this randomized controlled trial suggest that the beneficial association between physical activity and C-reactive protein levels is mediated in large part through beneficial changes in body weight.

▷ **EXERCISE AND** habitual moderately intense physical activity are associated with a favorable blood clotting profile and lower levels of markers for chronic low-grade inflammation that are predictors of sudden coronary death resulting from blood clots after ruptures of atheromas.

Responses to Acute Exercise

Though **acute exercise** increases blood coagulability, that effect appears to be offset by a co-occurring increase in fibrinolysis. Each of these responses increases with increasing intensity and duration of exercise (el-Sayed 1996). The increase in fibrinolysis after submaximal exercise is mainly explained by increases in tPA levels (about 40%) and tPA activity (about 150%), which return to resting levels within 30 min, and about a 25% decrease in PAI-1 activity that persists up to 1 h after exercise (e.g., DeSouza et al. 1997).

Adaptations After Chronic Exercise

Findings are not yet conclusive, but several studies suggest that **chronic exercise** diminishes increased coagulability during exercise while maintaining fibrinolytic activity. Cross-sectional population-based studies have indicated that physical activity is associated with lower levels of plasma fibrinogen in young adults (Folsom et al. 1993) and middle-aged men (Connelly, Cooper, and Meade 1992; Wannamethee et al. 2002). Also, physically active women have lower levels of fibrinogen, lower levels of tPA, and lower PAI-1 levels and activity, but higher tPA activity than sedentary women, regardless of age (DeSouza, Jones, and Seals 1998). In a study of 700 men and nearly 800 women ages 25 to 64 years, tPA activity was 30% higher in the most active men and 12% higher in the most active women, compared with their sedentary counterparts. PAI-1 activity was 40% and 30% lower among the most active men and women, respectively. Those differences remained after adjustment for age, BMI, and waist-to-hip ratio but not after further adjustment for triglyceride and insulin levels (Eliasson, Asplund, and Evrin 1996).

A clinical study showed that platelet stickiness and aggregability were temporarily increased by a single session of maximal cycling exercise but were decreased at rest and after exercise following eight weeks of cycling exercise for 30 min per day, five days per week, at an intensity of 60% of maximal aerobic capacity. Those training adaptations were reversed by 12 weeks of physical deconditioning (Wang, Jen, and Chen 1995). Similarly, increases in maximal power output of 12% in men and 18% in women after nine months of exercise training were accompanied by reductions in PAI-1 levels, independent of reduced plasma triglyceride levels (Ponjee et al. 1996).

Six months of exercise training that increased maximal oxygen uptake by about 20% was accompanied by a 140% increase in tPA level, a 40% increase in tPA activity, a 60% decrease in PAI-1 activity, and a 13% decrease in fibrinogen level in men ages 60 to 82 years, but not in men ages 24 to 30 years (Stratton et al. 1991). Finally, a study compared two groups of men already in an exercise program: those with and those without CHD, who were similar in age and amount of physical activity (Fernhall et al. 1997). The two groups showed similar increases in tPA activity and decreases in PAI-1 activity after a maximal exercise test but no changes in tPA or PAI-1 levels.

Thus, while there are some differences in individual findings across studies, the overall data suggest that chronic adaptations to physical activity result in decreased blood coagulability and maintained or increased fibrinolytic activity.

Electrical Stability of the Myocardium

Animal studies that induced myocardial ischemia by occluding a coronary artery have shown that the increased oxygen demand of the heart during acute exercise actually increases the risk of ventricular **fibrillation,** the leading cause of sudden cardiac death (Dawson, Leon, and Taylor 1979). In contrast, an increase in the ratio of oxygen supply to oxygen demand during exercise, which occurs after exercise training, should reduce the risk of ventricular fibrillation in people who have coronary artery disease. The reduction in sympathetic nervous system activity and catecholamine secretion during exercise of a fixed intensity, which occurs after exercise training, also should reduce myocardial irritability and the risk of ventricular fibrillation. However, exercise conditioning in CHD patients does not appear to change the frequency of irregular heartbeats originating outside the **sinoatrial node** (Laslett et al. 1983).

Dose Response

Another criterion that can help to determine whether a cause-and-effect relationship exists is dose response, that is, whether CHD risk decreases by a predictable dose–response pattern (e.g., linearly or curvilinearly) with increasing levels of physical activity or fitness, or whether there is a threshold level of activity or fitness above which further reductions in risk do not occur. The consensus from the Physical Activity Guidelines Advisory Committee (2008) is that a curvilinear dose–response relation between physical activity and CHD risk exists; a more recent meta-analysis also supports this (Sattelmair et al. 2011). For cardiorespiratory fitness, the association appears curvilinear as well (Kodama et al. 2009). In the following section, we discuss in more detail the nature of the dose–response relation, answering the question How much physical activity is needed to decrease CHD risk?

How Much Physical Activity Is Needed to Decrease Coronary Heart Disease Risk?

In addition to being one criterion for assessing causality, the amount of physical activity needed to decrease CHD risk also is important for public health, since this information is needed to make recommendations for physical activity. When considering how much physical activity is needed, we can investigate several specific dimensions of physical activity such as the total volume of energy expended on physical activity, the intensity, the duration, or the frequency. Each of these dimensions is discussed separately next.

As detailed in the preceding sections, data on the relation between physical activity and the primary prevention of CHD have come primarily from observational epidemiologic studies. Most of these studies used questionnaires to assess physical activity, and assessed one or more of these domains: occupational, leisure-time, household, and commuting activity. Most assessed mainly leisure-time physical activity of moderate or vigorous intensity. In analyses, investigators have typically combined the energy expended across all activities and then categorized subjects according to groups (generally three to five groups) based on their energy expenditure. Thus, most of the information available on how much physical activity is needed pertains to the volume of energy expended.

While many studies have provided information on the volume of energy expended, due to heterogeneity in the assessment of physical activity, as well as the groupings of subjects for analyses, it is difficult to combine physical activity data across studies. The Physical Activity Guidelines Advisory Committee qualitatively described the dose of physical activity for the dose–response relationship between physical activity and CHD risk (Physical Activity Guidelines Advisory Committee 2008). The expert panel defined three groups of different doses of physical activity (low, moderate, and high amounts) or intensity of physical activity without attempting to quantify what each of these levels translated to. Compared with men and women having "low" physical activity, on average, those with "moderate" physical activity had an approximately 20% to 25% reduced risk of CHD or CVD, and those with "high" physical activity had an approximately 30% to 35% risk reduction, suggesting a curvilinear relation (i.e., larger risk reduction from "low" to "moderate" than from "moderate" to "high"). A 2008 meta-analysis of prospective cohort studies assessing leisure-time physical activity used a similar approach. Investigators concluded that individuals with a moderate level of such activity had a relative risk of 0.88 (95% CI: 0.83-0.93) for CHD, compared with persons having low levels of leisure-time activity. For individuals with a high level of activity, the relative risk was 0.73 (0.66-0.80), suggesting a more linear inverse relation than that concluded by the 2008 Physical Activity Guidelines Advisory Committee. Again, these investigators did not attempt to translate what "low," "moderate," or "high" levels equated to (whether as energy expended or as time spent in physical activity). However, in both cases, it is clear that the three levels of physical activity represent increasing volumes of energy expended.

Individual studies have observed that the target set by the federal physical activity guidelines—an amount of energy expenditure equivalent to 150 min/week of moderate-intensity aerobic activity, or 75 min/week of vigorous-intensity aerobic activity, or a combination of the two that generates equivalent energy (U.S. Department of Health and Human Services 2008)—clearly is associated with reduction in rates of CHD. Additional reductions in CHD rates occur with the additional amounts of physical activity recommended by the 2008 federal guidelines—300 min/week of moderate-intensity, or 150 min/week of vigorous-intensity aerobic physical activity, or an equivalent combination of the two. For example, in an updated analysis from the Women's Health Study described previously, the multivariate relative risks for CHD associated with walking <1 h/week, 1 to 1.5 h/week, 2 to 3 h/week, and ≥4 h/week, compared with not walking, were 0.82 (0.67-1.00), 0.70 (0.56-0.88), 0.77 (0.60-0.97), and 0.65 (0.51-0.83), respectively; p, trend <0.001 (Weinstein et al. 2008).

While it is difficult to combine data across different studies, a recent meta-analysis attempted to do so for prospective cohort studies where the amount of energy expended on leisure-time physical activity could be estimated in kcal/week (Sattelmair et al. 2011). Although 33 identified studies published after 1995 allowed for qualitative estimations of the level of physical activity, only 9 provided sufficient data for quantitative estimates. Investigators calculated that individuals who expended 550 kcal/week in leisure-time physical activity (equivalent to 150 min/week of moderate-intensity activity, or current federal guidelines) had a 14% lower CHD risk compared with those reporting no leisure-time physical activity. And, expending 1100 kcal/week (300 min/week) was associated with a 20% lower risk. At higher levels of physical activity, risks continued to decline but more modestly, supporting a curvilinear relation. Persons who were physically active at levels lower than current guidelines also had a significantly lower risk of CHD, which supports federal guidelines that state that "some physical activity is better than none" and "additional benefits occur with more physical activity." (U.S. Department of Health and Human Services 2008).

With regard to dose response related to intensity of physical activity, the data have been limited. Several studies indeed have assessed physical activity of different intensities in relation to CHD risk. However, the interpretation of findings from these studies is not always straightforward because the intensity of physical activity is related to the total volume of energy expended. That is, when carried out for the same total duration, higher-intensity physical activities expend more total energy than do lower-intensity physical activities. Thus, if studies do not account for this correlation, it is unclear whether the significantly reduced risk associated with vigorous-intensity physical activity can be attributed to its intensity or whether it is merely due to the increase in the total volume of energy expended. It is clear from the discussion in the preceding paragraph that as volume of energy expended on physical activity increased, the risk of CHD decreased. Thus, the question of interest regarding intensity of physical activity is, For the same volume of energy expended, does vigorous-intensity activity confer additional benefits compared to moderate- or light-intensity activity? The data on this question are limited. Some studies, such as the Harvard Alumni Health Study, suggest that higher intensities of physical activity are associated with additional risk reductions, beyond their contribution to greater total volume of energy expended (Lee, Hiseh, and Paffenbarger 1995). But other studies, such as the Nurses' Health Study (Manson et al. 1999) and the Women's Health Initiative (Manson et al. 2002), suggest that equivalent energy expenditures, whether from walking (a moderate-intensity activity) or vigorous activities, are associated with similar risk reductions for CHD.

With regard to duration, longer duration of physical activity results in greater total volume of energy expended compared with shorter durations. However, just as with intensity, the duration of physical activity has the potential to be confounded by the total volume of energy expended. Therefore, the total volume must be taken into account in order to make conclusions regarding durations that are independent of the total volume of energy expended. The current federal physical activity guidelines allow physical activity to be accumulated in short bouts, lasting 10 min or more in duration, throughout the day (U.S. Department of Health and Human Services 2008). This allowance for accumulated short bouts of activity was based on the fact that in observational epidemiologic studies showing higher levels of physical activity associated with lower CHD risk, some subjects likely accumulated their activity throughout the day. Additionally, several randomized clinical trials now have shown that accumulated short bouts of physical activity during the day can improve cardiovascular risk factors (Murphy, Blair, and Murtagh 2009). Most of these trials investigated moderate-intensity physical activity, primarily walking. Typically, the trials have compared one long bout versus two or three accumulated bouts, totaling 20 to 30 min, five days a week. Thus, the short bouts tend to be bouts of 10 to 15 min. There are few data on bouts shorter than 10 min in duration.

The most common outcomes examined have been changes in cardiorespiratory fitness and body composition, with few data on other cardiovascular risk factors such as blood pressure, lipid profile, and glucose tolerance. The 2008 Physical Activity Guidelines Advisory Committee reviewed 11 randomized clinical trials that tested physical activity of different bout durations, all expending the same energy, and changes in cardiorespiratory fitness (Physical Activity Guidelines Advisory Committee 2008). In three studies, one single long bout produced superior changes in fitness compared with multiple short bouts; in two studies, multiple short bouts were superior to one single long bout; in five studies, long and short bouts produced equivalent changes in fitness; and in the last study, no improvements were observed with either one single long bout or multiple short bouts. Thus, the overall evidence suggests that comparable fitness responses can be achieved with different durations of physical activity when the energy expended is the same.

Murphy and colleagues reviewed 13 randomized controlled trials examining short versus long bouts of physical activity in relation to changes in body composition (Murphy, Blair, and Murtagh 2009). In one study, one single long bout produced larger changes in body composition compared with multiple short bouts expending the same energy; in another study, multiple short bouts were superior to one single long bout; in six studies, long and short bouts produced equivalent changes in body composition; and in the remaining five studies, no improvements were observed with either long bout or short bout regimens. Thus, these data also suggest comparable body composition changes with different physical activity durations that expend the same energy. Only one study has examined short versus long bouts of physical activity, controlling for the total energy expended in relation to CHD incidence. In an analysis of 7307 men from the Harvard Alumni Health Study with mean age 66 years, subjects were classified according to the longest duration reported per episode of activity, based on the various activities and different durations that they reported (Lee, Sesso, and Paffenbarger 2000). In multivariate analyses that also controlled for duration of activity bouts and the energy expended, duration of bouts was not predictive of CHD risk (P for trend = 0.25), but energy expenditure was (P for trend <0.05). These results indicate that it is the volume of energy expended that is important for decreasing CHD risk, and not the duration of physical activity, supporting current recommendations that allow activity to be accumulated in short bouts.

Indirect data supporting the concept of allowing accumulation of physical activity come from studies of commuting physical activity, which are suggestive of modest, inverse associations with cardiovascular end points (discussed in the earlier section "Other Kinds of Physical Activity and Coronary Heart Disease Risk"). A daily commute of 30 min by walking or cycling implies at least two bouts of physical activity: commuting to work and commuting from work.

Summary

The 2008 Physical Activity Guidelines Advisory Committee concluded that there is "strong evidence" that more active men and women have lower rates of CHD compared with less active persons (Physical Activity Guidelines Advisory Committee 2008). Data on the primary prevention of CHD with physical activity come only from observational epidemiologic studies. Experimental confirmation that physical inactivity directly causes CHD likely will never be obtained because the cost of randomized clinical trials is too great. It is also unethical to assign individuals to a sedentary control group given the strong and consistent evidence for a protective effect of increased physical activity against the risk for CHD, supported by plausible biological mechanisms. However, data do exist from randomized clinical trials of exercise-only cardiac rehabilitation programs in patients with CHD, showing that such programs decrease mortality rates. Public health policy in the United States is aggressively encouraging people to be more active because more than 60 epidemiologic studies published after 1996, including several reviewed in this chapter, consistently show that leisure-time physical activity is associated with lowered risks of CHD incidence and CHD mortality in both men and women regardless of age. The reduced risks are independent of several major risk factors for CHD, but the protective effect of physical activity can also operate through cardiovascular risk factors, by beneficially affecting risk factors for CHD such as blood pressure; body weight; blood lipids; and factors associated with atherosclerosis, blood coagulability, and inflammation.

Epidemiologic studies also suggest a dose–response relationship between physical activity and rates of CHD, but data on the shape of the association and the quantity of physical activity that provides optimal protection against the development of CHD are limited. This is largely due to methodological issues including the difficulty in measuring leisure-time physical activity precisely in population-based studies, the difficulty in comparing the amounts of physical activity estimated by different methods across studies, the lack of validation of self-reported physical activity with objective measures in several studies, and the fact that very few studies have quantified changes in physical activity or fitness in relation to changes in CHD incidence.

Nonetheless, there is general consensus among epidemiologists that current guidelines for physical activity from the federal government are sufficient to lower CHD risk. These guidelines encourage any amount of physical activity, and ideally require 150 min/week of moderate-intensity aerobic activity, or 75 min/week of vigorous-intensity physical activity, or the equivalent energy expenditure in a combination of moderate and vigorous activities. Physical activity can be accumulated in bouts of at least 10 min in duration to count toward the total. The guidelines further state that amounts of physical activity exceeding the target—300 min/week of moderate-intensity aerobic activity or 150 min/week of vigorous-intensity physical activity, or the equivalent energy expenditure in the two combined—are associated with additional risk reductions. Clinical experiments have shown that the recommended amounts of exercise provide enough of a stimulus to increase HDL cholesterol levels and fibrinolytic factors while helping to decrease blood pressure, triglycerides, body fat, and blood coagulability. Population studies also suggest a favorable effect of moderate physical activity on inflammatory features of atherogenesis and cardiac thrombosis.

Whether the dose–response relation between physical activity and lowered risk of CHD is linear or curvilinear is not clear. At present, most evidence supports a negatively accelerating decline in risk, where the largest reductions occur with moderate levels of activity or fitness as compared with those who are least active or fit, including data from a recent meta-analysis that attempted to combine data across different studies, quantitatively estimating kcal/week in leisure-time physical activity (Sattelmair et al. 2011). Risk continues to decline thereafter but to a diminishing degree. Whether more intense (e.g., vigorous) compared with less intense (e.g., moderate) activities provide additional protection against CHD risk, beyond merely contributing to higher volume of energy expenditure, also remains unclear.

In conclusion, there is a large body of epidemiologic evidence, supported by mechanistic studies, showing that physical activity lowers the risk of CHD in both men and women. Modest levels of physical activity, such as 150 min/week of brisk walking, which can be accumulated in bouts of at least 10 min, is sufficient to lower risk. And, for persons willing to do more, additional amounts of physical activity beyond that confer additional risk reductions.

· BIBLIOGRAPHY ·

Abramson, J.L., and V. Vaccarino. 2002. Relationship between physical activity and inflammation among apparently healthy middle-aged and older U.S. adults. *Archives of Internal Medicine* 162 (11): 1286-1292.

Adamopoulos, S., J. Parissis, C. Kroupis, M. Georgiadis, D. Karatzas, G. Karavolias, K. Koniavitou, A.J. Coats, and D.T. Kremastinos. 2001. Physical training reduces peripheral markers of inflammation in patients with chronic heart failure. *European Heart Journal* 22 (9): 791-797.

Albert, C.M., J. Ma, N. Rifai, M.J. Stampfer, and P.M. Ridker. 2002. Prospective study of C-reactive protein, homocysteine, and plasma lipid levels as predictors of sudden cardiac death. *Circulation* 105: 2595-2599.

Albert, C.M., N.R. Cook, J.M. Gaziano, E. Zaharris, J. MacFadyen, E. Danielson, J.E. Buring, and J.E. Manson. 2008. Effect of folic acid and B vitamins on risk of cardiovascular events and total mortality among women at high risk for cardiovascular disease: A randomized trial. *JAMA.* 299: 2027-2036.

Bijnen, F.C., C.J. Caspersen, E.J. Feskens, W.H. Saris, W.L. Mosterd, and D. Kromhout. 1998. Physical activity and 10-year mortality from cardiovascular diseases and all causes: The Zutphen Elderly Study. *Archives of Internal Medicine* 158: 1499-1505.

Bijnen, F.C., C.J. Caspersen, and W.L. Mosterd. 1994. Physical inactivity as a risk factor for coronary heart disease: A WHO and International Society and Federation of Cardiology position statement. *Bulletin of the World Health Organization* 72 (1): 1-4.

Bijnen, F., E. Feskens, C. Caspersen, S. Giampaoli, A. Nissinen, A. Menotti, W. Mosterd, and D. Kromhout. 1996. Physical activity and cardiovascular risk factors among elderly men in Finland, Italy, and the Netherlands. *American Journal of Epidemiology* 143: 553-661.

Bladbjerg, E.M., L. Moller, and J. Jespersen. 1998. Association of factor VII protein concentration with lifestyle factors. *Scandinavian Journal of Clinical and Laboratory Investigation* 58: 323-330.

Blair, S.N., J.B. Kampert, H.W. Kohl 3rd, C.E. Barlow, C.A. Macera, R.S. Paffenbarger Jr., and L.W. Gibbons. 1996. Influences of cardiorespiratory fitness and other precursors on cardiovascular disease and all-cause mortality in men and women. *Journal of the American Medical Association* 276: 205-210.

Blair, S.N., H.W. Kohl III, C.E. Barlow, R.S. Paffenbarger Jr., L.W. Gibbons, and C.A. Macera. 1995. Changes in physical fitness and all-cause mortality: A prospective study of healthy and unhealthy men. *Journal of the American Medical Association* 273: 1093-1098.

Blair, S.N., H.W. Kohl 3rd, R.S. Paffenbarger Jr., D.G. Clark, K.H. Cooper, and L.W. Gibbons. 1989. Physical fitness and all-cause mortality. A prospective study of healthy men and women. *Journal of the American Medical Association* 262: 2395-2401.

Blair, S., H. Kohl, R. Paffenbarger, D. Clark, K. Cooper, and L. Gibbons. 1989. Physical fitness and all-cause mortality: A prospective study of healthy men and women. *Journal of the American Medical Association* 262: 2395-2401.

Brunner, D., G. Manelis, M. Modan, and S. Levin. 1974. Physical activity at work and the incidence of myocardial infarction, angina pectoris and death due to ischemic heart disease: An epidemiological study in Israeli collective settlements (kibbutzim). *Journal of Chronic Diseases* 27: 217-233.

Cassell, J., S. Heyden, A.C. Bartel, B.H. Kaplan, H.A. Tyroler, J.C. Cornoni, and J.C. Hames. 1971. Occupation and physical activity and coronary heart disease. *Archives of Internal Medicine* 128: 920-928.

Chapman, J.M., and F.J. Massey. 1964. The inter-relationship of serum cholesterol, hypertension, body weight and risk of coronary heart disease: Results of the first ten years' follow-up in the Los Angeles Heart Study. *Journal of Chronic Diseases* 17: 933-947.

Church, T.S., C.E. Barlow, C.P. Earnest, J.B. Kampert, E.L. Priest, and S.N. Blair. 2002. Associations between cardiorespiratory fitness and C-reactive protein in men. *Arteriosclerosis, Thrombosis, and Vascular Biology* 22: 1869-1876.

Church, T.S., C.P. Earnest, J.S. Skinner, and S.N. Blair. 2007. Effects of different doses of physical activity on cardiorespiratory fitness among sedentary, overweight or obese postmenopausal women with elevated blood pressure: A randomized controlled trial. *Journal of the American Medical Association* 297: 2081-2091.

Clark, A.M., L. Hartling, B. Vandermeer, and F.A. McAlister. 2005. Meta-analysis: Secondary prevention programs for patients with coronary artery disease. *Annals of Internal Medicine* 143: 659-672.

Connelly, J.B., J.A. Cooper, and T.W. Meade. 1992. Strenuous exercise, plasma fibrinogen, and factor VII activity. *British Heart Journal* 67: 351-354.

Curfman, G. 1993. The health benefits of exercise: A critical appraisal. *New England Journal of Medicine* 328 (8): 574-575.

Currens, J.H., and P.D. White. 1961. Half century of running: Clinical, physiological, and pathological findings in the case of Clarence DeMar ("Mr. Marathon"). *New England Journal of Medicine* 265: 988-993.

Dawson, A.K., A.S. Leon, and H.L. Taylor. 1979. Effect of submaximal exercise on vulnerability to fibrillation in the canine ventricle. *Circulation* 60: 798-804.

DeSouza, C.A., D.R. Dengel, M.A. Rogers, K. Cox, and R.F. Macko. 1997. Fibrinolytic responses to acute physical activity in older hypertensive men. *Journal of Applied Physiology* 82: 1765-1770.

DeSouza, C.A., P.P. Jones, and D.R. Seals. 1998. Physical activity status and adverse age-related differences in coagulation and fibrinolytic factors in women. *Arteriosclerosis, Thrombosis, and Vascular Biology* 18: 362-368.

Division of Chronic Disease Control and Community Intervention. 1993. Public health focus: Physical activity and prevention of coronary heart disease. *Journal of the American Medical Association* 279: 1529-1530.

Dorn, J., J. Naughton, D. Imamura, and M. Trevisan. 1999. Results of a multicenter randomized clinical trial of exercise and long-term survival in myocardial infarction patients: The National Exercise and Heart Disease Project (NEHDP). *Circulation* 100 (17): 1764-1769.

Ekelund, L.G., W.L. Haskell, J.L. Johnson, F.S. Whaley, M.H. Criqui, and D.S. Sheps. 1988. Physical fitness as a predictor of cardiovascular mortality in asymptomatic North American men: The Lipid Research Clinics mortality follow-up study. *New England Journal of Medicine* 319: 1379-1384.

Eliasson, M., K. Asplund, and P.E. Evrin. 1996. Regular leisure time physical activity predicts high activity of tissue plasminogen activator: The Northern Sweden MONICA Study. *International Journal of Epidemiology* 25: 1182-1188.

el-Sayed, M.S. 1996. Effects of exercise on blood coagulation, fibrinolysis, and platelet aggregation. *Sports Medicine* 22: 282-298.

Epstein, L., G.T. Miller, F.W. Sitt, and J.N. Morris. 1976. Vigorous exercise in leisure-time, coronary risk factors, and resting electrocardiograms in middle-aged civil servants. *British Heart Journal* 38: 403-409.

Fernhall, B., L.M. Szymanski, P.A. Gorman, J. Milani, D.C. Paup, and C.M. Kessler. 1997. Fibrinolytic activity is similar in physically active men with and without a history of myocardial infarction. *Arteriosclerosis, Thrombosis, and Vascular Biology* 17: 1106-1113.

Fletcher, G.F., G. Balady, S.N. Blair, J. Blumenthal, C. Caspersen, B. Chaitman, S. Epstein, E.S. Sivarajan Froelicher, V.F. Froelicher, I.L. Pina, and M.L. Pollock. 1996. Statement on exercise: Benefits and recommendations for physical activity programs for all Americans. A statement for health professionals by the Committee on Exercise and Cardiac Rehabilitation of the Council on Clinical Cardiology, American Heart Association. *Circulation* 94 (4): 857-862.

Folsom, A.R., N. Aleksic, D. Catellier, H.S. Juneja, and K.K. Wu. 2002. C-reactive protein and incident coronary heart disease in the Atherosclerosis Risk in Communities (ARIC) study. *American Heart Journal* 144 (2): 233-238.

Folsom, A.R., H.T. Qamheih, J.M. Flack, J.E. Hilner, K. Liu, B.V. Howard, and R.P. Tracy. 1993. Plasma fibrinogen: Levels and correlates in young adults. The coronary artery risk development in young adults (CARDIA) study. *American Journal of Epidemiology* 138: 1023-1036.

Ford, E.S. 2002. Does exercise reduce inflammation? Physical activity and C-reactive protein among U.S. adults. *Epidemiology* 13 (5): 561-568.

Garcia-Palmieri, M.R., R. Costas Jr., M. Cruz-Vidal, P.D. Sorlie, and R.J. Havlik. 1982. Increased physical activity: A protective factor against heart attacks in Puerto Rico. *American Journal of Cardiology* 50: 749-755.

Geffken, D., M. Cushman, G. Burke, J. Polak, P. Sakkinen, and R. Tracy. 2001. Association between physical activity and markers of inflammation in a healthy elderly population. *American Journal of Epidemiology* 153 (3): 242-250.

Gulati, M., H.R. Black, L.J. Shaw, M.F. Arnsdorf, C.N. Merz, M.S. Lauer, T.H. Marwick, D.K. Pandey, R.H. Wicklund, and R.A. Thisted. 2005. The prognostic value of a nomogram for exercise capacity in women. *New England Journal of Medicine* 353: 468-475.

Haapanen-Niemi, N., I. Vuori, and M. Pasanen. 1999. Public health burden of coronary heart disease risk factors among middle-aged and elderly men. *Preventive Medicine* 28: 343-348.

Hakim, A.A., J.D. Curb, H. Petrovitch, B.L. Rodriguez, K. Yano, G.W. Ross, L.R. White, and R.D. Abbott. 1999. Effects of walking on coronary heart disease in elderly men: The Honolulu Heart Program. *Circulation* 100 (1): 9-13.

Hamer, M., and Y. Chida. 2008. Active commuting and cardiovascular risk: A meta-analytic review. *Preventive Medicine* 46: 9-13.

Hamer, M., and E. Stamatakis. 2009. Physical activity and mortality in men and women with diagnosed cardiovascular disease. *European Journal of Cardiovascular Prevention and Rehabilitation* 16: 156-160.

Hamilton, M.T., D.G. Hamilton, and T.W. Zderic. 2007. Role of low energy expenditure and sitting in obesity, metabolic syndrome, type 2 diabetes, and cardiovascular disease. *Diabetes* 56: 2655-2667.

Hamsten, A. 1995. Hemostatic function and coronary artery disease. *New England Journal of Medicine* 332: 677-678.

Heberden, W. 1818. *Commentaries on the history and cure of diseases.* Boston: Wells and Lilly.

Hellenius, M., U. Faire, B. Berglund, A. Hamsten, and I. Krakau. 1993. Diet and exercise are equally effective in reducing risk for cardiovascular disease: Results of a randomized controlled study in men with slightly to moderately raised cardiovascular risk factors. *Atherosclerosis* 103: 81-91.

Hennekens, C.H., J. Rosner, M.J. Jesse, M.E. Drolette, and F.E. Speizer. 1977. A retrospective study of physical activity and coronary deaths. *International Journal of Epidemiology* 6: 243-246.

Hinkle, L.E., L.A. Whitney, E.W. Lehman, J. Dunn, B. Benjamin, R. King, A. Plakun, and B. Flehiner. 1968. Occupation, education, and coronary heart disease. *Science* 161: 238-246.

Homocysteine Studies Collaboration. 2002. Homocysteine and risk of ischemic heart disease and stroke: A meta-analysis. *Journal of the American Medical Association* 288: 2015-2022.

Kampert, J., S.N. Blair, C.E. Barlow, and H.W. Kohl III. 1996. Physical activity, physical fitness, and all-cause and cancer mortality: A prospective study of men and women. *Annals of Epidemiology* 6: 452-457.

Kannel, W.B., and P. Sorlie. 1979. Some health benefits of physical activity: The Framingham Study. *Archives of Internal Medicine* 139: 857-861.

Karvonen, M.J. 1982. Physical activity in work and leisure time in relation to cardiovascular diseases. *Annals of Clinical Research* 14 (Suppl. 34): 118-123.

Katzmarzyk, P.T., T.S. Church, C.L. Craig, and C. Bouchard. 2009. Sitting time and mortality from all causes, cardiovascular disease, and cancer. *Medicine and Science in Sports and Exercise* 41: 998-1005.

Keys, A. 1980. *Seven countries: A multivariate analysis of death and coronary disease.* Cambridge, MA: Harvard University Press.

Kipple, K.F., ed. 1993. *The Cambridge world history of human disease.* New York: Cambridge University Press.

Kodama, S., K. Saito, S. Tanaka, M. Maki, Y. Yachi, M. Asumi, A. Sugawara, K. Totsuka, H. Shimano, Y. Ohashi, N. Yamada, and H. Sone. 2009. Cardiorespiratory fitness as a quantitative predictor of all-cause mortality and cardiovascular events in healthy men and women: A meta-analysis. *Journal of the American Medical Association* 301: 2024-2035.

Koenig, W., M. Sund, A. Doring, and E. Ernst. 1997. Leisure-time physical activity but not work-related physical activity is associated with decreased plasma viscosity: Results from a large population sample. *Circulation* 95: 335-341.

Kramsch, L.M., A.J. Aspen, B.M. Abramowitz, T. Kreimendal, and W.B. Hood Jr. 1981. Reduction of coronary artherosclerosis by moderate conditioning exercise in monkeys on an atherogenic diet. *New England Journal of Medicine* 305: 1483-1489.

LaCroix, A.Z., S.G. Leveille, J.A. Hecht, L.C. Grothaus, and E.H. Wagner. 1996. Does walking decrease the risk of cardiovascular disease hospitalizations and death in older adults? *Journal of the American Geriatrics Society* 44: 113-120.

Lakka, T.A., J.M. Venalainen, R. Rauramaa, R. Slagnen, J. Tuomilehto, and J.T. Salonen. 1994. Relation of leisure-time physical activity and cardiorespiratory fitness to the risk of acute myocardial infarction in men. *New England Journal of Medicine* 330: 1549-1554.

LaMonte, M.J., J.L. Durstine, F.G. Yanowitz, T. Lim, K.D. DuBose, P. Davis, and B.E. Ainsworth. 2002. Cardiorespiratory fitness and C-reactive protein among a tri-ethnic sample of women. *Circulation* 106 (4): 403-406.

Laslett, L., P.S. Baiser, L. Palmer, and E.A. Amsterdam. 1983. Ventricular ectopy frequency and complexity not altered in exercise training in coronary disease patients. *Cardiology* 70: 284-290.

Lee, I.M., C.C. Hsieh, and R.S. Paffenbarger Jr. 1995. Exercise intensity and longevity in men. The Harvard Alumni Health Study. *Journal of the American Medical Association* 273: 1179-1184.

Lee, I.M., and R.S. Paffenbarger Jr. 2000. Associations of light, moderate, and vigorous intensity physical activity and longevity: The Harvard Alumni Health Study. *American Journal of Epidemiology* 151: 293-299.

Lee, I.M., and R.S. Paffenbarger. 2001. Preventing coronary heart disease: The role of physical activity. *Physician and Sports-medicine* 29 (2): 37-52.

Lee, I.M., K.M. Rexrode, N.R. Cook, J.E. Manson, and J.E. Buring. 2001. Physical activity and coronary heart disease in women: Is "no pain, no gain" passe? *Journal of the American Medical Association* 285: 1447-1454.

Lee, I.M., H.D. Sesso, and R.S. Paffenbarger Jr. 2000. Physical activity and coronary heart disease risk in men: Does the duration of exercise episodes predict risk? *Circulation* 102: 981-986.

Lemaitre, R.N., D.S. Siscovick, T.E. Raghunathan, S. Weinmann, P. Arbogast, and D.Y. Lin. 1999. Leisure-time physical activity and the risk of primary cardiac arrest. *Archives of Internal Medicine* 159: 686-690.

Leon, A.S. 1972. Comparative cardiovascular adaptation to exercise in animals and man and its relevance to coronary heart disease. In *Comparative pathophysiology of circulatory disturbances,* edited by C.M. Bloor. New York: Plenum Press.

Leon, A.S., and H. Blackburn. 1977. The relationship of physical activity to coronary heart disease and life expectancy. *Annals of the New York Academy of Sciences* 301: 361-378.

Leon, A.S., and C.M. Bloor. 1977. The effects of complete and partial deconditioning on exercise-induced cardio-vascular changes in the rat. *Advances in Cardiology* 18: 81-92.

Leon, A.S., J. Connett, D.R. Jacobs Jr., and R. Rauramaa. 1987. Leisure-time physical activity levels and risk of coronary heart disease and death: The Multiple Risk Factor Intervention Trial. *Journal of the American Medical Association* 258: 2388-2395.

Leon, A.S., M.J. Myers, and J. Connett. 1997. Leisure time physical activity and the 16-year risks of mortality from coronary heart disease and all-causes in the Multiple Risk Factor Intervention Trial (MRFIT). *International Journal of Sports Medicine* 18 (Suppl. 3): S208-S215.

Libby, P., P.M. Ridker, and A. Maseri. 2002. Inflammation and atherosclerosis. *Circulation* 105: 1135-1143.

Lloyd-Jones, D., R.J. Adams, T.M. Brown, M. Carnethon, S. Dai, G. De Simone, T.B. Ferguson, E. Ford, K. Furie, C. Gillespie, A. Go, K. Greenlund, N. Haase, S. Hailpern, P.M. Ho, V. Howard, B. Kissela, S. Kittner, D. Lackland, L. Lisabeth, A. Marelli, M.M. McDermott, J. Meigs, D. Mozaffarian, M. Mussolino, G. Nichol, V.L. Roger, W. Rosamond, R. Sacco, P. Sorlie, R. Stafford, T. Thom, S. Wasserthiel-Smoller, N.D. Wong, and J. Wylie-Rosett. 2010. Heart disease and stroke statistics—2010 update: A report from the American Heart Association. *Circulation* 121: e46-e215.

Lloyd-Jones, D.M., M.G. Larson, A. Beiser, and D. Levy. 1999. Lifetime risk of developing coronary heart disease. *Lancet* 353 (9147): 89-92.

Magnus, K., A. Matroos, and J. Stracklee. 1979. Walking, cycling, or gardening with or without seasonal interruption in relation to acute coronary events. *American Journal of Epidemiology* 110: 724-733.

Manson, J.E., P. Greenland, A.Z. LaCroix, M.L. Stefanick, C.P. Mouton, A. Oberman, M.G. Perri, D.S. Sheps, M.B. Pettinger, and D.S. Siscovick. 2002. Walking compared with vigorous exercise for the prevention of cardiovascular events in women. *New England Journal of Medicine* 347: 716-725.

Manson, J.E., F.B. Hu, J.W. Rich-Edwards, G.A. Colditz, M.J. Stampfer, W.C. Willett, F.E. Speizer, and C.H. Hennekens. 1999. A prospective study of walking as compared with vigorous exercise in the prevention of coronary heart disease in women. *New England Journal of Medicine* 341 (9): 650-658.

Maresca, G., A. Di Blasio, R. Marchioli, and G. Di Minno. 1999. Measuring plasma fibrinogen to predict stroke and myocardial infarction: An update. *Arteriosclerosis, Thrombosis, and Vascular Biology* 19 (6): 1368-1377.

McCully, K.S. 1969. Vascular pathology of homocysteinemia: Implications for the pathogenesis of arteriosclerosis. *American Journal of Pathology* 56: 111-128.

McGrew, R.E. 1985. *Encyclopedia of medical history.* New York: McGraw-Hill.

Mitrani, Y., H. Karplus, and D. Bunner. 1970. Coronary atherosclerosis in cases of traumatic death. In *Physical activity and aging,* Vol. 4 of *Medicine and sport,* edited by D. Bruner and E. Jokl. Baltimore: University Park Press.

Mora, S., N. Cook, J.E. Buring, P.M. Ridker, and I.M. Lee. 2007. Physical activity and reduced risk of cardiovascular events: Potential mediating mechanisms. *Circulation* 116: 2110-2118.

Morris, J.N., S.P.W. Chave, C. Adams, C. Sirey, L. Epstein, and D.J. Sheehan. 1973. Vigorous exercise in leisure-time and the incidence of coronary heart disease. *Lancet* 1: 333-339.

Morris, J.N., D.G. Clayton, M.G. Everitt, A.M. Semmence, and E.H. Burgess. 1990. Exercise in leisure time: Coronary attack and death rates. *British Heart Journal* 63: 325-334.

Morris, J.N., and M.D. Crawford. 1958. Coronary heart disease and physical activity of work: Evidence of a national necropsy survey. *British Medical Journal* 2: 1488-1496.

Morris, J.N., M.D. Everitt, R. Pollard, S.P.W. Chave, and A.M. Semmence. 1980. Vigorous exercise in leisure-time: Protection against coronary heart disease. *Lancet* 2: 1207-1210.

Morris, J.N., J.A. Heady, P.A.B. Raffle, C.G. Roberts, and J.W. Parks. 1953. Coronary heart disease and physical activity of work. *Lancet* 2: 1053-1057, 1111-1120.

Mortensen, J.M., T.T. Stevensen, and L.H. Whitney. 1959. Mortality due to coronary heart disease analyzed by broad occupational groups. *Archives of Industrial Health* 19: 1-4.

Multiple Risk Factor Intervention Trial Research Group. 1982. Multiple Risk Factor Intervention Trial: Risk factor changes and mortality results. *Journal of the American Medical Association* 248: 1465.

Murphy, M.H., S.N. Blair, and E.M. Murtagh. 2009. Accumulated versus continuous exercise for health benefit: A review of empirical studies. *Sports Medicine* 39: 29-43.

National Heart, Lung, and Blood Institute. 1998. *Morbidity and mortality: 1998 chartbook on cardiovascular, lung, and blood diseases.* Rockville, MD: U.S. Department of Health and Human Services, National Institutes of Health.

O'Connor, G.T., J.E. Buring, S. Yusuf, S.Z. Goldhaber, E.M. Olmstead, R.S. Paffenbarger Jr., and C.H. Hennekens. 1989. An overview of randomized trials of rehabilitation with exercise after myocardial infarction. *Circulation* 80 (2): 234-244.

Paffenbarger, R.S. Jr., and W.E. Hale. 1975. Work activity and coronary heart disease mortality. *New England Journal of Medicine* 292: 545-550.

Paffenbarger, R.S. Jr., W.W. Hale, R.J. Brand, and R.T. Hyde. 1977. Work-energy level, personal characteristics, and fatal heart attack: A birth cohort effect. *American Journal of Epidemiology* 105: 200-213.

Paffenbarger, R.S. Jr., R.T. Hyde, A.L. Wing, I.M. Lee, D.L. Jung, and J.B. Kampert. 1993. The association of changes in physical-activity level and other lifestyle characteristics with mortality among men. *New England Journal of Medicine* 328: 538-545.

Paffenbarger, R.S. Jr., A. Wing, and R. Hyde. 1978. Physical activity as an index of heart attack risk in college alumni. *American Journal of Epidemiology* 108: 168-175.

Paffenbarger, R.S. Jr., A. Wing, and R. Hyde. 1981. Chronic disease in former college students: XVI. Physical activity as an index of heart attack risk in college alumni. *American Journal of Epidemiology* 108: 161-175.

Paul, O.M., M.H. Lepper, W.H. Phelan, G.W. Dupertuis, and G.W. Macmillan. 1963. A longitudinal study of coronary heart disease. *Circulation* 28: 20-31.

Perls, T.T., and R.C. Fretts. 2001. The evolution of menopause and human lifespan. *Annals of Human Biology* 28: 237-245.

Peters, R.K.L., L.D. Cady Jr., D.P. Bischoff, L. Berstein, and M.C. Pike. 1983. Physical fitness and subsequent myocardial infarction in healthy workers. *Journal of the American Medical Association* 249: 3052-3056.

Physical activity and cardiovascular health: NIH Consensus Development Panel on Physical Activity and Cardiovascular Health. 1996. *Journal of the American Medical Association* 276: 241-246.

Physical Activity Guidelines Advisory Committee. 2008. *Physical Activity Guidelines Advisory Committee report.* www.health.gov/paguidelines/.

Pomrehn, P.R., R.B. Wallace, and L.F. Burmeister. 1982. Ischemic heart disease mortality in Iowa farmers. The influence of life-style. *Journal of the American Medical Association* 248: 1073-1076.

Ponjee, G.A., E.M. Janssen, J. Hermans, and J.W. van Wersch. 1996. Regular physical activity and changes in risk factors for coronary heart disease: A nine month prospective study. *European Journal of Clinical Chemistry and Clinical Biochemistry* 34: 477-483.

Powell, K.E., and S.N. Blair. 1994. The public health burdens of sedentary living habits: Theoretical but realistic estimates. *Medicine and Science in Sports and Exercise* 26: 851-856.

Powell, K.E., P.D. Thompson, C.J. Caspersen, and J.S. Kendrick. 1987. Physical activity and the incidence of coronary heart disease. *Annual Review of Public Health* 8: 253-287.

Punsar, S., and M. Karvonen. 1976. Physical activity and coronary disease in populations from east and west Finland. *Advances in Cardiology* 18: 196-207.

Ridker, P.M., E. Danielson, F.A. Fonseca, J. Genest, A.M. Gotto, Jr., J.J. Kastelein, W. Koenig, P. Libby, A.J. Lorenzatti, J.G. MacFadyen, B.G. Nordestgaard, J. Shepherd, J.T. Willerson, and R.J. Glynn. 2008. Rosuvastatin to prevent vascular events in men and women with elevated C-reactive protein. *New England Journal of Medicine* 359: 2195-2207.

Rifai, N., and P.M. Ridker. 2002. Inflammatory markers and coronary heart disease. *Current Opinion in Lipidemiology* 13 (4): 383-389.

Rissanen, V. 1976. Occupational physical activity and coronary artery disease: A clinicopathologic appraisal. *Advances in Cardiology* 18: 113-121.

Rose, G. 1969. Physical activity and coronary heart disease. *Proceedings of the Royal Society of Medicine* 62: 1183-1188.

Ross, R., and J.A. Glomset. 1976. The pathogenesis of arteriosclerosis. *New England Journal of Medicine* 295: 369, 420.

Sattelmair, J.R., J. Pertman, E.L. Ding, H.W. Kohl III, W.L. Haskell, and I-M. Lee. 2011. Dose-response between physical activity and risk of coronary heart disease: A meta-analysis. *Circulation* 124 :789-795.

Sesso, H.D., R.S. Paffenbarger Jr., and I.M. Lee. 2000. Physical activity and coronary heart disease in men: The Harvard Alumni Health Study. *Circulation* 102: 975-980.

Shaper, A.G., G. Wannamethee, and R. Weatherall. 1991. Physical activity and ischaemic heart disease in middle-aged British men. *British Heart Journal* 66: 384-394.

Shapiro, S., E. Weinblatt, C.W. Frank, and R.V. Sager. 1969. Incidence of coronary heart disease in a population insured for medical care (HIP): Myocardial infarction, angina pectoris, and possible myocardial infarction. *American Journal of Public Health* 59 (Suppl. 2): 1-101.

Siscovick, D.S., N.S. Weiss, A.P. Hallstrom, T.S. Inui, and D.R. Peterson. 1982. Physical activity and primary cardiac arrest. *Journal of the American Medical Association* 248: 3113-3117.

Sofi, F., A. Capalbo, F. Cesari, R. Abbate, and G.F. Gensini. 2008. Physical activity during leisure time and primary prevention of coronary heart disease: An updated meta-analysis of cohort studies. *European Journal of Cardiovascular Prevention and Rehabilitation* 15: 247-257.

Spain, D.M., and V.A. Bradess. 1957. Sudden death from coronary atherosclerosis: Age, race, sex, physical activity, and alcohol. *Archives of Internal Medicine* 100: 228-231.

Spain, D.M., and V.A. Bradess. 1960. Occupational physical activity and the degree of coronary atherosclerosis in "normal" men: A postmortem study. *Circulation* 22: 239-242.

Stamler, J.D., D.M. Berkson, H.A. Lindberg, et al. 1970. Long term epidemiologic studies on the possible role of physical activity and physical fitness in the prevention of premature clinical coronary heart disease. In *Physical activity and aging,* Vol. 4 of *Medicine and sports,* edited by D. Brunner and E. Jokl. Baltimore: University Park Press.

Stamler, J., H.A. Lindberg, D.M. Berkson, A. Shaffer, W. Miller, and A. Poindexter. 1960. Prevalence and incidence of coronary heart disease in strata of the labor force of a Chicago industrial corporation. *Journal of Chronic Diseases* 11: 405-420.

Stratton, J.R., W.L. Chandler, R.S. Schwartz, M.D. Cerqueira, W.C. Levy, S.E. Kahn, V.G. Larson, K.C. Cain, J.C. Beard, and I.B. Abrass. 1991. Effects of physical conditioning on fibrinolytic variables and fibrinogen in young and old healthy adults. *Circulation* 83: 1692-1697.

Strong, K., C. Mathers, S. Leeder, and R. Beaglehole. 2005. Preventing chronic diseases: How many lives can we save? *Lancet* 366: 1578-1582.

Sui, X., S.P. Hooker, I.M. Lee, T.S. Church, N. Colabianchi, C.D. Lee, and S.N. Blair. 2008. A prospective study of cardiorespiratory fitness and risk of type 2 diabetes in women. *Diabetes Care* 31: 550-555.

Szymanski, L.M., R.R. Pate, and J.L. Durstine. 1994. Effects of maximal exercise and venous occlusion in fibrinolytic activity in physically active and inactive men. *Journal of Applied Physiology* 77: 2305-2310.

Tanasescu, M., M.F. Leitzmann, E.B. Rimm, W.C. Willett, M.J. Stampfer, and F.B. Hu. 2002. Exercise type and intensity in relation to coronary heart disease in men. *Journal of the American Medical Association* 288: 1994-2000.

Taylor, H.B., H. Blackburn, A. Keys, R.W. Parlin, C. Vasquez, and T. Puchner. 1970. Five-year follow-up of employees of selected U.S. railroad companies. *Circulation* 41 (Suppl. 1): 120-139.

Taylor, H.L., E. Klepetar, A. Keys, R.W. Parlin, and H. Blackburn. 1962. Death rates among physically active and sedentary employees of the railroad industry. *American Journal of Public Health* 52: 1697-1707.

Taylor, H.L., A. Mellotti, and V. Puddu. 1970. Five year follow-up of railroad men in Italy. *Circulation* 41 (Suppl.): 111-122.

Taylor, R.S., A. Brown, S. Ebrahim, J. Jolliffe, H. Noorani, K. Rees, B. Skidmore, J.A. Stone, D.R. Thompson, and N. Oldridge. 2004. Exercise-based rehabilitation for patients with coronary heart disease: Systematic review and meta-analysis of randomized controlled trials. *American Journal of Medicine* 116: 682-692.

Tunstall-Pedoe, H., K. Kuulasmaa, M. Mahonen, H. Tolonen, E. Ruokokoski, and P. Amouyel. 1999. Contribution of trends in survival and coronary-event rates to changes in coronary heart disease mortality: 10-year results from 37 WHO MONICA project populations. Monitoring trends and determinants in cardiovascular disease. *Lancet* 353 (9164): 1547-1557.

U.S. Department of Health and Human Services. 1996. *Physical activity and health: A report of the Surgeon General.* Atlanta: U.S. Department of Health and Human Services, Centers for Disease Control and Prevention, National Center for Chronic Disease Prevention and Health Promotion.

U.S. Department of Health and Human Services. 2008. *2008 Physical activity guidelines for Americans.* www.health.gov/paguidelines/.

Wang, J.S., C.J. Jen, and H.I. Chen. 1995. Effects of exercise training and deconditioning on platelet function in men. *Arteriosclerosis, Thrombosis, and Vascular Biology* 15: 1668-1674.

Wannamethee, S.G., G.D. Lowe, P.H. Whincup, A. Rumley, M. Walker, and L. Lennon. 2002. Physical activity and hemostatic and inflammatory variables in elderly men. *Circulation* 105 (15): 1785-1790.

Wei, M., J.B. Kampert, C.E. Barlow, M.Z. Nichaman, L.W. Gibbons, R.S. Paffenbarger Jr., and S.N. Blair. 1999. Relationship between low cardiorespiratory fitness and mortality in normal-weight, overweight, and obese men. *Journal of the American Medical Association* 282: 1547-1553.

Weinstein, A.R., H.D. Sesso, I.M. Lee, K.M. Rexrode, N.R. Cook, J.E. Manson, J.E. Buring, and J.M. Gaziano. 2008. The joint effects of physical activity and body mass index on coronary heart disease risk in women. *Archives of Internal Medicine* 168: 884-890.

Williams, M.A., W.L. Haskell, P.A. Ades, E.A. Amsterdam, V. Bittner, B.A. Franklin, M. Gulanick, S.T. Laing, and K.J. Stewart. 2007. Resistance exercise in individuals with and without cardiovascular disease: 2007 update: A scientific statement from the American Heart Association Council on Clinical Cardiology and Council on Nutrition, Physical Activity, and Metabolism. *Circulation* 116: 572-584.

Williams, P.T., P.D. Wood, W.L. Haskell, and K. Vranizan. 1982. The effects of running mileage and duration on plasma lipoprotein levels. *Journal of the American Medical Association* 247: 2674-2679.

World Health Organization. 2003. *The world health report 2002: Reducing risks, promoting healthy life.* Geneva: World Health Organization.

Zukel, W.J., R.H. Lewis, P.E. Enterline, R.C. Painter, and L.S. Ralston. 1959. A short-term community study of the epidemiology of coronary heart disease. *American Journal of Public Health* 49: 1630-1639.

CHAPTER 6

Cerebrovascular Disease and Stroke

Apoplexy is a stroke of God's hands.

· Oxford English Dictionary, 1599 ·

CHAPTER OBJECTIVES

▸ Describe the public health burden of cerebrovascular disease and stroke, including its prevalence, incidence, and mortality rates in population groups

▸ Identify the major modifiable and nonmodifiable risk factors of stroke

▸ Discuss the types and pathophysiology of stroke and how physical activity might alter the mechanisms of stroke

▸ Describe and evaluate the strength of evidence that physical activity reduces stroke risk

A stroke is the loss or impairment of bodily function resulting from injury or death of brain cells following insufficient blood supply. Hippocrates is credited with first describing stroke and its crippling effects. He used the Greek term *apolessein,* which means to be thunderstruck, because the disease was seen as a catastrophic, uncontrollable event of nature. Before the renaissance of medicine in the 16th century, the *Oxford English Dictionary* defined apoplexy (from *apoplexia,* the Latin derivation of *apolessein*) as "a stroke of God's hands," hence the modern usage of the term *stroke* to denote a cerebrovascular accident.

▷ **A STROKE IS** the loss or impairment of bodily function resulting from injury or death of brain cells consequent to insufficient blood supply.

See "Five Common Signs of Stroke" for warning signs. Not all of the common signs occur during a **stroke.** When they occur but last only a short while (e.g., a few minutes), they may indicate what is known as a **transient ischemic attack (TIA).** A TIA is not a stroke, but it can be a **prodromal** (i.e., early) **symptom;** TIAs precede about 15% of strokes and are a major risk factor for stroke, especially in older people. About a third of people who have had one or more TIAs have a stroke within five years. That rate is nearly 10 times greater than the rate of stroke among people of the same age and sex who have not had a TIA (American Heart Association 2002; Goldstein et al. 2001; Helgason and Wolf 1997; Mohr et al. 1997). One study showed that within 10 years after a TIA, the risk of a first stroke was 18%, and the risk of a myocardial infarction or death from coronary heart disease was 28% (Clark, Murphy, and Rothwell 2003). As many as 25% of stroke patients die within a year after a TIA (Kleindorfer et al. 2005).

▷ **WHEN SIGNS** of a stroke occur but last only a short while (e.g., a few minutes), they may indicate a transient ischemic attack.

Five Common Signs of Stroke

- Sudden numbness or weakness of the face, arm, or leg, especially on one side of the body
- Sudden confusion and trouble speaking or understanding
- Sudden trouble seeing in one or both eyes
- Sudden trouble walking, dizziness, or loss of balance or coordination
- Sudden, severe headache with no known cause

American Heart Association 2010.

Stroke is the common end point for cerebrovascular disease and is characterized by abrupt onset of persisting neurological symptoms that arise from injury or death of brain cells. About 85% of strokes are classified as primary ischemic or thromboembolic strokes (see figure 6.1*a*). They result from thrombosis (clotting in a vessel) or **stenosis** (narrowing of the artery), usually from atherosclerosis, or from **embolism** (occlusion of a vessel by a circulating atheroma or clot, often from the heart). Another 10% of all strokes result from bleeding in the brain and are classified as primary intracerebral hemorrhagic strokes (Broderick et al. 2007; Petrea et al. 2009), which account for nearly half of stroke deaths (Broderick et al. 1993). This type of stroke is illustrated in figure 6.1*b,* and images of a patient's brain after this type of stroke are shown in figure 6.2. The remaining 5% of strokes are subarachnoid hemorrhages, which occur when a vessel on the brain's surface ruptures and bleeds into the space between the brain and the cranium.

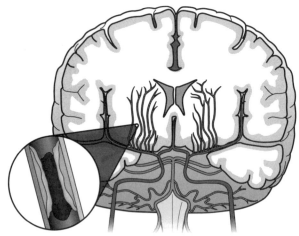

Blockage stops the flow of blood to an area of the brain

a

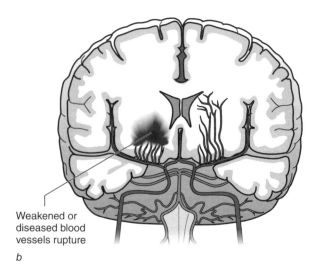

Weakened or diseased blood vessels rupture

b

Figure 6.1 Artist rendering of *(a)* ischemic stroke and *(b)* intracerebral hemorrhage.

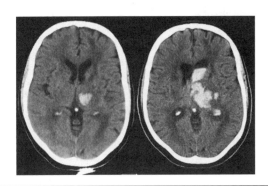

Figure 6.2 An intracerebral hemorrhage in the thalamus of the brain resulting from hypertension: 3 h after symptom onset (4 ml, left) and 1 h later (16 ml, right). Hematoma expansion in this case, ultimately lethal, was accompanied by clear neurological deterioration.

Reprinted from *Journal of the American College of Cardiology*, Vol. 56(9), "Stroke prevention and treatment," J.D. Marsh and S.G. Keyrouz, pgs. 683-691, copyright 2010, with permission of Elsevier.

Both ischemic and hemorrhagic types of stroke can lead to death or permanent brain damage, but people often recover lost brain function after a mild stroke.

▷ **ABOUT 85%** to 90% of strokes result from thrombosis (clotting in a vessel), stenosis (narrowing of the artery), or embolism (e.g., occlusion of a vessel by a circulating clot or atheroma). Other cases result from bleeding in or on the brain.

Magnitude of the Problem

Cerebrovascular disease (CVD) killed about 4.4 million people worldwide in 1990, second only to coronary heart disease, which caused 6.3 million deaths (Murray and Lopez 1997). A decade later, CVD was still number two, killing an estimated 5.4 million people worldwide, next to 7.06 million deaths from coronary heart disease (Lopez et al. 2006). Each year in the United States about 610,000 adults 20 years and older have a first stroke, another 185,000 have a recurrent stroke, and about 160,000 die from stroke-related causes (American Heart Association 2012). The cumulative prevalence of people with a history of stroke in 2006 was about 2.5 million men and 3.9 million women (Lloyd-Jones et al. 2010). Stroke incidence rates are greater in men than in women at younger ages but not at older ages. The male-to-female incidence ratio is 1.25 at ages 55 to 64, 1.50 for ages 65 to 74, 1.07 at 75 to 84, and 0.76 at 85 and older (American Heart Association 2010).

In 1990, the worldwide incidence of first-ever stroke was higher for females (120 per 100,000) than for males (110 per 100,000), and this difference between women and men was higher in developed countries, including the United States: 172 per 100,000 for females and 149 per 100,000 for males (Murray and Lopez 1997). The average age at onset also was higher for both women (72 years) and men (68 years) in developed nations than the worldwide averages for women (66 years) and men (63 years). Mortality rates from first-ever stroke worldwide are about 76 per 100,000 in males and 90 per 100,000 in females. In developed nations, those rates are about 82 per 100,000 for males and 115 per 100,000 for females.

▷ **BLACKS IN** the United States have almost twice the risk of first-ever stroke compared with whites. Age-adjusted rates per 1000 people aged 45 to 84 years are 6.6 in black males, 3.6 in white males, 4.9 in black females, and 2.3 in white females (American Heart Association 2010).

According to the Behavioral Risk Factor Surveillance System (BRFSS), managed by the Centers for Disease Control and Prevention, 2.4% of U.S. adults in 2009 said they had at some time been told by a health professional that they had had a stroke. Highest rates were in Alabama, Arkansas, Kentucky, Mississippi, Oklahoma, and West Virginia (figure 6.3).

▷ **ABOUT A** third of people who've had one or more transient ischemic attacks have a stroke within five years.

According to the National Heart, Lung, and Blood Institute, stroke has been the third leading cause of death in the United States since 1938, following coronary heart disease and cancer and just ahead of lung diseases. Similar to the reduction in heart attack deaths, the death rate from stroke in the United States has dropped sharply since 1950, from

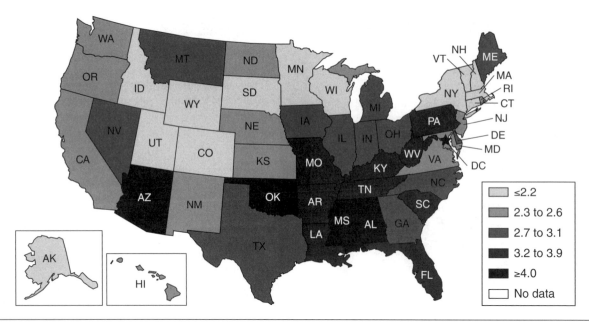

Figure 6.3 Map of strokes in the United States indicating adults who reported having had a stroke in 2009.
Reprinted from Centers for Disease Control 2010.

89 per 100,000 to a rate of approximately 45 per 100,000 in 2007. From 1998 to 2008, the stroke death rate fell 34.8%, and the actual number of stroke deaths declined 19.4%. Stroke accounted for 135,952 deaths in the United States in 2007 (54,111 males, 81,841 females), about 5% to 6% of all deaths (American Heart Association 2010). The 2007 final age-adjusted death rates per 100,000 people were 40.2 for white males and 67.1 for black males; 39.9 for white females and 55.0 for black females; and 34.4 for Hispanic or Latino males and 30.8 for females (Xu et al. 2010). Rates in 2006 were 39.8 for Asian or Pacific Islander males and 34.9 for females; they were 25.8 for American Indian/Alaska Native males and 30.9 for females (National Center for Health Statistics 2010) (figure 6.4). Because women live longer than men and stroke occurs at older ages, more women than men die of stroke each year. Women accounted for 60.6% of U.S. stroke deaths in 2006 (American Heart Association 2010).

▷ **AMONG PEOPLE** ages 45 to 64, 8% to 12% of ischemic strokes and 37% to 38% of hemorrhagic strokes result in death within 30 days, according to the Atherosclerosis Risk in Communities Study from the National Heart, Lung, and Blood Institute (Rosamond et al. 1999).

In addition to its contribution to total mortality, stroke is also the leading cause of adult disability in the United States. According to the National Institute of Neurological and Communicative Disorders and Stroke, nearly two-thirds of the 4.5 million U.S. stroke survivors alive in 2002 were disabled in some way. Disabilities include the loss of control over bodily functions; gait problems; impaired vision,

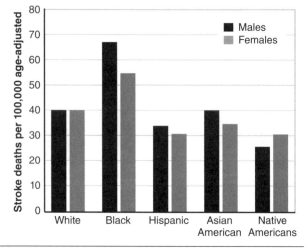

Figure 6.4 Stroke deaths in the United States according to sex and race or ethnicity.
Data from Xu et al. 2010 and National Center for Health Statistics 2009.

speech, or comprehension; depression; memory loss; and paralysis. The effects of stroke also place a significant burden on the survivor's family, friends, and caregivers. The direct and indirect economic cost of stroke in the United States for 2010 was estimated at $73.7 billion (American Heart Association 2010).

▷ **ACCORDING TO** the National Heart, Lung, and Blood Institute, stroke has been the third leading cause of death in the United States since 1938, following coronary heart disease and cancer.

Risk Factors for Stroke

Primary risk factors for stroke, in addition to TIA, include age over 55 years, female sex, cigarette smoking, alcohol abuse, hypertension, diabetes, coronary heart disease, and **cardiac arrhythmias** (e.g., atrial fibrillation) (Sacco, Wolf, and Gorelick 1999). In the WHO MONICA project, 12,224 strokes occurred in 18 populations in 11 countries during a three-year period in men and women ages 35 to 64. Smoking and high blood pressure accounted for 21% of stroke incidence in men and 42% in women (Stegmayr et al. 1997).

Obesity, hypercholesterolemia, and physical inactivity are considered secondary contributing risk factors to stroke (Goldstein et al. 2001). The primary risk factors, discussed in the preceding paragraph, have been clearly implicated in the pathogenesis of atherosclerosis. The secondary risk factors are equally important but are not as directly linked to the development of atherosclerosis.

The risk of recurrent stroke during the first year after an ischemic stroke is about 10%, which increases to about 50% after five years (Sacco et al. 1982). Most of the major risk factors for first stroke, with the exception of age, race, and sex, are either correctable or modifiable in all age groups by hygienic behaviors or medical treatment.

As we saw for coronary heart disease in chapter 5, lifestyle habits such as physical activity and a healthy diet also reduce the risk of stroke, especially ischemic stroke. Among nearly 44,000 men from the Health Professionals Study and more than 70,000 women from the Nurses' Health Study, it was found that 52% to 54% of ischemic strokes could potentially have been prevented by five lifestyle-related factors: not smoking, body mass index (BMI) <25 kg/m, an ounce or less of alcohol consumption each day, being in the top 40% of healthy eating, and 30 min or more of moderate physical activity each week (Chiuve et al. 2008).

In INTERSTROKE, a case–control study in 22 countries (Argentina, Australia, Brazil, Canada, Chile, China, Colombia, Croatia, Denmark, Ecuador, Germany, India, Iran, Malaysia, Mozambique, Nigeria, Peru, Philippines, Poland, South Africa, Sudan, and Uganda), 3000 cases of stroke were observed between 2007 and 2010 (2337 ischemic and 663 intracerebral hemorrhagic strokes). Cases were matched on age and sex with controls who had no history of stroke. The investigators found that 88% of ischemic stroke cases could be attributed to 11 risk factors. Only hypertension, smoking, waist-to-hip ratio, diet, and alcohol intake were significant risk factors for intracerebral hemorrhagic stroke (O'Donnell et al. 2010). Low physical activity was defined as less than 4 h each week of moderate (walking, cycling, or gardening) or vigorous exercise (jogging, football, and vigorous swimming). Table 6.1 shows the independent risk for each factor adjusted for other factors.

The following sections describe the association between the modifiable risk factors (hypertension, smoking, alcohol abuse, hypercholesterolemia, diabetes, and obesity) and stroke risk in more detail.

Selected Risk Factors for Stroke

- *Age.* Stroke risk doubles each decade after age 55. Two-thirds of strokes occur in people older than 65 years.
- *Sex.* Women have slightly higher stroke risk and are more likely to die from a stroke than men, but men die sooner than women from other causes, so there are more female (2.3 million) than male (2.2 million) stroke survivors in the United States.
- *Race.* Blacks have twice the risk of stroke of other Americans, possibly because they have more of the other key risk factors.
- *Atrial fibrillation.* Irregular contraction of the heart's atria causes an irregular heartbeat, which can lead to pooling of blood in the heart and contribute to clot formation and ischemic stroke.
- *Coronary heart disease.* Atherosclerosis underlies both coronary artery disease and carotid artery disease and is thus a main cause of ischemic stroke. Hence, people with coronary heart disease are at increased risk of stroke.

Hypertension

Hypertension is the primary risk factor for the development of stroke (Kannel et al. 1970), and stroke is a common consequence for people with hypertension. In the Framingham Heart Study, men with hypertension (over 160/95 mmHg) were about four times more likely to suffer a stroke than those who were normotensive (Kannel 1999; Kannel et al. 1970). In the Nurses' Health Study, the relative risk for stroke in women with hypertension was 4.2 compared with their normotensive counterparts (Fiebach et al. 1989). The elevated risk of stroke in these women occurred at all levels of BMI. Hence, hypertension appears to be an independent risk factor for stroke in middle-aged women. Even among young adults, the odds ratio of stroke was five times higher in those with hypertension (You et al. 1997). Effective control of hypertension appears to reduce the risk of stroke by about 40%.

Smoking

The risk of stroke is greater in persons who smoke, increases with the number of cigarettes smoked, and is lower among those who have given up smoking compared with current smokers. Mechanisms linking the components of tobacco smoke with arterial damage and the subsequent development

Table 6.1   Ischemic Stroke Risk Factors in 22 Countries

Risk factor	OR (95% CI)	Population attributable risk
History of hypertension	2.37 (2.00-2.79)	31.5%
Current smoking	2.32 (1.91-2.81)	21.4%
Waist-to-hip girth ratio (top vs. bottom third)	1.69 (1.38-2.07)	26.0%
Diet risk (top vs. bottom third)	1.34 (1.09-1.65)	17.3%
Low physical activity	**1.47 (1.10-1.96)**	**29.4%**
Diabetes	1.60 (1.29-1.99)	7.9%
Alcohol use (>30 drinks/month or binging)	1.41 (1.09-1.82)	1.0%
Perceived stress	1.30 (1.04-1.62)	4.7%
Depression	1.47 (1.19-1.83)	6.8%
Heart causes (atrial fibrillation, valve disease, prior myocardial infarction)	2.74 (2.03-3.72)	8.5%
Apo B:apo A1 ratio (top vs. bottom third)	2.40 (1.86-3.11)	35.2%

Data from O'Donnell et al. 2010.

of atherosclerosis have been identified. The Framingham Heart Study, for example, found about a 60% increase in the relative risk for stroke in female smokers compared with nonsmokers, independent of several other risk factors (Wolf et al. 1988). In eastern Finland, a decline in the prevalence of hypertension and smoking accounted for about 29% of the subsequent decline in stroke incidence during an eight-year follow-up of two population cohorts of men and women ages 30 to 59 years (Tuomilehto et al. 1991).

Alcohol Abuse

Alcohol consumption has been shown to both increase and decrease the risk for stroke. A prospective study of female nurses in the United States showed that among middle-aged women, moderate alcohol consumption decreased the risk of ischemic stroke (Stampfer et al. 1988). However, a report on the Honolulu Heart Program cohort showed that even light drinking in men significantly increased the risk of hemorrhagic stroke (Donahue et al. 1986). Despite the mixed evidence, it is generally accepted that moderate alcohol consumption may reduce the risk of thrombosis associated with atherosclerosis and ischemic stroke. If that effect is explainable by anticoagulability of blood, it paradoxically could pose a risk for hemorrhagic stroke because of a blood-thinning effect. This hypothesis would be consistent with information on the effects of drugs that inhibit platelet aggregation (e.g., aspirin) and that can reduce recurrent cerebrovascular accidents among people with CVD (Algra and van Gijn 1996; Antiplatelet Trialists' Collaboration 1994). However, aspirin is not recommended for the primary prevention of stroke because 325 to 500 mg daily has an unclear effect on reducing ischemic stroke and can double the risk of hemorrhagic stroke (Peto et al. 1988; Steering Committee of the Physicians' Health Study Research Group 1989).

Hypercholesterolemia

Elevated blood cholesterol has been associated only moderately with an increased risk for stroke. However, clinical trials have shown that statin drugs used to lower cholesterol have reduced the thickening of the carotid artery wall (Hodis et al. 1996) and reduced the frequency of strokes by about 30% (Cholesterol and Recurrent Events Trial Investigators 1996).

Obesity and Diabetes Mellitus

Overweight, as measured by BMI, is also an independent risk factor for stroke in both men and women (Lindenstrom, Boysen, and Nyboe 1993a, 1993b). Data from the third National Health and Nutrition Examination Survey (NHANES III) and the Framingham Heart Study indicate that the lifetime risk of stroke is elevated among middle-aged men and women who are obese (i.e., BMI >30; Thompson et al. 1999). Among young adults, the odds ratio of stroke is nearly 12 times higher in those with diabetes (You et al. 1997), possibly explainable by microvascular disease.

▷ **AMONG YOUNG** adults, the odds ratio of stroke is nearly 12 times higher in those with diabetes.

Etiology of Stroke

Much of the pathophysiology of stroke involves atherosclerotic disease and hemostatic dysfunction similar to that of coronary heart disease, discussed in chapter 5. The physiological mechanisms of stroke are classified as embolic, lacunar (i.e., brain cavities resulting from decreased perfusion in small, deep vessels), or thrombotic depending on the presence of risk factors for stroke and preexisting medical conditions (Mohr et al. 1997).

Embolic Stroke

Precipitating factors for embolic stroke include atrial fibrillation, sinoatrial disorder, recent myocardial infarction, bacterial endocarditis (inflammation of the heart), cardiac tumors, and valve disorders. Stroke occurs within weeks after about 2% of heart attacks, mainly from circulating clots from the wall of the left ventricle or from an atherosclerotic blood vessel. Medical risk factors for left ventricular thrombosis are large infarctions, dilation of the left ventricle (usually from congestive heart failure), and atrial fibrillation. Atherosclerotic plaques in the aortic arch are a main source of atherothrombosis (Vahedi and Amarenco 2000).

Lacunar: Reduced Perfusion

Stroke that results from reduced perfusion occurs with severe stenosis (greater than 70% narrowing) of the carotid and basilar arteries and with stenosis of small arteries deep in the brain. Inflammation from infections can also cause arterial stenosis. Strokes are commonly reported in patients with bacterial or tuberculous meningitis, cerebral cysticercosis (a cyst formed by tapeworm larvae), fungal infection, and herpes zoster (i.e., shingles). Lacunar infarcts result mainly from blockage of small arteries deep in the brain by small atherosclerotic plaques, cholesterol embolism, clots resulting from rheumatic heart disease or endocarditis, and arteriosclerosis of the cerebral arteries.

Thrombotic Stroke

Precipitating conditions for thrombotic stroke involve mainly abnormal regulation of hemostatic factors, such as anticlotting proteins, and of the fibrinolytic system that can occur at any age (see chapter 5). Genetic defects in regulatory hemostatic proteins are common in people who have vessel clots in their 20s or 30s. However, a causal link between hemostatic disease and stroke has not yet been established.

Physical Activity and Stroke Risk: The Evidence

The scientific advisory committee for the 2008 Physical Activity Guidelines for Americans concluded that physically active men and women generally have a lower risk of stroke incidence or mortality than the least active, with more active persons demonstrating a 25% to 30% lower risk for all strokes (including ischemic and hemorrhagic stroke); but the data on stroke subtypes are limited, and very little data exist for race and ethnicity groups other than whites of European ancestry (Physical Activity Guidelines Advisory Committee 2008).

In meta-analysis of 18 cohort studies (11 from the United States and one each from England, the Netherlands, Italy, Norway, Iceland, Sweden, and Japan), highly active people had a 25% lower risk of stroke incidence or mortality (both ischemic and hemorrhagic) (relative risk [RR] = 0.75; 95% CI: 0.69-0.82), and moderately active people had a 17% lower risk (RR = 0.83; 95% CI: 0.76-0.89), compared with people who had low physical activity (Lee, Folsom, and Blair 2003). Another meta-analysis that combined results of 24 prospective cohort studies and seven case–control studies similarly concluded that moderately active men and

---

Treatment for Stroke

Thrombolysis using intravenous injection of tissue plasminogen activator (tPA) is currently the only acute therapy (i.e., within 3 h of symptom onset) that is approved by the Food and Drug Administration for ischemic stroke. It improves clinical outcomes (odds ratio [OR] = 1.7; 95% confidence interval [CI]: 1.2-2.6), but not mortality rates, at three months after stroke (Marler et al. 2000). About a fourth of patients with strokes arrive at the hospital within 3 h of symptom onset (Demaerschalk and Yip 2005). However, thrombolysis by IV is used in only a small fraction of these patients (Demaerschalk and Yip 2005). This is probably the case because the rate of intracerebral hemorrhage within 36 h of stroke symptoms is six times higher after IV injection of tPA (Marler et al. 2000). In Europe,

thrombolysis is approved for up to 4.5 h after symptom onset, which has been recommended by the American Heart Association (del Zoppo et al. 2009). Other acute treatment and preventive interventions for ischemic stroke include the following:

- Statins for patients with diabetes and for those with prior strokes or TIAs
- Anticoagulation and antiplatelet therapy for stroke prevention in patients with atrial fibrillation or carotid stenting (implanting of a metal and mesh tube to extend and support the artery)
- Carotid endarterectomy (i.e., excision of plaques from carotid artery) for patients with greater than five-year life expectancy and 60% to 99% stenosis

Source: Marsh and Keyrouz, 2010.

women had lower rates of ischemic, hemorrhagic, and all strokes than people who were the least active (Wendel-Vos et al. 2004). Compared to low levels of leisure-time physical activity, moderate physical activity reduced the risk of all strokes by 15% (RR = 0.85; 95% CI: 0.78-0.93), and high levels of physical activity reduced risks by 20% to 25% for all strokes (RR = 0.78; 95% CI: 0.71-0.85), ischemic stroke (RR = 0.79; 95% CI: 0.69-0.91), and hemorrhagic stroke (RR = 0.74; 95% CI: 0.57-0.96).

A subsequent meta-analysis of 13 prospective cohort studies having an average follow-up of 14 years found that when compared to low physical activity, moderate physical activity was associated with an 11% reduction in risk of first stroke or stroke mortality, while high physical activity was associated with a 19% reduction in risk (Diep et al. 2010). Although results appeared stronger for men than women, the gender comparison was hampered by the few number of studies and smaller numbers of women, coupled with the problem of comparing levels of physical activity across population surveys.

▷ **ABOUT 25** prospective cohort studies and at least seven case–control studies show that regular participation in moderate-to-vigorous leisure-time physical activity reduces risks of ischemic and hemorrhagic stroke by 25% to 30% in middle-aged and older people.

Case–Control Studies

The following sections describe three case–control studies that assessed the association between physical activity and stroke. The evidence of a cause-and-effect association is also evaluated.

Birmingham, England

In one case–control study, 125 men and women ages 35 to 74 who had suffered a first stroke and 198 controls matched by age and sex were recruited over a two-year period from 11 general medical practices in west Birmingham, England (Shinton and Sagar 1993). The patients and controls were divided into groups by whether they reported engaging or not engaging in regular vigorous exercise (e.g., digging, running, swimming, cycling, tennis, squash, and keeping fit) during youth (ages 15 to 25), early middle age (ages 25 to 40), and late middle age (ages 40 to 55). When disability after the stroke prevented a response, the closest relative or friend of the subject was interviewed. Figure 6.5 shows that a history of vigorous exercise during ages 15 to 25 (OR adjusted for age and sex: 0.33; 95% CI: 0.20-0.60) and increasing years of participation in vigorous exercise between the ages of 15 and 55 was associated with an increasing reduction in the rate of stroke. This effect was independent of potential risk factors, including race; social class; peak BMI; subscapular skinfold thickness; cigarette smoking; alcohol consumption; dietary intake of saturated

fat; family history of stroke; and histories of hypertension, diabetes mellitus, and cardiac ischemia.

Among the 65 cases and 169 controls who were free of cardiac ischemia, peripheral vascular disease, and poor health, recent vigorous exercise and walking protected against stroke: The odds ratios were 0.41 (95% CI: 0.20-1.0) for recent vigorous exercise and 0.30 (0.10-0.70) for recent walking. The study suggested a dose–response relationship between more years of participation in vigorous exercise and decreased risk of stroke that was independent of other risk factors and consistent between sexes.

Northern Manhattan Stroke Study

The Northern Manhattan Stroke Study was a case–control study designed to investigate the association between leisure-time physical activity and ischemic stroke in an urban, multi-ethnic population (Sacco et al. 1998). Case subjects had experienced a first ischemic stroke; and for every case, two control subjects matched by age, sex, and race were recruited through random-digit dialing. Physical activity was assessed through a standardized in-person interview regarding the frequency and duration of 14 separate activities during the two weeks prior to the interview. Over a 30-month period, 369 case and 678 control subjects were enrolled. Their mean age was 70 years; 57% were women, 18% were white, 30% were black, and 52% were Hispanic. Results indicated that leisure-time physical activity is associated with a significantly reduced risk of stroke after adjustment for cardiac disease, peripheral vascular disease, hypertension, diabetes, smoking, alcohol use, obesity, medical reasons for limited activity, education, and season of enrollment. The protective effects of physical activity were observed in both younger and older groups, in men and women, and in whites, blacks, and Hispanics.

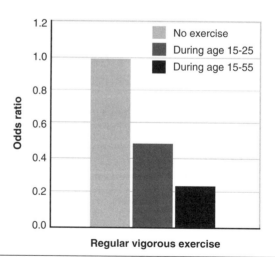

Figure 6.5 Physical activity and recurrent stroke in Birmingham, England. The numbers are adjusted for race; social class; peak BMI; skinfold thickness; smoking; alcohol consumption; dietary saturated fat; family history of stroke; and histories of hypertension, diabetes mellitus, and cardiac ischemia.

Adapted from Shinton and Sagar 1993.

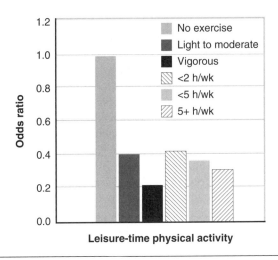

Figure 6.6 Physical activity and ischemic stroke in the Northern Manhattan Stroke Study, which included 369 cases of first stroke, 678 controls, mean age of 70 years, 57% women, 52% Hispanics, 30% blacks, and 18% whites, matched on age, sex, and race.

Adapted from Sacco et al. 1998.

Figure 6.6 shows a dose response for both intensity and duration of physical activity, regardless of age, sex, or ethnicity. Light- to moderate-intensity activities had an odds ratio of 0.39 (95% CI: 0.26-0.58), and heavy activity had an odds ratio of 0.23 (0.10-0.54). Duration of less than 2 h per week had an odds ratio of 0.42 (0.14-0.70), less than 5 h per week 0.35 (0.25-0.45), and more than 5 h per week 0.31 (0.25-0.59). Hence, there was a small linear gradient of decreased risk with increasing time spent in activity each week.

Guangdong Province, China

Physical activity exposure and other lifestyle traits were obtained from 374 incident ischemic stroke patients and 464 controls who were hospitalized for medical reasons other than stroke. Average age was 66 years (Liang et al. 2009). Stroke risk was inversely related to physical activity. After adjustment for stroke risk factors, the risk of ischemic stroke was 75% lower in people who said they regularly engaged in at least 22 MET-hours per week of leisure-time physical activity when compared to people who spent less than 10 MET-hours per week (OR = 0.25; 95% CI: 0.14-0.45).

Prospective Studies

The following sections describe some of the major prospective cohort studies that have assessed the association between physical activity and stroke.

Finnish Cohort

Beginning in 1972, Salonen, Puska, and Tuomilehto (1982) followed a randomly selected population sample from eastern Finland for seven years. Physical activity at work and during

leisure time were recorded for 3978 men and 3688 women. During the seven-year follow-up, 71 men and 56 women had a stroke. After controlling for age, total serum cholesterol, diastolic blood pressure, height, weight, and smoking, low physical activity at work was associated with a relative risk for stroke of 1.6 in men and 1.7 in women. The study showed an appropriate temporal sequence, independence of several confounders, and a moderately strong association between reduced occupational physical activity and increased stroke risk that was consistent between sexes.

Harvard Alumni Health Study

In the Harvard alumni cohort, the incidence of stroke was inversely related to self-reported weekly energy expenditure (figure 6.7; Paffenbarger et al. 1984). The stroke incidence rate for subjects expending less than 500 kcal each week was 6.5 per 10,000 person-years of observation; for those expending 500 to 1999 kcal each week it was 5.2, and for those expending more than 2000 kcal each week it was 2.4.

British Men

Physical activity levels were measured among 7630 British men ages 40 to 59, sampled randomly from general medical practices in 24 towns in England, Wales, and Scotland (Wannamethee and Shaper 1992). During a 9.5-year follow-up, 128 men suffered a major stroke. After statistical adjustment for age, social class, smoking, alcohol consumption, BMI, systolic blood pressure, and prevalence of ischemic heart disease or prior strokes, men who engaged in moderate activity and vigorous activity had 30% and 60% lower rates of stroke, respectively, compared with inactive men. The

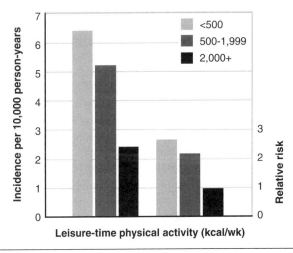

Figure 6.7 Findings on physical activity and stroke in the Harvard Alumni Study cohort include rate and relative risks of first stroke for more than 10,000 men who entered college in 1916 through 1950. Follow-ups were done in the 1960s and 1978. Study results were independent of blood pressure, age, smoking, body weight, and family history of cardiovascular disease.

Adapted from Paffenbarger 1984.

continued reduction in relative risk with increasing intensity of physical activity indicated a dose–response relationship.

Framingham Cohort

In a follow-up of the Framingham cohort, men and women were categorized into tertiles according to physical activity level (Kiely et al. 1994). Participants reporting medium or high levels of physical activity were compared with those reporting low levels of physical activity. The association between physical activity and the rate of stroke was analyzed twice over a 32-year follow-up period: first at 50 years of age among 1897 men and 2299 women, and again when the remaining 1361 men and 1862 women were 63 or 64 years old.

Among the men, physical activity (independent of age, systolic blood pressure, serum cholesterol, number of cigarettes smoked per day, glucose intolerance, total vital capacity, BMI, left ventricular hypertrophy, atrial fibrillation, vascular disease, history of congestive heart failure, history of ischemic heart disease, and occupation) was associated with a reduced risk for stroke. The lowest relative risk, 0.40 (95% CI: 0.24-0.69), was found among older men in the medium activity tertile. The highest level of physical activity did not confer an additional reduction in risk beyond that of the medium level. Physical activity level was not associated with a reduced risk of stroke among women in this cohort.

Honolulu Heart Study

The Honolulu Heart Study classified 7530 Hawaiian men of Japanese descent 45 to 68 years old as inactive, partially active, or active based on self-reports of 24-h physical activity at the time of study enrollment (Abbott et al. 1994). Risk of stroke during 22 years of follow-up was examined separately in younger (45 to 54 years) and older (55 to 68 years) men. Among the older men, the inactive men had a relative risk of 3.7 (95% CI: 1.3-10.4) for hemorrhagic stroke compared with active men; this risk was independent of hypertension, diabetes mellitus, and left ventricular hypertrophy. In older men who did not smoke cigarettes, the relative risk of thromboembolic stroke among inactive men was 2.8 compared with that for active men. The relative risk of partially active older men was 2.4 (95% CI: 1.0-5.7) compared with those who were active. Hence, an independent dose–response relationship was observed between increasing physical activity levels and decreasing risk for thromboembolic stroke. No associations were found between risk of stroke and either physical activity level or smoking in men ages 45 to 54, for whom the prevalence of stroke is low compared with that in older men.

NHANES I Cohort

As part of the NHANES I epidemiologic follow-up study, 5081 whites and 771 blacks 45 to 74 years of age who initially had no history of stroke were reassessed twice during a 12-year follow-up after initial measurements taken from 1971 to 1975 (Gillum, Mussolino, and Ingram 1996). Participants

rated their levels of habitual physical activity, both leisure time and nonleisure time, as low, moderate, or high. They were also categorized based on resting pulse rate. There were 249 cases of stroke among the white women, 270 among the white men, and 104 among the black men and women combined. The incidence of stroke was highest among those who were least active, regardless of sex or race. In addition, among white women ages 65 to 74, low nonleisure-time physical activity was independently associated with an increased risk of stroke (RR = 1.82; 95% CI: 1.10-3.02) after adjustment for age, smoking, history of diabetes, history of heart disease, education, systolic blood pressure, total serum cholesterol, BMI, and hemoglobin concentration.

Similar associations between low leisure-time physical activity and increased risk of stroke were seen for white men and for black men and women. A dose–response relation between activity level and reduced stroke incidence was observed among white women. Similarly, a linear relation was found between resting pulse rate and increased risk of stroke in blacks but not in whites. The study provided evidence for a consistent reduction in risk of stroke among middle-aged and older adults regardless of sex, age, and race. There was no uniform difference in the association between the amount of leisure-time physical activity with either total or nonhemorrhagic stroke in men or women aged 45 to 64 years compared to those who were 65 to 74 years at baseline. The strongest and most consistent association between activity level and reduced stroke risk in this study was observed in white women.

Atherosclerosis Risk in Communities Study (ARIC)

More recently, ischemic stroke incidence in more than 14,000 adults ages 45 to 64 years without history of stroke or coronary heart disease at study outset was observed for about seven years (Evenson et al. 1999). The risk ratios were about 0.80 to 0.90 (95% CI: 0.6-1.26) in the highest quartile of sport and leisure physical activity compared with the lowest quartile, after adjustment for age, sex, race, smoking, and education. These nonsignificant and modest reductions in risk were further diluted after adjustment for hypertension, diabetes, fibrinogen levels, and BMI, suggesting that the influence of physical activity on the risk of ischemic stroke is not direct but may operate indirectly through other key risk factors for stroke.

Icelandic Men

Agnarsson and colleagues (1999) reported on a study of 4484 men ages 40 to 80 years at baseline who were followed for approximately 11 years, during which 249 cases of stroke were identified. At baseline, participants responded to questions in a yes/no format about participation in regular physical activity during age periods 20 to 29, 30 to 39, 40 to 49, and 50 to 59 years. Those who responded affirmatively were asked to report the number of hours per week and the type of physical activity in which they participated. Results indicated that after adjustment for other known stroke risk factors, leisure-time physical activity maintained after 40 years of age was associated with 40% reductions in risks of ischemic and total stroke.

Physicians' Health Study

Lee and colleagues (1999) reported results from an 11-year follow-up of a Physicians' Health Study cohort of 21,823 men ages 40 to 80 years who were free of self-reported myocardial infarction, stroke, TIA, and cancer at baseline. During the follow-up period, 533 cases of stroke were reported. Physical activity level was measured in the baseline examination as the frequency of exercise vigorous enough to work up a sweat. After adjustment for age, smoking, alcohol intake, history of angina, and parental history of myocardial infarction, the relative risk of total stroke associated with vigorous exercise was reduced nearly 20% regardless of weekly frequency (i.e., even just one day). However, when the results were adjusted for potential mediators of the association between physical activity and stroke, such as BMI, history of hypertension, high cholesterol, and diabetes mellitus, the trend toward reduced risks was no longer significant.

Nurses' Health Study

In this study, 407 incident cases of stroke were observed during eight years of follow-up among 72,488 female nurses ages 40 to 65 years who were free from cardiovascular disease and cancer at baseline in 1986 and who completed physical activity questionnaires in 1986, 1988, and 1992 (Hu et al. 2000). Results indicated that after controlling for age, BMI, history of hypertension, and other covariates, increasing levels of physical activity were inversely associated with the risk for both total and ischemic stroke (figure 6.8). Walking

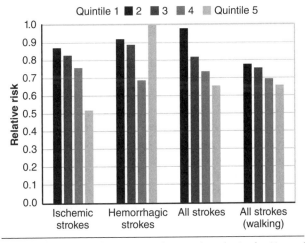

Figure 6.8 Physical activity and type of stroke in the Nurses' Health Study cohort according to level of vigorous physical activity and walking.

for exercise was also associated with reduced risk for total stroke. These results suggest that for women, participation in physical activity, including moderate-intensity activity such as walking, results in a reduction in risk for both total and ischemic stroke in a dose–response manner.

In a follow-up 10 years later in 2004, there had been a total of 1559 total strokes (853 ischemic, 278 hemorrhagic, 428 unspecified) among 71,243 women in the cohort (Chiuve et al. 2008). The most active 9% of the women, who said they spent 6 h or more each week in moderate or vigorous physical activity at baseline during 1980 and 1982 (i.e., walking at a 3 mph pace or faster; jogging; running; bicycling; swimming; rowing, calisthenics; or playing tennis, squash, or racquetball), had 40% lower risk of ischemic stroke and total strokes than the least-active women (24%), who said they did no exercise. After adjustments for age and several stroke risk factors, women who said they got 30 min or more of moderate or vigorous physical activity each day (24% of the cohort) had a 25% reduction in the risk of ischemic stroke and a 21% risk reduction for all strokes (figure 6.9a). About 20% of ischemic stroke cases and 17% of all strokes might have been prevented had all the women spent at least 30 min each day exercising.

U.S. Health Professionals Follow-Up Study

This was a cohort of 43,685 men who averaged 54 years of age at the 1984 baseline (Chiuve et al. 2008). There were 994 strokes (600 ischemic, 161 hemorrhagic) during 18 years of follow-up. The most active 17% of the men, who said they spent 6 h or more each week in moderate or vigorous physical activity at baseline during 1984 (defined in the same way as for the Nurses' Health Study), had about 40% lower risk of ischemic stroke and total strokes than the least-active men (37%), who said they did no exercise. After adjustments for age and several stroke risk factors, men who said they got 30 min or more of moderate or vigorous physical activity each day (29% of the cohort) had an 18% reduction in the risk of ischemic stroke and a 22% risk reduction for all strokes (figure 6.9b). About 14% of ischemic stroke cases and 17% of all strokes might have been prevented had all the men spent at least 30 min each day exercising.

After 20 years of follow-up, men who exercised vigorously ≥5 times/week had adjusted relative risk reductions of 33% for TIA but similar functional consequences of stroke compared to men who exercised vigorously less than once each week (Rist et al. 2011).

Japanese Men and Women

More than 31,000 men and 42,000 women aged 40 to 79 years with no history of stroke, coronary heart disease, or cancer were followed for an average of 9.7 years. Both sport participation and walking were inversely related to deaths from ischemic strokes and all strokes in both men and women (Noda et al. 2005). After adjustment for age,

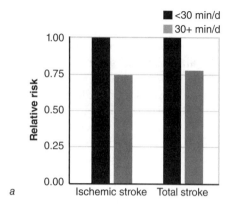

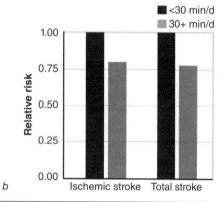

Figure 6.9 Physical activity and stroke in (a) the U.S. Nurses' Health Study and (b) the U.S. Health Professionals Study, which had similar study designs and showed notably similar results. The Nurses' Health Study was a cohort of 71,243 women free of cardiovascular disease in 1986, age range of 40 to 65 years. There were 1559 total strokes (853 ischemic, 278 hemorrhagic, 428 unspecified) during 18 years of follow-up. The U.S. Health Professionals Study was a cohort of 43,685 men who averaged 54 years of age at the 1984 baseline. There were 994 strokes (600 ischemic, 161 hemorrhagic) during 18 years of follow-up.

Data from Chiuve et al. 2008.

sex, and cardiovascular risk factors, people who walked an hour or more each day had 30% lower risk of ischemic stroke compared to those who spent half an hour each day walking.

Norwegian Men and Women, North Tröndelag Study

Among 34,868 women and 32,872 men without cardiovascular disease or diabetes who had a measure of weekly exercise at baseline, 719 women and 610 men died from stroke during 16 years of observation (Vatten et al. 2006). People were classified as active if they reported at least 30 min of moderate to vigorous activity two or more times a week. Adjustments were made for age and stroke risk factors. Women who said they infrequently or never exercised

had 45% higher risk of stroke death than active women. Men who said they never exercised had 35% higher risk of stroke death than active men.

Losartan Intervention for Endpoint Reduction in Hypertension (LIFE) Study

Physical activity was measured in 4961 women and 4232 men aged 55 to 80 years from 945 medical centers in Denmark, Finland, Iceland, Norway, Sweden, United Kingdom, and the United States who had hypertension and left ventricular hypertrophy. There were 541 incident strokes. Patients who said they got more than 30 min of exercise twice per week (52% of the patients) at the time they entered an antihypertensive drug intervention had nearly 25% lower risk of incident stroke during nearly five years of treatment, regardless of which drug they took and other risk factors for cardiovascular disease (Fossum et al. 2007).

U.S. National Runners' Health Study

The dose–response relation between vigorous exercise (daily running distance) and stroke risk was examined in 29,279 men and 12,123 women. One hundred men and 19 women said they had been told by a physician that they had had a stroke during 7.7 years of follow-up (Williams 2009). For each kilometer run each day, risk reductions were 8% and 7% after adjustment for age, smoking, diabetes, high cholesterol, hypertension, and BMI. Runners who averaged at least 4 km each day (i.e., met the 2008 Physical Activity Guidelines for Americans level) had nearly a 50% reduction in risk compared to those who ran less than 2 km, after adjustment for age and smoking (RR = 0.55; 95% CI: 0.32-0.99).

U.S. Women's Health Study

Participants were 39,315 healthy U.S. women 45 years of age or older who were randomly assigned in 1992 through 1995 to receive low-dose aspirin and vitamin E or placebo for preventive treatment against cardiovascular disease and cancer (Sattelmair et al. 2010). The women reported their physical activity then and again at 36, 72, 96, 125, and 149 months follow-up. There were 579 incident strokes (473 ischemic, 102 hemorrhagic, and four of unknown type) during nearly 12 years of observation. After adjustment for age and for being in the treatment or placebo group, the risks of ischemic strokes were reduced by 30% to 40% in women who reported spending the equivalent of 600 to 1499 kcal/week (28% of the women) or 1500 or more kcal/week (21% of the women) in leisure-time physical activity when compared to <200 kcal/week of physical activity. After further adjustment for confounding by stroke risk factors, those risk reductions were halved and no longer significant, indicating that physical activity did not have a protective effect on stroke that was independent of other stroke risk factors.

Prospective Studies of Cardiorespiratory Fitness and Stroke

Because physical activity in population surveys of stroke risk has been assessed mainly by people's recall, it is also important to show whether stroke risk is reduced among people who are more physically fit. As we saw in chapter 3, fitness can be an objectively measured surrogate of physical activity that can also suggest biological mechanisms for risk reduction.

Finnish Men

The association of low cardiorespiratory fitness measured by maximum oxygen consumption (i.e., $\dot{V}O_2$max) with incident stroke was examined in 2011 men without history of stroke or lung disease who lived in or near Kuopio, Finland (Kurl et al. 2003). During an average follow-up of 11 years, there were 110 strokes (87 were ischemic). The age-adjusted risk in the 25% lowest-fit men was more than tripled for ischemic stroke, compared with men in the highest 25% of fitness. The lower risk remained significant after further adjustment for stroke risk factors. The relative risk conferred by low cardiorespiratory fitness was similar to risks observed for systolic blood pressure, obesity, alcohol consumption, smoking, and low-density lipoprotein cholesterol level.

Aerobics Center Longitudinal Study

Cardiorespiratory fitness was measured by maximal treadmill endurance in 46,405 men and 15,282 women with no history of myocardial infarction or stroke (Hooker et al. 2008). During an average of 18 years follow-up, there were 527 nonfatal and 186 fatal strokes in men and 120 nonfatal and 55 fatal strokes in women. After adjustments were made for baseline age and stroke risk factors, men who were in the top 75% of fitness (at least 9.9 metabolic equivalents, METs) at baseline had about 50% lower risk of fatal stroke and 20% to 40% lower risk of nonfatal stroke when compared with the least-fit 25% of men. Results among women were similar to those for the men but were not statistically significant, mainly because of the smaller number of women and stroke cases. The highest rates of age-adjusted strokes occurred in men and women whose initial fitness levels were less than 8 METs.

Randomized Controlled Trials

There is an absence of randomized controlled trials of exercise on the primary or secondary prevention of stroke. A meta-analysis of 24 trials of 1147 participants who underwent cardiorespiratory training (11 trials, 692 participants), strength training (four trials, 158 participants), and mixed training interventions (nine trials, 360 participants) examined whether exercise reduces death, functional dependence, or disability (Saunders et al. 2009). A single death was reported during the period of the interventions, and eight deaths were reported among 627 participants who were followed up after exercise training. Graduated walking was effective in improving maximum walking speed and endurance (6.5 m/min for 6 min) and reduced the need for support during walking.

Studies of Peripheral Artery Disease

Peripheral artery disease (PAD) is the obstruction of blood flow in arteries other than those to the heart or brain, usually because of atherosclerosis. It is most commonly determined clinically by a resting ankle–brachial index (ABI) (i.e., the ratio of ankle to brachial systolic blood pressures) of less than 90% (Hirsch et al. 2001). About 10% to 30% of adults aged 55 years or older have PAD, and about half of people with PAD have symptoms of intermittent claudication (i.e., muscle pain) during leg exertion or leg pain while resting (Hankey, Norman, and Eikelboom 2006).

Although PAD is not included in guidelines for the prevention and treatment of stroke (Adams et al. 2007; European Stroke Organization Executive Committee 2008), there is evidence that PAD is a risk factor for stroke (Banerjee et al. 2010). For example, patients with PAD have increased stroke or TIA risk compared with patients without PAD (Criqui et al. 1997). A third to one half of stroke or TIA patients in large trials had a low ABI (Hooi et al. 1998; Weimar et al. 2007; Agnelli et al. 2006). Peripheral artery disease patients who have a decrease in ABI of 15% or more in five years have elevated risk of stroke (Criqui et al. 2008).

Among people in the REACH Registry, prior PAD predicted one-year stroke incidence independently of prior stroke, hyperglycemia, and hypercholesterolemia (Aichner et al. 2009). In Chinese patients with PAD, 25% had more than 70% stenosis of the carotid artery compared with 11% of patients with coronary artery disease (Cheng et al. 1999).

Common treatments for reducing PAD symptoms, including walking without pain, are smoking cessation, statins, and cilostazol (a vasodilating drug that also inhibits platelet aggregation). Three early randomized controlled trials showed that supervised exercise programs reduced PAD symptoms more than normal daily activity (Hiatt et al. 1990, 1994; Tisi et al. 1997). The supervised programs lasted approximately 60 min, three days a week, for four to 12 weeks. Patients participating in the exercise groups experienced significant improvements in both maximum and pain-free walking end points. In a later, long-term supervised exercise program, participants showed a 120% gain in maximum walking time and a 170% increase in pain-free walking time (Crowther et al. 2008).

A meta-analysis summarized 22 randomized controlled trials of exercise training at least two days a week, lasting for two weeks to two years, in a total 1200 people who had intermittent claudication because of PAD (Watson, Ellis, and Leng 2008). All trials used a treadmill walking test as an outcome. Most trials were small (i.e., about 20 to 50 patients). Fourteen trials compared exercise with usual care or placebo; patients with various medical conditions or other preexisting limitations to their exercise capacity were generally excluded. Compared with usual medical care or placebo, exercise improved maximal walking time by an average of 5 min (95% CI: 4.5-5.7), a range of improvement of about 50% to 200%, and the distance patients could walk without pain by 82 m (95% CI: 72-93 m). Despite those favorable clinical outcomes, exercise did not affect the ankle–brachial pressure index or mortality rates. However, not enough studies included those outcomes to permit a strong test of effects.

The most effective supervised exercise programs have used 30 to 45 min of treadmill walking at least three times a week for three to six months (Gardner and Poehlman 1995). The walking pace is selected to cause leg muscle pain within 3 to 5 min. Patients rest until pain subsides and then resume walking. Mechanisms that may explain improved walking performance and reduced ischemic pain after exercise training include increased capillary density, enhanced endothelial-mediated vasodilation, and improved hemostasis, which improve the delivery of oxygen to muscle, as well as increased mitochondria, which improves oxygen uptake by the muscle, and hypoalgesic effects of exercise (e.g., less sensitivity or increased tolerance to pain signals).

Strength of the Evidence

As described earlier, before determining whether an association between a risk factor and disease is causal, it is important to establish that the observed association is valid and not the result of selection bias, loss to follow-up, problems of measuring the independent and dependent variables, or other health factors. In general, both the case–control and prospective studies on physical activity and stroke risk have been well conducted and have used follow-up periods of sufficient length to reduce the effect of undiagnosed disease at study entry on the results, as well as to ensure an adequate number of stroke events for analysis. The physical activity assessment methods used in these studies vary considerably, from simply asking about the frequency of exercise-induced sweating to the use of more detailed activity histories. There is undoubtedly some degree of misclassification of physical activity using these methods that would potentially bias the results toward finding no association between physical activity and stroke risk. The independence of the association between physical activity and stroke risk is open to question.

Though several studies have shown a significant association of physical activity with stroke risk after adjustment for other major stroke risk factors, others have not. Additionally, at least two cohort studies have examined the association between physical fitness and stroke risk, but the association between changes in fitness or physical activity exposures and stroke risk has not been examined.

Although data on the association of physical activity with stroke risk are considerably fewer than those on its association with reduced risk of heart disease, about half the published studies on physical activity and stroke suggest a protective effect of physical activity, especially for ischemic stroke. In this section we evaluate the temporal sequence, strength of association, consistency, dose response, and biological plausibility of the evidence.

Temporal Sequence

About 25 studies included in our review used a prospective design in which the independent variable, physical activity, was assessed prior to knowledge of the outcome, stroke incidence or stroke deaths. The observation follow-ups ranged from two years to 32 years and averaged about 10 years. Therefore, these studies satisfy the criterion of temporal sequence.

Strength of Association

The degree of risk reduction for stroke associated with participation in physical activity is moderately strong and relatively consistent among studies. Because stroke incidence is low, the lower risk seen among active people did not reach statistical significance in nearly half the studies, especially those that had smaller cohorts. However, when averaged across all the studies, the risk reduction observed is in the range of 25% to 30% for ischemic and all strokes. Findings on hemorrhagic stroke reduction are less clear, in part because its incidence rate is lower than that of ischemic stroke.

Consistency

Though not all studies agree, most have shown that the risk of ischemic stroke among people who are physically active is less than that of their sedentary counterparts after adjustment for other stroke risk factors. Consistent results have been shown across different ages, in both sexes, and among several ethnic groups. However, most evidence is from whites of European descent. Studies have not sufficiently examined the association between physical activity and risk in African American men and women, who have higher stroke risk than other race or ethnic groups in the United States.

Dose Response

Evidence for a dose–gradient reduction in stroke risk with increasing weekly energy expenditure or higher intensity of physical activity is less clear than for coronary heart disease. Only about 60% of the studies examined three or more levels of physical activity, and about two-thirds of those studies showed a dose–response gradient of reduced stroke with increasing physical activity. Others showed a threshold or L-shaped effect; a certain minimum level of activity was associated with protection against stroke, but further increases in activity showed no greater decrease in risk. Three prospective cohort studies of leisure-time physical activity suggested an inverted-U relationship, in which a reduction in stroke risk was apparent only at moderate amounts of physical activity. The case–control Northern Manhattan Stroke Study reported a dose–response relationship between both intensity and duration of leisure physical activity and stroke risk that was consistent among ages, sexes, and races. In both the U.S. Nurses' Health and U.S. Health Professionals cohorts, 30 min per day of moderate-to-vigorous physical activity protected against ischemic and total strokes. The Nurses' Health Study also indicated a dose response to both total physical activity and walking for exercise for reducing total and ischemic strokes but not hemorrhagic stroke.

On balance, it appears that more physical activity each week confers more protection against all strokes and ischemic stroke, regardless of whether the intensity of the activity is moderate or vigorous.

Biological Plausibility

A possible explanation for the generally positive association between physical activity and reduced rate of ischemic stroke is that physical activity reduces risk of developing atherosclerosis and thrombosis. Ischemic stroke involves a pathophysiology similar to that of atherosclerotic disease, and arterial thrombosis develops similarly to coronary heart disease. Hence, the benefits of physical activity on reducing clotting risk, reducing blood lipids, and increasing high-density lipoprotein could explain a reduction in the risk of developing ischemic CVD.

Indeed, evidence has emerged that cardiorespiratory fitness may play a role in retarding the progression of carotid atherosclerosis in middle-aged men. The association of cardiorespiratory fitness and the progression of early carotid atherosclerosis was examined in a four-year follow-up study of 854 Finnish men 42 to 60 years of age (Lakka et al. 2001). After adjustments for age and cigarette smoking, there were inverse relationships between maximal aerobic capacity and surface roughness and thickness of the intima of the carotid artery and plaque height measured by ultrasonography. Those inverse associations were weakened but remained after additional adjustment for systolic blood pressure, serum levels of apolipoprotein B (a risk factor for atherosclerosis), diabetes,

and plasma fibrinogen levels. Men in the lowest quartile of maximal aerobic capacity (26 ml · kg^{-1} · min^{-1}) had twice the increase in mean thickness of the carotid artery intima and 31% greater increase in surface roughness compared with men in the highest quartile of maximal aerobic capacity (>36 ml · kg^{-1} · min^{-1}).

It is also possible that regular physical activity helps protect against stroke mortality by mitigating brain cell damage after a stroke. Convincing evidence from studies of rodents shows that moderate physical activity has a neurotroph effect on neurons in several brain regions (Cotman and Berchtold 2002); protects against ischemic stroke by upregulating nitric oxide synthase, thus enhancing endothelium-dependent vasodilation in the brain (Endres et al. 2003); and reduces brain damage (Wang, Yang, and Yu 2001) and mortality rate (Ang et al. 2003; Stummer et al. 1994) after stroke.

Summary

The scientific advisory committee for the 2008 Physical Activity Guidelines for Americans concluded that physically active men and women usually have a lower risk of stroke incidence or mortality than the least active. More active persons demonstrate a 25% to 30% lower risk for all strokes, including ischemic and hemorrhagic stroke. It appears that increased physical activity is associated with a reduced risk of atherosclerosis and blood clotting. Thus, an association between physical activity and decreased risk of ischemic stroke might be expected. Given that the incidence of stroke is relatively low, the association between activity and stroke can be evaluated only in large cohort studies, where the measures of physical activity often are not very precise and often do not allow an evaluation of a dose–response association. Better physical activity assessment techniques are necessary to allow clearer identification of the intensity and duration of physical activity associated with optimal reduction in stroke risk. Also, many studies did not classify the type of stroke, which is important because the mechanisms by which physical activity might protect against stroke could differ according to whether stroke results from ischemia, reduced perfusion, or embolism.

· BIBLIOGRAPHY ·

Abbott, R.D., B.L. Rodriguez, C.M. Burchfiel, and J.D. Curb. 1994. Physical activity in older middle-aged men and reduced risk of stroke: The Honolulu Heart Program. *American Journal of Epidemiology* 139: 881-893.

Adams, H.P. Jr., G. del Zoppo, M.J. Alberts, D.L. Bhatt, L. Brass, A. Furlan, R.L. Grubb, R.T. Higashida, E.C. Jauch, C. Kidwell, P.D. Lyden, L.B. Morgenstern, A.I. Qureshi, R.H. Rosenwasser, P.A. Scott, and E.F. Wijdicks. 2007. Guidelines for the early management of adults with ischemic stroke. *Circulation* 115: e478-534.

Agnarsson, U., G. Thorgeirsson, H. Sigvaldason, and N. Sigfusson. 1999. Effects of leisure-time physical activity and ventilatory function on risk for stroke in men: The Reykjavik Study. *Annals of Internal Medicine* 130: 987-990.

Agnelli, G., C. Cimminiello, G. Meneghetti, S. Urbinati, Polyvascular Atherothrombosis Observational Survey (PATHOS) investigators. 2006. Low ankle–brachial index predicts an adverse 1-year outcome after acute coronary and cerebrovascular events. *Journal of Thrombosis and Haemostasis* 4: 2599-2606.

Aichner, F.T., R. Topakian, M.J. Alberts, D.L. Bhatt, H.P. Haring, M.D. Hill, G. Montalescot, S. Goto, E. Touze, J.L. Mas, P.G. Steg, and J. Rother. 2009. High cardiovascular event rates in patients with asymptomatic carotid stenosis: The REACH Registry. *European Journal of Neurology* 16: 902-908.

Algra, A., and J. van Gijn. 1996. Aspirin at any dose above 30 mg offers only modest protection after cerebral ischaemia. *Journal of Neurological and Neurosurgical Psychiatry* 60 (2): 197-199.

Amarenco, P., A. Cohen, C. Tzourio, B. Bertrand, M. Hommel, G. Besson, C. Chauvel, P.J. Touboul, and M.G. Bousser. 1994. Atherosclerotic disease of the aortic arch and the risk of ischemic stroke. *New England Journal of Medicine* 331: 1474-1479.

American Heart Association. 1998. *1999 heart and stroke statistical update.* Dallas: American Heart Association.

American Heart Association. 2002. *Heart and stroke statistical update.* Dallas: American Heart Association.

American Heart Association. 2010. *Heart disease and stroke statistics - 2010 update.* Dallas, Texas: American Heart Association.

American Heart Association. 2012. Heart disease and stroke statistics - 2012 update: A report from the American Heart Association.*Circulation* 125 (1): e2-e220.

Ang, E.T., P.T. Wong, S. Moochhala, and Y.K. Ng. 2003. Neuroprotection associated with running: Is it a result of increased endogenous neurotrophic factors? *Neuroscience* 118: 335-345.

Antiplatelet Trialists' Collaboration. 1994. Collaborative overview of randomised trials of antiplatelet therapy: I. Prevention of death, myocardial infarction, and stroke by prolonged antiplatelet therapy in various categories of patients. *British Medical Journal* 308 (6921): 81-106. Erratum, *British Medical Journal* 308 (6943): 1540.

Banerjee A., F.G. Fowkes, and P.M. Rothwell. 2010. Associations between peripheral artery disease and ischemic stroke: implications for primary and secondary prevention. *Stroke* 41 (9): 2102-2107.

Barnett, H.J.M., J.P. Mohr, B.M. Stein, and F.M. Yatsu, eds. 1992. *Stroke: Pathophysiology, diagnosis, and management.* 2nd edition. New York: Churchill Livingstone.

Bijnen, F.C., C.J. Caspersen, E.J. Feskens, W.H. Saris, W.L. Mosterd, and D. Kromhout. 1998. Physical activity and 10-year mortality from cardiovascular diseases and all causes: The Zutphen Elderly Study. *Archives of Internal Medicine* 158 (14): 1499-1505.

Blair, S.H., C.L. Wells, R.D. Weathers, and R.S. Paffenbarger. 1994. Chronic disease: The physical activity dose–response controversy. In *Advances in exercise adherence,* edited by R.K. Dishman, pp. 31-54. Champaign, IL: Human Kinetics.

Broderick, J.P., T.G. Brott, J.E. Duldner, T. Tomsick, and G. Huster. 1993. Volume of intracerebral hemorrhage. A powerful and easy-to-use predictor of 30-day mortality. *Stroke* 24: 987-993.

Broderick, J., S. Connolly, E. Feldmann, et al. 2007. Guidelines for the management of spontaneous intracerebral hemorrhage in adults: 2007 update: A guideline from the American Heart Association/American Stroke Association Stroke Council, High Blood Pressure Research Council, and the Quality of Care and Outcomes in Research Interdisciplinary Working Group: The American Academy of Neurology affirms the value of this guideline as an educational tool for neurologists. *Stroke* 38: 2001-2023.

Cheng, S.W., L.L. Wu, H. Lau, A.C. Ting, and J. Wong. 1999. Prevalence of significant carotid stenosis in Chinese patients with peripheral and coronary artery disease. *ANZ Journal of Surgery* 69: 44-47.

Chiuve, S.E., K.M. Rexrode, D. Spiegelman, G. Logroscino, J.E. Manson, and E.B. Rimm. 2008. Primary prevention of stroke by healthy lifestyle. *Circulation* 118: 947-954.

Cholesterol and Recurrent Events Trial Investigators. 1996. The effect of pravastatin on coronary events after myocardial infarction in patients with average cholesterol levels. *New England Journal of Medicine* 335 (14): 1001-1009.

Clark, T.G., M.F.G. Murphy, and P.M. Rothwell. 2003. Long term risks of stroke, myocardial infarction, and vascular death in "low risk" patients with a non-recent transient ischaemic attack. *Journal of Neurology, Neurosurgery and Psychiatry* 74: 577-581.

Cotman, C.W., and N.C. Berchtold. 2002. Exercise: A behavioral intervention to enhance brain health and plasticity. *Trends in Neurosciences* 25: 295-301.

Criqui, M.H., J.O. Denenberg, R.D. Langer, and A. Fronek. 1997. The epidemiology of peripheral arterial disease: Importance of identifying the population at risk. *Vascular Medicine* 2: 221-226.

Criqui, M.H., J.K. Ninomiya, D.L. Wingard, M. Ji, and A. Fronek. 2008. Progression of peripheral arterial disease predicts cardiovascular disease morbidity and mortality. *Journal of the American College of Cardiology* 52: 1736-1742.

Crowther, R.G., W.L. Spinks, A.S. Leicht, K. Sangla, F. Quigley, and J. Golledge. 2008. Effects of a long-term exercise program on lower limb mobility, physiological responses, walking performance, and physical activity levels in patients with peripheral arterial disease. *Journal of Vascular Surgery* 47: 303-309.

del Zoppo, G.J., J.L. Saver, E.C. Jauch, and H.P. Adams Jr., on behalf of the AHA Stroke Council. 2009. Expansion of the time window for treatment of acute ischemic stroke with intravenous tissue plasminogen activator. A science advisory from the American Heart Association/American Stroke Association. *Stroke* 40: 2945-2948.

Demaerschalk, B.M., and T.R. Yip. 2005. Economic benefit of increasing utilization of intravenous tissue plasminogen activator for acute ischemic stroke in the United States. *Stroke* 36: 2500-2503.

Diep L., J. Kwagyan, J. Kurantsin-Mills, R. Weir, and A. Jayam-Trouth. 2010. Association of physical activity level and stroke outcomes in men and women: A meta-analysis. *Journal of Womens Health* (Larchmt) 19: 1815-1822.

Dobesh, P.P., Z.A. Stacy, and E.L. Persson. 2009. Pharmacologic therapy for intermittent claudication. Review. *Pharmacotherapy* 29 (5): 526-553.

Donahue, R.P., R.D. Abbott, D.M. Reed, and K. Yano. 1986. Alcohol and hemorrhagic stroke: The Honolulu Heart Program. *Journal of the American Medical Association* 255: 2311-2314.

Ellekjaer, H., J. Holmen, E. Ellekjaer, and L. Vatten. 2000. Physical activity and stroke mortality in women. Ten-year follow-up of the Nord-Trondelag health survey, 1984-1986. *Stroke* 31: 14-18.

Endres, M., K. Gertz, U. Lindauer, J. Katchanov, J. Schultze, H. Schröck, G. Nickenig, W. Kuschinsky, U. Dirnagl, and U. Laufs. 2003. Mechanisms of stroke protection by physical activity. Annals of Neurology 54 (5): 582-590.

European Stroke Organisation (ESO) Executive Committee; ESO Writing Committee. 2008. Guidelines for management of ischaemic stroke and transient ischaemic attack. Cerebrovascular Disease 25: 457-507.

Evenson, K.R., W.D. Rosamond, J. Cai, J.F. Toole, R.G. Hutchinson, E. Shahar, and A.R. Folsom. 1999. Physical activity and ischemic stroke risk: The Atherosclerosis Risk in Communities Study. Stroke 30: 1333-1339.

Fiebach, N.H., P.R. Hebert, M.J. Stampfer, G.A. Colditz, W.C. Willett, and B. Rosner. 1989. A prospective study of high blood pressure and cardiovascular disease in women. American Journal of Epidemiology 130: 646-654.

Folsom, A.R., R.J. Prineas, S.A. Kaye, and R.G. Munger. 1990. Incidence of hypertension and stroke in relation to body fat distribution and other risk factors in older women. Stroke 21: 701-706.

Fossum, E., G.W. Gleim, S.E. Kjeldsen, J.R. Kizer, S. Julius, R.B. Devereux, W.E. Brady, D.A. Hille, P.A. Lyle, and B. Dahlöf. 2007. The effect of baseline physical activity on cardiovascular outcomes and new-onset diabetes in patients treated for hypertension and left ventricular hypertrophy: The LIFE study. Journal of Internal Medicine 262 (4, October): 439-448.

Gardner, A.W., and E.T. Poehlman. 1995. Exercise rehabilitation programs for the treatment of claudication pain: A meta-analysis. Journal of the American Medical Association 274: 975-980.

Gillum, R.F., M.E. Mussolino, and D.D. Ingram. 1996. Physical activity and stroke incidence in women and men: The NHANES I epidemiological follow-up study. American Journal of Epidemiology 143: 860-869.

Goldstein, L.B., R. Adams, K. Becker, C.D. Furberg, P.B. Gorelick, G. Hademenos, M. Hill, G. Howard, V.J. Howard, B. Jacobs, et al. 2001. Primary prevention of ischemic stroke: A statement for healthcare professionals from the Stroke Council of the American Heart Association. Circulation 103: 163-182.

Haheim, L.L., I. Holme, I. Hjermann, and P. Leren. 1993. Risk factors of stroke incidence and mortality. A 12-year follow-up of the Oslo Study. Stroke 24: 1484-1489.

Hankey, G.J., P.E. Norman, and J.W. Eikelboom. 2006. Medical treatment of peripheral arterial disease. Journal of the American Medical Association 295 (5): 547-553.

Hardman, A.E. 1996. Exercise in the prevention of atherosclerotic, metabolic and hypertensive diseases: A review. Journal of Sports Sciences 14: 201-218.

Harmsen, P., G. Lappas, A. Rosengren, and L. Wilhelmsen. 2006. Long-term risk factors for stroke: Twenty-eight years of follow-up of 7457 middle-aged men in Göteborg, Sweden. Stroke 37 (7): 1663-1667.

Harmsen, P., A. Rosengren, A. Tsipogianni, and L. Wilhelmsen. 1990. Risk factors for stroke in middle-aged men in Göteborg, Sweden. Stroke 21: 223-229.

Helgason, C.M., and P.A. Wolf. 1997. American Heart Association Prevention Conference IV. Prevention and rehabilitation of stroke. Executive summary. Circulation 96 (2): 701-717.

Hiatt, W.R., J.G. Regensteiner, M.E. Hargarten, E.E. Wolfel, and E.P. Brass. 1990. Benefit of exercise conditioning for patients with peripheral arterial disease. Circulation 81: 602-609.

Hiatt, W.R., E.E. Wolfel, R.H. Meier, and J.G. Regensteiner. 1994. Superiority of treadmill walking exercise versus strength training for patients with peripheral arterial disease. Circulation 90: 1866-1874.

Higgins, M., W. Kannel, R. Garrison, J. Pinsky, and J. Stokes. 1988. Hazards of obesity: The Framingham experience. Acta Medica Scandinavica 723: 23-36.

Hirsch A.T., M.H. Criqui, D. Treat-Jacobson, J.G. Regensteiner, M.A. Creager, J.W. Olin, S.H. Krook, D.B. Hunninghake, A.J. Comerota, M.E. Walsh, M.M. McDermott, and W.R. Hiatt. 2001. Peripheral arterial disease detection, awareness, and treatment in primary care. JAMA 286 (11): 1317-1324.

Hodis, H.N., W.J. Mack, L. LaBree, R.H. Selzer, C. Liu, P. Alaupovic, H. Kwong-Fu, and S.P. Azen. 1996. Reduction in carotid arterial wall thickness using lovastatin and dietary therapy: A randomized clinical trial. Annals of Internal Medicine 124 (6): 548-556.

Hooi, J.D., H.E. Stoffers, A.D. Kester, P.E. Rinkens, V. Kaiser, J.W. van Ree, and J.A. Knottnerus. 1998. Risk factors and cardiovascular diseases associated with asymptomatic peripheral arterial occlusive disease. The Limburg PAOD Study. Peripheral Arterial Occlusive Disease. Scandinavian Journal of Primary Health Care 16: 177-182.

Hooker, S.P., X. Sui, N. Colabianchi, J. Vena, J. Laditka, M.J. LaMonte, and S.N. Blair. 2008. Cardiorespiratory fitness as a predictor of fatal and nonfatal stroke in asymptomatic women and men. Stroke 39: 2950-2957.

Hu, F.B., M.J. Stampfer, G.A. Coldwitz, A. Ascherio, K.M. Rexrode, W.C. Willett, and J.E. Manson. 2000. Physical activity and risk of stroke in women. Journal of the American Medical Association 283: 2961-2967.

Hypertension Detection and Follow-Up Program Cooperative Group. 1979. Five-year findings of the hypertension detection and follow-up program: I. Reduction in mortality in persons with high blood pressure, including mild hypertension. Journal of the American Medical Association 242 (23): 2562-2571.

Kannel, W.B. 1999. Historic perspectives on the relative contributions of diastolic and systolic blood pressure elevation to cardiovascular risk profile. American Heart Journal 138 (3 Pt 2): 205-210.

Kannel, W.B., and P. Sorlie. 1979. Some health benefits of physical activity: The Framingham Study. Archives of Internal Medicine 139: 857-861.

Kannel, W.B., P.A. Wolf, J. Verter, and P.M. McNamara. 1970. Epidemiologic assessment of the role of blood pressure in stroke: The Framingham Study. Journal of the American Medical Association 214: 301-310.

Kiely, D.K., P.A. Wolf, L.A. Cupples, A.S. Beiser, and W.B. Kannel. 1994. Physical activity and stroke risk: The Framingham Study. American Journal of Epidemiology 140: 860-869.

Kleindorfer, D., P. Panagos, A. Pancioli, J. Khoury, B. Kissela, D. Woo, A. Schneider, K. Alwell, E. Jauch, R. Miller, C. Moomaw, R. Shukla, and J.P. Broderick. 2005. Incidence and short-term prognosis of transient ischemic attack in a population-based study. *Stroke* 36 (4): 720-723.

Kohl, H.W. III. 2001. Physical activity and cardiovascular disease: Evidence for a dose response. *Medicine and Science in Sports and Exercise* 33 (Suppl. 6): S472-S483.

Kurl, S., J.A. Laukkanen, R. Rauramaa, T.A. Lakka, J. Sivenius, and J.T. Salonen. 2003. Cardiorespiratory fitness and the risk for stroke in men. *Archives of Internal Medicine* 163: 1682-1688.

Lakka, T.A., J.A. Laukkanen, R. Rauramaa, R. Salonen, H.M. Lakka, G.A. Kaplan, and J.T. Salonen. 2001. Cardiorespiratory fitness and the progression of carotid atherosclerosis in middle-aged men. *Annals of Internal Medicine* 134 (1): 12-20.

Lee, C.D., A.R. Folsom, and S.N. Blair. 2003. Physical activity and stroke risk: A meta-analysis. *Stroke* 34 (10): 2475-2481.

Lee, I.M., C.H. Hennekens, K. Berger, J.E. Bering, and J.E. Manson. 1999. Exercise and stroke risk in male physicians. *Stroke* 30: 1-6.

Lee, I.M., and R.S. Paffenbarger Jr. 1998. Physical activity and stroke incidence: The Harvard Alumni Health Study. *Stroke* 29: 2049-2054.

Lee, I.M., and P.J. Skerrett. 2001. Physical activity and all-cause mortality: What is the dose–response relation? *Medicine and Science in Sports and Exercise* 33 (Suppl. 6): S459-S470.

Leng, G.C., A.J. Lee, F.G. Fowkes, M. Whiteman, J. Dunbar, E. Housley, and C.V. Ruckley. 1996. Incidence, natural history and cardiovascular events in symptomatic and asymptomatic peripheral arterial disease in the general population. *International Journal of Epidemiology* 25: 1172-1181.

Liang, W., A.H. Lee, C.W. Binns, Q. Zhou, R. Huang, and D. Hu. 2009. Habitual physical activity reduces the risk of ischemic stroke: A case-control study in southern China. *Cerebrovascular Diseases* 28 (5): 454-459.

Lindenstrom, E., G. Boysen, and J. Nyboe. 1993a. Lifestyle factors and risk of cerebrovascular disease in women: The Copenhagen City Heart Study. *Stroke* 24: 1468-1472.

Lindenstrom, E., G. Boysen, and J. Nyboe. 1993b. Risk factors for stroke in Copenhagen, Denmark: II. Lifestyle factors. *Neuroepidemiology* 12: 43-50.

Lindsted, K.D., S. Tonstad, and J.W. Kuzma. 1991. Self-report of physical activity and patterns of mortality in Seventh Day Adventist men. *Journal of Clinical Epidemiology* 44: 355-364.

Lloyd-Jones, D., R.J. Adams, T.M. Brown, M. Carnethon, S. Dai, G. De Simone, T.B. Ferguson, E. Ford, K. Furie, C. Gillespie, A. Go, K. Greenlund, N. Haase, S. Hailpern, P.M. Ho, V. Howard, B. Kissela, S. Kittner, D. Lackland, L. Lisabeth, A. Marelli, M.M. McDermott, J. Meigs, D. Mozaffarian, M. Mussolino, G. Nichol, V.L. Roger, W. Rosamond, R. Sacco, P. Sorlie, V.L. Roger, T. Thom, S. Wasserthiel-Smoller, N.D. Wong, J. Wylie-Rosett; American Heart Association Statistics Committee and Stroke Statistics Subcommittee. 2010. Heart disease and stroke statistics—2010 update: A report from the American Heart Association. *Circulation* 121 (7): e46-e215.

Lopez, A.D., C.D. Mathers, M. Ezzati, D.T. Jamison, and C.J. Murray. 2006. Global and regional burden of disease and risk factors, 2001: Systematic analysis of population health data. *Lancet* 367: 1747-1757.

Marler, J.R., B.C. Tilley, M. Lu, et al. 2000. Early stroke treatment associated with better outcome: The NINDS rt-PA Stroke Study. *Neurology* 55: 1649-1655.

Marsh, J.D., and S.G. Keyrouz. 2010. Stroke prevention and treatment. *Journal of the American College of Cardiology* 56 (9): 683-691.

Mohr, J.P., G.W. Albers, P. Amarenco, V.L. Babikian, J. Biller, R.L. Brey, B. Coull, J.D. Easton, C.R. Gomez, C.M. Helgason, et al. 1997. American Heart Association Prevention Conference. IV. Prevention and rehabilitation of stroke. Etiology of stroke. *Stroke* 28 (7): 1501-1506.

Murray, C.J., and A.D. Lopez. 1997. Mortality by cause for eight regions of the world: Global Burden of Disease Study. *Lancet* 349 (9061): 1269-1276.

National Center for Health Statistics. 2007. *Health, United States, 2007 with chartbook on trends in the health of Americans.* Hyattsville, MD: National Center for Health Statistics.

National Center for Health Statistics. 2010. *Health, United States, 2009 with special feature on medical technology.* Hyattsville, MD: U.S. Department of Health and Human Services.

Noda, H., H. Iso, H. Toyoshima, C. Date, A. Yamamoto, S. Kikuchi, A. Koizumi, T. Kondo, Y. Watanabe, Y. Wada, Y. Inaba, A. Tamakoshi; JACC Study Group. 2005. Walking and sports participation and mortality from coronary heart disease and stroke. *Journal of the American College of Cardiology* 46 (9): 1761-1767.

O'Donnell, M.J., D. Xavier, L. Liu, H. Zhang, S.L. Chin, P. Rao-Melacini, S. Rangarajan, S. Islam, P. Pais, M.J. McQueen, C. Mondo, A. Damasceno, P. Lopez-Jaramillo, G.J. Hankey, A.L. Dans, T. Yusoff, T. Truelsen, H.C. Diener, R.L. Sacco, D. Ryglewicz, A. Czlonkowska, C. Weimar, X. Wang, S. Yusuf; INTERSTROKE investigators. 2010. Risk factors for ischaemic and intracerebral haemorrhagic stroke in 22 countries (the INTERSTROKE study): A case-control study. Lancet 376 (9735, July 10): 112-123.

Paffenbarger, R.S. Jr., R.T. Hyde, A.L. Wing, and C.H. Steinmetz. 1984. A natural history of athleticism and cardiovascular health. *Journal of the American Medical Association* 252: 491-495.

Peto, R., R. Gray, R. Collins, K. Wheatley, C. Hennekens, K. Jamrozik, C. Warlow, B. Hafner, E. Thompson, S. Norton, et al. 1988. Randomised trial of prophylactic daily aspirin in British male doctors. *British Medical Journal (Clinical Research Edition)* 296 (6618): 313-316.

Petrea, R.E., A.S. Beiser, S. Seshadri, M. Kelly-Hayes, C.S. Kase, and P.A. Wolf. 2009. Gender differences in stroke incidence and poststroke disability in the Framingham Heart Study. *Stroke* 40: 1032-1037.

Physical Activity Guidelines Advisory Committee. 2008. *Physical Activity Guidelines Advisory Committee report.* Washington, DC: U.S. Department of Health and Human Services.

Rist P.M., I.M. Lee, C.S. Kase, J.M. Gaziano, and T. Kurth. 2011. Physical activity and functional outcomes from cerebral vascular events in men. *Stroke* 42: 3352-3356.

Rosamond, W.D., A.R. Folsom, L.E. Chambless, C.H. Wang, P.G. McGovern, G. Howard, L.S. Copper, and E. Shahar. 1999. Stroke incidence and survival among middle-aged adults: 9-year follow-up of the Atherosclerosis Risk in Communities (ARIC) cohort. *Stroke* 30: 736-743.

Rosengren, A., and L. Wilhelmsen. 1997. Physical activity protects against coronary death and deaths from all causes in middle-aged men: Evidence from a 20-year follow-up of the primary prevention study in Goteborg. *Annals of Epidemiology* 7: 69-75.

Sacco, R., R. Gan, B. Boden-Albala, F. Lin, D. Kargman, A. Hauser, S. Shea, and M. Paik. 1998. Leisure-time physical activity and ischemic stroke: The Northern Manhattan Stroke Study. *Stroke* 29: 380-387.

Sacco, R.L., P.A. Wolf, and P.B. Gorelick. 1999. Risk factors and their management for stroke prevention: Outlook for 1999 and beyond. *Neurology* 53 (7 Suppl. 4): S15-S24.

Sacco, R.L., P.A. Wolf, W.B. Kannel, and P.M. McNamara. 1982. Survival and recurrence following stroke: The Framingham Study. *Stroke* 13 (3): 290-295.

Salonen, J.T., P. Puska, and J. Tuomilehto. 1982. Physical activity and risk of myocardial infarction, cerebral stroke, and death: A longitudinal study in eastern Finland. *American Journal of Epidemiology* 115: 526-537.

Sattelmair, J.R., T. Kurth, J.E. Buring, and I.M. Lee. 2010. Physical activity and risk of stroke in women. *Stroke* 41 (6): 1243-1250.

Saunders, D.H., C.A. Greig, G.E. Mead, and A. Young. 2009. Physical fitness training for stroke patients. *Cochrane Database of Systematic Reviews* (4): CD003316.

Shinton, R., and G. Sagar. 1993. Lifelong exercise and stroke. *British Medical Journal* 307: 231-234.

Stampfer, M.J., G.A. Colditz, W.C. Willett, F.E. Speizer, and C.H. Hennekens. 1988. A prospective study of moderate alcohol consumption and the risk of coronary disease and stroke in women. *New England Journal of Medicine* 319: 267-273.

Steering Committee of the Physicians' Health Study Research Group. 1989. Final report on the aspirin component of the ongoing Physicians' Health Study. *New England Journal of Medicine* 321 (3): 129-135.

Stegmayr, B., K. Asplund, K. Kuulasmaa, A.M. Rajakangas, P. Thorvaldsen, and J. Tuomilehto. 1997. Stroke incidence and mortality correlated to stroke risk factors in the WHO MONICA Project: An ecological study of 18 populations. *Stroke* 28 (7): 1367-1374.

Stummer, W., K. Weber, B. Tranmer, A. Baethmann, and O. Kempski. 1994. Reduced mortality and brain damage after locomotor activity in gerbil forebrain ischemia. *Stroke* 25: 1862-1869.

Thompson, D., J. Edelsberg, G.A. Colditz, A.P. Bird, and G. Oster. 1999. Lifetime health and economic consequences of obesity. *Archives of Internal Medicine* 159: 2177-2183.

Tisi, P.V., M. Hulse, A. Chulakadabba, P. Gosling, and C.P. Shearman. 1997. Exercise training for intermittent claudication: Does it adversely affect biochemical markers of the exercise-induced inflammatory response? *European Journal of Vascular and Endovascular Surgery* 14: 344-350.

Tuomilehto, J., R. Bonity, Q. Stewart, A. Nissinen, and J.T. Salonen. 1991. Hypertension, cigarette smoking and the decline in stroke incidence in eastern Finland. *Stroke* 22: 7-11.

U.S. Department of Health and Human Services. 1996. *Physical activity and health: A report of the Surgeon General.* Atlanta: U.S. Department of Health and Human Services, Centers for Disease Control and Prevention, National Center for Chronic Disease Prevention and Health Promotion.

Vahedi, K., and P. Amarenco. 2000. Cardiac causes of stroke. *Current Treatment Options in Neurology* 2: 305-318.

Vatten, L.J., T.I. Nilsen, P.R. Romundstad, W.B. Droyvold, and J. Holmen. 2006. Adiposity and physical activity as predictors of cardiovascular mortality. *European Journal of Cardiovascular Prevention and Rehabilitation* 13 (6): 909-915.

Wang, R.Y., Y.R. Yang, and S.M. Yu. 2001. Protective effects of treadmill training on infarction in rats. *Brain Research* 922: 140-143.

Wannamethee, G., and A.G. Shaper. 1992. Physical activity in British middle aged men. *British Medical Journal* 304: 597-601.

Watson, L., B. Ellis, and G.C. Leng. 2008. Exercise for intermittent claudication. *Cochrane Database Systematic Reviews* (4): CD000990.

Weimar, C., M. Goertler, J. Rother, E.B. Ringelstein, H. Darius, D.G. Nabavi, I.H. Kim, K. Theobald, and H.C. Diener. 2007. Systemic risk score evaluation in ischemic stroke patients (SCALA): A prospective cross sectional study in 85 German stroke units. *Journal of Neurology* 254: 1562-1568.

Wendel-Vos, G.C., A.J. Schuit, E.J. Feskens, H.C. Boshuizen, W.M. Verschuren, W.H. Saris, and D. Kromhout. 2004. Physical activity and stroke. A meta-analysis of observational data. *International Journal of Epidemiology* 33 (4): 787-798.

Williams, P.T. 2009. Reduction in incident stroke risk with vigorous physical activity: Evidence from 7.7-year follow-up of the national runners' health study. *Stroke* 40 (5): 1921-1923.

Wolf, P.A., R.B. D'Agostino, W.B. Kannel, R. Bonita, and A.J. Belanger. 1988. Cigarette smoking as a risk factor for stroke: The Framingham Study. *Journal of the American Medical Association* 259: 1025-1029.

Xu, J.Q., K.D. Kochanek, S.L. Murphy, and B. Tejada-Vera. 2010. Deaths: Final data for 2007. *National Vital Statistics Reports,* Vol. 58, No. 19. Hyattsville, MD: National Center for Health Statistics.

You, R.X., J.J. McNeil, H.M. O'Malley, S.M. Davis, A.G. Thrift, and G.A. Donnan. 1997. Risk factors for stroke due to cerebral infarction in young adults. *Stroke* 28: 1913-1918.

· PART THREE ·

Physical Activity and Risk Factors

A key objective of physical activity epidemiology is to determine whether physical activity exerts a protective effect on all-cause and cardiovascular disease (CVD) mortality that is independent of other risk factors, such as hypertension, dyslipidemia, and obesity. However, adjustment to control the confounding influences of such risk factors on mortality risk reduction might underestimate the protective effects of physical activity by obscuring its indirect influence on reducing risk factors that are biologically involved in the pathogenesis of CVD and other causes of premature death, such as diabetes and cancer. Moreover, hypertension, dyslipidemia, and obesity are regarded as diseases in themselves, in addition to being key risk factors for all-cause and CVD mortality. Hence, it is doubly important to determine whether physical activity has healthful effects by altering these conditions in positive ways. The chapters in this part of the book describe population-based studies and clinical experiments providing evidence that physical activity and exercise play a role in the primary and secondary prevention of hypertension, dyslipidemia, and obesity.

CHAPTER 7

Physical Activity
and Hypertension

The pulse is the diastole and systole of the heart and arteries. . . .

· Rufus of Ephesus, 200 AD ·

CHAPTER OBJECTIVES

▸ Describe the public health burden of hypertension, including its cost, prevalence, and trends in population groups and its role in the risk of cardiovascular diseases

▸ Describe the definition of prehypertension and hypertension

▸ Identify the major modifiable and nonmodifiable risk factors of hypertension

▸ Discuss the pathophysiology of primary hypertension

▸ Describe the known and hypothesized effects of physical activity on the regulation of blood pressure

▸ Describe and evaluate the strength of evidence that physical activity or exercise training protects against the development of hypertension or reduces blood pressure in people diagnosed with hypertension

Hypertension is a major risk factor for coronary heart disease and stroke. Ancient Egyptian and Chinese physicians observed "hardening of the pulse" 3000 years ago, and the Indian physician Sushruta made diagnoses based on pulse around 600 BC (Dwivedi and Dwivedi 2007). *Sphygmopalpation* (the word is derived from the Greek *sphygmos,* meaning "pulse," and Latin *palpare,* "feel") was taught by the Greek physician Praxagoras, a contemporary of Hippocrates, around 400 BC. However, it is Galen, the Turkish-born Greco-Roman physician, who is credited with taking these ideas to Arabia in the second century AD (Hajar 1999), where they were preserved by the Islamic physician Avicenna in his *Canon of Medicine* (Gruner 1930).

Hypertension has been recognized as a disease since the 1600s, when the English physician William Harvey properly described the motion of the heart and blood in animals in *De Motu Cordis,* published in 1628. However, a British theologian and science hobbyist named Stephen Hales was the first person to measure blood pressure (Ruskin 1956). In 1733, he placed a brass pipe in the carotid artery of a horse and attached the pipe to a flexible goose's trachea, which then was connected to a 12-foot-tall (3.7 m) glass tube. As his horse bled to death, the blood rose in the tube more than 9 feet (2.7 m). About 150 years later, the first sphygmomanometer was devised by Ritter von Basch. In 1905, Russian Nikolai Sergeyevich Korotkoff used a stethoscope to detect an arterial pulse during inflation of a blood pressure cuff, leading to the use of what are now known as Korotkoff sounds to determine the blood pressures that correspond with the systolic and diastolic phases of the heartbeat (Wain 1970).

The measurement of the pulse and blood pressure has a long history, but recognition of diseases associated with high blood pressure is relatively new. Until about the 1940s, high blood pressure was often referred to as benign essential hypertension, indicating a condition of unknown origin and of little consequence for health.

It is now known that elevated blood pressure is often deadly. Aggregated findings from 61 prospective observational studies of blood pressure and mortality among 1 million adults initially without vascular disease indicate that during middle and old age, elevations in usual blood pressure from 115 mmHg systolic or 75 mmHg diastolic are directly related to increased risk of death from both hemorrhagic or ischemic vascular disease and all causes (Lewington et al. 2002). During 12.7 million person-years of exposure to risk, there were about 56,000 vascular deaths (12,000 from stroke, 34,000 from coronary heart disease, 10,000 from other vascular events) and 66,000 other deaths at ages 40 to 89 years. The increased risk with elevations in pressure was the same for men and women and was proportional at every decade of age at the time of death (see figure 7.1). At ages 40 to 69 years, each difference of 20 mmHg systolic blood pressure (SBP)

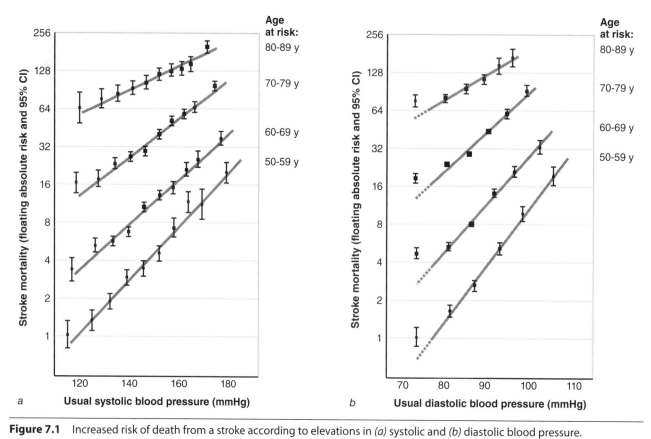

Figure 7.1 Increased risk of death from a stroke according to elevations in *(a)* systolic and *(b)* diastolic blood pressure.

or 10 mmHg diastolic blood pressure (DBP) was associated with a doubling of deaths from coronary artery disease and more than a doubling of deaths from stroke.

▶ AMONG PEOPLE who had hypertension, the 25-year odds of all-cause mortality, adjusted for age, education, race, smoking, alcohol, body mass index, and dyslipidemia, were doubled among men and nearly doubled in women who were in the lowest 20% of cardiorespiratory fitness compared to those in the top 20% of fitness (Evenson et al. 2004).

The Joint National Committee on Prevention, Detection, Evaluation, and Treatment of High Blood Pressure has defined hypertension as untreated SBP of 140 mmHg or greater or DBP of 90 mmHg or greater or as current use of antihypertensive medication (Joint National Committee 2003). Severity of hypertension is further categorized with the classification system shown in table 7.1.

Primary or essential hypertension, in which the cause is unknown or unpredictable, accounts for 90% to 95% of hypertension cases. Most cases of secondary hypertension, in which the cause is known, result from renal nephritis; hypersecretion of corticosteroids from the adrenal gland, including hyperaldosteronism; pheochromocytoma (a tumor in the **adrenal medulla,** which leads to hypersecretion of **catecholamines**); or malfunction of the renin–angiotensin–aldosterone system.

▶ PRIMARY OR essential hypertension, in which the cause is unknown or unpredictable, accounts for 90% to 95% of hypertension cases.

Table 7.1 Classification of Blood Pressure for Adults Ages 18 Years and Older

Category	Systolic, mmHg	Diastolic, mmHg
Normal	<120	<80
Prehypertension	120-139	80-89
Stage 1 hypertension	140-159	90-99
Stage 2 hypertension	≥160	≥100

Magnitude of the Problem

Though mortality rates from coronary heart disease and stroke have declined during the past 25 years, the prevalence of hypertension has remained high, at nearly 75 million Americans (American Heart Association 2012; National Center for Health Statistics 2008). During 30 years of prospective observation of participants in the Framingham Heart Study, two out of three middle-aged (45- to 54-year-old) people developed hypertension (Kannel, Garrison, and Dannenberg 1993). Analysis of data from the third National Health and Nutrition Examination Survey (NHANES III), conducted from 1999 to 2000, showed that the prevalence of high blood pressure had increased to an estimated 28.7% of U.S. adults 18 years and older (about 58 million people) (Hajjar and Kotchen 2003).

NHANES III showed that the prevalence of hypertension declined from 1960 to 1991 but rose again from a prevalence of about 25% among adults in 1991 to nearly 29% in 2000, an increase of about 8 million people. The Framingham Heart Study has estimated that the prevalence of stage 1 or 2 hypertension (>160/95 mmHg) has declined by two-thirds during the past 40 years. Some of that decline, however, can be explained by the fact that more people today have their hypertension normalized by antihypertensive medication. According to National Ambulatory Medical Care Surveys (National Center for Health Statistics 1995), hypertension was the most frequent principal diagnosis for patients visiting U.S. office-based physicians from 1980 to 1995. Hypertension accounted for 3.2% of all visits to office-based physicians in 1995, who mentioned at least one antihypertensive drug in nearly 80% of those visits (Nelson and Knapp 2000).

More recent estimates from NHANES are that 37.5 million men and 38.8 million women 20 years or older, 33.6% of noninstitutionalized adults in the United States, have high blood pressure, defined as untreated systolic pressure of 140 mmHg or higher, or diastolic pressure of 90 mmHg or higher, or current use of antihypertensive medicine, or having been diagnosed as hypertensive at least twice by a physician or other health professional (American Heart Association 2012).

Based on NHANES 2005-2006 data, it is estimated that another 25% of U.S. adults—32.4 million men and 21.2 million women—have prehypertension. About 10% to 15% of hypertension occurs in children or youths, and 70% of those cases are mild hypertension. According to NHANES, more men than women have high blood pressure until age 45. From ages 45 to 64, the rates in men and women are similar. After that, the percentage of hypertension is much higher in women (see table 7.2). The prevalence of diagnosed and undiagnosed hypertension after age 74 is about 80% for women and 65% for men (National Center for Health Statistics 2008).

The prevalence of hypertension is disproportionately higher among African Americans, and it's lower among Asian Americans, American Indians or Alaska Natives, and Mexican American men (see figure 7.2). About 43% of black men and 45% of black women have high blood pressure, compared to 34% of white men and 31% of white women. About 21% of Hispanics/Latinos and Asian Americans and 25% of American Indians or Alaska Natives have high blood pressure (American Heart Association 2012).

As with stroke, obesity, and diabetes, the prevalence of hypertension is highest in the southeastern region of the United States (figure 7.3). According to the 2009 Behavioral Risk Factor Surveillance System study, the percentage of

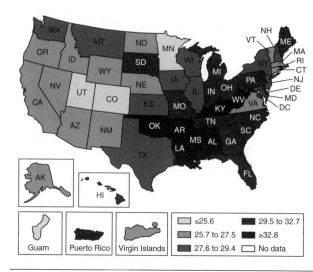

Figure 7.3　Regional differences in high blood pressure prevalence among U.S. adults.

Data from Centers for Disease Control. Available: http://www.cdc.gov/dhdsp/library/fs_bloodpressure.htm

Table 7.2　High Blood Pressure in U.S. Adults by Age Group

Age	Men (%)	Women (%)
20-34	9.2	2.2
35-44	21.1	12.6
45-54	36.2	36.2
55-64	50.2	54.4
65-74	64.1	70.8
75 and older	65.0	80.2
All	31.8	30.3

adults age 18 and older who had been told they had high blood pressure ranged from 22.4% in Colorado to 37.6% in West Virginia. The median percentage was 28.7%.

From 1996 to 2006, the age-adjusted death rate attributed to hypertension increased nearly 20% (American Heart Association 2012). The overall death rate attributed to hypertension in 2006 was 17.8% (24,382 males, 32,179 females). Death rates were 15.6% for white males, 51% for black males, 14.3% for white females, and 37.7% for black females.

▶ **ACCORDING TO** NHANES 2006, the total prevalence of hypertension among U.S. men and women ages 20 years or older was about 33%, nearly 75 million noninstitutionalized adults.

Compared with whites, blacks develop hypertension at a younger age and have higher lifetime blood pressures, resulting in elevated relative risks that are 30% higher for nonfatal stroke, 80% higher for fatal stroke, 50% higher for heart disease mortality, and four times greater for end-stage renal disease (ESRD), a condition that occurs when the kidneys can no longer function normally on their own. Hypertension is second only to diabetes as an attributable cause of ESRD. It is estimated that by 2015, more than 700,000 Americans will have ESRD or require chronic dialysis or kidney transplantation (Gilbertson et al. 2005).

Racial or ethnic differences in the rates of elevated blood pressure appear to be less pronounced among children and adolescents. Pediatric task force data from 11 studies of children and adolescents aged 1 to 17 years pooled blood pressures obtained from 58,698 children at 78,556 clinic visits (Rosner et al. 2009). Odds of body mass index (BMI)–

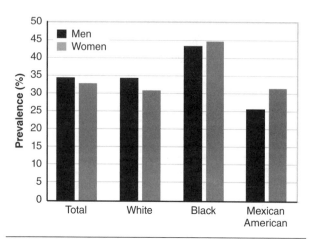

Figure 7.2　High blood pressure in Americans 20 years of age or older by sex and race.

Data from Centers for Disease Control 2006.

adjusted elevations in blood pressure were 20% higher in Hispanic boys than in white boys (odds ratio [OR]: 1.21; 95% confidence interval [CI]: 1.07-1.37) and were 14% higher among normal-weight (BMI: <85th percentile), but not overweight, black boys than among white boys (OR: 1.14; 95% CI: 1.03-1.27). No race or ethnic group differences in hypertension rates were observed among girls.

▶ **ACCORDING TO** the U.S. Renal Data System, the 2006 prevalence of ESRD was 506,256. That year, 110,854 new cases of ESRD were reported; 87,654 patients died from ESRD, and more than 18,000 kidney transplantations were performed (American Heart Association 2010).

The estimated direct and indirect cost of hypertension for 2010 was $76.6 billion in health care services, medications, and missed days of work (Lloyd-Jones et al. 2010).

Treating Hypertension

Ancient physicians observed that dietary salt "hardened the pulse" nearly 2000 years before the methods to measure blood pressure in humans were developed. Today, more than two-thirds of people in the United States diagnosed with high blood pressure use antihypertensive medications, which successfully control blood pressure to below 140/90 mmHg in nearly two-thirds of those cases (Ostchega et al. 2008).

Most of the drugs used to treat hypertension were developed in response to clinical observations that led to an evolving understanding of the etiology of hypertension. Drugs that block **sympathetic nervous system (SNS)** ganglions or deplete catecholamines were developed in the 1940s after it was observed that surgical lesioning of sympathetic nerves successfully lowered blood pressure. Diuretics were developed in the 1950s after a low-sodium diet was found to

Drug Treatment of Hypertension

Top five drugs	% of total hypertension prescriptions
Calcium channel blockers	21%
ACE inhibitors or SNS receptor blockers	18%
Diuretics	12%
SNS receptor blockers	8%
Combined (ACE inhibitor, plus SNS receptor blocker, plus diuretic)	7%

Data from Nelson and Knapp 2000.

lower blood pressure in some people. Renin was discovered in the kidneys in the late 1800s and found to be elevated in some people with high blood pressure, but the development of **angiotensin-converting enzyme (ACE)** inhibitors didn't occur until the 1980s.

Though drugs have high efficacy for managing hypertension and generally reducing mortality rates, it is often difficult to find the right combination for best effect, and hypertensive drugs haven't reduced mortality for white women in some studies (Anastos et al. 1991). Also, popular antihypertension drugs have serious side effects. For example, the Antihypertensive and Lipid-Lowering Treatment to Prevent Heart Attack Trial (ALLHAT), a randomized controlled trial conducted in the United States and Canada that included over 33,000 men and women aged 55 years or older with hypertension, showed that compared with patients taking a thiazide diuretic, patients taking other drugs had serious adverse events during a five-year follow-up. Specifically, an alpha-adrenergic blocking drug increased the incidence of heart attacks and strokes by 25%; a calcium channel blocker increased risk of heart failure by 38% (but not risks of fatal coronary heart disease or nonfatal heart attack); and an ACE inhibitor increased risk of stroke by 15% and risk of heart failure by 19% (Furberg et al. 2002). Subsequent evaluations of the ALLHAT trial have confirmed that the diuretic was usually superior as the first-step drug therapy for patients, especially blacks, who have diabetes, renal disease, metabolic syndrome, or more than one of these (Einhorn et al. 2010).

Similarly, a meta-analysis of seven randomized controlled trials including 27,433 patients found that beta-blockers reduced the risk of stroke by 19% when compared to placebo or no treatment; but 13 studies of nearly 106,000 patients taking beta-blockers showed that they had 16% higher risk compared to patients taking other antihypertensive drugs (Lindholm, Carlberg, and Samuelsson 2005). The Anglo-Scandinavian Cardiac Outcomes Trial–Blood Pressure Lowering Arm (ASCOT-BPLA), a randomized controlled trial of 19,257 patients with hypertension and at least three other cardiovascular risk factors, compared treatment with either a calcium channel blocker plus an ACE inhibitor as needed or a beta-blocker plus a diuretic as needed. The study was stopped early after about 5.5 years because the group receiving the beta-blocker had a 10% higher rate of heart attack or coronary death, a 30% higher rate of fatal or nonfatal stroke, and a 40% higher risk of developing diabetes (Dahlöf et al. 2005).

It is not clear whether the results of clinical trials have translated to change in evidence-based practice. For example, the Multi-Ethnic Study of Atherosclerosis (MESA), a prospective cohort study of 6814 adults from four ethnic groups, showed that after publication of ALLHAT, the percentage of new users of antihypertensive prescribed a diuretic rose from 32% to 44% in 2004 and was 39% in 2005 (Delaney et al. 2009). However, a search of the Maine

History of Hypertension Treatment

1940s
- Thiocyanates
- Ganglion-blocking agents
- Catecholamine depletors (*Rauwolfia* derivatives)

1950s
- Vasodilators (hydralazine)
- Peripheral sympathetic inhibitors (guanethidine)
- Monoamine oxidase inhibitors
- Diuretics

1960s
- Central α_2-agonists (SNS inhibitors)
- β-adrenergic inhibitors

1970s
- α-adrenergic inhibitors
- α-β-blockers

1980s
- ACE inhibitors
- Calcium channel blockers

1990s
- Angiotensin II receptor antagonists

2000s
- Gene therapy
- Physical activity?

Adapted from Moser 1997 and Opie 2009

Lifestyle Modifications for Primary Prevention of Hypertension

- Maintain normal body weight for adults (BMI: 18.5-24.9 kg/m²)
- Reduce dietary sodium intake to no more than 100 mmol/day (approximately 6 g of sodium chloride or 2.4 g of sodium per day)
- Engage in regular aerobic physical activity such as brisk walking (at least 30 min per day, most days of the week)
- Limit alcohol consumption to no more than 1 oz (30 ml) of ethanol (e.g., 24 oz [720 ml] of beer, 10 oz [300 ml] of wine, or 2 oz [60 ml] of 100-proof whiskey) per day in most men and to no more than 0.5 oz (15 ml) of ethanol per day in women and lighter-weight persons
- Maintain adequate intake of dietary potassium (>90 mmol [3500 mg] per day)
- Consume a diet that is rich in fruits and vegetables and in low-fat dairy products with a reduced content of saturated and total fat

Source: National High Blood Pressure Education Program (Whelton et al. 2002).

channel blockers, 6.4%; angiotensin receptor blockers, 1.6%; and others, 7.7% (Weiss, Buckley, and Clifford 2006). Thus, although diuretic prescriptions increased slightly, so did the use of beta-blockers; prescriptions of ACE inhibitors remained high despite their higher associated risks of stroke and heart failure.

For mild to moderate high blood pressure, frontline treatment often focuses on low-risk interventions including weight loss, reduction of dietary salt, and increased physical activity. In addition to age and race, high body fat, insulin resistance, dietary sodium, and alcohol use are known risk factors for hypertension (Fletcher and Bulpitt 1994). Thus, **primary prevention** of hypertension focuses on lifestyle changes, including decreasing salt intake, increasing potassium intake, losing weight, reducing stress, and increasing physical activity. About a decade ago, the Preventive Services Task Force appointed by the U.S. Office of Disease Prevention and Health Promotion concluded that the evidence was strong and independent of other risk factors that inactive men and women had about a one-third to a one-half greater risk of developing hypertension than active or fit people (Harris et al. 1989). That conclusion was based on observations of just two cohorts, the Harvard alumni and the Aerobics Center Longitudinal Study cohort, but other evidence agrees with that early view.

Hypertension Etiology

Theories about circulation have their origins in the writings of Hippocrates, who thought that arteries carried blood but that veins carried air, and Galen, who showed that arteries and veins each carried blood. Galen, though, believed that blood flowed from and to the heart in separate arterial and venous systems. It was not until 1616 that the British

Medicaid database of 5375 newly diagnosed hypertension patients followed for at least six months showed that in 2001, the proportional drug use was beta-blockers, 23.5%; diuretics, 17.5%; ACE inhibitors, 37.5%; calcium channel blockers, 9.5%; angiotensin receptor blockers, 3.8%; and others, 8.2%. By 2005, those proportions were beta-blockers, 27.8%; diuretics, 25.5%; ACE inhibitors, 30.9%; calcium

physician William Harvey concluded that blood circulation was a closed circuit, with capillaries connecting arteries and veins.

The basic determinants of blood pressure are described by Poiseuille's law, which states that laminar blood flow $(\dot{Q})$ through a vessel is limited by the difference in pressure along the length of the vessel (ΔP), the radius of the vessel (r), the viscosity of the blood (η), and vessel length (l) according to the following equation:

$$\dot{Q} = \frac{\Delta P \pi r^4}{8 \eta l}$$

Simplifying and solving the equation for pressure, we can determine that blood pressure is the algebraic product of blood flow (i.e., cardiac output) and **total peripheral resistance (TPR)** to flow. In practical terms, a person's blood pressure depends on the volume of blood, its rate of flow, and especially the diameter of blood vessels. Hypertension develops from an abnormal elevation in one or all of the factors that influence blood flow or resistance to flow; and the specific mechanisms that alter blood flow or resistance vary with age, race, and body composition.

▷ **BLOOD PRESSURE** is the algebraic product of blood flow (i.e., cardiac output) and total peripheral resistance to flow.

Autonomic Nervous System

Though the osmolality (i.e., concentrations of ions such as sodium) of the blood, **mineralocorticosteroids** such as aldosterone, and hemodynamic factors such as blood volume and viscosity influence blood pressure, so does the **autonomic nervous system (ANS).** The neurotransmitter **norepinephrine** (also called **noradrenaline**), released from sympathetic nerves, and the hormone **epinephrine** (also called **adrenaline**), secreted from the medulla of the adrenal gland, bind with **adrenergic receptors** (or adrenoreceptors) on cells of the heart to increase its rate and force of contraction; on the kidneys; and on smooth muscle cells in blood vessels, which then constrict to increase peripheral resistance. Hence, blood pressure increases during activity of the sympathetic nervous system (figure 7.4). A necessary step between the binding of norepinephrine or epinephrine (the "first messengers") with an adrenoreceptor and the contraction of muscle cells is activation of a "second messenger," cyclic adenosine monophosphate (cAMP), which regulates calcium channels that govern depolarization of the muscle cell (figure 7.5). Several drugs used to treat hypertension either inhibit sympathetic nerve activity (e.g., an α_2-agonist like clonidine), block β-adrenoreceptor binding (e.g., propranolol), or block calcium channels (e.g., verapamil).

In contrast to actions of the sympathetic nervous system, the neurotransmitter **acetylcholine,** released from the vagus nerve of the **parasympathetic nervous system,** binds with cholinergic receptors on the heart and blood vessels to slow the heart and relax muscle cells, thus lowering blood pressure, and on the kidneys. Systolic and diastolic blood pressures consequently depend on the balance of waxing and waning activity of the sympathetic and parasympathetic branches of the autonomic nervous system. An imbalance in favor of greater sympathetic activation can increase blood pressure by increasing cardiac output and total peripheral resistance through direct actions on the heart and blood vessels, or indirectly through the kidney by altering the regulation of the renin–angiotensin–aldosterone system. A key action of acetylcholine's binding with blood vessels is the release of vascular releasing factors, such as nitric

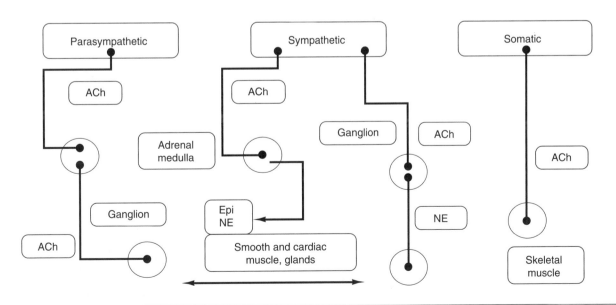

Figure 7.4 Autonomic nerves.

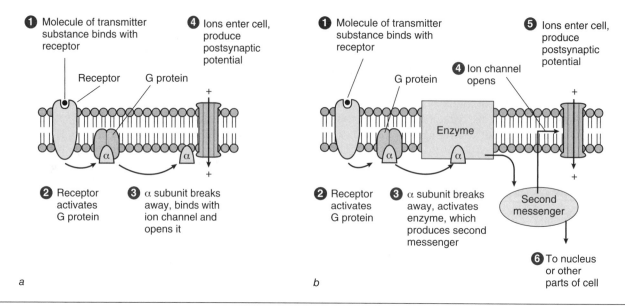

Figure 7.5   A receptor can open an ion channel *(a)* directly or *(b)* indirectly by a second messenger.

oxide, which are derived from endothelial cells that line blood vessels.

Physical Activity and Reduced Hypertension Risk: The Evidence

Both population-based epidemiologic studies and clinical experiments provide substantial evidence that moderate-intensity physical activity is associated with primary prevention and **secondary prevention** (i.e., treatment) of mild hypertension. In the following sections we describe that evidence and evaluate its strength for demonstrating causality.

▷ **BOTH POPULATION-BASED** epidemiologic studies and clinical experiments provide substantial evidence that moderate-intensity physical activity is associated with primary prevention and treatment of mild hypertension.

Cross-Sectional Studies

The following cross-sectional studies examined the association of physical activity and risk of hypertension.

North Carolina

The relationship of physical activity to hypertension was examined in a cross-sectional study of 1751 African American adults ages 20 to 50 years who lived in Pitt County, North Carolina (Ainsworth et al. 1991). Hypertension was defined as a diastolic pressure of 90 mmHg or higher or current use of antihypertensive medication. Sixty-five percent of women and 44% of men were classified as sedentary. Being sedentary was not associated with the prevalence of hypertension in men, but the odds ratio of hypertension for sedentary women (26% had hypertension) was 1.3 times that of active women (20% had hypertension). After adjustment for age, BMI, alcohol use, and waist-to-hip ratio, the odds ratio was 1.6.

Southern California

Nearly 650 white women ages 50 to 89 years living in Southern California were classified according to self-reported leisure-time physical activity into the categories light (58%), moderate (24%), heavy (6%), or no (12%) physical activity (Reaven, Barrett-Conner, and Edelstein 1991). The active and inactive women did not differ in alcohol or cigarette use or prevalence of coronary heart disease or diabetes, but the active women were younger, were lighter for their height, and had lower insulin levels. Age-adjusted systolic and diastolic blood pressures in the women who reported no physical activity were about 13 mmHg and 6 mmHg higher, respectively, than in women who reported heavy leisure physical activity during the past two weeks. After adjustments for age, BMI, and insulin levels, there was an overall linear trend for lower blood pressures with higher levels of physical activity.

Seventh Day Adventists

Among 114 African American Seventh Day Adventists about 55 years old, those who reported at least 20 min of vigorous exercise two or more times per week (mean four days a week) were classified as exercisers, and those who exercised once a week or less were classified as nonexercisers (Melby, Goldflies, and Hyner 1991). The groups had the same dietary intake of nutrients, but exercisers had lower BMI, waist circumference, and triceps skinfold thickness. After adjustment for age and sex, systolic and diastolic blood pressures were about 10 mmHg and 4 mmHg lower, respectively, among exercisers than among nonexercisers. After adjustment for the anthropometric differences, SBP was still about 8 mmHg lower in the exercisers. Forty-two percent of the nonexercisers had been diagnosed as hypertensive by a physician and were taking blood pressure medicine, compared with 20% of the exercisers.

Active Commuting in Finland

Four independent cross-sectional surveys of random national samples in Finland were carried out at five-year intervals from 1982 to 1997 as part of the Finnish cohort of the WHO MONICA study (Barengo et al. 2006). Stratified by sex and 10-year age categories, high leisure-time physical activity but not activity for commuting was associated with lower DBP among both men and women.

Active Commuting in CARDIA

This cross-sectional study included 2364 participants enrolled in the Coronary Artery Risk Development in Young Adults (CARDIA) study who worked outside the home during year 20 of the study (2005-2006) (Gordon-Larsen et al. 2009). Associations were examined between walking or biking to work (self-reported time, distance, and mode of commuting) with cardiorespiratory fitness, leisure-time physical activity measured by an accelerometer, BMI, and blood pressure. About 17% of participants reported active commuting to work. After adjustment for age, race, income, education, smoking, examination center, and physical activities other than walking, men with any active commuting, compared to none, had a 50% reduction in odds of having a BMI ≥ 30 kg/m^2 (OR: 0.50; 95% CI: 0.33-0.76) and had a DBP that was nearly 2 mmHg lower than in people who did not walk or bicycle to work (95% CI: −3.20 to −0.15).

Aerobics Center Longitudinal Study (ACLS)

Blood pressure, BMI, and cardiorespiratory fitness were measured in 35,061 patients (mean age 46 years, 70% white men) seen for an initial preventive health exam sometime between 1990 and 2010 (Chen et al. 2010). People were categorized into sex-specific quartiles on BMI as well as age-adjusted and sex-specific quintiles on cardiorespiratory fitness measured at that initial clinic visit. Normal-weight patients had a mean SBP 12 mmHg lower than obese patients (115 vs. 127 mmHg). People in the highest 20% of fitness had SBP 6 mmHg lower than those in lowest 20% of fitness (119 vs. 125 mmHg). When BMI and fitness were analyzed jointly, BMI had a stronger relation with SBP than did fitness. Normal-weight people, excluding those in the lowest 20% of fitness, had the lowest SBP.

Greek Schoolchildren

A school-based screening with anthropometric and blood pressure measurements was performed in adolescents aged 12 to 17 years on the island of Samos, Greece, in 2004 and also in 2007 (Kollias et al. 2009). A total of 446 adolescents were included in the analysis in 2004; 558 were included in 2007. Age-, sex- and BMI-adjusted blood pressures were higher in the 2007 sample (increase was 4 mmHg systolic and 11 mmHg diastolic). Lack of physical activity was associated with higher blood pressures independently of BMI, smoking, and diet.

Prospective Cohort Studies

The following prospective cohort studies examined the association of physical activity and risk of hypertension. Prospective studies help establish the temporal sequence of activity or inactivity and subsequent hypertension. Some of the studies show that physical activity or cardiorespiratory fitness protects against the risk of developing hypertension regardless of people's obesity and that the adverse effect of BMI on hypertension risk is modified favorably by cardiorespiratory fitness (Lee, Sui, and Blair 2009).

Aerobics Center Longitudinal Study (ACLS)

Nearly 5000 men and over 1200 women 20 to 65 years old who had a medical examination and treadmill fitness test at the Cooper Clinic in Dallas between 1970 and 1981 responded to a mail survey about their health in 1982 (Blair et al. 1984). People were classified as low or high in physical fitness according to their time to reach exhaustion during the treadmill test. During an average of four years of follow-up observation, 240 people developed high blood pressure, defined as greater than 140/90 mmHg. The relative risk for developing hypertension was 1.5 for the low-fitness group after adjustment for age, BMI, sex, and baseline blood pressure (figure 7.6). People in the low fitness category who had high normal systolic pressures (between 130 and 139 mmHg) and diastolic pressures (between 85 and 89 mmHg) had more than 10 times the risk of developing hypertension than those who were highly fit and had normal pressures (below 120/85 mmHg).

Of the people in the ACLS cohort, 1300 had a second clinic exam between 1970 and 1981. Hence, the association between altered fitness from the time of the first test until the second and changes in blood pressure could be examined. People who moved from the low-fitness group to the high-fitness group during that time had about half the risk of developing hypertension of those whose fitness remained low.

In a subsequent ACLS study, 16,601 men aged 20 to 82 years who had a baseline examination sometime between 1970 and 2002 were followed for an average of 18 years for incident cases of hypertension (Chase et al. 2009). There were 2346 men who developed hypertension. Adjusted for age and year of examination, rates were 86.2, 76.6, and 66.7 cases per

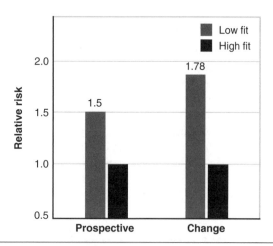

Figure 7.6 Fitness and hypertension in the Aerobics Center Longitudinal Study. Participants, including 4800 men and 1200 women aged 20 to 65 years, were classified by treadmill time in 1970 to 1980 and followed for approximately four years; 240 became hypertensive. Relative risk for the low-fitness group (i.e., prospective) was 1.50; for those who remained low in fitness compared to those who remained or became highly fit (i.e., changed positively), it was 1.78.

Adapted from Blair et al. 1984.

10,000 man-years of observation among men categorized, respectively, as sedentary, as a walker/jogger/runner, or as a regular participant in sports and fitness activities. Corresponding rates were 89.8, 78.4, and 64.6 for low, middle, and high levels of cardiorespiratory fitness. The protective associations of physical activity and fitness remained after adjustment for BMI, smoking, alcohol intake, resting SBP, baseline health status, and family history of diseases.

ACLS: HYPGENE Study

A systematic collection of blood samples from members of the ACLS cohort was begun in 2000 for the eventual purpose of studying the impact on health outcomes of interactions between people's genes and their fitness (Rankinen et al. 2007). At their first clinic visit, 1234 participants were healthy and normotensive. After a follow-up period averaging 8.7 years, 629 people developed hypertension. The other 605 people remained normotensive after a follow-up of about 10 years. The risk of developing hypertension was 19% less for each 1-MET (metabolic equivalent) level of cardiorespiratory fitness (95% CI: 12-24%) and 9% higher for each kg/m² unit of BMI (95% CI: 4-13%). The impact of higher BMI was cut by more than half (OR: 1.04 [95% CI: 0.99-1.09]) when it was jointly evaluated with fitness.

Harvard Alumni Health Study

About 15,000 male graduates of Harvard who entered college during the years 1916 to 1950 and were judged to have normal blood pressures at that time completed a question-naire in 1962 or 1966, when they were 35 to 74 years old, and again in 1972, for a six- to 10-year period of observation (Paffenbarger et al. 1983). During that time, the standard definition for hypertension was a systolic pressure of at least 160 mmHg or a diastolic pressure of at least 90 mmHg or both. Two-thirds of the men reported that they expended less than 2000 kcal per week in leisure-time physical activity. After adjustment for age, those men had a 30% greater risk of developing hypertension than those who reported expending more than 2000 kcal each week. In addition, the men who did not participate in vigorous recreational sports had a 35% higher risk of developing hypertension than those who were vigorously active. Those relative risks were independent of age, BMI over 36, a gain in BMI since college of at least 5, at least one hypertensive parent, and at least one parent with coronary heart disease.

A later analysis of nearly 17,000 Harvard male alumni from 1962 to 1985 found an inverse association between participation in vigorous recreational sports during middle age and the risk of developing hypertension that was independent of BMI, weight gain, or parental hypertension (Paffenbarger et al. 1991). In another analysis between 1977 and 1988, there were 885 cases of hypertension among 6390 men observed for 72,544 person-years. Moderately vigorous sport participation led to a reduced risk of hypertension, but walking, stair climbing, and light sports did not alter that risk (Paffenbarger and Lee 1997). Being overweight, parental hypertension, alcohol use, or cigarette use increased the risk of hypertension. The combination of all these factors accounted for one-quarter to one-half of the new cases of hypertension. The men who became active in vigorous sports between the 1960s and 1977 (Paffenbarger and Lee 1997) had a lower incidence of hypertension, independent of overweight, smoking, or alcohol use. The intensity of physical activity reduced the risk of hypertension more than total energy expenditure did.

University of Pennsylvania Alumni

Another study involving college alumni followed men who attended the University of Pennsylvania between the years 1931 and 1940 (Paffenbarger, Thorne, and Wing 1968). The time span between college and completion of a 1962 questionnaire was between 22 and 31 years. During this time, 9% of the 7685 subjects developed hypertension diagnosed by a physician. They were between 20 and 60 years old at the time of diagnosis. Activity level was assessed as less than or more than 5 h of sport participation per week. About 40% of those surveyed reported that they spent less than 5 h per week playing sports. They had a 30% higher age-adjusted risk of developing hypertension than men who spent 5 h or more in sports each week. However, systolic pressure over 130 mmHg (relative risk [RR] = 2.7), diastolic pressure over 80 mmHg (RR = 2.2), and parental history of hypertension (RR = 1.7) were better predictors of hypertension.

In a later analysis of the Penn cohort, nearly 740 of 5500 men developed hypertension between 1962 and 1985 (Paffenbarger et al. 1991). Participation in sports during college did not alter the incidence rate of hypertension. Neither did walking, stair climbing, or light recreational sports during middle age. However, participation in vigorous recreational sports in middle age reduced hypertension, independent of overweight, gain in weight, or history of parental hypertension. Vigorous sports did not reduce the death rate among those who had hypertension, but overweight and smoking increased their death rate.

Iowa Women

The two-year incidence of hypertension was examined in a cohort of nearly 42,000 women recruited from a random sample of all women aged 55 to 69 years on the 1985 Iowa driver's license list (Folsom et al. 1990). The relative risk of developing hypertension was 30% higher among women in the lowest third of leisure-time physical activity than in the most active upper third of the women sampled. However, that risk reduction was not independent of lower BMI, lower waist-to-hip ratio, less smoking, and younger age of the most active women.

The Northwestern Trial

Two groups of about 200 men and women ages 30 to 44 who were at high risk of developing hypertension (with high normal diastolic pressure, overweight, resting heart rate ≥80, or any combination of these) were observed for about five years (Stamler et al. 1989). One group was observed without intervention, while the other was instructed about changing lifestyle by (a) decreasing overweight by at least 4.5 kg (10 lb) or 5%, (b) decreasing sodium intake to no more than 1800 mg per day, (c) decreasing alcohol use to no more than two drinks a day, and (d) increasing moderate physical activity to 30 min at an intensity of 70% to 75% of maximum heart rate three days each week. The incidence of hypertension in the control group was twice that of the experimental intervention group (19.2% vs. 8.8%). About 75% of the intervention group reported an increase in physical activity and had increased fitness. Because several behaviors were changed at once, the study did not demonstrate an independent effect of exercise on the incidence of hypertension, but it did show the efficacy of nonpharmacologic interventions in people at high risk for developing hypertension.

Japanese Office Workers

Customary daily energy expenditure was estimated by a one-day activity record during an ordinary weekday in 2548 Japanese male office workers aged 35 to 59 years who initially had normal blood pressures, were not taking medication for hypertension, and had no history of cardiovascular disease. Blood pressures were then measured at annual health examinations over seven years (Nakanishi and Suzuki 2005).

After age, family history of hypertension, alcohol consumption, cigarette smoking, regular physical exercise at entry, and change in BMI during the follow-up period were controlled for, mean SBP and DBP in each follow-up year decreased according to higher levels of daily life energy expenditure measured at study entry. With additional adjustment for SBP at entry, the relative risks of hypertension or medication use for hypertension across quartiles of daily life energy expenditure relative to the least-active 25% of workers were 0.84, 0.75, and 0.54.

Finland

First-time use of free hypertension medicine was studied in a population-based cohort of 5935 men and 6227 women aged 25 to 64 years living in eastern and southwestern Finland who had no history of antihypertensive drug use, coronary heart disease, stroke, or heart failure at the start of observation (Barengo et al. 2005). After an average 11 years of follow-up observation, men with high leisure-time physical activity had a 20% reduction in risk of hypertension (RR: 0.79; 95% CI: 0.63-0.99) after adjustment for age, area and year of survey, education, smoking, alcohol intake, baseline SBP, BMI, commuting activity, and occupational physical activity. Women with high leisure-time physical activity had a reduced risk of hypertension after adjustment for age, area, and time of survey (RR: 0.65; 95% CI: 0.46-0.91), but not after further adjustments for the other covariates (RR: 0.73; 95% CI: 0.52-1.03). Commuting activity was not associated with risk of hypertension.

The joint association of physical activity and BMI with risk of hypertension was evaluated in another analysis from a larger sample from the cohort of 8302 men and 9139 women (Hu et al. 2004). Figure 7.7 shows that compared to people who said they got only light physical activity, risk ratios of hypertension associated with moderate and high physical activity were 0.60 and 0.59 in men and 0.80 and 0.72 in

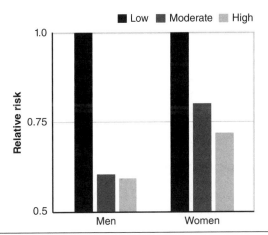

Figure 7.7 Lower hypertension risk according to levels of physical activity in Finnish men and women.

Data from Hu et al. 2004

women, regardless of initial SBP or whether people were overweight (BMI 25-29.9 kg/m²) or obese (BMI ≥30 kg/m²).

Copenhagen City Heart Study

This was a longitudinal study in a random sample of 19,698 people aged 20 years or older living in an area of Copenhagen, Denmark (Andersen and Jensen 2007). Three surveys were conducted between 1976 and 1994, with 74%, 70%, and 61% participation rates yielding a total of 37,056 mainly middle-aged people. More than half reported low leisure-time physical activity; 20% were sedentary; 25% said they got a moderate amount of activity; and only 2% were highly active. Systolic blood pressure averaged across the population dropped by 2 mmHg during the 15 years of observation. However, during that time, self-reports of physical activity at work and during leisure time did not change and remained low for most people, suggesting that physical activity had little impact on blood pressure measured at the level of a population. Nonetheless, the percentage of highly active men who used antihypertensive medication (5.4%) was lower than in sedentary men (8.7%). Also, those analyses didn't examine associations between naturally occurring change in physical activity and blood pressure. During the 15 years, 1029 of 4124 women and 815 of 2946 men who completed both the first and last surveys became more active, while 930 women and 930 men became less active. The women who increased their leisure-time physical activity had a 2 mmHg drop in SBP compared to those who either did not change their activity habits or became less active.

Migration in Tanzania

Migration from rural living to urban areas is common in many African nations. Investigators identified 103 men and 106 women 15 to 59 years old who planned to migrate for six months or more from the Morogoro rural region to Dar es Salaam in Tanzania. They were assessed at least one week but no more than one month before, and every few months after, they migrated; 132 were followed for a full year (Unwin et al. 2010). Participation rates in vigorous physical activity declined from about 80% to just more than 25% of men and from nearly 40% to 16% of women. Although weight increased by 5 lb in both men and women, SBP paradoxically dropped by 5 mmHg in men and 9 mmHg in women, which might have been explained by dietary changes including increased consumption of fresh fruit and vegetables.

Studies of Youths

The risk of developing hypertension increases with age during adulthood. However, blood pressure in children often tracks into adulthood, partly because of obesity. The epidemic of childhood obesity during the past 20 years has contributed to corresponding increases in childhood blood pressure. Hence, it is important to know whether physical activity can modify some of this increased risk in children.

New York City

A cohort of nearly 200 mainly Hispanic 5-year-olds who regularly visited an inner-city medical center was followed for 20 months (Shea et al. 1994). Age-related increases in blood pressure were inversely related to higher fitness. Children in the top 20% of fitness gains had a significantly smaller increase in SBP (3 mmHg per year) compared to children in the lowest 20% of fitness gains (5 mmHg per year).

The Northern Ireland Young Hearts Project

Cardiovascular risk factors were assessed in a random cohort of 229 boys and 230 girls when they were 12 years old and again when they were age 15. There was a significant relation between self-reports of physical activity and lower SBP over the three-year period among boys but not girls (Boreham et al. 1999).

Muscatine Iowa Study

A group of 125 children, 10 years old, were followed for five years (Janz, Dawson, and Mahoney 2002). After adjustment for age, sex, and rates of growth and maturation, physical activity during the first four years was examined as a predictor of cardiovascular health outcomes at year 5. Change in muscular strength during the first four years of the study explained 4% of differences between children in their year 5 SBP.

The Dietary Intervention Study in Childhood (DISC)

This was a randomized controlled trial to reduce saturated fat and cholesterol in the diets of 623 boys and girls, 8 to 10 years old, who had elevated low-density lipoprotein (LDL-C levels between the 80th and 98th percentiles for age and gender) but normal blood pressure (Gidding et al. 2006). Across three years of observation, there was a naturally occurring decrease in SBP of 1.15 mmHg for each 100 MET-hours per week of self-reported physical activity. The blood pressure change was accompanied by a nearly significant decrease in BMI of 0.2 kg/m² for every 10 h of vigorous physical activity. Because children's blood pressures normally increase 1 to 2 mmHg each year, the 1 mmHg decrease among active children during the three-year observation might be important for public health. However, a difference of 100 MET-hours between children is large (roughly 10 to 25 h of moderate-to-vigorous physical activity each week). It represents the difference between the 95% most active and 5% least-active children in the study, thus limiting its practical importance for most of the children.

Physical Activity and Treatment of Hypertension: The Evidence

A review of 25 clinical studies that were completed by 1988 concluded that regular exercise is effective for reducing SBP by about 11 mmHg and DBP by about 8 mmHg in men and women with mild hypertension (Hagberg 1990). Collectively, the reductions in mild hypertension observed in those studies differed according to several factors. People with mild hypertension benefited more than those diagnosed with severe hypertension or those with normal blood pressures. Women had larger reductions (–19/–14 mmHg) than men (–7/–5 mmHg). The drop in SBP was less in heavier people, but the reductions after exercise training were independent of weight change. The decreases in blood pressures were smaller when exercise intensity was higher. Drops in pressure were not consistent among studies when the intensity of exercise exceeded 75% of aerobic capacity. The reductions in DBP were greater the longer the exercise training program lasted. The reductions in blood pressure after exercise training were similar to or larger than those with other nonpharmacologic treatments of mild hypertension (Gordon et al. 1990).

Subsequent research showed that men with severe hypertension can also benefit from moderately intense exercise. After 16 weeks of cycling exercise for 45 min, three days a week, at an intensity of about 75% of maximum heart rate, African American men who had blood pressures over 180/110 mmHg when not medicated reduced their medicated diastolic pressure from 89 to 83 mmHg and reduced the size and thickness of their left ventricles (Kokkinos et al. 1995). (An enlarged left ventricle with thickened walls is a common side effect of chronic hypertension.)

A newer meta-analysis accumulated results of 72 randomized controlled trials of 3936 participants in 105 study groups who exercised mainly by walking, jogging, running, or cycling for at least four weeks (Cornelissen and Fagard 2005b). Results are summarized in figure 7.8. On average, peak oxygen uptake increased by 13%, and resting heart rate decreased by nearly 7%. After results were weighted by the size of the study (i.e., the number of participants who exercised), exercise training reduced systolic and diastolic pressures measured in a clinic by 3 mmHg and 2.4 mmHg, respectively, and daytime ambulatory systolic and diastolic pressures by 3.3 mmHg and 3.5 mmHg. The reduction of resting blood pressure was more pronounced in 30 groups of patients with mainly stage 1 hypertension (–6.9 mmHg systolic and –4.9 mmHg diastolic) than in normotensive groups (–1.9/–1.6 mmHg) (Fagard and Cornelissen 2007).

Those average changes were equivalent to reductions of about 5% each for SBP and DBP in people with hypertension and about 2% each in people who were prehypertensive or normotensive. Reductions of 3.3 mmHg (2%) SBP and 3.5

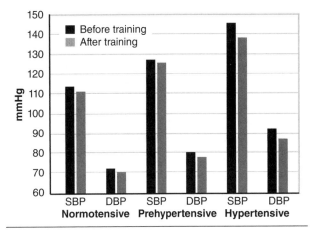

Figure 7.8 Cumulative results of 72 randomized controlled trials of chronic exercise and hypertension.

Data from Cornelissen and Fagard, 2005

mmHg (4%) DBP were also observed after exercise training when blood pressure was measured by automated recording during daytime activities outside a clinic setting (Fagard and Cornelissen 2007). Changes in both resting and ambulatory blood pressure were independent of changes in body weight (Cornelissen and Fagard 2005b).

▷ **A RECENT ANALYSIS** of results from more than 72 randomized controlled trials of aerobic exercise showed average reductions in SBP/DBP of about 7/5 mmHg among people with hypertension and about 3/2 mmHg among normotensives (Cornelissen and Fagard 2005b).

A meta-analysis of 48 trials of exercise-based cardiac rehabilitation, often combined with psychological or educational intervention, lasting at least six months and involving a total of 8940 patients with coronary heart disease, showed an average reduction in SBP of 3.2 mmHg (95% CI: –5.4 to –0.9 mmHg) but no change in DBP (Taylor et al. 2004).

There is also evidence to support the effectiveness of resistance exercise for reducing blood pressure. A meta-analysis of nine randomized controlled trials including 341 people in 12 study groups, using mostly dynamic resistance training, found cumulative net reductions in SBP of –6.0 mmHg (95% CI: –10.4 to –1.6) and DBP of –4.7 (95% CI: –8.1 to –1.4) mmHg (Cornelissen and Fagard 2005a). A handful of studies show that isometric handgrip exercise training also can lower resting blood pressure (Kelley and Kelley 2010). In 13 randomized controlled trials of people with abnormal glucose regulation, resistance exercise training reduced SBP by 6.19 mmHg (95% CI: 1.00-11.38) (Strasser, Siebert, and Schobersberger 2010).

Blood pressure reductions after either aerobic or resistance exercise training seem similar for men and women regardless of age (Kelley 1999; Kelley and Sharpe Kelley 2001). Also,

Table 7.3   Results of Meta-Analysis of Interventions to Reduce Blood Pressure

Intervention	Average decrease in blood pressure	Confidence interval
Improved diet	5 mmHg	95% CI: 3.1-7.0
Aerobic exercise	4.6 mmHg	95% CI: 2.0-7.1
Alcohol restriction	3.8 mmHg	95% CI: 1.4-6.1
Sodium restriction	3.6 mmHg	95% CI: 2.5-4.6
Fish oil supplements	2.3 mmHg	95% CI: 0.2-4.3

Data from Dickinson et al. 2006.

randomized controlled trials of physical activity interventions in children lasting up to several months typically have shown a 1% to 3% reduction in blood pressure after aerobic or resistance training or participation in games (Kelley, Kelley, and Tran 2003).

A meta-analysis of 105 trials of lifestyle interventions lasting at least eight weeks on nearly 7000 adults with elevated blood pressure found that aerobic exercise compared favorably to dietary changes, as shown in table 7.3. The evidence did not support the use of relaxation therapies or calcium, magnesium, or potassium supplements to reduce blood pressure (Dickinson et al. 2006).

Strength of the Evidence

When judged by the criteria of Mill's canons, the evidence is moderately strong that leisure-time physical activity is independently associated with reduced risk of developing hypertension and is effective in reducing blood pressure among adults who have mild hypertension.

Temporal Sequence

Large prospective cohort studies, which demonstrate the appropriate temporal sequence, have shown lowered risk of developing hypertension among people who are physically active.

Strength of Association

The cumulative evidence from nearly 20 observational studies using a prospective cohort design shows a 30% to 50% reduction in the risk of developing hypertension when active adults are compared with sedentary peers. Results from more than 70 randomized controlled trials have shown average reductions in systolic/diastolic blood pressure of about 7/6 mmHg among people with hypertension and about 3/2 mmHg among normotensives (Fagard 2001). Based on observational studies of elevated blood pressure and mortality risks (Lewington et al. 2002), those exercise effects on systolic and diastolic pressures, respectively, would hypothetically

reduce risks of deaths from CHD or stroke by 7% to 17% in people with prehypertension and by 10% to 30% in people who have hypertension.

Consistency

The majority of evidence has come from studies of white men of European ancestry. Nonetheless, a sufficient number of studies have been conducted with women and people of non-European ethnicities to suggest that physical activity reduces blood pressure equally regardless of age, sex, nation, or ethnicity.

Dose Response

A quantitative review of the cumulative evidence on aerobic or endurance physical activity and lowered blood pressure focused on dose response and included 72 studies involving 3936 adults aged 21 to 83 years (57% were men) published through 2003 (Cornelissen and Fagard 2005b). Outcomes were evaluated for normotensive, prehypertensive, and hypertensive participants. The reviewers concluded that there was no convincing evidence of a dose response to exercise training. Exercise intensities ranging from 30% to about 85% of aerobic capacity (average 65%), lasting between 15 min and 1 h (average 40 min) and performed one to seven times (average three times) each week for at least four weeks up to 52 weeks (average 16), were equally accompanied by reduced blood pressure.

Nine randomized controlled trials of people with normal blood pressures showed no average effect of walking on SBP, but six studies showed a reduction in DBP of 1.5 mmHg from an initial level of 78 mmHg, a 2% change, regardless of whether people walked less or more than 150 min per week (Murphy et al. 2007). Another nine studies of practitioners of qigong (pronounced chi-gung), a low-intensity Chinese healing system that uses breathing techniques, gentle movement, and meditation (tai chi is a popular form), showed average reductions in SBP and DBP that were similar to those in comparison groups participating in conventional aerobic exercise (Guo et al. 2008).

A recent study extended the dose–response question to blood pressures measured outside a clinical setting. This randomized trial of 18 sedentary men and 21 sedentary women, 55 years of age or older, addressed the effects of 10 weeks of endurance training (three times a week for 1 h each time at low [about one-third of aerobic capacity] and high [about two-thirds of aerobic capacity] intensities) on blood pressure determined at the medical office and during daily living using automated measures (Cornelissen et al. 2009). As would be expected, cardiorespiratory fitness was increased more after high-intensity training. Likewise, resting DBP measured in the medical office was decreased only after high-intensity training. However, SBP was decreased after either exercise intensity. Blood pressure measured during daily activities was unchanged by exercise training.

▶ **THERE IS** no clear evidence of a dose response to exercise training for lowering blood pressure. Exercise intensities ranging between 30% and 85% of exercise capacity, lasting between 15 min and 1 h, and performed a few or several times each week for at least four weeks appear equally effective for reducing blood pressure.

Biological Plausibility

Systolic/diastolic blood pressures can be temporarily lowered by about 19/8 mmHg in hypertensive people and 9/4 mmHg in normotensive people 2 to 4 h after a single session of moderately intense (>35% of maximal heart rate) running, walking, cycling, or swimming (Kenney and Seals 1993). Whether this acute hypotensive effect of exercise explains part of the long-term effects of regular exercise on lowering blood pressure is not known. However, it is likely that some of the same mechanisms that regulate blood pressure during and after exercise are altered by long-term physical activity habits. Because the hemodynamic profiles of people diagnosed with hypertension can vary, it is important to consider whether the effects of physical activity on cardiac output and total peripheral resistance differ in the primary and secondary prevention of hypertension.

In cardiogenic, or hyperdynamic, hypertension, which is usually seen in young people with borderline hypertension, resting cardiac output can be elevated by 10% to 20% despite normal total peripheral resistance (Weir 1991). Among older adults, hypertension is more commonly accompanied by decreased cardiac output but increased total peripheral vascular resistance. The suggested mechanisms for these changes are a decrease in maximum heart rate (i.e., a chronotropic response) and vascular stiffening and changes in central nervous system regulation of blood pressure that accompany aging. There seems to be a correlation between increasing age and increasing SBP in both men and women. The same relationship is seen with DBP until ages 50 to 60. After those ages, diastolic pressure typically levels off in men and women or declines slightly in men (Fletcher and Bulpitt 1994).

African Americans typically have increased peripheral resistance, decreased cardiac output, decreased renin production, and normal or expanded plasma volume compared with white people (Pickering 1994). People who are obese tend to have a high cardiac output, expanded plasma volume, increased sympathetic nervous system activity, and normal or slightly decreased peripheral resistance (Weir 1991).

▶ **EVIDENCE INDICATES** that exercise training can decrease resting blood pressure by reducing basal cardiac output or total peripheral resistance.

Cardiac Output

Cardiac output is the product of the stroke volume of the heart and heart rate, so a reduction in cardiac output must be explained by a reduction in one or both of those factors. In people with normal blood pressure, a common adaptation after exercise training is a reduced resting heart rate but a compensatory increase in stroke volume so that cardiac output is unchanged. The increased stroke volume results mainly from increased plasma volume and venous return to the left heart. A different response to chronic exercise may result for people with hypertension. Some studies have shown no change in heart rate despite reduced blood pressure after exercise training (Krotkiewski et al. 1979). That outcome might be explained by a reduction in plasma volume, which has been observed after 10 weeks of exercise training in obese people with hypertension (Weir 1991).

Total Peripheral Resistance

Changes in total peripheral resistance (TPR) in response to acute exercise have been studied in both normotensive and hypertensive patients. Cleroux and colleagues (1992) reported that a 27% reduction in TPR and a 20% reduction in plasma norepinephrine accompanied postexercise hypotension in people with mild hypertension who exercised for 30 min at an intensity of 50% $\dot{V}O_2max$. The effect continued for up to 90 min after cessation of exercise, despite a 30% increase in cardiac output after exercise. A common finding in a number of studies is a reduction in plasma norepinephrine levels, suggesting reduced sympathetic nervous system activity with exercise training (Arakawa 1993). This could favorably affect cardiac output as well as peripheral resistance.

Exercise and Hypertension: Plausible Mechanisms

Decreased cardiac output	Decreased total peripheral resistance
Decreased SNS nerve activity?	Decreased SNS nerve activity?
Increased cardiac **vagal tone?**	Decreased resting catecholamine levels?
Decreased resting catecholamine levels?	Increased α_2-receptors?
Decreased β_1-**receptors?**	Decreased α_1-**receptors?**
Increased α_2-**receptors?**	Decreased insulin?
Renal effects: increased sodium excretion?	Endothelial relaxers?

Randomized controlled trials that showed an average reduction in blood pressure after aerobic endurance training have also reported concurrent reductions in systemic vascular resistance (7%), plasma noradrenaline (29%), and plasma renin activity (20%). Thus, aerobic endurance training appears to decrease blood pressure by lowering systemic vascular resistance associated with less activation of the sympathetic nervous system and the renin–angiotensin system. Decreases in body fatness and insulin resistance seen in those studies may also have contributed indirectly to lowered vascular resistance (Cornelissen and Fagard 2005b).

In a recent randomized controlled trial, a 25% energy deficit in overweight adults achieved by diet alone or by equal contributions of diet (12.5% decrease in intake) and exercise (12.5% increase in expenditure) led to similar losses of total and intra-abdominal fat mass and SBP in each group (Larson-Meyer et al. 2010). However, only people in the diet and exercise group had a reduction in DBP and low-density lipoprotein (LDL) cholesterol and improved insulin sensitivity.

One study showed that people with hypertension had about 30% lower levels of taurine than did normotensive peers (Arakawa 1993). Taurine is an amino acid that has antihypertensive properties and is found in high concentrations in the myocardium, brain, and skeletal muscle. Exercise training three times a week for 10 weeks at an intensity of 40% to 60% $\dot{V}O_2$max increased serum taurine concentrations by 26% in Japanese men and women with hypertension, with accompanying reductions in plasma levels of norepinephrine and blood pressure (Tanabe et al. 1989).

Insulin

Insulin resistance and hyperinsulinemia have also been implicated in the development of hypertension. People with hypertension are commonly insulin resistant, hyperinsulinemic, and hyperglycemic, whether the hypertension is treated or not. There seems to be a direct relationship between plasma insulin concentration and blood pressure, and hyperinsulinemia has been shown to precede development of hypertension (Reaven 1988). It appears that blood pressure can be regulated by changes in insulin metabolism, thus explaining why weight loss, which enhances insulin sensitivity and decreases plasma insulin levels, can decrease blood pressure in those with hypertension (Gilders, Voner, and Dudley 1989). Also, blood pressure was decreased in obese patients after exercise training without any change in weight, but only in those who were hyperinsulinemic before training (Kiyonaga et al. 1985). The mechanism explaining the relationship between hyperinsulinemia and blood pressure may be related to increased sympathetic nervous system activity in obese as well as nonobese people or to promotion of sodium reabsorption by the renal tubes that leads to increased plasma volume (Reaven 1995). It is possible that one mechanism of preventing hypertension with exercise is preventing obesity, as obesity is related to insulin resistance and has been shown

to be an independent direct risk factor for cardiovascular disease and primary hypertension.

Postexercise Hypotension

Postexercise hypotension (PEH) is a prolonged decrease in resting blood pressure in the minutes and hours following acute exercise. Reduced cardiac output (particularly decreased stroke volume of the heart in people who have hypertension) and decreased resistance to blood flow in small arterioles in the muscles that were exercised can each explain PEH, but specific explanations for those likely causes are as yet unknown (MacDonald 2002). Postexercise hypotension varies widely among people with normal blood pressure, but it is common among people who are prehypertensive or hypertensive.

During endurance exercise like cycling or running, increased cardiac output and constriction of vessels supplying organs that are not involved in exercise lead to increases in SBP that can exceed 200 mmHg. At the same time, dilation of vessels supplying the contracting muscles dilate, usually leading to no change in DBP from resting levels or a small decrease. In contrast, during resistance exercise (e.g., weightlifting or isometric maneuvers), SBP can rise to 300 to 500 mmHg and DBP can increase to 200 to 350 mmHg because of additional mechanical compression on vessels to the contracting muscles involved in the exercise but also increased chest pressures during breath holding. Unlike what occurs during endurance exercise, increases in blood pressure during resistance exercise rise and fall with the rhythm of the resistance.

When a session of either endurance or resistance exercise ends, blood pressures usually fall to levels that are lower than they were just prior to the beginning of the exercise, partly because of reduced peripheral resistance to blood flow and pooling of blood in the dilated vessels in the muscles that were exercised and, among people who have hypertension, because of lowered stroke volume and cardiac output. Those drops in pressure often are returned to normal within 10 min or so, but they can last for an hour or more, especially when the exercise is intense (especially heavy resistance exercise). Postexercise hypotension has not as yet been explained, but it may contribute to the overall, cumulative reductions in blood pressures that are seen in exercise training programs, either by eliciting more longer-lasting changes in systems that regulate blood pressure or simply by adding more periods of reduced pressures during the day—if that can be shown to happen during periods of increased physical activity that naturally occur during the day in physically active people (MacDonald 2002).

In one study, ambulatory blood pressures were recorded for 12 h after the accumulation of lifestyle physical activity during a day at home (brisk walking, lawn mowing, and gardening) in eight people who had normal blood pressure, 10 who were prehypertensive, and 10 who had mild, stage 1 hypertension (Padilla, Wallace, and Park 2005). There were no effects of daily physical activity on DBP. However, figure 7.9 shows that drops in SBP across 6-8 h after the

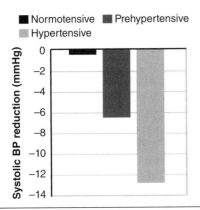

Figure 7.9 Postexercise hypotension in people with prehypertension or mild hypertension.

Data from Padilla, Wallace, and Park 2005.

Prescription of Physical Activity for People With Hypertension

Frequency: On most, preferably all, days of the week

Intensity: Moderate intensity (40-60% of aerobic capacity reserve)

Time: 30 min of continuous or accumulated physical activity per day

Type: Primarily endurance physical activity supplemented by resistance exercise

Source: The American College of Sports Medicine. 2004

cessation of physical activity were about 7 ± 2 mmHg in people with prehypertension and 13 ± 4 mmHg in people with hypertension. Those drops were unrelated to the estimated total energy cost of the physical activity. However, other evidence suggests that the accumulation of several shorter sessions of physical activity is more effective for eliciting postexercise hypotension during the day than is a single, long session. In one study, SBP and DBP were lowered for 10 to 11 h after four 10-min walks at an intensity of 50% of aerobic capacity, each separated by about an hour, but both pressures were lowered for 7 h after a single 40-min walk at the same intensity (Park, Rink, and Wallace 2006).

Stress Reactivity

Several prospective studies have shown that exaggerated blood pressure responses during the cold pressor test (i.e., submersion of the hand or foot in ice water) predicts the development of hypertension, but others have not (e.g., Carroll et al. 1996; Kasagi 1994; Menkes et al. 1989). Those studies did not control for cardiorespiratory fitness, which is inversely related to the risk of future hypertension (Blair et al. 1984). Several studies have shown that cardiorespiratory fitness level mitigates the increases in SBP (Dishman, Jackson, and Nakamura 2002; Dishman et al. 2003; Jackson and Dishman 2002) during the cold pressor test among women, but not men, and suggest that fitness is associated with altered vascular responses (Jackson and Dishman 2002) or either blunted sympathetic, or augmented parasympathetic, nervous system responses during some types of stress. In general, though, aerobic endurance training has not altered blood pressure responses during mental stress tests (Jackson and Dishman 2006), even though postexercise hypotension after a single session of moderately intense aerobic exercise extends to a blunted blood pressure response to those types of tests (Hamer, Taylor, and Steptoe 2006).

Though there are several potential mechanisms whereby exercise might help reduce or prevent high blood pressure, it is not yet clear which of those mechanisms are most reliably affected by physical activity or whether the same mechanisms that reduce blood pressure in hypertensive people also prevent hypertension in people with normal blood pressure.

▷ **TEN OF** 15 randomized controlled trials found reductions of 3 to 5 mmHg in blood pressure responses to mental stress after at least 30 min of moderately intense exercise (50% of aerobic capacity or higher) (Hamer, Taylor, and Steptoe 2006).

Summary of the Evidence

Longitudinal and cross-sectional studies have demonstrated the protective effects of exercise training and physical fitness on the primary and secondary prevention of hypertension. Those effects are independent of age and body mass. However, diet was not well controlled in many studies, mainly because of the impracticality of measuring diet in population studies that last many years. Also, population studies have not provided enough evidence to allow conclusions about whether there is a dose–response relationship between physical activity and primary prevention of hypertension. Often, only one level of physical fitness or physical activity was reported.

Clinical studies of treatment of mild hypertension have suggested that there is no relation between intensity of exercise, expressed as a percentage of $\dot{V}O_2$max, and reduced blood pressure after exercise training. On balance, it appears that regular physical activity of moderate intensity offers some protection against primary hypertension (American College of Sports Medicine 2004). This type of exercise training should be considered one of the nonpharmacologic methods for prevention and treatment of hypertension.

▷ **WHEN JUDGED** by the criteria of Mill's canons, the evidence is moderately strong that leisure-time physical activity is independently associated with reduced risk of developing hypertension and is effective in reducing blood pressure among adults who have mild hypertension.

Summary

On balance, observational epidemiologic studies and randomized controlled trials in clinical settings have shown that regular physical activity has potential for reducing or preventing mild hypertension. Clinical studies have the advantage of experimental control, but it is difficult to separate the independent effects of physical activity from those of dietary and weight changes in many studies, especially as hypertension, dyslipidemia, and obesity are intricately related to each other. Also, it is virtually impossible to prevent fat loss during increased physical activity without increasing caloric intake, which can influence hypertension and dyslipidemia if micronutrients also change with the altered food intake. Nonetheless, many studies have indicated that much of the benefit of moderate physical activity appears sufficiently independent of weight change and other risk factors for hypertension, consistent across types of people, temporally logical, and biologically plausible to support the current public health position that physical activity represents an effective adjuvant in the prevention and treatment of hypertension. At present, evidence does not support a linear dose–response gradient for typical middle-aged or older adults who have been sedentary and embark on a new physical activity program. Some emerging evidence suggests that a dose response may exist among recreational runners who perform at a level substantially above that likely to be a feasible goal for people who currently are sedentary, who constitute a large part of the population of the United States and other countries. Randomized controlled trials of either resistance or aerobic exercise training among people diagnosed with stage 1 hypertension show an average reduction in resting systolic blood pressure of about 6-7 mmHg for systolic blood pressure and 5-6 mmHg for diastolic blood pressure (Cornelissen and Fagard 2005a, 2005b). Reductions of this magnitude are potentially important for public health, as population-based evidence in the United States has led to an estimate that a 5 mmHg reduction of SBP would be accompanied by a 14% reduction in the population risk of stroke mortality, a 9% reduction in CHD mortality, and a 7% reduction in all-cause mortality (Whelton et al. 2002).

· BIBLIOGRAPHY ·

Ainsworth, B.E., N.L. Keenan, D.S. Strogatz, J.M. Garrett, and S.A. James. 1991. Physical activity and hypertension in black adults: The Pitt County study. *American Journal of Public Health* 81: 1477-1479.

American College of Sports Medicine. 2004. American College of Sports Medicine position stand: Exercise and hypertension. *Medicine and Science in Sports and Exercise* 36: 533-553.

American Heart Association. 2002. *Heart and stroke statistical update.* Dallas: American Heart Association.

American Heart Association. 2012. Heart disease and stroke statistics - 2012 update: A report from the American Heart Association. *Circulation* 125 (1): e2-e220.

Anastos, K., P. Charney, R.A. Charon, E. Cohen, C.Y. Jones, C. Marte, D.M. Swiderski, M.E. Wheat, and S. Williams. 1991. Hypertension in women: What is really known? The Women's Caucus, Working Group on Women's Health of the Society of General Internal Medicine. *Annals of Internal Medicine* 115 (4): 287-293.

Andersen, U.O., and G. Jensen. 2007. Decreasing population blood pressure is not mediated by changes in habitual physical activity. Results from 15 years of follow-up. *Blood Pressure* 16 (1): 28-35.

Arakawa, K. 1993. Antihypertensive mechanisms of exercise. *Journal of Hypertension* 11: 223-229.

Barengo, N.C., G. Hu, M. Kastarinen, T.A. Lakka, H. Pekkarinen, A. Nissinen, and J. Tuomilehto. 2005. Low physical activity as a predictor for antihypertensive drug treatment in 25-64-year-old populations in eastern and south-western Finland. *Journal of Hypertension* 23 (2): 293-299.

Barengo, N.C., M. Kastarinen, T. Lakka, A. Nissinen, and J. Tuomilehto. 2006. Different forms of physical activity and cardiovascular risk factors among 24-64-year-old men and women in Finland. *European Journal of Cardiovascular Prevention and Rehabilitation* 13 (February): 51-59.

Blair, S.N., N.N. Goodyear, L.W. Gibbons, and K.H. Cooper. 1984. Physical fitness and incidence of hypertension in healthy normotensive men and women. *Journal of the American Medical Association* 252: 487-490.

Blumenthal, J.A., W.C. Siegel, and M. Appelbaum. 1991. Failure of exercise to reduce blood pressure in patients with mild hypertension: Results of a randomized controlled trial. *Journal of the American Medical Association* 266 (15): 2098-2104.

Boreham, C., J. Twisk, W. van Mechelen, M. Savage, J. Strain, and G. Cran. 1999. Relationships between the development of biological risk factors for coronary heart disease and lifestyle parameters during adolescence: The Northern Ireland Young Hearts Project. *Public Health* 113: 7-12.

Burt, V.L., J.A. Cutler, M. Higgins, M.J. Horan, D. Labarthe, P. Whelton, C. Brown, and E.J. Roccella. 1995. Trends in the prevalence, awareness, treatment, and control of hypertension in the adult US population. Data from the health examination surveys, 1960 to 1991. *Hypertension* 26: 60-69.

Burt, V.L., P. Whelton, E.J. Roccella, C. Brown, J.A. Cutler, M. Higgins, M.J. Horan, and D. Labarthe. 1995. Prevalence of hypertension in the US adult population. Results from the Third National Health and Nutrition Examination Survey, 1988-1991. *Hypertension* 25: 305-313.

Carlson, N. 1994. *Physiology and behavior.* 5th edition. Boston: Allyn & Bacon.

Carroll, D., G.D. Smith, D. Sheffield, G. Willemsen, P.M. Sweetnam, J.E. Gallacher, and P.C. Elwood. 1996. Blood pressure reactions to the cold pressor test and the prediction of future blood pressure status: Data from the Caerphilly study. *Journal of Human Hypertension* 10: 777-780.

Chase, N.L., X. Sui, D.C. Lee, and S.N. Blair. 2009. The association of cardiorespiratory fitness and physical activity with incidence of hypertension in men. *American Journal of Hypertension* 22: 417-424.

Chen, J., S. Das, C.E. Barlow, S. Grundy, and S.G. Lakoski. 2010. Fitness, fatness, and systolic blood pressure: Data from the Cooper Center Longitudinal Study. *American Heart Journal* 160 (1, July): 166-170.

Cleroux, J., N. Kouame, A. Nadeau, D. Coulombe, and Y. Lacourciere. 1992. Aftereffects of exercise on regional and systemic hemodynamics in hypertension. *Hypertension* 19: 183-191.

Cornelissen, V.A., J. Arnout, P. Holvoet, and R.H. Fagard. 2009. Influence of exercise at lower and higher intensity on blood pressure and cardiovascular risk factors at older age. *Journal of Hypertension* 27: 753-762.

Cornelissen, V.A., and R.H. Fagard. 2005a. Effect of resistance training on resting blood pressure: A meta-analysis of randomized controlled trials. *Journal of Hypertension* 23: 251-259.

Cornelissen, V.A., and R.H. Fagard. 2005b. Effects of endurance training on blood pressure, blood pressure-regulating mechanisms, and cardiovascular risk factors. *Hypertension* 46: 667-675.

Dahlöf, B., P.S. Sever, N.R. Poulter, H. Wedel, D.G. Beevers, M. Caulfield, R. Collins, S.E. Kjeldsen, A. Kristinsson, G.T. McInnes, J. Mehlsen, M. Nieminen, E. O'Brien, J. Ostergren; ASCOT investigators. 2005. Prevention of cardiovascular events with an antihypertensive regimen of amlodipine adding perindopril as required versus atenolol adding bendroflumethiazide as required, in the Anglo-Scandinavian Cardiac Outcomes Trial-Blood Pressure Lowering Arm (ASCOT-BPLA): A multicentre randomised controlled trial. *Lancet* 366: 895-906.

Delaney, J.A., R.L. McClelland, C.D. Furberg, R. Cooper, S. Shea, G. Burke, and B.M. Psaty. 2009. Time trends in the use of anti-hypertensive medications: Results from the Multi-Ethnic Study of Atherosclerosis. *Pharmacoepidemiology and Drug Safety* 18: 826-832.

Dickinson, H.O., J.M. Mason, D.J. Nicolson, F. Campbell, F.R. Beyer, J.V. Cook, B. Williams, and G.A. Ford. 2006. Lifestyle interventions to reduce raised blood pressure: A systematic review of randomized controlled trials. *Journal of Hypertension* 24: 215-233.

Dishman, R.K., E.M. Jackson, and Y. Nakamura. 2002. Influence of fitness and gender on blood pressure responses during active or passive stress. *Psychophysiology* 39: 568-576.

Dishman, R.K., Y. Nakamura, E.M. Jackson, and C.A. Ray. 2003. Blood pressure and muscle sympathetic nerve activity during cold pressor stress: Fitness and gender. *Psychophysiology* 40: 370-380.

Dwivedi, G., and S. Dwivedi. 2007. Sushruta – the clinician-teacher par excellence. *Indian Journal of Chest Diseases and Allied Sciences* 49: 243-244.

Einhorn, P.T., B.R. Davis, J.T. Wright Jr., M. Rahman, P.K. Whelton, S.L. Pressel; ALLHAT Cooperative Research Group. 2010. ALLHAT: Still providing correct answers after 7 years. *Current Opinion in Cardiology* 25: 355-365.

Evenson, K.R., J. Stevens, R. Thomas, and J. Cai. 2004. Effect of cardiorespiratory fitness on mortality among hypertensive and normotensive women and men. *Epidemiology* (5, September 15): 565-572.

Fagard, R.H. 2001. Exercise characteristics and the blood pressure response to dynamic physical training. *Medicine and Science in Sports and Exercise* 33 (Suppl. 6): S484-S492.

Fagard, R.H. 2006. Exercise is good for your blood pressure: Effects of endurance training and resistance training. *Clinical and Experimental Pharmacology and Physiology* 33: 853-856.

Fagard, R.H., and V.A. Cornelissen. 2007. Effect of exercise on blood pressure control in hypertensive patients. *European Journal of Cardiovascular Prevention and Rehabilitation* 14 (1, February): 12-17.

Fletcher, A., and C. Bulpitt. 1994. Epidemiology of hypertension in the elderly. *Journal of Hypertension* 12 (Suppl. 6): S3-S5.

Folsom, A.R., R.J. Prineas, S.A. Kaye, and R.G. Munger. 1990. Incidence of hypertension and stroke in relation to body fat distribution and other risk factors in older women. *Stroke* 21 (5): 701-706.

Furberg, C.D., J.T. Wright Jr., B.R. Davis, J.A. Cutler, M. Alderman, H. Black, W. Cushman, R. Grimm, L.J. Haywood, F. Leenen, et al. 2002. Major outcomes in high-risk hypertensive patients randomized to angiotensin-converting enzyme inhibitor or calcium channel blocker vs diuretic: The Antihypertensive and Lipid-Lowering Treatment to Prevent Heart Attack Trial (ALLHAT). *Journal of the American Medical Association* 288: 2981-2997.

Gidding, S.S., B.A. Barton, J.A. Dorgan, S.Y. Kimm, P.O. Kwiterovich, N.L. Lasser, A.M. Robson, V.J. Stevens, L. Van Horn, and D.G. Simons-Morton. 2006. Higher self-reported physical activity is associated with lower systolic blood pressure: The Dietary Intervention Study in Childhood (DISC). *Pediatrics* 118 (6, December): 2388-2393.

Gilbertson, D.T., J. Liu, J.L. Xue, T.A. Louis, C.A. Solid, J.P. Ebben, and A.J.Collins. 2005. Projecting the number of patients with end-stage renal disease in the United States to the year 2015. *Journal of the Amercian Society of Nephrology* 16: 3736-3741.

Gilders, R.M., C. Voner, and G.A. Dudley. 1989. Endurance training and blood pressure in normotensive and hypertensive adults. *Medicine and Science in Sports and Exercise* 21: 629-636.

Gordon, N.F., C.B. Scott, W.J. Wilkinson, J.J. Duncan, and S.N. Blair. 1990. Exercise and mild essential hypertension: Recommendations for adults. *Sports Medicine* 10 (6): 390-404.

Gordon-Larsen, P., J. Boone-Heinonen, S. Sidney, B. Sternfeld, D.R. Jacobs Jr., and C.E. Lewis. 2009. Active commuting and cardiovascular disease risk: The CARDIA study. *Archives of Internal Medicine* 169: 1216-1223.

Gruner, C.O., trans. 1930. *A treatise on The Canon of Medicine of Avicenna,* pp. 283-322. London: Luzac & Co.

Guo, X., B. Zhou, T. Nishimura, S. Teramukai, and M. Fukushima. 2008. Clinical effect of qigong practice on essential hypertension: A meta-analysis of randomized controlled trials. *Journal of Alternative and Complementary Medicine* 14 (1, January-February): 27-37.

Haffner, S.M., E. Ferrannini, H.P. Hazuda, and M.P. Stern. 1992. Clustering of cardiovascular risk factors in confirmed prehypertensive individuals. *Hypertension* 20: 38-45.

Hagberg, J.M. 1990. Exercise, fitness, and hypertension. In *Exercise, fitness, and health: A consensus of current knowledge,* edited by C. Bouchard, R.J. Shephard, T. Stephens, J.R. Sutton, and B.D. McPherson, pp. 455-466. Champaign, IL: Human Kinetics.

Hajar, R. 1999. The Greco-Islamic pulse. *Heart Views* 1 (4): 136-140.

Hajjar, I., and T.A. Kotchen. 2003. Trends in prevalence, awareness, treatment, and control of hypertension in the United States, 1988-2000. *Journal of the American Medical Association* 290: 199-206.

Hamer, M., A. Taylor, and A. Steptoe. 2006. The effect of acute aerobic exercise on stress related blood pressure responses: A systematic review and meta-analysis. *Biological Psychology* 71 (2): 183-190. [Epub, June 23, 2005]

Harris, S.S., C.J. Caspersen, G.H. DeFriese, and E.H. Estes Jr. 1989. Physical activity counseling for healthy adults as a primary preventive intervention in the clinical setting: Report for the U.S. Preventive Services Task Force. *Journal of the American Medical Association* 261: 3588-3598.

Hu, G., N.C. Barengo, J. Tuomilehto, T.A. Lakka, A. Nissinen, and P. Jousilahti. 2004. Relationship of physical activity and body mass index to the risk of hypertension: A prospective study in Finland. *Hypertension* 43 (1): 25-30.

Hubert, H.B., M. Feinleib, P.M. McNamara, and W.P. Castelli. 1983. Obesity as an independent risk factor for cardiovascular disease: A 26 year follow-up of participants in the Framingham Heart Study. *Circulation* 67: 968-977.

Jackson, E.M., and R.K. Dishman. 2002. Hemodynamic responses to stress among black women: Fitness and parental hypertension. *Medicine and Science in Sports and Exercise* 34: 1097-1104.

Jackson, E.M., and R.K. Dishman. 2006. Cardiorespiratory fitness and laboratory stress: A meta-regression analysis. *Psychophysiology* 43: 57-72.

Janz, K.F., J.D. Dawson, and L.T. Mahoney. 2002. Increases in physical fitness during childhood improve cardiovascular health during adolescence: The Muscatine Study. *International Journal of Sports Medicine* 23 (Suppl. 1): S15-S21.

Joint National Committee on Prevention, Detection, Evaluation, and Treatment of High Blood Pressure. 2003. *The seventh report of the Joint National Committee on Prevention, Detection, Evaluation, and Treatment of High Blood Pressure.* U.S. Department of Health and Human Services. NIH Publication No. 03-5233. Bethesda, MD: NHLBI.

Kannel, W.B., R.J. Garrison, and A.L. Dannenberg. 1993. Secular blood pressure trends in normotensive persons: The Framingham study. *American Heart Journal* 125: 1154-1158.

Kasagi, F. 1994. Prognostic value of the cold pressor test for hypertension based on 28-year follow-up. *Hiroshima Journal of Medical Sciences* 43 (3): 93-103.

Kelley, G.A. 1999. Aerobic exercise and resting blood pressure among women: A meta-analysis. *Preventive Medicine* 28 (3): 264-275.

Kelley, G.A., and K.S. Kelley. 2010. Isometric handgrip exercise and resting blood pressure: A meta-analysis of randomized controlled trials. *Journal of Hypertension* 28 (3): 411-418.

Kelley, G.A., K.S. Kelley, and Z.V. Tran. 2003. The effects of exercise on resting blood pressure in children and adolescents: A meta-analysis of randomized controlled trials. *Preventive Cardiology* 6: 8-16.

Kelley, G.A., and K. Sharpe Kelley. 2001. Aerobic exercise and resting blood pressure in older adults: A meta-analytic review of randomized controlled trials. *Journals of Gerontology Series A: Biological Sciences and Medical Sciences* 56 (5): M298-303.

Kenney, M.J., and D.R. Seals. 1993. Postexercise hypotension: Key features, mechanisms, and clinical significance. *Hypertension* 22 (5): 653-664.

Kiyonaga, A., K. Arakawa, H. Tanaka, and M. Shindo. 1985. Blood pressure and humoral response to aerobic exercise. *Hypertension* 7: 125-131.

Kokkinos, P.F., P. Narayan, J.A. Colleran, A. Pittaras, A. Notargiacomo, D. Reda, and V. Papademetriou. 1995. Effects of regular exercise on blood pressure and left ventricular hypertrophy in African-American men with severe hypertension. *New England Journal of Medicine* 333 (22): 1462-1467.

Kollias, A., P. Antonodimitrakis, E. Grammatikos, N. Chatziantonakis, E.E. Grammatikos, and G.S. Stergiou. 2009. Trends in high blood pressure prevalence in Greek adolescents. *Journal of Human Hypertension* 23 (6): 385-390.

Krotkiewski, M., K. Mandroukas, L. Sjostrom, L. Sullivan, H. Wetterqvist, and P. Bjorntorp. 1979. Effects of long-term physical training on body fat, metabolism, and blood pressure in obesity. *Metabolism* 28: 650-658.

Larson-Meyer, D.E., L. Redman, L.K. Heilbronn, C.K. Martin, and E. Ravussin. 2010. Caloric restriction with or without exercise: The fitness versus fatness debate. *Medicine and Science in Sports and Exercise* 42: 152-159.

Lee, D.C., X. Sui, and S.N. Blair. 2009. Does physical activity ameliorate the health hazards of obesity? *British Journal of Sports Medicine* 43: 49-51.

Lewington, S., R. Clarke, N. Qizilbash, R. Peto, and R. Collins; Prospective Studies Collaboration. 2002. Age-specific relevance of usual blood pressure to vascular mortality: A meta-analysis of individual data for one million adults in 61 prospective studies. *Lancet* 360: 1903-1913.

Lindholm, L.H., B. Carlberg, and O. Samuelsson. 2005. Should beta blockers remain first choice in the treatment of primary hypertension? A meta-analysis. *Lancet* 366 (9496, October 29-November 4): 1545-1553.

Lloyd-Jones, D., R.J. Adams, T.M. Brown, et al. 2010. Heart disease and stroke statistics—2010 update. A report from the American Heart Association Statistics Committee and Stroke Statistics Subcommittee. *Circulation* 121: e1-e170.

Lyons, S.A., and R.J. Petrucelli. 1987. *Medicine: An illustrated history.* New York: Abradale Press.

MacDonald, J.R. 2002. Potential causes, mechanisms, and implications of post exercise hypotension. *Journal of Human Hypertension* 16: 225-236.

Melby, C.L., D.G. Goldflies, and G.C. Hyner. 1991. Blood pressure and anthropometric differences in regularly exercising and non-exercising black adults. *Clinical and Experimental Hypertension* A13: 1233-1248.

Menkes, M.S., K.A. Matthews, D.S. Krantz, U. Lundberg, L.A. Mead, B. Qaqish, K. Liang, C.B. Thomas, and T.A. Pearson. 1989. Cardiovascular reactivity to the cold pressor test as a predictor of hypertension. *Hypertension* 14: 524-530.

Moser, M. 1997. Evolution of the treatment of hypertension from the 1940s to JNC V. *American Journal of Hypertension* 10: 2S-8S.

Murphy, M.H., A.M. Nevill, E.M. Murtagh, and R.L. Holder. 2007. The effect of walking on fitness, fatness and resting blood pressure: A meta-analysis of randomised, controlled trials. *Preventive Medicine* 44: 377-385.

Nakanishi, N., and K. Suzuki. 2005. Daily life activity and the risk of developing hypertension in middle-aged Japanese men. *Archives of Internal Medicine* 165 (2, January 24): 214-220.

Naqvi, N.H., and M.D. Blaufox. 1998. *Blood pressure measurement: An illustrated history*, pp. 9-27. London: Parthenon Publishing Group.

National Center for Health Statistics. 1995. *National Ambulatory Medical Care Survey summaries: 1995. Advance data from vital health statistics*. Publication No. 286. Hyattsville, MD: National Center for Health Statistics.

National Center for Health Statistics. 1997. *Health: United States, 1996*. Hyattsville, MD: U.S. Public Health Service.

National Center for Health Statistics. 2008. *Health, United States, 2008*. Hyattsville, MD: National Center for Health Statistics.

Nelson, C.R., and D.A. Knapp. 2000. Trends in antihypertensive drug therapy of ambulatory patients by US office-based physicians. *Hypertension* 36: 600-603.

Opie, L.H. 2009. Hypertension, the changing pattern of drug usage. *Cardiovascular Journal of Africa* 20: 52-56.

Ostchega, Y., S.S. Yoon, J. Hughes, and T. Louis. 2008. *Hypertension awareness, treatment, and control—continued disparities in adults: United States, 2005-2006*. NCHS Data Brief No. 3. Hyattsville, MD: National Center for Health Statistics.

Padilla, J., J.P. Wallace, and S. Park. 2005. Accumulation of physical activity reduces blood pressure in pre- and hypertension. *Medicine and Science in Sports and Exercise* 37: 1264-1275.

Paffenbarger, R.S. Jr. 1982. Energy imbalance and hypertension risk. In *Diet and exercise: Synergisms in health maintenance*, edited by P.L. White and T. Mondeika, pp. 115-125. Chicago: American Medical Association.

Paffenbarger, R.S. Jr., D.L. Jung, R.W. Leung, and R.T. Hyde. 1991. Physical activity and hypertension: An epidemiological view. *Annals of Medicine* 23: 319-327.

Paffenbarger, R.S. Jr., and I.M. Lee. 1997. Intensity of physical activity related to incidence of hypertension and all-cause mortality: An epidemiological view. *Blood Pressure Monitoring* 2 (3): 115-123.

Paffenbarger, R.S. Jr., M.C. Thorne, and A.L. Wing. 1968. Chronic disease in former college students: VIII. Characteristics in youth predisposing to hypertension in later years. *American Journal of Epidemiology* 88: 25-32.

Paffenbarger, R.S., A.L. Wing, R.T. Hyde, and D.L. Jung. 1983. Physical activity and incidence of hypertension in college alumni. *American Journal of Epidemiology* 117: 245-257.

Park, S., L.D. Rink, and J.P. Wallace. 2006. Accumulation of physical activity leads to a greater blood pressure reduction than a single continuous session, in prehypertension. *Journal of Hypertension* 24 (9): 1761-1770.

Pickering, T.G. 1994. Hypertension in blacks. *Current Opinion in Nephrology and Hypertension* 3: 207-212.

Rankinen, T., T.S. Church, T. Rice, C. Bouchard, and S.N. Blair. 2007. Cardiorespiratory fitness, BMI, and risk of hypertension: The HYPGENE study. *Medicine and Science in Sports and Exercise* 39: 1687-1692.

Reaven, G.M. 1988. Role of insulin resistance in human disease. *Diabetes* 37: 1595-1607.

Reaven, G.M. 1995. Are insulin resistance and/or compensatory hyperinsulinemia involved in the etiology and clinical course of patients with hypertension? *International Journal of Obesity* 19 (Suppl. 1): S2-S5.

Reaven, P.D., E. Barrett-Conner, and S. Edelstein. 1991. Relation between leisure-time physical activity and blood pressure in older women. *Circulation* 83: 559-565.

Rosenthal, M., W.L. Haskell, R. Solomon, A. Widstrom, and G.M. Reaven. 1983. Demonstration of a relationship between level of physical training and insulin stimulated glucose utilization in normal humans. *Diabetes* 32: 408-411.

Rosner, B., N. Cook, R. Portman, S. Daniels, and B. Falkner. 2009. Blood pressure differences by ethnic group among United States children and adolescents. *Hypertension* 54: 502-508.

Ruskin, A. 1956. *Classics in arterial hypertension*. Springfield, IL: Charles C Thomas.

Shea, S., C.E. Basch, B. Gutin, A.D. Stein, I.R. Contento, M. Irigoyen, and P. Zybert. 1994. The rate of increase in blood pressure in children 5 years of age is related to changes in aerobic fitness and body mass index. *Pediatrics* 94: 465-470.

Stamler, R., J. Stamler, F.C. Gosch, J. Civinelli, J. Fishman, P. McKeever, A. McDonald, and A.R. Dyer. 1989. Primary prevention of hypertension by nutritional hygienic means: Final report of a randomized clinical trial. *Journal of the American Medical Association* 262: 1801-1807.

Stamler, J., R. Stamler, and J.D. Neaton. 1993. Blood pressure, systolic and diastolic, and cardiovascular risks: U.S. population data. *Archives of Internal Medicine* 153: 598-615.

Strasser, B., U. Siebert, and W. Schobersberger. 2010. Resistance training in the treatment of the metabolic syndrome: A systematic review and meta-analysis of the effect of resistance training on metabolic clustering in patients with abnormal glucose metabolism. *Sports Medicine* 40: 397-415.

Tanabe, Y., H. Urata, A. Kiyonaga, M. Ikeda, H. Tanaka, M. Shindo, and K. Arakawa. 1989. Changes in serum concentrations of taurine and other amino acids in clinical antihypertensive exercise therapy. *Clinical and Experimental Hypertension* A11: 149-165.

Taylor, R.S., A. Brown, S. Ebrahim, J. Jolliffe, H. Noorani, K. Rees, B. Skidmore, J.A. Stone, D.R. Thompson, and N. Oldridge. 2004. Exercise-based rehabilitation for patients with coronary heart disease: Systematic review and meta-analysis of randomized controlled trials. *American Journal of Medicine* 116 (10, May 15): 682-692.

Unwin, N., P. James, D. McLarty, H. Machybia, P. Nkulila, B. Tamin, M. Nguluma, and R. McNally. 2010. Rural to urban migration and changes in cardiovascular risk factors in Tanzania: A prospective cohort study. *BMC Public Health* 10 (May 24): 272.

Wain, H. 1970. *A history of medicine.* Springfield, IL: Charles C Thomas.

Weir, M.R. 1991. Impact of age, race, and obesity on hypertensive mechanisms and therapy. *American Journal of Medicine* 90 (Suppl. 5A): 3S-14S.

Weiss, R., K. Buckley, and T. Clifford. 2006. Changing patterns of initial drug therapy for the treatment of hypertension in a Medicaid population, 2001-2005. *Journal of Clinical Hypertension* 8: 706-712.

Whelton, P.K., J. He, L.J. Appel, J.A. Cutler, S. Havas, T.A. Kotchen, E.J. Roccella, R. Stout, C. Vallbona, M.C. Winston, and J. Karimbakas. 2002. Primary prevention of hypertension: Clinical and public health advisory from the National High Blood Pressure Education Program. *Journal of the American Medical Association* 288: 1882-1888.

Wolz, M., J. Cutler, E.J. Roccella, F. Rohde, T. Thom, and V. Burt. 2000. Statement from the National High Blood Pressure Education Program: Prevalence of hypertension. *American Journal of Hypertension* 13: 103-104.

CHAPTER 8

Physical Activity
and Dyslipidemia

Their heart is as fat as grease.

· *The Holy Bible* ·
Psalms 119:70

CHAPTER OBJECTIVES

▸ Describe the public health burden of dyslipidemia, including its prevalence in population groups and its role in the risk of cardiovascular diseases

▸ Identify and describe the function of key lipoproteins

▸ Identify the major modifiable and nonmodifiable risk factors of dyslipidemia

▸ Describe the known and hypothesized effects of physical activity on lipoproteins and their functions

▸ Describe and evaluate the strength of evidence that physical activity and exercise training improve lipoprotein levels and function

Cholesterol is a waxy substance found in all cell membranes, including those in the brain, nerves, muscle, skin, liver, intestines, and heart. Cholesterol is needed to produce many hormones, vitamin D, and the bile acids that help emulsify insoluble lipids (e.g., from eating food high in saturated fats) so they can be used for cellular metabolism. Because it is insoluble in blood, cholesterol also transports vitamin A and E, which too are insoluble. Too much cholesterol in the blood contributes to atherosclerosis, the disease process that hardens and blocks arteries and leads to coronary heart disease (CHD) and ischemic stroke. **Hyper-cholesterolemia** commonly refers to levels of total serum cholesterol that exceed the population average of 200 mg/dl among adults. Dyslipidemia refers to hypercholesterolemia or high triglycerides (a key energy store that includes fat), or both, or low levels of **high-density lipoprotein cholesterol (HDL-C,** the "good" cholesterol).

After describing dyslipidemia and its impact on public health, this chapter presents the evidence that physical activity is associated with lowered blood lipids, decreased **low-density lipoprotein cholesterol (LDL-C,** the "bad" cholesterol), and increased HDL-C—changes that can help explain part of the protective effect that physical activity confers against cardiovascular disease and mortality.

▷ **AN ESTIMATED** 102.2 million American adults have total blood cholesterol levels of 200 mg/dl and higher, which is above desirable levels. Of these, 35.7 million have levels of 240 mg/dl or higher, which is considered high risk for heart disease (American Heart Association 2012).

Though hypercholesterolemia is associated with increased risk of CHD (see table 8.1), lipoprotein fractions, which transport cholesterol, are better predictors of CHD risk (see table 8.2). A low level of HDL-C (<40 mg/dl) is a major risk factor for CHD; the incidence of CHD is about 18% among people having an HDL-C level below 25 mg/dl. Average levels of HDL-C are 40 to 50 mg/dl in men and 50 to 60 mg/dl in women. General rules are a 2% change in risk for a 1% change in total cholesterol, a 2% to 3% change in risk for a 1% change in LDL-C. Epidemiological studies show that a 1 mg/dl increase in HDL-C level is associated with a reduction in coronary artery disease of 2% in men and 3% in women (Gordon et al. 1989). However, randomized controlled trials of fibrates have shown a 3% to 5% reduction in coronary deaths, as well as a 2% mortality reduction in heart patients, for each 1 mg/dl increase in HDL-C (Frick et al. 1987; Robins et al. 2001; Rubins et al. 1999). A high ratio of total serum cholesterol to HDL-C is a better predictor of increased risk than is either component alone (see table 8.3).

High levels of LDL-C (>160 mg/dl) and triglycerides (>200 mg/dl) also are associated with a high risk of CHD (figure 8.1). Generally, an LDL-C level less than 130 mg/dl is predictive of a total cholesterol of less than 200 mg/dl and is normal; LDL-C levels of 130 to 159 mg/dl are considered borderline risk; and levels greater than 160 mg/dl are predictive of a total cholesterol greater than 240 mg/dl and

Table 8.2   HDL and CHD Risk: Framingham Heart Study

HDL (mg/dl)	Relative risk	
	Men	Women
25	2.00	—
30	1.80	—
35	1.50	—
40	1.22	1.94
45	1.00	1.55
50	0.82	1.25
55	0.67	1.00
60	0.55	0.80
65	0.45	0.64
70	—	0.52
75	Protection threshold against CHD?	

Table 8.1   Total Cholesterol and CHD Risk: Framingham Heart Study

Cholesterol (mg/dl)	Relative risk
300	3.0
260	2.0
235	1.4 (average level of CHD cases)
225	1.0 (average)
220	0.95 (average level of people without CHD)
200	0.90
185	0.80
150	Likely protection threshold against CHD

Table 8.3   HDL Ratios and CHD Risk: Framingham Heart Study

RR	Total/HDL	LDL/HDL
Men		
0.50	3.43	1.00
1.00	4.97	3.55
2.00	9.55	6.35
3.00	24.00	8.00
Women		
0.50	3.27	1.47
1.00	4.44	3.22
2.00	7.05	5.00
3.00	11.04	6.14

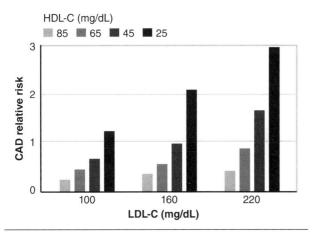

Figure 8.1 HDL cholesterol and LDL cholesterol as risk factors for coronary artery disease.

Data from Castelli 1988.

National Cholesterol Education Program Guidelines for Hypercholesterolemia

TOTAL CHOLESTEROL (MG/DL)

Optimal <200; borderline high 200-239; high ≥240

LDL-C (MG/DL)

Optimal <100; near optimal 100-129; borderline high 130-159; high 160-189; very high ≥190

TRIGLYCERIDES (MG/DL)

Normal <150; borderline high 150-199; high 200-499; very high ≥500

HDL-C (MG/DL)

Low <40; high >60
Values are based on blood levels after fasting.

Third Report of the National Cholesterol Education Program Expert Panel on Detection, Evaluation, and Treatment of High Blood Cholesterol in Adults (Adult Treatment Panel III). National Cholesterol Education Program; National Heart, Lung, and Blood Institute; National Institutes of Health. NIH Publication No. 01-3670. May 2001.

---

are regarded as high risk. Blood levels of triglycerides above 145 mg/dl elevate the risk of CHD by about 12.5%. Averaged across 17 prospective cohort studies totaling 46,413 men and 10,864 women, every 1 mmol/L (88.5 mg/dl) increase in fasting triglycerides increased risk of cardiovascular disease by 32% in men (14% adjusted for HDL-C) and 76% in women (32% adjusted for HDL-C). A 1% change in triglycerides was associated with about a 0.5% change in CHD risk in men and a 1.3% change in CHD risk in women (Hokanson and Austin 1996).

The sidebar gives guidelines for determining **hyperlipidemia** from the National Cholesterol Education Program Adult Treatment Panel III (ATP III).

Since the publication of Adult Treatment Panel III, results of several major clinical trials of drug therapy led to modifications in treatment options and goals for people who were at high risk. The current recommended LDL-C goal is <100 mg/dl; but when risk is very high, an LDL-C goal of <70 mg/dl is a clinical treatment option that also applies to patients who have LDL-C <100 mg/dl but are otherwise at very high risk (Grundy et al. 2004).

Magnitude of the Problem

Estimates from the National Health and Nutrition Examination Survey (NHANES) and the National Center for Health Statistics show that nearly 36 million U.S. adults aged 20

years or older have high CHD and stroke risk because they have total cholesterol levels of 240 mg/dl or higher. Another 66.5 million have borderline high levels between 200 and 240. Ten percent of youths 12 to 19 years of age have levels over 200 mg/dl. About 18% of white women have levels of 240 mg/dl or higher. Nearly 43% of Mexican American men have elevated risk because they have LDL-C levels of 130 mg/dl or higher. The prevalence of low HDL-C is about half as great in black men compared to white and Mexican American men, and it is 40% and 80% higher among Mexican American women than in white and black women, respectively (American Heart Association 2010).

Figure 8.2 shows the prevalence rates of high LDL-C and low HDL-C among Americans ages 20 and older by sex and selected racial and ethnic groups.

According to data from NHANES 2005-2006, between 1999-2000 and 2005-2006, mean serum total cholesterol levels in adults age 20 and older declined from 204 mg/dl to 199 mg/dl (American Heart Association 2010). That 2.5% decline in total cholesterol levels could account for a 5% to

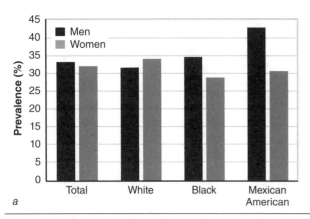
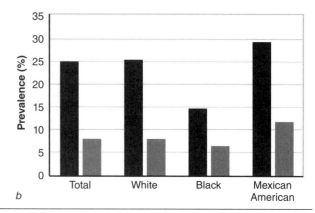

Figure 8.2   Age-adjusted prevalence of Americans age 20 and older with *(a)* LDL cholesterol of 130 mg/dl or higher and *(b)* HDL cholesterol of 40 mg/dl or lower, by race/ethnicity and sex. United States, 2006.

National Health and Nutrition Examination Survey (NHANES) 2003-2006. American Heart Association 2010.

7% reduction in the incidence of CHD (Centers for Disease Control and Prevention 2000).

What Are Lipoproteins?

Cholesterol and other fats (i.e., lipids) are not soluble, so they are carried in the blood by binding with proteins. Such lipoproteins include **chylomicrons,** LDL, very low density lipoprotein, and HDL; they differ in their relative composition of cholesterol, lipids, **phospholipids,** and proteins. They also differ in size and density such that higher concentrations of lipids are found in lipoprotein molecules that are larger and less dense (see figure 8.3 and table 8.4).

Triglyceride is the major form of biological fat; it is formed when a glycerol molecule is esterified by three fatty acid molecules. (An ester is formed via removal of water between the hydroxyl groups of an alcohol and an acid.) Dietary triglycerides make up about 98% of chylomicrons, which are formed by enterocytes in the intestines and enter

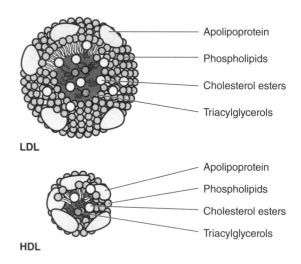

Figure 8.3   LDL and HDL molecules differ in size as well as their composition by triglycerides, phospholipids, cholesterol, and apolipoproteins.

Table 8.4   Characteristics of Lipoproteins

Characteristic	HDL	LDL	VLDL	Chylomicrons
Density (g/ml)	1.21-1.06	1.06-1.006	1.006-0.95	<0.95
Size (Å)	50-100	215-220	300-800	400-10,000
Lipid (% of total)	~50%	~75%	~90%	~98%
Triglyceride	4-10	10	50-70	85-95
Cholesterol	25-35	45-60	10-20	2-10
Phospholipid	30-50	20-30	10-20	4-12
Major apoprotein	A1, A2	B	B, C3, E	A1, A2, A4, B48, E
Source: Major	Intestine	Plasma	Liver	Intestine
Source: Minor	Liver		Intestine	

Triglycerides

Triglycerides are the most abundant lipids in the human body. They consist of a glycerol molecule combined with three fatty acids. High levels of triglycerides are closely associated with hypercholesterolemia and can be used to predict VLDL levels if one assumes that VLDL = triglycerides/5. Levels of VLDL exceeding 40 mg/dl indicate lipoproteinemia. Levels of LDL-C can be estimated using Friedewald's equation: LDL-C = Total cholesterol − HDL − VLDL.

the blood circulation via the thoracic duct (also known as the left lymphatic duct or the chyliferous duct). Triglycerides are hydrolyzed (i.e., split by water) into monoacylglycerol and two fatty acids by the enzyme **lipoprotein lipase (LPL)** for use in cellular oxidative respiration (e.g., as fuel during muscle contraction). Lipoprotein lipase is found in the capillary endothelium of the heart, skeletal muscle, and adipose tissue. **Hydrolysis of** triglycerides helps to clear chylomicrons from blood circulation. Chylomicron remnants that remain after hydrolysis can be atherogenic, but LPL can reduce the adhesion of chylomicron remnants to endothelial cells and promote their re-esterification in the liver. **Very low density lipoprotein (VLDL)** is mainly responsible for the transport of triglycerides synthesized in liver cells to adipose cells for storage. After entering the circulation, VLDL is converted into LDL (Tortora and Grabowski 1993). Low-density lipoprotein is the main transporter of cholesterol in the blood. High-density lipoprotein removes cholesterol from extrahepatic (outside the liver) tissue by the process of **reverse cholesterol transport.** Efflux of cellular cholesterol toward apo A1 is catalyzed by adenosine triphospate (ATP)-binding cassette (ABC) transporter 1 to form HDL. Reverse transport involves **esterification** and storage of cholesterol in the core of the HDL molecule by the enzyme **lecithin:cholesterol acyltransferase (LCAT)** and a cofactor protein named apolipoprotein A1 (or apo A1). The transfer of cholesterol ester from newly formed HDL (which is designated HDL3) to LDL, VLDL, and chylomicrons in exchange for triglycerides is regulated by **cholesterol ester transfer protein (CETP).** The ultimate fate of the less dense forms, HDL2 and HDL1, is their recycling as nascent HDL in the liver, which is regulated by the enzymes **hepatic lipoprotein lipase (HPL)** and acyl-CoA:cholesterol acyltransferase (ACAT-2).

HDL Structure and Function

High-density lipoprotein consists of a family of molecules that differ in size, density, their composition of lipids and apolipoproteins, and likely their function (Von Eckardstein, Huang, and Assmann 1994). They range in density from approximately 1.06 to 1.21 g/ml. High-density lipoprotein has a high phospholipid content relative to other lipoproteins in the blood. The majority of HDL phospholipid is **lecithin.** High-density lipoprotein also has the largest surface area, about 80% greater than that of other lipoproteins in the blood.

High-density lipoprotein molecules are classified according to increasing density into three subclasses or fractions: HDL1, HDL2, and HDL3 (Eisenberg 1984). The most abundant fractions are HDL2 and HDL3. There are several major differences between the HDL fractions (Eisenberg 1984). First, the core diameter of the particle increases from HDL3 to HDL1. The core of HDL1 is about 50% larger than that of HDL3, and the cholesterol ester content and triglyceride content of HDL1 are three to four times greater than those of HDL3. HDL2 has about twice the surface area of HDL3 and 50% more protein (apolipoproteins [apo] A, C, and E) than HDL3. HDL1 has less protein than HDL2, but the protein is of only one class, apo E. HDL1 has the most apo E of any HDL fraction, which enhances its uptake by apo E receptors in the liver.

High-density lipoprotein can also be classified as containing only apo A1 (LpA1), which has about 35% of the total apo A1 bound in HDL, and apo A1 combined with apo A2 (LpA1:A2), which accounts for the remaining 65% of HDL apo A1. LpA1 is mainly found in HDL2, and LpA1:A2 is most abundant in HDL3. Levels of LpA1 vary widely among people. Levels of HDL 2 and LpA1 are increased by lipoprotein lipase and reduced by hepatic lipase. Because LpA1 accepts cholesterol efflux from cells but LpA1:A2 does not, LpA1 and HDL2 appear especially important for reverse transport of cholesterol and protection against atherogenesis. However, it remains unclear whether lower LpA1 alone or lower levels of both LpA1 and LpA1:A2 increase risk for CHD (Asztalos et al. 2006).

It is controversial whether apolipoproteins predict CHD better than traditional lipid levels. In a 15-year follow-up of 3322 middle-aged white men and women from the Framingham Offspring cohort without cardiovascular disease, the apo B:apo A1 ratio conferred elevations in risk (about 40%) similar to those associated with total cholesterol:HDL-C (40%) and LDL-C:HDL-C (35%). And, the apo B:apo A1 ratio did not add to the prediction of risk when it was added to the Framingham risk score beyond total cholesterol and HDL-C (Ingelsson et al. 2007). However, in a multiethnic sample of 7594 middle-aged U.S. adults from the third NHANES mortality study, risks of death from CHD were nearly doubled by high apo B and halved by high apo A1, compared to a smaller risk elevation for total cholesterol (17%) and a smaller risk reduction for HDL-C (32%). Only apo B and the apo B:apo A1 ratio were associated with CHD death after adjustment for cardiovascular risk factors (Sierra-Johnson et al. 2009).

HDL-C Formation

There are three main sources of new HDL molecules: (1) secretion from the liver or small intestine; (2) lipid and protein fragments from the hydrolysis of other lipoproteins rich in triglycerides, such as VLDL and chylomicrons; and (3) those from chemical interactions between phospholipids and apopoproteins. New HDL molecules secreted by the liver are disc shaped (Hamilton et al. 1976) and contain surface apo E, C, and A1 proteins, in that order of density (Marsh 1976). In contrast, in HDL in the blood, apo A1 is most predominant and apo E the least predominant. The discrepancy probably results from the actions of the enzyme LCAT on new HDL molecules (Eisenberg 1984). In contrast to the liver, the intestine secretes new HDL-C molecules that have high apo A1. A second source of new HDL is from hydrolyzed chylomicrons and VLDL (Shepherd and Packard 1989; Winkler and Marsh 1989). The molecules that are shed during lipolysis from the surface of chylomicrons and VLDL contain apo A1, apo C, phospholipids, and free cholesterol (Eisenberg 1976; Tall and Small 1978) and interact with LCAT. The third source of new HDL is the binding of unbound apoproteins, especially apo A1, and phospholipids in the plasma (Eisenberg 1984).

Apo A1 is the key in all three types of new HDL formation. The liver and intestine secrete apo A1 at about the same rate (Wu and Windmueller 1979). Apo A1 is the main coenzyme for LCAT reactions and is essential for the formation of other HDL fractions. The pool of free, secreted apo A1 can be transformed into new HDL, excreted in urine, or absorbed into LDLs (Eisenberg 1984). Apo A1 also regulates the removal of excess cholesterol from tissues outside the liver (Barbaras et al. 1986; Mahlberg and Rothblat 1992).

HDL3 Formation

Formation of a spherical HDL3 molecule from new HDL depends on the activity of LCAT (Norum 1984). In the plasma, LCAT binds to the new HDL and a lower-density lipoprotein and catalyzes the esterification of free cholesterol. The esterification involves the transfer of a free fatty acid from a phospholipid (lecithin), located on the shell of an HDL molecule, to another cholesterol molecule (Norum 1984). The esterified cholesterol is hydrophobic (i.e., repels water molecules) and moves to the core of the HDL-C molecule. The esterified cholesterol leaves a gap, or space, on the surface of the HDL molecule, which is filled by cholesterol from cell membranes, such as endothelial cells, or from other lipoproteins (Tall and Small 1978; Eisenberg 1984; Tall 1990). The transfer of cholesterol from other lipoproteins or cell surfaces to HDL is the first part of the reverse cholesterol transport mediated by HDL. Over time, the core of the new HDL enlarges and the molecule becomes HDL3.

HDL2 Formation

As HDL3 accumulates cholesterol esters, its diameter increases and its density decreases. The addition of esterified cholesterol to the core of HDL3 also increases the surface region of HDL3, which is thus transformed to HDL2. As the surface region of the HDL increases, it is able to accept more apolipoprotein, in particular, apo A1. An important characteristic of HDL2 is the capacity to transfer cholesterol ester to LDL-C directly (Eisenberg 1984) or to exchange it for triglycerides in VLDL and chylomicrons through the action of CETP (Tall 1986). The CETP reaction depends on the apopoprotein present on the surface of the lipoproteins. The magnitude of the transfer, though, is determined by the relative proportions of cholesterol ester and triglyceride in the lipoproteins and is proportional to the surface area of the lipoproteins (Deckelbaum et al. 1982). The exchange of cholesterol ester for triglyceride by the CETP reaction reduces the HDL2 core content of cholesterol. After more CETP and LCAT reactions, HDL2 is transformed into a larger, less dense HDL1 molecule, which contains mainly triglycerides and apo E absorbed from VLDL and chylomicrons (figure 8.4; Daerr and Greten 1982).

Risk Factors

Only 1 in 500 people has the genetic form of hypercholesterolemia known as the heterozygous familial type. Less than 1 in a million have the homozygous version. Hence, almost everyone has some control over whether blood cholesterol or its components rise to the level that exaggerates risk for CHD. Though nearly 70% of the variation in blood cholesterol level is explained by endogenous production by the liver, dietary intake of cholesterol from meats, poultry, fish, seafood, and dairy products explains most of the fluctuation in each person's serum cholesterol level.

Fruits, vegetables, grains, nuts, and seeds have no cholesterol. Though the national goal for dietary cholesterol is less than 300 mg per day, the average American daily intake is 450 mg among men and 320 mg among women. Although a large egg has 200 mg, eggs also contain lecithin, which limits absorption of dietary cholesterol.

Cigarette smoking, diabetes mellitus, obesity, alcohol, androgenic and anti-inflammatory steroids, and emotional stress also negatively influence blood lipid levels, especially increasing triglyceride and LDL-C levels (table 8.5). Obesity and cigarette smoking reduce HDL-C. Total cholesterol, LDL-C, and triglyceride levels are elevated in people with diabetes mellitus, but levels tend to normalize when blood glucose levels are controlled (Conti and Tonnessen 1992).

Sex and Estrogen

Before menopause, women usually have total cholesterol levels that are lower than those of men of the same age. As

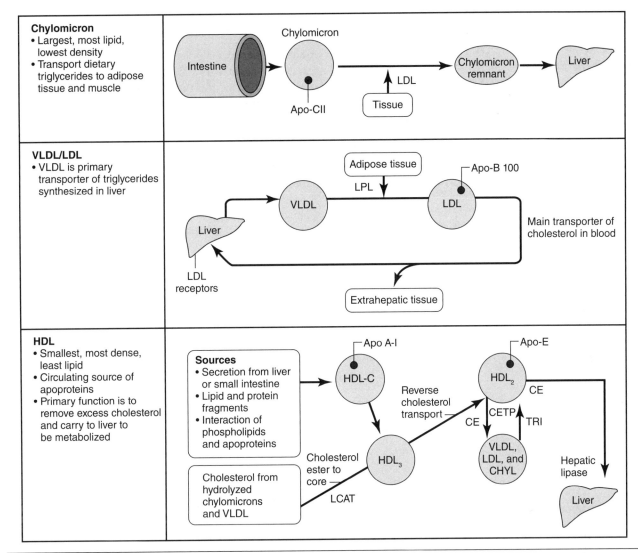

Chylomicron
- Largest, most lipid, lowest density
- Transport dietary triglycerides to adipose tissue and muscle

VLDL/LDL
- VLDL is primary transporter of triglycerides synthesized in liver

HDL
- Smallest, most dense, least lipid
- Circulating source of apoproteins
- Primary function is to remove excess cholesterol and carry to liver to be metabolized

Figure 8.4 Lipoprotein metabolism. Plausible sites whereby exercise might increase HDL-C levels are noted for ACAT and HPL activity at the liver; regulation of reverse transport by HDL through esterification by LCAT and apo A1; CETP regulation of triglyceride exchange with chylomicrons and VLDL; and increasing the activity of LPL.

Table 8.5 What Influences Lipoproteins?

Factor	Effect
Sex	Total is lower and HDL-C is higher in premenopausal women.
Age	Total increases and HDL-C decreases with age.
% Body fat	Total and LDL-C are higher, but HDL-C is lower, among overweight and obese people.
Diet	Total, LDL-C, and triglycerides are higher with fat and cholesterol intake.
Diabetes	Total, LDL-C, and triglycerides are elevated, but normalized when glucose is controlled.
Alcohol	Moderate use increases HDL-C.
Smoking	HDL-C decreases.
Steroids	HDL-C decreases.
Stress	Total increases and HDL-C decreases.
Exercise	HDL-C increases and LDL-C and triglycerides decrease.

women and men get older, until about 60 to 65 years of age, their blood cholesterol levels rise. In women, menopause often causes an increase in LDL-C and a decrease in HDL-C, and after the age of 50, women often have higher total cholesterol levels than men of the same age. Some women may benefit from hormone replacement therapy (also called estrogen replacement therapy) after menopause because estrogen lowers LDL and raises HDL.

Alcohol Use

Alcohol intake increases HDL-C but does not lower LDL-C. However, drinking too much alcohol can damage the liver and heart muscle and lead to high blood pressure and elevated triglycerides, so alcoholic beverages should not be used as a way to prevent heart disease.

▷ **STUDIES AMONG** people with heart disease have shown that lowering blood cholesterol can reduce the risk of dying from heart disease, having a nonfatal heart attack, and needing bypass surgery or angioplasty.

Drug Treatment

When proper diet, regular physical activity, and weight loss aren't sufficient to lower high blood lipids, cholesterol drugs are the treatment of choice. Drug therapy is medically indicated in some children and adolescents with hyperlipidemia, particularly those whose parents have high cholesterol levels (McCrindle et al. 2007). Table 8.6 shows situations in which drug therapy may be indicated.

The drugs commonly used to lower LDL-C levels include the **statin** drugs (e.g., atorvastatin, lovastatin, pravastatin, simvastatin, fluvastatin, rosuvastatin), which inhibit an enzyme named HMG-CoA reductase, and bile acid sequestrants (e.g., cholestyramine, colestipol, colesevelam) or nicotinic acid (i.e., niacin), which is preferred for patients with triglycerides over 250 mg/dl because bile acid sequestrants can elevate triglycerides. Other popular drugs used to lower triglycerides include fibrates (e.g., gemfibrozil and fenofibrate) and cholesterol absorption inhibitors (e.g., ezetimibe). See table 8.7. Combination therapy is often used in patients with extreme hyperlipidemia, but this requires careful monitoring because of the increased occurrence of side effects

Lifestyle Changes in LDL-Lowering Therapy

Lifestyle Risk Factors for Dyslipidemia

- Obesity (BMI ≥30)
- Physical inactivity
- Atherogenic diet

Therapeutic Lifestyle Changes

- Therapeutic Lifestyle Changes Diet
  - Reduced intake of cholesterol-raising nutrients
  - Saturated fats <7% of total calories
  - Polyunsaturated fat up to 10% of total calories

- Monounsaturated fat up to 20% of total calories
- Carbohydrate 50% to 60% of total calories
- Protein approximately 15% of total calories
- Dietary cholesterol <200 mg per day
- LDL-lowering therapeutic options
- Plant stanols/sterols (2 g per day)
- Viscous (soluble) fiber (10-25 g per day)
- Weight reduction
- Increased physical activity

Source: Adult Treatment Panel III (ATP III) Guidelines. National Cholesterol Education Program.

Table 8.6   Guidelines for Drug Therapy to Reduce Cholesterol

LDL cholesterol	Level for drug consideration	Goal of therapy
No CHD and fewer than two CHD risk factors	190 mg/dl or higher*	Less than 130 mg/dl
No CHD but two or more CHD risk factors	160 mg/dl or higher*	Less than 130 mg/dl
Diagnosis of CHD	130 mg/dl or higher**	100 mg/dl or less

* In men less than 35 years old and premenopausal women with levels of 190 to 219 mg/dl, drug therapy should be delayed except in high-risk patients (e.g., those with diabetes).

** In CHD patients with levels of 100 to 129 mg/dl, drug treatment depends on the clinical judgment of the physician.

Drug therapy may not be appropriate for some patients who meet the preceding criteria, including the elderly.

Reprinted from the National Heart, Lung, and Blood Institute 2002.

Table 8.7   Cholesterol Drugs

Statin drugs		
Generic names	**Brand names**	**How they work**
atorvastatin lovastatin pravastatin simvastatin fluvastatin rosuvastatin	Lipitor Altocor Prevachol Zocor Lescol Crestor	Reduce the production of cholesterol in the liver by inhibiting the rate-limiting enzyme, 3-hydroxy-3-methyl-glutaryl-CoA (or HMG-CoA) reductase. Cells then sense low cholesterol and express more LDL receptors, which remove circulating LDL-C. Lower LDL-C by: • Lowering LDL-C by 20% to 60% • Lowering triglycerides 10% to 40% depending on level • Increasing HDL by 10%

Drugs that may be used with a statin			
Type	**Generic names**	**Brand names**	**How they work**
Bile acid sequestrants	cholestyramine colestipol colesevelam	Questran Colestid Welchol	• Bind with cholesterol-containing bile acids in the intestines and are excreted. • Lower LDL-C by 10% to 20%.
Fibric acid derivatives	gemfibrozil fenofibrate	Lopid Tricor	• Activate lipoprotein lipase, which decreases apolipoprotein C3. • Reduce VLDL-C and triglycerides by 20% to 50%. • Increase HDL-C by 10% to 15%.
Nicotinic acid	niacin (vitamin B_3)	Niacor Niaspan Nicolar	• Blocks lipolysis, so less fatty acid is delivered to the liver for VLDL synthesis. • Also spares apo A1 when cholesteryl esters are removed from HDL in liver. • Reduces LDL-C by 10% to 20%. • Reduces triglycerides by 20% to 50%. • Raises HDL-C by 15% to 35%.
Cholesterol absorption inhibitor	Ezetimibe	Zetia	• Inhibits Niemann-Pick C1-Like 1 (NPC1L1) protein thus blocking absorption of dietary cholesterol in the liver and the small intestine • Lowers LDL-C by 15% to 20%.

Reprinted from the National Heart, Lung, and Blood Institute 2002.

such as constipation, cramping, flushing, stomach pain, and edema, which can be deadly for some patients with heart or vessel disease (American Heart Association 2012).

Some patients on statins complain of muscle pain during exercise. In one study, however, physically inactive people with high cholesterol who received rosuvastatin (10 mg/day) plus three days of endurance exercise for 20 weeks (including resistance exercise for the last 10 weeks) had similar reductions in LDL-C and greater reductions in oxidized LDL-C, compared to those on statin treatment only, without sustained elevations in creatine kinase (a marker of muscle damage) or reports of muscle pain (Coen et al. 2009).

The LDL-C target of 100 mg/dl (2.6 mmol/L) can result in undertreatment in people who have other risk factors for coronary heart disease, stroke, and peripheral vascular disease. The joint European Societies treatment targets are 2 mmol/L (77 mg/dl) for LDL-C and 4 mmol/L (155 mg/dl) for total cholesterol. The Heart Protection Study (HPS) showed that

LDL-C reduction to levels as low as 1.7 mmol/L (66 mg/dl) was associated with clinical benefits for patients with type 2 diabetes mellitus or peripheral and cerebrovascular disease, regardless of initial cholesterol levels. A 1 mmol/L (39 mg/dl) reduction in LDL-C results in a 25% reduction in CVD events, regardless of baseline LDL-C levels (Fourth Joint Task Force 2007).

Statins typically reduce LDL-C levels by 50%. Ezetimibe, a selective cholesterol absorption inhibitor, added to statin therapy further reduces total cholesterol by 16%, decreases LDL-C by 24%, and increases HDL-C (1.7%) (Mikhailidis et al. 2007).

When a high-risk patient has high triglycerides or low HDL-C, consideration can be given to combining a fibrate or nicotinic acid with an LDL-lowering drug. For moderately high-risk persons (two or more risk factors and 10-year risk 10% to 20%), the recommended LDL-C goal is <130 mg/dl, but an LDL-C goal <100 mg/dl is a therapeutic option on the

The Metabolic Syndrome as a Secondary Target of Therapy

Risk of cardiovascular disease is exaggerated when dyslipidemia co-occurs with abdominal obesity, high blood pressure, insulin resistance, and systemic inflammation. This collection of risk factors is collectively referred to as metabolic syndrome.

General Features of the Metabolic Syndrome

- Abdominal obesity
- Atherogenic dyslipidemia
  - Elevated triglycerides
  - Small LDL particles
  - Low HDL-C
- Raised blood pressure
- Insulin resistance (with or without glucose intolerance)
- Prothrombotic state
- Pro-inflammatory state

basis of recent trial evidence. The latter option extends also to moderately high-risk persons with a baseline LDL-C of 100 to 129 mg/dl. When LDL-lowering drug therapy is employed in high-risk or moderately high-risk persons, it is advised that intensity of therapy be sufficient to achieve at least a 30% to 40% reduction in LDL-C levels. Moreover, any person at high risk or moderately high risk who has lifestyle-related risk factors (e.g., obesity, physical inactivity, elevated triglycerides, low HDL-C, or metabolic syndrome) is a candidate for intervention to modify these risk factors regardless of LDL-C level (Grundy et al. 2004). The sidebar shows major risk factors that influence drug treatment options, and table 8.8 gives recommended LDL goals based on risk category.

The medical significance of statins for cardiovascular health has expanded beyond their role in cholesterol synthesis, including their anti-inflammatory properties (Arnaud, Veillard, and Mach 2005; Sorrentino and Landmesser 2005). Anti-inflammatory effects of lipid-lowering drugs may provide additional reductions in CVD risk by retarding atherogenesis, even in people with normal LDL-C. The Justification for the Use of Statins in Prevention: An Intervention Trial Evaluating Rosuvastatin (JUPITER) study found that statin therapy reduced vascular events in healthy men and women with low levels of LDL-C (average of 104 mg/dl) who were nonetheless at elevated risk because of high C-reactive protein, a marker of inflammation (Ridker et al.

2009). Among 17,802 trial participants, rosuvastatin resulted in a 44% reduction in vascular events, a 54% reduction in myocardial infarction, a 48% reduction in stroke, a 46% reduction in arterial revascularization procedures, and a 20% reduction in all-cause mortality. All participants benefited, including women, nonsmokers, and those with low Framingham risk scores. Risk reductions were similar to those seen when statins are used to treat people with high LDL-C (Ridker 2009).

Fibrates reduce the number of nonfatal heart attacks, but do not improve all-cause mortality, and are therefore indicated only in those not tolerant to statins. Although less effective in lowering LDL, fibrates improve HDL and triglyceride levels and seem to improve insulin resistance when the dyslipidemia is associated with other features of the metabolic syndrome (hypertension and type 2 diabetes). The combination of a cholesterol absorption inhibitor (i.e., ezetimibe) with a statin (e.g., Vytorin) has not been shown to further reduce atherosclerosis, despite a 25% greater reduction in LDL-C (Kastelein et al. 2008), and ezetimibe appears inferior to niacin for reducing atherosclerosis (Taylor et al. 2009).

▷ **STUDIES AMONG** people without heart disease have shown that lowering blood cholesterol can reduce the risk of developing heart disease, including heart attacks and deaths related to heart disease. This is true for those with high blood cholesterol levels and even for those with average levels.

Table 8.8 Treatment Goals for LDL Levels

Risk category	LDL goal (mg/dl)
CHD or equivalent risks	<100 mg/dl
Multiple (two or more) major risk factors	<130 mg/dl
Zero to one major risk factor	<160 mg/dl

Equivalent risks are peripheral artery disease, symptomatic carotid artery disease, abdominal aorta aneurism, diabetes, multiple risk factors that confer 10-year risk of CHD >20%.

Reprinted from the National Heart, Lung, and Blood Institute 2002.

Low levels of HDL-C are a stronger predictor of CHD than are elevated levels of LDL-C. High-density lipoprotein has important antiatherogenic effects, including reverse cholesterol transport, inhibition of LDL-C oxidation, and antiplatelet and anti-inflammatory actions. First-line therapy for low HDL-C generally includes lifestyle intervention to increase physical activity and lose weight. Common drug therapy options include statins, fibrates, and nicotinic acid, as well as emerging approaches to augment HDL-C and reverse cholesterol transport (Cardenas et al. 2008).

Major Risk Factors (Exclusive of LDL-C) That Modify LDL Goals

Established Risks

- Cigarette smoking
- Hypertension (BP ≥140/90 mmHg or on anti-hypertensive medication)
- Low HDL-C (<40 mg/dl)[†]
- Family history of premature CHD
- CHD in male first-degree relative <55 years
- CHD in female first-degree relative <65 years
- Age (men ≥45 years; women ≥55 years)

Emerging Risk Factors

- Lipoprotein (a)
- Homocysteine
- Prothrombotic factors
- Pro-inflammatory factors
- Impaired fasting glucose
- Subclinical atherosclerosis

[†] HDL cholesterol ≥60 mg/dl counts as a "negative" risk factor; its presence removes one risk factor from the total count.

Source: Adult Treatment Panel III (ATP III) Guidelines. National Cholesterol Education Program.

About half of CHD patients who do not respond to lipid therapy are at elevated risk for CVD events because they have low HDL-C. For example, in the United Kingdom General Practice Research Database, 6823 of 19,843 patients treated with statins had elevated LDL-C despite having been treated for an average of two years. Among them, 3115 (46%) also had low HDL-C or high triglycerides. Those patients had 24% higher risk of a vascular event in the heart or brain compared to patients with high LDL-C but normal HDL-C or triglycerides (Sazonov et al. 2010).

In the Framingham Offspring Study participants who underwent lipid drug treatment from 1975 through 2003, there was 21% (95% confidence interval [CI]: 7-33%) reduction in risk for cardiovascular events over eight years of follow-up for each 5 mg/dl increase in HDL-C (Grover et al. 2009). The risk reduction was strongest when pretreatment LDL-C was low, and it was independent of changes in LDL-C, triglycerides, and pretreatment lipid levels, as well as smoking status, weight, and the use of beta-blockers. It held across types of patients and drug classes. For these reasons, drugs are being developed and tested that affect both LDL-C and HDL-C metabolism. Examples of drug targets are inhibitors of acyl-coenzyme A-cholesterol acyl transferase (ACAT2) and cholesterol ester transfer protein (CETP).

CETP can contribute to an atherogenic lipoprotein profile by redistributing cholesteryl esters from HDL toward apolipoprotein B-containing lipoproteins, especially when VLDL and chylomicron levels are high. Drugs that inhibit CETP, such as dalcetrapib and anacetrapib, can lower LDL-C and double HDL-C (Kappelle et al. 2010), so they might reduce cardiovascular risk (Ansell and Hobbs 2006). However, it is controversial whether raising HDL-C by inhibiting CETP activity actually lowers cardiovascular risk.

A clinical trial of the CETP inhibitor torcetrapib, which increased HDL-C by 60% and decreased LDL-C by 20% more than the statin Lipitor in 15,000 heart patients, was stopped because it increased systolic blood pressure by 5 mmHg, didn't slow atherosclerosis, and led to a 25% increase in cardiovascular events and a 60% higher than expected mortality rate, possibly by hypertensive effects following activation of the rennin–angiotensin–aldosterone system (Barter et al. 2007; Nissen et al. 2007). Dalcetrapib is a less potent CETP inhibitor, raising HDL-C by 25% to 30%, but it does not appear to increase blood pressure or raise aldosterone levels (Robinson 2010).

It is equally likely that CETP has protective effects against atherogenesis. Observational studies show that higher CETP levels are associated with lower cardiovascular risk, and experimental studies show that CETP stimulates the reverse cholesterol transport pathway that removes cholesterol from macrophages prior to its metabolism in the liver and excretion as bile. Clinical trials are under way to test whether CETP inhibition has favorable effects on atherosclerosis and cardiovascular events (Kappelle et al. 2010).

Dyslipidemia Etiology and Physical Activity

Primary causes of dyslipidemia are single- or polygene mutations that result in either overproduction or defective clearance of triglycerides and LDL-C, or in underproduction or excessive clearance of HDL-C (see table 8.9). Most cases of dyslipidemia are secondary to behavior or other medical conditions. The most important secondary cause in developed nations is a sedentary lifestyle with excessive dietary intake of saturated fat, cholesterol, and trans fats (i.e., polyunsaturated or monounsaturated fatty acids that have been hydrogenated during food processing). Other common secondary causes include diabetes mellitus; alcohol overuse; chronic kidney disease; hypothyroidism; primary biliary cirrhosis and other cholestatic liver diseases; and drugs such as thiazides (diuretics used to treat edema and hypertension),

Table 8.9   Primary Genetic Dyslipidemias

Disorder	Genetic defect	Mechanism	Prevalence
Familial hypercholesterolemia	LDL receptor defect	Impaired LDL clearance	Common among French Canadians, Christian Lebanese, and Afrikaners
Familial defective apo B100	LDL apo B receptor binding defect	Impaired LDL clearance	1 per 700 in population
Polygenic hypercholesterolemia	Unknown	Nonspecific	Common
LPL (lipoprotein lipase) deficiency	Endothelial LPL defect	Impaired chylomicron clearance	Rare but worldwide
Apo C2 deficiency	Apo C2 defect	LPL functional impairment	Less than 1 per million population

Adapted from http://www.merckmanuals.com/media/professional/pdf/Table_159-3.pdf.

beta-blockers, retinoids (vitamin A derivatives), antiretroviral agents, estrogen and progestins, and glucocorticoids.

Dietary intake of cholesterol and fat has a strong influence on blood levels of cholesterol and lipids, even when a person's synthesis and metabolism of lipoproteins are normal. Cholesterol-lowering drugs are designed to alter various aspects of the synthesis and metabolism of lipoproteins. Likewise, it is believed that regular physical activity has metabolic effects, in addition to promoting weight loss, that can positively affect the regulatory physiology of lipid and cholesterol. The most consistent and fully studied effects of regular exercise on cholesterol fractions are a decrease in triglycerides and an increase in HDL-C, with a somewhat smaller lowering of LDL-C. To better understand how those effects might be biologically plausible, it is necessary to understand the basic physiology of lipoproteins, especially the metabolism of HDL-C.

▶ **A 10% DECREASE** in total blood cholesterol levels may result in an estimated 20% to 30% reduction in the incidence of CHD.

The risk of heart attack in both men and women overall is highest at lower HDL-C levels and higher total blood cholesterol levels. However, people with lower levels of HDL-C (37 mg/dl or lower in men and 47 mg/dl or lower in women) are at a high risk regardless of their total blood cholesterol levels. Conversely, those with high levels of total blood cholesterol have a lower risk of heart attack when they also have higher levels of HDL-C (53 mg/dl or greater in men and 67 mg/dl or greater in women).

An increase in HDL-C after exercise training probably doesn't tell the whole story of the antiatherogenic effects of exercise (Leaf 2003). Exercise training increases the size or content of HDL-C (Kraus et al. 2002), and it can result in

increases in HDL2-C and decreases in HDL3-C that yield no net change in total HDL-C (Nye et al. 1981). Exercise training also elevates apo A1 levels (Couillard et al. 2001; Kiens et al. 1980; Thompson et al. 1997) or increases its biological half-life (possibly by increased lipoprotein lipase activity in skeletal muscle) (Thompson 1990) to promote HDL2 survival and enhance cholesterol retrieval from peripheral tissues and the delivery of cholesterol ester to the liver for removal (Leaf 2003).

Though hydrolysis of HDL-C is regulated by hepatic lipase activity, the concentration of HDL2 in plasma is regulated by lipoprotein lipase (LPL). The primary fate of HDL2 is the hydrolysis of its triglyceride and phospholipid content by hepatic lipase (Eisenberg 1984; Shepherd and Packard 1989; Durstine and Haskell 1994). The net effect of hepatic lipase is the conversion of HDL2 back to recycled, nascent HDL in the liver. Increased activity of LPL increases the hydrolysis of VLDL and chylomicrons, increasing the formation of lower-density lipoprotein remnants, which can be cleared by the liver or can yield cholesterol more easily to HDL (Eisenberg 1984; Eisenberg and Deckelbaum 1989). LCAT and LPL activity may exert a protective effect against atherosclerosis, beyond that of increasing HDL2 molecules, by reducing blood levels of triglycerides and cholesterol. Lipoprotein lipase also can attach to chylomicron remnants that remain after triglycerides are hydrolyzed to fatty acids for cell fuel and aid the uptake of these remnants by the liver. This is important because it is thought that chylomicron remnants can penetrate endothelial cells and contribute to atherogenesis.

The protective effect of decreased hepatic lipase activity against atherosclerosis is more difficult to understand. Hepatic lipase hydrolyzes triglyceride and phospholipid from HDL2 and returns an HDL3 molecule back into the circulation. In addition, hepatic lipase may remove HDL-C from the circulation via the **phospholipase** activity of hepatic lipase (Tall 1990). Decreasing hepatic lipase activity causes an increase in HDL2 molecules, but an

Key Steps in Reverse Transport of Cholesterol

Step 1: Cholesterol Efflux

- Cholesterol is removed from extrahepatic cells by HDL3 particles.
- Cellular efflux is catalyzed by ATP-binding cassette (ABC) transporter 1.

Step 2: HDL Growth

- Apo A1 catalyzes LCAT to esterify cholesterol for storage in the core of the maturing HDL2-C molecule.
- Cholesteryl ester transfer protein (CETP) regulates the transfer of cholesterol ester from the HDL2-C particle to chylomicrons, VLDL-C, and LDL-C in exchange for triglycerides.

- Lipoprotein lipase in skeletal muscle accelerates this process by hydrolysis of triglycerides from lipoprotein components of HDL2-C.

Step 3: Clearance in the Liver

- HDL binds to HDL receptor for clearance.
- Hepatic lipase readies HDL-C for receptor binding by hydrolysis of triglycerides and phospholipids from HDL-C.
- HDL docks at scavenger receptor type B class I (SR-BI) for removal of cholesterol esters and then recirculates.
- Cholesterol ester carried by LDL is cleared by LDL receptors.

---

elevated HDL2 fraction alone would not necessarily exert a protective effect against atherosclerosis. However, apo A1 is required for the uptake of cholesterol by HDL (Barbaras et al. 1986; Mahlberg and Rothblat 1992). Hepatic lipase causes the release of apo A1 (Melchior et al. 1994). Thus, decreasing hepatic lipase activity can enhance the capacity of HDL to accept cholesterol from extrahepatic tissue and from other lipoproteins. Also, a reduction in hepatic lipase reduces hydrolysis of HDL2, so HDL2 molecules can become larger HDL1 molecules, which contain primarily apo E. HDL1 molecules, then, would be cleared by apo E receptors in the liver.

▷ **FOR SEDENTARY** people, it appears that moderate physical activity, such as brisk walking 8 to 15 miles (13-24 km) a week for six to nine months, increases HDL levels and lowers triglyceride levels in the blood. Among recreational runners (i.e., those who run 15-60 miles, or 24-97 km, a week), HDL levels are higher in those who run faster, regardless of distance.

Physical Activity and Lipoprotein Levels: The Evidence

Exercise is recommended as an adjuvant, along with a low-fat, high-fiber diet, to lipid therapy (National Cholesterol Education Program [NCEP] Expert Panel 2002).

Most of the studies of physical activity and lipoproteins done so far, including the earliest in 1957, were clinical studies of exercise training among people with normal or borderline high cholesterol levels. Those studies mainly involved white men and have limited application to the general population of people at risk for CHD. Though prospective cohort studies have not yet been reported, several observational, population-based studies and many randomized controlled trials have been published in the past 20 years. Summaries of some of these studies and some specific examples follow.

Cross-Sectional Studies

In cross-sectional comparisons of small clinical samples, male and female endurance athletes of the same age had 20% to 30% higher levels of HDL-C than untrained peers, and a dose–response relationship was seen between more physical activity and greater HDL-C (Durstine and Haskell 1994). However, moderate intensities of exercise were not as effective for increasing HDL-C in young and middle-aged women as in men. Cross-sectional studies have shown 2 to 3 mg/dl elevations in HDL-C that were dose dependent and 8 to 20 mg/dl reductions in triglycerides when physical activity exposures ranged from 15 to 20 miles (24 to 32 km) per week of brisk walking or jogging or expended 1200 to 2200 kcal/week (Durstine et al. 2001). See figures 8.5 and 8.6.

Healthy, Nonsmoking Men

Weekly running distance was associated with HDL-C and other blood lipid levels among nearly 3000 healthy, nonsmoking men ages 30 to 64 years (Kokkinos et al. 1995). After adjustments for body mass index (BMI) and alcohol consumption, there was an increase in HDL-C of about 0.3 mg/dl for each mile run. LDL-C and triglyceride levels were positively associated with BMI and inversely correlated with the distance run per week, the frequency of exercise per week, and the duration of the exercise sessions. Those who ran 11 to 14 miles (17.7-22.5 km) per week had 11% higher

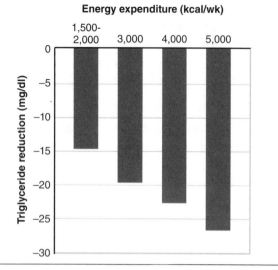

Figure 8.5 Summary of dose-dependent relation of physical activity and triglyceride levels from cross-sectional studies.

Data from Durstine et al. 2001.

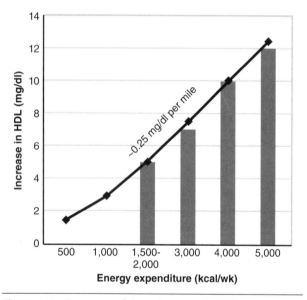

Figure 8.6 Summary of dose-dependent relation of physical activity and HDL-C levels from cross-sectional studies.

Data from Durstine et al. 2001.

HDL-C and 8% lower LDL-C compared with nonrunners. Higher HDL-C levels were observed among men who ran 7 to 14 miles (11.3-22.5 km) per week at paces of 10 to 11 min per mile (about 6-7 min/km).

Marathon Study

Leisure-time physical activity was quantified from self-reports for the past year in 537 healthy men ages 20 to 60 years (Marrugat et al. 1996). After adjustments for age, alcohol consumption, smoking, and BMI, each 100 kcal expended per day in leisure-time physical activity at an intensity greater

than 7 kcal/min during the previous year was associated with an increase of 2.09 mg/dl (0.054 mmol/L) in HDL-C. Intensities of 9.5 to 12 kcal/min were associated with lower levels of total cholesterol, non-HDL-C, and triglycerides. Better physical fitness was associated with physical activities requiring at least 5 kcal/min. There was a threshold in the intensity of exercise associated with serum lipid profile (7 kcal/min) and physical fitness (5 kcal/min).

Boston Area Health Study

A case–control study matched 340 patients (266 men, 74 women) who survived a first myocardial infarction with 340 controls by sex, age, and place of residence (O'Connor et al. 1995). Total energy expenditure was not associated with blood lipids or apolipoproteins, but moderate to vigorous participation in recreational sports was directly related to HDL-C and HDL2.

Strong Heart Study

Total physical activity (leisure plus occupational) and blood lipoproteins were studied in about 4500 American Indian men and women ages 45 to 74 years who were selected from 13 communities in Arizona, Oklahoma, and the Dakotas (Yurgalevitch et al. 1998). Among diabetic men and non-diabetic men and women, physical activity was associated positively with levels of apo A1; several other factors, such as age, BMI, smoking, alcohol use, and waist-to-hip ratio, were controlled for.

U.S. Worksite Study

The association of strength training and blood lipids was examined among 8500 working men with a mean age of 40 years (Tucker and Silvester 1996). After adjustment for smoking, alcohol use, BMI, age, and other types of physical activity, the odds ratio of hypercholesterolemia among men who spent 4 to 7 h each week strength training was half that observed in nonlifters. Spending less than 4 h a week in strength training conferred no protection against high cholesterol levels.

Aerobics Center Longitudinal Study

In contrast, another study suggested that strength is associated with unfavorable lipid profiles. A cross-sectional analysis in the Aerobics Center Longitudinal Study examined the association between muscular strength and serum lipid and lipoprotein status in a group of 1193 women and 5460 men (Kohl et al. 1992). After adjustments for age, body composition, and cardiovascular fitness, there was no association between muscular strength and total cholesterol or LDL-C for either men or women. However, triglycerides were higher in stronger men, who also had lower HDL-C. The findings suggest that strength is associated with a less favorable lipid profile. However, most of the people studied were not involved in regular resistance training, so other unknown factors common to inherent muscular strength and lipids, or other factors not controlled in the study, probably explain the findings.

Postmenopausal Women

The association between physical activity and HDL-C was examined in 255 white postmenopausal women with a mean age of 58 years (Cauley et al. 1986). After adjustment for several factors, physical activity was independently and positively associated with higher HDL-C and HDL2. There was a nearly linear relationship between frequency of sport activity and level of HDL2.

Spanish Men

The association of physical activity with serum apo A protein was examined in 332 healthy Spanish men ages 20 to 60 years (Martin et al. 1999). Among men with a family history of CHD, the odds of having above-average levels of apo A of men who expended more than 300 kcal each day in leisure physical activity was less than 15% that of men who expended less than 300 kcal a day. The results suggest that regular daily physical activity is helpful for controlling apo A protein levels in men who have a family history of CHD.

Tanzania

A cross-sectional comparison of nearly 1000 adults living in Tanzania showed that those who lived in rural areas reported higher physical activity levels, had lower BMI, and had lower levels of total cholesterol, LDL-C, triglycerides, and apolipoproteins A1 and B (Mbalilaki et al. 2007). However, the rural Tanzanians also had lower HDL-C, so their otherwise favorable lipid profile might also have been influenced by their diet, which is known to be lower in fat and higher in complex carbohydrates when compared to that of urban dwellers. However, Masai people living in Tanzania have a low-risk lipid profile despite their high-fat diet, which might be attributable to their high physical activity levels (2565 kcal/day). These levels are nearly twice those of rural Bantu people (1500 kcal/day), who have a low-fat diet, and three times higher than those of urban Bantu (891 kcal/day), who have a high-fat diet (Mbalilaki et al. 2010).

FINMONICA

Cross-sectional national surveys, conducted in Finland at five-year intervals in 1982, 1987, 1992, and 1997, found that leisure-time physical activity, physical activity during commuting, and occupational physical activity were positively related to HDL-C in both men and women (Barengo et al. 2006). However, part of those effects might have been explained by lower BMI and waist circumference among active people.

Los Angeles Atherosclerosis Study

The relation between physical activity, HDL-C, and three-year progression of carotid atherosclerosis, which can be estimated by intima media thickness of an artery, was examined in a cohort of 500 men and women 40 to 60 years of age initially without cardiovascular disease (Nordstrom et al. 2003). There was a linear trend of increased HDL-C across physical activity groups. Adjusted for age, sex, smoking, alcohol use, dietary fat and antioxidant vitamin supplements, blood pressure and cholesterol drugs, and diabetes, rates of increased intima media thickness (microns per year) measured by ultrasound in the common carotid arteries were 14.6, 10, and 5.8 in sedentary, moderately active, and highly active (aerobic activity 3.5 or more times per week) people, respectively.

Atherosclerosis Risk in Communities (ARIC) Study

Minority groups have been underrepresented in population-based studies of physical activity and lipids. The ARIC Study examined the longitudinal association of changes in physical activity with changes in plasma lipids and lipoproteins across nine years of follow-up in 8764 African American and white participants aged 45 to 64 at baseline (Monda, Ballantyne, and North 2009). For each age- and smoking-adjusted increase in physical activity of 180 MET-minutes per week (e.g., 45-60 min of brisk walking), HDL-C increased by 3 to 4.9 mg/dl in all participants; LDL decreased by 4 to 10.6 mg/dl in women; total cholesterol decreased by 7.4 mg/dl in African American women; and triglycerides decreased by 9 to 12.9 mg/dl in white participants. Associations with BMI were inconsistent.

Exercise Training Studies

Clinical studies have examined the effects of exercise training on cholesterol and blood lipid levels from as early as 1957. Since then, around half of the more than 70 studies of men and women have reported an association of aerobic or resistance exercise with decreased triglycerides and increased HDL-C. Results have generally been more favorable among men, possibly because estrogen appears to influence lipid metabolism in women. Fluctuations in sex hormone levels in women during the menstrual cycle produce variations in blood lipoprotein levels that must be considered in studies on premenopausal women. The effects on LDL-C and total cholesterol have been less consistent.

Aerobic endurance training increases HDL-C levels by 4% to 22% and decreases triglyceride levels by 4% to 37% (Durstine et al. 2001; Leon and Sanchez 2001). Durstine and colleagues (2001) concluded that exercise training programs that expend 1200 to 2200 kcal/week typically elevate HDL-C levels by 2 to 8 mg/dl and lower triglyceride levels by 5 to 38 mg/dl. Although reductions in total cholesterol or LDL-C were not usually found, they were reported when studies used the higher amounts of exercise.

Another review examined 51 exercise training studies published since 1987 involving about 4700 adults (60% were men) ages 18 to 80 years (mean age 47 years; Leon and Sanchez 2001). The studies lasted at least 12 weeks and consisted mainly of structured group exercise among healthy, sedentary white people; a few studies monitored lifestyle or home exercise or used resistance exercise. Twenty-eight of the studies were randomized controlled trials. Only nine studies involved people with high total cholesterol levels (>240 mg/dl). There were just two studies of African Americans and two studies of Asians.

Generally, the exercise intensities were moderate to vigorous, with weekly energy expenditures ranging from about 500 kcal to 4800 kcal. The most consistent outcome of physical activity, independent of dietary intervention, was a mean increase in HDL-C of about 5%. Decreases in LDL-C (about 5%) and triglycerides (about 4%) were less consistently seen, and total cholesterol was unchanged by exercise training. Those changes were independent of the age or sex of the participants and the weekly energy expenditure. Only a handful of studies used more than one intensity of exercise, so there was not enough evidence to judge whether a dose response occurred with increasing exercise intensity.

In most of the studies, diets were not manipulated, and weight loss on average was negligible (mean less than 1 kg, ranging from no loss to a 7.2 kg loss) after exercise. Fifteen studies of overweight or obese people combined exercise and dietary restriction. In these studies, weight loss ranged from 7 to 18 kg, so changes in lipoproteins in those people could have been confounded or moderated by weight loss.

The cumulative results of 31 randomized clinical trials of aerobic or resistance exercise training, conducted for at least four weeks and involving over 1800 participants with and without hyperlipidemia, indicated that aerobic exercise training led to small but statistically significant decreases of about 3.8 mg/dl each in total cholesterol, LDL-C, and triglycerides and an increase in HDL-C of 1.9 mg/dl (0.05 mmol/L; Halbert et al. 1999). An exercise frequency exceeding three times a week was not more beneficial. The evidence for the effects of resistance exercise training was inconclusive. Since that review, there have been a host of similar quantitative summaries supportive of favorable effects of exercise training on lipoproteins and lipids.

Averaged across 25 randomized controlled trials, the effect of exercise training on HDL-C level was 2.53 mg/dl (0.065 mmol/L) (Kodama et al. 2007). The thresholds for increasing HDL-C level were about 120 min of exercise each week or a weekly energy expenditure of about 900 kcal. For each 10 minutes of exercise there was a 1.4 mg/dl (0.036 mmol/L) increase in HDL-C level. The intensity or weekly frequency of exercise was unrelated to HDL-C changes. People with a BMI less than 28 and total cholesterol level of 220 mg/

dl (5.7 mmol/L) or more had a 2.1 mg/dl (0.054 mmol/L) larger increase in HDL-C level than people with a BMI of 28 or more and total cholesterol level less than 220 mg/dl (5.7 mmol/L). Exercise was more effective in subjects with initially high total cholesterol levels or low BMI. In another quantitative review, an increase in HDL2-C of 11% (2.6 mg/dl; 95% CI: 1.0-4.4 mg/dl) was observed when averaged across 19 randomized controlled trials of aerobic exercise lasting eight weeks or more in a total of 984 adults (Kelley and Kelley 2006a). The increase in HDL2-C was independent of decreases in body weight and percent body fat.

Benefits of exercise do not appear to be limited to vigorous aerobic endurance training. Twenty-nine randomized controlled trials of progressive resistance training lasting four or more weeks in a total of 1329 adults were evaluated (Kelley and Kelley 2009). On average, reductions were seen for total cholesterol (−5.5 mg/dl or 2.7%), total cholesterol/HDL-C (−0.5 or 11.6%), non-HDL-C (−8.7 mg/dl or 5.6%), LDL-C (−6.1 mg/dl or 4.6%), and triglycerides (−8.1 mg/dl or 6.4%). A small average increase in HDL-C (0.7 mg/dl or 1.4%) was not significant. Also, 22 randomized controlled trials of walking for exercise representing 948 adults reported an average reduction of 4% (−8.8 to −2.4 mg/dl) in non-HDL-C (Kelley, Kelley, and Tran 2005c).

During the past several years George Kelley, a professor of Community Medicine at the University of West Virginia, and his colleagues have provided a series of systematic reviews of randomized controlled trials on aerobic exercise and lipids in various populations. The reviews give quantitative estimates of the average efficacy of exercise as a first-line treatment, or adjuvant to diet, which can be judged by comparison with the efficacy of drug therapy described earlier in the chapter.

Averaging the results from studies conducted on very different types of people with varying (and often normal) lipoprotein levels, using different types and amounts of exercise, prevents strong conclusions about the efficacy of exercise for altering blood lipids in specific circumstances. So, it is informative to examine some individual studies that represent some of those differing circumstances, especially in people who have dyslipidemia.

Aerobic Exercise Training

Probably because early studies of heart disease focused on aerobic types of endurance exercise, most studies of the effects of exercise training on blood lipoprotein levels also have used aerobic exercise and physical activities of moderate-to-vigorous intensities. Usually the studies have shown positive benefits for elevated HDL-C levels and lowered levels of triglycerides, with less clear effects on LDL-C and total cholesterol. Whether the effects of exercise and physical activity are independent of, or additive with, changes in diet and body fatness has not been clear in many of the studies.

Meta-Analyses of Randomized Controlled Trials of Exercise and Lipids

MEN

In 49 trials of aerobic exercise lasting eight or more weeks that included 2990 men, average improvements were seen for total cholesterol (−2%), LDL-C (−3%), HDL-C (2%), and triglycerides (−9%) (Kelley and Kelley 2006b).

WOMEN

Trials in which aerobic exercise was the main intervention led to improvements in total cholesterol (2%, −4.3 mg/dl), HDL-C (3%, 1.8 mg/dl), LDL-C (3%, −4.4 mg/dl), and triglycerides (5%, −4.2 mg/dl) (Kelley, Kelley, and Tran 2004).

PATIENTS WITH CARDIOVASCULAR DISEASE

Ten trials of aerobic exercise lasted at least four weeks in a total of 1260 adults with cardiovascular disease (Kelley, Kelley, and Franklin 2006). There was an average increase of 9% in HDL-C (3.7 mg/dl) and a decrease of 11% in triglycerides (−19.3 mg/dl), but no decreases were seen in total cholesterol (95% CI: −22.3 to 4.7 mg/dl) or LDL-C (95% CI: −19.5 to 4.2 mg/dl).

ADULTS WITH TYPE 2 DIABETES

Averaged across seven trials of 220 adults with type 2 diabetes, results showed a reduction of about 5% for LDL-C but no changes in total cholesterol, HDL-C, total cholesterol/HDL-C, or triglycerides (Kelley and Kelley 2007b).

OVERWEIGHT OR OBESE ADULTS

In 13 trials of aerobic exercise lasting eight or more weeks in a total of 613 people with BMI ≥25 kg/m², triglycerides were decreased by 11% (16 mg/dl) (Kelley, Kelley, and Tran 2005a). Increases in HDL-C and decreases in LDL-C were dependent on decreases in body weight.

OLDER ADULTS

This analysis included 28 outcomes of aerobic exercise among 1427 adults 50 years of age or older. Improvements were observed for HDL-C (5.6%, 2.5 mg/dl) and total cholesterol/HDL-C (7.1%, −0.8) (Kelley, Kelley, and Tran 2005b).

YOUTHS

There were 12 outcomes from trials of aerobic exercise lasting four or more weeks representing 389 boys and girls 5 to 19 years of age. A decrease of 12% was found for triglycerides (−1.0 mg/dl), including in children who were overweight. The average changes were not statistically significant for HDL-C or LDL-C, but decreases in LDL-C were greater with increased training intensity and in older ages, while increases in HDL-C were larger when initial HDL-C levels were lower (Kelley and Kelley 2007a)

Washington University, St. Louis, Missouri

The effects of endurance exercise training on plasma lipoprotein lipids were determined in 10 men aged 46 to 62 years with coronary artery disease who maintained their body weight and their diets during the study (Heath et al. 1983). Training increased $\dot{V}O_2max$ by 30% and HDL-C by 11% while reducing plasma cholesterol by 8%, LDL-C by 9%, and triglycerides by 13%. Changes in LDL-C and $\dot{V}O_2max$ were inversely correlated ($r = -0.73$), while the changes in LDL-C and HDL-C each were correlated inversely with the levels measured before training. Thus, the authors concluded that protective effects of exercise against atherogenic risk seemed to be the result of a training effect, since they correlated best with changes in $\dot{V}O_2max$ and were greatest in patients who initially had low $\dot{V}O_2max$, high LDL-C, and low HDL-C levels.

Stanford, California

In a randomized study, 48 sedentary, healthy men ages 30 to 55 were assigned to a running program that lasted a year, while another 33 remained sedentary (Wood et al. 1983). The group of runners increased their cardiorespiratory fitness and lost body fat, but the changes in lipoprotein levels were not statistically different from the control values. However, the 25 men who ran an average of at least 8 miles (12.9 km) per week had an increase in HDL-C of 4.4 mg/dl and an increase in HDL2 of 3.3 mg/dl. Increases in HDL-C and HDL2 and decreases in LDL-C were directly related to weekly running distance. Because lost body fat also was related to increased HDL-C, part of the effects of running on HDL might have been explained by fat loss.

In another Stanford study, the effects of exercise and of the National Cholesterol Education Program (NCEP) diet, which restricts fat and cholesterol, were studied in 180 postmenopausal women ages 45 to 64 years and nearly 200 men ages 30 to 64 years who had below-average levels of HDL-C (<60 mg/dl in women, <44 mg/dl in men) and elevated LDL-C (125-210 mg/dl in women, 125 to 190 mg/dl in men) (Stefanick et al. 1998). They were randomly assigned to aerobic exercise, the NCEP diet, diet plus exercise, or a control group that received no intervention. After a year, dietary intake of fat and cholesterol, as well as body weight, decreased in both women and men in both the diet group and the diet plus exercise group. HDL-C, triglyceride levels, and the ratio of total cholesterol to HDL-C were not affected by diet or exercise. However, LDL-C was reduced by 14.5 mg/dl among women and 20 mg/dl among men in the diet plus exercise group. The diet did not change LDL-C in either women or men unless they also participated in exercise.

The effects of weight loss through dieting or through running on apo A1, apo A2, and HDL were studied in sedentary, moderately overweight men randomly assigned to three groups: (1) running about 10 miles (16 km) a week without reducing caloric intake, (2) eating about 350 fewer kilocalories each day, and (3) making no change in eating or exercise habits (Williams et al. 1992). After one year, body weight was reduced by 7 kg in dieters and 4 kg in runners. The runners and dieters each had a decrease in HDL3 and an increase in HDL2. The runners also had increases in plasma apo A1 levels. However, when the lipoprotein changes were adjusted for how much weight was lost, they disappeared, so the favorable effects of exercise were not independent of weight loss.

Overweight Men

Changes in total cholesterol, HDL-C, LDL-C, and triglycerides were examined in 51 sedentary, overweight men after nine months of endurance exercise training (treadmill walking, jogging, and stationary cycling) consisting of 45 min at 70% to 80% of maximal oxygen uptake three days each week (about 1000 kcal/week). The men had normal total cholesterol levels but were on the American Heart Association Step I Diet to lose weight. To determine whether genetic factors influenced the outcome, the men were classified according to their isoform of the apo E regulatory protein for lipid metabolism: apo E2 (n = 6), apo E3 (n = 33), or apo E4 (n = 12). The men of all genotypes had similar age, body weight and composition, and plasma lipoprotein and lipid profiles at the beginning of the study. Men with the apo E2 genotype had a larger mean increase in plasma HDL-C and HDL2-C with exercise training than the other two groups (HDL-C increase was 8 mg/dl, 3 mg/dl, and 2 mg/dl for the apo E2, E3, and E4 groups, respectively; HDL2-C increase was 5, 1, and 1 mg/dl, respectively). That effect remained even after adjustment for body weight changes. Though based on a very small group of men, these findings suggest that the gene for apo E—which regulates uptake of LDL by extrahepatic tissues, uptake of chylomicron remnants by the liver, and, to a lesser extent, the function of HDL-C molecules—may moderate the effects of exercise training on HDL-C responses.

Premenopausal Women

Duncan, Gordon, and Scott (1991) studied 102 sedentary premenopausal women to determine the effects of 24 weeks of walking. Three groups of subjects walked the same distance five days per week, but their speeds differed; the groups

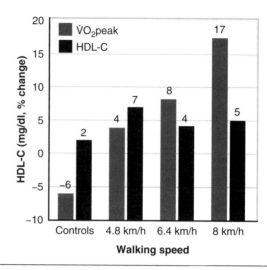

Figure 8.7 An HDL dose response study included premenopausal women who walked five days per week for 24 weeks.
Adapted from Duncan, Gordon, and Scott 1991.

walked 3 miles (4.8 km) in 36, 45, or 60 min by week 14 and thereafter. Figure 8.7 shows that aerobic fitness increased in a dose–response manner; however, increases in HDL-C were similar among the three groups and did not follow a dose-dependent pattern with increasing walking speed.

In contrast, 50 healthy middle-aged women (mean age, 50 years) were randomly assigned to 12 weeks of walking and jogging or 12 weeks of resistance exercise (Blumenthal et al. 1991). Peak oxygen uptake was increased by 18%, from 26.7 to 31.4 ml · kg^{-1} · min^{-1}, after aerobic exercise but unchanged after resistance training. Both exercise groups had small reductions in total cholesterol and HDL-C, increases in apo A1, and no change in triglycerides. Because both premenopausal and postmenopausal women were included, it was not possible to determine whether the exercise responses were independent of reproductive hormone status. In another study, 40 obese women (BMI = 33) ages 21 to 60 years (mean = 43) participated in a 16-week randomized controlled trial that combined a low-fat 1200-kcal diet with either a structured step aerobics exercise training program or a moderate lifestyle physical activity program (weekly energy cost of about 1500 kcal; Andersen et al. 1999). Changes in body weight, body composition, cardiovascular risk profiles, and physical fitness were compared after 16 weeks and one year later. Mean (±SD) 16-week weight losses were about 8 kg (±4) for both groups. A year later, the aerobic group had regained 1.6 kg on average, while the lifestyle activity group regained half that amount, 0.8 (±4.6) kg. Reductions in triglyceride (16%) and total cholesterol (10%) levels were seen after 16 weeks of the weight loss program regardless of the type of exercise but returned to near the initial levels a year later. The two forms of exercise seemed equivalent and would have accounted for about 40% of the weight loss after 16 weeks. However because they each were combined with diet, it wasn't possible to directly determine the relative importance of exercise compared with the diet for reducing the cholesterol and triglyceride levels.

Postmenopausal Women

Seals and colleagues (1984) reported that six months of high-intensity endurance training resulted in increased HDL-C and decreased triglyceride levels in elderly women. Other evidence suggests that estrogen replacement optimizes the effects of regular exercise on blood lipids in postmenopausal women. Lindheim and colleagues (1994) studied the effects of a six-month moderate exercise program with and without oral estrogen replacement on blood lipid and lipoprotein levels in postmenopausal women. One hundred healthy, sedentary, postmenopausal women ages 42 to 59 were randomly assigned to one of the following four groups: exercise, estrogen replacement, exercise and estrogen replacement, and a control group that received neither estrogen nor exercise. Exercise consisted of treadmill walking or cycling for about 30 min at least three times a week. Women in the exercise group had a 5% decrease in total cholesterol and a 10% decrease in LDL-C. The exercise group showed a 20% reduction in triglycerides but no change in HDL-C. However, both the sedentary and the exercising groups that got estrogen therapy had a nearly 10% increase in HDL-C levels.

African American Men With Hypertension

Sufficiently intense exercise also can improve lipid metabolism in patients with hypertension. Thirty-six African American men ages 35 to 76 years with essential hypertension were randomly assigned to no exercise or to cycling exercise at 60% to 80% of maximum heart rate, three times per week for 16 weeks (Kokkinos et al. 1998). Peak oxygen uptake in the exercise group improved nearly 10%, but body weight was unchanged. Though changes in HDL-C among the exercisers did not exceed those in the control group, they nonetheless were greater in men who exercised at higher intensities. Ten men who exercised at 75% of maximal heart rate or higher had a 10% increase (from 42 to 46 mg/dl) in HDL-C. Thus, low- to moderate-intensity aerobic exercise might not provide a sufficient stimulus to alter blood lipid levels in African American men with severe hypertension.

HERITAGE Family Study

Recent evidence suggests that the impact of aerobic exercise training on blood lipids is independent of changes in cardiorespiratory fitness and is more related to energy expenditure and reduced body fat (Katzmarzyk et al. 2001). Men (77 black and 218 white) and women (131 black and 224 white), ages 17 to 65 years, participated in five months of endurance cycling training that led to a 17.5% increase in maximal oxygen uptake and a 3.3% decrease in body fat mass. After controlling for age, the change in fitness was unrelated to changes in blood lipids, regardless of race. In contrast, changes in fat mass among men were correlated inversely with changes in HDL-C and HDL2-C and positively with the ratio of total cholesterol to HDL; among women, they were correlated positively with total cholesterol, LDL-C, and the ratio of total cholesterol to HDL. Hence, the changes in blood lipids after endurance exercise training were unrelated to changes in cardiorespiratory fitness but were related to changes in body fat mass. This suggests that the metabolic influences of physical activity on blood lipids depend more on energy expenditure or fat loss than on fitness changes.

The HERITAGE Family Study also showed that HDL-C changes after exercise training vary widely among people (Leon et al. 2000). There was a mean increase of about 1.55 mg/dl (0.04 mmol/L), but the standard deviation was three times greater than the mean, and nearly half the participants had no change or a decrease. Part of the variation was explained by level of HDL-C before training. People with HDL-C less than 35 mg/dl had nearly twice the increase (2.0 mg/dl) that others did (1.2 mg/dl). Initial levels of triglycerides had a bigger influence, though. When participants were divided into four groups based on the 50th percentiles of triglycerides (119 mg/dl) and HDL-C (36 mg/dl) as cutpoints, HDL-C levels increased by an average of 4.9% in the high triglyceride and low HDL-C group but only by 0.4% in the low triglyceride and low HDL-C group (Couillard et al. 2001). Thus, increases in plasma HDL-C are larger in people who have elevated triglycerides. Figure 8.8 shows the pattern of individual variation in blood lipid change that has been seen after exercise training.

Associations between genetic variation in CETP and changes in HDL-C after 20 weeks of exercise training were also investigated in the HERITAGE Family Study (Spielmann et al. 2007). Plasma HDL-C, HDL2-C, HDL3-C, and apo A1 levels were measured, and 13 CETP single nucleotide polymorphisms (SNPs) were genotyped in 265 blacks and 486 whites. One of the CETP variants was independently associated with higher initial levels of HDL-C and apo A1 in

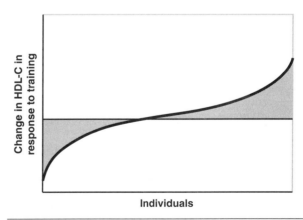

Figure 8.8 Heterogeneity of training responses of HDL cholesterol, showing individual differences in response to regular physical activity.

whites. When combined with APO E genotype, it accounted for nearly 10% of the variation seen in initial HDL-C levels. White women homozygous on that CETP variant had greater increases in HDL3-C and apo A1 after exercise training (Spielmann et al. 2007).

Available evidence supports the hypothesis that endurance exercise training at both moderate and vigorous intensities has a favorable influence on the blood lipid profile. The most frequently observed change is an increase in the HDL-C. It is estimated that for every 1 mg/dl increase in HDL-C, the risk of a CHD event is reduced by 3% in men and about 4% in women. Reduction in total blood cholesterol, LDL-C, and triglycerides also may occur with endurance exercise. In general, a 1% reduction in LDL-C is associated with a 2% to 3% lower risk of heart disease.

Studies of Targeted Risk Reduction Interventions Through Defined Exercise (STRRIDE)

Sedentary, overweight men ($n = 49$) and women ($n = 35$) with mild-to-moderate dyslipidemia (either LDL-C of 130-190 mg/dl or HDL-C <40 mg/dl in men or <45 in women) were randomly assigned to participate for six months in a control group or for eight months in one of three exercise groups: (1) high amount–high intensity: the equivalent of jogging 20 miles (32.0 km) per week at 65% to 80% of aerobic capacity (about 23 kcal · kg^{-1} · week^{-1}); (2) low amount–high intensity: the equivalent of jogging 12 miles (19.2 km) per week at 65% to 80% of aerobic capacity (about 14 kcal · kg^{-1} · week^{-1}); or (3) low amount–moderate intensity: the equivalent of walking 12 miles per week at 40% to 55% of aerobic capacity (about 14 kcal · kg^{-1} · week^{-1}). Exercise training had no effect on total cholesterol or LDL-C levels. HDL-C was increased by 9.7% (4.3 mg/dl) after high-amount–high-intensity exercise only. Triglycerides were decreased after exercise by 10% to 25% (13.1 to 51.6 mg/dl) regardless of dose.

University of Maryland

The effects of six months of aerobic exercise training were evaluated in a trial of 100 healthy 50- to 75-year-old men and women who had one or more lipid abnormalities (cholesterol >200 mg/dl, HDL-C <40 mg/dl, triglycerides >200 mg/dl) and who ate a standardized diet throughout the trial. There was no control comparison group, but aerobic fitness was increased by 15%. Reductions in total cholesterol (−2.1 mg/dl), triglycerides (−17 mg/dl), and LDL-C (−0.7 mg/dl) and increases in HDL3-C (1.9 mg/dl) and HDL2-C (1.2 mg/dl) were observed that were independent of diet. Changes in HDL-C and HDL2-C were slightly dependent on change in body fatness.

Postmenopausal Women: Unsupervised Exercise

Although most studies show that exercise has efficacy for improving lipid profiles, other studies suggest that the effectiveness of exercise (i.e., its impact in unsupervised settings) may be less predictable. For example, 170 sed-

entary women aged 50 to 75 years of age who had low fitness, were overweight or obese, and had dyslipidemia were randomly assigned to an exercise intervention or a stretching control group (Mohanka et al. 2006). The exercise intervention included 12 months of facility- and home-based (45 min, five days a week) moderate-intensity sports or recreational exercise. Exercisers averaged 176 min/week of moderate- to vigorous-intensity exercise, expending about 900 kcal/week. Even though the exercisers increased aerobic fitness by 11% and lost more body weight and fat mass than did the women in the control group, there were no effects of exercise on total cholesterol, LDL-C, HDL-C, or triglycerides.

Postprandial Lipemia

Endurance-trained people exhibit low levels of postprandial lipemia (i.e., increased triglycerides in the blood after a meal), which can also be blunted after a single exercise session, depending on energy expenditure. These effects are explainable by increased lipoprotein lipase activity and reduced triglyceride secretion by the liver (Gill and Hardman 2003). With values averaged across 29 studies involving 555 people, exercising before a meal reduced postprandial triglyceride levels by more than a half standard deviation compared to no exercise, and the reduction appeared related to energy expenditure (Petitt and Cureton 2003).

Effects of prior exercise on the concentrations and compositions of lipoprotein subfractions were investigated in 20 middle-aged men after a high-fat (80 g) meal. Before the meal, men walked on a treadmill for 90 min or rested. Prior exercise reduced postprandial triglycerides by 29%, concentrations of chylomicrons by 28.6% (14.6 mg/dl), large VLDL1 by 34.4% (39.7 mg/dl), and small VLDL2 by 23% (9.6 mg/dl) (Gill et al. 2006). Over 95% of VLDL1 and VLDL2 molecules were composed of apolipoprotein (apo) B100–containing particles. Postprandial apo C3/apo B and apo E/apo B ratios in VLDL1 were lower after exercise. Postprandial cholesteryl ester/triglyceride ratios were lower in VLDL1 and VLDL2 and higher in HDL2 after exercise. Thus, the effect of prior moderately intense exercise on VLDL1 is quantitatively greater than its effect on chylomicrons and causes changes in lipoprotein composition that likely reduce their atherogenic properties.

Egg Beaters

Six weeks of moderately intense endurance exercise training (four or five days a week, 60 min/session) increased HDL-C by 10% and decreased LDL-C and apo B levels by about 20% even when unfit men and women increased their dietary cholesterol by eating 12 eggs each week for two months (Vislocky et al. 2009).

Resistance Exercise Training

Studies of the effects of resistance exercise training on blood lipoprotein levels have produced conflicting results. Most cross-sectional studies have reported a reduced HDL-C level or an elevated total cholesterol-to-HDL ratio in resistance-trained athletes compared with endurance-trained athletes. Because of selection biases in many of these studies, there has been poor control for other factors that might influence lipids and lipoproteins, such as age, body composition, diet, and anabolic or androgenic steroid use. In contrast, most clinical studies found that resistance exercise training led to favorable changes in lipoprotein and lipid levels. However, many of those studies had no control group and took a single blood sample before and after training. Many also involved people with normal levels of lipoproteins and lipids and did not verify that diet was controlled during the exercise training (Hurley 1989). When those factors are controlled, resistance exercise training does not appear to alter lipoprotein or lipid levels among individuals who have hypercholesterolemia.

Men at Risk

Changes in lipoprotein and lipid levels and activity of lipoprotein lipase and hepatic lipase were examined in 16 untrained, middle-aged men who had high total cholesterol (about 230 mg/dl), high LDL-C (140 mg/dl), high triglycerides (190 mg/dl), low HDL-C (35 mg/dl), and two or more other risk factors for CHD (Kokkinos et al. 1991). At least two blood samples were taken on separate days before the exercise began. After 20 weeks of resistance exercise training, the exercisers had a 50% increase in upper body strength, a 37% increase in lower body strength, and no change in $\dot{V}O_2$max or percent body fat. There also were no changes in blood levels of triglycerides, total cholesterol, HDL-C, and LDL-C or in the activity of lipoprotein lipase and hepatic lipase. Though diet was reportedly not changed, possible effects of smoking, alcohol use, and blood glucose or insulin levels were not controlled in this study.

Premenopausal Women

Twenty-four healthy but sedentary premenopausal women with normal levels of cholesterol and lipoproteins were randomly assigned either to participate in 45- to 50-min resistance exercise sessions at 85% of 1-repetition maximum (1RM) three days a week or to remain sedentary (Prabhakaran et al. 1999). After 14 weeks, the exercisers had increased their strength, lost body fat, and decreased total cholesterol from 180 to 164 mg/dl, LDL-C from 115 to 99 mg/dl, and the ratio of total cholesterol to HDL-C from 4.2 to 3.6. Triglycerides and HDL-C were not changed by the resistance exercise training.

Obese Women

Sixteen sedentary obese women ages 22 to 57 years performed three sets of six to eight repetitions at 60% to 70% of 1RM three times a week. Six others remained sedentary (Manning et al. 1991). The women reported that their diets remained unchanged. After 12 weeks, body weight, BMI, and caloric intake remained unchanged. Though strength increased by 58%, blood levels of total cholesterol, HDL-C, LDL-C, triglycerides, apo A1, and apo B100 and the ratio of total cholesterol to HDL-C were unchanged. Apo B is the primary apolipoprotein constituent of LDL-C. Thus, resistance exercise training in the absence of body fat loss does not appear to alter lipoprotein levels among sedentary obese women. Though six of the women were postmenopausal, their lipoprotein levels at the beginning of the study were not different from those of the younger women, so it was unlikely that estrogen status affected the study outcomes. However, the levels of total cholesterol (200 mg/dl), HDL-C (59 mg/dl), LDL-C (120 mg/dl), and triglycerides (110 mg/dl) were normal at the beginning of the study, so there was little room for improvement regardless of the intervention used.

Postprandial Lipemia

To determine whether reductions in postprandial lipemia after resistance exercise depend on intensity, 10 healthy men performed resistance exercises at a moderate or hard intensity but of equal work (repetitions and sets were varied to equate work) and ate a high-fat meal 15 1/2 h later (Singhal et al. 2009). Fasting triglycerides were reduced by about 35% after hard exercise and about 25% after moderate exercise. Fat oxidation 3 h after the meal was increased by 39% after hard exercise and 18% after moderate exercise.

Exercise and Plant Sterols

Plant sterols decrease both total and LDL-C levels by reducing the absorption of dietary cholesterol in the intestine. In contrast, exercise appears to decrease triglyceride levels by reducing hepatic VLDL secretion and increasing the activity of lipoprotein lipase activity in skeletal muscle. Also, exercise training seems to increase HDL-C by altering HDL subfractions (e.g., increasing HDL2) while also changing reverse cholesterol transport enzyme activities (Marinangeli, Varady, and Jones 2006).

In an eight-week randomized controlled trial without dietary control in adults with high total cholesterol, plant sterols combined with moderate-to-vigorous aerobic exercise (25-40 min, three days per week) resulted in reductions in total cholesterol (7.7%) and triglycerides (11.8%) and an increase in HDL-C (7.5%) (Varady, Houweling, and Jones 2007). Exercise alone decreased triglycerides by 16.6% and increased HDL-C by 9.5%. Percent body fat was reduced in each group by about 4%. Cholesterol absorption was reduced by 18% by plant sterols but was not affected by exercise.

▷ **IN A** randomized study of 30 middle-aged adults, nine months of aerobic exercise training that increased $\dot{V}O_2$peak by 24% was accompanied by an 18% reduction in apolipoprotein B (Ring-Dimitriou et al. 2007).

Strength of the Evidence

The overall evidence that regular aerobic or endurance exercise can improve lipoprotein profiles is encouraging (Durstine and Thompson 2001).

Temporal Sequence

The population-based observational studies have so far been mainly limited to cross-sectional studies, which lack the proper sequence to establish causality: physical activity measurements before lipid outcome measurements. However, a few prospective cohort studies support that physical activity increases HDL-C and reduces atherosclerosis.

Strength of Association

The cumulative evidence from more than 50 randomized controlled trials indicates that aerobic and endurance exercise training increase HDL-C by about 5%. Similar reductions of about 5% for LDL-C and 4% for triglycerides have been reported, but in fewer studies and less consistently than for HDL-C levels. Population-based cross-sectional studies and a limited number of prospective cohort studies have shown similar effects.

Consistency

Improvements in lipoprotein profiles after exercise generally have been similar for men and women regardless of age or CVD risk. Though results have been encouraging for ethnic minorities, the vast majority of studies have been conducted on white men of European ancestry. People with lower HDL-C levels before exercise training had greater increases after exercise, but only a dozen or so studies examined the effects of exercise among people with dyslipidemia. Those studies used varying methods. Hence, it is premature to conclude whether the benefits of exercise have been underestimated or whether they occur reliably in people who have high levels of LDL-C or triglycerides or low HDL-C.

Dose Response

Based on the collective evidence, it appears that aerobic exercise expending between about 1200 and 2400 kcal each week for at least 12 weeks and conducted at moderate or vigorous intensities yields favorable changes in lipoproteins. Changes do not appear to depend on changes in fitness. There have not been enough randomized controlled trials comparing different intensities or amounts of physical activity to determine experimentally the dose response. However, the best available evidence suggests that increases in HDL and decreases in triglycerides and LDL in people with dyslipidemia are dose dependent on total energy expenditure, more so than exercise intensity, occurring after thresholds of 10 to 13 MET-hours per week of physical activity (e.g., 12 miles of brisk walking) (Kodama et al. 2007; Slentz et al. 2007; Wood et al. 1983).

Biological Plausibility

The blood lipid improvements most consistently reported with exercise are increased HDL-C (mainly HDL2) and decreased triglycerides, which do not seem explainable by cholesterol exchange across contracting skeletal muscle (Jacobs et al. 2006). One mechanism by which exercise is responsible for lowered triglycerides and increased HDL-C is the increased use of triglycerides as energy during prolonged exercise, although free fatty acids and intramuscular triglycerides remain secondary to carbohydrates as fuels during moderate-to-vigorous intensity exercise (Bergman et al. 1999).

The enzyme LPL, found in extrahepatic tissues, is responsible for breaking down triglycerides into fatty acids that are then used as fuel during prolonged exercise at moderate intensities. As triglycerides are hydrolyzed, VLDL molecules shrink and lose surface cholesterol to HDL molecules for reverse transport to the liver for excretion as bile salts (Gibbons and Mitchell 1995). Gene transcription, protein synthesis, and activity of LPL have been shown to persist for up to 48 h after acute endurance exercise (Ferguson et al. 1998; Seip et al. 1997). Increased LPL activity after exercise might explain the blunting effect of acute exercise on postprandial lipemia (i.e., high triglycerides after a meal). A recent quantitative review of the evidence accumulated from 555 people in 29 studies indicated that people who exercise before a meal have an attenuation of the triglyceride increase after a meal of one-half standard deviation, regardless of their sex or age; the type of meal; or the intensity, duration, or timing of the exercise (Stewart and Cureton 2003).

A second mechanism by which exercise increases HDL-C is through another enzyme called lecithin:cholesterol acyltransferase (LCAT). It is known that exercise increases LCAT activity. LCAT is responsible for transferring free fatty acids in the blood and for esterification of cholesterol to yield HDL2 cholesterol. However, LCAT is not a rate-limiting enzyme, so increased LCAT activity after exercise may merely indicate higher lipid availability as a result of increased LPL activity. A third mechanism thought to be responsible for the increase in HDL-C levels with exercise involves the decreased activity of yet another enzyme, hepatic lipase. Hepatic lipase, an enzyme found in the liver, is responsible for HDL2 catabolism. Exercise can decrease the activity of hepatic lipase. This results in less HDL-C catabolism, leading to more HDL-C remaining in the blood. Several studies also indicate that regular exercise can favorably affect apo A1, a cofactor of LCAT; apo B100, which is a ligand for LDL receptors; and levels of cholesterol ester transfer protein (CETP), which regulates the transfer of cholesterol ester from HDL molecules to other lipoproteins for reverse transport of cholesterol from extrahepatic tissues. It is not yet established whether exercise training affects CETP or the activity of **diacylglycerol O-acyltransferase (DGAT)**

1 and 2 (which influence esterification of diacylglycerol to yield triglycerides) or **microsomal triglyceride transfer protein (MTP),** which is necessary for the assembly and secretion of apolipoprotein B–containing lipoproteins.

Table 8.10 summarizes lipoprotein enzyme changes that accompany exercise.

Although the effects of exercise training on LDL-C levels in the blood have been small and inconsistent in many studies, some evidence suggests that exercise protects against oxidation of LDL-C. In a small uncontrolled study of 13 people who had coronary artery disease, running just twice weekly for two months was associated with a reduced rate of LDL-C oxidation despite no change in LDL-C levels (Ziegler et al. 2006). In another uncontrolled study of 17 healthy, young medical students, 16 weeks of vigorous aerobic exercise training (50 min/day, five days a week) improved LDL resistance to oxidation and reduced oxidized LDL by 16% after a 25-min session of moderate-to-vigorous cycling exercise (Elosua et al. 2003).

Table 8.10   Lipoprotein Enzyme Changes That Accompany Exercise

Enzyme	Single exercise session	Exercise training
LPL activity	Increased ~4 h after exercise	Increased
HL activity	Unchanged	Unchanged unless weight loss
Apo A1	Unchanged	Increased
LCAT activity	Increased or unchanged	Increased or unchanged
CETP activity	Not studied	Increased or unchanged
CETP mass	Increased or decreased	Increased or decreased

Adapted from Durstine and Thompson 2001; Leaf 2003.

Summary

The American Heart Association and the World Health Organization have concluded that high levels of total cholesterol, LDL-C, and triglycerides and low levels of HDL-C are primary risk factors for developing CHD and atherosclerosis. Though weight loss, reduced dietary fat and cholesterol, and the statin drugs remain the frontline interventions for the primary and secondary prevention of dyslipidemia, physical activity also is recommended. Randomized controlled trials and population-based studies have generally agreed that physical activity can help increase HDL-C levels and decrease triglyceride levels, with less consistent reduction in LDL-C. Those effects appear to be largely independent of age, sex, and weight loss. Though the biological mechanisms are not fully understood, physical activity has a favorable effect on several features of fat and cholesterol metabolism, including increases in regulatory apolipoproteins, CETP, and enzymes such as LPL and LCAT. It appears that regular exercise of moderate-to-vigorous intensities aids the reverse transport of cholesterol to the liver in ways that are independent of, but can augment, diet or drug therapy. In clinical practice, a few randomized trials show that a prudent diet plus exercise is more effective than exercise alone for reducing total cholesterol and LDL-C but that exercise alone reduces triglycerides (Kelley et al. 2011).

· BIBLIOGRAPHY ·

Acton, S., A. Rigotti, K.T. Landschulz, S. Xu, H.H. Hobbs, and M. Krieger. 1996. Identification of scavenger receptor SR-BI as a high density lipoprotein receptor. *Science* 271: 518-520.

American College of Sports Medicine. 1993. *The American College of Sports Medicine's resource manual for guidelines for exercise testing and prescription.* 2nd edition. Philadelphia: Lea & Febiger.

American Heart Association. 2002. *Heart and stroke statistical update.* Dallas: American Heart Association.

American Heart Association. 2012. Heart disease and stroke statistics-2012 update: A report from the American Heart Association. Circulation. 125 (1): e2-e220.

Andersen, R.E., T.A. Wadden, S.J. Bartlett, B. Zemel, T.J. Verde, and S.C. Franckowiak. 1999. Effects of lifestyle activity vs. structured aerobic exercise in obese women: A randomized trial. *Journal of the American Medical Association* 281 (4): 375-376.

Anderson, D.W., A.V. Nichols, S.S. Pan, and F.T. Lindgren. 1978. High lipoprotein distribution: Resolution and determination of three major components in a normal population sample. *Atherosclerosis* 29: 161-179.

Ansell, B., and F.D. Hobbs. 2006. The potential for CETP inhibition to reduce cardiovascular disease risk. *Current Medical Research and Opinion* 22: 2467-2478.

Arnaud, C., N.R. Veillard, and F. Mach. 2005. Cholesterol-independent effects of statins in inflammation, immunomodulation and atherosclerosis. *Current Drug Targets in Cardiovascular and Haematological Disorders* 5: 127-134.

Assmann, G., and H. Schulte. 1992. Relation of high-density lipoprotein cholesterol and triglycerides to incidence of atherosclerotic coronary artery disease (the PROCAM experience). Prospective Cardiovascular Munster study. *American Journal of Cardiology* 70: 733-737.

Asztalos, B.F., S. Demissie, L.A. Cupples, D. Collins, C.E. Cox, K.V. Horvath, H.E. Bloomfield, S.J. Robins, and E.J. Schaefer. 2006. LpA-I, LpA-I:A-II HDL and CHD-risk: The Framingham Offspring Study and the Veterans Affairs HDL Intervention Trial. *Atherosclerosis* 188: 59-67.

Backer, J.M., and E.A. Dawidowicz. 1981. Mechanism of cholesterol exchange between phospholipid vesicles. *Biochemistry* 20 (13): 3805-3810.

Ball, M., and J. Mann. 1994. *Lipids and heart disease: A guide for the primary care team.* 2nd edition. New York: Oxford University Press.

Barbaras, R., P. Grimaldi, R. Negrel, and G. Ailhaud. 1986. Characterization of high-density lipoprotein binding and cholesterol efflux in cultured mouse adipose cells. *Biochimica et Biophysica Acta* 888: 143-156.

Barengo, N.C., M. Kastarinen, T. Lakka, A. Nissinen, and J. Tuomilehto. 2006. Different forms of physical activity and cardiovascular risk factors among 24-64-year-old men and women in Finland. *European Journal of Cardiovascular Prevention and Rehabilitation* 13: 51-59.

Barter, P.J., M. Caulfield, M. Eriksson, S.M. Grundy, J.J.P. Kastelein, M. Komajda, J. Lopez-Sendon, L. Mosca, J.C. Tardif, D.D. Waters, C.L. Shear, J.H. Revkin, K.A. Buhr, M.R. Fisher, A.R. Tall, and B. Brewer. 2007. Effects of torcetrapib in patients at high risk for coronary events. *New England Journal of Medicine* 357: 2109-2122.

Bergman, B.C., G.E. Butterfield, E.E. Wolfel, G.A. Casazza, G.D. Lopaschuk, and G.A. Brooks. 1999. Evaluation of exercise and training on muscle lipid metabolism. *American Journal of Physiology* 276: E106-E117.

Bisgaier, C.L., and R.M. Glickman. 1983. Intestinal synthesis, secretion, and transport of lipoproteins. *Annual Review of Physiology* 45: 625-636.

Blumenthal, J.A., K. Matthews, M. Fredrikson, N. Rifai, S. Schniebolk, D. German, J. Steege, and J. Rodin. 1991. Effects of exercise training on cardiovascular function and plasma lipid, lipoprotein, and apolipoprotein concentrations in premenopausal and postmenopausal women. *Arteriosclerosis and Thrombosis* 11: 912-917.

Cardenas, G.A., C.J. Lavie, V. Cardenas, R.V. Milani, and P.A. McCullough. 2008. The importance of recognizing and treating low levels of high-density lipoprotein cholesterol: A new era in atherosclerosis management. *Reviews in Cardiovascular Medicine* 9: 239-258.

Carr, M.C., A.F. Ayyobi, S.J. Murdoch, S.S. Deeb, and J.D. Brunzell. 2002. Contribution of hepatic lipase, lipoprotein lipase, and cholesteryl ester transfer protein to LDL and HDL heterogeneity in healthy women. *Arteriosclerosis, Thrombosis, and Vascular Biology* 22: 667-673.

Castelli, W.P. 1988. Cholesterol and lipids in the risk of coronary artery disease: The Framingham Heart Study. *Canadian Journal of Cardiology* 4 (Suppl. A): 5A-10A.

Cauley, J.A., R.E. LaPorte, R.B. Sandler, T.J. Orchard, C.W. Slemenda, and A.M. Petrini. 1986. The relationship of physical activity to high density lipoprotein cholesterol in postmenopausal women. *Journal of Chronic Diseases* 39 (9): 687-697.

Centers for Disease Control and Prevention. 2000. State-specific cholesterol screening trends – 1991. *Morbidity and Mortality Weekly Report* 49 (33): 750-755.

Chajek, T., L. Aron, and C.J. Fielding. 1980. Interaction of lecithin:cholesterol acyltransferase and cholesteryl ester transfer protein in the transport of cholesteryl ester into sphingomyelin liposomes. *Biochemistry* 19: 3673-3677.

Coen, P.M., M.G. Flynn, M.M. Markofski, B.D. Pence, and R.E. Hannemann. 2009. Adding exercise training to rosuvastatin treatment: Influence on serum lipids and biomarkers of muscle and liver damage. *Metabolism* 58 (7): 1030-1038.

Conti, C.R., and D. Tonnessen. 1992. *Heart disease and high cholesterol: Beating the odds.* Reading, MA: Addison-Wesley.

Couillard, C., J-P. Despres, B. Lamarche, J. Bergeron, J. Gagnon, A.S. Leon, D.C. Rao, J.S. Skinner, J.H. Wilmore, and C. Bouchard. 2001. Effects of endurance exercise training on plasma HDL cholesterol levels depend on the levels of triglycerides: Evidence from men of the HERITAGE family study. *Arteriosclerosis, Thrombosis, and Vascular Biology* 21: 1226-1232.

Daerr, W.H., and H. Greten. 1982. In vitro modulation of the distribution of normal human plasma high density lipoprotein subfractions through the lecithin:cholesterol acyltransferase reaction. *Biochimica et Biophysica Acta* 710 (2): 128-133.

Deckelbaum, R.J., S. Eisenberg, Y. Oschry, E. Butbul, I. Sharon, and T. Olivecrona. 1982. Reversible modification of human plasma low density lipoproteins toward triglyceride-rich precursors. *Journal of Biological Chemistry* 257: 6509-6517.

Deckelbaum, R.J., S. Eisenberg, Y. Oschry, E. Granot, I. Sharon, and G. Bengtsson-Olivecrona. 1986. Conversion of human plasma high density lipoprotein-2 to high density lipoprotein-3. *Journal of Biological Chemistry* 261: 5201-5208.

Deckelbaum, R.J., T. Olivecrona, and S. Eisenberg. 1984. Plasma lipoproteins in hyperlipidemia: Roles of neutral lipid exchange and lipase. In *Treatment of hyperlipoproteinemia,* edited by L.A. Carlson and A.G. Olsson, pp. 85-93. New York: Raven Press.

Duncan, J.J., N.F. Gordon, and C.B. Scott. 1991. Women walking for health and fitness. How much is enough? *Journal of the American Medical Association* 266 (23): 3295-3299.

Durstine, J.L., P.W. Grandjean, P.G. Davis, M.A. Ferguson, N.L. Alderson, and K.D. DuBose. 2001. Blood lipid and lipoprotein adaptations to exercise: A quantitative analysis. *Sports Medicine* 31: 1033-1062.

Durstine, J.L., and W.L. Haskell. 1994. Effects of exercise training on plasma lipids and lipoproteins. *Exercise and Sport Sciences Reviews* 22: 477-521.

Durstine, J.L., and P.D. Thompson. 2001. Exercise in the treatment of lipid disorders. *Cardiology Clinics* 19: 471-488.

Eisenberg, S. 1976. Metabolism of very low density lipoprotein. In *Lipoprotein metabolism,* edited by H. Greten, pp. 32-43. Heidelberg: Springer-Verlag.

Eisenberg, S. 1984. High density lipoprotein metabolism. *Journal of Lipid Research* 25: 1017-1058.

Eisenberg, S., and R. Deckelbaum. 1989. Intravascular lipoprotein remodelling: Neutral lipid transfer proteins. In *Human plasma lipoproteins,* edited by J.C. Fruchart and J. Shepherd. New York: de Gruyter.

Elosua, R., L. Molina, M. Fito, A. Arquer, J.L. Sanchez-Quesada, M.I. Covas, J. Ordoñez-Llanos, and J. Marrugat. 2003. Response of oxidative stress biomarkers to a 16-week aerobic physical activity program, and to acute physical activity, in healthy young men and women. *Atherosclerosis* 167: 327-334.

Ferguson, M.A., N.L. Alderson, S.G. Trost, D.A. Essig, J.R. Burke, and J.L. Durstine. 1998. Effects of four different single exercise sessions on lipids, lipoproteins, and lipoprotein lipase. *Journal of Applied Physiology* 85: 1169-1174.

Fidge, N.H. 1999. High density lipoprotein receptors, binding proteins and ligands. *Journal of Lipid Research* 40: 187-201.

Fielding, C.J., and P.E. Fielding. 1981. Regulation of human plasma lecithin:cholesterol acyltransferase activity by lipoprotein acceptor cholesteryl ester content. *Journal of Biological Chemistry* 256: 2102-2104.

Fielding, P.E., and C.J. Fielding. 1980. A cholesteryl ester transfer complex in human plasma. *Proceedings of the National Academy of Sciences* 77: 3327-3330.

Fourth Joint Task Force of the European Society of Cardiology and Other Societies on Cardiovascular Disease Prevention in Clinical Practice. 2007. European guidelines on cardiovascular disease prevention in clinical practice: Executive summary. *European Heart Journal* 28: 2375-2414.

Fransischini, G. 2001. Epidemiologic evidence for high-density lipoprotein cholesterol as a risk factor for coronary artery disease. *American Journal of Cardiology* 88 (12, Suppl. 1): 9-13.

Frick, M.H., O. Elo, K. Haapa, O.P. Heinonen, P. Heinsalmi, P. Helo, J.K. Huttunen, P. Kaitaniemi, P. Koskinen, V. Manninen, et al. 1987. Helsinki Heart Study: Primary prevention trial with gemfibrozil in middle-aged men with dyslipidemia. *New England Journal of Medicine* 317: 1237-1246.

Gibbons, L.W., and T.L. Mitchell. 1995. HDL cholesterol and exercise. *Your Patient and Fitness* 9 (4): 6-13.

Gill, J.M., A. Al-Mamari, W.R. Ferrell, S.J. Cleland, N. Sattar, C.J. Packard, J.R. Petrie, and M.J. Caslake. 2006. Effects of a moderate exercise session on postprandial lipoproteins, apolipoproteins and lipoprotein remnants in middle-aged men. *Atherosclerosis* 185: 87-96.

Gill, J.M., and A.E. Hardman. 2003. Exercise and postprandial lipid metabolism: An update on potential mechanisms and interactions with high-carbohydrate diets. *Journal of Nutritional Biochemistry* 14: 122-132.

Glomset, J.A., and K.R. Norum. 1973. The metabolic role of lecithin:cholesterol acyltransferase: Perspectives from pathology. *Advances in Lipid Research* 11: 1-65.

Gordon, D.J., J.L. Probstfield, R.L. Garrison, J.D. Neaton, W.P. Castelli, J.D. Knoke, D.R. Jacobs Jr., S. Bangdiwala, and H.A. Tyroler. 1989. High density lipoprotein cholesterol and cardiovascular disease: Four prospective American studies. *Circulation* 79: 8-20.

Green, P.H.R., and R.M. Glickman. 1981. Intestinal lipoprotein metabolism. *Journal of Lipid Research* 22: 1153-1173.

Grover, S.A., M. Kaouache, L. Joseph, P. Barter, and J. Davignon. 2009. Evaluating the incremental benefits of raising high-density lipoprotein cholesterol levels during lipid therapy after adjustment for the reductions in other blood lipid levels. *Archives of Internal Medicine* 169 (19, October 26): 1775-1780.

Grundy, S.M., J.I. Cleeman, C.N. Merz, H.B. Brewer Jr., L.T. Clark, D.B. Hunninghake, R.C. Pasternak, S.C. Smith Jr., N.J. Stone; National Heart, Lung, and Blood Institute; American College of Cardiology Foundation; American Heart Association. 2004. Implications of recent clinical trials for the National Cholesterol Education Program Adult Treatment Panel III guidelines. *Circulation* 110: 227-239.

Hagberg, J.M., R.E. Ferrell, L.I. Katzel, D.R. Dengel, J.D. Sorkin, and A.P. Goldberg. 1999. Apolipoprotein E genotype and exercise training–induced increases in plasma high-density lipoprotein (HDL)- and HDL2-cholesterol levels in overweight men. *Metabolism* 48 (8): 943-945.

Halbert, J.A., C.A. Silagy, P. Finucane, R.T. Withers, and P.A. Hamdorf. 1999. Exercise training and blood lipids in hyperlipidemic and normolipidemic adults: A meta-analysis of randomized, controlled trials. *European Journal of Clinical Nutrition* 53: 514-522.

Halverstadt, A., D.A. Phares, K.R. Wilund, A.P. Goldberg, and J.M. Hagberg. 2007. Endurance exercise training raises high-density lipoprotein cholesterol and lowers small low-density lipoprotein and very low-density lipoprotein independent of body fat phenotypes in older men and women. *Metabolism* 56 (4): 444-450.

Hamilton, R.L., M.C. Williams, C.J. Fielding, and R.J. Havel. 1976. Discoidal bilayer structure of nascent high density lipoproteins from perfused rat liver. *Journal of Clinical Investigation* 58: 667-680.

Haskell, W.L. 1984. The influence of exercise on the concentrations of triglyceride and cholesterol in human plasma. In *Exercise and sport sciences reviews,* edited by R.L. Terjung, pp. 205-244. Lexington, MA: D.C. Heath.

Heath, G.W., A.A. Ehsani, J.M. Hagberg, J.M. Hinderliter, and A.P. Goldberg. 1983. Exercise training improves lipoprotein lipid profiles in patients with coronary artery disease. *American Heart Journal* 105 (6): 889-895.

Hokanson, J.E., and M.A. Austin. 1996. Plasma triglyceride is a risk factor for cardiovascular disease independent of high-density lipoprotein cholesterol: A meta-analysis of population-based prospective studies. *Journal of Cardiovascular Risk* 3: 213-219.

Horowitz, B.S., I.J. Goldberg, J. Merab, T.M. Vanni, R. Ramakrishnan, and H.N. Ginsberg. 1993. Increased plasma and renal clearance of an exchangeable pool of apolipoprotein A-1 in subjects with low levels of high density lipoprotein cholesterol. *Journal of Clinical Investigation* 91: 1743-1752.

Hurley, B.F. 1989. Effects of resistive training on lipoprotein-lipid profiles: A comparison to aerobic exercise training. *Medicine and Science in Sports and Exercise* 6: 689-693.

Ingelsson, E., E.J. Schaefer, J.H. Contois, J.R. McNamara, L. Sullivan, M.J. Keyes, M.J. Pencina, C. Schoonmaker, P.W. Wilson, R.B. D'Agostino, and R.S. Vasan. 2007. Clinical utility of different lipid measures for prediction of coronary heart disease in men and women. *Journal of the American Medical Association* 298 (7, August 15): 776-785.

Jacobs, K.A., R.M. Krauss, J.A. Fattor, M.A. Horning, A.L. Friedlander, T.A. Bauer, T.A. Hagobian, E.E. Wolfel, and G.A. Brooks. 2006. Endurance training has little effect on active muscle free fatty acid, lipoprotein cholesterol, or triglyceride net balances. *American Journal of Physiology, Endocrinology, and Metabolism* 291: E656-665.

Kappelle, P.J., A. van Tol, B.H. Wolffenbuttel, and R.P. Dullaart. 2010. Cholesteryl ester transfer protein inhibition in cardiovascular risk management: Ongoing trials will end the confusion. *Cardiovascular Therapeutics,* July 14. [Epub ahead of print]

Kastelein, J.J., F. Akdim, E.S. Stroes, A.H. Zwinderman, M.L. Bots, A.F. Stalenhoef, F.L. Visseren, E.J. Sijbrands, M.D. Trip, E.A. Stein, D. Gaudet, R. Duivenvoorden, E.P. Veltri, A.D. Marais,

E. de Groot; ENHANCE investigators. 2008. Simvastatin with or without ezetimibe in familial hypercholesterolemia. *New England Journal of Medicine* 358: 1431-1443.

Katzmarzyk, P.T., A.S. Leon, T. Rankinen, T. Gagnon, J.S. Skinner, J.H. Wilmore, D.C. Rao, and C. Bouchard. 2001. Changes in blood lipids consequent to aerobic exercise training related to changes in body fatness and aerobic fitness. *Metabolism* 50: 841-848.

Kekki, M. 1980. Lipoprotein–lipase action determining plasma high density lipoprotein cholesterol level in adult normolipaemics. *Atherosclerosis* 37: 143-150.

Kelley, G.A., and K.S. Kelley. 2006a. Aerobic exercise and HDL2-C: A meta-analysis of randomized controlled trials. *Atherosclerosis* 184: 207-215.

Kelley, G.A., and K.S. Kelley. 2006b. Aerobic exercise and lipids and lipoproteins in men: A meta-analysis of randomized controlled trials. *Journal for Men's Health and Gender* 3 (1): 61-70.

Kelley, G.A., and K.S. Kelley. 2007a. Aerobic exercise and lipids and lipoproteins in children and adolescents: A meta-analysis of randomized controlled trials. *Atherosclerosis* 191: 447-453.

Kelley, G.A., and K.S. Kelley. 2007b. Effects of aerobic exercise on lipids and lipoproteins in adults with type 2 diabetes: A meta-analysis of randomized-controlled trials. *Public Health* 121: 643-655.

Kelley, G.A., and K.S. Kelley. 2009. Impact of progressive resistance training on lipids and lipoproteins in adults: A meta-analysis of randomized controlled trials. *Preventive Medicine* 48: 9-19.

Kelley, G.A., K.S. Kelley, and B. Franklin. 2006. Aerobic exercise and lipids and lipoproteins in patients with cardiovascular disease: A meta-analysis of randomized controlled trials. *Journal of Cardiopulmonary Rehabilitation* 26: 131-139.

Kelley, G.A., K.S. Kelley, S. Roberts, and W. Haskell. 2011. Comparison of aerobic exercise, diet, or both on lipids and lipoproteins in adults: A meta-analysis of randomized controlled trials. *Clinical Nutrition* Dec 9. [Epub ahead of print]

Kelley, G.A., K.S. Kelley, and Z.V. Tran. 2004. Aerobic exercise and lipids and lipoproteins in women: A meta-analysis of randomized controlled trials. *Journal of Women's Health (Larchmt)* 13: 1148-1164.

Kelley, G.A., K.S. Kelley, and Z.V. Tran. 2005a. Aerobic exercise, lipids and lipoproteins in overweight and obese adults: A meta-analysis of randomized controlled trials. *International Journal of Obesity (Lond)* 29: 881-893.

Kelley, G.A., K.S. Kelley, and Z.V. Tran. 2005b. Exercise, lipids, and lipoproteins in older adults: A meta-analysis. *Preventive Cardiology* 8: 206-214.

Kelley, G.A., K.S. Kelley, and Z.V. Tran. 2005c. Walking and non-HDL-C in adults: A meta-analysis of randomized controlled trials. *Preventive Cardiology* 8: 102-107.

Kiens, B., I. Jörgensen, S. Lewis, G. Jensen, H. Lithell, B. Vessby, S. Hoe, and P. Schnohr. 1980. Increased plasma HDL-cholesterol and apo A-I in sedentary middle-aged men after physical conditioning. *European Journal of Clinical Investigation* 10: 203-209.

Kodama, S., S. Tanaka, K. Saito, M. Shu, Y. Sone, F. Onitake, E. Suzuki, H. Shimano, S. Yamamoto, K. Kondo, Y. Ohashi, N. Yamada, and H. Sone. 2007. Effect of aerobic exercise training on serum levels of high-density lipoprotein cholesterol: A meta-analysis. *Archives of Internal Medicine* 167: 999-1008.

Kohl, H.W. III, N.F. Gordon, C.B. Scott, H. Vaandrager, and S.N. Blair. 1992. Musculoskeletal strength and serum lipid levels in men and women. *Medicine and Science in Sports and Exercise* 24: 1080-1087.

Kokkinos, P.F., J.C. Holland, P. Narayan, J.A. Colleran, C.O. Dotson, and V. Papademetriou. 1995. Miles run per week and high-density lipoprotein cholesterol levels in healthy, middle-aged men. *Archives of Internal Medicine* 155 (4): 415-420.

Kokkinos, P.F., B.F. Hurley, M.A. Smutok, C. Farmer, C. Reece, R. Shulman, C. Charabogos, J. Patterson, S. Will, J. Devane-Bell, and A.P. Goldberg. 1991. Strength training does not improve lipoprotein–lipid profiles in men at risk for CHD. *Medicine and Science in Sports and Exercise* 23 (10): 1134-1139.

Kokkinos, P.F., P. Narayan, J. Colleran, R.D. Fletcher, R. Lakshman, and V. Papademetriou. 1998. Effects of moderate intensity exercise on serum lipids in African-American men with severe systemic hypertension. *American Journal of Cardiology* 81 (6): 732-735.

Kraus, W.E., J.A. Houmard, B.D. Duscha, K.J. Knetzger, M.B. Wharton, J.S. McCartney, C.W. Bales, S. Henes, G.P. Samsa, J.D. Otvos, K.R. Kulkarni, and C.A. Slentz. 2002. Effects of the amount and intensity of exercise on plasma lipoproteins. *New England Journal of Medicine* 347: 1483-1492.

Kuusi, T., P. Saarinen, and E.A. Nikkila. 1980. Evidence for the role of hepatic endothelial lipase in the metabolism of plasma high density lipoprotein2 in man. *Atherosclerosis* 36: 589-593.

Leaf, D.A. 2003. The effect of physical exercise on reverse cholesterol transport. *Metabolism* 52: 950-957.

Leon, A.S., T. Rice, S. Mandel, J.P. Despres, J. Bergeron, J. Gagnon, D.C. Rao, J.S. Skinner, J.H. Wilmore, and C. Bouchard. 2000. Blood lipid response to 20 weeks of supervised exercise in a large biracial population: The HERITAGE Family Study. *Metabolism* 49: 513-520.

Leon, A.S., and O.A. Sanchez. 2001. Response of blood lipids to exercise training alone or combined with dietary intervention. *Medicine and Science in Sports and Exercise* 33 (Suppl. 6): S502-S515.

Lindheim, S.R., M. Notelovitz, E.B. Feldman, S. Larsen, F.Y. Khan, and R.A. Lobo. 1994. The independent effects of exercise and estrogen on lipids and lipoproteins in postmenopausal women. *Obstetrics and Gynecology* 83 (2): 167-171.

Mahlberg, F.H., and G.H. Rothblat. 1992. Cellular cholesterol efflux. *Journal of Biological Chemistry* 267: 4541-4550.

Mahley, R.W., and T.L. Innearity. 1983. Lipoprotein receptors and cholesterol homeostasis. *Biochimica et Biophysica Acta* 737: 197-222.

Manning, J.M., C.R. Dooly-Manning, K. White, I. Kampa, S. Silas, M. Kesselhaut, and M. Ruoff. 1991. Effects of a resistive training program on lipoprotein-lipid levels in obese women. *Medicine and Science in Sports and Exercise* 23: 1222-1226.

Marinangeli, C.P., K.A. Varady, and P.J. Jones. 2006. Plant sterols combined with exercise for the treatment of hypercholesterolemia: Overview of independent and synergistic mechanisms of action. *Journal of Nutritional Biochemistry* 17: 217-224.

Marrugat, J., R. Elosau, M. Covas, L. Molina, J. Rubies-Prat, and the Marathon investigators. 1996. Amount and intensity of physical activity, physical fitness, and serum lipids in men. *American Journal of Epidemiology* 143 (6): 562-569.

Marsh, J.B. 1976. Apoproteins of the lipoproteins in a nonrecirculating perfusate of rat liver. *Journal of Lipid Research* 17: 85-90.

Martin, S., R. Elosua, M.I. Covas, M. Pavesi, J. Vila, and J. Marrugat. 1999. Relationship of lipoprotein(a) levels to physical activity and family history of coronary heart disease. *American Journal of Public Health* 89: 383-385.

Mbalilaki, J.A., M.L. Hellènius, Z. Masesa, A.T. Høstmark, J. Sundquist, and S.B. Strømme. 2007. Physical activity and blood lipids in rural and urban Tanzanians. *Nutrition, Metabolism, and Cardiovascular Disease* 17: 344-348.

Mbalilaki, J.A., Z. Masesa, S.B. Strømme, A.T. Høstmark, J. Sundquist, P. Wändell, A. Rosengren, and M.L. Hellenius. 2010. Daily energy expenditure and cardiovascular risk in Masai, rural and urban Bantu Tanzanians. *British Journal of Sports Medicine* 44: 121-126.

McCrindle, B.W., E.M. Urbina, B.A. Dennison, M.L. Jacobson, J. Steinberger, A.P. Rocchini, L.L. Hayman, S.R. Daniels; American Heart Association Atherosclerosis, Hypertension, and Obesity in Youth Committee; American Heart Association Council of Cardiovascular Disease in the Young; American Heart Association Council on Cardiovascular Nursing. 2007. Drug therapy of high-risk lipid abnormalities in children and adolescents: A scientific statement from the American Heart Association Atherosclerosis, Hypertension, and Obesity in Youth Committee, Council of Cardiovascular Disease in the Young, with the Council on Cardiovascular Nursing. *Circulation* 115: 1948-1967.

McGoon, M.D. 1993. *Mayo Clinic heart book.* New York: Morrow.

Melchior, G.W., C.K. Castle, R.W. Murray, W.L. Blake, D.M. Dinh, and K.R. Marotti. 1994. Apolipoprotein A-1 metabolism in cholesterol ester transfer protein transgenic mice. *Journal of Biological Chemistry* 269: 8044-8051.

Mikhailidis, D.P., G.C. Sibbring, C.M. Ballantyne, G.M. Davies, and A.L. Catapano. 2007. Meta-analysis of the cholesterol-lowering effect of ezetimibe added to ongoing statin therapy. *Current Medical Research and Opinion* 23: 2009-2026.

Mohanka, M., M. Irwin, S.R. Heckbert, Y. Yasui, B. Sorensen, J. Chubak, S.S. Tworoger, C.M. Ulrich, and A. McTiernan. 2006. Serum lipoproteins in overweight/obese postmenopausal women: A one-year exercise trial. *Medicine and Science in Sports and Exercise* 38: 231-239.

Monda, K.L., C.M. Ballantyne, and K.E. North. 2009. Longitudinal impact of physical activity on lipid profiles in middle-aged adults: The Atherosclerosis Risk in Communities Study. *Journal of Lipid Research* 50: 1685-1691.

National Center for Health Statistics. 1995. *Health: United States.* Hyattsville, MD: Public Health Service.

National Cholesterol Education Program (NCEP) Expert Panel on Detection, Evaluation, and Treatment of High Blood Cholesterol in Adults (Adult Treatment Panel III). 2002. Third report of the National Cholesterol Education Program (NCEP) Expert Panel on Detection, Evaluation, and Treatment of High Blood Cholesterol in Adults (Adult Treatment Panel III) final report. *Circulation* 106: 3143-3421.

National Heart, Lung, and Blood Institute. 2002, September. *Third report of the National Cholesterol Education Program Expert Panel on the Detection, Evaluation, and Treatment of High Blood Cholesterol Levels in Adults (Adult Treatment Panel III).* National Cholesterol Education Program, National Heart, Lung, and Blood Institute, National Institutes of Health. NIH Publication No. 02-5215.

Nissen, S.E., J.C. Tardif, S.J. Nicholls, J.H. Revkin, C.L. Shear, W.T. Duggan, W. Ruzyllo, W.B. Bachinsky, G.P. Lasala, and E.M. Tuzcu. 2007. Effect of torcetrapib on the progression of coronary atherosclerosis. *New England Journal of Medicine* 356: 1304-1316.

Nordstrom, C.K., K.M. Dwyer, C.N. Merz, A. Shircore, and J.H. Dwyer. 2003. Leisure time physical activity and early atherosclerosis: The Los Angeles Atherosclerosis Study. *American Journal of Medicine* 115: 19-25.

Norum, K.R. 1984. Familial lecithin:cholesterol acyltransferase deficiency. In *Clinical and metabolic aspects of high density lipoproteins,* edited by N.E. Miller and G.J. Miller, pp. 297-318. Amsterdam: Elsevier.

Nye, E.R., K. Carlson, P. Kirstein, and S. Rössner. 1981. Changes in high density lipoprotein subfractions and other lipoproteins induced by exercise. *Clinica Chimica Acta* 113: 51-57.

O'Connor, G.T., C.H. Hennekens, W.C. Willett, S.Z. Goldhaber, R.S. Paffenbarger Jr., J.L. Breslow, I.M. Lee, and J.E. Buring. 1995. Physical exercise and reduced risk of nonfatal myocardial infarction. *American Journal of Epidemiology* 142 (11): 1147-1156.

Oschry, Y., and S. Eisenberg. 1982. Rat plasma lipoproteins: Re-evaluation of a lipoprotein system in an animal devoid of cholesteryl ester transfer activity. *Journal of Lipid Research* 23: 1099-1106.

Petitt, D.S., and K.J. Cureton. 2003. Effects of prior exercise on postprandial lipemia: A quantitative review. *Metabolism* 52: 418-424.

Prabhakaran, B., E.A. Dowling, J.D. Branch, D.P. Swain, and B.C. Leutholtz. 1999. Effect of 14 weeks of resistance training on lipid profile and body fat percentage in premenopausal women. *British Journal of Sports Medicine* 33: 190-195.

Ridker, P.M. 2009. Moving toward new statin guidelines in a post-JUPITER world: Principles to consider. *Current Atherosclerosis Reports* 11: 249-256.

Ridker, P.M., J.G. MacFadyen, F.A. Fonseca, J. Genest, A.M. Gotto, J.J. Kastelein, W. Koenig, P. Libby, A.J. Lorenzatti, B.G. Nordestgaard, J. Shepherd, J.T. Willerson, R.J. Glynn; JUPITER Study Group. 2009. Number needed to treat with rosuvastatin to prevent first cardiovascular events and death among men and women with low low-density lipoprotein cholesterol and elevated high-sensitivity C-reactive protein: Justification for the use of statins in prevention: An intervention trial evaluating rosuvastatin (JUPITER). *Circulatory and Cardiovascular Quality Outcomes* 2: 616-623.

Ring-Dimitriou, S., S.P. von Duvillard, B. Paulweber, M. Stadlmann, L.M. Lemura, K. Peak, and E. Mueller. 2007. Nine months aerobic fitness induced changes on blood lipids and lipoproteins in untrained subjects versus controls. *European Journal of Applied Physiology* 99: 291-299.

Robins, S.J., D. Collins, T. Wittes, V. Papademetriou, P.C. Deedwania, E.J. Schaefer, J.R. McNamara, M.L. Kashyap, J.M. Hershman, L.F. Wexler, H.B. Rubins; VA-HIT Study Group. 2001. Veterans Affairs High-Density Lipoprotein Intervention Trial. Relation of gemfibrozil treatment and lipid levels with major coronary events: VA-HIT: A randomized controlled trial. *Journal of the American Medical Association* 285: 1585-1591.

Robinson, J.G. 2010. Dalcetrapib: A review of phase II data. *Expert Opinion on Investigational Drugs* 19: 795-805.

Rubins, H.B., S.J. Robins, D. Collins, C.L. Fye, J.W. Anderson, M.B. Elam, F.H. Faas, E. Linares, E.J. Schaefer, G. Schectman, T.J. Wilt, and J. Wittes. 1999. Gemfibrozil for the secondary prevention of coronary heart disease in men with low levels of high-density lipoprotein cholesterol. Veterans Affairs High-Density Lipoprotein Cholesterol Intervention Trial Study Group. *New England Journal of Medicine* 341: 410-418.

Sazonov, V., J. Beetsch, H. Phatak, C. Wentworth, and M. Evans. 2010. Association between dyslipidemia and vascular events in patients treated with statins: Report from the UK General Practice Research Database. *Atherosclerosis* 208: 210-216.

Seals, D.R., J.M. Hagberg, B.F. Hurley, A.A. Ehsani, and J.O. Holloszy. 1984. Endurance training in older men and women. I. Cardiovascular responses to exercise. *Journal of Applied Physiology: Respiratory, Environmental and Exercise Physiology* 57 (4): 1024-1029.

Seip, R.L., K. Mair, T.G. Cole, and C.F. Semenkovich. 1997. Induction of human skeletal muscle lipoprotein lipase gene expression by short-term exercise is transient. *American Journal of Physiology* 272 (2 Pt 1): E255-E261.

Shepherd, J., and C.J. Packard. 1989. Lipoprotein metabolism. In *Human plasma lipoproteins,* edited by J.C. Fruchart and J. Shepherd. New York: de Gruyter.

Shepherd, J., C.J. Packard, J.M. Stewart, B.D. Vallance, T.D.V. Lawrie, and H.G. Morgan. 1980. The relationship between the cholesterol content and subfraction distribution of plasma high-density lipoproteins. *Clinica Chimica Acta* 101: 57-62.

Sierra-Johnson, J., R.M. Fisher, A. Romero-Corral, V.K. Somers, F. Lopez-Jimenez, J. Ohrvik, G. Walldius, M.L. Hellenius, and A. Hamsten. 2009. Concentration of apolipoprotein B is comparable with the apolipoprotein B/apolipoprotein A-I ratio and better than routine clinical lipid measurements in predicting coronary heart disease mortality: Findings from a multi-ethnic US population. *European Heart Journal* 30: 710-717.

Singhal, A., J.L. Trilk, N.T. Jenkins, K.A. Bigelman, and K.J. Cureton. 2009. Effect of intensity of resistance exercise on postprandial lipemia. *Journal of Applied Physiology* 106: 823-829.

Slentz, C.A., J.A. Houmard, J.L. Johnson, L.A. Bateman, C.J. Tanner, J.S. McCartney, B.D. Duscha, and W.E. Kraus. 2007. Inactivity, exercise training and detraining, and plasma lipoproteins. STRRIDE: A randomized, controlled study of exercise intensity and amount. *Journal of Applied Physiology* 103: 432-442.

Sorrentino, S., and U. Landmesser. 2005. Nonlipid-lowering effects of statins. *Current Treatment Options in Cardiovascular Medicine* 7: 459-466.

Spielmann, N., A.S. Leon, D.C. Rao, T. Rice, J.S. Skinner, C. Bouchard, and T. Rankinen. 2007. CETP genotypes and HDL-cholesterol phenotypes in the HERITAGE Family Study. *Physiological Genomics* 31: 25-31.

Stefanick, M.L., S. Mackey, M. Sheehan, N. Ellsworth, W.L. Haskell, and P.D. Wood. 1998. Effects of diet and exercise in men and postmenopausal women with low levels of HDL cholesterol and high levels of LDL cholesterol. *New England Journal of Medicine* 339: 12-20.

Stewart, D.J., and K.J. Cureton. 2003. Effects of prior exercise on post-prandial lipemia: A quantitative review. *Metabolism* 52: 418-424.

Tall, A.R. 1986. Plasma lipid transfer proteins. *Journal of Lipid Research* 27: 361-367.

Tall, A.R. 1990. Plasma high density lipoproteins. *Journal of Clinical Investigation* 86: 379-384.

Tall, A.R., X. Jiang, Y. Luo, and D. Silver. 2000. 1999 George Lyman Duff Memorial Lecture: Lipid transfer proteins, HDL metabolism, and atherogenesis. *Arteriosclerosis, Thrombosis, and Vascular Biology* 20: 1185-1188.

Tall, A.R., and D.S. Small. 1978. Plasma high density lipoproteins. *New England Journal of Medicine* 299: 1232-1236.

Taylor, A.J., T.C. Villines, E.J. Stanek, P.L. Devine, L. Griffen, M. Miller, N.J. Weissman, and M. Turco. 2009. Extended-release niacin or ezetimibe and carotid intima-media thickness. *New England Journal of Medicine* 361: 2113-2122.

Thompson, P.D. 1990. What do muscles have to do with lipoproteins? *Circulation* 81: 1428-1430.

Thompson, P.D., E.M. Cullinane, S.P. Sady, M.M. Flynn, D.N. Bernier, M.A. Kantor, A.L. Saritelli, and P.N. Herbert. 1988. Modest changes in high-density lipoprotein concentration and metabolism with prolonged exercise training. *Circulation* 78: 25-34.

Thompson, P.D., S.M. Yurgalevitch, M.M. Flynn, J.M. Zmuda, D. Spannaus-Martin, A. Saritelli, L. Bausserman, and P.N. Herbert. 1997. Effect of prolonged training without weight loss on high-density lipoprotein metabolism in overweight men. *Metabolism* 46: 217-223.

Tortora, G.J., and S.R. Grabowski. 1993. *Principles of anatomy and physiology.* 7th edition. New York: Harper-Collins College.

Tran, Z.V., A. Weltman, G.V. Glass, and D.P. Mood. 1983. The effects of exercise on blood lipids and lipoproteins: A meta-analysis of studies. *Medicine and Science in Sports and Exercise* 15 (5): 393-402.

Tucker, L.A., and L.J. Silvester. 1996. Strength training and hypercholesterolemia: An epidemiological study of 8499 employed men. *American Journal of Health Promotion* 11 (1): 35-41.

Varady, K.A., A.H. Houweling, and P.J. Jones. 2007. Effect of plant sterols and exercise training on cholesterol absorption and synthesis in previously sedentary hypercholesterolemic subjects. *Translational Research* 149: 22-30.

Vislocky, L.M., M.A. Pikosky, K.H. Rubin, S. Vega-López, P.C. Gaine, W.F. Martin, T.L. Zern, I.E. Lofgren, M.L. Fernandez, and N.R. Rodriguez. 2009. Habitual consumption of eggs does not alter the beneficial effects of endurance training on plasma lipids and lipoprotein metabolism in untrained men and women. *Journal of Nutritional Biochemistry* 20: 26-34.

Von Eckardstein, A., Y. Huang, and G. Assmann. 1994. Physiological role and clinical relevance of high-density lipoprotein subclasses. *Current Opinion in Lipidology* 5: 404-416.

Williams, P.T., R.M. Krauss, K.M. Vranizan, J.J. Albers, and P.D. Wood. 1992. Effects of weight-loss by exercise and by diet on apolipoproteins A-I and A-II and the particle-size distribution of high-density lipoproteins in men. *Metabolism* 41 (4): 441-449.

Williams, P.T., M.L. Stefanick, K.M. Vranizan, and P.D. Wood. 1994. The effects of weight loss by exercise or by dieting on plasma high-density lipoprotein (HDL) levels in men with low, intermediate, and normal-to-high HDL at baseline. *Metabolism* 43 (7): 917-924.

Windmueller, H.G., and A.L. Wu. 1981. Biosynthesis of plasma apolipoproteins by rat small intestine without dietary or biliary fat. *Journal of Biological Chemistry* 256: 3013-3016.

Winkler, K.E., and J.B. Marsh. 1989. Characterization of nascent high density lipoprotein subfractions from perfusates of rat liver. *Journal of Lipid Research* 30: 979-996.

Wood, P.D., W.L. Haskell, S.N. Blair, P.T. Williams, R.M. Krauss, F.T. Lindgren, J.J. Albers, P.H. Ho, and J.W. Farquhar. 1983. Increased exercise level and plasma lipoprotein concentrations: A one-year, randomized, controlled study in sedentary, middle-aged men. *Metabolism* 32: 31-39.

Wu, A.L., and H.G. Windmueller. 1979. Relative contributions by liver and intestine to individual plasma apolipoproteins in the rat. *Journal of Biological Chemistry* 254: 7316-7322.

Yurgalevitch, S.M., A.M. Kriska, T.K. Welty, O. Go, D.C. Robbins, and B.V. Howard. 1998. Physical activity and lipids and lipoproteins in American Indians ages 45-74. *Medicine and Science in Sports and Exercise* 30: 543-549.

Ziegler, S., G. Schaller, F. Mittermayer, J. Pleiner, J. Mihaly, A. Niessner, B. Richter, S. Steiner-Boeker, M. Penak, B. Strasser, and M. Wolzt. 2006. Exercise training improves low-density lipoprotein oxidability in untrained subjects with coronary artery disease. *Archives of Physical Medicine and Rehabilitation* 87: 265-269.

Physical Activity and Obesity

I am resolved to grow fat, and look young till forty.

• John Dryden (1631-1700) •

The Maiden Queen, Act III, Scene 1

What have I done to merit these cruel sufferings? Many things;
you have ate and drank too freely, and too much indulged those legs of yours
in their indolence . . . the quantity of meat and drink proper for a man,
who takes a reasonable degree of exercise, would be too much for another,
who never takes any.

• Benjamin Franklin (1706-1790) •

Dialogue Between Franklin and the Gout Midnight, 22 October, 1780 (Matthews 1914)

CHAPTER OBJECTIVES

▸ Describe the public health burden of obesity, including its cost, prevalence, and trends in population groups and its role in the risk of cardiovascular diseases and diabetes

▸ Identify and discuss the components of energy balance

▸ Identify the major health risks of obesity

▸ Discuss the methods used to measure body fatness in clinical and population studies

▸ Describe the known and hypothesized effects of physical activity on adiposity

▸ Describe and evaluate the strength of evidence that physical activity and exercise training reduce the health risks associated with obesity, protect against excess weight gain, contribute to fat loss, and help maintain weight loss after dieting

Overweight and **obesity** are characterized by excess body fat resulting from a positive energy balance (i.e., an energy intake greater than energy expenditure). As early as the 10th century, the Persian physician Avicenna viewed obesity as a health hazard, devoting an entire chapter to it in his *Canon of Medicine* (Bassem 1992). Although being overweight was socially valued during the economic austerity of 17th-century Europe, as portrayed by the English dramatist John Dryden in the quotation that opens this chapter, it has become a 21st-century burden to the public health of developed nations. Obesity now co-occurs with undernutrition in many developing nations.

▶ **THE WORLD** Health Organization (WHO) has coined the term "globesity" to refer to the global epidemic of overweight and obesity.

The scientific advisory committee for the Dietary Guidelines for Americans concluded that most Americans consume more calories than they need, and this excess consumption is not likely to change in the near future (Dietary Guidelines Advisory Committee 2005).

Environments in many nations today are "obesogenic" largely because of relentless advertising of food that cues the desire to eat, easy access to affordable high-energy foods, and sedentary lifestyles. Thus, overweight and obesity in modern humans who are genetically prone to gain weight are biologically normal, though unhealthy. Experts agree that so-called "thrifty genes" have evolved in humans to defend against fat loss. Food restriction and fat depletion led to a "hungry brain" that is motivated to increase energy intake and reduce energy expenditure through decreased activity (Zheng et al. 2009).

Obesity experts usually attribute excess weight gain to overeating more than to insufficient physical activity, but the relative importance of eating less or exercising more as a means to stall or reverse global obesity is not yet known. Both are undoubtedly necessary to close the *energy gap,* which is the change in energy expenditure relative to energy intake needed to reverse excess body weight in a population (Hill et al. 2003). The energy gap was initially estimated to be about 100 kilocalories (kcal) per day among young U.S. adults. However, studies that used doubly labeled water to estimate energy expenditure in nearly 1000 children aged 4 to 18, as well as 1400 adults aged 18 to 98, found that each 10% increase in energy intake was associated with an increase in body weight of about 4.5% in children and 7.1% in adults (Swinburn et al. 2006, 2009). That translates to an energy gap of 400 kcal/day needed to reverse the population weight gain by U.S. adults during the past 40 years (Heymsfield 2009). However, two-thirds of the weight gain in those studies was fat-free, that is lean, mass (3.1%/4.5% in children and 4.8%/7.1% in adults) (Swinburn et al. 2009). The goal of public health is to reduce excess body fat, not lean mass. Physical activity is uniquely suited to that purpose because it can preserve fat-free mass while burning excess calories.

Estimates are that our prehistoric ancestors who relied on hunting and gathering for their subsistence expended about 1200 kcal a day in physical activity (nearly 22 kcal/kg of body weight) while consuming about 2900 kcal. Thus, their *subsistence efficiency* (energy consumption divided by energy expended in daily living) was about 2.4:1 (i.e., 2900 kcal/1200 kcal). Today, sedentary humans in wealthy societies typically consume about 2030 kcal each day but expend only about 580 kcal (less than 9 kcal/kg), a subsistence efficiency of 3.5:1 (Cordain, Gotshall, and Eaton 1998; Eaton and Eaton 2003). One theory is that a return to a ratio near 2:1, achievable by increasing daily physical activity by 500 kcal, would slow worldwide obesity by resetting resting metabolic rate (RMR) at the rate of our prehistoric ancestors; they had a RMR believed to be 15% higher than that of today's sedentary adults (Eaton and Eaton 2003). Most people could accomplish this by adding an extra hour of moderate-to-vigorous physical activity each day (Saris et al. 2003). The WHO recommendation that people's daily physical activity level (PAL) should be 1.75 times their RMR when averaged across the day comes close to achieving this level. Among adults, the highest measured PAL occurring under normal life conditions is about 2.5 (Westerterp and Plasqui 2004). Most adults achieve their PAL by moderately intense physical activities such as walking, while children achieve theirs by a combination of high- and low-intensity physical activities. Sedentary adults in the United States have a RMR of about 1450 kcal, so adding an extra 500 kcal in physical activity each day to their current expenditure of 580 kcal would yield a PAL of nearly 1.75 (Eaton and Eaton 2003). This would require, though, nearly a doubling of people's current physical activity levels! We'll see in chapter 17 why this is unlikely to happen without drastic social or environmental change.

The concept of *subsistence efficiency* complements the hypothesis of *high energy flux* stemming from research conducted by world-renowned nutritionist Jean Mayer over 50 years ago. Based on his study of male jute mill workers in India, Mayer observed that food intake was high in sedentary clerks and supervisors, who were heavy, but also in laborers, who were lean (Mayer, Roy, and Mitra 1956). His observation led to the hypothesis that healthy body weight is best maintained at high levels of both energy intake and energy expenditure (i.e., high energy flux or throughput). Some research has suggested that during aging, people who maintain a high energy flux with high physical activity have higher RMR because of higher body density (i.e., more muscle and less fat) or elevated activity by the sympathetic nervous system (Bell et al. 2004). Although it is possible to maintain body weight at low energy flux, most people are not able or willing to restrict their eating enough to do this. Because RMR naturally decreases as people get smaller, the optimal way to reduce obesity and maintain a high energy flux is to increase physical activity as people lose body weight (Hill 2006).

The U.S. National Institutes of Health (NIH) regards obesity as a chronic disease that develops from an interaction of a person's genotype (i.e., the DNA), the environment, and the person's dietary and physical inactivity habits (National Heart, Lung, and Blood Institute 1998). Excess weight gain manifests its health risks mostly during adulthood, contributing to chronic but reversible diseases. People who are overweight or obese have higher risks of developing hypertension; hypercholesterolemia; type 2 diabetes; coronary heart disease (CHD); stroke; gallbladder disease; osteoarthritis; and cancers of the breast (in postmenopausal women), uterus, esophagus, colon, pancreas, and kidney. In adolescents, obesity (body mass index [BMI] ≥95th percentile) roughly triples the risks for high levels of blood sugar, blood pressure, and triglycerides and low levels of high-density lipoprotein cholesterol (HDL-C), the "good" cholesterol (Cook et al. 2003). Similarly in younger children, obesity doubles or triples the risk of high blood pressure and low HDL-C (Messiah et al. 2008). White and Hispanic, but not black, adolescents who have a large waist circumference (another index of obesity) are more likely to also have high triglycerides, high blood sugar (boys only), and low HDL-C (Johnson et al. 2009).

Based on cumulative data from the National Health and Nutrition Examination Survey III and the Framingham Heart Study, moderately obese (BMI >32.5 kg/m^2) middle-aged men and women have about double the risk of hypertension, triple the risk of type 2 diabetes, and a one-year reduction in life expectancy compared with their nonobese peers (Thompson et al. 1999). After adjustment for other risk factors, the risk of type 2 diabetes among U.S. adults aged 18 to 44 years increases by 6% for each 5 to 8 lb of body mass (Hillier and Pedula 2001). According to data from the Behavioral Risk Factor Surveillance System (BRFSS) maintained by the Centers for Disease Control and Prevention, obese U.S. adults with a BMI of 40 or higher (6% of U.S. adults in 2006) have about seven times higher risk of diabetes, six times higher risk of hypertension, double the risk of high cholesterol, and four times the risk of self-rated fair or poor health compared to adults with normal weight (Mokdad et al. 2003). Obese persons also have five to six times the risk

of developing gallstones (Erlinger 2000). Finally, obese men and women are more likely to die younger from any cause, compared with persons of normal weight (Berrington de Gonzalez et al. 2010).

Obesity cost the United States an estimated $147 billion in 2008, nearly 10% of all medical costs (Finkelstein et al. 2009). In a simulation model of population data, medical costs of obesity were higher than for smoking until people reached their mid 50s, after which smokers had higher costs. However, lifetime costs were still higher in people who were obese because smokers died at younger ages (van Baal et al. 2008).

The number of annual deaths in the United States among adults aged 18 years or older attributable to obesity in 1991 was estimated to be approximately 280,000 (Allison et al. 1999). The number of deaths in the United States attributed to obesity seems to have declined since then (Flegal et al. 2005, 2007), perhaps in part because of better disease prevention. Except for diabetes, major risk factors for cardiovascular disease (high cholesterol, hypertension, and smoking) have declined in U.S. adults during the past 30 years, even more so in people who are obese (Gregg et al. 2005). We also now know that early studies likely overestimated mortality risk attributable to obesity because they did not adequately account for other mortality risk factors that differ according to people's weight status. For example, after adjustment for age, sex, race, smoking, and alcohol use, obesity (BMI ≥30) was associated with only about 112,000 excess deaths in 2000 when compared with the number for normal-weight people (BMI 18.5 to 25) (Flegal et al. 2005). However, there is not agreement among researchers about the true number of deaths attributable to obesity each year.

Obesity risks also differ by disease. In 2004, obesity was associated with over 112,000 excess deaths from cardiovascular diseases and nearly 14,000 excess deaths combined from colon, breast, uterine, ovarian (obesity isn't strongly linked to ovarian cancer), kidney, and pancreatic cancers; but it was not linked with other cancers or other causes of death. When overweight and obese groups were combined, they had about 61,000 more deaths from diabetes and kidney disease than did people of normal weight (Flegal et al. 2007). None of the national studies have controlled for other mortality risks associated with overweight or obesity such as hypertension, dyslipidemia, weight loss or gain, and physical inactivity. However, among patients who have coronary artery disease, only underweight (BMI <20) and very obese (BMI ≥35) patients have increased risks for dying from cardiovascular disease (Romero-Corral et al. 2006).

A recent review of 10 prospective cohort studies of intentional weight loss by adults in the United States, Great Britain, and Finland found that mortality risk was reduced only among obese people who were also unhealthy (i.e., had chronic disease or risk factors other than obesity) at baseline (relative risk [RR] 0.84; 95% confidence interval [CI]: 0.73-0.97). Weight loss did not affect mortality risk among those who were otherwise healthy or were just overweight (Harrington, Gibson, and Cottrell 2009). Most of the studies adjusted for physical activity levels. However, they did not examine whether physical activity or fitness modified the effect of weight loss on mortality. No randomized controlled trials have examined whether weight loss through diet, exercise, or both among overweight or obese adults will prolong life expectancy. However, as we'll discuss later in the chapter, physical activity and physical fitness each cut mortality risk in people who are overweight. So, being fit

may protect the health of people who are as much as 30 lb (13.6 kg) overweight.

Magnitude of the Problem

According to a recent summary of global statistics from the WHO, 1.6 billion people aged 15 or older were overweight in 2005; 400 million were obese. About 20 million children under the age of 5 years were overweight. Other estimates show that between 1980 and 2008, mean BMI worldwide increased by 0.4 kg/m² per decade among men and 0.5 kg/m² per decade among women. The United States had the highest BMI of high-income countries. In 2008, 205 million men and 297 million women worldwide were judged to be obese (Finucane 2011). The past decade was the first time in recorded history that the number of people who were overweight equaled the number of people who were underfed and underweight worldwide (see figure 9.1). For example, Saudi Arabia and the United Kingdom have the 4th and 22nd highest rates of adult obesity worldwide, but they also rank in the top 20 nations in the percentage of the population that is underweight. Overweight and obesity are not problems just in wealthy nations; they have emerged as health threats in

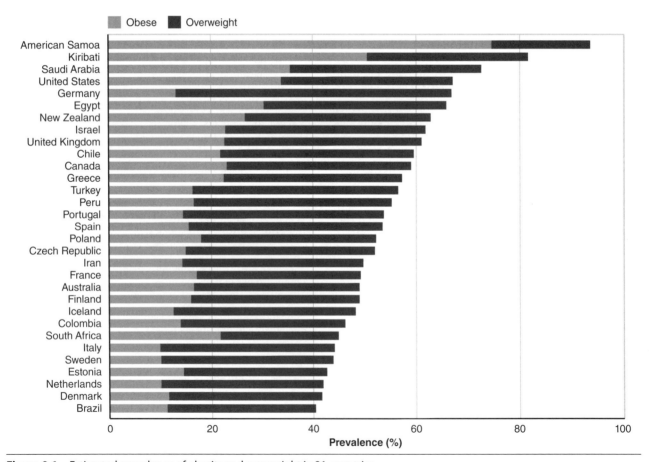

Figure 9.1   Estimated prevalence of obesity and overweight in 31 countries.

Data from WHO 2006.

low- and middle-income nations, especially in urban areas. The WHO projects that by 2015, 2.3 billion adults will be overweight and more than 700 million will be obese.

In the United States, 68% of adults 20 years or older are overweight, based on measured weight, including the 34% of adults who are considered obese; 15% of children ages 6 to 11 and 18% of youths 12 to 19 years are obese (Flegal et al. 2010; National Center for Health Statistics 2009). The prevalence of overweight and obesity in the United States increased steadily after the 1970s, finally leveling off at record highs during the past 10 years in women and the past five years in men (Flegal et al. 2010). Just 15 years ago, half as many American adults were classified as obese. Figure 9.2 illustrates the epidemic of obesity in the United States, spreading from the South to the West and North from 2004 to 2010. Between 2008-2010, only one state (Colorado) had a prevalence of obesity less than 20%. Thirty-two states had a rate of at least 25%; 12 states (Alabama, Arkansas, Kentucky, Louisiana, Michigan, Missouri, Mississippi, Oklahoma, South Carolina, Tennessee, Texas, and West Virginia) had a

rate of 30% or more. These estimates from the BRFSS come from people's self-reported weights, which are underestimates compared to measured weights.

The ongoing National Health and Nutrition Examination Survey (NHANES), a series of cross-sectional national surveys conducted every five years or so since 1960 and now conducted yearly, estimated that during the period from 1976 to 1980, about 24% of men and 27% of women were 20% or more above desirable weight based on 1983 Metropolitan Life Insurance Company actuarial height and weight tables. **Desirable weight** on those tables was the weight that predicted normal life expectancy according to body frame, age, and sex. In the period between 1988 and 1991, those rates had increased by nearly 30%, up to 31.3% for men and 34.1% for women (Kuczmarski 1992; Kuczmarski et al. 1994; Williamson 1993). Thus, compared with those in past surveys, adults had gained about 3.6 kg of body weight. Desirable weight has been replaced by BMI for use in contemporary surveys.

The rates of obesity are highest in groups of people who have less formal education and lower income and in some

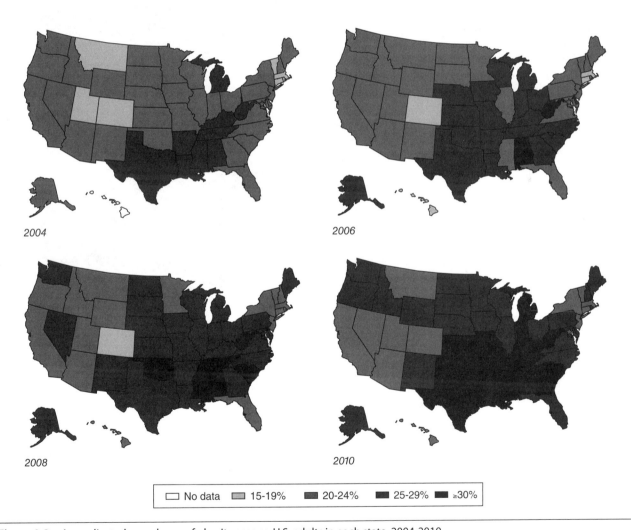

2004

2006

2008

2010

☐ No data   ▨ 15-19%   ▨ 20-24%   ■ 25-29%   ■ ≥30%

Figure 9.2 Age-adjusted prevalence of obesity among U.S. adults in each state, 2004-2010.

Reprinted from Centers for Disease Control. Available: http://www.slideshare.net/nrcpara/cdc-obesity-maps

minority groups, especially American Indians or Alaska Natives and African American and Mexican American women (see figures 9.3 and 9.4).

The National Longitudinal Survey of Youth, a prospective cohort study of 8270 children aged 4 to 12 years conducted from 1986 to 1998, reported steady increases in the prevalence of obesity (defined as greater than the 95th percentile of age- and sex-specific BMI using 1970s-era norms) during that time, doubling the prevalence rates to 21.5% in African American and to 21.8% in Hispanic youth and rising by half to 12.3% in white youth (Strauss and Pollack 2001). According to the NHANES, the prevalence rate of obesity in youth was 10.4% among 2- to 5-year-olds, 15.3% among 6- to 11-year-olds, and 15.5% among 12- to 19-year-olds in 1999 to 2000 compared to rates of 7.2%, 11.3%, and 10.5%, respectively, in 1988 to 1994. Gains were comparatively largest among non-Hispanic black and Mexican American adolescents (Ogden et al. 2002). In contrast, obesity rates in American Indian youths 5 to 17 years of age increased from 24% in 1995-1996 to 28% in 2002-2003 (Zephier et al. 2006). Among U.S. 4-year-old children in 2005, the rate of obesity in American Indian or Native Alaskans (31%) was double the rates in non-Hispanic white (16%) or Asian (13%) children and half again higher than the rates in non-Hispanic black (21%) and Hispanic (22%) children (Anderson and Whitaker 2009). According to the Pediatric Nutrition Surveillance System (PedNSS) of the Centers for Disease Control and Prevention (CDC), the prevalence of obesity in low-income, preschool-aged children increased from 12.4% in 1998 to 14.5% in 2003 (Centers for Disease Control and Prevention 2009). It leveled off at 14.6% in 2008 except among

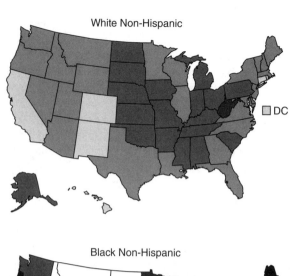

White Non-Hispanic

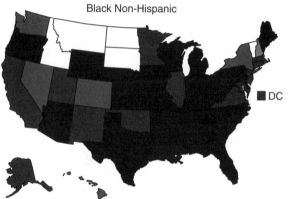

Black Non-Hispanic

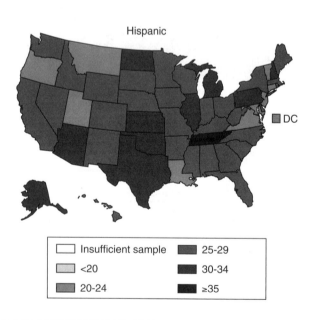

Hispanic

Insufficient sample	25-29
<20	30-34
20-24	≥35

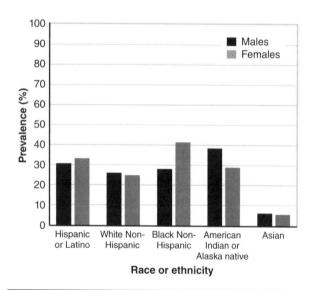

Figure 9.3 Age-adjusted prevalence of obesity in U.S. adults ages 18 and over by sex and race.

Data from Centers for Disease Control 2009.

Figure 9.4 Age-adjusted state-specific prevalence of U.S. adults considered obese, by black/white race or Hispanic ethnicity, based on data from the 2006-2008 Behavioral Risk Factor Surveillance System.

Reprinted from the Centers for Disease Control 2009.

American Indian or Alaska Native children, who had the highest prevalence (21.2%) compared to Hispanic (18.5%), non-Hispanic white (12.6%), non-Hispanic black (11.8%), and Asian or Pacific Islander (12.3%) children.

Childhood obesity (BMI ≥95th percentile) tracks into adulthood. The Bogalusa Heart Study observed nearly 2400 children aged 5 to 14 for 17 years into young adulthood. Among the obese children, 65% of white girls and 84% of black girls were obese (BMI ≥30) as adults. Those rates were 71% for white boys and 82% for black boys (Freedman et al. 2005). See figure 9.5.

It is discouraging that the U.S. population failed to meet the *Healthy People 2010* objective of lowering obesity to only 15% of adults and 5% of children and youth 6 to 19 years of age. However, the growth in rates of overweight and obesity in adults appears to have leveled off during the past few years (Ogden et al. 2006, 2007a). Likewise, overweight among American schoolchildren has hit a plateau of about 32% (Ogden, Carroll, and Flegal 2008).

▷ **SIXTY-SEVEN PERCENT** of adults and 32% of youths in the United States are overweight; the prevalence of obesity nearly tripled the past 20 years to 34% in adults and 17% in youths. The economic burden of obesity is $147 billion a year, nearly 10% of the national health care budget.

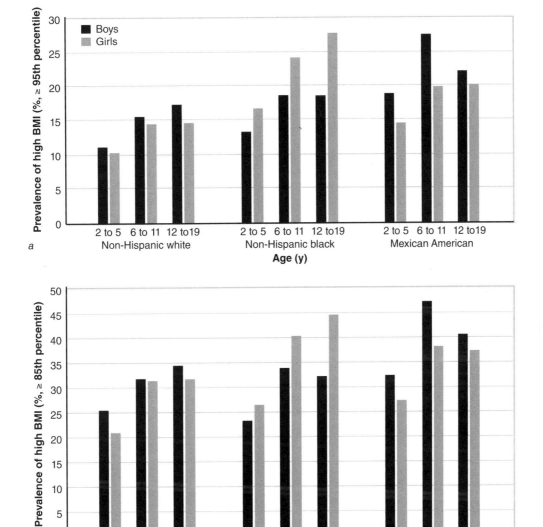

Figure 9.5 Prevalence of (a) obesity and (b) overweight in children and adolescents by sex, age, and race/ethnicity. United States: 2003-2006.

Data from Ogden, Carroll, and Flegal 2008.

Health Risks of Obesity

Hypertension

Gallbladder disease

Hypercholesterolemia

Osteoarthritis

Type 2 diabetes

Cancer (uterus, prostate, breast, colon)

Coronary heart disease

Stroke

Treatment of Overweight and Obesity

As yet unknown interactions between genes, behaviors, and the environment are surely important influences on obesity (Agurs-Collins and Bouchard 2008; Rankinen et al. 2009). Nonetheless, most obesity is the result of overeating and too little physical activity. Those behaviors are mainly under people's control, but preventing and treating obesity by changing people's habits is challenging.

Improvements in chronic disease risk factors can occur with just a 2% to 3% reduction in excess body weight. The average weight loss in dietary interventions with people who are obese is about 10 kg (22 lb) over an average period of 18 weeks; two-thirds of the loss is maintained for one year, but pretreatment weight is regained within three to five years (Foreyt and Goodrich 1994). Clinical weight loss trials show that obesity drugs are effective only when used in combination with a healthy diet and regular exercise, resulting in at best an additional loss of 5 lb (2.3 kg) or so beyond that with diet and exercise alone. The only drug currently approved by the Food and Drug Administration (FDA) in the long-term treatment of obesity is orlistat, a lipase inhibitor that reduces the digestion and absorption of fat and is marketed in the United States as Xenical and Alli (an over-the-counter version). The FDA continues to monitor reports of liver disease and pancreas inflammation in people taking orlistat. Sibutramine, which blocks reuptake of monoamines in the brain and suppresses appetite, was marketed in the United States as Meridia but was withdrawn from the market by the FDA in October 2010 because of adverse cardiovascular events (heart attacks, stroke, and elevated blood pressure). The use of the serotonin agonists dexfenfluramine and fenfluramine, alone or combined with the stimulant phentermine, is not recommended by the FDA because of evidence suggesting increased risk of pulmonary hypotension and valvular heart disease. A decision by the FDA about approval of Qnexa, an anti-seizure drug that combines phentermine with topiramate, also suppresses appetite and is under review by the FDA.

The NIH expert panel on obesity and overweight (National Heart, Lung, and Blood Institute 1998) reached these conclusions, though updates are expected in the near future:

- Physical activity is a clinically accepted approach to weight loss, as are low-calorie diets and lower-fat diets, behavior therapy, pharmacotherapy, surgery, and combinations of these techniques.

- For most overweight people, the initial goal of a prudent weight loss program is to lose about 10% of weight over a period of six months. Among people with BMIs in the range of 27 to 35, that goal can be achieved by a decrease of 300 to 500 kcal per day, which will result in weight losses of about 0.5 to 1 lb (0.2-0.5 kg) per week. For obese people with BMIs over 35, deficits of up to 500 to 1000 kcal per day are required to achieve those goals. After six months, the rate of weight loss usually declines, and weight tends to stabilize at a plateau because of the reduction in basal metabolic rate that results from the lower body mass.

- Lost weight is usually regained unless a weight maintenance program consisting of dietary therapy, physical activity, and behavior therapy is continued indefinitely. After six months of successful weight loss, efforts to maintain weight loss should be undertaken.

▷ **WITHOUT SUSTAINED** physical activity, the average weight loss after dieting among people who are obese is about 10 kg (22 lb); one-third is gained back within a year, and nearly all is gained back within three to five years.

Assessing and Defining Overweight and Obesity

Though the most accurate methods of assessing body fat require laboratory equipment, Quetelet's **body mass index (BMI)** and relative weight are typically used to estimate overweight and obesity in epidemiologic studies because they are easy to assess in large numbers of subjects. Relative weight is calculated by dividing body weight by the midpoint of desirable weight for a person judged to have a medium frame as recommended in the 1959 or 1983 Metropolitan Life tables. For many years, a body weight of 20% or more above desirable body weight was viewed as the threshold for health risk. That equates to a BMI of 27.8 for men and 27.3 for women (Kuczmarski 1992). More recently, the NIH defined people as overweight when BMI is in the range of 25 to 29.9 kg/m^2 and as obese when BMI equals or exceeds 30 kg/m^2 (National Heart, Lung, and Blood Institute 1998). Hence, someone can be overweight but not obese, but an obese person is also overweight. Obesity is further categorized as class I (BMI, 30-34.9), class II (BMI, 35-39.9), and class III (BMI, equal to or greater than 40). Weight classifications by BMI are shown in table 9.1. Table 9.2 converts selected heights and weights to BMI. For example, a BMI of 30 equates to being about 30 lb (13.6 kg) overweight.

Table 9.1   Classification of Overweight and Obesity by BMI

	Obesity class	BMI (kg/m^2)
Underweight		>18.5
Normal		18.5-24.9
Overweight		25.0-29.9
Obesity	I	30.0-34.9
	II	35.0-39.9
Extreme obesity	III	≥40

Reprinted from National Institutes of Health 1998.

Table 9.2   Selected BMI Units Categorized by Inches (cm) and Pounds (kg)

Height in inches (cm)	BMI 25 kg/m^2	BMI 27 kg/m^2	BMI 30 kg/m^2
	Body weight in pounds (kg)		
58 (147.32)	119 (53.98)	129 (58.51)	143 (64.86)
59 (149.86)	124 (56.25)	133 (60.33)	148 (67.13)
60 (152.40)	128 (58.06)	138 (62.60)	153 (69.40)
61 (154.94)	132 (59.87)	143 (64.86)	158 (71.67)
62 (157.48)	136 (61.69)	147 (66.68)	164 (74.39)
63 (160.02)	141 (63.96)	152 (68.95)	169 (76.66)
64 (162.56)	145 (65.77)	157 (71.22)	174 (78.93)
65 (165.10)	150 (68.04)	162 (73.48)	180 (81.65)
66 (167.64)	155 (70.31)	167 (75.75)	186 (84.37)
67 (170.18)	159 (72.12)	172 (78.02)	191 (86.64)
68 (172.72)	164 (74.39)	177 (80.29)	197 (89.36)
69 (175.26)	169 (76.66)	182 (82.56)	203 (92.08)
70 (177.80)	174 (78.93)	188 (85.28)	207 (93.90)
71 (180.34)	179 (81.19)	193 (87.54)	215 (97.52)
72 (182.88)	184 (83.46)	199 (90.27)	221 (100.25)
73 (185.42)	189 (85.73)	204 (92.53)	227 (102.97)
74 (187.96)	194 (86.00)	210 (95.26)	233 (105.69)
75 (190.50)	200 (90.72)	216 (97.98)	240 (108.86)
76 (193.04)	205 (92.99)	221 (100.25)	246 (111.59)

Metric conversion formula = weight (kg)/height (m)^2	Nonmetric conversion formula = [weight (lb)/height (in.)^2] × 704.5
Example of BMI calculation: A person who weighs 78.93 kg and is 177 cm tall has a BMI of 25: weight (78.93 kg)/height (1.77 m)^2 = 25	Example of BMI calculation: A person who weighs 164 lb and is 68 in. (or 5 ft 8 in.) tall has a BMI of 25: [weight (164 lb)/height (68 in.)^2] × 704.5 = 25

Patterning of Body Fat and Disease Risk

Excess fat in the abdomen out of proportion to total body fat is another risk factor for chronic diseases associated with obesity. **Waist circumference** is positively correlated with abdominal fat content and provides a clinically acceptable measurement for assessing a patient's abdominal fat content before and during weight loss treatment. Girth at the waist greater than 102 cm (40 in.) for men and 88 cm (35 in.) for women is considered risky. For children ages 6 to 19, a girth (either the narrowest waist circumference or midway between the iliac crest and the floating rib) at the 90th percentile is commonly used to define high risk. Several risk factors for cardiovascular disease are doubled or tripled in children who are overweight (BMI 85th to 94th percentile) and who have high a waist-to-height ratio (Freedman et al. 2009). Table 9.3 illustrates the additive risk of increased abdominal fat to the risk of BMI in the development of obesity-associated diseases in adults with a BMI of 25 to 34.9 kg/m^2. Waist circumference does not add to the accuracy of predicting disease risk in people who have a BMI of 35 kg/m^2 or more.

The **waist-to-hip ratio** predicts the patterning of visceral fat. Excess fat above the waist, so-called androidal fat, increases risk for CHD more than does excess fat below the waist, so-called gynoidal fat. The American Heart Association (2001) suggests that the desirable waist-to-hip ratio is less than 1.00 for men and less than 0.80 for women.

Some evidence indicates that extra fat stored above the waist indicates high visceral fat, which is believed to be more biologically active, that is, more readily mobilized from **adipose** cells into the bloodstream, where it can contribute to atherosclerosis. Other evidence indicates that intra-abdominal adipose cells are more likely to secrete inflammatory factors that lead to vessel and organ damage. Trunk fat increases risk for CHD independently of serum lipids. For example, in the Paris Prospective Study, subcutaneous fat distribution and incidence of CHD was examined among 6718 men ages 42 to 53 after a follow-up period of 6.6 years (Ducimetiere, Richard, and Cambien 1986). Fat distribution was described as the measurement of 13 skinfold thicknesses (five on the trunk, four at the triceps level, four at midthigh). The trunk measurements were correlated with BMI (r ~0.50) but were better predictors of myocardial infarction and angina pectoris, independent of their moderate correlations with systolic blood pressure, serum cholesterol, and serum triglycerides.

Precise measurement of the percentage of body mass that is fat and its regional distribution requires laboratory measurements that estimate the four tissue components constituting body mass: water, mineral, protein, and fat. Body fat cannot be measured directly, so it is calculated from estimates of mineral content of bone, body water, and body density. Most commonly, mineral content is measured by dual-energy X-ray absorptiometry (DXA); body water is measured by dilution with deuterium; and body density is measured by underwater weighing. Based on the relative portions of these four components measured directly in cadavers, predictive equations have been developed that have a standard accuracy for estimating body fat percentage of ±2% to ±3%,

Table 9.3　Classification of Overweight and Obesity by BMI, Waist Circumference, and Associated Disease Risks

	BMI (kg/m²)	Obesity class	Disease risk relative to normal weight and waist circumference	
			Men ≤102 cm (≤40 in.) Women ≤88 cm (≤35 in.)	>102 cm (>40 in.) >88 cm (>35 in.)
Underweight	<18.5		—	—
Normal	18.5-24.9		—	—
Overweight	25.0-29.9		Increased	High
Obesity	30.0-34.9	I	High	Very high
	35.0-39.9	II	Very high	Very high
Extreme obesity	≥40	III	Extremely high	Extremely high

Reprinted from National Institutes of Health 1998.

compared with ±5% to ±7% for BMI. Also, total fat mass (including subcutaneous abdominal fat and intra-abdominal or visceral fat) can be measured by computer-assisted tomography and compared with waist circumference as an index of body fatness. These more direct measures show that the accuracy of BMI and measures of waist girth as estimates of body fatness can differ across age, sex, and race-ethnicity. This is the case mainly because BMI and girth scores used to define overweight and obesity were derived using data primarily from white adults.

For example, the relation between BMI and percent body fat in 665 black and white men and women 17 to 65 years of age from the HERITAGE Family Study cohort was quadratic, not linear, for both men and women (Jackson et al. 2002). At a BMI under 20 or over 35, percent fat was lower than would be expected from a linear relation. After adjusting the relation to be linear, the percent body fat at each BMI was 10.4% higher for women than men. The relation also differed according to age and BMI among men and according to age, BMI, and race among women. Regardless of age, BMI underestimated percent fat in black women by 2% and overestimated percent fat in white women by 0.8%, but only when BMI was less than 25 kg/m². Regardless of race, BMI underestimated percent fat by 3.3% in men who were younger than 30 years and who had a BMI greater than 30. Also, at any age, BMI, or waist circumference, abdominal fat mass was higher in white men and women than in black men and women (Stanforth et al. 2004).

In a study of 30- to 65-year-old residents of Canada, men and women of European ancestry were compared with minority groups of Aboriginal, Chinese, and South Asian origin (Lear et al. 2007a, 2007b). At each BMI, percent body fat was similar between people of Chinese origin and those with European ancestry. However, BMI underestimated percent fat in people of South Asian origin by 3.9%. Compared with Europeans at a BMI of 25 or 30, Chinese had less total body fat but more intra-abdominal fat, while South Asians had more total body fat and more intra-abdominal fat. At each BMI, intra-abdominal fat was higher in all the non-European groups.

Among college students 17 to 35 years of age who were attending the University of Houston, percent body fat was higher in women than in men at any BMI, and the size of the discrepancy differed according to race-ethnicity (Jackson et al. 2009). Among women, percent body fat at any BMI was 1.76% lower in non-Hispanic blacks but higher in Hispanics (by 1.65%), Asians (by 2.65%), and Asian Indians (by 6%) when compared to non-Hispanic whites. Among men, at any BMI, percent body fat was lower by 4.6% in non-Hispanic blacks, was higher by 4.6% in Asian Indians, and was similar in Hispanics and Asians when compared to non-Hispanic whites.

Similarly, the accuracy of BMI for estimating body fatness in children and adolescents varies widely depending on the level of BMI used to define overweight or obesity (Neovius and Rasmussen 2008). When BMI reaches or exceeds the 95th percentile of age- and sex-specific norms judged by CDC standards (1970s-era norms), BMI has high specificity (about 95%) and moderately high (70% to 80%) sensitivity and predictive value for detecting excess body fatness (Freedman and Sherry 2009). Errors are greater when the 85th percentile is used to define overweight. Accuracy also differs according to race-ethnicity. In a study of 1100 black, white, Hispanic, and Asian boys and girls aged 5 to 18 years, overweight was defined as the 95th percentile of BMI, and excess body fatness was defined as ~85th percentile of percent body fat measured by DXA (Freedman et al. 2009). At the 95th percentile of equivalent age- and sex-specific BMI levels, percent body fat was 2.5% lower in black girls and 1.5% lower in Hispanic and Asian girls compared to white girls. Among girls classified as having excess body fatness, 89% (24/27) of black girls, but only 50% (8/16) of Asian girls, were judged to overweight according to BMI. The proportion of overweight girls who had excess body fatness varied from 62% (8/13) among Asians to 100% (13/13) among whites. In contrast, there were not racial–ethnic differences in percent body fat among the boys at the 95th percentile of BMI, where sensitivity and predictive values for detecting excess body fat ranged between 65% and 83%.

Medical technology such as DXA provides a relatively accurate assessment of body fat and its distribution in laboratory or clinical settings. It has mainly been used to validate the accuracy of BMI, girth, or other anthropometric measures that are feasible to use with large numbers of people in population-based studies of disease risk and in smaller clinical trials designed to change total or regional body fatness. However, these techniques have not as yet been widely used in large population-based studies of physical activity to determine whether they provide better estimates of CHD morbidity and mortality than do BMI and waist girth measurements. For example, among nearly 13,000 adults from the NHANES, BMI and waist circumference were more closely related to each other than each was to percent body fat measured by DXA, and those relations differed between men and women and according to age and race-ethnicity (Flegal et al. 2009). Despite this, attributable risks of all-cause mortality and obesity-related causes of death were similar when either BMI or comparable levels of waist circumference or percent body fat were used to classify people as overweight (Flegal and Graubard 2009). Nonetheless, it is important to remember throughout this chapter that BMI and girth measurements are not equivalent indexes of body fatness or abdominal fatness among men and women of differing ages, race, or ethnicity.

The Consensus About Obesity

In 1995, the National Heart, Lung, and Blood Institute's Obesity Education Initiative and the National Institute of Diabetes and Digestive and Kidney Diseases assembled an expert panel charged with the identification, evaluation, and treatment of overweight and obesity in adults. Their guidelines, which appeared in 1998, were based on a review of 236 studies of randomized clinical trials indexed by the National Library of Medicine from January 1980 to September 1997 (National Heart, Lung, and Blood Institute 1998). These studies lasted at least four months, with the exception of a few three-month studies of dietary therapy and pharmacotherapy. Long-term outcomes from the studies were followed for a year or longer.

These are some main conclusions of the review:

- Treatment of overweight is recommended only when patients have two or more risk factors or a high waist circumference. Treatment should focus on altering dietary and physical activity patterns to prevent development of obesity and to produce moderate weight loss.

- Cardiovascular risk factors among obese people do not differ from those for people of normal weight.

- Obese people who have at least three major CHD risk factors usually require medical treatment aimed at risk reduction. Their CHD risk is increased further if they are physically inactive and have high serum triglycerides (>200 mg/dl), though the increased risk has not been quantified.

- There is strong evidence that weight loss among people who are overweight or obese reduces risk factors for diabetes and cardiovascular disease (CVD). Weight loss reduces blood pressure in both hypertensive and nonhypertensive overweight individuals, reduces serum triglycerides, increases HDL-C, and

somewhat reduces total serum cholesterol and low-density lipoprotein cholesterol (LDL-C). Weight loss reduces blood glucose levels in overweight and obese people with and without diabetes and can reduce glycosylated hemoglobin (HbA1c) in people with type 2 diabetes.

Metabolic Syndrome

Though obesity is considered a disease, there is controversy about whether it is an independent cause of premature death or whether it is deadly because of the constellation of risk factors for mortality that accompanies it. For example, the co-occurrence of obesity with diabetes or prediabetes, hypertension, and dyslipidemia partly define the **metabolic syndrome,** an absolute risk for CHD and cardiovascular mortality that was introduced in chapter 8.

The age-adjusted prevalence of metabolic syndrome among men and women aged 20 years or older estimated from NHANES III was nearly 24%, about 47 million people (Ford, Giles, and Dietz 2002). The prevalence rate was highest among Mexican Americans (32%). Though rates were similar for men and women averaged across ethnic groups, African American women had about a 57% higher prevalence and Mexican American women about a 26% higher prevalence than did their male counterparts. The age-adjusted prevalence of metabolic syndrome among U.S. adults is now estimated to be 34% (Ervin 2009). In men, the rate in non-Hispanic whites was twice as high as in non-Hispanic blacks and nearly a third higher than in Mexican Americans. That was reversed in women; non-Hispanic whites had 33% lower risk.

There are no well-accepted criteria for diagnosing the metabolic syndrome. The criteria proposed by the National Cholesterol Education Program (NCEP) Adult Treatment Panel III (ATP III), with minor modifications, are currently recommended and widely used (Alberti et al. 2009). The American Heart Association and the National Heart, Lung, and Blood Institute recommend that the metabolic syndrome be identified as the presence of three or more of these components (specific to population; U.S. shown):

- Elevated waist circumference:
    Men—equal to or greater than 40 in. (102 cm)
    Women—equal to or greater than 35 in. (88 cm)
- Elevated triglycerides:
    Equal to or greater than 150 mg/dl
- Reduced HDL ("good") cholesterol:
    Men—less than 40 mg/dl
    Women—less than 50 mg/dl
- Elevated blood pressure:
    Equal to or greater than 130/85 mmHg
- Elevated fasting glucose:
    Equal to or greater than 100 mg/dl

Etiology of Overweight and Obesity: Set Point or Settling Point?

Weight gain resulting from excess storage of fat is ultimately explained by an intake of calories that exceeds those expended. However, the physiological mechanisms that govern the metabolic balance of food consumption and energy extraction with the energy costs of basal metabolism, digestion, and physical exertion are complex and incompletely understood. The factors that influence the behaviors of eating and physical activity, which determine energy balance and gains or loss of body fat, are even less well understood. Two common theories about the etiology of overweight and obesity, set point and settling point, address how physical activity can play a role in the treatment or prevention of overweight and obesity. The concept of reasonable weight, discussed later in this chapter, provides an alternative view of weight goals for obese people.

Set Point Theory

Set point theory hypothesizes that the body has an internal control mechanism, that is, a set point, located in the lateral hypothalamus of the brain, that regulates metabolism to maintain a certain level of body fat. Though evidence in rats has supported the **theory,** there is no scientific consensus that such a metabolic set point exists in humans for fat maintenance. Though weight losses after the use of stimulant drugs, nicotine, and exercise seem consistent with the concept of an altered set point, these effects can also be explained by the alteration of basal metabolism in ways that do not require a change in the set point. Studies using mainly dietary restriction have shown that weight loss is accompanied by a decrease in fat-free body mass and basal energy expenditure (Sum et al. 1994). Severe caloric restriction has been shown to depress resting metabolism by as much as 45% (McArdle, Katch, and Katch 1991).

Settling Point Theory

Interventions designed to alter diet and reduce weight have used principles of behavior therapy with modest success, particularly among the obese (Foreyt and Goodrich 1993). The most successful weight loss programs incorporate physical activity (Pavlou, Krey, and Steffee 1989; Perri et al. 1986). The **settling point theory** was proposed by obesity researcher James Hill of the University of Colorado to help explain why overweight and obesity are more than problems of metabolism (Hill, Pagliassotti, and Peters 1994). His idea is that weight loss and gain in most humans are more related to the patterns of diet and physical activity that people "settle" into as habits based on the interaction of their genetic dispositions, learning, and environmental cues to behavior.

Evidence suggests that obese people are more sensitive to food-related stimuli in the social and physical environment, which influence their energy intake, than to the stimuli for energy expenditure.

▶ **THE IDEA** of a settling point recognizes that overweight and obesity are more than metabolic problems for most overweight and obese people. People who have settled into weight gain habits appear more sensitive to food-related cues than to opportunities for physical activity.

The Role of Physical Activity

Physical activity has an important role in the prevention and treatment of overweight and obesity, even if that role is not yet completely understood.

The association between moderate-to-vigorous physical activity and the prevalence of overweight and obesity was estimated from self-reports in a cross-sectional survey of 137,593 youth (10-16 years of age) from 34 countries (including a number in Europe, as well as Israel, Canada, and the United States) that participated in the 2001-2002 Health Behaviour in School-Aged Children Study (Janssen et al. 2005). The international child BMI standards were used to project youth as overweight (BMI ≥25) or obese (BMI ≥30) at age 18. Overweight and obesity prevalence was particularly high in countries located in North America, Great Britain, and southwestern Europe (Greece, Italy, Malta, Portugal, and Spain). The two countries with the highest prevalence of obese and overweight youth were Malta (7.9% and 25.4%) and the United States (6.8% and 25.1%). Physical activity levels were lower in overweight youth in 30 of 34 countries. After adjustments for age, gender, TV watching, computer use, current attempts to lose weight, and dietary factors (intake of fruit, vegetables, sweets, and soft drinks), each day of weekly physical activity reduced the odds of being overweight or obese rather than normal weight. Odds ranged from 0.80 (95% CI: 0.76-0.85) in Austria to 0.95 (95% CI: 0.90-1.00) in Greece and were 0.90 (95% CI: 0.87-0.94) in the United States.

The relation of physical activity with body fatness in adolescents is complex, though. A study of over 600 black and white U.S. teens 14 to 18 years of age found that regardless of age or race, boys and girls with the lowest percent body fat spent the most time in vigorous physical activities but also had the highest daily intake of calories (Stallmann-Jorgensen et al. 2007). Also, the vigorously active consumed about 440 kcal a day more than those who said they got no vigorous activity, but their moderate physical activity and TV watching were the same. So, the researchers speculated that the lower percent body fat in those who were vigorously active resulted from elevated metabolic rate and fat oxidation, similar to the concepts of *energy flux* and *subsistence efficiency* introduced at the beginning of this chapter. If this is true, the study suggests that prevention of obesity in children should focus on increasing vigorous physical activity rather than restricting energy intake (Gutin 2008).

The scientific advisory committee for the 2005 Dietary Guidelines for Americans concluded that moderate physical activity for an hour each day can increase energy expenditure by about 150 to 200 calories, which can be helpful in preventing unhealthy weight gain if the extra calories used aren't offset by an equal increase in calorie intake. The committee also concluded that adults who've lost weight may need 60 to 90 min of daily activity to help avoid regaining weight and that children and adolescents need at least 60 min of moderate-to-vigorous physical activity most days of the week for healthy weight gain as they mature (Dietary Guidelines Advisory Committee 2005). Likewise, the scientific advisory committee for the 2008 Physical Activity Guidelines for Americans recognized that recommendations about the amount of physical activity needed for weight maintenance, weight loss, or prevention of weight regain after weight loss must allow for energy intake. The committee also noted that in most weight loss studies that included dieting, the contribution of physical activity to the overall calorie reduction and weight loss was small. Finally, the committee noted that increased use of labor-saving tools at work and home, as well as more time spent in sedentary activities (e.g., Internet use and online social networking) during discretionary leisure, has shifted downward the energy cost of activities of daily living in ways that put extra importance on planned physical activities above daily routines in order to achieve energy balance (Physical Activity Guidelines Advisory Committee 2008).

The American College of Sports Medicine (ACSM) recommends that adults participate in at least 150 min/week of moderate-intensity physical activity to protect against excessive weight gain and reduce chronic disease risk factors, especially in adults with a BMI ≥25 or a waist circumference above 88 cm (35 in.) in women and 102 cm (40 in.) in men. The ACSM recommends a weight loss of 5% to 10% of body weight for those people, with additional health benefits expected for those who sustain weight loss of more than 10%. Overweight and obese individuals will likely benefit from 250 or more minutes each week to experience greater weight reduction and prevent weight regain. The ACSM also recommends strength training to increase or maintain fat-free mass and further reduce health risks. Although resistance exercise added to aerobic exercise doesn't typically enhance weight loss, it can increase basal metabolic rate by retarding loss of muscle (sarcopenia) during aging and dieting.

Even among people who are considered sedentary during their work or leisure, there can be meaningful differences in daily energy expenditure that results from the routine activities of daily living, maintaining an upright posture (e.g., standing rather than sitting), and spontaneously arising movements (e.g., pacing or fidgeting), which has been termed non-exercise activity thermogenesis, or NEAT (Levine, Eberhardt, and Jensen 1999). People vary widely in weight gain when they overeat. A groundbreaking study measured changes in weight gain and naturally occurring energy expenditure in young, nonobese adults who were fed 1000 kilocalories more than they needed for weight maintenance each day for eight weeks. Body fatness was measured with DXA, and total daily energy expenditure was measured using doubly labeled water. Exercise was estimated by accelerometer counts and interviews and did not change during overfeeding. On average, 432 of the extra calories were stored as fat, and 531 calories were burned by increased NEAT. Fat gain varied among people by 10-fold, ranging from a gain of about 0.40 kg to 4 kg. The amount gained was inversely related to how much people increased their NEAT, which also varied widely from 298 to 1692 calories each day. The average increase in NEAT was 336 calories a day, which accounted for two-thirds of the increase in daily energy expenditure. The authors surmised that when people overeat, some increase NEAT to preserve leanness, while others are vulnerable to weight gain because they do not naturally increase NEAT.

A related laboratory study showed that NEAT is substantially reduced by the common use of labor-saving devices (Lanningham-Foster et al. 2003). Not surprisingly, the energy cost (kcal/day) of several household chores and work-related transportation was less when they were carried out using a machine instead of by hand (washing clothes: 27 vs. 45; washing dishes: 54 vs. 80) or by foot (riding instead of walking nearly a mile to work: 25 vs. 83; taking an elevator instead of climbing stairs while at work: 3 vs. 11). The total energy cost of daily physical activities lost to the use of labor-saving devices was about 110 kcal a day!

Evidence shows that regular physical activity or physical fitness can (1) reduce health risks in people who are overweight, (2) protect against excessive weight gain, (3) help overweight and obese people lose weight, and (4) help people maintain stable weight after they lose it.

Physical Activity and Fitness and the Health Risks of Obesity: The Evidence

The results from studies of physical fitness differ somewhat from those relating to physical activity (Fogelholm 2010). Studies of physical fitness generally have observed that being fit can remove the excess risk of all-cause or cardiovascular mortality associated with being overweight or obese (Lee, Sui, and Blair 2009). In contrast, studies of physical activity generally have shown that each risk factor (i.e., inactivity or overweight/obesity) is associated with increased risk of all-cause or mortality or CVD, of approximately equal magnitude, and that being physically active does not remove the excess risk associated with increased adiposity. This difference may reflect that the two attributes, lack of fitness and inactivity, do not represent identical characteristics. Also, physical fitness tends to be more precisely measured than physical activity. In this section we describe some studies in more detail.

With regard to type 2 diabetes, the findings from studies of physical fitness and physical activity have been more similar, showing that adiposity drastically increases the risk associated with type 2 diabetes and that neither physical fitness nor physical activity removes the excess risk associated with being overweight or obese (Fogelholm 2010; Sui et al. 2008).

Physical Activity

Studies on the joint association of self-reported physical activity and high BMI typically show that each is an independent risk factor for all-cause mortality and mortality from CVD and cancer. The mortality risk of obesity is not eliminated by physical activity, but it was usually reduced substantially in population cohorts that did not initially have a chronic disease.

Harvard Alumni Health Study

Results from nearly 17,000 male Harvard alumni ages 34 to 74 indicated that being physically active can reduce risk of death even in the presence of obesity (Paffenbarger et al. 1986). The 25% to 33% reduction in all-cause deaths among men who expended at least 2000 kcal/week was still present regardless of smoking, high BMI, or gains in body weight during the years of follow-up. Low net weight gain since the college years was associated with a 33% increase in relative risk, though that finding might be explained by smoking or wasting diseases such as cancer, which were not controlled for.

Nurses' Health Study

The prospective associations of BMI and physical activity with subsequent death were followed for 24 years in 116,564 women who were 30 to 55 years of age and free of known CVD and cancer at the beginning of the study (Hu et al. 2004). There were 10,282 deaths: 2370 from CVD, 5223 from cancer, and 2689 from other causes. Figure 9.6 shows that higher levels of physical activity reduced, but did not eliminate, the elevated risk of death associated with high BMI. Compared to the reference group of women who had low BMI (<25) and were active (≥3.5 h of moderate-to-vigorous exercise each week, an average of 30 min or more a day), relative risks of death from all causes were 1.55 for inactive women with low BMI; 1.91 for women who were obese (BMI ≥30) but active, and 2.42 for obese, inactive women. Protection against mortality was strongest for cardiovascular deaths (Li et al. 2006). Thus, 30 or more minutes of moderate-to-vigorous physical activity each day reduced CVD mortality risk by about 40% to 50% at each level of BMI. In contrast, that amount of physical activity reduced cancer mortality risk by 25% but only in women with low BMI. The attributable risk of a combination of excess

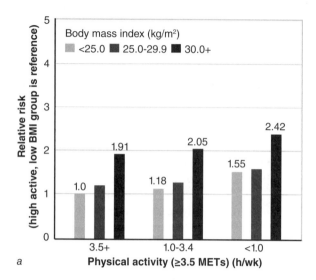

a

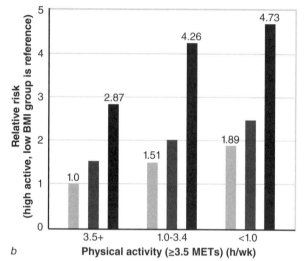

b

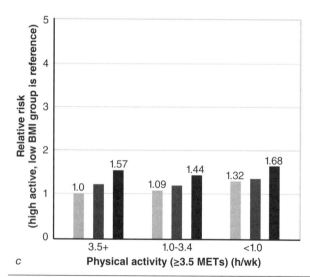

c

Figure 9.6 Results of the Nurses' Health Study showed that physical activity reduced *(a)* all-cause mortality, *(b)* cardiovascular disease mortality, and *(c)* cancer mortality. Results were adjusted for age, smoking, parental history of coronary heart disease, menopause and hormone use, and alcohol use.

Data from Hu et al. 2004.

weight (BMI ≥25) and physical inactivity was about 30% of all premature deaths, 60% of cardiovascular deaths, and 20% of cancer deaths among women who were not smokers.

Women's Health Study

The combined association of leisure-time physical activity (≥1000 kcal/week) and BMI with CHD incidence (nonfatal heart attack, coronary artery bypass, angioplasty, or CHD death) was examined in 38,987 women who were initially free of CVD, cancer, and diabetes (Weinstein et al. 2008). A total of 948 cases of CHD occurred during an average of 11 years of follow-up. High BMI and physical inactivity were each related to elevated risk of CHD. Compared with risk for active normal-weight women, the relative risks were 1.54 for overweight and physically active, 1.87 for obese and physically active, 1.08 for normal weight and physically inactive, 1.88 for overweight and physically inactive, and 2.53 for obese and physically inactive women. The risk of CHD associated with high BMI was reduced but not eliminated by physical activity.

Kuopio and North Karelia, Finland

In a study of 22,528 men and 24,684 women aged 25 to 64 years at baseline, 7394 deaths occurred during an average follow-up of nearly 18 years (Hu et al. 2005). Self-reported physical activity during leisure and occupation had an independent dose relation with lowered mortality rates. Physically active men and women had lower age-adjusted mortality rates from all causes (~25-40% reduction) and from CVD (~20-45% reduction) and cancer (~15-20% reduction), even after adjustment for BMI and other CVD risk factors. Those who were obese (BMI ≥30) also had higher cardiovascular and all-cause mortality than those who were normal weight, but that was explained partly by their higher rates of other obesity-related risk factors. Figure 9.7 shows that obese men and women who were sedentary during leisure and in their occupation had elevated mortality risks compared to those who were nonobese and reported being moderately or highly active.

Norway

In a cohort of 34,868 women and 32,872 men initially without CVD or diabetes, 3026 women and 3526 men had died from cardiovascular causes after 16 years of follow-up (Vatten et al. 2006). In middle age, obesity (BMI ≥30 kg/m^2) was associated with increased risk of cardiovascular death. At all ages, a low level of physical activity was associated with high cardiovascular mortality. Among men and women who were obese, cardiovascular mortality was lower in those who said they got 30 or more minutes of moderate-to-vigorous activity more than once a week compared to those who reported no regular physical activity. Also, the mortality risk of obese women was not higher than for normal-weight women if they participated in that much activity. In contrast, active

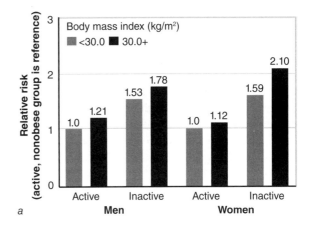

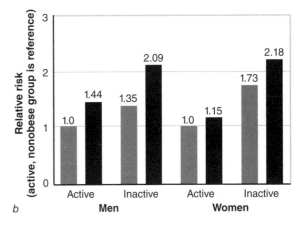

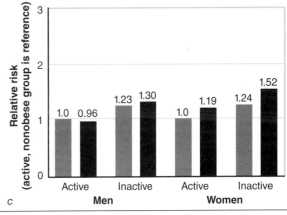

Figure 9.7 Results of the study in Kuopio and North Karelia, Finland, showed that inactive, obese adults had elevated risk of (a) all-cause mortality, (b) cardiovascular disease mortality, and (c) cancer mortality. Results were adjusted for age, survey year, education, smoking, systolic blood pressure, cholesterol, and diabetes.

Data from Hu et al. 2005.

obese men had higher cardiovascular mortality than active, normal-weight men (RR = 1.62; 95% CI: 1.09-2.40). Thus, being highly active protected against the risk of cardiovascular death in obese women, but the mortality risk of obese men who were highly active remained elevated compared to that in equally active men who had normal body weight.

Physical Fitness

Similar to the studies of self-reported physical activity, studies of the joint association of physical fitness and overweight or obesity (measured by BMI, waist girth, or percent body fat) with mortality risks usually show that cardiorespiratory fitness and also muscular strength are independent influences on risk of all-cause mortality and mortality from CVD and cancer. However, in contrast to what is seen in the studies of physical activity, fitness typically reduces mortality risks associated with overweight and eliminates this excess risk in some cohorts that were initially healthy.

Lipid Research Clinics Mortality Study

In the Lipid Research Clinics Mortality Study, 4276 men ages 30 to 69 years were observed for an average of 8.5 years (Ekelund et al. 1988). Fitness was determined by time to exhaustion and submaximal heart rate during treadmill walking. Body mass index was not an independent risk factor for mortality. However, among the lowest levels of physical fitness, the relative risks were 2.7 to 3.0 for CVD deaths and 2.8 to 3.2 for CHD deaths after adjustment for age, systolic blood pressure, high-density lipoproteins, glucose level, smoking, resting heart rate, regular physical activity, and BMI.

In a later study, the prospective associations of cardiorespiratory fitness (maximal treadmill performance) and BMI with cancer mortality risk were compared in 2585 women and 2890 men who were followed for 22 to 26 years (Evenson et al. 2003). Gender-specific risk ratios (HR) were adjusted for age, education, smoking, alcohol intake, diet, and menopause (women only). Cancer mortality was lower by half in the most fit quintile relative to the other four quintiles for men but not for women (HR = 0.84; 95% CI: 0.52-1.36). Cancer mortality was 50% higher in the highest BMI quintile relative to the other four BMI quintiles for women but not for men (HR = 1.05; 95% CI: 0.77-1.43). In this investigation, high fitness was a stronger predictor of cancer mortality than was high BMI in men, but high BMI was a stronger predictor of cancer mortality than was high fitness in women.

Another Lipid Research Clinics study further examined the prospective associations of fitness and BMI with mortality risk in 1359 Russian men and 1716 U.S. men aged 40 to 59 years who were followed for 18 to 23 years (Stevens et al. 2002). Risk ratios were adjusted for age, education, smoking, alcohol intake, and diet. In Russian men, fitness was associated with all-cause and CVD mortality, but fatness was not. Men who were fit and fat had the same mortality risk as those who were fit and not fat, but the risk ratios were about 75% higher in unfit men regardless of fatness. Among U.S. men, low fitness and fatness each increased mortality risks by about 40% to 50%. Thus, fitness eliminated the risks of obesity in Russian men; but in American men, fitness

and fatness were associated with mortality independently of each other.

Aerobics Center Longitudinal Study (ACLS)

The most convincing evidence for a positive health benefit of fitness, independent of fatness, has come from the Cooper Clinic cohort in Dallas. Several other ACLS studies measured percent body fat, as well as BMI or girth, and reported that moderate to high fitness eliminates the elevated risk of all-cause, CVD, and cancer mortality associated with obesity. In an initial eight-year follow-up of 21,925 men aged 30 to 83 years, there were 428 deaths (144 from CVD, 143 from cancer, and 141 from other causes) (Lee, Blair, and Jackson 1999). After adjustment for age, examination year, cigarette smoking, alcohol intake, and parental history of ischemic heart disease, unfit (low cardiorespiratory fitness as determined by maximal exercise testing), lean men had twice the risk of all-cause mortality compared to fit, lean men. Unfit, lean men also had a higher risk of all-cause and CVD mortality than did men who were fit and obese. Additionally, unfit men had a higher risk of all-cause and CVD mortality than did fit men regardless of total fat mass and fat-free mass. Similarly, unfit men with low waist girths (<87 cm) had greater risk of all-cause mortality than did fit men with high waist girths (≥99 cm). In a subsequent analysis, 38,410 healthy men were followed for an average of 17 years (Farrell et al. 2007); 1037 cancer deaths occurred. There were linear increases in mortality risk across levels of each measure of fatness and decreased risks across quintiles of fitness (RR = 1.0, 0.70, 0.67, 0.70, and 0.49). Adjustment for fitness level eliminated the trend in mortality risk across percent body fat groups and attenuated the trend in risk across BMI and waist circumference groups, independently of the measures of fatness.

Figure 9.8 shows results of eight years of follow-up of nearly 22,000 men, ages 30 to 83, from the Dallas cohort. The relative risk of all-cause and CVD mortality among low-fit men was twice that of fit men, whether BMI indicated normal weight or overweight (>27.8).

In another ACLS report, the prospective associations of fitness and CVD mortality across levels of BMI were observed for an average of 16 years in 2316 men with diabetes but no history of CVD (Church et al. 2005). There were 179 CVD deaths during 36,710 man-years of exposure. Mortality risk was adjusted for age and CVD risk factors. Men in the lowest 20% of fitness had higher mortality risk at all BMI levels: normal weight (2.7), overweight (2.7), and class 1 obesity (2.8) compared with normal-weight men in the top 40% of fitness level.

In an ACLS cohort of older adults, obese people who were fit had no increased risk of CVD or all-cause mortality. The prospective association of cardiorespiratory fitness (maximal treadmill performance) with mortality rates was observed for an average of 12 years in a cohort of 2603

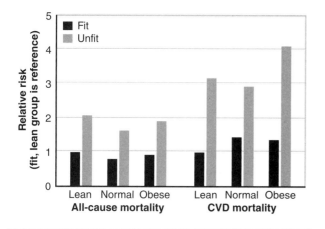

Figure 9.8 Aerobics Center Longitudinal Study with 21,856 men followed for approximately eight years. A total of 21,925 men aged 33 to 83 years were followed and men with abnormal ECG or history of myocardial infarction, stroke, or cancer excluded. Results were adjusted for age, examination year, smoking, alcohol intake, and parental history of coronary heart disease.

Percent body fat groups: Lean, <16.7%; Normal, 16.7% to <25%; Obese, ≥25%; Unfit, lowest 20% of age-specific norms. Reference group is fit, lean group.

Data from Lee et al. 1999.

adults aged 60 years or older (Sui et al. 2007). There were 450 deaths. After adjustment for age, sex, and examination year, mortality rates were about 1.30 and 2.30 for stage 1 (BMI 30.0-34.9) and stage 2 (BMI ≥35.0) obesity compared to normal weight and nearly 1.4 for high waist circumference (≥88 cm in women; ≥102 cm in men). Mortality risks declined linearly across quintiles of fitness (0.51, 0.39, 0.38, and 0.25). Lower mortality risk in higher fitness groups remained after adjustment for smoking; baseline health; and either BMI, waist circumference, or percent bodyfat. The association between waist circumference and mortality was eliminated after adjustment for fitness.

Muscular strength (1-repetition maximum for leg and chest press combined) and mortality from all causes, CVD, and cancer was examined in 8762 men aged 20 to 80 from the ACLS cohort (Ruiz et al. 2008). During an average follow-up of 18.9 years, 503 deaths occurred (145 CVD, 199 cancer). Age-adjusted death rates per 10,000 person-years across age-specific tertiles of muscular strength were 38.9, 25.9, and 26.6 for all causes; 12.1, 7.6, and 6.6 for CVD; and 6.1, 4.9, and 4.2 for cancer. After adjustment for age, physical activity, smoking, alcohol intake, BMI, baseline medical conditions, and family history of CVD, men in the lowest third of strength had about 40% higher risks for deaths from CVD, cancer, and all causes. The elevated risks for all-cause and cancer mortality, but not for CVD, were independent of cardiorespiratory fitness.

Women's Ischemia Syndrome Evaluation (WISE)

From 1996 to 2000, 936 women were enrolled at four U.S. academic medical centers when clinical evaluation and angiography indicated they had myocardial ischemia (Wessel et al. 2004). At enrollment, 76% were overweight (BMI ≥25), 70% had low functional capacity (7 METs [metabolic equivalents] or less) based on a validated self-report measure of fitness, and 39% had coronary artery disease (CAD). They had a follow-up clinical exam about four years later. During follow-up, 337 (38%) women had a first cardiovascular event; 118 (13%) had a major cardiovascular event; and 68 (8%) died. Overweight women were more likely than normal-weight women to have CAD risk factors, but BMI and girth measures were not associated with CAD or cardiovascular events after adjustment for other risk factors. In contrast, women with lower fitness scores at entry were 80% more likely to have CAD risk factors and obstructive CAD at the time of enrollment. Each 1-MET level of estimated fitness was associated with an 8% decrease in the risk of major adverse cardiovascular events during follow-up independently of CAD risk factors.

Are Overweight and Obesity Risk Factors Independent of Physical Activity?

Although bariatric surgery (i.e., gastric bypass or banding) increases long-term survival in morbidly obese patients (Adams et al. 2007; Pontiroli and Morabito 2011), large-scale randomized clinical trials have not been conducted to determine whether weight loss after diets reduces mortality among people who are obese. Neither have such studies been done for physical inactivity. Dr. Glenn Gaesser (1996, 2002), an exercise physiologist at the University of Virginia, challenged the consensus view that being fat is life threatening and that being thin guarantees health. He proposed that any person can have good health regardless of body weight by achieving and maintaining metabolic fitness, which we defined in chapter 3. In contrast to the NIH expert panel's consensus (National Heart, Lung, and Blood Institute 1998), Gaesser argued that the scientific evidence is not sufficiently strong to allow the conclusion that overweight and obesity are directly responsible for early death.

However, a recent large study using pooled data from 19 prospective studies of 1.46 million white adults, 19 to 84 years of age, observed that after taking biases from smoking and ill health into consideration and adjusting for physical activity, there was a J-shaped relationship between BMI and all-cause mortality (Berrington de Gonzalez et al. 2010). The highest mortality rates occurred at BMI of 40.0 to 49.9 kg/m² and the lowest generally at 20.0 to 24.9 kg/m². The relation between adiposity and all-cause mortality also may differ among persons of different race–ethnic groups, with a recent analysis of 1.1 million Asians showing that the excess risk of death associated with a high BMI was seen among East Asians but not among Indians and Bangladeshis (Zheng et al. 2011). In any case, the evidence is clear that physical activity can favorably modify the impact of overweight and moderate obesity on several health risk factors, including metabolic syndrome.

▶ **MODERATE PHYSICAL** activity can help lower blood pressure among overweight and obese people even when they do not lose weight.

▶ **HIGH BODY** fat contributes to impaired glucose tolerance and diabetes risk by impairing insulin receptor function in muscle, liver, and fat cells. Physical activity can improve insulin sensitivity and glucose tolerance in people who are overweight or obese.

Reducing Health Risks in People Who Are Overweight

In a cross-sectional analysis of 3458 U.S. adults from the 2003-2004 NHANES, people who met federal recommendations for total weekly amount of physical activity measured by accelerometer counts had lower odds of clinical elevations of blood pressure, blood glucose levels, triglyceride levels, and BMI, along with low levels of high-density lipoproteins—all risk factors related to metabolic syndrome (Metzger et al. 2010). In the Health Worker Cohort Study in Mexico, odds of metabolic syndrome were about 25% lower in men who said they got 30 or more min/day of leisure-time physical activity and in women who reported at least 3 h/day of workplace physical activity (Méndez-Hernández et al. 2009).

After adjustments for age and education levels, household income, smoking status, and alcohol consumption, the prevalence of metabolic syndrome among nearly 12,000 Koreans 30 to 79 years of age who said they got no leisure-time physical activity was 25% to 30% higher in men and 50% to 85% higher in women compared to people in the top two-thirds of physical activity (Cho et al. 2009). Among 6400 men residing in Oslo, Norway, those who said they engaged in moderate-to-vigorous leisure-time physical activity in 1972 had 35% lower age-adjusted risk of developing metabolic syndrome 28 years later (Holme et al. 2007). The risk reduction was mainly explained by the active men's lower glucose and triglyceride levels, BMI, and blood pressure in 1972.

A quantitative review of 43 randomized controlled trials including 3476 overweight or obese adults found that exercise combined with diet resulted in a small added weight loss compared with diet alone (−1.1 kg; 95% CI: −1.5 to −0.6) (Shaw et al. 2006). Although exercise training alone resulted in small weight losses across studies, it led to significant reductions in diastolic blood pressure (−2 mmHg; 95% CI: −4 to −1), triglycerides (−0.2 mmol/L; 95% CI: −0.3 to −0.1), and fasting glucose (−0.2 mmol/L; 95% CI: −0.3 to −0.1). Thus, exercise was accompanied by improvements in several CVD risk factors even when no weight was lost.

In a recent randomized controlled trial, a 25% energy deficit in overweight adults achieved by diet alone or by equal contributions of diet (12.5% decrease in intake) and exercise (12.5% increase in expenditure) led to similar losses of total and intra-abdominal fat mass in each group (Larson-Meyer et al. 2010). However, only people in the diet and exercise group had improvements in metabolic fitness, indicated by drops in diastolic blood pressure and LDL-C and by improved insulin sensitivity.

Because metabolic syndrome is defined by the presence of several health risk factors, it is important to determine which of its components are positively affected by diet or exercise. In the HERITAGE Family Study, 105 people (17%) had metabolic syndrome before exercise training. After 20 weeks of training, 32 people no longer had metabolic syndrome: 43% decreased triglycerides, 16% improved HDL-C, 38% decreased blood pressure, 9% improved fasting plasma glucose, and 28% decreased their waist circumference (Katzmarzyk et al. 2003).

In the STRRIDE trial of overweight men and women who had dyslipidemia (i.e., risky levels of cholesterol) (Johnson et al. 2007), 69 (40%) had metabolic syndrome. After eight months of exercise training, that percentage was decreased to 28%. Vigorous-intensity (65-80% of aerobic capacity) activities that expended 23 kcal/kg each week (e.g., jogging 20 miles/week) were most effective for improving all components of metabolic syndrome except blood glucose levels, and results were generally more favorable in men than women.

Elderly German women with metabolic syndrome were randomly assigned to exercise training or control. After 12 months of exercise, there were favorable changes in total body fat, abdominal fat, hip circumference, triglycerides, and HDL-C, but blood pressure and glucose levels were no better than values in controls (Kemmler et al. 2009).

In a one-year randomized controlled trial, 179 men and 149 postmenopausal women who had dyslipidemia were assigned to control, diet, exercise, or diet plus exercise (Camhi et al. 2009). Change in metabolic syndrome was more favorable after diet or diet plus exercise in men and after diet, exercise, or diet plus exercise in women compared to control. After adjustment for change in percent body fat, those differences were eliminated. Thus, improvement in metabolic syndrome from either diet or exercise depended on the loss of body fat.

Physical Activity and Prevention of Excess Weight Gain: The Evidence

Current opinion is that an increase of 3% or more of body weight in adults is excess weight gain and more than 5% is risky for health (Stevens et al. 2006, 2009). For someone weighing 165 lb, a 5-lb gain would be excess weight, and 8 lb or more might be unhealthy. During the 1980s and 1990s, it was estimated that more than half of U.S. adults gained more than 5 lb across periods of three and four years (Sherwood et al. 2000; St. Jeor et al. 1997).

A review of 11 prospective cohort studies concluded that physical activity or increased fitness measured by maximal treadmill endurance is associated with minimizing weight gain or with a reduction in the risk of large weight gains (e.g., 5-10 kg) among adults over periods ranging from two to 10 years (DiPietro 1999). More recently, the scientific advisory committee for the Physical Activity Guidelines for Americans located nine prospective cohort studies published since 1995, with follow-ups of at least one year to more than six years, that showed an inverse association between physical activity and a body weight outcome. The committee concluded that the optimal amount of physical activity needed for weight maintenance (<3% change in body weight) over the long term is unclear, but that many people may need more than 150 min of moderate-intensity activity each week to maintain their weight at a stable level (Physical Activity Guidelines Advisory Committee 2008).

In contrast, a review of 38 prospective cohort studies of physical activity exposure and body fatness outcomes measured one to 30 years later concluded that physical activity was not inversely associated with excess weight gain (Summerbell et al. 2009). However, the review did not average the studies' effects or weigh them by quality or study size (which ranged from less than a hundred to several thousand). Notwithstanding the overall conclusion, the review acknowledged that studies published since 2000 seemed to show an inverse relation between physical activity and weight gain.

▷ **PHYSICAL ACTIVITY** contributes to weight loss and helps minimize the weight gain that commonly occurs as people age.

Though the studies used different methods to measure physical activity, different definitions of weight change, and poor control of confounders such as smoking and diet that also affect weight change, they generally agreed that being physically active has potential efficacy as an intervention for slowing the weight gain commonly associated with aging during the early and middle adult years. However, low physical activity can be both a cause and a consequence of weight gain. An observational study that defines physical activity exposure only at follow-up or only as change from baseline to follow-up, without showing that baseline activity was related to lower initial weight or predicted subsequent weight gain, would be misleading if people with high initial weight become less active. This would suggest "reverse causality"—that is, that higher weight led to lower activity rather than that higher weight resulted from low activity. Of course, randomized controlled trials are necessary to determine causal effects. Nonetheless, more prospective studies with several measures of both physical activity and body weight over time are needed to fully describe the temporal relationship between physical activity and weight change in the general population.

Finnish Cohort

Predictors of weight gain were studied for an average of about five and a half years in 12,669 Finnish adults who were examined twice during that period (Rissanen et al. 1991). Risk factors associated with the prevalence of obesity (BMI >30 kg/m^2) were also examined in another cross-sectional survey of 5673 adults. The risk of gaining 5 kg or more was elevated in people with little leisure-time physical activity, as well as in those with a low level of education, chronic diseases, or heavy alcohol use. Having children and total calorie consumption also predicted weight gain in women.

NHANES I Follow-Up Study

Data from the 1982 to 1984 epidemiologic follow-up to the NHANES I survey (conducted from 1971 to 1975) were used to examine the relationship between leisure physical activity level (low, medium, or high) and weight change among a representative U.S. sample of 3515 men and 5810 women ages 25 to 74 years (Williamson et al. 1993). A low level of physical activity reported in the follow-up survey was strongly related to major weight gain. The relative risk of major weight gain (>13 kg) for the lowest physical activity category in the follow-up survey compared with the high-activity category was 3.1 (95% CI: 1.6-6.0) for men and 3.8 (2.3-6.5) for women. The relative risk for people who reported low physical activity at both the initial and follow-up surveys was 2.3 (0.9-5.8) in men and 7.1 (2.2-23.3) in women.

Nurses' Health Study

Among a cohort of 121,700 women, the mean two-year weight gain in 1476 women who stopped smoking was 3 kg compared to 0.6 kg in 7832 women who continued smoking (Kawachi et al. 1996). Women who had smoked up to a pack of cigarettes a day and quit without changing their physical activity levels gained an average of 2.3 kg more (95% CI: 1.9-2.6) than women who continued smoking. By comparison, women who quit smoking but increased their physical activity by 8 to 16 MET-hours per week gained 1.8 kg (95% CI: 1.0-2.5); weight gain was only 1.3 kg (0.7-1.9) in women who increased exercise by more than 16 MET-hours per week.

The Coronary Artery Risk Development in Young Adults (CARDIA) Study

Weight change was studied prospectively over seven years in a U.S. cohort of black and white men (n = 1823) and women (n = 2083) ages 18 to 30 years (Lewis et al. 1997). Weight increased an average of 5.2 kg (SE = 0.2, n = 811) in white women, 8.5 kg (SE = 0.3, n = 882) in black women, 4.8 kg (SE = 1.0, n = 711) in black men, and 2.6 kg (SE = 0.8, n = 944) in white men. Decreased physical fitness was strongly associated with weight gain in both sexes. Each 1-min decrease in maximal treadmill endurance time predicted a 1.5 kg weight gain for men and a 2.1 kg gain for women.

A follow-up examined long-term associations between changes in physical activity and changes in body weight, adjusting for secular trend, age, clinic site, education, smoking, alcohol intake, parity, percentage energy intake from fat, and changes in these variables over time (Schmitz et al. 2000). Analyses were conducted for three separate five-year intervals: baseline to year 5 (n = 3641), years 2 to 7 (n = 3160), and years 5 to 10 (n = 2617). Change in physical activity was inversely related to change in body weight within all four race and sex subgroups. The predicted weight change associated with change in physical activity was four to five times larger in participants who were overweight at baseline compared with those who were not overweight. Compared to people who decreased their physical activity, the average five-year weight gain was blunted by 0.8 to 2.8 kg among those who increased physical activity by at least 2 h each week, six or more months each year, during the first two to three years of follow-up.

U.S. Male Health Professionals

The influences of habitual physical activity, TV watching, smoking, and diet on weight change were observed over four years in 19,478 men, ages 40 to 75 in 1986, who were free of cancer, CHD, stroke, and diabetes (Coakley et al. 1998). Weight gain was adjusted for initial age, hypertension, and hypercholesterolemia. Middle-aged men who increased their vigorous physical activity, decreased TV viewing, and stopped eating between meals lost an average weight of 1.4 kg (95% CI: 1.6-1.1 kg), compared with a weight gain of 1.4 kg in the total cohort. Each 1.5-h increase in weekly vigorous physical activity predicted a 2 kg weight loss in men ages 45 to 54.

American Cancer Society: Cancer Prevention Study I and II

A cohort of healthy, non-Hispanic white men (n =35,156) and women (n = 44,080) aged 50 to 74 years who had self-reported BMI (kg/m^2) of 18 to 32 were questioned in 1982 and 1992 about their weight and participation in 10 leisure-time physical activities and home chores (Kahn et al. 1997). People who reported diuretic use, cancer history, diabetes, or a 10-year change in BMI greater than 8 (i.e., 3%) were excluded from analysis. The average 10-year increase in BMI (kg/m^2) was 0.6 (SD = 1.7) in men and 1.4 (SD = 1.9) in women. Adjustments were made for age, education, region of the United States, initial BMI, change in marital status, total calorie intake, smoking, and alcohol use, and also for menopause, estrogen replacement, and parity in women. The increase in BMI was 0.22 to 0.34 kg/m^2 less among men who had said they jogged or did aerobics/calisthenics either 1 to 3 h or 4 or more hours per week in 1982 (or when they were age 40) and also in 1992 compared to men who said they didn't engage in those activities. Women who said they jogged 1 to 3 h per week or did 4 or more hours per week of aerobics/calisthenics at both of those times had 0.27 to 0.29 kg/m^2 less gain in BMI than women who did not report doing those activities. Walking 4 or more hours per week was associated with modest protection (0.08 and 0.16 kg/m^2 less) against BMI gain in both men and women. Figure 9.9 also shows that men and women who jogged 1 to 3 h or walked 4 or more hours each week were less likely than the inactive participants to gain weight and say they gained weight at the waist. A subsequent analysis of that cohort between 1992 and 1999 (Blanck et al. 2007) examined seven-year weight gain among 18,583 women aged 40 to 69 years who were postmenopausal and had no history of chronic diseases including diabetes, heart disease, stroke, and cancer. The odds of weight gain greater than 10 lb were 12% lower for normal-weight women (BMI <25) who reported more than 18 MET-hours per week of leisure-time physical activity (n = 2609) compared with those who reported 4 or fewer MET-hours per week (n = 2278). Physical activity did not protect against weight gains between 5 and 9 lb or weight gain greater than 10 lb in women who were initially overweight (BMI ≥25).

Study of Women's Health Across the Nation (SWAN)

This was a prospective study of the associations of weight and waist circumference with physical activity around the period of menopausal transition among 3064 racially and ethnically diverse U.S. women aged 42 to 52 years at the start of the observation period (Sternfeld et al. 2004). Over three years of follow-up (1996-1997 to 1999-2000), mean weight increased by 2.1 kg ± 4.8 kg (about 3% ± 6.5%), and mean waist circumference increased by 2.2 cm ± 5.4 cm (about 2.8% ± 6.3%). Change in menopausal status was not associated with weight gain or increases in waist circumference. A

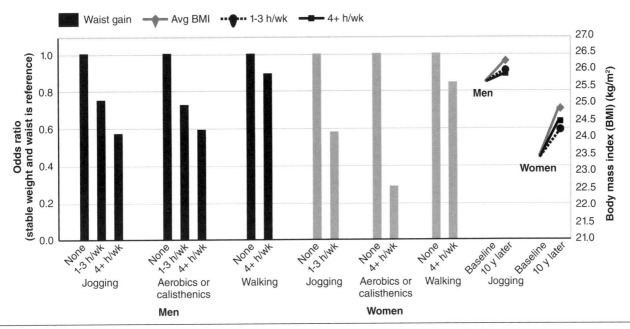

Figure 9.9 Consistent leisure-time physical activity and 10-year body mass gain in normal-weight Americans.

Data from Kahn et al. 1997.

standard deviation increase in self-reported level of sports/ exercise was longitudinally related to decreases of 0.32 kg in weight but not to change in waist circumference. Similar inverse relations (a decrease of 0.21 kg; 95% CI = −0.01 to 0.41 kg) were observed for daily routine physical activity (biking and walking for transportation and less television viewing). Thus, maintaining or increasing physical activity levels helped protect against midlife increases in body weight and girth that women commonly experience.

Sweden

The association of moderate-to-vigorous exercise two or more days a week with BMI was examined over eight years of follow-up in a random sample of 1972 women and 1871 men, aged 25 to 74 years, living in Sweden (Sundquist and Johansson 1998). About one-third of the sample changed their physical activity level. In both men and women, those who did not exercise had an increase in BMI of 0.30 kg/m² (95% CI: ~0.17-0.45). After adjustment for age, men who said they exercised at baseline but not at follow-up had a 0.28 kg/ m² larger increase in BMI than men who exercised at both baseline and at follow-up. Women who did not exercise at either baseline or follow-up had an increase in BMI of 0.37 kg/m² compared to women who exercised both at baseline and follow-up.

Norway Nord-Trøndelag Health Study: HUNT 1 and HUNT 2

This longitudinal study of an entire county in Norway examined whether leisure-time physical activity (walks, skiing, swimming, or working out) reported during 1984-1986

could predict change in BMI measured 11 years later in 9357 women, aged 20 to 49 years (Drøyvold et al. 2004a), and 6749 men, aged 20 to 69 years (Drøyvold et al. 2004b), who initially had a normal body weight and were free of CVD, diabetes, or long-term illnesses that limited activities of daily living. People were then classified as highly active (e.g., 30-60 min of moderate-to-vigorous activity nearly every day), moderately active (e.g., 16-30 min of moderate-to-vigorous activities two or three times a week), or inactive (less than once a week or never). About 50% of men and 60% of women gained at least 11 lb (5 kg); only 1% to 2% lost that much. After adjustment for age, education, smoking (in men), and BMI measured at baseline, women in the highly active group had gained 0.18 kg/m² less than those who were inactive. Weight gain among moderately active and inactive groups was the same. Men who were moderately active gained 0.12 kg/m² less than the inactive men. Body mass index change in highly active men did not differ from that in inactive men. Thus, as shown in figure 9.10, weight gain was greater among inactive men and women, but physical activity had a modest impact on slowing weight gain in healthy, normal-weight adults.

Aerobics Center Longitudinal Study

Change in fitness was used as an index of physical activity among 4599 men and 724 women (mean age 43 years) who had three or more measurements of body weight and fitness (maximal treadmill endurance time) between 1970 and 1994 (DiPietro et al. 1998). Change in fitness between the first two measurements (after about two years) predicted weight gain or loss over the average period of 7.5 years between the first and last measurements of body weight. During that

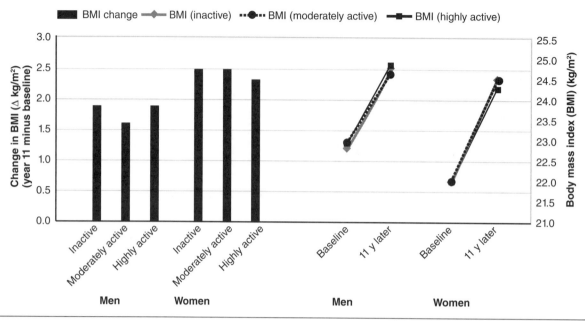

Figure 9.10   Leisure-time physical activity and 11-year weight gain in normal-weight Norwegian adults.

Adapted from Drøyvold et al. 2004.

time, men gained an average of 0.6 kg, and women gained an average of 1.5 kg. However, there was wide variation in weight change (the standard deviation was about 5 kg) that was linearly dependent on the changes in fitness. Among both men and women, each minute of improved treadmill endurance reduced weight gain by 0.6 kg; it reduced the risk of a weight gain of 5 kg or more by 14% in men and 9% in women and reduced the risk of a weight gain of 10 kg or more by 21% in both men and women.

A five-year follow-up analyzed the prospective association of weight change with leisure-time physical activity level (PAL), expressed as average daily energy expenditure in METs per 24 h, in 2500 healthy men ages 20 to 55 years from the ACLS cohort who had four or more clinic examinations between 1970 and 1998 (DiPietro, Dziura, and Blair 2004). There was a curvilinear weight gain over the follow-up among the men who maintained their physical activity level between the first and third clinic visit. The acceleration in weight gain was greater among men who decreased their PAL. A shift from a low PAL (<1.45 METs per 24 h) to a moderate (1.45-1.60 METs per 24 h) or high (>1.60 METs per 24 h) PAL was necessary for weight loss over time. Men with initially the lowest PAL had the greatest benefit from increasing activity to levels that can be achieved by incorporating 45 to 60 min of brisk walking, gardening or yard work, or cycling into the daily routine.

The Framingham Children's Study (FCS)

This longitudinal study of childhood cardiovascular risk behaviors began in 1987 with a small cohort of 106 healthy children aged 3 to 5 years who were third- and fourth-generation offspring of the initial Framingham Study cohort. Total physical activity was measured by an accelerometer three to five consecutive days on two occasions each year. An eight-year follow-up of 94 children found that boys and girls in the highest one-third of average daily activity from ages 4 to 11 years had smaller gains in BMI and skinfold thickness throughout childhood than the other children (Moore et al. 2003). The difference was most pronounced in girls. By age 11, BMI was about 7% lower and skinfold thickness about 20% lower in the most active children.

American Indian Schoolchildren— PATHWAYS

A cohort of 454 American Indian schoolchildren was followed for three years from 2nd to 5th grade (Stevens et al. 2004). Skinfolds and bioelectrical impedance were used to estimate percent body fat. After adjustment for body composition measures in 2nd grade, higher levels of total physical activity (recorded from accelerometry counts) predicted lower percentage body fat by 5th grade among normal-weight children but not overweight children. Among overweight children, higher physical activity was unrelated to change in percent body fat and was paradoxically associated with increases in BMI. Although an objective measure of physical activity was used in this study, it was performed for only one day of observation. Also, skinfolds, bioelectrical impedance, and BMI are imprecise measures of body fatness.

Avon Longitudinal Study of Parents and Children (ALSPAC)

This is an ongoing birth cohort study with data collected between 2003 and 2007 that examined associations between children's physical activity at age 12 and their body fatness at age 14 (Riddoch et al. 2009). In 1991 to 1992, 14,541 pregnant women living in the former County of Avon (United Kingdom) were recruited into the study. At age 12, 1964 boys and 2186 girls attended the clinic and provided information on exposure, outcome, and confounding variables. Total and moderate-to-vigorous physical activity (measured by an accelerometer for seven days) at age 12 was predictive of body fat mass (measured by DXA) at age 14. An extra 15 min of moderate-to-vigorous physical activity per day at age 12 was associated with lower fat mass at age 14 in boys (by 11.9% [95% CI: 9.5-14.3%]) and girls (by 9.8% [6.7-12.8%]).

The Women's Health Study (WHS)

The WHS was a randomized trial testing low-dose aspirin and vitamin E for preventing CVD and cancer among healthy women, conducted between 1992 and 2004. At the end of the trial, women continued in an observational follow-up study. A recent analysis examined the association of different amounts of physical activity with long-term weight changes among women consuming a usual diet (Lee et al. 2010). This analysis included 34,079 healthy U.S. women aged 54 years on average who consumed a usual diet, who were followed from 1992 to 2007. At the beginning of the study and at updates approximately every three years, women reported their physical activity. Body weight also was regularly reported throughout the study. Women were classified as expending <7.5 (equivalent to 150 min/week of moderate-intensity physical activity), 7.5 to <21 (equivalent to 60 min/day, or 420 min/week of moderate-intensity physical activity), and ≥21 MET-hours/week of activity at each time. Analyses examined physical activity and weight change over intervals averaging three years.

Women gained an average of 5.7 lb throughout the study. Compared with women who engaged in ≥21 MET-hours/week, those performing 7.5 to <21 MET-hours/week of activity, as well as those engaging in <7.5 MET-hours/week, gained significantly more weight, with no difference in weight gain between the two less active groups. The two less active groups also were significantly more likely to gain at least 5 lb over any three-year period than the most active women. More physical activity was associated with less weight gain only among women with normal BMI. Among heavier women, there was no association between physical activity and weight change. A small group of women—about 13%—started the study with a normal BMI (<25 kg/m²) and maintained their body weight throughout the study, gaining <5 lb at any time. Their mean physical activity level was approximately equivalent to 60 min/day

of moderate-intensity physical activity, sustained over the duration of the study.

The findings from this large study with long follow-up provide support for the conclusion of the scientific advisory committee for the Physical Activity Guidelines for Americans—that many individuals may need more than 150 min of moderate-intensity activity each week to maintain their weight at a stable level (Physical Activity Guidelines Advisory Committee 2008).

Physical Activity and Weight Loss: The Evidence

It is paradoxical that at the same time the prevalence of obesity in the United States was increasing, more adults were engaging in voluntary weight loss (Serdula et al. 1999; Williamson et al. 1992). In the 1950s and the early 1960s, only 7% of men and 14% of women were trying to lose weight, whereas in 1989, a national survey indicated that approximately 25% of men and 40% of women were trying to lose weight. The average man wanted to lose 30 lb (13.6 kg) and weighed 178 lb (80.7 kg). The average woman wanted to lose 31 lb (14.1 kg) and weighed 133 lb (60.3 kg). These trends were seen regardless of age, sex, and ethnicity. Most overweight individuals who are attempting to lose weight are not successful, especially in the long term. This means that a large majority of the adult population engages in weight cycling.

A recent systematic, quantitative review evaluated 18 prospective cohort studies of mortality risk after intentional weight loss by change in diet or physical activity (Harrington, Gibson, and Cottrell 2009). Intentional weight loss had a small benefit for people with obesity-related risk factors (RR = 0.87; 95% CI: 0.77-0.99), especially when they were also obese (RR = 0.84; 95% CI: 0.73-0.97). However, weight loss was associated with a small increase in mortality risk among people without obesity-related risk factors (RR = 1.11; 95% CI: 1.00-1.22) and people who were overweight but not obese (RR = 1.09; 95% CI: 1.02-1.17). There was no apparent benefit of weight loss among obese people who were otherwise healthy. Fourteen of the studies adjusted for physical activity, but the studies did not clarify the relative contributions of diet or physical activity to weight loss or to mortality risk. The authors concluded that there was a need for well-designed studies to identify the independent and interactive effects of physical activity, diet, and body composition in populations most likely to increase longevity through weight loss.

Weight Cycling: Aerobics Center Longitudinal Study (ACLS)

Some evidence from the ACLS suggests that physical activity or fitness can offset some of the risk of weight fluctuation or unhealthy diet. Weight gain associated with weight cycling across six years was observed in a clinic-based study of an ACLS cohort (Van Wye et al. 2007). Healthy, normal-weight men ($n = 797$) and women ($n = 141$), 20 to 78 years of age, completed at least four medical exams between 1987 and 2003. Weight loss history was reported, and body weight was measured at all examinations. Weight cycling status was defined as five or more episodes of losing at least 2.3 kg. Baseline BMI was 23 and 21 kg/m^2 among cycling and noncycling women and was 27 and 25 kg/m^2 among cycling and noncycling men. After adjustment for initial BMI, age, and smoking, weight gain was similar between men and women who weight cycled and those who didn't weight cycle. Even though a history of weight cycling did not increase the risk of long-term weight gain, cardiorespiratory fitness at baseline and increased fitness over the follow-up were associated with less weight gain in both women and men. For each extra 1 min of endurance on a maximal treadmill test at baseline, or for each 1-min increase in endurance between clinic visits (a difference of 7% in women and 5% in men), initial weight or weight gain was 0.2 kg lower for women and 0.55 kg lower for men.

▶ **REGULAR PHYSICAL** activity can help offset the weight fluctuations, loss of nonfat body mass, and subsequent health risk of restrictive yo-yo dieting.

Exercise Training Studies

Although physical activity has great potential efficacy for reducing body fat mass, studies have found that its actual effectiveness is small. Among normal-weight men and women, exercise training studies that followed the ACSM guidelines for increasing or maintaining cardiorespiratory fitness showed that on average, body weight was lowered by 1.5 kg (3.3 lb) and fat mass was lowered by 2.2% (American College of Sports Medicine 1983). The American Dietetic Association recently concluded that few studies have used a large enough "dose" of physical activity to achieve a 5% weight loss with a physical activity intervention alone. Also, it is common for some people to naturally eat more calories when they start exercising more. This increase in energy intake can negate the effects of extra exercise on negative energy balance in short-term studies that do not keep dietary calories constant. There is emerging evidence, though, that regular physical activity can have favorable effects on abdominal obesity and excess fat stored in the liver and skeletal muscle when its effects on body weight or total fat mass are minimal (Janisnewski and Ross 2007; Ross et al. 2000).

Exercise Only

The scientific advisory committee for the Physical Activity Guidelines for Americans located four randomized controlled trials that had enough participants to allow detection of a significant effect of physical activity on both body weight and body composition. They lasted between eight and 16 months, and the amount of physical activity ranged from 180 min of moderate-intensity physical activity per week to 360 min of moderate- to vigorous-intensity physical activity per week (Physical Activity Guidelines Advisory Committee 2008). Some other well-designed trials have shown benefits of exercise on abdominal obesity or have combined physical activity with diet for favorable weight-related outcomes.

A recent meta-analysis evaluated 14 aerobic exercise trials that lasted three to 12 months and involved 1847 obese or overweight patients. Six-month and 12-month programs similarly were associated with modest reductions in weight of 1.6 and 1.7 kg and waist circumference of about 2 cm (Thorogood et al. 2011).

The Midwest Exercise Trial

This 16-month randomized controlled trial tested whether supervised, moderate-intensity exercise without dieting was effective for losing weight or preventing weight gain in young adults who were overweight (BMI 25 to 34.9 kg/m^2) and sedentary (Donnelly et al. 2003). One hundred thirty-one adults aged 17 to 35 years were randomly assigned to a control group ($n = 44$) that maintained usual activity and eating habits or to the exercise group ($n = 87$). The exercise group was asked to walk on a treadmill or use a stationary exercise cycle or elliptical trainer at an intensity of 55% to 70% of aerobic capacity for 45 min a day, five days each week. Thirty-three controls and 41 exercisers finished the trial and participated in 90% of the sessions. Participants ate as they wished throughout the study, and there were no changes in energy intake during the study or between the groups. Strengths of the study were the use of underwater weighing and computer-assisted tomography to estimate body composition and fat mass, doubly labeled water to estimate energy expenditure, and a maximal exercise test to confirm that exercise adherence was sufficient to increase fitness. At 16 months, men expended about 670 kcal (6.7 kcal/kg of body weight), and women expended about 440 kcal (5.4 kcal/kg) each session.

Exercise prevented weight gain in women and produced weight loss in men. Figure 9.11 shows that men who exercised had reductions (mean ± SD) in weight (5.2 ± 4.7 kg), BMI (1.6 ± 1.4 kg/m^2), and fat mass (4.9 ± 4.4 kg) compared with controls. Women who exercised maintained their initial weight, BMI, and fat mass, while controls had increases in weight (2.9 ± 5.5 kg), BMI (1.1 ± 2.0 kg/m^2), and fat mass (2.1 ± 4.8 kg). The study confirmed that adherence to a regular, moderate-intensity exercise program is effective for managing weight without dieting in overweight young adults if it is sustained for 16 months. However, because more than half the exercisers dropped out of the program, the study also shows that the public health effectiveness of exercise in weight management is limited by people's willingness or ability to sustain a regular exercise program.

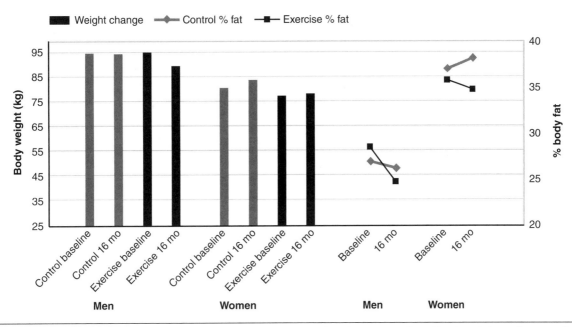

Figure 9.11 Results of the Midwest Exercise Trial showed that 16 months of exercise reduced body weight and percent body fat without dieting in overweight men and women.

Adapted from Donnelly et al. 2003.

Fred Hutchinson Cancer Research Center—Seattle

This 12-month trial examined the effect of moderate-to-vigorous aerobic exercise (60 min/day, three days a week using treadmills, stationary cycles, elliptical machines, and rowers at the clinic or health clubs and three days a week at home) on body weight and body composition in sedentary men ($n = 102$) and women ($n = 100$) 40 to 75 years of age (McTiernan et al. 2007). Men actually averaged 370 min/week, and women averaged 295 min/week. Women who exercised lost 1.4 kg of body weight and 1.9 kg of fat mass, while women in the nonexercising control group gained 0.7 kg of body weight. The authors estimated that the extra physical activity should have led to a weight loss of 7.8 kg had caloric intake remained stable, so the study shows that people tend to eat more when they exercise more, a practical problem of using exercise alone for short-term weight loss.

Another 12-month trial tested the effects of three or four days per week of moderate-intensity exercise (mainly walking) on total and intra-abdominal body fat among sedentary postmenopausal women aged 50 to 75 years who were overweight (body fat >33%) (Irwin et al. 2003). Women in the exercise group ($n = 87$) averaged three or four days a week and nearly 180 min/week in activity. Compared to a control group ($n = 86$) that met once a week for 45 min of stretching, the intervention group increased their aerobic capacity by about 11% and had decreases in body weight (−1.4 kg), percent body fat (−1.0%), intra-abdominal fat mass (−8.6 g/cm²), and subcutaneous abdominal fat mass (−28.8 g/cm²).

Duke University—STRRIDE Trial

One hundred seventy-five sedentary, overweight men and women (average BMI of 30 kg/m²) with dyslipidemia (i.e., risky levels of cholesterol) were randomly assigned to participate for six months in a control group or for eight months in one of three exercise groups that used treadmills, elliptical machines, or stationary cycles: (1) moderate intensity at 40% to 55% of aerobic capacity to expend 14 kcal/kg each week (e.g., walking 12 miles/week), (2) vigorous intensity at 65% to 80% of aerobic capacity to expend 14 kcal/kg each week (e.g., jogging 12 miles/week), or (3) vigorous intensity to expend 23 kcal/kg each week (e.g., jogging 20 miles/week) (Slentz et al. 2005). People in the control group had a 1% increase in body weight and an 8.6% increase in intra-abdominal fat, while the two exercise groups that expended about 14 kcal/kg each week had about a 1% decrease in body weight. The highest dose of exercise (i.e., about 23 kcal/kg each week) produced a nearly 3% decrease in weight and 7% decreases in intra-abdominal fat and subcutaneous abdominal fat without changes in caloric intake.

Minnesota Strength Training in Women Study

Sixty middle-aged women who had a BMI between 20 and 35 kg/m² were randomly assigned to 15 weeks of twice-weekly supervised strength training, followed by six months of unsupervised training, or to a no-intervention control group (Schmitz et al. 2003). At 39 weeks of follow-up, there was no effect of strength training on weight change, but the exercise group had changed the composition of their body weight. They gained 0.89 kg more fat-free mass, lost 1.0 kg more fat mass, and lost 1.63% more percent body fat compared to the control group who did not exercise. This study shows not only that resistance training can be effective in helping women lose body fat but also why it is wrong to judge the effectiveness of exercise by body weight alone. There is also evidence that aerobic exercise and resistance exercise can preserve fat-free mass while people lose weight by dieting.

University of Virginia

The effects of exercise training intensity on abdominal fat and body composition were tested in 27 middle-aged obese women (BMI = 34 ± 6 kg/m^2) with metabolic syndrome (Irving et al. 2008). Women were randomly assigned to one of three 16-week conditions: (1) control group (seven women who maintained their existing physical activity); (2) low-intensity exercise (11 who exercised five days each week at an intensity at or below lactate threshold), or (3) high-intensity exercise (nine participants who exercised three days each week at an intensity above lactate threshold and two days each week at or above lactate threshold). Session duration was manipulated to equate caloric expenditure during exercise training to about 400 kcal each session. Computed tomography scans were used to determine abdominal fat. Percent body fat was assessed by air displacement plethysmography. High-intensity training, but not low-intensity training, reduced total abdominal fat, subcutaneous abdominal fat, and intra-abdominal fat.

Weight Gain After Pregnancy

A review of six randomized controlled trials or quasi-experimental clinical trials including 245 women showed that exercise alone did not contribute to weight loss (a single study of 33 women), but that averaged across four trials including 169 women, diet plus exercise led to nearly 3 kg (95% CI: −4.83 to −0.95 kg) greater weight loss than usual medical care (Adegboye, Linne, and Lourenco 2007).

Exercise Plus Diet

The scientific advisory committee for the Physical Activity Guidelines for Americans concluded that adults who want to lose more than 5% of their body weight through an exercise program must also keep their food intake constant or restrict it through diet (Physical Activity Guidelines Advisory Committee 2008). Several studies have shown that this can be effective in people who are overweight or obese.

Women's Healthy Lifestyle Project

This was a five-year randomized controlled trial of a dietary and physical activity lifestyle intervention conducted from 1992 to 1999 that enrolled 535 healthy premenopausal women 44 to 50 years of age at study entry. Of these, 509 finished the trial (Simkin-Silverman et al. 2003). The diet plus physical activity group set weight loss goals of 5 to 15 lb (2.3-6.8 kg), depending on initial body weight. They were asked to eat 1300 to 1500 kcal/day (25% total fat, 7% saturated fat, 100 mg dietary cholesterol) and to increase their physical activity to at least 1000 to 1500 kcal/week. The intervention included 15 group meetings during the first 20 weeks and less frequent sessions later, when participants learned behavior change skills and took cooking lessons, exercise classes, and group walks. A control group underwent assessments only, with no experimental change in lifestyle. Women in the lifestyle intervention group were more physically active and reported eating fewer calories than controls during the study period (see figure 9.12). After 4.5 years, 55% of intervention participants but just 26% of control participants were at or below their initial body weight. The mean weight change in the diet plus physical activity group was 0.2 lb (0.1 kg, SD = 5.2 kg) below their entry weight, compared with an average gain of 5.2 lb (2.4 kg, SD = 4.9 kg) in the control group. Body mass index (kg/m^2) averaged 25 in each group at the beginning of the study. It increased to 26 in the control participants but did not change in the intervention group. However, percent body fat measured by skinfolds and DXA decreased by 0.5% (SD = 4%) in the diet plus physical activity group while increasing by 1% (SD = 4%) in the control group. Waist circumference decreased more in the intervention group (M = −2.9 cm, SD = 5.3) than in controls (M = −0.5 cm, SD = 5.6).

St. Luke's–Roosevelt Hospital, New York City

Moderately obese patients aged 19 to 48 years received weekly nutrition counseling and were randomly assigned to one of three groups for eight months: diet plus strength training (progressive resistance for arms and legs), diet plus aerobic training (leg and arm cycling), or diet only (Geliebter et al. 1997). Twenty-five men and 40 women finished the trial. Their formula diet had an energy content that was 70% of their RMR (about 1230 ± 255 kcal/day). Three weekly supervised exercise sessions were roughly equivalent in energy expenditure. All groups lost about 9.0 kg. The strength training group lost less fat-free mass than the aerobic and diet-only groups but nonetheless had a similar drop in RMR. Thus, strength training protected lean mass during dieting but did not prevent the decline in RMR commonly seen when overweight people lose weight.

Behavioral Factors

The Dose-Response to Exercise in Women (DREW) trial randomly assigned 464 postmenopausal overweight women who said they did not exercise regularly into three groups that exercised with a personal trainer at half their aerobic capacity for an average of 72, 136, or 194 min (about 4, 8, or 12 kcal · kg^{-1} · week^{-1}) each for six months or to a control group that maintained their usual exercise habits and completed a symptom questionnaire each month (Church et al. 2009).

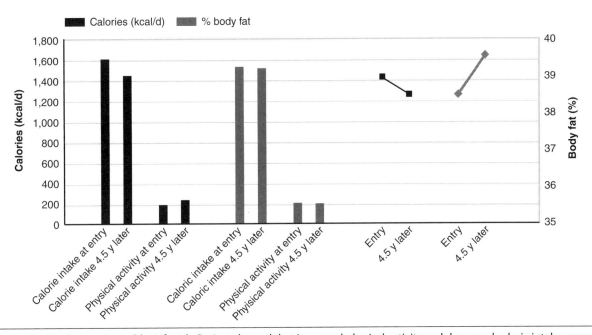

Figure 9.12 The Women's Healthy Lifestyle Project showed that increased physical activity and decreased calorie intake prevented five-year weight gain in perimenopausal women.

Source: Simkin-Silverman et al. 2003; Kuller et al. 2001; Simkin-Silverman et al. 1995.

Waist circumference was reduced in all exercise groups; and all the groups, including the controls, lost 1 to 2 kg. Weight loss by the 4 and 8 kcal · kg^{-1} · week^{-1} groups was about what would be expected based on the energy expended and no change in calorie intake from diet. However, the loss by the 12 kcal · kg^{-1} · week^{-1} group was about half that expected. Even though the exercisers were asked to keep their normal diet, most of the women who exercised ate more than they had before starting the trial. It is also possible that they compensated for their extra exercise by becoming less active in their daily routines than they had been before they entered the program. This study illustrates the practical problems of gauging the impact of exercise on weight loss, as people may eat more than normal or decrease daily nonexercise activities when they undertake a new exercise program. It doesn't take much extra consumption to offset the negative energy balance from a single exercise session. Eating a healthy bran muffin and drinking a bottle of fruit juice can more than replenish the 200 or 300 calories burned in a typical exercise session.

Although there is a general view that an increase in physical activity will increase hunger and eating to offset any benefit of exercise for weight loss, the actual evidence for that view is scant (e.g., Woo, Garrow, and Pi-Sunyer 1982). Exercise studies lasting up to two weeks, with a negative energy balance up to 1000 kcal/day, show that increased food intake follows initial weight loss but is only about 30% of the energy expended by exercise. And, some people show no compensation by extra eating. On the other hand, when active people become sedentary, they typically don't eat less to balance off the decrease in energy expenditure (Blundell et al. 2003).

Exercise and Appetite

The brain senses blood levels of glucose and insulin and regulates hunger between meals. Low glucose stimulates appetite, while high levels of glucose and insulin inhibit appetite. Exercise lowers insulin and glucose levels, so it might affect appetite. Whether exercise stimulates or inhibits appetite in the short term has not as yet been clearly determined, but studies generally show that appetite is suppressed shortly after an exercise session (Martins, Morgan, and Truby 2008). Recent studies have begun to examine the effect of exercise on leptin and ghrelin, two hormones that regulate energy balance, in part by affecting appetite in ways similar to glucose and insulin. Leptin is the primary energy balance hormone released from fat cells, partly in response to insulin. Together with other energy-regulating hormones released from the gut, fat cells, and skeletal muscle, low leptin levels activate peripheral and brain systems to restore energy balance. High levels suppress eating and increase energy expenditure. Leptin induces feelings of satiety by binding with receptors in the hypothalamus that affect appetite, mainly by suppressing secretion of neuropeptide Y by cells in the arcuate nucleus—in the same way that insulin does. It also activates other brain systems involved in finding food, smelling and tasting food, and in regulating the rewarding effects of food (Lenard and Berthoud 2008). Levels of leptin in the blood are proportional to body fat, so people who are obese typically have high levels, suggesting that they are resistant to the normal effect of leptin to suppress energy intake. Their levels return to normal after weight loss. Ghrelin is secreted mainly by the stomach and by epsilon cells in the pancreas to stimulate appetite, mainly by stimulating neuropeptide Y secretion. It increases in the blood before meals and decreases after meals.

Blood levels of leptin are not changed after exercise lasting less than an hour or expending less than 800 kcal, but are decreased after longer sessions that stimulate release of free fatty acids in the blood or expend more than 800 kcal (Bouassida et al. 2008). Ghrelin levels are not affected by acute sessions of moderate to vigorous aerobic exercise (Kraemer and Castracane 2007); but hypothetically, leptin should be decreased after chronic exercise that leads to weight loss. Leptin levels and waist circumference were reduced in sedentary, obese women after 14 weeks of resistance exercise three days per week or a 1200 kcal/day diet (Kerksick et al. 2009). In a study of obese teens, eight months of moderate or vigorous exercise training did not change leptin levels on average, but youths who had the lowest increase in cardiovascular fitness tended to have the highest increase in leptin levels (Barbeau et al. 2003). Other proteins produced in the hypothalamus (e.g., orexin A and neuropeptide Y) stimulate eating and contribute to obesity. Orexin A also stimulates physical activity and is elevated in obesity-resistant rats (Teske et al. 2006), but the effects of exercise on orexin A and neuropeptide Y in humans are not known.

Exercise training programs that allow people who are overweight to eat as they wish frequently lead to fat loss in men but not women, possibly because of sex differences in the way energy-regulating hormones and appetite respond to increased energy expenditure (Hagobian and Braun 2010). One small study had overweight men and women exercise with or without extra dietary calories to balance the energy cost of the exercise (Hagobian et al. 2009). Ghrelin levels were not affected by exercise in men, but they were elevated after exercise in women regardless of whether energy cost was balanced with more intake. Appetite was inhibited in the men after energy-balanced exercise, but exercise did not change women's appetite. One interpretation of the results is that mechanisms to maintain body fat are more effective in women than in men. In a separate study, women's feelings of hunger were suppressed during a session of walking that expended 550 kcal, but they were not affected between meals despite an increase in ghrelin and a delayed and short-term decrease in leptin after exercise (Borer et al. 2009).

Genetic Factors

At least 22 genes have been supported in descriptive studies as influences on obesity (Rankinen et al. 2006), but they each account for a small portion (less than 1%) of variation among people. A stronger association has been found for the FTO (fat mass and obesity associated) gene. People of European ancestry who inherit a risky variation in the FTO gene from one or both parents (30-50% of the populations studied) weigh on average 1 to 4 kg more and have a 15% to 65% increased risk of having high BMI, perhaps because the gene contributes to eating more or storing more fat (Loos and Bouchard 2008). The population attributable risk of

obesity from variations in the FTO gene has been shown to be about 20%.

Physical activity has been associated with lower BMI in people who have a risky version of the FTO gene in several studies, but not all. In a group of 700 Pennsylvania Amish adults, who by tradition lead an active lifestyle, an FTO variant was associated with high BMI only in those in the bottom 25% of age- and sex-adjusted physical activity measured by an accelerometer for seven days (about 2600 and 3100 kcal/day) (Rampersaud et al. 2008). There was no increased risk of being overweight or obese in people with the risky FTO gene if they were in the top 25% in physical activity (about 3600 and 4000 kcal/day). However, even the least-active Amish were spending about 3 to 4 h each day in moderate physical activity, a level much higher than that of the typical American who has a more sedentary lifestyle.

Another FTO variant was studied in a cohort of 20,374 British men and women aged 39 to 79 years from the European Prospective Investigation into Cancer and Nutrition–Norfolk Study (Vimaleswaran et al. 2009). People with the risky version of the FTO gene who said they had a sedentary job and got no leisure-time physical activity had 75% higher risk of elevated BMI and 60% higher risk of greater waist circumference than those who said they got at least some physical activity during a typical week. In 17,162 middle-aged adults living in Denmark, people with a different GTO variant commonly related to obesity risk in white Europeans had about 20 to 30 greater odds of being overweight or obese and had higher waist circumference, fat mass, and fasting serum leptin levels. People who inherited the variant from both parents and were also physically inactive had the highest BMI (Andreasen et al. 2008). However, physical activity did not modify the risk of high BMI associated with that FTO variant in cohorts from Sweden and Finland (Jonsson et al. 2009).

A few exercise training studies have examined whether people with a risky form of FTO lose less or more fat after exercise training. After a 20-week endurance training program in 481 sedentary white participants in the HERITAGE Family Study, men and women who had a nonrisky variant of the FTO gene lost three to four times more body weight, fat mass, and percent body fat than people who got the risky variant from both parents rather than just one parent. The FTO genotype explained 2% of the variation in fat loss. FTO was not associated with weight loss among 259 black participants (Rankinen et al. 2009). The same FTO variant was examined in the Dose-Response to Exercise in Women (DREW) trial of 234 white, postmenopausal women (Mitchell et al. 2009). The women who inherited the risky variant from both parents had higher BMI before starting the exercise program than those who lacked the risky gene, but they lost a similar amount of weight after six months of moderate-intensity exercise. However, among women who met or exceeded the amount of physical activity recommended for weight loss, those who were homozygous for the risky FTO variant lost twice as much weight (about 3 kg) as women without the risky variant or women who got it from only one parent.

Despite the likelihood that physical activity will interact with people's genes to influence obesity-related outcomes, some studies seem to show that physical activity habits during adulthood influence obesity just as strongly as, or more strongly than, genetic inheritance or childhood habits. In a classic experimental study of genetic influence on weight loss, seven pairs of young adult male identical twins exercised twice a day, nine out of 10 days, while their daily energy and nutrient intake remained unchanged (Bouchard et al. 1994). The total energy deficit above RMR caused by exercise was about 58,000 kcal. Average fat loss was 11 lb (5.0 kg). Although the difference in weight loss between sets of twins was six times greater than the average difference within each pair of twins, about one-fourth of the weight loss couldn't be explained by the fact that twins had the same DNA. In a 30-year observational study of 89 pairs of twins from the Finnish Twin cohort, 42 twin pairs differed in their self-reported physical activity in 1975, 1981, and 2005. Weight gain between 1975 and 2005 was 5.4 kg less, and waist circumference in 2005 was 8.4 cm less, in the active compared to inactive twins. The differences were similar for identical and fraternal twin pairs and did not appear between twin pairs that reported similar physical activity. Though limited to self-reports, this study suggests that persistent physical activity reduces odds of weight gain even after genes and childhood environment are partially controlled for (Waller, Kaprio, and Kujala 2008).

Children and Adolescents

A quantitative review summarized 14 randomized controlled trials of physical activity that typically lasted 16 weeks and were designed to reduce weight in a total of 481 overweight or obese boys and girls from the United States, Australia, Austria, Canada, Sweden, and Hong Kong (Atlantis, Barnes, and Singh 2006). On average, the studies reported reductions in body weight (−2.7 kg, 95% CI: −6.1 to −0.8 kg) and percent body fat (−0.4%, 95% CI: −0.7 to −0.01%). Although those effects are modest in size, they are clinically meaningful. And they were dose related, with larger effects generally seen after 155 to 180 min each week than after 120 to 150 min each week. However, the studies had many weaknesses. Only four reported dietary intake of calories. Also, despite presumed randomization, differences between the exercise and control groups at the beginning of the study were often larger than the effects of exercise, making it difficult to show benefits. Finally, no study used more than 200 min of weekly physical activity, which is far below current public recommendations that school-age children get 60 min of moderate-to-vigorous physical activity each day (i.e., 420 min each week). Some more recent studies have used improved methods and obtained stronger results.

A quantitative review of 18 school-based physical activity interventions that lasted six months to three years (Harris et al. 2009), as well as another review of 14 interventions last-

ing seven weeks to six years (Dobbins et al. 2009), reported no average effect of physical activity on BMI. This might be explained by an insufficient amount of physical activity, poor adherence to the planned interventions, failure to control diet, and the use of BMI as the outcome rather than a more accurate measure of body fatness. Body weight typically doesn't change after increased physical activity when the study was not designed with weight or fat loss as the primary outcome (Webber et al. 2008). The studies also did not focus on children who are overweight or obese or on the importance of physical activity in preventing weight gain in children who initially have normal weight. Fighting obesity in children will no doubt require coordinated efforts to change environments and behaviors that put children at risk for excess weight gain (see the sidebar Treating Childhood Obesity).

Nonetheless, well-executed research such as the FitKid Project at the Medical College of Georgia has shown positive effects of physical activity for weight loss in children. In this project, a 10-month randomized controlled trial tested the effect of a daily after-school program consisting of 30 min of schoolwork and healthy snack time and 80 min of moderate-to-vigorous physical activity (MVPA) (25 min of skills instruction, 35 min of aerobic physical activity, and 20 min of strengthening/stretching) on body composition in 118 black girls aged 8 to 12 years. Another 83 girls were measured only on outcomes (Barbeau et al. 2007). Outcomes were waist circumference, BMI, percent body fat measured by DXA, and abdominal fat mass measured by magnetic resonance imaging. Girls in the control group had gotten fatter or had stayed about the same 10 months later. Girls in the intervention stayed about the same or lost body fat. After adjustment for age, initial scores on the outcome measures, and a doctor's rating of sexual maturation, the intervention group showed larger decreases in percent body fat (−2%, 95% CI: −3 to −1%), BMI (−0.45 kg/m², 95% CI: −0.79 to −0.12 kg/m²), and abdominal fat mass (−14.6 cm³, 95% CI: −24.2 to −5.1 cm³) but not waist circumference, even though average attendance was just 54% of the sessions. Higher attendance was associated with greater decreases in percent body fat and BMI. Also, girls who exercised more vigorously during the sessions had greater decreases in percent body fat.

An eight-month randomized controlled trial tested the FitKid Project (40 min of homework and healthy snacks plus about an hour of physical activity [20 min of warm-up and skills instruction; 40 min of moderate-to-vigorous physical activity, about 200 kcal; and 10 min of cool-down]) in 600 3rd-grade girls and boys (61% black, 31% white, 3% Asian or Hispanic) from 18 public schools. Children who attended at least 40% of the daily sessions (n = 182) decreased their percent body fat by 0.76% (95% CI: −1.42 to −0.09%) compared to the children in the control group (n = 265), who did not change (Yin et al. 2005). Results were not different according to race, sex, or school (including the percentage of students receiving a free or reduced-price lunch). Among these children, 164 students from the control group and 42 students who attended at least 40% of all sessions were still attending the same schools two years later. Each year the

Treating Childhood Obesity

- Change family lifestyle.
- Parents should be "agents of change" for young children.
- Use behavior modification to support long-term change in behavior, including modifying the environment (e.g., removing cues to eat and adding cues to be active), monitoring behavior, setting and checking goals, and rewarding positive change.
- Change dietary intake and eating patterns: Parents should model healthy food choices and have children eat lower-fat and lower-energy foods, increase fruits and vegetables, decrease portion sizes, and drink fewer sweetened beverages.

- Increase physical activity: Have children do more unstructured outdoor play; have them use active transport (e.g., walking or bicycling) to school and parks; provide transportation for sport participation when needed; parents should model an active lifestyle.
- Decrease time spent in sedentary behavior (e.g., limit television viewing and computer use to less than 2 h each day).
- Use nonconventional treatments, including weight loss drugs, as an adjuvant to support long-term lifestyle changes in adolescents who are obese.

Adapted from Baur 2009.

children attending the FitKid program had a reduction in percent body fat while the control children had an increase. This occurred despite a larger increase in BMI among the intervention children. The intervention children returned to the level of the controls during the summers when the program was not offered, suggesting the need for year-round physical activity programming during elementary school (Gutin et al. 2008).

A review that compared lifestyle and drug treatments for obesity in children and adolescents found that 12 interventions, centered on increasing physical activity or reducing sedentary behaviors, had on average a significant effect on reducing BMI after six or 12 months. The effect was small compared to treatment with the drugs orlistat or sibutramine, but the drugs had adverse side effects in the children (Oude Luttikhuis et al. 2009).

Restricting Caloric Intake and Increasing Physical Activity

The American Dietetic Association concluded that weight loss studies have shown only small reductions in body weight with physical activity treatment compared to no-treatment control groups. This likely reflects the fact that energy deficits that can be induced through physical activity alone—at least, in amounts tolerable for most individuals—are relatively small. However, the amount of weight loss with physical activity is additive to the loss that follows a reduction in calorie intake with a diet. Depending on body size, fitness level, and exercise intensity, adults can easily expend an extra 1000 kcal per week by exercising 30 min five days a week. By comparison, a person on a diet can easily consume an extra 1000 kcal each week by miscalculating portion sizes or

by have a few extra snacks or beverages (American Dietetic Association 2009).

Food restriction produces a decline in basal energy expenditure that accompanies the decline in body weight. Basal metabolic rate (BMR) and the thermic effect of food are reduced during food restriction. Basal metabolic rate declines as total mass and fat-free mass decline. Because physical activity, especially resistance exercise, can decrease the percentage of body mass that is fat while increasing fat-free mass, it has the potential to retard the reduction in BMR common during restrictive diets. Initial body fat influences the changes in **body composition** after chronic exercise. People with more body fat have some protection against the loss of fat-free mass during early weight loss. They lose only about 0.25 kg of fat-free mass for each kilogram of body weight lost (Forbes 1992).

There is consensus that an exercise program cannot prevent some loss of fat-free mass during substantial weight loss, even when caloric intake remains the same as it was prior to the beginning of the exercise program. Exercise can lead to a small gain in fat-free mass as body fat is reduced; this occurs when body weight does not change during the exercise program. Hence, people who desire to increase or maintain fat-free mass during an exercise program must have a diet of sufficient calories to balance the increased energy expenditure.

In one study of obese women (You et al. 2006), adding either low-intensity (nearly an hour at 50% of aerobic capacity) or high-intensity (30 min at about 70% of capacity) walking three days a week to a 20-week diet to yield a 2800 kcal/week energy deficit produced reductions in body weight (11-13%), fat mass (17-20%), fat-free mass (6-8%), waist girth (9-10%), and percent body fat (7-10%) similar to those with diet alone. However, only diet plus exercise, not diet alone, decreased the size of subcutaneous fat cells in the abdomen, a risk factor for type 2 diabetes.

Physical Activity and Weight Maintenance: The Evidence

Lost body weight is usually regained when diets are used alone, but diet combined with increased exercise seems to yield better maintenance of weight loss, especially if the exercise program is maintained after the diet ends. Figure 9.13 illustrates the results of an eight-week diet among obese adults (Pavlou, Krey, and Steffee 1989). Not only was exercise as effective as diet for weight loss, but adding an exercise program at the end of the diet also prevented participants from regaining weight eight and 18 months later. The amount of physical activity needed to keep weight off after a diet is not fully known, but experts have suggested it may be as much as 2500 to 2800 kcal/week, two to three times as much as recommended for reducing other health risks (Johannsen, Redman, and Ravussin 2007).

If a change in body weight less than 3% is used as the standard for weight maintenance and a change of 5% or more is judged as clinically meaningful for reducing health risks (Stevens et al. 2006), an obese person weighing 200 lb (91 kg) would need to lose and keep off 6 lb (2.7 kg) to reduce excess weight and lose and keep off 10 lb (4.5 kg) for a health benefit.

The American Dietetics Association concluded physical activity seems crucial for preventing weight regain after initial weight loss (American Dietetic Association 2009). Many correlation studies show a strong association between physical activity at follow-up and maintenance of a weight loss (Kayman, Bruyold, and Stern 1990). For example, in one study, overweight or obese women recruited from a hospital-based weight loss center were asked to increase physical activity by 1000 to 2000 kcal/week and told to reduce intake to 1200 to 1500 kcal/day. After six months, physical activity had increased on average by about 1200 kcal/week, but that increase dropped to about 700 kcal/week after 24 months. The women who maintained a loss of 10% or more of initial body weight after 24 months reported more physical activity (an increase of 275 min/week) than those who sustained a weight loss of less than 10% (increases of 75 to 125 min/week) (e.g., Jakicic et al. 2008).

A systematic, quantitative review of 25 years of weight loss interventions published through 1994 reported that studies had focused on middle-aged adults who had class 1 obesity (BMI = 33.2 ± 0.5 kg/m² ; percent body fat 33.4 ± 0.7%) using short-term interventions (15.6 ± 0.6 weeks) (Miller, Koceja, and Hamilton 1997). The average diet or diet plus exercise intervention each resulted in a weight loss of about 11 kg. About 6.6 ± 0.5 and 8.6 ± 0.8 kg of weight loss was maintained after one year following diet only or diet plus exercise, respectively.

A subsequent systematic review of six randomized clinical trials lasting 10 to 52 weeks compared maintenance of long-term weight loss (at least one year) in overweight and obese adults (BMI >25 kg/m²) after a diet plus exercise intervention with a diet-only intervention (Curioni and Lourenco 2005). Differences were small in each study, but when the studies were averaged together, diet plus exercise resulted in 20% greater initial weight loss (13 kg ± 10 kg) than diet alone (−9.9 kg ± 9.6 kg) and a 20% greater sustained weight loss after one year (6.7 kg ± 8.3 kg) than diet alone (4.5 kg ± 11.3). Nonetheless, nearly half of the initial weight loss was regained after one year, regardless of whether the program included extra physical activity. Similarly, a recent systematic, quantitative review of 18 randomized controlled trials lasting at least six months compared the effect of diet plus

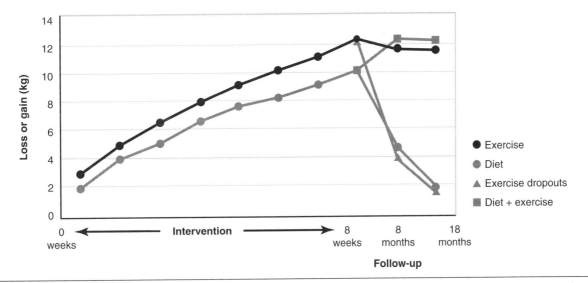

Figure 9.13 Study on moderately obese people illustrates not only that exercise was as effective for weight loss as an eight-week diet among adults, but also that adding an exercise program at the end of a diet prevented participants from regaining weight later.

Adapted from Pavlou et al. 1989.

Reasonable Weight

It is important to recognize behavioral factors and a person's history when implementing a successful weight loss or maintenance program. Yale psychologist and weight loss expert Kelly Brownell has popularized the notion of **reasonable weight** rather than "desirable" weight (Wilfley and Brownell 1994). His view is that desirable weight has been judged by normative (i.e., averaged among many people) weights associated with risks for disease and mortality rather than by the impact of weight gain on individuals, their unique histories, and the circumstances that contribute to their settling point and to their likelihood of successful maintenance of weight loss.

Wilfley and Brownell 1994.

What Is a Reasonable Weight Goal?

Clinical questions:

Is there a history of excess weight in your parents or grandparents?

What is the lowest weight you have maintained as an adult for at least one year?

What is the largest size of clothes about which you would say, "I look pretty good considering where I have been"?

At what weight would you wear these clothes?

What does a friend or family member of your age and frame weigh who looks "normal" to you?

At what weight can you live with the required changes in eating and exercise?

---

exercise interventions with diet-only interventions on weight loss in obese or overweight adults (Wu et al. 2009). Results favored the combination of diet and exercise. The average weight loss was 1.14 kg (95% CI: 0.21-2.07) and the average reduction in BMI was 0.50 kg/m² (95% CI: 0.21-0.79) greater after diet plus exercise than after diet alone. Again, much of the lost weight was regained after the interventions ended.

The scientific advisory committee of the Physical Activity Guidelines for Americans concluded that many people may need more than 300 min of moderate-intensity activity each week to meet their weight control goals (Physical Activity Guidelines Advisory Committee 2008). A doubly labeled water study of women who had lost about 12 kg to achieve a target BMI of 20 to 30 kg/m² estimated that a daily energy expenditure from physical activity of 11 to 12 kcal/kg might be needed to prevent weight regain after weight loss (Schoeller, Shay, and Kushner 1997).

Data from the National Weight Control Registry also indicate that a high level of daily physical activity may be necessary to prevent weight regain (Klem et al. 1997). The National Weight Control Registry is a registry of more than 3000 individuals who have successfully maintained at least a 30-lb (13.6 kg) weight loss for a minimum of one year. These individuals have reported using a variety of methods to lose weight initially, but more than 90% report exercise as crucial to their long-term weight loss maintenance. They report expending, on average, 2682 kcal per week in exercise, an energy equivalent of walking 4 miles (6.4 km) seven days a week.

Strength of the Evidence

Both population-based epidemiological studies and clinical trials support the claim that regular physical activity and

exercise training are useful for reducing the primary and secondary risk of excess weight gain during adulthood and for helping obese or overweight people keep off most of the weight they lose after a weight loss intervention. The usefulness of physical activity for short-term weight loss depends in part on a person's initial fatness and diet.

Temporal Sequence

Nearly 20 prospective cohort studies agree that increases in physical activity or fitness (defined as increased maximal treadmill endurance) predict weight loss or an attenuation of weight gain over periods of two to 10 years.

Strength of Association

A quantitative review evaluated 22 nonrandomized and nine randomized clinical trials published between 1966 and 2000 that studied the effect of exercise training on weight or fat loss (Ross and Janssen 2001). Twenty short-term studies lasting four months or less increased energy expenditure by an average of 2200 kcal/week and reported mean reductions in body weight of 0.18 kg/week and fat weight of 0.21 kg/week. Eleven long-term studies lasting 6.5 months or more increased energy expenditure by an average of 1100 kcal/week and reported mean reductions in body weight of 0.06 kg/week and fat weight of 0.06 kg/week. On average, physical activity that expends 13 to 26 kcal $\cdot$ kg^{-1} $\cdot$ week^{-1} (about 180 min of moderate exercise or 115 min of vigorous exercise) will lead to small weight losses of 1% to 3% (Slentz et al. 2005). Though modest for weight loss purposes, those amounts can be very useful for helping people keep their weight stable as they age and for maintaining weight loss after a diet.

Consistency

Population-based observational studies that included men and women from nationally representative cohorts in the United States and a few nations in Europe generally agree that physical activity is associated with less weight gain, regardless of age, sex, or race. Physical activity and fitness level also reduce mortality risk in people who are overweight. However, most studies were of people of European descent. Similarly, randomized controlled trials have shown that exercise training contributes to weight and fat loss in both men and women regardless of race, though most studies were limited to white people.

Dose Response

Fat loss is proportional to the amount of energy expenditure in short-term exercise studies but not long-term studies (Ross and Janssen 2001). The weight loss during short-term studies is about 85% of what would be predicted based on energy expenditure, assuming a controlled diet. In contrast, weight loss is only about 30% of that expected in long-term studies, suggesting poor adherence by the participants to either the prescribed physical activity or the prescribed diet. Only a few studies of women had them expend more than 1500 kcal/week, so it was not clear whether the dose response occurred in women. Also, studies generally did not compare results between men and women or among people of different races. Based on available evidence, it does not seem that high intensities of exercise lead to greater losses in weight or total fat than moderate intensities when time is adjusted to keep energy expenditure the same for each. The ACSM concluded that there is a dose response that is effective between about 2.5 to 4.5 h of moderate-intensity exercise (55-69% of maximal heart rate or about 3 to 6 METs depending on age) that results in an energy expenditure of at least 1200 to 2000 kcal/week. That amount of activity, combined with reduced calorie intake of 1000 to 1500 kcal/week, will yield healthful weight loss (1 to 2 lb/week [0.5-1 kg]). Intermittent periods of physical activity (e.g., 10-min sessions that accumulate to 30 to 40 min per day) seem to be as effective as continuous sessions.

The scientific advisory committee of the Physical Activity Guidelines for Americans further concluded that physical activity equivalent to 13 to 26 MET-hours/week is associated with a 1% to 3% weight loss in the absence of dieting. The low end of that range could be achieved by 150 min of brisk walking each week. Physical activity that expends 26 kcal/kg of body weight or more each week (1500+ MET-minutes) is needed for weight loss of 5% or greater. Most people could achieve that by brisk walking daily for about 45 to 70 min or jogging 20 to 25 min each day. The committee also concluded that many adults need about 60 min of walking or 30 min of jogging daily (about 4.4 kcal/kg daily) to prevent substantial weight regain over periods of six months or longer (Physical Activity Guidelines Advisory Committee 2008).

Biological Plausibility

Physical activity can contribute to energy expenditure in three main ways.

First, energy expenditure during exercise can be elevated to two to 20 times resting metabolism, depending on the duration and intensity of the exercise and the person's fitness. This effect contributes to an increase in total daily energy expenditure unless the added exercise is followed by a compensatory and equivalent decline in physical activity during the rest of the day. Second, exercise can produce both temporary and persistent increases in RMR. Resting metabolic rate is the largest component of most people's total daily energy expenditure (about 60% to 75%). Thus, temporary increases in RMR after single exercise sessions and persistent increases after exercise training could accumulate to contribute to weight loss or maintenance over time, in addition to the direct energy cost of muscular work. Third, long-term exercise training that increases or preserves lean mass produces a persistent increase in RMR even when fat mass and body mass are each reduced by strict diets or by old age.

Energy expenditure does not return to preexercise resting levels immediately after exercise ends. As people recover, their oxygen consumption, and thus their RMR, remains elevated. This is known as the *excess postexercise oxygen consumption* (EPOC), which results from higher body temperature, breathing, and circulation and acts to replenish oxygen in tissues, to resynthesize ATP (adenosine triphosphate) and creatine phosphate in muscle, and to replenish glycogen stores in muscle and the liver. The period of EPOC can be a few minutes or 24 h, depending on the intensity and duration of the exercise (Hill, Drougas, and Peters 1994). EPOC shows a rapid, steep decline within the first 2 h after exercise that is followed by a longer-lasting gradual decline, which can last for 24 h or so depending on the person's fitness level and how strenuous the exertion was (Børsheim and Bahr 2003). An increased rate of triglyceride to fatty acid cycling and a shift from carbohydrate to fat as fuel can contribute to the prolonged component of EPOC. EPOC is proportional to the duration of exercise at intensities above 50% to 60% of aerobic capacity. A prolonged EPOC (3-24 h) can follow durations of 50 min or more at vigorous intensities of at least 70% of aerobic capacity, but even prolonged EPOC durations yield only 6% to 15% of oxygen cost of the exercise (LaForgia, Withers, and Gore 2006). The U.S. Institute of Medicine estimated that EPOC is 15% of energy expenditure during exercise, but recent simulations of daily physical activities by men under laboratory conditions showed that it was 5% to 6% of the total energy expended during moderately or vigorously strenuous days (Ohkawara et al. 2008). So, adults who follow public health recommendations to increase their physical activity by 500 kcal each day might burn as many as 75 extra kilocalories after the exercise ends if they are vigorously active. For most people, though, 25 to 30 extra kilocalories is more likely.

Many studies, but not all, show that long-term exercise training that increases or preserves lean mass produces a persistent increase in RMR even when fat mass and body mass are each reduced (Speakman and Selman 2003). How big a contribution can that be? Resting muscle cells require about three times more energy at rest than fat cells (about 6 vs. 2 kcal per lb per day) (Wang et al. 2001). So, a person weighing 180 lb (82 kg) who loses 5 lb (2.3 kg) of fat and increases lean mass by 5 lb after a three-month exercise program would increase RMR by a net of 20 kcal per day even though body weight did not change. This is not a big difference, but it is one that could contribute substantially to fat loss or weight maintenance in the long term (about a 10-lb [4.5 kg] impact over a five-year period).

However, most investigators have found that aerobic exercise training in people who are not obese has little persistent effect on RMR. This is not surprising because training in nonobese subjects generally has a very small effect on fat-free mass, the major determinant of RMR. The intensity and duration of exercise needed to produce long-lasting elevations in RMR by increasing lean mass, or to elicit a prolonged EPOC after a single exercise session, exceed what most people choose, or are able, to do. Hence, the cumulative energy expended during exertion seems to be the main contribution of exercise and physical activity to weight loss and maintenance.

It is also plausible that regular exercise might have healthful effects on hormones that regulate energy balance. One of those hormones, adiponectin, is secreted by fat cells to help regulate the metabolism of glucose and fatty acids. Higher levels of adiponectin are associated with reduced risks of metabolic diseases such as type 2 diabetes, atherosclerotic diseases, nonalcoholic fatty liver disease, and metabolic syndrome. Although acute exercise does not seem to affect the level of adiponectin in the blood, the long-term effects of regular physical activity are not yet known (Bouassida et al. 2008).

Resistance Exercise

Weight loss after resistance exercise training is usually less than 1 kg, but that can be misleading when the training produces an increase in fat-free mass. Studies have shown that weight training led to reductions in body fat only slightly less than those produced by aerobic exercise and that weight training also produced more substantial increases in fat-free mass, which may have the added benefit of increasing energy expenditure. Exercise might increase RMR by increasing fat-free body mass or RMR per unit of fat-free mass (i.e., of cells other than fat). Because the energy needs of internal organs exceed those of skeletal muscle, it remains unclear whether increases in muscle mass explain the increase in RMR reported after resistance exercise training. In one study, RMR was increased by about 10%, or 180 kcal per day, 15 h after a session of resistance exercise (Melby, Scholl, and Bullough 1993).

▷ **RESISTANCE EXERCISE** training can increase basal metabolic rate by an extra 50 to 75 kcal on average. Most of the increase is explained by increased nonfat body mass, not by extra use of protein as fuel.

Metabolic Fitness

The potential importance of the concept of metabolic fitness introduced in chapter 3 is highlighted by the high failure rates of dietary weight loss programs and the clinical and epidemiologic evidence in favor of physical activity for maintaining weight loss and reducing the health risks that accompany overweight and obesity. It is also recommended that all individuals, regardless of BMI, pursue at least a moderate level of daily physical activity in addition to a prudent diet low in fat, high in complex carbohydrates, and moderate in total calories.

Physical activity reduces obesity-related risks for CHD, hypertension, dyslipidemia, and type 2 diabetes independently of body weight loss. Moreover, as insulin resistance appears to be a key catalyst that induces the cascade of risks associated with metabolic syndrome, the demonstrated protective role of physical activity against impaired glucose tolerance assumes special importance for people who are overweight. Improvements in diet and physical activity patterns can improve health outcomes independent of weight loss. Increased physical activity and better nutrition have been shown to normalize glucose and lipid blood profiles in the absence of significant weight loss in many individuals. The mechanism responsible for this metabolic change is an increased insulin sensitivity because of an **upregulation** of receptors on muscle and liver cells. In addition, the insulin-

---

How Does Exercise Help People Lose Body Fat?

- Increases energy expenditure
- Retards loss of muscle mass, hence maintaining BMR
- Increases metabolic rate during and after exercise
- Possibly increases SNS activity in people who have abnormally low tonic activity of the sympathetic nervous system (i.e., hypostress syndrome)
- Possibly suppresses appetite acutely after exercise, though overall appetite tends to increase with chronic increases in physical activity
- Offsets effects of weight cycling (yo-yo dieting)
- Has positive psychological effects that help people adhere to dietary or exercise programs

Adapted from Grilo, Brownell, and Stunkard 1993.

like effect of exercise increases blood glucose clearance in the absence of insulin because of the action of the glucose transporter GLUT4.

The Ultimate Goal: Weight Loss or Risk Reduction?

Most individuals judge the success of diet and exercise by scale weight. Rates of weight loss with a successful program average approximately 1 kg per week, which is viewed by many as frustratingly slow progress. Hence, dropout rates can be high within the first three to six months of a weight loss or exercise program. A change from preoccupation with scale weight to healthful management of blood pressure, blood glucose, and blood lipid levels through a prudent diet and regular physical activity in pursuit of moderate physical fitness is perhaps a more important health goal for most people who are overweight but not obese.

Summary

Overweight and obesity have reached pandemic status in the United States and several other developed nations. Despite some scientific debate, the general consensus remains that people who are overweight or obese have increased risks, independent of physical inactivity, of developing hypertension; hypercholesterolemia; type 2 diabetes; CHD; stroke; gallbladder disease; osteoarthritis; and cancers of the uterus, breast (postmenopausal women), esophagus, colon, pancreas, and kidney. The co-occurrence of obesity with prediabetes, hypertension, and dyslipidemia defines metabolic syndrome, which constitutes an absolute risk for coronary artery disease and premature death. An estimated 100,000 deaths in the United States are attributed each year to obesity, which mainly results from overeating and physical inactivity.

This chapter describes the evidence that physical activity, as the most variable aspect of energy balance, has great potential for helping people avoid becoming overweight and obese. Though the effects of exercise training on weight loss are often modest because most individuals are willing to perform only modest amounts of physical activity, they can be similar to the effects of caloric intake restriction. The best methods for losing weight and maintaining weight loss over the long term include prudent reduction in caloric intake and increased physical activity, including resistance exercise. Finally, regular physical activity and an above-average level of cardiorespiratory fitness each substantially reduce the risk of mortality among people who are overweight. On balance, epidemiologic and clinical studies have shown that regular physical activity has potential for reducing the primary and secondary risk of becoming overweight or obese. Clinical studies have the advantage of experimental control in most instances, but it is difficult to separate the independent effects of physical activity from those of dietary and weight changes in many studies, especially as hypertension, dyslipidemia, and obesity are intricately related to each other. Also, it is difficult to prevent fat loss during increased physical activity without increasing caloric intake, which can influence hypertension and dyslipidemia if nutrients change with altered food intake. Nonetheless, many studies have indicated that much of the benefit of moderate physical activity appears to be sufficiently strong, consistent, temporally logical, and biologically plausible to support the current public health position that physical activity represents an effective adjuvant in the prevention and treatment of overweight and obesity.

At present, evidence does not support a linear dose–response gradient between the intensity of exercise and fat reduction among typical middle-aged or older adults who have been sedentary and embark on a new physical activity program. Weight and fat loss are linearly related to total energy expenditure from increased physical activity in programs that last about four months or less. However, that relationship is lost in longer-lasting programs, probably because people have difficulty adhering to a diet and exercise program for long periods of time.

In sum, not only does regular physical activity independently reduce the risk of all-cause, cancer, and CVD mortality; it also can help protect against CVD indirectly by favorably affecting its major risk factors—hypertension, dyslipidemia, and hyperglycemia—in overweight people even when they don't lose weight. Those factors also pose elevated risk for other prevalent and deadly diseases such as type 2 diabetes and cancer. The evidence that physical activity reduces risk of those diseases is addressed in subsequent chapters of this book.

· BIBLIOGRAPHY ·

Adams, T.D., R.E. Gress, S.C. Smith, R.C. Halverson, S.C. Simper, W.D. Rosamond, M.J. Lamonte, A.M. Stroup, and S.C. Hunt. 2007. Long-term mortality after gastric bypass surgery. *New England Journal of Medicine* 357 (8): 753-761.

Agurs-Collins, T., and C. Bouchard. 2008. Gene-nutrition and gene-physical activity interactions in the etiology of obesity. Introduction. *Obesity (Silver Spring)* 16 (Suppl. 3): S2-4.

Alberti, K.G., R.H. Eckel, S.M. Grundy, P.Z. Zimmet, J.I. Cleeman, K.A. Donato, J.C. Fruchart, W.P. James, C.M. Loria, S.C. Smith Jr. 2009. Harmonizing the metabolic syndrome: A joint interim statement of the International Diabetes Federation Task Force on Epidemiology and Prevention; National Heart, Lung, and Blood Institute; American Heart Association; World Heart Federation; International Atherosclerosis Society; and Inernational Association for the Study of Obesity. *Circulation* 120 (16): 1640-1645.

Allison, D.B., K.R. Fontaine, J.E. Manson, J. Stevens, and T.B. Van Itallie. 1999. Annual deaths attributable to obesity in the United States. *Journal of the American Medical Association* 282: 1530-1538.

American College of Sports Medicine. 1983. Proper and improper weight loss programs. *Medicine and Science in Sports and Exercise* 15 (1): ix-xiii.

American Dietetic Association. 2009. Position of the American Dietetic Association: Weight management. *Journal of the American Dietetic Association* 109: 330-346.

American Heart Association. 2001. *2002 Heart and stroke statistical update.* Dallas: American Heart Association.

Amorim Adegboye, A.R., Y.M. Linee, and P.M.C. Lourenco. 2007. Diet or exercise, or both, for weight reduction in women after childbirth. *Cochrane Database of Systematic Reviews,* July 18 (3): CD005627.

Anderson, S.E., and R.C. Whitaker. 2009. Prevalence of obesity among US preschool children in different racial and ethnic groups. *Archives of Pediatric and Adolescent Medicine* 163 (4): 344-348.

Andreasen, C.H., K.L. Stender-Petersen, M.S. Mogensen, S.S. Torekov, L. Wegner, G. Andersen, A.L. Nielsen, A. Albrechtsen, K. Borch-Johnsen, S.S. Rasmussen, J.O. Clausen, A. Sandbaek, T. Lauritzen, L. Hansen, T. Jørgensen, O. Pedersen, and T. Hansen. 2008. Low physical activity accentuates the effect of the FTO rs9939609 polymorphism on body fat accumulation. *Diabetes* 57: 95-101.

Anonymous. 1968. General findings of the International Atherosclerosis Project. *Laboratory Investigation* 18 (5): 498-502.

Applegate, W.B., J.P. Hughes, and R.V. Zwagg. 1991. Case–control study of coronary heart disease risk factors in the elderly. *Journal of Clinical Epidemiology* 44: 409-415.

Atlantis, E., E.H. Barnes, and M.A. Singh. 2006. Efficacy of exercise for treating overweight in children and adolescents: A systematic review. *International Journal of Obesity (Lond)* 30 (7): 1027-1040.

Barbeau, P., B. Gutin, M.S. Litaker, L.T. Ramsey, W.E. Cannady, J. Allison, C.R. Lemmon, and S. Owens. 2003. Influence of physical training on plasma leptin in obese youths. *Canadian Journal of Applied Physiology* 28: 382-396.

Barbeau, P., M. Johnson, C. Howe, J. Allison, C. Davis, B. Gutin, and C. Lemmon. 2007. Ten months of exercise improves general and visceral adiposity, bone, and fitness in black girls. *Obesity* 15: 2077-2085.

Barnard, R.J., T. Jung, and S.B. Inkeles. 1994. Diet and exercise in the treatment of NIDDM. *Diabetes Care* 17: 1469-1471.

Barnard, R.J., E.J. Ugianskis, D. Martin, and S.B. Inkeles. 1992. Role of diet and exercise in the management of hyperinsulinemia and associated atherosclerotic risk factors. *American Journal of Cardiology* 69: 440-444.

Barrett-Connor, E. 1985. Obesity, atherosclerosis, and coronary artery disease. *Annals of Internal Medicine* 103: 1010-1019.

Bassem, N. 1992. A medieval medical view on obesity. *Obesity Surgery* 2: 217-218.

Baur, L.A. 2009. Tackling the epidemic of childhood obesity *Canadian Medical Association Journal* 180: 701-702.

Befort, C.A., E.E. Stewart, B.K. Smith, C.A. Gibson, D.K. Sullivan, and J.E. Donnelly. 2008. Weight maintenance, behaviors and barriers among previous participants of a university-based weight control program. *International Journal of Obesity (Lond)* 32 (3): 519-526.

Bell, C., D.S. Day, P.P. Jones, D.D. Christou, D.S. Petitt, K. Osterberg, C.L. Melby, and D.R. Seals. 2004. High energy flux mediates the tonically augmented β-adrenergic support of resting metabolic rate in habitually exercising older adults. *Journal of Clinical Endocrinology and Metabolism* 89: 3573-3578.

Berdanier, C.D. 1995. Carbohydrates. In *Advanced nutrition: Macronutrients,* pp. 160-208. Boca Raton, FL: CRC Press.

Berrington de Gonzalez, A., P. Hartge, J.L. Cerhan, et al. 2010. Body-mass index and mortality among 1.46 million white adults. *New England Journal of Medicine* 363 (23): 2211-2219.

Blair, S.N., J.B. Kampert, H.W. Kohl, C.E. Barlow, C.A. Macera, R.S. Paffenbarger, and L.W. Gibbons. 1996. Influences of cardiorespiratory fitness and other precursors on cardiovascular disease and all-cause mortality in men and women. *Journal of the American Medical Association* 276: 205-210.

Blair, S.N., and J.N. Morris. 2009. Healthy hearts—and the universal benefits of being physically active: Physical activity and health. *Annals of Epidemiology* 19: 253-256.

Blair, S.N., J. Shaten, K. Brownell, G. Collins, and L. Lissner. 1993. Body weight change, all-cause mortality, and cause-specific mortality in the Multiple Risk Factor Intervention Trial. *Annals of Internal Medicine* 117: 749-757.

Blanck, H.M., M.L. McCullough, A.V. Patel, C. Gillespie, E.E. Calle, V.E. Cokkinides, D.A. Galuska, L.K. Khan, and M.K. Serdula. 2007. Sedentary behavior, recreational physical activity, and 7-year weight gain among postmenopausal U.S. women. *Obesity (Silver Spring)* 15 (6): 1578-1588.

Blundell, J.E., R.J. Stubbs, D.A. Hughes, S. Whybrow, and N.A. King. 2003. Cross talk between physical activity and appetite control: Does physical activity stimulate appetite? *Proceedings of the Nutrition Society* 62: 651-661.

Borer, K.T., E. Wuorinen, K. Ku, and C. Burant. 2009. Appetite responds to changes in meal content, whereas ghrelin, leptin, and insulin track changes in energy availability. *Journal of Clinical Endocrinology and Metabolism* 94: 2290-2298.

Borkan, G.A. 1986. Body weight and coronary disease risk: Patterns of risk factor change associated with long-term weight change. *American Journal of Epidemiology* 124: 410-419.

Børsheim, E., and R. Bahr. 2003. Effect of exercise intensity, duration and mode on post-exercise oxygen consumption. *Sports Medicine* 33: 1037-1060.

Bouassida, A., K. Chamari, M. Zaouali, Y. Feki, A. Zbidi, and Z. Tabka. 2008. Review on leptin and adiponectin responses and adaptations to acute and chronic exercise. *British Journal of Sports Medicine,* October 16. [Epub ahead of print]

Bouchard, C., and S.N. Blair. 1999. Introductory comments to the consensus on physical activity and obesity. *Medicine and Science in Sports and Exercise* 31 (Suppl. 11): S502-S508.

Bouchard, C., A. Tremblay, J.P. Després, G. Thériault, A. Nadeau, P.J. Lupien, S. Moorjani, D. Prudhomme, and G. Fournier. 1994. The response to exercise with constant energy intake in identical twins. *Obesity Research* 2: 400-410.

Cambien, F., J.M. Chretien, P. Ducimetiere, L. Guize, and J.L. Richard. 1985. Is the relationship between blood pressure and cardiovascular risk dependent on body mass index? *American Journal of Epidemiology* 122: 434-442.

Cambien, F., J.M. Warnet, E. Eschwege, A. Jacqueson, J.L. Richard, and G. Rosselin. 1987. Body mass, blood pressure, glucose, and lipids: Does plasma insulin explain their relationships? *Arteriosclerosis* 7 (2): 197-202.

Camhi, S.M., M.L. Stefanick, P.T. Katzmarzyk, and D.R. Young. 2009. Metabolic syndrome and changes in body fat from a low-fat diet and/or exercise randomized controlled trial. *Obesity (Silver Spring)*, October 1. [Epub ahead of print]

Centers for Disease Control and Prevention. 2002. *National diabetes fact sheet: General information and national estimates on diabetes in the United States, 2000.* Atlanta: U.S. Department of Health and Human Services, Centers for Disease Control and Prevention.

Centers for Disease Control and Prevention. 2008. State-specific prevalence of obesity among adults—United States, 2007. *Morbidity and Mortality Weekly Report* 57 (36): 765-768.

Centers for Disease Control and Prevention. 2009. Obesity prevalence among low-income, preschool-aged children—United States, 1998–2008. *Morbidity and Mortality Weekly Report* 58 (28): 769-773.

Cho, E.R., A. Shin, J. Kim, S.H. Jee, and J. Sung. 2009. Leisure-time physical activity is associated with a reduced risk for metabolic syndrome. *Annals of Epidemiology* 19: 784-792.

Church, T.S., M.J. LaMonte, C.E. Barlow, et al. 2005. Cardiorespiratory fitness and body mass index as predictors of cardiovascular disease mortality among men with diabetes. *Archives of Internal Medicine* 165: 2114-2120.

Church, T.S., C.K. Martin, A.M. Thompson, C.P. Earnest, C.R. Mikus, and S.N. Blair. 2009. Changes in weight, waist circumference and compensatory responses with different doses of exercise among sedentary, overweight postmenopausal women. *PLoS One* 4 (2): e4515. [Epub, February 18]

Coakley, E.H., E.B. Rimm, G. Colditz, I. Kawachi, and W. Willett. 1998. Predictors of weight change in men: Results from the Health Professionals Follow-Up Study. *International Journal of Obesity and Related Metabolic Disorders* 22 (2): 89-96.

Cook, S., M. Weitzman, P. Auinger, M. Nguyen, and W.H. Dietz. 2003. Prevalence of a metabolic syndrome phenotype in adolescents: Findings from the third National Health and Nutrition Examination Survey, 1988-1994. *Archives of Pediatric and Adolescent Medicine* 157 (8): 821-827.

Cordain, L., R.W. Gotshall, and S.B. Eaton. 1998. Physical activity, energy expenditure and fitness: An evolutionary perspective. *International Journal of Sports Medicine* 19: 328-335.

Couzin, J. 2002. Nutrition research. IOM panel weighs in on diet and health. *Science* 297 (5588): 1788-1789.

Curioni, C.C., and P.M. Lourenco. 2005. Long-term weight loss after diet and exercise: A systematic review. *International Journal of Obesity (Lond)* 29 (10): 1168-1174.

Dietary Guidelines Advisory Committee. 2005. *Report of the Dietary Guidelines Advisory Committee on the Dietary Guidelines for Americans, 2005.* Washington, DC: U.S. Department of Agriculture. Agricultural Research Service.

DiPietro, L. 1999. Physical activity in the prevention of obesity: Current evidence and research issues. *Medicine and Science in Sports and Exercise* 31 (11 Suppl.): S542-S546.

DiPietro, L., J. Dziura, and S.N. Blair. 2004. Estimated change in physical activity level (PAL) and prediction of 5-year weight change in men: The Aerobics Center Longitudinal Study. *International Journal of Obesity and Related Metabolic Disorders* 28: 1541-1547.

DiPietro, L., H.W. Kohl III, C.E. Barlow, and S.N. Blair. 1998. Improvements in cardiorespiratory fitness attenuate age-related weight gain in healthy men and women: The Aerobics Center Longitudinal Study. *International Journal of Obesity and Related Metabolic Disorders* 22 (1): 55-62.

Dobbins, M., K. De Corby, P. Robeson, H. Husson, and D. Tirilis. 2009. School-based physical activity programs for promoting physical activity and fitness in children and adolescents aged 6-18. *Cochrane Database of Systematic Reviews,* January 21 (1): CD007651.

Donnelly, J.E., S.N. Blair, J.M. Jakicic, M.M. Manore, J.W. Rankin, and B.K. Smith BK. 2009. American College of Sports Medicine. American College of Sports Medicine position stand. Appropriate physical activity intervention strategies for weight loss and prevention of weight regain for adults. *Medicine and Science in Sports and Exercise* 41 (2): 459-471.

Donnelly, J.E., J.O. Hill, D.J. Jacobsen, J. Potteiger, D.K. Sullivan, S.L. Johnson, K. Heelan, M. Hise, P.V. Fennessey, B. Sonko, T. Sharp, J.M. Jakicic, S.N. Blair, Z.V. Tran, M. Mayo, C. Gibson, and R.A. Washburn. 2003. Effects of a 16-month randomized controlled exercise trial on body weight and composition in young, overweight men and women: The Midwest Exercise Trial. *Archives of Internal Medicine* 163 (11): 1343-1350.

Drøyvold, W.B., J. Holmen, O. Kruger, and K. Midthjell. 2004a. Leisure time physical activity and change in body mass index: An 11-year follow-up study of 9357 normal weight healthy women 20-49 years old. *Journal of Women's Health* 13: 55-62.

Drøyvold, W.B., J. Holmen, K. Midthjell, and S. Lydersen. 2004b. BMI change and leisure time physical activity (LTPA): An 11-y follow-up study in apparently healthy men aged 20-69 y with normal weight at baseline. *International Journal of Obesity* 28: 410-417.

Ducimetiere, P., J. Richard, and F. Cambien. 1986. The pattern of subcutaneous fat distribution in middle-aged men and the risk of coronary heart disease: The Paris Prospective Study. *International Journal of Obesity* 10 (3): 229-240.

Dustan, H.P. 1985. Obesity and hypertension. *Annals of Internal Medicine* 103: 1047-1049.

Eaton, S.B., and S.B. Eaton. 2003. An evolutionary perspective on human physical activity: Implications for health. *Comparative Biochemistry and Physiology Part A: Molecular and Integrative Physiology* 136 (1): 153-159.

Ekelund, L.G., W.L. Haskell, J.L. Johnson, F.S. Whaley, M.H. Criqui, and D.S. Sheps. 1988. Physical fitness as a predictor of cardiovascular mortality in asymptomatic North American men. *New England Journal of Medicine* 319: 1379-1384.

Erlinger, S. 2000. Gallstones in obesity and weight loss. *European Journal of Gastroenterology and Hepatology* 12 (12): 1347-1352.

Ervin, R.B. 2009. Prevalence of metabolic syndrome among adults 20 years of age and over, by sex, age, race and ethnicity, and body mass index: United States, 2003-2006. *National Health Statistics Reports,* No. 13, pp 1-8. Hyattsville, MD: National Center for Health Statistics.

Evenson, K.R., J. Stevens, J. Cai, et al. 2003. The effect of cardiorespiratory fitness and obesity on cancer mortality in women and men. *Medicine and Science in Sports and Exercise* 35: 270-277.

Farrell, S.W., G.M. Cortese, M.J. LaMonte, and S.N. Blair. 2007. Cardiorespiratory fitness, different measures of adiposity, and cancer mortality in men. *Obesity (Silver Spring)* 15: 3140-3149.

Finkelstein, E.A., J.G. Trogdon, J.W. Cohen, and W. Dietz. 2009. Annual medical spending attributable to obesity: Payer-and service-specific estimates. *Health Affairs* 28 (5): w822-831.

Finucane, M.M., G.A. Stevens, M.J. Cowan, G. Danaei, J.K. Lin, C.J. Paciorek, G.M. Singh, H.R. Gutierrez, Y. Lu, A.N. Bahalim, F. Farzadfar, L.M. Riley, M. Ezzati M; Global Burden of Metabolic Risk Factors of Chronic Diseases Collaborating Group (Body Mass Index). 2011. National, regional, and global trends in body-mass index since 1980: Systematic analysis of health examination surveys and epidemiological studies with 960 country-years and 9.1 million participants. *Lancet* 377 (9765): 557-567.

Flegal, K.M., M.D. Carroll, C.L. Ogden, and L.R. Curtin. 2010. Prevalence and trends in obesity among US adults, 1999-2008. *Journal of the American Medical Association* 303: 235-241.

Flegal, K.M., and B.I. Graubard. 2009. Estimates of excess deaths associated with body mass index and other anthropometric variables. *American Journal of Clinical Nutrition* 89: 1213-1219.

Flegal, K.M., B.I. Graubard, D.F. Williamson, and M.H. Gail. 2005. Excess deaths associated with underweight, overweight, and obesity. *Journal of the American Medical Association* 293 (15): 1861-1867.

Flegal, K.M., B.I. Graubard, D.F. Williamson, and M.H. Gail. 2007. Cause-specific excess deaths associated with underweight, overweight, and obesity. *Journal of the American Medical Association* 298 (17): 2028-2037.

Flegal, K.M., J.A. Shepherd, A.C. Looker, B.I. Graubard, L.G. Borrud, C.L. Ogden, T.B. Harris, J.E. Everhart, and N. Schenker. 2009. Comparisons of percentage body fat, body mass index, waist circumference, and waist-stature ratio in adults. *American Journal of Clinical Nutrition* 89 (2): 500-508.

Fogelholm, M. 2010. Physical activity, fitness and fatness: Relations to mortality, morbidity and disease risk factors. A systematic review. *Obesity Review* 11 (3): 202-221.

Forbes, G.B. 1992. Exercise and lean weight: The influence of body weight. *Nutrition Reviews* 50 (6): 157-161.

Ford, E.S., W.H. Giles, and W.H. Dietz. 2002. Prevalence of the metabolic syndrome among US adults: Findings from the third National Health and Nutrition Examination Survey. *Journal of the American Medical Association* 287: 356-359.

Foreyt, J.P., and G.K. Goodrich. 1993. Evidence for success of behavior modification in weight loss and control. *Annals of Internal Medicine* 119: 698-701.

Foreyt, J.P., and G.K. Goodrich. 1994. Impact of behavior therapy on weight loss. *American Journal of Health Promotion* 8: 466-468.

Freedman, D.S., W.H. Dietz, S.R. Srinivasan, and G.S. Berenson. 2009. Risk factors and adult body mass index among overweight children: The Bogalusa Heart Study. *Pediatrics* 123 (3): 750-757.

Freedman, D.S., L.K. Khan, M.K. Serdula, W.H. Dietz, S.R. Srinivasan, and G.S. Berenson. 2005. Racial differences in the tracking of childhood BMI to adulthood. *Obesity* 13 (5): 928-935.

Freedman, D.S., and B. Sherry. 2009. The validity of BMI as an indicator of body fatness and risk among children. *Pediatrics* 124 (Suppl. 1): S23-34.

Freedman, D.S., J. Wang, J.C. Thornton, Z. Mei, R.N. Pierson Jr., W.H. Dietz, and M. Horlick. 2008. Racial/ethnic differences in body fatness among children and adolescents. *Obesity (Silver Spring)* 16 (5): 1105-1111.

Gaesser, G.A. 1996. Obesity a killer disease? A closer look at the evidence. In *Big fat lies,* pp. 59-78. New York: Ballantine.

Gaesser, G.A. 2002. *Big fat lies: The truth about your weight and your health.* Updated edition. Carlsbad, CA: Gürze Books.

Gardner, G., and B. Halweil. 2000. *Underfed and overfed: The global epidemic of malnutrition.* Washington, DC: Worldwatch Institute.

Geliebter, A., M.M. Maher, L. Gerace, B. Gutin, S.B. Heymsfield, and S.A. Hashim. 1997. Effects of strength or aerobic training on body composition, resting metabolic rate, and peak oxygen consumption in obese dieting subjects. *American Journal of Clinical Nutrition* 66: 557-563.

Gibbons, L.W., S.N. Blair, K.H. Cooper, and M. Smith. 1983. Association between coronary heart disease risk factors and physical fitness in healthy adult women. *Circulation* 67: 977-983.

Gregg, E.W., Y.J. Cheng, B.L. Cadwell, G. Imperatore, D.E. Williams, K.M. Flegal, K.M. Narayan, and D.F. Williamson. 2005. Secular trends in cardiovascular disease risk factors according to body mass index in US adults. *Journal of the American Medical Association* 293 (15): 1868-1874.

Grilo, C.M., K.D. Brownell, and A.J. Stunkard. 1993. The metabolic and psychological importance of exercise in weight control. In A.J. Stunkard and T. Wadden (Eds.), Obesity: Theory and therapy (2nd ed.) (pp. 253-273). New York: Raven Press.

Gutin, B. 2008. Child obesity can be reduced with vigorous activity rather than restriction of energy intake. *Obesity* 16: 2193-2196.

Gutin, B., Z. Yin, M. Johnson, and P. Barbeau. 2008. The Medical College of Georgia FitKid Project – preliminary findings for fatness and fitness. *International Journal of Pediatric Obesity* 3: 3-9.

Hagobian, T.A., and B. Braun. 2010. Physical activity and hormonal regulation of appetite: Sex differences and weight control. *Exercise and Sport Sciences Reviews* 38: 25-30.

Hagobian, T.A., C.G. Sharoff, B.R. Stephens, G.N. Wade, J.E. Silva, S.R. Chipkin, and B. Braun. 2009. Effects of exercise on energy-regulating hormones and appetite in men and women. *American Journal of Physiology* 296: R233-242.

Harrington, M., S. Gibson, and R.C. Cottrell. 2009. A review and meta-analysis of the effect of weight loss on all-cause mortality risk. *Nutrition Research Reviews* 22 (1): 93-108.

Harris, K.C., L.K. Kuramoto, M. Schulzer, and J.E. Retallack. 2009. Effect of school-based physical activity interventions on body mass index in children: A meta-analysis. *Canadian Medical Association Journal* 180: 719-726.

Héroux, M., I. Janssen, M. Lam, D.C. Lee, J.R. Hebert, X. Sui, and S.N. Blair. 2009. Dietary patterns and the risk of mortality: Impact of cardiorespiratory fitness. *International Journal of Epidemiology,* April 20. [Epub ahead of print]

Heymsfield, S.B. 2009. How large is the energy gap that accounts for the obesity epidemic? *American Journal of Clinical Nutrition* 89: 1717-1718.

Higgins, M., R.D. D'Agostino, W. Kannel, and J. Cobb. 1993. Benefits and adverse effects of weight loss: Observations from the Framingham study. *Annals of Internal Medicine* 119: 758-763.

Hill, J.O. 2006. Understanding and addressing the epidemic of obesity: An energy balance perspective. *Endocrine Reviews* 27 (7): 750-761.

Hill, J.O., H.J. Drougas, and J.C. Peters. 1994. Physical activity, fitness, and moderate obesity. In *Exercise, fitness, and health: A consensus of current knowledge,* edited by C. Bouchard, R.J. Shephard, T. Stephens, J.R. Sutton, and B.D. McPherson, pp. 684-695. Champaign, IL: Human Kinetics.

Hill, J.O., M.J. Pagliassotti, and J.C. Peters. 1994. Nongenetic determinants of obesity and fat topography. In *Genetic determinants of obesity,* edited by C. Bouchard, pp. 35-48. Boca Raton, FL: CRC Press.

Hill, J.O., H.R. Wyatt, G.W. Reed, and J.C. Peters. 2003. Obesity and the environment: Where do we go from here? *Science* 299: 853-855.

Hillier, T.A., and K.L. Pedula. 2001. Characteristics of an adult population with newly diagnosed type 2 diabetes. *Diabetes Care* 24: 1522-1527.

Holme, I., S. Tonstad, A.J. Sogaard, P.G. Larsen, and L.L. Haheim. 2007. Leisure time physical activity in middle age predicts the metabolic syndrome in old age: Results of a 28-year follow-up of men in the Oslo study. *BMC Public Health* 7: 154.

Hu, F.B., W.C. Willett, T. Li, et al. 2004. Adiposity as compared with physical activity in predicting mortality among women. *New England Journal of Medicine* 351: 2694-2703.

Hu, G., J. Tuomilehto, K. Silventoinen, et al. 2005. The effects of physical activity and body mass index on cardiovascular, cancer and all-cause mortality among 47,212 middle-aged Finnish men and women. *International Journal of Obesity (Lond)* 29: 894-902.

Hubert, H.B., M. Feinleib, P.M. McNamara, and W.P. Castelli. 1983. Obesity as an independent risk factor for cardiovascular disease: A 26-year follow-up of participants in the Framingham Heart Study. *Circulation* 67: 968-976.

Irving, B.A., C.K. Davis, D.W. Brock, J.Y. Weltman, D. Swift, E.J. Barrett, G.A. Gaesser, and A. Weltman. 2008. Effect of exercise training intensity on abdominal visceral fat and body composition. *Medicine and Science in Sports and Exercise* 40: 1863-1872.

Irwin, M.L., Y. Yasui, C.M. Ulrich, D. Bowen, R.E. Rudolph, R.S. Schwartz, M. Yukawa, E. Aiello, J.D. Potter, and A. McTiernan. 2003. Effect of exercise on total and intra-abdominal body fat in postmenopausal women: A randomized controlled trial. *Journal of the American Medical Association* 289 (3): 323-330.

Jackson, A.S., K.J. Ellis, B.K. McFarlin, M.H. Sailors, and M.S. Bray. 2009. Body mass index bias in defining obesity of diverse young adults: The Training Intervention and Genetics of Exercise Response (TIGER) study. *British Journal of Nutrition* 102: 1084-1090.

Jackson, A.S., P.R. Stanforth, J. Gagnon, T. Rankinen, A.S. Leon, D.C. Rao, J.S. Skinner, C. Bouchard, and J.H. Wilmore. 2002. The effect of sex, age and race on estimating percentage body fat from body mass index: The Heritage Family Study. *International Journal of Obesity and Related Metabolic Disorders* 26: 789-796.

Jakicic, J.M. 1998. Treating obesity with exercise. *Physician and Sportsmedicine* 12 (4): 13-20.

Jakicic, J.M. 2002. The role of physical activity in prevention and treatment of body weight gain in adults. *Journal of Nutrition* 132: 3826S-3829S.

Jakicic, J.M., K. Clark, E. Coleman, J.E. Donnelly, J. Foreyt, E. Melanson, J. Volek, and S.L. Volpe. 2001. American College of Sports Medicine position stand. Appropriate intervention strategies for weight loss and prevention of weight regain for adults. *Medicine and Science in Sports and Exercise* 33: 2145-2156.

Jakicic, J.M., B.H. Marcus, W. Lang, and C. Janney. 2008. Effect of exercise on 24-month weight loss maintenance in overweight women. *Archives of Internal Medicine* 168: 1550-1559.

Janiszewski, P.M., and R. Ross. 2007. Physical activity in the treatment of obesity: Beyond body weight reduction. *Applied Physiology, Nutrition, and Metabolism* 32 (3): 512-522.

Janssen, I., P.T. Katzmarzyk, W.F. Boyce, C. Vereecken, C. Mulvihill, C. Roberts, C. Currie, W. Pickett; Health Behaviour in School-Aged Children Obesity Working Group. 2005. Comparison of overweight and obesity prevalence in school-aged youth from 34 countries and their relationships with physical activity and dietary patterns. *Obesity Reviews* 6 (2): 123-132.

Johannsen, D.L., L.M. Redman, and E. Ravussin. 2007. The role of physical activity in maintaining a reduced weight. *Current Atherosclerosis Reports* 9: 463-471.

Johnson, J.L., C.A. Slentz, J.A. Houmard, G.P. Samsa, B.D. Duscha, et al. 2007. Exercise training amount and intensity effects on metabolic syndrome (from Studies of a Targeted Risk Reduction Intervention through Defined Exercise). *American Journal of Cardiology* 100: 1759-1766.

Johnson, W.D., J.J. Kroon, F.L. Greenway, C. Bouchard, D. Ryan, and P.T. Katzmarzyk. 2009. Prevalence of risk factors for metabolic syndrome in adolescents: National Health and Nutrition Examination Survey (NHANES), 2001-2006. *Archives of Pediatric and Adolescent Medicine* 163 (4): 371-377.

Jonsson, A., F. Renström, V. Lyssenko, E.C. Brito, B. Isomaa, G. Berglund, P.M. Nilsson, L. Groop, and P.W. Franks. 2009. Assessing the effect of interaction between an FTO variant (rs9939609) and physical activity on obesity in 15,925 Swedish and 2,511 Finnish adults. *Diabetologia* 52: 1334-1338.

Kahn, H.S., L.M. Tatham, C. Rodriguez, E.E. Calle, M.J. Thun, and C.W. Heath Jr. 1997. Stable behaviors associated with adults' 10-year change in body mass index and likelihood of gain at the waist. *American Journal of Public Health* 87: 747-754.

Katzmarzyk, P.T., A.S. Leon, J.H. Wilmore, J.S. Skinner, D.C. Rao, et al. 2003. Targeting the metabolic syndrome with exercise: Evidence from the HERITAGE Family Study. *Medicine and Science in Sports and Exercise* 35: 1703-1709.

Kawachi, I., R.J. Troisi, A.G. Rotnitzky, E.H. Coakley, and G.A. Colditz. 1996. Can physical activity minimize weight gain in women after smoking cessation? *American Journal of Public Health* 86 (7): 999-1004.

Kayman, S., W. Bruvold, and J.S. Stern. 1990. Maintenance and relapse after weight loss in women: Behavioral aspects. *American Journal of Clinical Nutrition* 52: 800-807.

Kemmler, W., S. Von Stengel, K. Engelke, and W.A. Kalender. 2009. Exercise decreases the risk of metabolic syndrome in elderly females. *Medicine and Science in Sports and Exercise* 41: 297-305.

Kerksick, C., A. Thomas, B. Campbell, L. Taylor, C. Wilborn, B. Marcello, M. Roberts, E. Pfau, M. Grimstvedt, J. Opusunju, T. Magrans-Courtney, C. Rasmussen, R. Wilson, and R.B. Kreider. 2009. Effects of a popular exercise and weight loss program on weight loss, body composition, energy expenditure and health in obese women. *Nutrition and Metabolism (Lond)* 6: 23.

Klem, M.L., R.R. Wing, M.T. McGuire, H.M. Seagle, and J.O. Hill. 1997. A descriptive study of individuals successful at long-term maintenance of substantial weight loss. *American Journal of Clinical Nutrition* 66: 239-246.

Kraemer, R.R., and V.D. Castracane. 2007. Exercise and humoral mediators of peripheral energy balance: Ghrelin and adiponectin. *Experimental Biology and Medicine (Maywood)* 232: 184-194.

Kuczmarski, R.J. 1992. Prevalence of overweight and weight gain in the United States. *American Journal of Clinical Nutrition* 55 (Suppl. 2): 495S-502S.

Kuczmarski, R.J., K.M. Flegal, S.M. Campbell, and C.L. Johnson. 1994. Increasing prevalence of overweight among U.S. adults. *Journal of the American Medical Association* 272: 205-211.

LaForgia, J., R.T. Withers, and C.J. Gore. 2006. Effects of exercise intensity and duration on the excess post-exercise oxygen consumption. *Journal of Sports Sciences* 24: 1247-1264.

Lanningham-Foster, L., L.J. Nysse, and J.A. Levine. 2003. Labor saved, calories lost: The energetic impact of domestic labor-saving devices. *Obesity Research* 11: 1178-1181.

Larson-Meyer, D.E., L. Redman, L.K. Heilbronn, C.K. Martin, and E. Ravussin. 2010. Caloric restriction with or without exercise: The fitness versus fatness debate. *Medicine and Science in Sports and Exercise* 42: 152-159.

Lear, S.A., K.H. Humphries, S. Kohli, and C.L. Birmingham. 2007a. The use of BMI and waist circumference as surrogates of body fat differs by ethnicity. *Obesity (Silver Spring)* 15 (11): 2817-2824.

Lear, S.A., K.H. Humphries, S. Kohli, A. Chockalingam, J.J. Frohlich, and C.L. Birmingham. 2007b. Visceral adipose tissue accumulation differs according to ethnic background: Results of the Multicultural Community Health Assessment Trial (M-CHAT). *American Journal of Clinical Nutrition* 86: 353-359.

Lee, C.D., S.N. Blair, and A.S. Jackson. 1999. Cardiorespiratory fitness, body composition, and all-cause and cardiovascular disease mortality in men. *American Journal of Clinical Nutrition* 69 (3): 373-380.

Lee, C.D., A.S. Jackson, and S.N. Blair. 1998. US weight guidelines: Is it also important to consider cardiorespiratory fitness? *International Journal of Obesity and Related Metabolic Disorders* 22 (Suppl. 2): S2-S7.

Lee, D.C., X. Sui, and S.N. Blair. 2009. Does physical activity ameliorate the health hazards of obesity? *British Journal of Sports Medicine* 43 (1): 49-51.

Lee, I.M., L. Djousse, H.D. Sesso, L. Wang, and J.E. Buring. 2010. Physical activity and weight gain prevention. *Journal of the American Medical Association* 303 (12): 1173-1179.

Lemmens, V.E., A. Oenema, K.I. Klepp, H.B. Henriksen, and J. Brug. 2008. A systematic review of the evidence regarding efficacy of obesity prevention interventions among adults. *Obesity Reviews* 9: 446-455.

Lenard, N.R., and H.R. Berthoud. 2008. Central and peripheral regulation of food intake and physical activity: Pathways and genes. *Obesity (Silver Spring)* 16 (Suppl. 3): S11-22.

Leon, A.S., J. Connett, D.R. Jacobs, and R. Rauramaa. 1987. Leisure-time physical activity levels and risk of coronary heart disease and death. *Journal of the American Medical Association* 258: 2388-2395.

Levine, J.A., N.L. Eberhardt, and M.D. Jensen. 1999. Role of nonexercise activity thermogenesis in resistance to fat gain in humans. *Science* 283 (5399): 212-214.

Lewis, C.E., D.E. Smith, D.D. Wallace, O.D. Williams, D.E. Bild, and D.R. Jacobs Jr. 1997. Seven-year trends in body weight and associations with lifestyle and behavioral characteristics in black and white young adults: The CARDIA study. *American Journal of Public Health* 87 (4): 635-642.

Li, T.Y., J.S. Rana, J.E. Manson, W.C. Willett, M.J. Stampfer, G.A. Colditz, K.M. Rexrode, and F.B. Hu. 2006. Obesity as compared with physical activity in predicting risk of coronary heart disease in women. *Circulation* 113: 499-506.

Loos, R.J., and C. Bouchard. 2008. FTO: The first gene contributing to common forms of human obesity. *Obesity Reviews* 9: 246-250.

Manson, J.E., W.C. Willet, M.J. Stampfer, G.A. Colditz, D.J. Hunter, S.E. Hankinson, C.H. Hennekens, and F.E. Spetzer. 1995. Body weight and mortality among women. *New England Journal of Medicine* 333: 677-685.

Martins, C., L. Morgan, and H. Truby. 2008. A review of the effects of exercise on appetite regulation: An obesity perspective. *International Journal of Obesity (Lond)* 32: 1337-1347.

Matthews, B., ed. 1914. Dialogue between Franklin and the gout. *The Oxford book of American essays.* New York: Oxford University Press.

Mayer, J., P. Roy, and K.P. Mitra. 1956. Relation between caloric intake, body weight and physical work: Studies in an industrial male population in West Bengal. *American Journal of Clinical Nutrition* 4: 169-175.

McArdle, W.D., F.I. Katch, and V.L. Katch. 1991. *Exercise physiology: Energy, nutrition and human performance.* 3rd edition. Philadelphia: Lea & Febiger.

McGinnis, J.M., and W.H. Foege. 1993. Actual causes of death in the United States. *Journal of the American Medical Association* 270: 2207-2212.

McTiernan, A., B. Sorensen, M.L. Irwin, A. Morgan, Y. Yasui, R.E. Rudolph, C. Surawicz, J.W. Lampe, P.D. Lampe, K. Ayub, and J.D. Potter. 2007. Exercise effect on weight and body fat in men and women. *Obesity (Silver Spring)* 15: 1496-1512.

Melby, C.L., C. Scholl, and R.C. Bullough. 1993. Effect of acute resistance exercise on postexercise energy expenditure and resting metabolic rate. *Journal of Applied Physiology* 75: 1847-1853.

Méndez-Hernández, P., Y. Flores, C. Siani, M. Lamure, L.D. Dosamantes-Carrasco, E. Halley-Castillo, G. Huitrón, J.O. Talavera, K. Gallegos-Carrillo, and J. Salmerón. 2009. Physical activity and risk of metabolic syndrome in an urban Mexican cohort. *BMC Public Health* 9 (July 31): 276.

Messiah, S.E., K.L. Arheart, B. Luke, S.E. Lipshultz, and T.L. Miller. 2008. Relationship between body mass index and metabolic syndrome risk factors among US 8- to 14-year-olds, 1999 to 2002. *Journal of Pediatrics* 153 (2): 215-221.

Metzger, J.S., D.J. Catellier, K.R. Evenson, M.S. Treuth, W.D. Rosamond, and A.M. Siega-Riz. 2010. Associations between patterns of objectively measured physical activity and risk factors for the metabolic syndrome. *American Journal of Health Promotion* 24: 161-169.

Miller, W.C., D.M. Koceja, and E.J. Hamilton. 1997. A meta-analysis of the past 25 years of weight loss research using diet, exercise or diet plus exercise intervention. *International Journal of Obesity and Related Metabolic Disorders* 21: 941-947.

Mitchell, J.A., T.S. Church, T. Rankinen, C.P. Earnest, X. Sui, and S.N. Blair. 2009. FTO genotype and the weight loss benefits of moderate intensity exercise. *Obesity (Silver Spring),* October 1. [Epub ahead of print]

Mokdad, A.H., E.S. Ford, B.A. Bowman, W.H. Dietz, F. Vinicor, V.S. Bales, and J.S. Marks. 2003. Prevalence of obesity, diabetes, and obesity-related health risk factors, 2001. *Journal of the American Medical Association* 289: 76-79.

Mokdad, A.H., M.K. Serdula, W.H. Dietz, B.A. Bowman, J.S. Marks, and J.P. Koplan. 1999. The spread of the obesity epidemic in the United States, 1991–1998. *Journal of the American Medical Association* 282 (16): 1519-1522.

Mokdad, A.H., M.K. Serdula, W.H. Dietz, B.A. Bowman, J.S. Marks, and J.P. Koplan. 2000. The continuing epidemic of obesity in the United States. *Journal of the American Medical Association* 284 (13): 1650-1651.

Mole, P.A., J.S. Stern, C.L. Schultz, E.M. Bernauer, and B.J. Holcomb. 1989. Exercise reverses depressed metabolic rate produced by severe caloric restriction. *Medicine and Science in Sports and Exercise* 21: 29-33.

Moore, L.L., D. Gao, M.L. Bradlee, L.A. Cupples, A. Sundarajan-Ramamurti, M.H. Proctor, M.Y. Hood, M.R. Singer, and R.C. Ellison. 2003. Does early physical activity predict body fat change throughout childhood? *Preventive Medicine* 37: 10-17.

National Center for Health Statistics. 2009. *Health, United States, 2008.* Hyattsville, MD: National Center for Health Statistics.

National Heart, Lung, and Blood Institute of the National Institutes of Health. 1998. *Clinical guidelines on the identification, evaluation, and treatment of overweight and obesity in adults: The evidence report.* NIH Publication No. 98-408. Bethesda, MD: National Institutes of Health.

National Institutes of Health Development Panel on the Health Implications of Obesity. 1985. Health implications of obesity. *Annals of Internal Medicine* 103: 1073-1077.

National Task Force on the Prevention and Treatment of Obesity. 1994. Weight cycling. *Journal of the American Medical Association* 272: 1196-1201.

Neovius, M., and F. Rasmussen. 2008. Evaluation of BMI-based classification of adolescent overweight and obesity: Choice of percentage body fat cutoffs exerts a large influence. The COMPASS study. *European Journal of Clinical Nutrition* 62 (10): 1201-1207.

Ogden, C.L., M.D. Carroll, L.R. Curtin, M.A. McDowell, C.J. Tabak, and K.M. Flegal. 2006. Prevalence of overweight and obesity in the United States, 1999-2004. *Journal of the American Medical Association* 295: 1549-1555.

Ogden, C.L., M.D. Carroll, and K.M. Flegal. 2008. High body mass index for age among U.S. children and adolescents, 2003-2006. *Journal of the American Medical Association* 299: 2401-2405.

Ogden, C.L., M.D. Carroll, M.A. McDowell, and K.M. Flegal. 2007a. Obesity among adults in the United States—no statistically significant change since 2003-2004. *NCHS Data Brief* (1, November): 1-8.

Ogden, C.L., K.M. Flegal, M.D. Carroll, and C.L. Johnson. 2002. Prevalence and trends in overweight among US children and adolescents, 1999–2000. *Journal of the American Medical Association* 288: 1728-1732.

Ogden, C.L., S.Z. Yanovski, M.D. Carroll, and K.M. Flegal. 2007b. The epidemiology of obesity. *Gastroenterology* 132 (6): 2087-2102.

Ohkawara, K., S. Tanaka, K. Ishikawa-Takata, and I. Tabata. 2008. Twenty-four-hour analysis of elevated energy expenditure after physical activity in a metabolic chamber: Models of daily total energy expenditure. *American Journal of Clinical Nutrition* 87: 1268-1276.

Oude Luttikhuis, H., L. Baur, H. Jansen, V.A. Shrewsbury, C. O'Malley, R.P. Stolk, and C.D. Summerbell. 2009. Interventions for treating obesity in children. *Cochrane Database of Systematic Reviews,* January 21 (1): CD001872.

Paffenbarger, R.S., R.T. Hyde, A.L. Wing, and C.C. Hsieh. 1986. Physical activity, all-cause mortality, and longevity of college alumni. *New England Journal of Medicine* 314: 605-613.

Patel, Y.C., D.A. Eggen, and J.P. Strong. 1980. Obesity, smoking and atherosclerosis. *Atherosclerosis* 36: 481-490.

Pavlou, K.N., S. Krey, and W.P. Steffee. 1989. Exercise as an adjunct to weight loss and maintenance in moderately obese subjects. *American Journal of Clinical Nutrition* 49: 1115-1123.

Perri, M.G., W.G. Macadoo, D.A. Mcallister, J.B. Lauer, and D.Z. Yancey. 1986. Enhancing the efficacy of behavior therapy for obesity: Effects of aerobic exercise and a multicomponent maintenance program. *Journal of Consulting and Clinical Psychology* 54: 670-675.

Physical Activity Guidelines Advisory Committee. 2008. *Physical Activity Guidelines Advisory Committee report,* pp. 1-163. Washington, DC: U.S. Department of Health and Human Services.

Pontiroli, A.E., and A. Morabito. 2011. Long-term prevention of mortality in morbid obesity through bariatric surgery. A systematic review and meta-analysis of trials performed with gastric banding and gastric bypass. *Annals of Surgery* 253 (3): 484-487.

Rampersaud, E., B.D. Mitchell, T.I. Pollin, M. Fu, H. Shen, J.R. O'Connell, J.L. Ducharme, S. Hines, P. Sack, R. Naglieri, A.R. Shuldiner, and S. Snitker. 2008. Physical activity and the association of common FTO gene variants with body mass index and obesity. *Archives of Internal Medicine* 168: 1791-1797.

Rankinen, T., T. Rice, M. Teran-Garcia, D.C. Rao, and C. Bouchard. 2009. FTO genotype is associated with exercise training-induced changes in body composition. *Obesity (Silver Spring)*, June 18. [Epub ahead of print]

Rankinen, T., A. Zuberi, Y.C. Chagnon, et al. 2006. The human obesity gene map: The 2005 update. *Obesity (Silver Spring)* 14: 529-644.

Riddoch, C.J., S.D. Leary, A.R. Ness, S.N. Blair, K. Deere, C. Mattocks, A. Griffiths, G. Davey Smith, and K. Tilling. 2009. Prospective associations between objective measures of physical activity and fat mass in 12-14 year old children: The Avon Longitudinal Study of Parents and Children (ALSPAC). *British Medical Journal* 339: b4544. doi: 10.1136/bmj.b4544.

Rissanen, A.M., M. Heliovaara, P. Knekt, A. Reunanen, and A. Aromaa. 1991. Determinants of weight gain and overweight in adult Finns. *European Journal of Clinical Nutrition* 45 (9): 419-430.

Romero-Corral, A., V.M. Montori, V.K. Somers, J. Korinek, R.J. Thomas, T.G. Allison, F. Mookadam, and F. Lopez-Jimenez. 2006. Association of bodyweight with total mortality and with cardiovascular events in coronary artery disease: A systematic review of cohort studies. *Lancet* 368 (9536): 666-678.

Ross, R., D. Dagnone, P.J. Jones, H. Smith, A. Paddags, R. Hudson, and I. Janssen. 2000. Reduction in obesity and related comorbid conditions after diet-induced weight loss or exercise-induced weight loss in men. A randomized, controlled trial. *Annals of Internal Medicine* 18 (133): 92-103.

Ross, R., and I. Janssen. 2001. Physical activity, total and regional obesity: Dose–response considerations. *Medicine and Science in Sports and Exercise* 33 (6 Suppl.): S521-S527.

Ruiz, J.R., X. Sui, F. Lobelo, J.R. Morrow Jr., A.W. Jackson, M. Sjöström, and S.N. Blair. 2008. Association between muscular strength and mortality in men: Prospective cohort study. *British Medical Journal* 337: a439. doi: 10.1136/bmj.a439.

Saris, W.H., S.N. Blair, M.A. van Baak, S.B. Eaton, P.S. Davies, L. Di Pietro, M. Fogelholm, A. Rissanen, D. Schoeller, B. Swinburn, A. Tremblay, K.R. Westerterp, and H. Wyatt. 2003. How much physical activity is enough to prevent unhealthy weight gain? Outcome of the IASO 1st Stock Conference and consensus statement. *Obesity Reviews* 4 (2): 101-114.

Schmitz, K.H., D.R. Jacobs Jr., A.S. Leon, P.J. Schreiner, and B. Sternfeld. 2000. Physical activity and body weight: Associations over ten years in the CARDIA Study. *International Journal of Obesityand Related Metabolic Disorders* 24: 1475-1487.

Schmitz, K.H., M.D. Jensen, K.C. Kugler, R.W. Jeffery, and A.S. Leon. 2003. Strength training for obesity prevention in midlife women. *International Journal of Obesity and Related Metabolic Disorders* 27: 326-333.

Schoeller, D.A., K. Shay, and R.F. Kushner. 1997. How much physical activity is needed to minimize weight gain in previously obese women? *American Journal of Clinical Nutrition* 66: 551-556.

Serdula, M.K., A.H. Mokdad, D.F. Williamson, D.A. Galuska, J.M. Mendlein, and G.W. Heath. 1999. Prevalence of attempting weight loss and strategies for controlling weight. *Journal of the American Medical Association* 282: 1353-1358.

Shah, M., and R.W. Jeffery. 1991. Is obesity due to overeating and inactivity, or to a defective metabolic rate? A review. *Annals of Behavioral Medicine* 13 (2): 73-81.

Shaw, K., H. Gennat, P. O'Rourke, and C. Del Mar. 2006. Exercise for overweight or obesity. *Cochrane Database of Systematic Reviews*, October 18 (4): CD003817.

Sherwood, N.E., R.W. Jeffery, S.A. French, P.J. Hannan, and D.M. Murray. 2000. Predictors of weight gain in the Pound of Prevention study. *International Journal of Obesity and Related Metabolic Disorders* 24: 395-403.

Simkin-Silverman, L.R., R.R. Wing, M.A. Boraz, L.H. Kuller. 2003. Lifestyle intervention can prevent weight gain during menopause: Results from a 5-year randomized clinical trial. *Annals of Behavioral Medicine* 26: 212-220.

Slentz, C.A., L.B. Aiken, J.A. Houmard, C.W. Bales, J.L. Johnson, C.J. Tanner, B.D. Duscha, and W.E. Kraus. 2005. Inactivity, exercise, and visceral fat. STRRIDE: A randomized, controlled study of exercise intensity and amount. *Journal of Applied Physiology* 99: 1613-1618.

Speakman, J.R., and C. Selman. 2003. Physical activity and resting metabolic rate. *Proceedings of the Nutrition Society* 62: 621-634.

Stallmann-Jorgensen, I.S., B. Gutin, J.L. Hatfield-Laube, M.C. Humphries, M.H. Johnson, and P. Barbeau. 2007. General and visceral adiposity in black and white adolescents and their relation with reported physical activity and diet. *International Journal of Obesity (Lond)* 31 (4): 622-629.

Stanforth, P.R., A.S. Jackson, J.S. Green, J. Gagnon, T. Rankinen, J.P. Després, C. Bouchard, A.S. Leon, D.C. Rao, J.S. Skinner, and J.H. Wilmore. 2004. Generalized abdominal visceral fat prediction models for black and white adults aged 17-65 y: The HERITAGE Family Study. *International Journal of Obesity and Related Metabolic Disorders* 28: 925-932.

Sternfeld, B., H. Wang, C.P. Quesenberry Jr., B. Abrams, S.A. Everson-Rose, G.A. Greendale, K.A. Matthews, J.I. Torrens, and M. Sowers. 2004. Physical activity and changes in weight and waist circumference in midlife women: Findings from the Study of Women's Health across the Nation. *American Journal of Epidemiology* 160: 912-922.

Stevens, J., J. Cai, K.R. Evenson, et al. 2002. Fitness and fatness as predictors of mortality from all causes and from cardiovascular disease in men and women in the lipid research clinics study. *American Journal of Epidemiology* 156: 832-841.

Stevens, J., C. Suchindran, K. Ring, C.D. Baggett, J.B. Jobe, M. Story, J. Thompson, S.B. Going, and B. Caballero. 2004. Physical activity as a predictor of body composition in American Indian children. *Obesity Research* 12: 1974-1980.

Stevens, J., K.P. Truesdale, J.E. McClain, and J. Cai. 2006. The definition of weight maintenance. *International Journal of Obesity (Lond)* 30: 391-399.

Stevens, J., K.P. Truesdale, C.H. Wang, and J. Cai. 2009. Prevention of excess gain. *International Journal of Obesity (Lond)* 33: 1207-1210.

St. Jeor, S.T., R.L. Brunner, M.E. Harrington, B.J. Scott, S.A. Daugherty, G.R. Cutter, K.D. Brownell, A.R. Dyer, and J.P. Foreyt. 1997. A classification system to evaluate weight maintainers, gainers, and losers. *Journal of the American Dietetic Association* 97: 481-488.

Story, M., J. Stevens, J. Himes, E. Stone, B.H. Rock, B. Ethelbah, and S. Davis. 2003. Obesity in American-Indian children: Prevalence, consequences, and prevention. *Preventive Medicine* 37 (6 Pt 2): S3-S12.

Strauss, R.S., and H.A. Pollack. 2001. Epidemic increase in childhood overweight, 1986–1998. *Journal of the American Medical Association* 286: 2845-2848.

Sui, X., S.P. Hooker, I.M. Lee, et al. 2008. A prospective study of cardiorespiratory fitness and risk of type 2 diabetes in women. *Diabetes Care* 31 (3): 550-555.

Sui, X., M.J. LaMonte, J.N. Laditka, J.W. Hardin, N. Chase, S.P. Hooker, and S.N. Blair. 2007. Cardiorespiratory fitness and adiposity as mortality predictors in older adults. *Journal of the American Medical Association* 298 (21): 2507-2516.

Sum, C.F., K.W. Wang, D.C. Choo, C.E. Tan, A.C. Fok, and E.H. Tan. 1994. The effect of a 5-month supervised program of physical activity on anthropometric indices, fat-free mass, and resting energy expenditure in obese male military recruits. *Metabolism* 43: 1148-1152.

Summerbell, C.D., W. Douthwaite, V. Whittaker, L.J. Ells, F. Hillier, S. Smith, S. Kelly, L.D. Edmunds, and I. Macdonald. 2009. The association between diet and physical activity and subsequent excess weight gain and obesity assessed at 5 years of age or older: A systematic review of the epidemiological evidence. *International Journal of Obesity (Lond)* 33 (Suppl. 3): S1-92.

Sundquist, J., and S.E. Johansson. 1998. The influence of socioeconomic status, ethnicity and lifestyle on body mass index in a longitudinal study. *International Journal of Epidemiology* 27: 57-63.

Swinburn, B.A., D. Jolley, P.J. Kremer, A.D. Salbe, and E. Ravussin. 2006. Estimating the effects of energy imbalance on changes in body weight in children. *American Journal of Clinical Nutrition* 83: 859-863.

Swinburn, B.A., G. Sacks, S.K. Lo, K.R. Westerterp, E.C. Rush, M. Rosenbaum, A. Luke, D.A. Schoeller, J.P. DeLany, N.F. Butte, and E. Ravussin. 2009. Estimating the changes in energy flux that characterize the rise in obesity prevalence. *American Journal of Clinical Nutrition* 89: 1723-1728.

Teske, J.A., A.S. Levine, M. Kuskowski, J.A. Levine, and C.M. Kotz. 2006. Elevated hypothalamic orexin signaling, sensitivity to orexin A, and spontaneous physical activity in obesity-resistant rats. *American Journal of Physiology* 291: R889-899.

Thompson, D., J. Edelsberg, G.A. Colditz, A.P. Bird, and G. Oster. 1999. Lifetime health and economic consequences of obesity. *Archives of Internal Medicine* 159: 2177-2183.

Thorogood, A., S. Mottillo, A. Shimony, K.B. Filion, L. Joseph, J. Genest, L. Pilote, P. Poirier, E.L. Schiffrin, and M.J. Eisenberg. 2011. Isolated aerobic exercise and weight loss: a systematic review and meta-analysis of randomized controlled trials. *American Journal of Medicine* 124: 747-755.

U.S. Department of Health and Human Services. 1988. *The Surgeon General's report on nutrition and health.* DHHS Publication No. 88-50210. Washington, DC: U.S. Government Printing Office.

van Baal, P.H.M., J.J. Polder, G.A. de Wit, R.T. Hoogenveen, T.L. Feenstra, et al. 2008. Lifetime medical costs of obesity: Prevention no cure for increasing health expenditure. *PLoS Medicine* 5 (2): e29. doi:10.1371/journal. pmed.0050029.

Van Itallie, T.B. 1985. Health implications of overweight and obesity in the United States. *Annals of Internal Medicine* 103: 983-988.

Van Wye, G., J.A. Dubin, S.N. Blair, and L. Di Pietro. 2007. Weight cycling and 6-year weight change in healthy adults: The Aerobics Center Longitudinal Study. *Obesity (Silver Spring)* 15 (3): 731-739.

Vatten, L.J., T.I. Nilsen, P.R. Romundstad, W.B. Drøyvold, and J. Holmen. 2006. Adiposity and physical activity as predictors of cardiovascular mortality. *European Journal of Cardiovascular Prevention and Rehabilitation* 13: 909-915.

Vimaleswaran, K.S., S. Li, J.H. Zhao, J. Luan, S.A. Bingham, K.T. Khaw, U. Ekelund, N.J. Wareham, and R.J. Loos. 2009. Physical activity attenuates the body mass index-increasing influence of genetic variation in the FTO gene. *American Journal of Clinical Nutrition* 90: 425-428.

Wadden, T.A., and A.J. Stunkard. 1985. Social and psychological consequences of obesity. *Annals of Internal Medicine* 103: 1062-1067.

Waller, K., J. Kaprio, and U.M. Kujala. 2008. Associations between long-term physical activity, waist circumference and weight gain: A 30-year longitudinal twin study. *International Journal of Obesity (Lond)* 32: 353-361.

Wang, Z., S. Heshka, K. Zhang, C.N. Boozer, and S.B. Heymsfield. 2001. Resting energy expenditure: Systematic organization and critique of prediction methods. *Obesity Research* 9: 331-336.

Warnes, C.A., and W.C. Roberts. 1984. The heart in massive (more than 300 pounds or 136 kilograms) obesity: Analysis of 12 patients studied at necropsy. *American Journal of Cardiology* 54: 1087-1091.

Webber, L.S., D.J. Catellier, L.A. Lytle, D.M. Murray, C.A. Pratt, D.R. Young, J.P. Elder, T.G. Lohman, J. Stevens, J.B. Jobe, R.R. Pate; TAAG Collaborative Research Group. 2008. Promoting physical activity in middle school girls: Trial of Activity for Adolescent Girls. *American Journal of Preventive Medicine* 34: 173-184.

Wei, M., J.B. Kampert, C.E. Barlow, M.Z. Nichaman, L.W. Gibbons, R.S. Paffenbarger Jr., and S.N. Blair. 1999. Relationship between low cardiorespiratory fitness and mortality in normal-weight, overweight, and obese men. *Journal of the American Medical Association* 282: 1547-1553.

Weinsier, R.L., R.J. Fuchs, T.D. Kay, J.H. Triebwasser, and M.C. Lancaster. 1976. Body fat: Its relationship to coronary heart disease, blood pressure, lipids and other risk factors measured in a large male population. *American Journal of Medicine* 61: 815-823.

Weinstein, A.R., H.D. Sesso, I.M. Lee, et al. 2008. The joint effects of physical activity and body mass index on coronary heart disease risk in women. *Archives of Internal Medicine* 168: 884-890.

Wessel, T.R., C.B. Arant, M.B. Olson, et al. 2004. Relationship of physical fitness vs body mass index with coronary artery disease and cardiovascular events in women. *Journal of the American Medical Association* 292: 1179-1187.

Westerterp, K.R., and G. Plasqui. 2004. Physical activity and human energy expenditure. *Current Opinion in Clinical Nutrition and Metabolic Care* 7: 607-613.

Wilfley, D.E., and K.D. Brownell. 1994. Physical activity and diet in weight loss. In *Advances in exercise adherence,* edited by R.K. Dishman, pp. 351-383. Champaign, IL: Human Kinetics.

Williamson, D.F. 1993. Descriptive epidemiology of body weight and weight change in U.S. adults. *Annals of Internal Medicine* 119 (7 Pt 2): 646-649.

Williamson, D.F., J. Madans, R.F. Anda, J.C. Kleinman, H.S. Kahn, and T. Byers. 1993. Recreational physical activity and 10-year weight change in a U.S. national cohort. *International Journal of Obesity* 17: 279-286.

Williamson, D.F., M.K. Serdula, R.F. Anda, A. Levy, and T. Byers. 1992. Weight loss attempts in adults: Goals, duration, and rate of weight loss. *American Journal of Public Health* 82: 1251-1257.

Winkleby, M.A., H.C. Kraemer, D.K. Ahn, and A.N. Varady. 1998. Ethnic and socioeconomic differences in cardiovascular risk factors for women from the Third National Health and Nutrition Examination Survey, 1988–1994. *Journal of the American Medical Association* 280: 356-362.

Woo, R., J.S. Garrow, and F.X. Pi-Sunyer. 1982. Effect of exercise on spontaneous calorie intake in obesity. *American Journal of Clinical Nutrition* 36: 470-477.

Wu, T., X. Gao, M. Chen, and R.M. van Dam. 2009. Long-term effectiveness of diet-plus-exercise interventions vs. diet-only interventions for weight loss: A meta-analysis. *Obesity Reviews* 10: 313-323.

Yin, Z., B. Gutin, M.H. Johnson, J. Hanes Jr., J.B. Moore, M. Cavnar, J. Thornburg, D. Moore, and P. Barbeau. 2005. An environmental approach to obesity prevention in children: Medical College of Georgia FitKid Project year 1 results. *Obesity Research* 13: 2153-2161.

You, T., K.M. Murphy, M.F. Lyles, J.L. Demons, L. Lenchik, and B.J. Nicklas. 2006. Addition of aerobic exercise to dietary weight loss preferentially reduces abdominal adipocyte size. *International Journal of Obesity* 30: 1211-1216.

Zephier, E., J.H. Himes, M. Story, and X. Zhou. 2006. Increasing prevalences of overweight and obesity in Northern Plains American Indian children. *Archives of Pediatric and Adolescent Medicine* 160 (1): 34-39.

Zheng, H., N.R. Lenard, A.C. Shin, and H.R. Berthoud. 2009. Appetite control and energy balance regulation in the modern world: Reward-driven brain overrides repletion signals. *International Journal of Obesity (Lond)* 33 (Suppl. 2): S8-13.

Zheng, W., D.F. McLerran, B. Rolland, X. Zhang, M. Inoue, K. Matsuo, et al. 2011. Association between body-mass index and risk of death in more than 1 million Asians. *New England Journal of Medicine* 364 (8): 719-729.

· PART FOUR ·

Physical Activity and Chronic Diseases

The chapters in this section deal with two chronic diseases that are increasing in prevalence worldwide but are nonetheless underdiagnosed: type 2 diabetes and osteoporosis. The latest data compiled by the World Health Organization showed that 220 million people suffered from diabetes mellitus worldwide in 2005 and that this number might double by the year 2030. Much of this increase is predicted to occur in developing countries, resulting from an aging population, unhealthy diets, obesity, and a sedentary lifestyle. In the United States, diabetes is the leading cause of adult blindness, end-stage kidney failure, and nontraumatic amputations. Diabetes is the seventh leading cause of death in the United States, and it increases the risk of coronary heart disease, hypertension, and stroke two to four times. The first chapter in this section discusses the clear evidence that physical activity can help reduce the risk of type 2 diabetes.

The prevalence of osteoporosis is also increasing, especially among women of European descent. Twenty percent of U.S. women 50 years old or older who are non-Hispanic white or Asian have osteoporosis. Recent estimates are that more than 50 million women and men 50 years old or older in the United States have low bone mass or osteoporosis. By 2020 the prevalence is expected to be 61 million. The public health impact of this trend is perhaps most clearly seen in the increased risk of fractures among people with low bone mass. For example, a woman's risk of hip fracture is equal to her combined risk of breast, uterine, and ovarian cancer, and about one in five people who fracture a hip, most after age 75, dies in the year following the fracture; 50% of the survivors become dependent on others for care. Though part of the increasing risk of osteoporosis and fractures can be explained by increased longevity, which leads to more older people, it is also becoming clear that physical inactivity contributes to bone loss and that some types of vigorous exercise that load bones with mechanical stress can promote peak bone mass in adolescents and young adults and retard the bone loss that accompanies aging.

CHAPTER 10

Physical Activity and Diabetes

A melting of the flesh and limbs to urine.

• Aretaeus of Cappodocia, AD 150 •

CHAPTER OBJECTIVES

▸ Describe the public health burden of type 2 diabetes, including its prevalence in population groups, its costs, and its role in the risk of cardiovascular diseases and early mortality

▸ Discuss common diagnostic tests used to identify diabetes and identify the major modifiable and nonmodifiable risk factors for type 2 diabetes

▸ Describe and explain key aspects of insulin-dependent and insulin-independent glucose metabolism

▸ Describe the known and hypothesized effects of skeletal muscle action on glucose uptake and insulin sensitivity

▸ Describe and evaluate the strength of evidence that physical activity and exercise training improve glucose use and lower risk of type 2 diabetes

Diabetes mellitus is a chronic disease caused by a deficiency in the production of insulin or in its use to transport glucose from the blood into other tissues. The result is excess glucose in the blood, **hyperglycemia,** which is toxic. According to death certificates, diabetes was the seventh leading cause of death in the United States in 2006, was the underlying cause of 72,507 deaths, and contributed to a total of nearly 234,000 deaths (National Institute of Diabetes and Digestive and Kidney Diseases 2008). The World Health Organization estimates that diabetes accounts for 3 million deaths each year worldwide. World Diabetes Day is celebrated by the International Diabetes Federation (IDF) and the World Health Organization on November 14 each year (the birthday of Frederick Banting, codiscoverer of insulin) to raise global awareness of diabetes. Diabetes is the leading cause of adult blindness, end-stage kidney failure, and nontraumatic amputations in the United States. It increases the risk of hypertension, stroke, and coronary heart disease mortality two to four times each.

The economic burden of diabetes in the United States is great, $174 billion in 2007: $116 billion in direct medical costs and another $58 billion for disability and work loss ($39 billion) and premature death ($19 billion). If ancillary costs associated with undiagnosed diabetes, prediabetes, and gestational diabetes are added, the total cost of diabetes in the United States in 2007 approximated $218 billion annually (Centers for Disease Control and Prevention 2008). Expressed per patient, the lifetime costs of the medical complications of diabetes have been estimated at about $47,000, with the following proportional costs: diseases of large blood vessels (52%), kidney (21%), peripheral nerves (17%), and retina of the eye (10%) (Caro, Ward, and O'Brien 2002).

According to the American Diabetes Association (2008), 20% of health care dollars in the United States are spent on people with diabetes, and another 10% are spent on medical conditions that accompany diabetes. Per capita, health care costs are 2.3 times higher for people with diabetes, an excess cost per person of about $6500 each year. The hallmark symptoms of diabetes are excessive secretion of urine (polyuria), persistent thirst (polydipsia), increased hunger (polyphasia), and chronic fatigue or apathy. Hindu writings from around 1500 BC first described a baffling disease that caused intense thirst and excessive urine excretion. It was first noticed when ants and flies were drawn to the urine of people suffering from diabetes. Around 600 BC, the Indian physician Sushruta described *madhumeha*—honey-like urine—as a disease of excess urine that was sweet in taste (Dwivedi and Dwivedi 2007). The term diabetes, from the Greek prefix *dia-* ("across") and the Greek verb *bainen* ("to walk") and a noun derived later meaning "siphon," was first used around 250 BC to indicate that urine excretion seemed to be greater than the amount of fluids that sufferers could take in. The Latin word *mellitus* ("sweetened with honey") was added later to describe the urine. About AD 150, Greek

physicians wrote how diabetes "melted the flesh" (Gordon 1960). In 1798, the English physician John Rollo was the first to detect excessive sugar in the blood of diabetics. Though centuries earlier, Greco-Roman physicians had prescribed exercise for the treatment of diabetes, Rollo ironically recommended bed rest. This chapter describes diabetes and its public health impact and then presents strong evidence that the Greeks were right and Rollo was wrong about exercise for diabetes.

Magnitude of the Problem

The world prevalence of diabetes among adults (aged 20–79 years) was estimated to be 6.4% (285 million people) in 2010 and predicted to increase to 7.7% (439 million people) by 2030 (Shaw et al. 2010). The International Diabetes Federation now estimates that 4.6 million people 20-79 years of age died from diabetes in 2011 (a 13% increase over estimates in 2010), accounting for 8.2% of global all-cause mortality of people those ages (International Diabetes Federation 2011). The United States has the third highest number of cases (about 26 million) and the second highest prevalence rate of diabetes among adults 20 to 79 years old in the world (figure 10.1). That is more than half the cases in India (51 million) and China (43 million), nations that each have about four times as many people.

According to estimates by the U.S. Centers for Disease Control and Prevention, nearly 19 million American children and adults say they have been told by a doctor that they have diabetes, but another 7 million people who have diabetes have not yet been diagnosed (Centers for Disease Control and Prevention 2011). Approximately 1.9 million new cases of adult diabetes are diagnosed annually in the United States. The number of persons diagnosed with diabetes increased sixfold from 1.6 million in 1958 to 10 million in 1997 and then nearly doubled to the current figure. Of people diagnosed with diabetes, a large portion report being physically inactive. Figure 10.2 shows trends in obesity and diabetes, and figure 10.3 shows rates of diabetic patients who are inactive.

According to the Behavioral Risk Factor Surveillance System, the prevalence of diagnosed diabetes in U.S. adults increased from 6.5% in 1998 to 6.9% in 1999 (Mokdad et al. 2001), a 6% increase in a single year. The rate continues to grow. From 2000 to 2001, prevalence increased from 7.3% to 7.9%, an 8% increase (Mokdad et al. 2003). Since then, prevalence has stabilized to about 8%, probably because the prevalence of overweight and obesity leveled off over the past five to 10 years.

Other estimates predict that diabetes prevalence in the United States, if uncontrolled, will increase to about 10% by 2030 and 12%, or about 48 million people, by 2050 (Narayan et al. 2006). Diabetes and its complications occur among Americans of all ages and racial and ethnic groups,

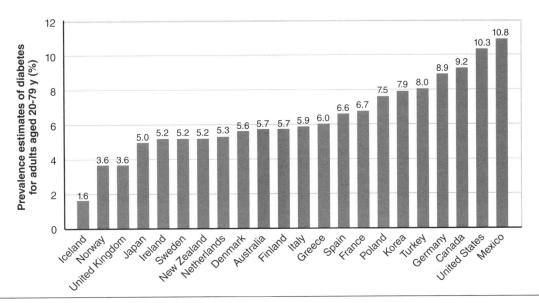

Figure 10.1 Prevalence of diabetes worldwide.

Prevalence estimates of diabetes, adults aged 20-79 years, 2010, © OECD, 2009, *Health at a glance,* pg. 39. Available: http://www.oecd.org/dataoecd/55/2/44117530.pdf

but the elderly and certain racial and ethnic groups are more commonly affected than others. The annual incidence of diabetes in U.S. adults over 65 years increased by 23% to more than 40,000 people between 1994-1995 and 2003-2004, and prevalence increased by 65%; about 27% of Americans over 65 have diabetes (Centers for Disease Control 2011;Sloan et al. 2008).

▷ **IF OBESITY** and physical inactivity remain unchecked, it is predicted that diabetes prevalence in the United States will increase to about 10% by 2030 and to 12%, about 48 million people, by 2050.

Demographics of Diabetes

The Centers for Disease Control and Prevention (2011) estimated that in 2010 the prevalence of diabetes in the United States was about 12.6 million women, 13 million men, 215,000 children and adolescents (less than 20 years of age), and 10.9 million older adults (65 years of age or older). Although prevalence rates are similar for men (11.8%) and women (10.8%) in the United States, they differ according to race or ethnic groups after adjustment for age. Among adults 20 years or older, 10.2% of non-Hispanic whites (15.7 million people) have diabetes, compared to 18.7% of non-Hispanic blacks (4.9 million people) (Centers for Disease Control 2011).

After adjustment for population age differences, 2007-2009 national survey data for people diagnosed with diabetes aged 20 years or older included the following prevalences by race-ethnicity (Centers for Disease Control 2011):

- 7.1% of non-Hispanic whites
- 8.4% of Asian Americans
- 12.6% of non-Hispanic blacks
- 11.8% of Hispanics
    - 7.6% for Cubans
    - 13.3% for Mexican Americans
    - 13.8% for Puerto Ricans

Obesity (BMI ≥30 kg/m²)

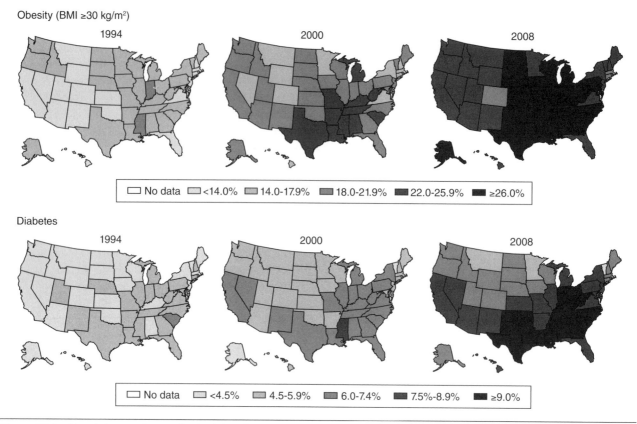

No data | <14.0% | 14.0-17.9% | 18.0-21.9% | 22.0-25.9% | ≥26.0%

No data | <4.5% | 4.5-5.9% | 6.0-7.4% | 7.5%-8.9% | ≥9.0%

Figure 10.2 Trends in prevalence of U.S. adults who were obese or were diagnosed with diabetes from 1994 to 2008.

Reprinted from the Centers for Disease Control Division of Diabetes Translation.

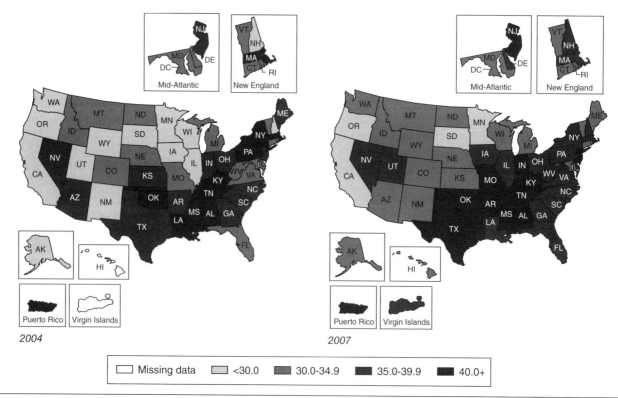

Missing data | <30.0 | 30.0-34.9 | 35.0-39.9 | 40.0+

Figure 10.3 Prevalence of U.S. adults diagnosed with diabetes who were physically inactive in 2004 and 2007.

Reprinted from the Centers for Disease Control Division of Diabetes Translation.

Elderly and minorities in United States

African Americans

Hispanic Americans

Native Americans

Asian and Pacific Island Americans

The prevalence of type 2 diabetes is more than doubled among black and Mexican American women ages 25 to 64 who have not completed high school. At about 16% among those who receive care from the Indian Health Service (IHS), the prevalence of diabetes in American Indians and Alaska Natives is the highest of any cultural group in the United States. It approaches 50% in women among certain tribal groups.

The SEARCH for Diabetes in Youth Study estimated that 154,000 U.S. youth had diagnosed diabetes in 2001. Among ages 10 to 19, black and non-Hispanic white youths had the highest rates (0.32%), followed by American Indian youth (0.23%), Hispanic youth (0.22%), and Asian/Pacific Islander youth (0.13%). Among older youth, the proportion of diabetes that was type 2 ranged from 6% for non-Hispanic white youth to 76% for American Indian youth (SEARCH for Diabetes in Youth Study Group 2006). See figure 10.4.

Clinical Features

There are two principal forms of diabetes: **type 1,** also known as insulin-dependent diabetes mellitus (IDDM) or juvenile diabetes, and **type 2,** also known as non-insulin-dependent diabetes mellitus (NIDDM). In type 1 diabetes, the pancreas

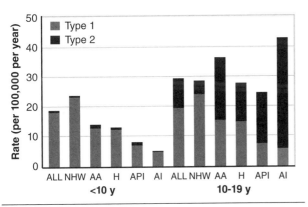

Figure 10.4 Incidence rates of diabetes among U.S. youth according to race and ethnicity. NHW = Non-Hispanic White; AA = African American; H = Hispanic-Latino; API = Asian or Pacific Islander; AI = Asian Indian.

Reprinted from Centers for Disease Control and Prevention 2008.

fails to produce insulin, which is essential for survival. This form develops most frequently in children and adolescents but is being increasingly noted later in life. About 90% of diabetes in children and adolescents is type 1 diabetes. Type 2 diabetes is much more common among adults and accounts for about 90% of all diabetes cases worldwide and in the United States (about 10.7% of adults age 20 years or older, or 23.5 million people).

About 2 million U.S. adolescents (1 in every 6 who are overweight) have prediabetes (e.g., elevated fasting blood glucose or impaired ability to clear extra glucose from the blood), the penultimate risk factor for developing type 2 diabetes. Type 2 diabetes occurs mostly in adults over age 40 and results initially from insulin resistance—that is, an inadequate response to rising insulin in the blood, which normally lowers blood glucose after a meal. Eventually, normal insulin production is also impaired in type 2 diabetes. A little more than half of cases of type 2 diabetes occur after age 60, with risk continuing to increase as people age.

About half of the cases of type 2 diabetes can normalize after weight reduction from increased physical activity and diet, and the remaining half can normalize after an increase in dietary carbohydrates that have a low glycemic index (e.g., fruits, vegetables, and pasta, which do not cause blood glucose levels to spike). The focus of this chapter is on type 2 diabetes because it is highly preventable by diet, weight loss, and physical activity. Though some evidence suggests that physical activity can help manage blood glucose levels in people with type 1 diabetes, there are special safety concerns regarding exercise by people in this group (e.g., preventing hypoglycemia and injuries to extremities because of microcirculation problems) that are appropriately addressed in a book on clinical medicine rather than epidemiology.

Insulin, discovered by Canadians Frederick Banting and Charles Best in 1921, is a hormone produced by beta cells located in the islets of Langerhans of the pancreas (so named for the German medical student, Paul Langerhans, who discovered them in 1869). Insulin regulates blood glucose and is required by all tissues except the brain and intestines (but mainly by muscle, liver, and adipose cells) for glucose to be transported from the blood across the cell membrane. Deficiencies in the normal production of insulin or in its transport into cells leads to hyperglycemia and **ketosis,** which damages tissues, especially the blood vessels and nerves.

▷ **ABOUT 90%** of diabetes cases in the United States and worldwide are non-insulin dependent, or type 2, which results from the development of insensitivity of muscle and fat cells to insulin, leading to high blood glucose levels. Increased physical activity and weight loss can normalize blood glucose in 50% of the cases.

Normal blood glucose is 80 to 100 mg/dl postabsorptively (i.e., well after the last meal has been digested) and is normally elevated postprandially (i.e., after a meal). In

Clinical Tests for Diabetes

- *Glucose tolerance test:* Detects elevated serum glucose usually 2 h after oral ingestion of typically 75 mg of glucose. A positive test indicates inadequate insulin response or insulin insensitivity, but this test is not always accurate because it is influenced by preexamination diet.
- *Home glucose monitoring:* Is usually done over four to seven days and is more reliable than a glucose tolerance test.

- *Glycosylated hemoglobin:* Measures the binding of glucose with the iron in red blood cells—that is, glycosylated hemoglobin (HbA1c). This is the most accurate test because it is not affected by acute plasma changes and is related to long-term exposure (i.e., two to three months) of red blood cells to glucose during their 120-day life span in the circulation.

Table 10.1 Glucose Diagnostic Criteria for Diabetes

Indication	Oral glucose tolerance test	Fasting blood glucose test	Glycosylated hemoglobin
Normal	<140 mg/dl	<100 mg/dl	<5.6%
Impaired	140-199 mg/dl	100-125 mg/dl	5.6-6.9%
Diabetes	≥200 mg/dl	≥126 mg/dl	≥7.0%

Data from American Diabetes Association, 2010, "Standards of medical care in diabetes-2010," *Diabetes Care* 33 (suppl 1): S11-S61; American Diabetes Association, 2010, "Summary of revisions for the 2010 clinical practice recommendations," *Diabetes Care* 33 (suppl 1): S3.

unregulated diabetics, blood glucose typically is about 300 to 400 mg/dl but can be as high as 1000 mg/dl. When blood glucose is over 180 to 200 mg/dl, there is sugar exudate (i.e., overflow) into urine. Diagnostic criteria for diabetes based on blood tests are shown in table 10.1. The most common tests to measure blood glucose levels are oral glucose tolerance tests and blood glucose tests. Both tests are done after people have fasted for 8 to 12 h. The oral test involves measuring the change in blood glucose levels 2 h after a glucose drink. The blood glucose test is done without any additional glucose load to the blood.

▶ **THE AMERICAN** Diabetes Association (2012) recommends that patients with impaired glucose tolerance, impaired fasting glucose, or an HbA1c of 5.7% to 6.9% lose 5% to 10% of their body weight and increase their moderate physical activity by at least 150 min each week.

Health Burden of Diabetes

Chronic complications of uncontrolled diabetes include coronary heart disease, nerve diseases, blindness, kidney failure, and amputation of the limbs. Cardiovascular disease is two to four times more common among persons with diabetes; the risk of stroke is two to four times higher; 75%

of people with diabetes use hypertension drugs or have blood pressures of 130/80 or higher; and 60% to 70% have mild to severe diabetic nerve damage. Nearly 75% of the deaths among diabetics living in economically developed nations can be attributed to heart or blood vessel disease. Also, premenopausal women with diabetes do not have the same degree of protection against coronary heart disease as other women their age. The following are some statistics about the complications and health impact of uncontrolled diabetes (Centers for Disease Control 2007).

- *Diabetic neuropathy.* About half the people with diabetes have diabetic neuropathy, which can result in loss of sensations in the limbs. Diabetes is a common cause of impotence in men. Nerve damage and poor circulation to the limbs cause tissue damage in the extremities, especially the foot, which can lead to ulceration. Diabetes is the leading cause of nontraumatic amputation of lower limbs.

- *Diabetic retinopathy.* Diabetic retinopathy results from damage to the small blood vessels in the eye and is the leading cause of incident blindness (12,000 to 24,000 new cases each year) in adults aged 20 to 74 years. On average, about 2% of people with diabetes go blind, and 10% have vision problems after 15 years of diabetes. The risks of glaucoma and cataracts are increased among diabetics.

- *Loss of limbs.* More than 60% of nontraumatic lower limb amputations occur in people diagnosed with diabetes. In 2004, about 71,000 nontraumatic lower limb amputations were performed in diabetic patients.

- *Renal disease.* The risk of kidney failure is directly related to the severity and duration of diabetes and is retarded by controlling blood glucose levels and blood pressure and by restricting protein in the diet. Diabetes accounted for 44% of new cases of kidney failure in 2005. A total of 46,739 people with diabetes began treatment for end-stage kidney disease, and 178,689 people with end-stage kidney disease because of diabetes were living on chronic dialysis or with a kidney transplant in the United States and Puerto Rico.

Gestational Diabetes

A diagnosis of gestational diabetes requires at least two of the following plasma glucose values:

- Fasting: ≥92 mg/dL (5.1 mmol/L)
- OR the following glucose levels after a glucose tolerance test
- 1 h: ≥180 mg/dL (10.0 mmol/L)
- 2 h: ≥153 mg/dL (8.5 mmol/L)

Source: American Diabetes Association 2012

- *Complications in pregnancy.* The risks for birth defects and prenatal mortality are increased among women who have diabetes. Women who have **gestational diabetes** (temporary glucose elevations during pregnancy among nondiabetic women) have 35% to 60% odds of developing diabetes in the following 1 to 20 years (Centers for Disease Control 2011) and have increased risks of pregnancy. Gestational diabetes occurs in up to 10% of pregnancies and costs an estimated $623 million in 2007 (American Diabetes Association 2008).

Risk Factors

Diabetes mellitus is partly a hereditary disease. Certain genetic markers are known to indicate risk of developing type 1 diabetes, but such markers have not been determined as yet for type 2 diabetes, though it is strongly familial and differs according to race and ethnicity in the United States. Other than age, race, and ethnicity, which are not modifiable, several risk factors for diabetes can be modified by physical activity to help in primary and secondary prevention of type 2 diabetes. These include excess body weight, insulin resistance, high blood pressure, high cholesterol, and gestational diabetes.

▷ **RISK FACTORS** for type 2 diabetes that are modifiable by physical activity include insulin resistance, excess body weight, high blood pressure, high cholesterol, and gestational diabetes.

Prospective cohort studies show that both physical inactivity and weight gain are risk factors for developing type 2 diabetes. Randomized clinical trials have not been conducted to confirm experimentally that changing body weight, fat distribution, diet, or physical activity independently decreases the risk of type 2 diabetes. However, follow-up analysis of successful interventions that combined physical activity with diet to achieve weight loss have found that people who become more active reduce their risk even when they don't achieve significant weight loss.

Insulin and Glucose Transport

Around 1813, the French physiologist Claude Bernard concluded that diabetes was a disease caused by abnormal metabolism of glycogen. Then in 1888, Oskar Minkowski and Joseph von Mering at the University of Strasbourg found that removal of the pancreas led to the development of diabetes mellitus in dogs (Luft 1989). A decade later, a Johns Hopkins medical student, Eugene Opie, showed that diabetics had pancreatic degeneration in the islets of Langerhans, which produce insulin (Opie 1900).

Movement of glucose from the blood into a cell mainly depends on the binding of insulin to an insulin receptor on the cell membrane and the subsequent movement of glucose transporter (GLUT) proteins from the cytoplasm to the cell membrane via second-messenger–mediated phosphorylation of a glucose "channel." The most common glucose transporter in adipose tissue and skeletal muscle is GLUT4. After an insulin molecule binds with the receptor and has effected its action, it is degraded by enzyme action in the liver within about an hour after its initial release into circulation.

The insulin receptor is a tyrosine kinase, an enzyme that transfers phosphates from adenosine triphosphate (ATP) onto tyrosine residues found on target proteins that regulate cellular actions. It is made up of two alpha subunits that bind with an insulin molecule and then cause two beta subunits to phosphorylate themselves and protrude into the cell to activate insulin receptor substrates (IRS) that have different forms in different tissues. For example, IRS-1 is prominent in skeletal muscle and adipose tissue, and IRS-2 is found there but also in the liver and brain.

Insulin receptor signaling involves two major enzyme pathways: (1) a phosphatidylinositol-3-kinase (PI3-K) to protein kinase B (Akt) pathway that increases glucose uptake and glycogen synthesis, suppresses gluconeogenesis and lipid metabolism, and protects against cell death; and (2) a mitogen-activated protein kinase (MAPK) pathway that regulates gene expression and works with the PI3-K to Akt pathway to control protein synthesis and cell turnover.

The activated IRS acts as a second messenger within the cell to begin a cascade of enzyme actions. First guanosine diphosphate (GDP) is replaced with guanosine triphosphate (GTP) on a G-protein named guanine nucleotide binding protein (Ras). This begins a phosphorylation cascade that ends in the activation of MAPK and the enzyme pathway from PI3-K to PI3-K-dependent serine/threonine kinases (PDK1) to Akt, which regulates cell signaling to mobilize glucose transporters to the cell membrane. These steps are necessary for the recruitment of insulin-dependent glucose transporters to the plasma membrane, but the mechanism connecting Akt to GLUT4 mobilization is not yet known. See figure 10.5.

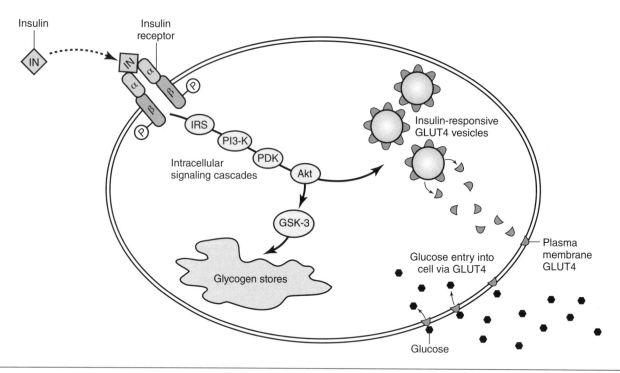

Figure 10.5 Mobilization of glucose transporters by insulin. Insulin signaling cascade involved in stimulating glucose transport. Phosphorylation of the insulin receptor substrate (IRS) on tyrosine residues, activation of phosphatidylinositol 3-kinase (PI3-K), activation of PI3-K-dependent serine/threonine kinase (PDK) and protein kinase B (Akt) from cytoplasm to the plasma membrane.

Glycogen synthase kinase 3 (GSK-3) also is a key factor in insulin signaling and glucose metabolism. When insulin is absent, GSK-3 is active and inhibits glycogen synthase. Insulin binding to the receptor inhibits GSK-3 via inhibitory phosphorylation by Akt. As a result, insulin activates glycogen synthase (thus increasing conversion of glucose to glycogen in the cell). Insulin also stimulates glycogen synthesis indirectly in the liver by activating hexokinase and inhibiting glucose-6-phosphatase, so that glucose is sequestered in the cells. Insulin also inhibits gluconeogenesis, preserving amino acids and further reducing glucose output from the liver. Additionally it inhibits breakdown of fat in adipose tissue by inhibiting the intracellular lipase that hydrolyzes triglycerides to release fatty acids. Thus, insulin not only promotes the use of glucose above fatty acids as the fuel of choice for energy production; it also contributes to the storage of fat in adipose tissue. However, when the liver is saturated to about 5% of its mass with glycogen, additional glucose taken up by liver cells is used to synthesize fatty acids, which are exported from the liver as lipoproteins used by adipose cells to synthesize and store triglycerides.

Other enzymes inhibit insulin action. Protein tyrosine phosphatases (PTPase) catalyze dephosphorylation of the insulin receptor and IRS, thus blunting insulin action. Also, phosphatidylinositol-3-phosphatases can decrease the activity of the PI3-kinase pathway, which dampens or terminates insulin signaling.

Although neurons can use only glucose as fuel, adipose, muscle, and liver cells use fatty acids and protein as fuels when insulin is not available. When insulin levels in the blood fall, glycogen synthesis in the liver is reduced and enzymes that break down glycogen are activated. Glycogen breakdown is stimulated not only by the absence of insulin but also by the presence of glucagon, which is secreted by alpha cells in the pancreas when blood glucose levels fall below the normal range. Glucagon essentially reverses the actions of insulin by stimulating glycogenolysis, gluconeogenesis, and glucose output from the liver, as well as hydrolysis of free fatty acids from triglycerides. We will see later how insulin secretion is decreased during exercise so that skeletal muscle has an advantage over other tissues during exercise for using glucose and fat as fuel.

Etiology of Type 2 Diabetes

The 19th-century French physician Lancereaux distinguished between fat diabetes, *diabete gras,* and thin diabetes, *diabete maigre* (Lancereaux 1880). Before the discovery of insulin therapy, most children and some adults died of diabetes within months, while overweight patients often survived for years (Harley 1866). Elliot P. Joslin, founder of the Joslin Diabetes Center, now affiliated with Harvard University, attributed the increasing prevalence of diabetes in the United States during the 1930s to obesity (Pincus, Joslin, and White 1934).

Today it is understood that the pathogenesis of type 2 diabetes begins with some degree of insulin resistance, mainly in skeletal muscle, adipose tissue, and liver (figure 10.6). Compensatory initial responses include increased glucose output from the liver, followed by hyperinsulinemia in response to increased blood glucose. If high insulin levels compensate for the insulin resistance, the person maintains normal glucose tolerance; otherwise, early stages of progressive **impaired glucose tolerance (IGT)** begin. Type 2 diabetes develops in about 40% to 50% of patients with IGT; the rate of progression to overt disease is about 1% to 5% each year after the development of IGT. The transition from IGT to diabetes occurs when insulin resistance becomes severe and is associated with elevated basal hepatic glucose output and subsequently a marked deterioration of insulin secretion—that is, beta cell dysfunction. Studies have found a 50% reduction in beta cell mass in people with type 2 diabetes. Also, the secretion of proinsulin (the biologically inactive precursor of insulin) is increased relative to insulin.

▷ **NEARLY HALF** of people with IGT develop type 2 diabetes within five to 20 years. The most effective treatment for reducing the progression of IGT into diabetes is weight loss through diet and increased physical activity.

Insulin resistance or insensitivity (i.e., a decrease in insulin receptor signaling) leads to type 2 diabetes because cells in adipose tissue, liver, and skeletal muscle are unable to take up glucose. This results in hyperglycemia (an increase in circulating glucose). Insulin resistance also increases free fatty acid levels in the blood and fat storage in the liver and muscle, which contribute to impaired insulin action and elevated glucose output by the liver.

People who have type 2 diabetes or are obese have impairments in insulin receptor activity and insulin signaling after insulin binding to the receptor (i.e., reduced IRS phosphorylation and PI3-kinase activation) in skeletal muscle, adipose, and liver cells (Caro et al. 1986, 1987; Goodyear et al. 1995;

Krook et al. 1998; Sinha et al. 1987). Some evidence suggests that insulin resistance in skeletal muscle results from decreases in insulin receptors and their activity in people who are obese but not diabetic, but that it results from poor insulin signaling downstream of insulin receptor binding in people who have type 2 diabetes (Caro et al. 1987).

The exact mechanisms that explain the development of insulin resistance during prediabetes or after a diagnosis of type 2 diabetes are not fully known. However, adipose cells have a key role. High free fatty acids secreted by fat cells promote insulin resistance by inhibiting glucose uptake and glycogen synthesis in cells and by increasing glycolysis and glucose output from the liver. High free fatty acids also seem to impair IRS-1 phosphorylation and PI3-kinase activation after insulin binding. Insulin resistance is also associated with triglyceride and fatty acids stored in skeletal muscle, which is reversible by fat loss.

Adipose tissue also acts as an endocrine organ by secreting proteins such as leptin and adiponectin that act like hormones to modify the effects of insulin. Leptin, which acts in the brain to influence satiety, also acts in the liver and skeletal muscle to help regulate the action of insulin. Deficiencies in leptin levels or signaling are linked with insulin resistance. Leptin replacement in people who have lipodystrophy and leptin deficiency can improve their regulation of blood glucose. Adiponectin increases the use of fatty acids as fuel in skeletal muscle, can contribute to weight loss, and is inversely associated with insulin resistance and hyperinsulinemia. People who are obese or have type 2 diabetes often have low levels of adiponectin in their blood.

Nearly 20 years ago, investigators found that tumor necrosis factor-alpha (TNF-α), a cytokine secreted by macrophages during inflammation, causes insulin resistance by suppressing phosphorylation of the insulin receptor and IRS-1 (Feinstein et al. 1993; Hotamisligil, Shargill, and Spiegelman 1993). Since then, TNF-α and other inflammatory cytokines (known as adipokines) that are secreted by macrophages when they enter adipose tissue, including in the liver, have been linked to insulin resistance in people who are obese (Hotamisligil

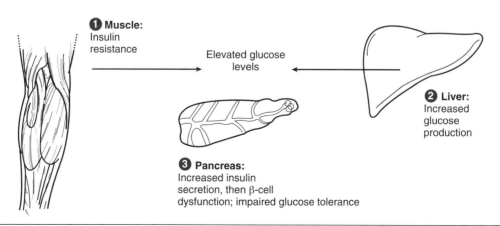

Figure 10.6 Pathogenesis of type 2 diabetes.

2006; Hevener et al. 2010). Conversely, anti-inflammatory cytokines such as interleukin-10 (IL-10) enhance insulin sensitivity.

Glucostatic Medication for Type 2 Diabetes

The evidence shown later in the chapter is clear that insulin sensitivity is improved, while type 2 diabetes is prevented or delayed, in most people when they lose body fat or when they increase their amount of moderate-to-vigorous physical activity even when they don't lose much weight. Hence, diet and exercise are part of frontline medical therapy in the prevention and care of type 2 diabetes. Nonetheless, drugs that regulate glucose are often needed in the treatment of people with type 2 diabetes. Understanding the mechanisms of glucostatic drugs is also helpful for the study and interpretation of biological responses to exercise that explain how skeletal muscle action regulates glucose use.

Thiazolidinediones (Glitazones)

Rosiglitazone (marketed as Avandia) and pioglitazone (marketed as Actos) were approved by the United States in 1999 to reduce insulin resistance in skeletal muscle, liver, and adipose tissue. With proper dosing they can lower fasting blood glucose levels by about 20% and can reduce HbA1c by about 1% after a month or two of treatment. Avandia and Actos are believed to work by affecting proteins that modify genes to increase the activity of the insulin receptor and IRS-1 tyrosine phosphorylation and PI3-kinase activity, and possibly by reducing levels of inflammatory cytokines like TNF-α. The drugs are not recommended for people with kidney or liver disease, enlarged heart, congestive heart failure, or edema or during pregnancy.

Some evidence indicates that Avandia, but not Actos (Lincoff et al. 2007), increases the risk of heart attacks, congestive heart failure, or cardiovascular deaths (Home et al. 2009; Nissen and Wolski 2007, 2010) and bone fractures in women (Home et al. 2009). Whether Avandia increases cardiovascular risk more than the other most popular diabetes drug, metformin, is controversial (Home et al. 2009; Komajda et al. 2010); but Avandia prescriptions in the United States dropped by 80% from 2007 to 2010 while its safety was under intense scrutiny by the Food and Drug Administration. In September 2010, sales of Avandia were halted in Europe and restricted in the United States to use as the drug of last choice when both doctor and patient attest that all other diabetes drugs have been ineffective and that the patient fully accepts the risks Avandia poses to the heart.

Metformin

Metformin (marketed as Glucophage) was developed in 1957 in France by pharmacist Jan Aron and physician Jean Stern, but because of concerns about adverse health risks it was held off the market until it was used in France in 1979. Metformin is a derivative of the French lilac plant, which was observed over 100 years ago to lower blood sugar but was toxic. Metformin was not approved in the United States for treatment of type 2 diabetes until 1994. With proper dosing, it can lower fasting blood glucose levels by about 20% mainly by reducing glucose output by the liver, and it can lower HbA1c by about 1% to 3% after a month or two of treatment. Averaged across 31 trials with 4570 patients, metformin reduced BMI (body mass index) by 5.3%, fasting glucose by 4.5%, fasting insulin by 14.4%, triglycerides by 5.3%, and low-density lipoprotein cholesterol by 5.6%. It increased high-density lipoprotein cholesterol by 5.0% compared with placebo or no treatment. The incidence of new-onset diabetes was reduced by 40% (Salpeter et al. 2008). It is not recommended for people who have diabetic ketoacidosis, kidney or liver disease, congestive heart failure or heart attack or for alcoholics or binge drinkers, people over age 80, or pregnant women. Metformin is the most commonly used drug worldwide for treating type 2 diabetes. Randomized controlled trials have shown that metformin helps prevent type 2 diabetes (Crandall et al. 2008; Knowler et al. 2002), improves regulation of blood glucose, and lowers cardiovascular deaths in overweight people who have type 2 diabetes (Rotella, Monami, and Mannucci 2006). Evidence indicates that metformin works mainly by inhibiting gluconeogenesis and thus reducing glucose output by the liver (Bailey and Turner 1996). It is now accepted that metformin impairs ATP production, thus activating 5'-adenosine monophosphate–activated protein kinase (AMPK), which is sensitive to change in energy balance (i.e., when ATP production is decreased by restricted energy intake or ATP consumption is increased by elevated energy expenditure). Activated AMPK switches cells from an anabolic to a catabolic state, shutting down the ATP-consuming synthetic pathways and restoring energy balance.

AMPK is a drug target for the treatment of obesity and type 2 diabetes because it is a key sensor of energy depletion in adipose tissue, skeletal muscle, the liver, and the central nervous system. Both acute and chronic hyperglycemia reduce AMPK activation in muscle and the liver, and there is a strong correlation between low AMPK activation, which mainly results from overeating and lack of exercise, and metabolic disorders associated with insulin resistance and obesity (Ruderman and Prentki 2004). In a recent study, insulin sensitivity was increased by 50% and AMPK activity in skeletal muscle was increased by 200% 4 h after a single 40-min session of moderate-to-hard exercise. However, those changes did not occur when the same exercise followed two to three weeks of metformin treatment (Sharoff et al. 2010).

How Does Exercise Improve Glucose Use?

Weight loss and thiazolidinediones improve glucose control in part by increasing insulin-stimulated insulin receptor and IRS-1 tyrosine phosphorylation and PI3-kinase activity. In contrast, regular exercise and metformin improve whole-body glucose use with only small effects on insulin signaling (Musi and Goodyear 2006). Nonetheless, exercise training, like metformin, may activate enzyme pathways downstream of the insulin receptor (e.g., AMPK) and the protein kinase B (Akt) substrate AS160 to improve glucose transport in skeletal muscle. Also, increased use of fat as fuel and increased mitochondria in skeletal muscle could indirectly increase insulin sensitivity (Hawley and Lessard 2008).

Insulin-Like Effect of Muscle Contraction

The contraction of skeletal muscle results in several metabolic events that increase glucose uptake without the use of insulin. The main proteins suspected to be most involved are AMPK, LKB1, Ca^{2+}/calmodulin-dependent protein kinases (CaMKs), PKCs, and AS160 (Röckl, Wotczak, and Goodyear 2008; figure 10.7).

AMP-Activated Protein Kinase

AMPK is activated in contracting skeletal muscle during exercise because of an increase in the adenosine monophosphate (AMP)-to-ATP ratio associated with energy turnover in the muscle (McBride and Hardie 2009; McGee et al.

2003). In rats, exercise also increases AMPK activity in the liver and adipose tissue—tissues that do not have increased energy demand during exercise (Kelly et al. 2009). That effect appears to depend on the glucostatic cytokine, IL-6, which is released by skeletal muscle and acts as a hormone to increase insulin sensitivity and total-body uptake of glucose (Ruderman et al. 2006).

It is also believed that AMPK helps determine muscle fiber type and the generation of mitochondria and GLUT4 protein in skeletal muscle (McGee and Hargreaves 2010). Also, similar to the recent evidence on the action of metformin, studies have shown that glucose transport in contracting skeletal muscle is unaffected or only partially diminished when activity in AMPK or its primary activator, serine/threonine kinase 11 (commonly known as LKB1), is blocked (Röckl, Witczak, and Goodyear 2008). Thus, whether AMPK explains increased GLUT4 levels and glucose transport after exercise, or depends on muscle glycogen levels (McBride and Hardie 2009), has not yet been confirmed.

Protein Kinase C

There are three main types of PKC in mammals: (1) conventional PKCs (cPKCs) that depend on Ca^{2+} and diacylglycerol for activation, (2) novel PKCs (nPKCs) that depend on diacylglycerol for activation, and (3) atypical PKCs (aPKCs) that are activated without Ca^{2+} or diacylglycerol. Drugs that block cPKCs and nPKCs also impair glucose uptake during skeletal muscle contraction, but muscle contraction during exercise does not appear to increase cPKC or nPKC activity. The effects of AMPK on glucose transport may be mediated by activation of extracellular signal–regulated kinase (ERK) and aPKCs.

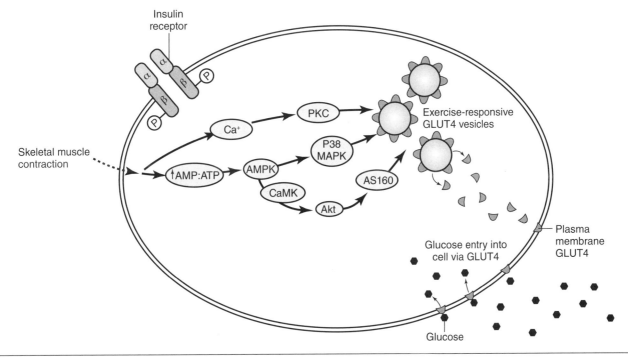

Figure 10.7 Plausible steps explaining the insulin-like effect of skeletal muscle contraction on glucose uptake.

Ca²⁺/Calmodulin-Dependent Protein Kinases

Skeletal muscle contraction depends on increases in intracellular Ca^{2+} levels, and studies suggest that Ca^{2+}/calmodulin (*cal*cium *modul*ated prote*in*) signaling and Ca^{2+}/calmodulin-dependent protein kinases (CaMK) are part of GLUT4 mobilization during muscle contraction. It is currently being debated whether CaMK signaling can stimulate muscle glucose uptake without changes in AMPK activity.

MAPK

The MAPK family of proteins in skeletal muscle includes (1) extracellular signal–regulated kinases (ERK) and (2) p38 mitogen-activated protein kinase (p38 MAPK), which are activated by cytokines, growth factors, and cellular stress, including exercise (Röckl, Witczak, and Goodyear 2008). P38 MAPK is activated by insulin, inflammatory cytokines (e.g., response to muscle injury), and high-intensity muscle contraction during exercise (Kramer and Goodyear 2007), but its response to acute exercise may depend on training history (Gibala et al. 2009; Yeo et al. 2010).

Akt Substrate of 160 kDa (AS160)

The Akt substrate of 160 kDa (AS160) is a protein that regulates insulin-stimulated GLUT4 translocation in adipose tissue and rat skeletal muscle. AMPK phosphorylates AS160 in response to skeletal muscle contraction (Kramer et al. 2006), and Akt appears to regulate insulin-stimulated AS160 phosphorylation in skeletal muscle. Although AS160 phosphorylation is important for insulin-stimulated GLUT4 translocation, it is unclear whether AS160 phosphorylation is responsible for glucose transport during exercise (Cartee and Wojtaszewski 2007).

Effects of Physical Activity on Diabetes Risk: The Evidence

Exercise appears to have been first recommended to treat diabetes by the Indian physician Sushruta around 600 BC. It also was recommended by the Roman physician and philosopher Celsus at the beginning of the first millennium. Greco-Roman physicians were still prescribing exercise around the year 1000 for diabetic patients, but they preferred horseback riding because they incorrectly believed it reduced urination through the mild friction between rider and horse. A tradition of exercise treatment persisted until the later part of the 18th century, when the British physician John Rollo recommended bed rest as the preferred treatment. The tradition of rest, drugs, and dietary restrictions on sugar and starchy foods persisted in Europe for nearly 100 years. However, some doctors also recommended muscular exercise.

In his history of the treatment of diabetes, the English physician William Morgan concluded that "active muscular exercise daily, in the open air, may be considered as a valuable addenda to our code of treatment of Diabetes Mellitus" (Morgan 1877, p. 169). Morgan gave accounts of other physicians of the day who used exercise as treatment, noting that M. Bouchardat, a professor of hygiene in the faculty of medicine in Paris, urged his patients "to go through a daily course of exercise at a gymnasium, or to engage in work or exercise sufficiently active to throw them into a good perspiration. By this, he is of opinion, that a return of power of appropriating the starchy and saccharine elements of food is promoted" (p. 169). Likewise, Morgan recounted that Dr. Külz of Marburg "observed 8 cases of diabetes mellitus in which active exercise was of decided value; but such exercise must consist of vigorous movement in the open air; simple in-door gymnastics are scarcely of the slightest use . . . provided the patients are fond of such exercise and can support the necessary exertion, he strongly recommends this treatment in lieu of drugs, provided that careful preliminary experiments have shown that exercise diminishes the excretion of sugar. . ." (p. 170).

The true role of exercise, though, in the primary and secondary prevention of type 2 diabetes has emerged only during the past 15 years or so (American College of Sports Medicine 2000; American College of Sports Medicine and the American Diabetes Association 2010; Physical Activity Guidelines Advisory Committee 2008). Physical activity could potentially contribute to primary (reducing initial occurrence), secondary (reversal), and tertiary (delay of medical complications) prevention and treatment of diabetes (King and Kriska 1992). Metabolic studies suggest that the major effect of physical activity is improved glucose transport and insulin sensitivity, some of which may be indirect effects of weight loss (Goodyear and Kahn 1998). Therefore, it may have the greatest benefit in primary prevention and in early treatment of diabetes.

Cross-sectional and prospective population-based studies have provided evidence consistent with such a protective benefit. There is also some evidence that exercise positively influences metabolic control of glucose and the prevention or delay of chronic medical complications in patients with type 2 diabetes.

Cross-Sectional Cultural Studies

Several studies have addressed whether a decline in physical activity resulting from naturally occurring changes in culture is associated with increased risk for type 2 diabetes. Some populations that have traditionally led physically active lifestyles become sedentary after their society becomes more urban. In South Pacific island cultures, Zimmet and colleagues (1990) found a significant association between an abandonment of traditional lifestyles, which were physically demanding, in favor of more sedentary lifestyles and an increased incidence of type 2 diabetes mellitus.

Other investigators observed individuals who migrated from a rural region to a more urban region. Individuals from a population subgroup who migrated were compared with individuals who remained in their homeland. For example, Kawate and colleagues (1979) found that type 2 diabetes was twice as prevalent among Japanese immigrants to the United States as among those who remained in Japan. Both types of studies have assumed that the adoption of a more urban lifestyle leads to increased risk of diabetes because of a decrease in physical activity. Of course, the effects of dietary changes are often difficult to isolate from the effects of urbanization.

Kiribati

A population-based survey of 2938 Micronesians living on the Pacific islands of the Republic of Kiribati found that the age-adjusted prevalence of type 2 diabetes was nearly three times as high in urban as in rural samples (King et al. 1984). The rural population was leaner and engaged in more physical activity. The higher prevalence of diabetes among the urban sample was not fully explainable by greater obesity. Among women, obesity, urbanization, and physical inactivity were each independently associated with higher rates of diabetes. A later study included Melanesians and Indians in Fiji and Melanesians in Vanuatu (Taylor et al. 1992). Urban participants were more obese than rural ones and had higher prevalence rates of diabetes. Rural participants were leaner, suffered less from diabetes, and had greater total energy intakes than urban dwellers. Rural people ate a greater proportion of carbohydrates, while urban people ate proportionally more protein and fat. Rural participants in all three studies had higher levels of physical activity.

Mauritius

The island nation of Mauritius, located in the southwest Indian Ocean, has a high prevalence of type 2 diabetes among all of its ethnic groups (Hindu and Muslim Indians, African-origin Creoles, and Chinese). The high rates of this disease among groups who differ in ethnic and genetic backgrounds illustrate the importance of environmental factors in the development of type 2 diabetes, and these groups provide a unique population in which to study behaviors that add to risk. A random sample of 4658 Asian, Indian, Creole, and Chinese adults ages 25 to 74 years were categorized as active or inactive based on an interview conducted in 1987 about leisure and occupational physical activity. People with diabetes were excluded. Fasting glucose levels and 2-h plasma glucose and serum insulin levels after a glucose tolerance test were lower in active subjects of both sexes, independently of BMI and waist-to-hip ratio. In a subsequent study of Mauritius, total physical activity was associated with lower 2-h blood glucose levels after a glucose tolerance test among middle-aged Hindu, Creole, Chinese, and Muslim males and among Hindu and Creole females, even after adjustment for BMI, waist-to-hip ratio, age, and family history of type 2 diabetes (Pereira et al. 1995).

Pima Indians

The Pima Indians have the highest known incidence of type 2 diabetes in the United States. Among 1054 Pima Indians ages 15 to 59 years who lived in Arizona, current (during the most recent calendar year) and lifetime leisure plus occupational physical activity were measured by questionnaire (Kriska et al. 1993). Current physical activity was inversely associated with fasting glucose levels and 2-h glucose levels after a glucose tolerance test. However, active people also had lower BMIs and waist-to-thigh ratios in most sex and age groups, which could confound the association between physical activity and diabetes risk. Even so, after adjustments for age, BMI, and waist-to-thigh ratio, 2-h glucose levels were still lower among men who were physically active, and people who reported low levels of lifetime physical activity had a higher rate of diabetes. In both males and females, the age-adjusted prevalence of type 2 diabetes was lower among people classified in the middle and top leisure physical activity groups than among those who had the lowest level of leisure physical activity during the past year.

A follow-up study compared oral glucose tolerance between adult Pima Indian, as well as non-Pima populations living in the Sierra Madre Mountains of Mexico, and Pima Indians living in Arizona (Schulz et al. 2006). The findings supported that environmental influences on lifestyle behaviors, including physical activity, were stronger influences on diabetes risk than were genetic factors. The Pima populations were genetically similar. However, the prevalence of type 2 diabetes in the Mexican Pima Indians was about 7%, similar to the rate among non-Pima Mexicans but less than one-fifth the rate of 38% observed among Pima Indians living in the United States. The prevalence of obesity was similar in the Mexican Pima Indians (7% in men and 20% in women) and non-Pima Mexicans (9% in men and 27% in women) but was much lower than in the U.S. Pima Indians (64% in men and 75% in women). Conversely, time spent in physical activity by Pima and non-Pima Mexican men and women, respectively, was 2.5 times and 7.5 times more than that spent by U.S. Pima men and women.

Prospective Cohort Studies

A systematic review of 10 prospective cohort studies, including 301,221 participants and 9367 incident cases, showed that the mean relative risk of type 2 diabetes was 0.69 (95% confidence interval [CI]: 0.58-0.83) for regular participation in physical activity of at least moderate intensity as compared with being sedentary (Jeon et al. 2007). In this section we examine several prospective cohort studies.

University of Pennsylvania Alumni Study

Nearly 6000 male alumni of the University of Pennsylvania were observed for 14 years. A dose-dependent reduction in risk of developing type 2 diabetes mellitus was associated with higher levels of leisure-time physical activity (Helmrich

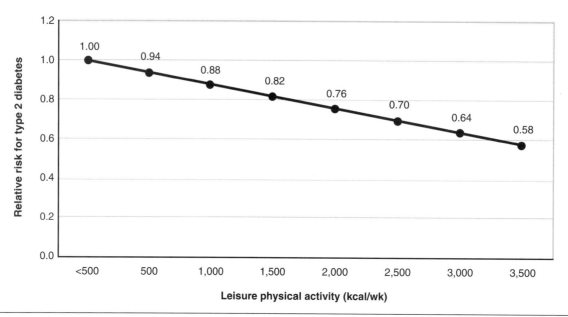

Figure 10.8 University of Pennsylvania alumni study examining leisure physical activity with relative risk for type 2 diabetes. The study included 5990 males who were followed for 14 years; age-adjusted risk for type 2 diabetes decreased by 6% for each 500 kcal/week increase in leisure-time physical activity up to 3500 kcal/week.

Adapted from Helmrich et al. 1991.

et al. 1991). Figure 10.8 shows that the age-adjusted risk of type 2 diabetes decreased by 6% for each 500 kcal/week increase in leisure-time physical activity up to 3500 kcal/week. The risk reduction remained after adjustments for obesity, hypertension, and parental history of diabetes.

Nurses' Health Study

This is an ongoing prospective cohort study that obtained survey reports of physical activity from female nurses located in 11 U.S. states who had no history of diabetes, cardiovascular disease, or cancer at baseline. Participants were surveyed first in 1986 and periodically afterward. The women were asked to report the average time spent per week on the following activities: walking, jogging, running, bicycling, lap swimming, playing tennis or squash, and participating in calisthenics. In an initial period, approximately 87,000 participants were observed for eight years, during which 1300 new cases of type 2 diabetes were confirmed (Manson et al. 1991). Women who had engaged in at least one vigorous activity per week had an age-adjusted relative risk that was one-third lower than that for women who had not participated in at least one vigorous activity. Figure 10.9 shows that when adjusted for BMI, the risk reduction conferred by vigorous activity was cut in half, to a relative risk of 0.84. Nonetheless, this reduced risk was still significantly different from that for women who had not exercised at least once per week. No dose response was observed, though. Up to five days of vigorous activity each week was no more beneficial than one day. When just the first two years of the study were analyzed, a period that was closer to the time when physical activity

levels were measured, the age-adjusted relative risk of those who exercised was 0.5, and age- and BMI-adjusted relative risk was 0.69. In general, the protective effects of physical activity were seen in obese and normal-weight women and remained regardless of age and family history of diabetes.

After 16 years of follow-up observation, there were 4030 incident cases of type 2 diabetes among 68,907 participants

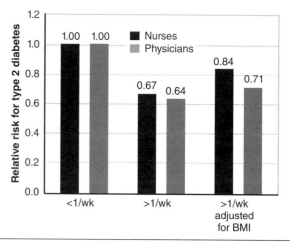

Figure 10.9 U.S. Nurses' and U.S. Physicians' Health studies examining vigorous physical activity and relative risk for type 2 diabetes. The studies included 87,253 women who were followed for eight years and 21,000 men followed for five years. The relative risk is independent of weekly frequency of activity, age, BMI, and family history.

Data from Manson et al. 1991; Manson et al. 1992.

(Rana et al. 2007). After adjustment for age, smoking, and other diabetes risk factors, risk of type 2 diabetes increased with increasing BMI and waist circumference and with decreasing physical activity levels. Compared to risks for normal-weight women (BMI <25 kg/m^2) who were active at least 21.8 MET-hours per week, the relative risks of type 2 diabetes were 16.75 (95% CI: 13.99-20.04) for women who were obese and inactive (i.e., exercised less than 2.1 MET-hours per week), 10.74 (8.74-13.18) for women who were active but obese, and 2.08 (1.66-2.61) for normal-weight women who were inactive. Thus, although obesity and physical inactivity were each independent risk factors for the development of type 2 diabetes, the risk conferred by obesity was greater than the risk of physical inactivity.

Physicians' Health Study

The Physicians' Health Study was designed as a randomized controlled trial of aspirin and beta-carotene in the primary prevention of cardiovascular disease and cancer. The original cohort of 22,071 U.S. male physicians aged 40 to 84 years who were free of diabetes, myocardial infarction, cerebrovascular disease, and cancer at enrollment has been followed continuously since 1982 via annual questionnaires.

Over 21,000 of the men were observed five years after their initial level of self-reported frequency of vigorous exercise and other risk factors were determined (Manson et al. 1992). During 105,141 person-years of follow-up, 285 new cases of type 2 diabetes were reported. The age-adjusted incidence was 369 cases per 100,000 person-years in men who were active less than once a week and 214 cases per 100,000 person-years in those who exercised at least five times a week. Men who exercised at least once per week had an age-adjusted relative risk (RR) that was one-third less than the risk of those who were physically inactive. The age-adjusted RR of diabetes decreased with increasing frequency of exercise: 0.77 for once weekly, 0.62 for two to four times per week, and 0.58 for five or more times per week. The protective effect of physical activity remained after adjustments for age, smoking, hypertension, and BMI. Though the overall protective effects of physical activity were independent of BMI, the association of exercise with reduced risk of type 2 diabetes was especially strong among overweight men.

A subsequent analysis examined the independent and joint associations between self-reports of vigorous activity and BMI and incident cases of diabetes in 20,757 men without diabetes at baseline (Siegel et al. 2009). After a median follow-up of 23.1 years, there were 1836 cases of incident diabetes. Compared with active (any weekly vigorous activity) participants with normal BMIs, active but overweight and obese men had risk ratios of 2.39 (95% CI: 2.11-2.71) and 6.22 (95% CI: 5.12-7.56). Inactive men with normal, overweight, or obese BMIs had adjusted risk ratios of 1.41 (95% CI: 1.19-1.67), 3.14 (95% CI: 2.73-3.62), and 6.57

(95% CI: 5.25-8.21). Active men who were normal weight or overweight had lower risks of developing diabetes than inactive men. However, activity did not protect men who were obese.

British Men

A cohort of 5159 men ages 40 to 59 years with no history of coronary heart disease, type 2 diabetes, or stroke were selected from general medical practices in 18 British towns (Wannamethee, Shaper, and Alberti 2000). During an average follow-up period of 16.8 years, there were 196 new cases of type 2 diabetes. After adjustment for potential confounders (lifestyle characteristics and preexisting disease), physical activity was inversely related to risk of type 2 diabetes, blood insulin levels, and γ-glutamyltransferase level, a marker of insulin resistance in the liver. Adjustment for insulin and γ-glutamyltransferase level explained most of the reduction in risk of type 2 diabetes associated with physical activity, suggesting that physical activity reduces risk of type 2 diabetes mainly by improving insulin sensitivity (Heath et al. 1983).

Aerobics Center Longitudinal Study (ACLS)

This was a prospective analysis of 14,006 men (7795 men for analyses of impaired fasting glucose) without overt cardiovascular disease, cancer, or diabetes (Lee et al. 2009). There were 3612 incident cases of impaired fasting glucose and 477 incident cases of type 2 diabetes. Compared with risk for the least-fit 20%, risks of developing impaired fasting glucose levels or type 2 diabetes were 14% and 52% lower, respectively, in the most fit 20%. The highest risks were found in men who were both obese and unfit. Obese men in the lowest 20% of fitness had nearly six times higher risk for type 2 diabetes than normal-weight men in the other 80% of fitness level. Similar trends were found for joint associations of BMI and fitness with impaired fasting glucose. Low fitness and obesity similarly increased the risks of impaired fasting glucose and type 2 diabetes. Fitness blunted but did not eliminate the increased risks associated with obesity.

A subsequent analysis of 23,444 men 20 to 85 years of age without cardiovascular disease (CVD), cancer, or diabetes at baseline examined the joint effects of fitness and self-reported physical activity on the risk of 589 incident cases of self-reported diabetes during an average of 18 years of follow-up (Sieverdes et al. 2010). After adjustment for age and other risk factors, men who either walked, jogged or ran regularly for exercise or who participated in vigorous sports or fitness activities had a 40% and 28% lower risk, respectively, of developing diabetes than sedentary men. Similarly, moderate and high fitness groups had 38% and 63% lower risk compared with the low fitness group.

As in men, there was an independent, protective effect of fitness in women from the ACLS study who had elevated risk of diabetes because they were overweight or obese, but fitness did not eliminate the elevated risk (Sui et al. 2008). During an average 17-year follow-up, there were 143 cases of type 2 diabetes in a cohort of 6249 women aged 20 to 79 years without CVD, cancer, or diabetes at baseline. After adjustment for BMI and other risk factors, the risk was 0.86 (0.59-1.25) for the middle third and 0.61 (0.38-0.96) for the upper third of fitness compared to the lowest third. After adjustment for fitness and other risk factors, the risk was 2.34 (1.55-3.54) for overweight individuals and 3.70 (2.12-6.44) for obese individuals, compared with normal-weight women (figure 10.10). Overweight/obese women who were also in the lowest one-third of fitness had higher risk of diabetes than normal-weight women in the upper two-thirds of fitness.

Malmo, Sweden

Among nearly 7000 men ages 47 to 49 who were screened for diabetes, over 4600 men without diabetes were given an oral glucose tolerance test and a submaximal $\dot{V}O_2$ test of cardiorespiratory fitness (Eriksson and Lindgarde 1996). During the next six years, 116 men developed type 2 diabetes. Those men had 11% higher mean BMIs, more family history of diabetes (31% vs. 18%), 16% lower mean physical activity, 16% lower mean estimated maximal oxygen uptake, and nearly three times higher mean 2-h insulin levels after

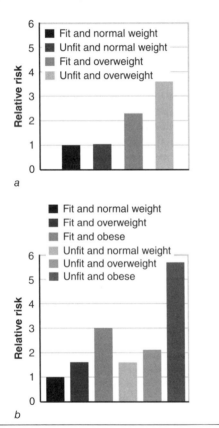

Figure 10.10 Relative risk of diabetes according to cardiorespiratory fitness level and normal or overweight BMI among (a) women and (b) men in the Aerobics Center Longitudinal Study.

Data for (a) from Sui et al. 2008; data for (b) from Lee et al. 2009

the glucose tolerance test. Men with higher physical fitness had lower 2-h insulin response to the glucose tolerance test. Hyperinsulinemia, BMI, and fasting blood glucose level were independent risk factors for type 2 diabetes. Among 278 men who had IGT at baseline, 44 developed type 2 diabetes, which was predicted only by fasting glucose levels. Both physical fitness and the level of physical activity were associated with lowered risk of developing type 2 diabetes.

Women's Health Initiative Study

During nearly a half million person-years of observation of 86,907 women, incident rates of self-reported diabetes were 2.2% of non-Hispanic white, 6.2% of African American, 4.5% of Hispanic, 3% of Asian, and 5.7% of American Indian women during 458,018 woman-years of follow-up between 1994-1998 and 2002 (Hsia et al. 2005). After adjustment for age, BMI, alcohol use, education, smoking, hypertension, high cholesterol, dietary fiber, and dietary carbohydrates, white women had a 20% to 33% reduction in risk if they were in the top 60% of total physical activity and a 25% reduction in risk if they were in the top 40% of walking when compared with the 20% least-active women. Similar trends of lower risk with higher physical activity were found among African American and Hispanic women after adjusting for age and BMI, but there were not enough women in the minority groups to provide a strong test of whether race or ethnicity modifies the effect of physical activity on reducing the risk of developing type 2 diabetes.

▷ **OBSERVATIONAL STUDIES,** but no randomized controlled trials, have shown a 50% lower risk of gestational diabetes among women who spent about 30 min a day in moderate physical activity before or during early pregnancy (Dempsey, Butler, and Williams 2005).

Women's Health Study

In a prospective cohort study of 37,878 U.S. female health care professionals without CVD, cancer, or diabetes at baseline, 1361 incident cases of self-reported diabetes were observed during nearly seven years of follow-up (Weinstein et al. 2004). Women who were classified as active expended more than 1000 kcal per week in leisure-time physical activities and had a 15% reduction in diabetes risk after adjustment for several other risk factors, including age, family history of diabetes, hypertension, high cholesterol, hormone replacement therapy, and diet. However, the benefit of physical activity was not independent of obesity. Compared to normal-weight women who were active, those who were overweight and obese had nearly four times and 12 times the risk of developing diabetes, respectively, regardless of whether they were active. Walking 2 to 3 h each week reduced risk by more than one-third in overweight and obese women, but not in women who were normal weight.

Losartan Intervention for Endpoint Reduction in Hypertension (LIFE) Study

Physical activity was measured in 4961 women and 4232 men aged 55 to 80 years from 945 medical centers in Denmark, Finland, Iceland, Norway, Sweden, United Kingdom, and the United States who had hypertension and left ventricular hypertrophy. Patients who said they got more than 30 min of exercise twice per week (52% of the patients) at entry into an antihypertensive drug intervention had 25% to 40% lower risk of incident diabetes during nearly five years of treatment, regardless of which drug they took. Compared to patients who said they never exercised, relative risks were 0.74 (95% CI: 0.55-0.99) for women and 0.60 (95% CI: 0.44-0.81) for men (Fossum et al. 2007). The risk reduction was independent of age, smoking, alcohol use, race, severity of ventricular hypertrophy, and other risk factors for CVD.

Walking and Mortality Risk in People With Diabetes

A cross-sectional study of adults with diabetes from the National Health Interview Survey showed that compared with inactive adults, people who walked at least 2 h/week had a 39% lower all-cause mortality rate (2.8% vs. 4.4% per year) and a 34% lower rate of cardiovascular deaths (1.4% vs. 2.1% per year), regardless of sex, age, race, BMI, smoking, hypertension, cancer, and disability (Gregg et al. 2003). It was estimated that one death each year might be prevented for every 61 people who were previously inactive but then walked 2 or more hours each week.

Effects of Obesity Versus Physical Activity on Risk

A recent review concluded that having high BMI (30-35 kg/m^2) even with high physical activity was a greater risk for the incidence of type 2 diabetes and diabetes risk factors than having normal BMI and low physical activity (Fogelholm 2010). Notwithstanding those results, a review of five cohort studies published between 1999 and 2008 that examined the joint effects of obesity and physical activity on the risk of type 2 diabetes concluded that the joint effect of obesity and low physical activity was, on average, additive and sometimes more than the sum of their individual effects (Qin et al. 2010). That is, being inactive and obese carries exponential risk. The implication of that finding is that preventing obesity or physical inactivity will not only reduce diabetes risk by the amount of each factor's independent effect but also prevent cases associated with the interaction between the two factors. Of course, the test of that hypothesis requires experimental manipulation of physical activity with or without weight loss using randomized controlled trials.

Clinical Studies

Several studies conducted in the late 1980s and early 1990s examined the combined benefits of diet and physical activity on blood glucose levels among type 2 diabetics or people with IGT.

The Zuni Diabetes Project was initiated in 1983 to reduce rates of obesity and provide primary and secondary prevention of type 2 diabetes. After two years of follow-up, diabetic participants in an exercise program compared with diabetic nonparticipants experienced weight loss, a drop in fasting blood glucose values, and reductions in the use of hypoglycemic medications (Heath et al. 1991).

From the Malmo, Sweden, cohort discussed earlier in this chapter, 41 who had early-stage type 2 diabetes mellitus and 181 with IGT participated in a six-month intervention consisting of dietary treatment, increased physical activity, or both, followed by annual checkups for five years (Eriksson and Lindgarde 1991). After the intervention, body weight was reduced by 2.3% to 3.7%, maximal oxygen uptake was increased by 10% to 14%, and glucose tolerance was normalized in more than half the men who initially had IGT. Men who initially had IGT but participated in the clinical exercise program had half the relative risk of developing type 2 diabetes compared with matched patients who received standard care but remained sedentary. More than half the diabetic patients were in remission after a mean follow-up of six years. Improvement in glucose tolerance was associated with both weight reduction and increased fitness, and mortality was a third lower than in the rest of the cohort who were not treated.

Other large-scale clinical trials, including randomized controlled studies, have confirmed the benefits of increased physical activity and weight loss in reducing the progression of IGT to diabetes.

Da Qing, China

Physical activity was included in a randomized controlled study that compared diet with exercise for reducing the development of diabetes among adults in Da Qing, China, who had IGT (Pan et al. 1997). Nearly 111,000 men and women from 33 health care clinics in the city of Da Qing were screened for IGT and type 2 diabetes. The 577 patients classified as having IGT were randomly assigned by clinic either to a control group or to one of three active treatment groups: diet only, exercise only, or diet plus exercise. Follow-up examinations were conducted at two-year intervals over a six-year period to identify people who developed type 2 diabetes. After six years of follow-up, those who exercised had half the rate of diabetes (8 cases per 100 person-years of observation) of those who maintained their normal physical activity levels (16 cases per 100 person-years). The cumulative incidence of diabetes at six years was 67.7% (95% CI: 59.8-75.2) in the control group compared with 43.8% (35.5-52.3) in the diet group, 41.1% (33.4-49.4) in the exercise group, and 46.0% (37.3-54.7) in the diet plus exercise group. All the intervention groups had lower rates of diabetes than the control group, regardless of whether participants were normal weight or overweight (BMI ≥25 kg/m²). Weight loss was similar after diet or exercise. After adjustment for baseline BMI and fasting glucose, the risks of diabetes were reduced by 31%, 46%, and 42% with the diet, exercise, and diet plus exercise treatments, respectively (see figure 10.11). Hence, exercise was as effective as diet alone for reducing the six-year risk of diabetes in people with IGT.

When compared with control participants nearly 15 years after the intervention ended, people in the combined lifestyle intervention groups had a 43% lower age- and clinic-adjusted incidence (0.57; 0.41-0.81) of diabetes over the 20-year period of exposure. Cumulative incidence during that time was 80% (7% each year) in the intervention participants and 95% (11% each year) in the control group. Participants in the intervention group spent an average of 3.6 fewer years with diabetes than those in the control group (Li et al. 2008).

The Finnish Diabetes Prevention Study

Middle-aged, overweight men and women with IGT (*n* = 522) were randomized into an intensive lifestyle modification intervention that included leisure-time physical activity, weight reduction, and dietary counseling or into a minimal intervention control group (Eriksson et al. 1999; Tuomilehto et al. 2001). The average time people stayed in the intervention period was four years. The physical activity prescription was for 30 min a day of moderate exercise for a total of more than 4 h per week. People in the intervention lost nearly 3 kg more body weight after three years and had about half the incidence of diabetes after four years compared to the control group (11% vs. 23%) (Lindström et al. 2003).

Weight loss was the main driver of reduced diabetes risk. However, follow-up analysis of 107 new cases of diabetes in 487 of the participants, four years after the trial ended, found

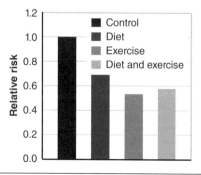

Figure 10.11 The Da Qing, China, six-year controlled clinical trial showed reduced risk for type 2 diabetes among patients with impaired glucose tolerance after diet or exercise or exercise plus diet intervention. Adjusted for body mass index and fasting glucose.

Data from Pan et al. 1997.

that yearly physical activity helped prevent diabetes (Laaksonen et al. 2005). People who had the biggest increases (top third) in moderate-to-vigorous physical activity or strenuous, structured exercise were 50% to 60% less likely to develop diabetes than people in the bottom third, even after adjustment for changes in diet and body weight during the study.

Even three years after the trial ended, people who had been in the lifestyle intervention were about 40% less likely to develop type 2 diabetes (4.3 vs. 7.4 incident cases per 100 person-years of observation). The amount of risk reduction was about 50% for people who met the weight loss goal and nearly 40% for people who met the physical activity goal. When simultaneously adjusted for all goals, only the risk reduction associated with meeting the weight loss goal was statistically significant (Lindström et al. 2006).

U.S. Diabetes Prevention Program

The U.S. Diabetes Prevention Program was a randomized clinical trial of 3234 adults ages 25 to 85 years (mean age 51) from 27 medical centers across the United States; it cost over $174 million (Knowler et al. 2002). Forty-five percent of the participants were ethnic minorities. All had IGT as measured by an oral glucose tolerance test, and all were overweight, with a mean BMI of 34. They were randomly assigned for three years to one of three groups: (1) lifestyle change aiming to reduce weight by 7% through a low-fat diet and exercising 150 min per week, (2) treatment with the oral hypoglycemic (i.e., reduces blood sugar) drug metformin (850 mg twice a day) plus information on diet and exercise, or (3) a control group that took a placebo pill and also received information about diet and exercise. Figure 10.12 shows the results; after an average of three years, 29% of the placebo group had developed diabetes, while 22% of the metformin group (about a 30% risk reduction) and just 14% of the exercise and diet group (more than a 50% risk reduction) developed diabetes.

The relative risks depicted are based on crude incidence rates of 11, 7.8, and 4.8 cases per 100 person-years for the placebo, metformin, and the diet plus exercise groups, respectively. Diet and exercise led to an average weight loss of 15 lb (6.8 kg) in the first year of the study, or 7% of the group's initial average BMI; a 5% weight loss was maintained throughout the three years of the intervention. The lifestyle intervention was effective in men and women and all ethnic groups, including people 60 years old and older. The drug was effective, too, but not in older people or in those who were less overweight.

Weight loss was the dominant predictor of a reduced incidence of diabetes. However, nearly half the people in the lifestyle intervention failed to meet the weight loss goal in the first year. Those people still had nearly a 50% reduction in risk of diabetes if they had met the physical activity goal of at least 150 min each week of moderate activity (Hamman et al. 2006). After three years of treatment, the prevalence of the metabolic syndrome increased from 55% at baseline to 61% in the placebo group, did not change from 54% in the

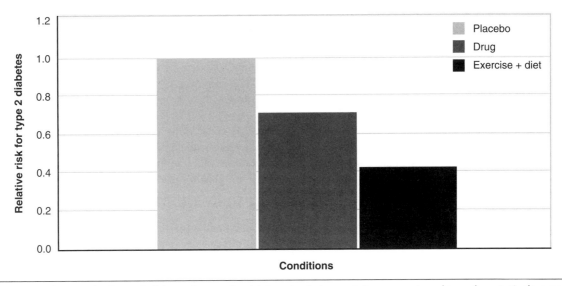

Figure 10.12 Relative risk of type 2 diabetes in people with impaired glucose tolerance assigned to a glucostatic drug or exercise and diet compared to a placebo group.

Data from Knowler et al. 2002.

metformin group, and decreased from 51% to 43% in the diet plus exercise group. The incidence of metabolic syndrome in the diet plus exercise condition was about 40% lower than in the placebo group and nearly 25% lower than in the group that received metformin (Orchard et al. 2005).

Enhanced Glycemic Control in People With Type 2 Diabetes

A meta-analysis of randomized and nonrandomized controlled trials included 12 studies of an aerobic training group that met on average 3.4 times a week for 18 weeks and two studies of a resistance training group that met 2.5 times per week for 15 weeks. HbA1c was lowered by 0.66% after exercise training compared to the controls, independently of changes in BMI (Boulé et al. 2001).

A subsequent meta-analysis of 14 randomized controlled trials that lasted eight weeks to 12 months compared exercise to no exercise in a total of 377 patients with type 2 diabetes. On average, exercise decreased HbA1c by 0.3% to 0.9% and improved insulin levels during a glucose tolerance test without affecting body mass (Thomas et al. 2006). In 13 randomized controlled trials of people with abnormal glucose regulation, resistance exercise training reduced HbA1c by 0.48% (95% CI: −0.76 to −0.21) and systolic blood pressure by 6.19 mmHg (95% CI: −1.00 to −11.38) (Strasser, Siebert, and Schobersberger 2010).

A meta-analysis of 23 randomized controlled trials including 8538 patients found that both aerobic and resistance exercise training accompanied declines in HbA1c levels of 0.7% and 0.6%, respectively, when compared with control patients (Umpierre et al. 2011). Those reductions were larger, nearly 0.9%, when patients spent 150 minutes or more exercising each week.

Look AHEAD Trial

The Look AHEAD (Action for HEAlth in Diabetes) study was a multicenter, randomized controlled trial of 5145 overweight adults (45-74 years old) with type 2 diabetes designed to compare a lifestyle intervention to achieve and maintain weight loss through diet and increased physical activity with a diabetes support and education condition (Look AHEAD Research Group 2007). After one year of the intervention, people in the weight loss group lost an average 8% of their weight and had reductions in diabetes, hypertension, and lipid-lowering medicines. Mean HbA1c dropped from 7.3% to 6.6%. Triglycerides and high-density lipoprotein cholesterol also improved.

DARE (Diabetes Aerobic and Resistance Exercise) Trial

A six-month randomized controlled trial conducted at eight community exercise facilities in Ottawa, Canada, assigned 251 inactive, middle-aged people with type 2 diabetes to supervised exercise sessions three times per week using either aerobic training (45 min/session at 75% maximum heart rate), resistance training (two or three sets at 7- to 9-repetitions maximum at seven stations), aerobic plus resistance training, or no exercise. Energy intake was controlled to approximate 90% of weight maintenance. Compared to no exercise, HbA1c levels were reduced by aerobic training (−0.51%) and resistance training (−0.38). Combined training led to bigger drops (−0.83%). Aerobic training but not resistance exercise reduced body weight and waist circumference more than no exercise. There was no effect of exercise on levels of triglyceride or high- or low-density lipoprotein cholesterol (Sigal et al. 2007). Because the combined group exercised twice as much as the aerobic or resistance training groups, it is not possible to know whether the additive effect of the combined exercises on reducing HbA1c is explainable by different features of aerobic and resistance modes or by the extra work that was done.

▷ **THE FIRST** randomized trial in youths with type 2 diabetes is ongoing. The Treatment Options for Type 2 Diabetes in Adolescents and Youth (TODAY) study will follow 800 youths ages 10 to 17 for two or more years, comparing the effects of metformin with those of metformin plus a weight loss intervention of diet and exercise (Today Study Group 2007, 2010).

Strength of the Evidence

Many population-based studies and a few large, well-controlled clinical studies show that moderate-to-vigorous physical activity is associated with lower risk of developing type 2 diabetes. That apparent protective effect is temporally correct, large, consistent across sexes and among ages and ethnic groups, dose-dependent, and biologically plausible.

Temporal Sequence

A substantial number of cross-sectional studies that lack the proper temporal sequence have been succeeded by a growing number of prospective cohort studies lasting four to 16 years and randomized controlled trials lasting from three months to six years. All these studies agree that physical activity reduces risk of type 2 diabetes and improves glucose control in people with IGT or type 2 diabetes. Combining physical activity with diet to achieve weight loss is more effective than the world's most widely prescribed glucostatic drug, metformin, in reducing incidence of type 2 diabetes in people with IGT. Physical activity reduced their risk even when they didn't meet their weight loss goals.

Strength of Association

A limited number of prospective cohort studies and randomized controlled trials consistently agree that regular, vigorous physical activity is associated with a 25% to 50% reduction in the risk of development of type 2 diabetes.

Averaged across 10 prospective cohort studies, including 301,221 participants, regular participation in moderate-to-vigorous physical activity reduced the risk of developing type 2 diabetes by 30% compared to that for people who were sedentary (Jeon et al. 2007). A larger number of nonrandomized and randomized controlled clinical trials show increases of about 10% on average (ranging from 5% to 50%) in glucose tolerance in people with IGT and a 0.5% to 1% reduction in glycosylated hemoglobin in people with type 2 diabetes.

Consistency

The cross-sectional, prospective cohort, and randomized clinical trials that examined physical activity and risk of type 2 diabetes included samples of men and women from several nations who represented diverse racial and ethnic groups (Jeon et al. 2007). There is good agreement that physical activity reduces the risk of type 2 diabetes in middle-aged and older men and women, including those who have IGT, regardless of initial fitness level, race, or ethnic background.

Dose Response

A review of prospective cohort studies and randomized controlled trials concluded that 30 min/day of moderate- or high-level physical activity is an effective and safe way to prevent type 2 diabetes in all the populations studied in nations in North America, Europe, and Asia (Hu et al. 2007). Risk reduction averaged for five prospective studies of regular walking (typically 2.5 h/week or more of brisk walking), compared with low levels of walking, was 30%, the same as for overall physical activity (Jeon et al. 2007).

There are not enough controlled clinical studies to permit a clear consensus about the amount or intensity of physical activity that improves glucose control among people with type 2 diabetes (Kelley and Goodpaster 2001). However, clinical exercise training studies suggest that increases in insulin sensitivity and reductions in HbA1c reliably occur after exercise at intensities of 60% to 80% of $\dot{V}O_2$max. In contrast, some studies have reported increased insulin sensitivity and decreased HbA1c levels after exercise training at low to moderate intensities of 50% to 60% $\dot{V}O_2$max (e.g., Trovati et al. 1984), but increases in maximal oxygen uptake after aerobic exercise performed near that intensity appear unrelated to changes in blood glucose and insulin levels measured at rest or after an oral glucose tolerance test (e.g., Wilmore et al. 2001). The normal HbA1c levels at the beginning of the Trovati study suggested that the participants had IGT but had not yet developed type 2 diabetes. Hence, different levels of disease (e.g., IGT or type 2 diabetes) could moderate the intensity or amount of physical activity required to induce a meaningful change in glucose control.

Nonetheless, a multicultural cross-sectional study of nearly 1500 men and women ages 40 to 69 of African American (29%), Hispanic (34%), and non-Hispanic white (38%) ethnicities found that insulin resistance measured by oral glucose tolerance test was inversely related to the usual weekly frequency of self-reported vigorous physical activity and to quintiles of weekly total energy expenditure estimated by a recall interview about physical activity during the past year (Mayer-Davis et al. 1998). Figure 10.13 shows that after adjustment for age, sex, ethnicity, dietary fat, alcohol intake, and smoking, insulin sensitivity among people who reported vigorous physical activity five or more times a week was significantly higher (1.59, 95% CI: 1.39-1.79) than that

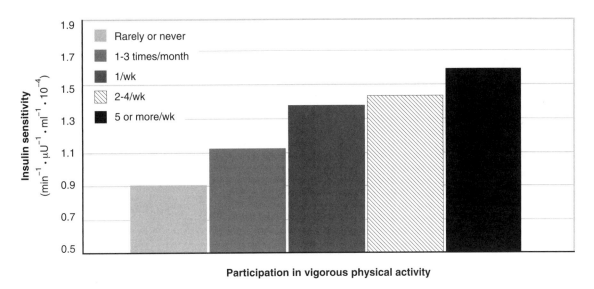

Figure 10.13 Insulin sensitivity according to frequency of self-reported participation in vigorous physical activity. Adjusted for ethnicity, clinic, age, sex, alcohol intake, smoking, dietary fat, and hypertension.

Data from Mayer-Davis et al. 1998.

of people who reported that they rarely or never participated in vigorous physical activity (0.90, 95% CI: 0.83-0.97). The effect of physical activity was reduced but not removed after adjustment for BMI.

Biological Plausibility

The hallmark features of type 2 diabetes are impaired insulin sensitivity and insufficient insulin secretion. The sequence of the pathophysiology of type 2 diabetes still is not fully understood, but five events are key: a decrease in insulin receptor number, impaired chemical signaling for insulin, impaired transport of glucose transporters to the cell membrane, impaired glucose transporter function, and impaired enzyme action. These features provide the framework for examining the biological plausibility that regular physical activity can prevent or normalize type 2 diabetes. Because high fat mass decreases insulin sensitivity, it is understandable that studies suggest that about half the effects of lowered risk of type 2 diabetes and improved insulin sensitivity can be explained by lowered fat mass among physically active people. However, physical activity also appears to exert an effect on insulin sensitivity and glucose control beyond its indirect effect of contributing to fat weight loss.

Among 1783 U.S. adolescents (11% Mexican American, 14% non-Hispanic black, 63% non-Hispanic white, and 12% other) aged 12 to 19 years who were examined in the 1999-2002 National Health and Nutrition Examination Survey, self-reported physical activity (MET-hours per week) and estimated aerobic fitness from treadmill testing were each positively related to insulin sensitivity in boys, but not girls

(Imperatore et al. 2006). Among girls, insulin sensitivity was inversely related to BMI.

Glucose Use During Exercise

Skeletal muscle is the main tissue that determines total-body glucose use, so it is plausible that changes in the metabolism of glucose after exercise training could alter the sensitivity of muscle cells to insulin. At the beginning of an exercise session, the energy for muscular contraction is provided by ATP. The body's natural response to compensate for ATP depletion is the recruitment of glycogen and triglycerides. The preferential recruitment of these two fuels depends on the intensity and duration of the exercise. During long sessions of low- to moderate-intensity exercise, the lipolysis of triglyceride is most important because more ATP can be derived from its oxidation than from the oxidation of glycogen. However, during high-intensity exercise, ATP can be generated faster from the metabolism of glycogen than of triglycerides. Thus, glycogen is the preferred fuel during high-intensity exercise.

Physiological evidence suggests that insulin efficiency is most likely to be increased during the metabolism of glycogen. Therefore, the preferred fuel metabolized during high-intensity exercise, glycogen, could provide a potential mechanism for increased insulin efficiency (Little et al. 2011).

Increased Insulin Sensitivity After Exercise

After an acute bout of exercise, insulin stimulation of glucose transport is greatly enhanced. This postexercise increase in insulin sensitivity does not seem to involve activation of the insulin signaling pathway, but it may be related to reduced

Skeletal Muscle Action and GLUT4

Muscle cell contraction recruits a pool of intracellular GLUT4 to the plasma membrane and an increase in glucose transport that does not involve the insulin signaling pathway. Muscle action may recruit GLUT4 by the following mechanisms:

INTRACELLULAR CALCIUM

Muscle contraction requires an influx of calcium into the cell (needed to permit cross-bridge formation of actin and myosin proteins). This extra intracellular calcium activates protein kinase C (PKC) and Ca^{2+}/ calmodulin-dependent protein kinases (CaMK), which may stimulate GLUT4.

AMPK

Muscle contraction alters the ratio of AMP to ATP, which stimulates AMP-activated protein kinase (AMPK), leading to an increase in glucose transport, through several possible mechanisms. AMPK can also lead to the phosphorylation of p38 MAPK (mitogen-activated protein kinase), which may be involved in the GLUT4 translocation response.

---

glycogen stores or increased AMPK activity after exercise (Wojtaszewski, Nielsen, and Richter 2002).

Insulin Resistance

Exercise benefits glucose control by aiding glucose transport for use as fuel during muscle contraction and by enhancing insulin sensitivity when people are not exercising.

Regular aerobic exercise increases glucose transporter 4 (GLUT4) protein levels and mitochondrial enzyme content, and alters fiber types in skeletal muscle that promote glucose transport and use (Röckl, Witczak, and Goodyear 2008). Muscle fiber types are classified as fast-twitch fibers (type IIb, IIx, and IIa) that fatigue quickly and slow-twitch fibers (type I) that are fatigue resistant. Type IIb and type IIx fibers produce ATP mainly from anaerobic glycolysis, and type IIa and type I fibers are mostly oxidative. Type I fibers have the most mitochondria, and type IIb fibers have the least. Aerobic exercise training increases mitochondria in each fiber type but also can transform type IIb to IIx and IIa fibers so that they are more oxidative. Regular exercise also increases GLUT4 protein, especially in slow oxidative fiber types. People who have insulin resistance or type 2 diabetes have fewer than normal slow oxidative muscle fibers and low GLUT4 levels in those fibers (Gaster et al. 2001; Nyholm et al. 1997).

Nearly 20 controlled clinical studies have indicated that exercise training improves glucose tolerance by increasing sensitivity to insulin. Improvements in insulin sensitivity, inferred from lowered blood glucose levels, have been observed 12 h after a single exercise session. However, blood glucose levels typically return to preexercise levels 48 to 72 h after exercise. Long-term improvements, averaging about 10%, are most consistently seen after high-intensity exercise training five or more days a week.

Though exercise may improve glucose use and insulin action in fat cells, most of its effects occur in skeletal muscle. The uptake of glucose by a cell requires the function of a glucose transporter. Normally, glucose transporters lie inside the cell membrane and can help with the uptake of glucose into the cell only if they are situated on the cell membrane.

There is evidence that glucose transport systems are altered in people with type 2 diabetes because of decreased movement of glucose transporters to the cell membrane. Muscle contraction has an insulin-like effect of promoting the transport of glucose from the blood through the muscle cell membrane (Holloszy and Hansen 1996).

Insulin increases the number of glucose transporters in plasma membranes. At least six glucose transporters have been discovered, two of which (GLUT1 and GLUT4) are found in skeletal muscle. Because glucose transporters, GLUT4 in particular, appear to be essential for insulin-mediated glucose transport in muscle, it appears plausible that an increase in the number or function of these transporters could help explain decreased insulin resistance after exercise training (Henriksen 2001). Recent evidence also suggests that reactive oxygen species and nitric oxide that are increased in contracting skeletal muscle act to increase glucose uptake in muscle in ways that are independent of other signaling pathways (Merry and McConell 2009).

Weight Loss

Regular physical activity also might prevent or retard the development of type 2 diabetes indirectly by helping to reduce body fat, including intra-abdominal fat, which is

Chronic Effects of Exercise on Diabetes

- Lowers circulating insulin
- Improves glucose tolerance
- Reduces insulin resistance
- Increases number of insulin receptors in skeletal muscle in people with type 2 diabetes
- Increases insulin-like effect of muscle contraction, increases GLUT4 transporter
- Increases insulin sensitivity in people with type 2 diabetes

Acute Effects of Exercise

- Increased hepatic glucose
- Increased glucose uptake in muscle
- Increased lipolysis of free fatty acids from adipose cells
- Decreased insulin secretion due to
  - increased epinephrine secretion from adrenal medulla,
  - increased glucagon (secreted by alpha cells of pancreas, it activates glycogenolysis in the liver and yields 75% of the glucose from the liver),
  - increased growth hormone, and
  - increased cortisol from the adrenal cortex.

associated with insulin resistance. About 80% of patients with type 2 diabetes are also obese, which contributes to the development of the disease. Although exercise may promote metabolic improvements in obese individuals, severe obesity can limit the types and intensities of physical activity that can be performed safely. However, lower-intensity physical activity, possibly insufficient to make big changes in glucose metabolism, may lead to weight loss and thus indirectly improve insulin resistance. For example, in the Look AHEAD trial of weight loss by diet (500 fewer kilocalories per day) and exercise ($\geq$175 min/week) in obese men and women with type 2 diabetes, overall body fat loss and fat loss in the liver contributed to lowering of fasting glucose and insulin sensitivity (Albu et al. 2010).

In CALERIE, a small randomized controlled trial of overweight men and women without diabetes, people lost the same amount of fat during six months through a 25% reduction in energy intake and a 12.5% reduction in energy intake combined with a 12.5% increase in energy expenditure via exercise (Larsen-Mayer et al. 2010). However, only diet plus exercise led to a significant improvement in insulin sensitivity (more than 50% better than after diet only).

Among 1079 participants in the lifestyle intervention arm of the Diabetes Prevention Program, weight loss was the main predictor of reduced diabetes incidence (Hamman et al. 2006). There was a 16% reduction in risk for every kilogram of weight loss, regardless of how much individuals changed their diet and physical activity. However, among 495 participants who did not meet the weight loss goal (7% reduction) after a year of intervention, those who had achieved the physical activity goal (at least 150 min of moderate intensity) had a 44% reduction in the incidence of diabetes.

On balance, most studies suggest that vigorous physical activity three or more times a week provides most of the independent benefits of glucose control. Additional benefits of improved insulin sensitivity with daily moderate physical activity can occur through fat weight loss.

Summary

Population-based studies and a few controlled clinical studies indicate that moderate physical activity is associated with a dose-dependent reduction in the risk of developing type 2 diabetes. That apparent protective effect is temporally correct, consistent across sexes and among ages and ethnic groups, and biologically plausible. The U.S. Diabetes Prevention Program, a multicultural randomized controlled trial of 3234 obese adults ages 25 to 85 years with IGT, confirmed that a three-year program combining 150 min per week of exercise and a low-fat diet led to a 5% weight loss and reduced the risk of developing diabetes by nearly 60% compared to placebo, which was superior to the approximately 30% reduction in risk after treatment with an oral hypoglycemic drug. It is not yet clear whether the effect of physical activity is wholly independent of BMI, fat loss, and diet. Though physical activity can indirectly help lower diabetes risk by contributing to weight loss, physical activity improves glucose tolerance and insulin sensitivity, and muscle contraction has an insulin-like effect on the transport of glucose from the blood. The effect of lowered glucose after acute exercise lasts about 48 h, so exercising every other day each week may be sufficient to help maintain normalized blood glucose levels. The University of Pennsylvania alumni study showed a dose-dependent reduction in risk for each additional 500 kcal of weekly leisure-time physical activity. Current recommendations call for people at risk or those who have type 2 diabetes to get at least 150 min of moderate-to-vigorous physical activity in their leisure time each week.

· BIBLIOGRAPHY ·

Albu, J.B., L.K. Heilbronn, D.E. Kelley, S.R. Smith, K. Azuma, E.S. Berk, F.X. Pi-Sunyer, E. Ravussin; Look AHEAD Adipose Research Group. 2010. Metabolic changes following a 1-year diet and exercise intervention in patients with type 2 diabetes. *Diabetes* 59: 627-633.

American College of Sports Medicine. 2000. Exercise and type 2 diabetes. *Medicine and Science in Sports and Exercise* 32: 1345-1360.

American College of Sports Medicine and the American Diabetes Association. 2010. Exercise and type 2 diabetes: Joint position statement. *Medicine and Science in Sports and Exercise* 42: 2282-2303.

American Diabetes Association. 1998. Economic consequences of diabetes mellitus in the U.S. in 1997. *Diabetes Care* 21: 296-309.

American Diabetes Association. 2008. Economic costs of diabetes in the U.S. in 2007. *Diabetes Care* 31: 596-615.

American Diabetes Association. 2012. Standards of medical care in diabetes—2012. *Diabetes Care* 35 (Suppl. 1): S11-S63.

Bailey, C.J., and R.C. Turner. 1996. Metformin. *New England Journal of Medicine* 334: 574-579.

Barnard, R.J., E.J. Ugianskis, D.A. Martin, and S.B. Inkeles. 1992. Role of diet and exercise in the management of hyperinsulinemia and associated atherosclerotic risk factors. *American Journal of Cardiology* 69: 440-444.

Barre, L., C. Richardson, M.F. Hirshman, J. Brozinick, S. Fiering, B.E. Kemp, L.J. Goodyear, and L.A. Witters. 2007. Genetic model for the chronic activation of skeletal muscle AMP-activated protein kinase leads to glycogen accumulation. *American Journal of Physiology: Endocrinology and Metabolism* 292: E802-E811.

Bliss, M. 1982. *The discovery of insulin.* Chicago: University of Chicago Press.

Boulé, N.G., E. Haddad, G.P. Kenny, G.A. Wells, and R.J. Sigal. 2001. Effects of exercise on glycemic control and body mass in type 2 diabetes mellitus: A meta-analysis of controlled clinical trials. *Journal of the American Medical Association* 286: 1218-1227.

Burstein, R., Y. Epstein, Y. Shapiro, I. Charuzi, and E. Karnieli. 1990. Effect of an acute bout of exercise on glucose disposal in human obesity. *Journal of Applied Physiology* 69 (1): 299-304.

Burstein, R., C. Polychronakos, C.J. Toews, H.J. MacDougall, and B.I. Posner. 1985. Acute reversal of the enhanced insulin action in trained athletes. *Diabetes* 34: 756-760.

Caro, J.F., O. Ittoop, W.J. Pories, D. Meelheim, E.G. Flickinger, F. Thomas, M. Jenquin, J.F. Silverman, P.G. Khazanie, and M.K. Sinha. 1986. Studies on the mechanism of insulin resistance in the liver from humans with noninsulin-dependent diabetes. Insulin action and binding in isolated hepatocytes, insulin receptor structure, and kinase activity. *Journal of Clinical Investigation* 78: 249-258.

Caro, J.F., M.K. Sinha, S.M. Raju, O. Ittoop, W.J. Pories, E.G. Flickinger, D. Meelheim, and G.L. Dohm. 1987. Insulin receptor kinase in human skeletal muscle from obese subjects with and without noninsulin dependent diabetes. *Journal of Clinical Investigation* 79: 1330-1337.

Caro, J.J., A.J. Ward, and J.A. O'Brien. 2002. Lifetime costs of complications resulting from type 2 diabetes in the U.S. *Diabetes Care* 25: 476-481.

Cartee, G.D., and J.F. Wojtaszewski. 2007. Role of Akt substrate of 160 kDa in insulin-stimulated and contraction-stimulated glucose transport. *Applied Physiology, Nutrition and Metabolism* 32: 557-566.

Castaneda, C., J.E. Layne, L. Munoz-Orians, P.L. Gordon, J. Walsmith, M. Foldvari, R. Roubenoff, K.L. Tucker, and M.E. Nelson. 2002. A randomized controlled trial of resistance exercise training to improve glycemic control in older adults with type 2 diabetes. *Diabetes Care* 25: 2335-2341.

Centers for Disease Control and Prevention. 2002. *National diabetes fact sheet: General information and national estimates on diabetes in the United States, 2000.* Atlanta: U.S. Department of Health and Human Services, Centers for Disease Control and Prevention.

Centers for Disease Control and Prevention. 2003. Deaths: Preliminary data for 2001. *National Vital Statistics Reports* 51 (5): 1-48.

Centers for Disease Control and Prevention. 2008. *National diabetes fact sheet: General information and national estimates on diabetes in the United States, 2007.* Atlanta: U.S. Department of Health and Human Services, Centers for Disease Control and Prevention.

Centers for Disease Control and Prevention. 2011. National diabetes fact sheet: National estimates and general information on diabetes and prediabetes in the United States, 2011. Atlanta, GA: U.S. Department of Health and Human Services, Centers for Disease Control and Prevention.

Crandall, J.P., et al. 2008. The prevention of type 2 diabetes. *Nature Clinical Practice Endocrinology and Metabolism* 4: 382-393.

Dempsey, J.C., C.L. Butler, and M.A. Williams. 2005. No need for a pregnant pause: Physical activity may reduce the occurrence of gestational diabetes mellitus and preeclampsia. *Exercise and Sport Sciences Reviews* 33: 141-149.

Devlin, J.T., M. Hirshman, E.D. Horton, and E.S. Horton. 1987. Enhanced peripheral and splanchnic insulin sensitivity in NIDDM men after single bout of exercise. *Diabetes* 36: 444-449.

Douen, A.G., T. Ramlal, S. Rastogi, P.J. Bilan, G.D. Cartee, M. Vranic, J.O. Holloszy, and A. Klip. 1990. Exercise induces recruitment of the insulin-responsive glucose transporter. *Journal of Biological Chemistry* 265 (23): 13427-13430.

Durak, E.P., L. Jovanovic-Peterson, and C.M. Peterson. 1990. Randomized crossover study of effect of resistance training on glycemic control, muscular strength, and cholesterol in type I diabetic men. *Diabetes Care* 13: 1039-1043.

Dwivedi, G., and S. Dwivedi. 2007. Sushruta – the clinician-teacher par excellence. *Indian Journal of Chest Diseases and Allied Sciences* 49: 243-244.

Eriksson, K.F., and F. Lindgarde. 1991. Prevention of type 2 (non-insulin-dependent) diabetes mellitus by diet and physical exercise: The 6-year Malmo feasibility study. *Diabetologia* 34: 891-898.

Eriksson, K.F., and F. Lindgarde. 1996. Poor physical fitness, and impaired early insulin response but late hyperinsulinaemia, as predictors of NIDDM in middle-aged Swedish men. *Diabetologia* 39: 573-579.

Eriksson, J., J. Lindstrom, T. Valle, S. Aunola, H. Hamalainen, P. Ilanne-Parikka, S. Keinanen-Kiukaanniemi, M. Laakso, M. Lauhkonen, P. Lehto, A. Lehtonen, A. Louheranta, M. Mannelin, V. Martikkala, M. Rastas, J. Sundvall, A. Turpeinen, T. Viljanen, M. Uusitupa, and J. Tuomilehto. 1999. Prevention of type II diabetes in subjects with impaired glucose tolerance: The Diabetes Prevention Study (DPS) in Finland. Study design and 1-year interim report on the feasibility of the lifestyle intervention programme. *Diabetologia* 42: 793-801.

Feinstein, R., P. Kanety, M.Z. Papa, B. Lunenfeld, and A. Karasik. 1993. Tumor necrosis factor-alpha suppresses insulin-induced tyrosine phosphorylation of insulin receptor and its substrates *Journal of Biological Chemistry* 268: 26055-26058.

Fogelholm, M. 2010. Physical activity, fitness and fatness: Relations to mortality, morbidity and disease risk factors. A systematic review. *Obesity Reviews* 11 (3): 202-221.

Foretz, M., S. Hébrard, J. Leclerc, E. Zarrinpashneh, M. Soty, G. Mithieux, K. Sakamoto, F. Andreeli, and B. Viollet. 2010. Metformin inhibits hepatic gluconeogenesis in mice independently of the LKB1/AMPK pathway via a decrease in hepatic energy state. *Journal of Clinical Investigation* 120 (7): 2355-2369. doi: 10.1172/JCI40671. [Epub ahead of print]

Fossum, E., G.W. Gleim, S.E. Kjeldsen, J.R. Kizer, S. Julius, R.B. Devereux, W.E. Brady, D.A. Hille, P.A. Lyle, and B. Dahlöf. 2007. The effect of baseline physical activity on cardiovascular outcomes and new-onset diabetes in patients treated for hypertension and left ventricular hypertrophy: The LIFE study. *Journal of Internal Medicine* 262 (4, October): 439-448.

Gaster, M., P. Staehr, H. Beck-Nielsen, B.D. Schroder, and A. Handberg. 2001. Glut4 is reduced in slow muscle fibers of type 2 diabetic patients: Is insulin resistance in type 2 diabetes a slow, type 1 fiber disease? *Diabetes* 50: 1324-1329.

Gibala, M.J., S.L. McGee, A.P. Garnham, K.E. Howlett, R.J. Snow, and M. Hargreaves. 2009. Brief intense interval exercise activates AMPK and p38 MAPK signaling and increases the expression of PGC-1alpha in human skeletal muscle. *Journal of Applied Physiology* 106: 929-934.

Goodyear, L.J., F. Giorgino, L.A. Sherman, J. Carey, R.J. Smith, and G.L. Dohm. 1995. Insulin receptor phosphorylation, insulin receptor substrate-1 phosphorylation, and phosphatidylinositol 3-kinase activity are decreased in intact skeletal muscle strips from obese subjects. *Journal of Clinical Investigation* 95: 2195-2204.

Goodyear, L.J., and B.B. Kahn. 1998. Exercise, glucose transport, and insulin sensitivity. *Annual Reviews in Medicine* 49: 235-261.

Gordon, B.L. 1960. *Medieval and Renaissance medicine.* New York: Philosophical Library.

Gregg, E.W., R.B. Gerzoff, C.J. Caspersen, D.F. Williamson, and K.M. Narayan. 2003. Relationship of walking to mortality among US adults with diabetes. *Archives of Internal Medicine* 163: 1440-1447.

Gudat, U., M. Berger, and P.J. Lefebvre. 1993. Physical activity, fitness, and non-insulin-dependent (type II) diabetes mellitus. In *Exercise, fitness, and health,* 2nd edition, edited by C. Bouchard, R.J. Shephard, T. Stephens, J.R. Sutton, and B.D. McPherson. Champaign, IL: Human Kinetics.

Hamman, R.F., R.R. Wing, S.L. Edelstein, J.M. Lachin, G.A. Bray, J. Delahanty, M. Hoskin, A.M. Kriska, E.J. Mayer-Davis, X. Pi-Sunyer, J. Regensteiner, B. Venditti, and J. Wylie-Rosett. 2006. Effect of weight loss with lifestyle intervention on risk of diabetes. *Diabetes Care* 29 (9): 2102-2107.

Harley, G. 1866. *Diabetes: Its various forms and different treatments.* London: Walton and Mabberley.

Harris, M.I., W.C. Hadden, W.C. Knowler, and P.H. Bennett. 1987. Prevalence of diabetes and impaired glucose tolerance and plasma glucose levels in US population aged 20 to 74 years. *Diabetes* 36: 523-534.

Hawley, J.A., and S.J. Lessard. 2008. Exercise training-induced improvements in insulin action. *Acta Physiologica (Oxford)* 192: 127-135.

Heath, G.W., J.R. Gavin III, J.M. Hinderliter, J.M. Hagberg, S.A. Bloomfield, and J.O. Holloszy. 1983. Effects of exercise and lack of exercise on glucose tolerance and insulin sensitivity. *Journal of Applied Physiology* 55 (2): 512-517.

Heath, G.W., R.H. Wilson, J. Smith, and B.E. Leonard. 1991. Community-based exercise and weight control: Diabetes risk reduction and glycemic control in Zuni Indians. *American Journal of Clinical Nutrition* 53 (6 Suppl.): 1642S-1646S.

Helmrich, S.P., D.R. Ragland, R.W. Leung, and R.S. Paffenbarger. 1991. Physical activity and reduced occurrence of noninsulin-dependent diabetes mellitus. *New England Journal of Medicine* 325: 147-152.

Henriksen, E.J. 2001. Invited review: Effects of acute exercise and exercise training on insulin resistance. *Journal of Applied Physiology* 93: 788-796.

Hevener, A.L., M.A. Febbraio; the Stock Conference Working Group. 2010. The 2009 Stock Conference report: Inflammation, obesity and metabolic disease. *Obesity Review.* [Epub ahead of print]

Hollander, P.A., and J. Nordstrom. 1991. Exercise and diabetes: Great for type II, good for type I. *Your Patient and Fitness* 5 (3): 6-13.

Holloszy, J.O., and P.A. Hansen. 1996. Regulation of glucose transport into skeletal muscle. *Reviews of Physiology, Biochemistry, and Pharmacology* 128: 99-193.

Holmes, B.E., E.J. Kurth-Kraczek, and W.W. Winder. 1999. Chronic activation of 5'-AMP-activated protein kinase increases GLUT4, hexokinase, and glycogen in muscle. *Journal of Applied Physiology* 87: 1990-1995.

Home, P.D., S.J. Pocock, H. Beck-Nielsen, et al.; RECORD Study Team. 2009. Rosiglitazone evaluated for cardiovascular outcomes in oral agent combination therapy for type 2 diabetes (RECORD): A multicentre, randomised, open-label trial. *Lancet* 373 (9681): 2125-2135.

Hotamisligil, G.S. 2006. Inflammation and metabolic disorders. *Nature* 444: 860-867.

Hotamisligil, G.S., N.S. Shargill, and B.M. Spiegelman. 1993. Adipose expression of tumor necrosis factor-alpha: Direct role in obesity-linked insulin resistance. *Science* 259: 87-91.

Hsia, J., L. Wu, C. Allen, A. Oberman, W.E. Lawson, J. Torrens, M. Safford, M.C. Limacher, and B.V. Howard. 2005. Physical activity and diabetes risk in postmenopausal women. *American Journal of Preventive Medicine* 28 (1): 19-25.

Hu, F.B., R.J. Sigal, J.W. Rich-Edwards, G.A. Colditz, C.G. Solomon, W.C. Willett, F.E. Speizer, and J.E. Manson. 1999. Walking compared with vigorous physical activity and risk of type 2 diabetes in women: A prospective study. *Journal of the American Medical Association* 282 (15): 1433-1439.

Hu, G., T.A. Lakka, T.O. Kilpeläinen, and J. Tuomilehto. 2007. Epidemiological studies of exercise in diabetes prevention. *Applied Physiology, Nutrition, and Metabolism* 32: 583-595.

Hu, G., J. Lindström, T.T. Valle, J.G. Eriksson, P. Jousilahti, K. Silventoinen, Q. Qiao, and J. Tuomilehto. 2004. Physical activity, body mass index, and risk of type 2 diabetes in patients with normal or impaired glucose regulation. *Archives of Internal Medicine* 164 (8): 892-896.

Imperatore, G., Y.J. Cheng, D.E. Williams, J.E. Fulton, and E.W. Gregg. 2006. Physical activity, cardiovascular fitness, and insulin sensitivity among U.S. adolescents: The National Health and Nutrition Examination Survey, 1999-2002. *Diabetes Care* 29 (7): 1567-1572.

International Diabetes Federation. 2011. *The IDF diabetes atlas, fifth edition.* Brussels: International Diabetes Federation.

Jeon, C.Y., R.P. Lokken, F.B. Hu, and R.M. van Dam. 2007. Physical activity of moderate intensity and risk of type 2 diabetes: A systematic review. *Diabetes Care* 30 (3): 744-752.

Kawate, R., M. Yamakido, Y. Nishimoto, P.H. Bennett, R.F. Garnman, and W.C. Knowler. 1979. Diabetes and its vascular complications in Japanese migrants on the island of Hawaii. *Diabetes Care* 2: 161-170.

Kelley, D.E., and B.H. Goodpaster. 2001. Effects of exercise on glucose homeostasis in type 2 diabetes mellitus. *Medicine and Science in Sports and Exercise* 33 (Suppl. 6): S495-S501.

Kelly, M., M.S. Gauthier, A.K. Saha, and N.B. Ruderman. 2009. Activation of AMP-activated protein kinase by interleukin-6 in rat skeletal muscle: Association with changes in cAMP, energy state, and endogenous fuel mobilization. *Diabetes* 58: 1953-1960.

King, H., and A.M. Kriska. 1992. Prevention of type II diabetes by physical training: Epidemiological considerations and study methods. *Diabetes Care* 15: 1794-1799.

King, H., R. Taylor, P. Zimmet, K. Pargeter, L.R. Raper, T. Beriki, and J. Tekanene. 1984. Non-insulin-dependent diabetes (NIDDM) in a newly independent Pacific nation: The Republic of Kiribati. *Diabetes Care* 7: 409-415.

Knowler, W.C., E. Barrett-Connor, S.E. Fowler, R.F. Hamman, J.M. Lachin, E.A. Walker, and D. Nathan. 2002. Reduction in the incidence of type 2 diabetes with lifestyle intervention or metformin. *New England Journal of Medicine* 346 (6): 393-403.

Kohl, H.W., N.F. Gordon, J.A. Villegas, and S.N. Blair. 1992. Cardiorespiratory fitness, glycemic status, and mortality risk in men. *Diabetes Care* 15 (2): 184-192.

Kolaczynski, J.W., and J.F. Caro. 1998. Insulin resistance: Site of the primary defect or how the current and the emerging therapies work. *Journal of Basic and Clinical Physiology and Pharmacology* 9: 281-294.

Komajda, M., J.J. McMurray, H. Beck-Nielsen, R. Gomis, M. Hanefeld, S.J. Pocock, P.S. Curtis, N.P. Jones, and P.D. Home. 2010. Heart failure events with rosiglitazone in type 2 diabetes: Data from the RECORD clinical trial. *European Heart Journal* 31: 824-831.

Kramer, H.F., and L.J. Goodyear. 2007. Exercise, MAPK, and NF-kappaB signaling in skeletal muscle. *Journal of Applied Physiology* 103: 388-395.

Kramer, H.F., E.B. Taylor, C.A. Witczak, N. Fujii, M.F. Hirshman, and L.J. Goodyear. 2007. The calmodulin-binding domain of AS160 regulates contraction- but not insulin-stimulated glucose uptake in skeletal muscle. *Diabetes* 56: 2854-2862.

Kramer, H.F., C.A. Witczak, N. Fujii, N. Jessen, E.B. Taylor, D.E. Arnolds, K. Sakamoto, M.F. Hirshman, and L.J. Goodyear. 2006. Distinct signals regulate AS160 phosphorylation in response to insulin, AICAR, and contraction in mouse skeletal muscle. *Diabetes* 55: 2067-2076.

Kriska, A. 1997. Physical activity and the prevention of type II (non-insulin-dependent) diabetes. *President's Council on Physical Fitness and Sports Research Digest* 2 (10): 1-7.

Kriska, A.M., S.N. Blair, and M.A. Pereira. 1994. The potential role of physical activity in the prevention of non-insulin-dependent diabetes mellitus: The epidemiological evidence. *Exercise and Sport Sciences Reviews* 22: 121-143.

Kriska, A.M., R.E. LaPorte, S.L. Patrick, L.H. Kuller, and T.J. Orchard. 1991. The association of physical activity and diabetic complications in individuals with insulin-dependent diabetes mellitus: The Epidemiology of Diabetes Complications Study VII. *Journal of Clinical Epidemiology* 44: 1207-1214.

Kriska, A.M., R.E. LaPorte, D.J. Pettitt, M.A. Charles, R.G. Nelson, L.H. Kuller, P.H. Bennett, and W.C. Knowler. 1993. The association of physical activity with obesity, fat distribution and glucose intolerance in Pima Indians. *Diabetologia* 36: 863-869.

Krook, A., R.A. Roth, X.J. Jiang, J.R. Zierath, and H. Wallberg-Henriksson. 1998. Insulin-stimulated Akt kinase activity is reduced in skeletal muscle from NIDDM subjects. *Diabetes* 47: 1281-1286.

Laaksonen, D.E., J. Lindström, T.A. Lakka, J.G. Eriksson, L. Niskanen, K. Wikström, S. Aunola, S. Keinänen-Kiukaanniemi, M. Laakso, T.T. Valle, P. Ilanne-Parikka, A. Louheranta, H. Hämäläinen, M. Rastas, V. Salminen, Z. Cepaitis, M. Hakumäki, H. Kaikkonen, P. Härkönen, J. Sundvall, J. Tuomilehto, M. Uusitupa; Finnish diabetes prevention study. 2005. Physical activity in the prevention of type 2 diabetes: The Finnish diabetes prevention study. *Diabetes* 54 (1): 158-165.

Lancereaux, E. 1880. Le diabete maigre: Ses symptomes, son evolution, son prognostie et son traitement. *Un Med Paris* 20: 205-211.

Larson-Meyer, D.E., L. Redman, L.K. Heilbronn, C.K. Martin, and E. Ravussin. 2010. Caloric restriction with or without exercise: The fitness versus fatness debate. *Medicine and Science in Sports and Exercise* 42 (1): 152-159.

Lee, D.C., X. Sui, T.S. Church, I.M. Lee, and S.N. Blair. 2009. Associations of cardiorespiratory fitness and obesity with risks of impaired fasting glucose and type 2 diabetes in men. *Diabetes Care* 32 (2): 257-262.

Li, G., P. Zhang, J. Wang, E.W. Gregg, W. Yang, Q. Gong, H. Li, H. Li, Y. Jiang, Y. An, Y. Shuai, B. Zhang, J. Zhang, T.J. Thompson, R.B. Gerzoff, G. Roglic, Y. Hu, and P.H. Bennett. 2008. The long-term effect of lifestyle interventions to prevent diabetes in the China Da Qing Diabetes Prevention Study: A 20-year follow-up study. *Lancet* 371: 1783-1789.

Lincoff, A.M., K. Wolski, S.J. Nicholls, and S.E. Nissen. 2007. Pioglitazone and risk of cardiovascular events in patients with type 2 diabetes mellitus: A meta-analysis of randomized trials. *Journal of the American Medical Association* 298 (10): 1180-1188.

Lindström, J., P. Ilanne-Parikka, M. Peltonen, S. Aunola, J.G. Eriksson, K. Hemiö, H. Hämäläinen, P. Härkönen, S. Keinänen-Kiukaanniemi, M. Laakso, A. Louheranta, M. Mannelin, M. Paturi, J. Sundvall, T.T. Valle, M. Uusitupa, J. Tuomilehto; Finnish Diabetes Prevention Study Group. 2006. Sustained reduction in the incidence of type 2 diabetes by lifestyle intervention: Follow-up of the Finnish Diabetes Prevention Study. *Lancet* 368 (9548): 1673-1679.

Lindström J., A. Louheranta, M. Mannelin, M. Rastas, V. Salminen, J. Eriksson, M. Uusitupa, J. Tuomilehto; Finnish Diabetes Prevention Study Group. 2003. The Finnish Diabetes Prevention Study (DPS): Lifestyle intervention and 3-year results on diet and physical activity. *Diabetes Care* 26: 3230-3236.

Lindström, J., M. Peltonen, J.G. Eriksson, S. Aunola, H. Hämäläinen, P. Ilanne-Parikka, S. Keinänen-Kiukaanniemi, M. Uusitupa, J. Tuomilehto; Finnish Diabetes Prevention Study (DPS) Group. 2008. Determinants for the effectiveness of lifestyle intervention in the Finnish Diabetes Prevention Study. *Diabetes Care* 31 (5): 857-862.

Little, J.P., J.B. Gillen, M.E. Percival, A. Safadar, M.A. Tarnopolsky, Z. Punthakee, M.E. Jung, M.J. Gibala. 2011. Low-volume high-intensity interval training reduces hyperglycemia and increases muscle mitochondrial capacity in patients with type 2 diabetes. *Journal of Applied Physiology* 111 (6): 1554-1560.

Look AHEAD Research Group, X. Pi-Sunyer, G. Blackburn, F.L. Brancati, G.A. Bray, R. Bright, J.M. Clark, J.M. Curtis, M.A. Espeland, J.P. Foreyt, K. Graves, S.M. Haffner, B. Harrison, J.O. Hill, E.S. Horton, J. Jakicic, R.W. Jeffery, K.C. Johnson, S. Kahn, D.E. Kelley, A.E. Kitabchi, W.C. Knowler, C.E. Lewis, B.J. Maschak-Carey, B. Montgomery, D.M. Nathan, J. Patricio, A. Peters, J.B. Redmon, R.S. Reeves, D.H. Ryan, M. Safford, B. Van Dorsten, T.A. Wadden, L. Wagenknecht, J. Wesche-Thobaben, R.R. Wing, and S.Z. Yanovski. 2007. Reduction in weight and cardiovascular disease risk factors in individuals with type 2 diabetes: One-year results of the look AHEAD trial. *Diabetes Care* 30: 1374-1383.

Luft, R. 1989. Oskar Minkowski: Discovery of the pancreatic origin of diabetes, 1889. *Diabetologia* 32 (7): 399-401.

Manson, J.E., D.M. Nathan, A.S. Krolewski, M.J. Stampfer, W.C. Willett, and C.H. Hennekens. 1992. A prospective study of exercise and incidence of diabetes among US male physicians. *Journal of the American Medical Association* 268: 63-67.

Manson, J.E., E.B. Rimm, M.J. Stampfer, G.A. Colditz, W.C. Willett, A.S. Krolewski, B. Rosner, C.H. Hennekens, and F.E. Speizer. 1991. Physical activity and incidence of noninsulin-dependent diabetes mellitus in women. *Lancet* 338: 774-778.

Manson, J.E., and A. Spelsberg. 1994. Primary prevention of non-insulin-dependent diabetes mellitus. *American Journal of Preventive Medicine* 10 (3): 172-184.

Mayer-Davis, E.J., R. D'Agostino, A.J. Karter, S.M. Haffner, M.J. Rewers, M. Saad, and R.N. Bergman. 1998. Intensity and amount of physical activity in relation to insulin sensitivity: The Insulin Resistance Atherosclerosis Study. *Journal of the American Medical Association* 279: 669-674.

McBride, A., and D.G. Hardie. 2009. AMP-activated protein kinase—a sensor of glycogen as well as AMP and ATP? *Acta Physiologica (Oxford)* 196: 99-113.

McConell, G.K., R.S. Lee-Young, Z.P. Chen, N.K. Stepto, N.N. Huynh, T.J. Stephens, B.J. Canny, and B.E. Kemp. 2005. Short-term exercise training in humans reduces AMPK signalling during prolonged exercise independent of muscle glycogen. *Journal of Physiology* 568 (Pt 2): 665-676.

McGee, S.L., and M. Hargreaves. 2006. Exercise and skeletal muscle glucose transporter 4 expression: Molecular mechanisms. *Clinical and Experimental Pharmacology and Physiology* 33: 395-399.

McGee, S.L., and M. Hargreaves. 2010. AMPK-mediated regulation of transcription in skeletal muscle. *Clinical Science (Lond)* 118: 507-518.

McGee, S.L., K.F. Howlett, R.L. Starkie, D. Cameron-Smith, B.E. Kemp, and M. Hargreaves. 2003. Exercise increases nuclear AMPK alpha2 in human skeletal muscle. *Diabetes* 52: 926-928.

Merry, T.L., and G.K. McConell. 2009. Skeletal muscle glucose uptake during exercise: A focus on reactive oxygen species and nitric oxide signaling. *IUBMB Life* 61: 479-484.

Miller, R.A., and M.J. Birnbaum. 2010. An energetic tale of AMPK-independent effects of metformin. *Journal of Clinical Investigation* 120 (7): 2267-2270. doi: 10.1172/JCI43661.

Mokdad, A.H., E.S. Ford, B.A. Bowman, W.H. Dietz, F. Vinicor, V.S. Bales, and J.S. Marks. 2003. Prevalence of obesity, diabetes, and obesity-related health risk factors, 2001. *Journal of the American Medical Association* 289: 76-79.

Mokdad, A.H., E.S. Ford, B.A. Bowman, D.E. Nelson, M.M. Engelgau, F. Vinicor, and J.S. Marks. 2001. The continuing increase of diabetes in the US. *Diabetes Care* 24: 412.

Morgan, W. 1877. *Diabetes mellitus: Its history, chemistry, anatomy, pathology, physiology, and treatment,* 1st edition, pp. 1-184. London: Homeopathic Publishing Company.

Moy, C.S., T.J. Songer, R.E. LaPorte, J.S. Dorman, A.M. Kriska, T.J. Orchard, D.J. Becker, and A.L. Drash. 1993. Insulin-dependent diabetes mellitus, physical activity, and death. *American Journal of Epidemiology* 137: 74-81.

Musi, N., and L.J. Goodyear. 2006. Insulin resistance and improvements in signal transduction. *Endocrine* 29: 73-80.

Narayan, K.M., J.P. Boyle, L.S. Geiss, J.B. Saaddine, and T.J. Thompson. 2006. Impact of recent increase in incidence on future diabetes burden: U.S., 2005–2050. *Diabetes Care* 29 (9): 2114-2116.

National Institute of Diabetes and Digestive and Kidney Diseases. 2008. *National diabetes statistics, 2007 fact sheet.* Bethesda, MD: U.S. Department of Health and Human Services, National Institutes of Health.

Nissen, S.E., and K. Wolski. 2007. Effect of rosiglitazone on the risk of myocardial infarction and death from cardiovascular causes [published correction appears in *New England Journal of Medicine,* 2007, 357 (1): 100]. *New England Journal of Medicine* 356: 2457-2471.

Nissen, S.E., and K. Wolski. 2010. Rosiglitazone revisited: An updated meta-analysis of risk for myocardial infarction and cardiovascular mortality. *Archives of Internal Medicine,* June. doi:10.1001/archinternmed.2010.207.

Nyholm, B., Z. Qu, A. Kaal, S.B. Pedersen, C.H. Gravholt, J.L. Andersen, B. Saltin, and O. Schmitz. 1997. Evidence of an increased number of type IIb muscle fibers in insulin-resistant first-degree relatives of patients with NIDDM. *Diabetes* 46: 1822-1828.

Olefsky, J.M., O.G. Kolterman, and J.A. Scarlett. 1982. Insulin action and resistance in obesity and noninsulin-dependent type II diabetes mellitus. *American Journal of Physiology: Endocrinology and Metabolism* 6: E15-E30.

Opie, E.L. 1900. On the histology of the islands of Langerhans of the pancreas. *Bulletin of the Johns Hopkins Hospital* 11: 205-209.

Orchard, T.J., M. Temprosa, R. Goldberg, S. Haffner, R. Ratner, S. Marcovina, S. Fowler; Diabetes Prevention Program Research Group. 2005. The effect of metformin and intensive lifestyle intervention on the metabolic syndrome: The Diabetes Prevention Program randomized trial. *Annals of Internal Medicine* 142: 611-619.

Pan, X.R., G.W. Li, Y.H. Hu, J.X. Wang, W.Y. Yang, Z.X. An, Z.X. Hu, J. Lin, J.Z. Xiao, H.B. Cao, et al. 1997. Effects of diet and exercise in preventing NIDDM in people with impaired glucose tolerance: The Da Qing IGT and Diabetes Study. *Diabetes Care* 20 (4): 537-544.

Paternostro-Bayles, M., R.R. Wing, and R.J. Robertson. 1989. Effect of lifestyle activity of varying duration on glycemic control in type II diabetic women. *Diabetes Care* 12: 34-37.

Pedersen, O., J.F. Bak, P.H. Andersen, S. Lund, D.E. Moller, J.S. Flier, and B.B. Kahn. 1990. Evidence against altered expression of GLUT1 or GLUT4 in skeletal muscle of patients with obesity or NIDDM. *Diabetes* 39: 865-870.

Pereira, M.A., A.M. Kriska, M.L. Joswiak, G.K. Dowse, V.R. Collins, P.Z. Zimmet, H. Gareeboo, P. Chitson, F. Hemraj, A. Purran, et al. 1995. Physical inactivity and glucose intolerance in the multiethnic island of Mauritius. *Medicine and Science in Sports and Exercise* 27 (12): 1626-1634.

Physical Activity Guidelines Advisory Committee. 2008. *Physical Activity Guidelines Advisory Committee report,* pp. 1-683. Washington, DC: U.S. Department of Health and Human Services.

Pincus, G., E.P. Joslin, and P. White. 1934. Age-incidence relations in diabetes mellitus. *American Journal of Medical Science* 188: 116-121.

Qin, L., M.J. Knol, E. Corpeleijn, and R.P. Stolk. 2010. Does physical activity modify the risk of obesity for type 2 diabetes: A review of epidemiological data. *European Journal of Epidemiology* 25 (1): 5-12.

Rana, J.S., T.Y. Li, J.E. Manson, et al. 2007. Adiposity compared with physical inactivity and risk of type 2 diabetes in women. *Diabetes Care* 30 (1): 53-58.

Reitman, J.S., B. Vasquez, I. Klimes, and M. Nagulesparan. 1984. Improvement of glucose homeostasis after exercise training in noninsulin-dependent diabetes. *Diabetes Care* 7: 434-441.

Richter, E.A., L. Turcotte, P. Hespel, and B. Kiens. 1992. Metabolic responses to exercise. *Diabetes Care* 15 (Suppl. 4): 1767-1776.

Röckl, K.S.C., M.F. Hirshman, J. Brandauer, N. Fujii, L.A. Witters, and L.J. Goodyear. 2007. Skeletal muscle adaptation to exercise training: AMP-activated protein kinase mediates muscle fiber type shift. *Diabetes* 56: 2062-2069.

Röckl, K.S., C.A. Witczak, and L.J. Goodyear. 2008. Signaling mechanisms in skeletal muscle: Acute responses and chronic adaptations to exercise. *IUBMB Life* 60: 145-153.

Rogers, M.A., C. Yamamoto, D.S. King, J.M. Hagberg, A.A. Ehsani, and J.O. Holloszy. 1988. Improvement in glucose tolerance after one week of exercise in patients with mild NIDDM. *Diabetes Care* 11 (8): 613-618.

Rotella, C.M., M. Monami, and E. Mannucci. 2006. Metformin beyond diabetes: New life for an old drug. *Current Diabetes Reviews* 2 (3): 307-315.

Ruderman, N.B., C. Keller, A.M. Richard, A.K. Saha, Z. Luo, X. Xiang, M. Giralt, V.B. Ritov, E.V. Menshikova, D.E. Kelley, J. Hidalgo, B.K. Pedersen, and M. Kelly. 2006. Interleukin-6 regulation of AMP-activated protein kinase. Potential role in the systemic response to exercise and prevention of the metabolic syndrome. *Diabetes* 55 (Suppl. 2): S48-S54.

Ruderman, N., and M. Prentki. 2004. AMP kinase and malonyl-CoA: Targets for therapy of the metabolic syndrome. *National Review of Drug Discovery* 3: 340-351.

Salpeter, S.R., N.S. Buckley, J.A. Kahn, and E.E. Salpeter. 2008. Meta-analysis: Metformin treatment in persons at risk for diabetes mellitus. *American Journal of Medicine* 121: 149-157.

Schneider, S.H., L.F. Amorosa, A.K. Khachadurian, and N.B. Ruderman. 1984. Studies on the mechanism of improved glucose control during regular exercise in type 2 (noninsulin-dependent) diabetes. *Diabetologia* 26: 355-360.

Schneider, S.H., A.K. Khachadurian, L.F. Amorosa, L. Clemow, and N.B. Ruderman. 1992. Ten-year experience with an exercise-based outpatient life-style modification program in the treatment of diabetes mellitus. *Diabetes Care* 15 (4): 1800-1810.

Schulz, L.O., P.H. Bennett, E. Ravussin, J.R. Kidd, K.K. Kidd, J. Esparza, and M.E. Valencia. 2006. Effects of traditional and western environments on prevalence of type 2 diabetes in Pima Indians in Mexico and the U.S. *Diabetes Care* 29 (8): 1866-1871.

SEARCH for Diabetes in Youth Study Group, A.D. Liese, R.B. D'Agostino Jr., R.F. Hamman, P.D. Kilgo, J.M. Lawrence, L.L. Liu, B. Loots, B. Linder, S. Marcovina, B. Rodriguez, D. Standiford, and D.E. Williams. 2006. The burden of diabetes mellitus among US youth: Prevalence estimates from the SEARCH for Diabetes in Youth Study. *Pediatrics* 118 (4): 1510-1518.

Segal, K.R., A. Edano, A. Abalos, J. Albu, L. Blando, M.B. Tomas, and F.X. Pi-Sunyer. 1991. Effects of exercise training on insulin sensitivity and glucose metabolism in lean, obese and diabetic men. *Journal of Applied Physiology* 71 (6): 2402-2411.

Sharoff, C.G., T.A. Hagobian, S.K. Malin, S.R. Chipkin, H. Yu, M.F. Hirshman, L.J. Goodyear, and B. Braun. 2010. Combining short-term metformin treatment and one bout of exercise does not increase insulin action in insulin-resistant individuals. *American Journal of Physiology: Endocrinology and Metabolism* 298: E815-823.

Siegel, L.C., H.D. Sesso, T.S. Bowman, I.M. Lee, J.E. Manson, and J.M. Gaziano. 2009. Physical activity, body mass index, and diabetes risk in men: A prospective study. *American Journal of Medicine* 122 (12): 1115-1121.

Sieverdes, J.C., X. Sui, D.C. Lee, T.S. Church, A. McClain, G.A. Hand, and S.N. Blair. 2010. Physical activity, cardiorespiratory fitness and the incidence of type 2 diabetes in a prospective study of men. *British Journal of Sports Medicine* 44 (4): 238-244.

Sigal, R.J., G.P. Kenny, N.G. Boulé, G.A. Wells, D. Prud'homme, M. Fortier, R.D. Reid, H. Tulloch, D. Coyle, P. Phillips, A. Jennings, and J. Jaffey. 2007. Effects of aerobic training, resistance training, or both on glycemic control in type 2 diabetes: A randomized trial. *Annals of Internal Medicine* 147: 357-369.

Shaw J.E., R.A. Sicree, and P.Z. Zimmet. 2010. Diabetes Atlas Global estimates of the prevalence of diabetes for 2010 and 2030. *Diabetes Research and Clinical Practice* 87: 4-14.

Sinha, M.K., W.J. Pories, E.G. Flickinger, D. Meelheim, and J.F. Caro. 1987. Insulin-receptor kinase activity of adipose tissue from morbidly obese humans with and without NIDDM. *Diabetes* 36: 620-625.

Sloan, F.A., M.A. Bethel, D. Ruiz Jr., A.M. Shea, and M.N. Feinglos. 2008. The growing burden of diabetes mellitus in the US elderly population. *Archives of Internal Medicine* 168 (2, January 28): 192-199.

Strasser, B., U. Siebert, and W. Schobersberger. 2010. Resistance training in the treatment of the metabolic syndrome: A systematic review and meta-analysis of the effect of resistance training on metabolic clustering in patients with abnormal glucose metabolism. *Sports Medicine* 40 (5, May 1): 397-415.

Sui, X., S.P. Hooker, I.M. Lee, T.S. Church, N. Colabianchi, C.D. Lee, and S.N. Blair. 2008. A prospective study of cardiorespiratory fitness and risk of type 2 diabetes in women. *Diabetes Care* 31 (3): 550-555.

Taylor, R., J. Badcock, H. King, K. Pargeter, P. Zimmet, T. Fred, M. Lund, H. Ringrose, F. Bach, R.L. Wang, et al. 1992. Dietary intake, exercise, obesity and noncommunicable disease in rural and urban populations of three Pacific Island countries. *Journal of the American College of Nutrition* 11 (3): 283-293.

Thomas, D.E., E.J. Elliott, and G.A. Naughton. 2006. Exercise for type 2 diabetes mellitus. *Cochrane Database of Systematic Reviews,* July 19 (3): CD002968.

TODAY Study Group. 2010. Design of a family-based lifestyle intervention for youth with type 2 diabetes: The TODAY study. *International Journal of Obesity (Lond)* 34: 217-226.

TODAY Study Group, P. Zeitler, L. Epstein, M. Grey, K. Hirst, F. Kaufman, W. Tamborlane, and D. Wilfley. 2007. Treatment options for type 2 diabetes in adolescents and youth: A study of the comparative efficacy of metformin alone or in combination with rosiglitazone or lifestyle intervention in adolescents with type 2 diabetes. *Pediatric Diabetes* 8: 74-87.

Trovati, M., Q. Carta, F. Cavalot, S. Vitali, C. Banaudi, P.G. Luchhina, F. Fiocchi, G. Emanuelli, and G. Lenti. 1984. Influence of physical training on blood glucose control, glucose tolerance, insulin secretion, and insulin action in non-insulin-dependent diabetic patients. *Diabetes Care* 7 (5): 416-420.

Tuomilehto, J., J. Lindstrom, J.E. Eriksson, T.T. Valle, H. Hamalainen, P. Ilanne-Parikka, S. Keinanen-Kiukaanniemi, M. Laakso, A. Louheranta, M. Rastas, V. Salminen, and M. Uusitupa. 2001. Prevention of type 2 diabetes mellitus by changes in lifestyle among subjects with impaired glucose tolerance. *New England Journal of Medicine* 344 (18): 1343-1350.

Umpierre, D., P.A. Ribeiro, C.K. Kramer, C.B. Leitão, A.T. Zucatti, M.J. Azevedo, J.L. Gross, J.P. Ribeiro, and B.D. Schaan. 2011. Physical activity advice only or structured exercise training and association with HbA1c levels in type 2 diabetes: A systematic review and meta-analysis. *JAMA* 4;305: 1790-1799.

Uusitupa, M., M. Peltonen, J. Lindström, S. Aunola, P. Ilanne-Parikka, S. Keinänen-Kiukaanniemi, T.T. Valle, J.G. Eriksson, J. Tuomilehto; Finnish Diabetes Prevention Study Group. 2009. Ten-year mortality and cardiovascular morbidity in the Finnish Diabetes Prevention Study—secondary analysis of the randomized trial. *PLoS One* 4 (5): e5656.

Vanninen, E., M. Uusitupa, O. Siitonen, J. Laitinen, and E. Lansimies. 1992. Habitual physical activity, aerobic capacity, and metabolic control in patients with newly diagnosed type 2 (non-insulin-dependent) diabetes mellitus: Effect of a 1-year diet and exercise intervention. *Diabetologia* 4: 340-346.

Wallberg-Henriksson, H. 1992. Interaction of exercise and insulin in type II diabetes mellitus. *Diabetes Care* 15 (4): 1777-1782.

Wannamethee, S.G., A.G. Shaper, and G.M.M. Alberti. 2000. Physical activity, metabolic factors, and the incidence of coronary heart disease and type 2 diabetes. *Archives of Internal Medicine* 160 (14): 2108-2116.

Weinstein, A.R., H.D. Sesso, I.M. Lee, N.R. Cook, J.E. Manson, J.E. Buring, and J.M. Gaziano. 2004. Relationship of physical activity vs. body mass index with type 2 diabetes in women. *JAMA* 292: 1188-1194.

Wilmore, J.H., J.S. Green, P.R. Stanforth, J. Gagnon, T. Rankinen, A.S. Leon, D.C. Rao, J.S. Skinner, and C. Bouchard. 2001. Relationship of changes in maximal and submaximal aerobic fitness to changes in cardiovascular disease and non-insulin-dependent diabetes mellitus risk factors with endurance training: The HERITAGE Family Study. *Metabolism* 50 (11): 1255-1263.

Wojtaszewski, J.F., J.N. Nielsen, and E.A. Richter. 2002. Invited review: Effect of acute exercise on insulin signaling and action in humans. *Journal of Applied Physiology* 93: 384-392.

World Health Organization. 1998. *The world health report 1998. Life in the 21st century—a vision for all.* Geneva: World Health Organization.

World Health Organization. 2009. Global health risks: Mortality and burden of disease attributable to selected major risks. Geneva: World Health Organization.

Yeo, W.K., S.L. McGee, A.L. Carey, C.D. Paton, A.P. Garnham, M. Hargreaves, and J.A. Hawley. 2010. Acute signalling responses to intense endurance training commenced with low or normal muscle glycogen. *Experimental Physiology* 95: 351-358.

Zimmet, P.Z., V.R. Collins, G.K. Dowse, K.G. Alberti, J. Tuomilehto, H. Gareeboo, and P. Chitson. 1991. The relation of physical activity to cardiovascular disease risk factors in Mauritians: Mauritius Noncommunicable Disease Study Group. *American Journal of Epidemiology* 134: 862-875.

Zimmet, P., G. Dowse, C. Finch, S. Serjeantson, and H. King. 1990. The epidemiology and natural history of NIDDM: Lessons from the South Pacific. *Diabetes Metabolic Review* 6: 91-124.

CHAPTER 11

Physical Activity and Osteoporosis

My strength faileth because of mine iniquity and my bones are consumed.

· *The Holy Bible* ·
Psalms 31:10

CHAPTER OBJECTIVES

▸ Describe the public health burden of osteoporosis including its prevalence in population groups, its costs, and its role in functional health and late-life mortality

▸ Discuss common methods used to measure bone mineral and define osteopenia and osteoporosis

▸ Describe the processes of osteogenesis and bone involution

▸ Identify the major modifiable and nonmodifiable risk factors of osteoporosis

▸ Describe the ways bone loading is believed to be affected by different types of physical activities

▸ Describe and evaluate the strength of evidence that physical activity and exercise training improve bone health and lower risks of osteoporosis and osteoporotic fractures

steoporosis, or "porous bone," is a disease characterized by abnormally low bone mass and microstructural deterioration of bone tissue that leads to brittle bones and increased risk of fractures. People's bone mineral can be compared to norms that are specific to age, sex, and race, but the World Health Organization (WHO) has defined **osteoporosis** as a bone mineral density (BMD) measurement more than 2.5 standard deviations below the average in young white adults (WHO Study Group 1994; table 11.1). Based on this definition, bone is considered osteoporotic if it is unable to withstand the stress of normal physical activities or if a person has a history of spontaneous, non- or low-trauma fractures such as compression or crush fractures of the vertebrae. For each standard deviation decrease in bone mass, there is a 50% to 100% increase in the risk of fracture (Hui, Slemenda, and Johnston 1989). A standard deviation loss of bone mass in the neck of the femur at the hip joint increases the risk of hip fracture by 300%.

Bone mineral density between 1 and 2.5 standard deviations below that of young adults aged 20 to 29 years indicates **osteopenia** (i.e., low bone mass), which is a direct risk factor for osteoporosis (WHO Study Group 1994). According to the WHO, physical inactivity is also a risk factor for osteoporosis. World Osteoporosis Day, celebrated by the International Osteoporosis Foundation on October 20, 2005, was dedicated to exercise. After describing osteoporosis and its public health impact, this chapter presents the evidence that physical activity contributes to peak bone mass during youth and young adulthood, retards bone loss with aging, and can help reduce the risks of osteoporotic fractures.

▶ **FOR EACH** standard deviation decline in bone mass in the hip, the risk of fracture increases threefold. A woman's lifetime risk of hip fracture is equal to her combined risk of breast, uterine, and ovarian cancer.

Like the other chronic diseases discussed in this book, osteoporosis has existed since antiquity. As recorded in the Bible, King David, the ruler of Israel from about 990 to 970 BC, probably suffered from osteoporosis in his later years (Ben-Noun 2002); and judging by the quotation that opened this chapter, he linked his bone loss to bad habits and failing strength. Bone archaeologists found a case of severe osteo-

porosis in the remains of a sixth-century female, discovered in the Negev desert of southern Israel, who had compression fractures in two thoracic vertebrae and bone mineral densities at various sites that were 5 to 8 standard deviations below the values expected for young adults (Foldes and Popovtzer 1996). A case of hip fracture attributed to osteoporosis was documented in a mummy excavated from Lisht, Upper Egypt, that was dated to the XIIth Dynasty (1990-1786 BC) (Dequeker et al. 1997).

Even in ancient times, women had lower BMD and greater risk of osteoporosis than men, even though both men and women would have been physically active because of their nomadic or agrarian lifestyles. In a group of skeletons excavated in Unterhautzental, Austria, dated to the Bronze Age (i.e., 2200 to 1600 BC), the average (mean ± SD) BMD in the neck of the femur of 14 women about 45 years old was 0.98 ± 0.15 g/cm^2, significantly lower than the average for five men (1.2 ± 0.26 g/cm^2) found at the site (Frigo and Lang 1995).

Other archaeological evidence suggests that osteoporosis has become a more prevalent health problem in the 21st century, as the incidence rate of osteoporotic hip fractures has become higher in the United States and Europe than would be expected merely from increased numbers of people living longer. During restoration of Christ Church at Spitalfields, London, skeletons of 87 white women ages 15 to 89 years who died between 1729 and 1852 were exhumed (Lees et al. 1993). The rate of bone mineral loss in their femoral necks was significantly less than found in a comparative sample of 294 modern-day women between 42 and 48 years old, before or after menopause. The authors suggested that the results might be explainable by the lower prevalence of daily physical activity in modern-day women compared with the Spitalfields sample, who were known to have worked typically 14 to 16 h a day operating weaving looms and walking for transportation. Other changes during the past 200 years that could contribute to greater loss of bone mass include lower consumption of dairy products, which contain calcium, and more tobacco smoking. All these factors are modifiable risks for the development of osteoporosis.

▶ **ABOUT ONE** in five patients who fracture a hip, most after age 75, dies in the year following the fracture, and 50% of the survivors become dependent on others for care.

Table 11.1   World Health Organization Diagnostic Criteria for Osteoporosis

Category	Diagnostic criteria
Normal	BMD within 1 SD of the mean of a young adult reference population
Osteopenia or low bone mass	BMD between 1.0 and 2.5 SD below the mean of a young adult reference population
Osteoporosis	BMD 2.5 or more SD below the mean of a young adult reference population
Severe osteoporosis	Osteoporosis with one or more fragility fractures

Magnitude of the Problem

The annual prevalence of diagnosed osteoporosis in the United States is about 10 million people; 80% are women. It is estimated that 44 million Americans ages 50 or older, 55% of adults, have either osteoporosis or osteopenia (National Osteoporosis Foundation 2010). Compared to rates observed in population-based cohorts in other regions of the world (table 11.2), osteoporosis in people aged 80 years or older is lower in U.S. men but higher in U.S. women (Kanis et al. 2008).

Bone mass is generally lowest among women who are white or Asian, thin framed, and sedentary (Robitaille et al. 2008). Twenty percent of U.S. women ages 50 years or older who are non-Hispanic white or of Asian descent have osteoporosis. Black women and overweight or obese women have higher bone mass and thus are at comparatively lower risk of developing osteoporosis. Five percent of non-Hispanic black women and men ages 50 years or older have osteoporosis; another 35% and 19%, respectively, have osteopenia. Ten percent of Latina women 50 years or older have osteoporosis, and another 49% have osteopenia. The prevalence of osteoporosis is expected to continue to increase in nations that have increasing life expectancies and hence an increasing number of older people. Based on trends of increasing incidence prior to 2002, it was predicted that more than 61 million women and men 50 years old or older in the United States would have low bone mass or osteoporosis by the year 2020 (National Osteoporosis Foundation 2002). Figure 11.1 illustrates the projected trends for osteoporosis and osteopenia among U.S. women and men. In 2005-2006, 5.3 million U.S. men and women aged 50 years or older had osteoporosis, and 34.5 million had osteopenia, at the neck of the femur (Looker et al. 2010). The risk of hip fracture increases 2.6 times for every standard deviation drop in BMD at the femur neck (Marshall, Johnell, and Wedel 1996). Hip fractures are associated with 10%-20% excess mortality within one year (U.S. Department of Health and Human Services 2004) and are associated with a 2.5 times increase in risk of future fractures (Colón-Emeric et al. 2003).

Table 11.2 Prevalence (Percentage) Estimates of WHO-Defined Osteoporosis in the United States and Other Regions of the World

Nation	Age (years)				
	50	60	70	80	90
Men					
United States	1.0	2.0	4.1	8.2	15.7
Europe	0.6	1.4	3.7	9.2	21.0
Canada	0.5	1.5	4.3	11.6	27.9
Australia	0.5	1.4	4.1	11.4	28.2
Japan	0.9	2.2	5.1	11.4	23.5
Women					
United States	1.9	6.2	18.8	44.8	73.9
Europe	3.8	8.5	17.9	33.9	54.6
Canada	2.9	7.8	19.1	39.8	64.9
Australia	3.6	8.8	20.0	39.1	62.2
Japan	5.6	10.7	19.5	32.8	49.7

Used with permission of the WHO Collaborating Centre for Metabolic Bone Diseases, University of Sheffield. FRAX® is registered to Professor JA Kanis, University of Sheffield.

Fractures and Mortality

Osteoporosis or osteopenia is responsible for more than 2 million fractures in the United States each year, including approximately 300,000 hip fractures, 550,000 vertebral crush fractures, 400,000 wrist fractures, and 300,000 fractures at other sites (National Osteoporosis Foundation 2002). Annual fracture incidence is expected to be more than 3 million by the year 2025. Currently, about half of hip fractures worldwide occur in Europe and North America, but it has been estimated that by the year 2050 those regions will contribute only one-fourth of total fractures, as incidence rates are predicted to increase markedly in Asia and Latin America (Riggs and Melton 1995). In the United States and worldwide, the lifetime risk for a fracture of the hip, spine, or forearm that is related to osteoporosis is 40% to 50% in women and 13% to 22% in men over age 50 (Johnell and Kanis 2005). A woman's risk of hip fracture is equal to her combined risk of breast, uterine,

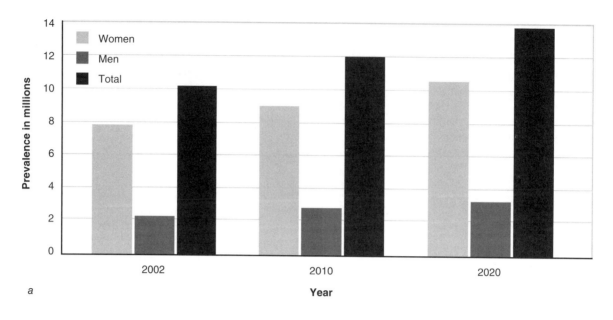

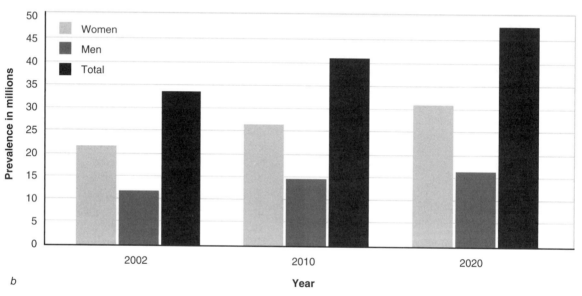

Figure 11.1 *(a)* Osteoporosis trends projected from 2002 to 2020 in the United States for adults 50 years and older. *(b)* Osteopenia trends projected from 2002 to 2020 in the United States for adults 50 years and older. Projections based on NHANES III data.

Data from the National Osteoporosis Foundation 2002.

Incidence of Fractures

According to estimates, more than 2 million fractures were attributable to osteoporosis or osteopenia in the U.S. in 2005, including the following:

- 297,000 hip fractures
- 547,000 vertebral fractures
- 397,000 wrist fractures
- 135,000 pelvic fractures
- 675,000 fractures at other sites

Source: American Osteoporosis Foundation. 2010.

and ovarian cancer. Osteoporotic fractures are an important cause of disability and mortality in the elderly. About 20% of patients who fracture a hip die in the year following the fracture, and 50% of the survivors become dependent on others for care. Though men have fewer incidents of hip fracture, they have twice the risk of mortality after a fracture.

The lifetime risk for hip fracture has been estimated at 17.5% in white women and 6.0% in white men. Lower risks have been estimated for black women and men: 5.6% and 2.8%, respectively. White women have about a 16% lifetime risk for developing either vertebral or distal radius fractures. The lifetime risk for white females for fracture of the proximal femur, radius, or vertebrae is 40%. Vertebral fractures, including microcompression or crush fractures, account for half of all fractures. One in four people older than 70 years has some compression fractures of the vertebrae that can lead to **kyphosis** of the thoracic spine ("dowager's hump"). White women lose an average of 6.4 cm (2.5 in.) of height after menopause if they do not receive medical treatment. Complications of osteoporosis represent an economic burden to public health. The direct cost of treating osteoporotic fractures of the proximal femur, radius, and vertebrae was about $19 billion in 2005. By the year 2025, it is predicted to be $25 billion. Risk is rising the fastest among Hispanics, especially women, who are expected to incur treatment costs of $2 billion by 2025 (National Osteoporosis Foundation 2010).

Etiology of Osteopenia and Osteoporosis

There are two main categories of osteoporosis. Primary osteoporosis includes age-related (type I, or senile) bone loss and postmenopausal (type II) bone loss (Garnero and Delmas 1997). Secondary osteoporosis is caused by another disease but may not be independent of age or menopause. This chapter deals mainly with primary osteoporosis because it can be positively affected by physical activity, especially through increasing peak bone mass during adolescence and young adulthood or through retarding bone loss during aging. Osteoporosis results mainly from loss of trabecular bone mass (i.e., trabeculae and their interconnections) and microdamage within the bone (Johnston and Slemenda 1995). Twin studies have demonstrated that several genes appear to regulate the fragility of bone, but the specific genes have not yet been identified fully (Slemenda et al. 1996). Dietary calcium and vitamin D, as well as regular physical activity, contribute to peak bone mass, particularly before age 20. Bone loss among women is related to estrogen levels and,

to a lesser extent, androgen levels, and bone loss accelerates after menopause. Although their dietary and lifestyle risk factors are the same, men lose bone at about half the rate of women, and the mechanisms for primary bone loss in men are poorly understood. Biologically available testosterone (the fraction not bound to globulin) declines about 60% in men between ages 20 and 80 years, but it appears that estrogen (converted from testosterone by the enzyme aromatase) has a greater effect on bone than does testosterone in men (Olszynski et al. 2004).

Sex Differences

The rate of bone loss differs between men and women as they age. At all ages, men have more bone mass than women, and men's natural bone loss is more gradual. Bone loss in men is thought to begin at age 40 to 45 years, proceeds at a rate of about 0.5% per year, then accelerates substantially after age 60 to a rate of up to 4% per decade until age 90 (Menkes et al. 1993). Women lose bone at a rate of about 1% to 2% beginning around age 35 (Whitfield and Morley 1998). During lactation, there is a slight, transient increase in bone loss to 7% in the first six months after childbirth, which returns to the normal rate of loss at the resumption of menses (Sowers, Corton, and Shapiro 1993). In addition, women can lose up to 20% of their bone mass in the five to seven years after menopause (Riggs and Melton 1986). The larger and faster decreases in bone mass in women explain most of the difference in prevalence of osteoporotic fractures between women and men. The onset of osteoporosis in late life among women differs according to bone health soon after menopause ends. A recent study reported evidence from repeated bone scanning in a cohort of postmenopausal women in the United States who had normal BMD when they were first scanned at age 65. The time between subsequent screenings when at least 10% of the women developed osteoporosis was 15 years for those who initially had normal bone density or mild osteopenia, 5 years for those with moderate osteopenia, and 1 year for women with advanced osteopenia (Gourlay et al. 2012).

It is believed that the marked decline in levels of estrogen after menopause accounts for the greater bone loss experienced by women; 75% or more of the bone loss that occurs in women during the first 15 years after menopause is attributable to estrogen deficiency. Men lose bone mass at an accelerated rate after about age 60; bone loss can be associated with a decline in gonadal function in some men (WHO Study Group 1994).

▷ **MOST OF** the higher prevalence of osteoporotic fractures among women compared to men occurs after menopause. Without hormone replacement therapy, women can lose up to 20% of their bone mass within five to seven years after menopause.

Generalized Secondary Osteoporosis Causes

Hypogonadism	Hyperadrenocorticism
Thyrotoxicosis	Anorexia nervosa
Hyperprolactinemia	Diabetes mellitus
Pregnancy	Vitamin D deficiency
Chronic liver disease	Alcoholism
Chronic heparin use	Anticonvulsants
Osteogenesis	Homocystinuria
Rheumatoid arthritis	Myeloma

Bone Renewal and Involution

To understand how **bone involution** might be retarded by physical activity, it is necessary to understand the basics of bone renewal. The **endosteum** is the layer of cells lining the inner surface of bone in the central medullary cavity. The **exosteum** refers to bone cells that are outside the central medullary cavity. After about age 30 to 40, endosteal bone is lost at a faster rate than exosteal bone is deposited. This is called bone involution, which results in osteopenia and is a risk factor for osteoporosis. One-third of women who have bone involution develop osteoporosis. See figure 11.2.

There are two types of bone: **cortical bone** and **trabecular bone.** Cortical, or compact, bone is found mainly in the shaft of long bones and accounts for about 80% of all bone. Trabecular bone is spongy tissue, has a lattice or honeycomb design, and is found in the vertebrae, pelvis, flat bones, and ends of the long bones. See figure 11.3.

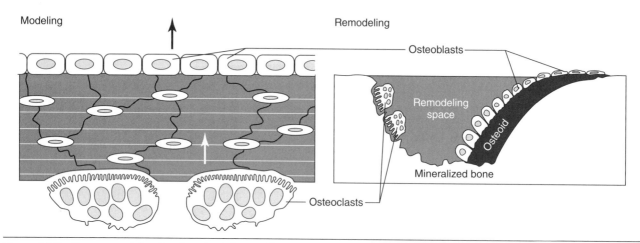

Figure 11.2   Bone remodeling involves the balance of bone loss by osteoclasts with bone renewal by osteoblasts. When these two processes are no longer in balance and bone loss exceeds bone renewal, bone involution occurs.

Reprinted from Office of the Surgeon General, 2004, *The basics of bone in health and disease. Bone health and osteoporosis: A Report of the Surgeon General* (Rockville, MD: Office of the Surgeon General).

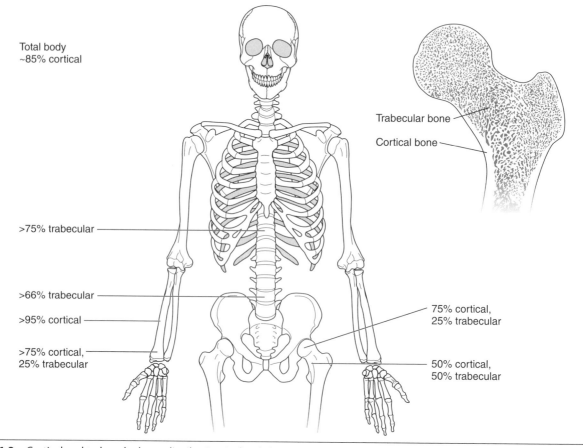

Figure 11.3   Cortical and trabecular bone distribution in the skeleton.

Trabecular bone has more surface area per volume and is more metabolically active (e.g., a higher flux of minerals occurs between bone and blood) than cortical bone; the formation and resorption of trabecular bone occur about six times faster than in cortical bone. Thus, trabecular bone is more susceptible to osteoporotic disease (figure 11.4).

White women lose an average of 50% of trabecular bone and 30% of cortical bone over their lifetimes (mainly after menopause), while men lose about 15% of trabecular and 12% of cortical bone mass (Sowers 1997). The loss of vertebral bone in the spine begins in the 20s but is usually negligible until after menopause. Bone density in the neck of the femur peaks in the mid-to-late 20s and starts to decline around age 30. Without intervention, about 5% of trabecular bone and 1% to 1.5% of total bone mass are lost each year during the 10 to 15 years after menopause. The rate of loss is slower among black women.

Bone remodeling is a continuous process involving hormonal and local regulation of three types of cells: **osteoclasts, osteoblasts,** and **osteocytes.** Osteoclasts are phagocytes that digest old bone cells and thus are involved in bone resorption (i.e., breakdown). Osteoblasts rebuild by forming new bone cells (i.e., osteocytes) from collagen to make an **osteoid matrix.** The osteoid matrix provides the infrastructure for the mineralization of bone (e.g., by calcium and phosphorus) and, along with trabecular bone, gives bone its mechanical, elastic, and tensile strength.

Increases (during growth) and decreases (with age) in BMD depend on the balance of activity of osteoclasts and osteoblasts. During growth and maturation of skeletal bone in youth and young adulthood, osteoblastic activity exceeds osteoclastic activity, so bones grow and increase their mineral density. After peak bone mass is attained, the activity of osteoclasts gradually outpaces that of osteoblasts, leading to an accumulation of cavities in the bone's osteoid matrix (figure 11.5).

During normal aging (i.e., without lifestyle intervention), women lose both endosteal and periosteal bone. In contrast, aging men have less net bone loss because their periosteal bone remains more stable, which can partly compensate for their endosteal bone loss to help retard loss of bone strength. Elderly men's bones are larger than women's also because they were larger in youth (Szulc and Delmas 2007).

Hormonal Influences

Parathyroid hormone contributes to bone remodeling by stimulating resorption of calcium from the

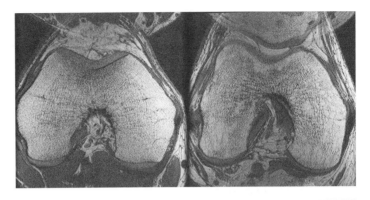

Figure 11.4 High-resolution cross-sectional images of osteoporotic distal femur bone of a spinal cord–injured subject on the right and an able-bodied control on the left. Notice the fewer black lines (bone) and more white (marrow) in the image of the spinal cord–injured subject.

Courtesy of Dr. Christopher Modlesky.

bone, while **calcitonin** inhibits resorption. It is not yet fully understood how reproductive hormones such as estrogen and testosterone help protect against bone loss. Low levels of 25-hydroxy (25- OH) **vitamin D** is a risk factor for osteoporosis, which is monitored in the population by NHANES. 25-OH is converted in the kidney to the biologically active metabolite 1,25-dihydroxyvitamin D, which enhances the absorption of dietary calcium by bone. Also, the presence of receptors for estrogen on osteoblasts indicates that estrogen can have a direct effect on osteogenesis. Estrogen stimulates several bone growth factors (e.g., insulin-like growth factors I and II) and inhibits the **lymphokines** interleukin-1 and interleukin-6 (cells that regulate the immune response during inflammation), which promote osteopenia. Estrogen also stimulates the synthesis of calcitonin, which inhibits bone resorption and increases vitamin D receptors in osteoblasts,

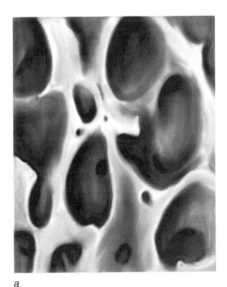
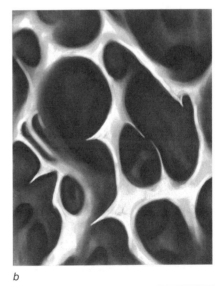

a   *b*

Figure 11.5 Structure of *(a)* normal trabecular bone and *(b)* osteoporotic trabecular bone showing loss of osteoid matrix and minerals.

Reprinted, by permission, from American College of Sports Medicine, 2011, *ACSM's complete guide to fitness and health* (Champaign, IL: Human Kinetics), 360.

thus influencing the activity of 1,25-dihydroxyvitamin D in bone (Speroff, Glass, and Case 1994).

Risk Factors and Prevention

Twin and family studies show that BMD and other risk factors for fracture (e.g., death and replacement of bone cells and bone geometry) are partly inherited. However, most of genes that regulate bone are as yet undiscovered. Both genetic and family influences are modified by age (e.g., increased risk of falling as people become older) and environmental factors such as diet and exercise (Ralston and Uitterlinden 2010).

Several medical conditions that mainly occur in later life (e.g., Cushing's disease, Paget's disease, hypogonadism, acromegaly, thyroid or parathyroid disease, rheumatoid arthritis, and cancer) can lead to osteoporosis. Also, several drugs have been associated with decreased bone mass and increased risk of osteoporotic fractures. These drugs include glucocorticosteroids, anticonvulsants, thyroxin in excessive doses, and some antitumor drugs used to treat cancer.

The development of osteoporosis is inversely related to the maximum amount of bone accumulated during growth and positively related to the rate and duration of bone loss that occurs with aging, which accelerates after menopause among women. The lower the peak bone mass or the greater the rate of bone loss, the greater the risk of osteoporosis. Key unmodifiable and modifiable risk factors, including physical inactivity, are listed in the sidebar.

Dietary Calcium and Vitamin D

A diet containing an adequate amount of calcium, vitamin D, and protein is recommended to promote bone health and reduce the risks of osteopenia and osteoporosis. Calcium is the main component of bone, which stores 99.5% of the body's calcium and supplies calcium to meet the body's metabolic needs (e.g., nerve conductance and muscle contraction) via the blood. Inadequate calcium is a risk factor for osteopenia

---

Steps to Prevent Osteoporosis

A comprehensive program that can help prevent osteoporosis includes

- a balanced diet rich in calcium and vitamin D,
- weight-bearing aerobic and resistance exercise,
- a healthy lifestyle with limited alcohol intake and no smoking, and
- bone density testing and prescribed medication when appropriate.

---

and osteoporosis. The recommended calcium intake during adolescence and adulthood, depending on age, is between 1000 and 1300 mg per day. This is not a problem for some populations. The Hunza, for example, live in a high mountain pass between China and Pakistan and are renowned for being among the longest-living people in the world. Much of their longevity has been attributed to their water, called "Glacial Milk," which comes from the nearby Ultar Glacier and contains mineral-rich rock ground by the glacier, including 11,500 mg of calcium per liter (Wallach and Lan 1994). An 8-oz (237 ml) glass of cow's milk contains about 300 mg of calcium. However, most Americans do not have a calcium-rich water source, so their calcium intake is determined by dietary choice, which often leads to insufficient intake, especially by adolescent girls and women, who commonly consume less than half (mean of about 700 mg per day) of their recommended daily allowance (Alaimo et al. 1994).

Vitamin D is necessary for the body to absorb calcium from food. Its synthesis depends on sun exposure. Though sufficient amounts of vitamin D can be synthesized in the skin with 10 to 15 min of direct exposure of the face and extremities to sunlight two or three days each week, the biosynthesis of vitamin D is less in dark-skinned people and lessens as people age. Thus, vitamin D deficiency is common without

---

Risk Factors for Osteoporosis

Modifiable	Unmodifiable
Cigarette smoking	Heredity
Excessive alcohol intake	Small body frame
Low testosterone levels	Female sex
Vitamin D intake	Race (European or Asian)
Physical inactivity	Age
Calcium intake	Postmenopause
Anorexia or bulimia	Amenorrhea
Amenorrhea	Premature menopause
Medications (e.g., benzodiazepenes)	

Recommended Daily Allowance of Calcium

Children and adolescents (ages 9-18)	1300 mg
Women (ages 19-50)	1000 mg
Men (ages 19-50)	1000 mg
Women and men older than 50	1200 mg

Institute of Medicine 2003.

dietary supplementation and results in resorption of stored calcium from bone. The recommended daily dietary intake of vitamin D is between 400 and 800 international units (IU). Dietary supplementation with calcium (500 mg a day) and vitamin D (700 IU a day) has been shown to reduce by 50% the three-year risk of developing osteoporosis among men and women over age 65 years (Dawson-Hughes et al. 1997).

Hormone Replacement Therapy

A report from the National Institutes of Health Women's Health Initiative on a randomized clinical trial of 16,608 postmenopausal women ages 50 to 79, recruited by 40 U.S. clinical centers in 1993 to 1998, showed that hormone replacement therapy (HRT) combining estrogen and progestin reduced the risk of hip fracture (RR = 0.66; 95% CI [confidence interval]: 0.45-0.98) and all fractures (RR = 0.76; 0.69-0.85) (Rossouw et al. 2002). Notwithstanding the favorable effect of HRT on postmenopausal bone health, the trial was stopped by the National Heart, Lung, and Blood Institute because of the number of adverse events during the study. The investigators concluded that the overall health risks exceeded benefits across an average 5.2-year follow-up and that the regimen of estrogen plus progestin should not be initiated or continued for primary prevention of coronary heart disease (CHD)—in contrast with many epidemiological studies that consistently showed reduced incidence of CHD and all-cause mortality among postmenopausal women using HRT (Mosca 2000). In the Women's Health Initiative study, increased risks (95% CI) after HRT were observed for total cardiovascular disease (CVD), 1.22 (1.09-1.36); CHD, 1.29 (1.02-1.63); stroke, 1.41 (1.07-1.85); and breast cancer, 1.26 (1.00-1.59).

A decreased risk after HRT was observed for colorectal cancer, 0.63 (0.43-0.92). Though all-cause mortality was not affected by HRT, absolute excess risks per 10,000 person-years attributable to estrogen plus progestin were seven more CHD events, eight more strokes, and eight more invasive breast cancers, while absolute risk reductions per 10,000 person-years were six fewer colorectal cancers and five fewer hip fractures. Key risk factors for fractures in postmenopausal women are shown in figure 11.6.

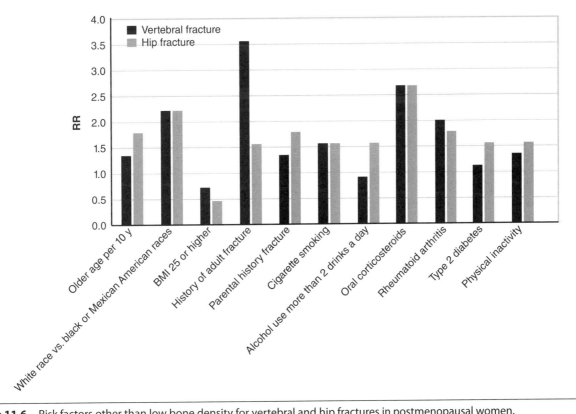

Figure 11.6   Risk factors other than low bone density for vertebral and hip fractures in postmenopausal women.

*Risk compared to Black or Mexican-American race.

▶ **THE WORLD** Health Organization concluded more than a decade ago that women who take estrogen for at least seven years between the onset of menopause and the age of 75 have a 50% reduction in risk of fractures as well as CHD (WHO Study Group 1994). However, some studies have shown increased risk of breast cancer and CVD after estrogen or estrogen plus progestin replacement therapy.

The WHO developed the FRAX algorithm to estimate the risk of fracture (www.sheffield.ac.uk/FRAX/) to better predict and prevent fractures in people who are at risk even if they don't yet have osteoporosis. It estimates 10-year risk of hip or other major osteoporotic fracture (wrist, humerus,or spinal crush fracture) using several risk factors, BMD in the femoral neck, and nation-specific data on fracture and mortality. The National Osteoporosis Foundation of the United States recommends that physicians and patients consider drug therapy if the 10-year risk of hip fracture exceeds 3% or if the risk of major osteoporotic fracture exceeds 20% (www.nof.org/professionals/clinical-guidelines) (Siris, Baim, and Nattiv 2010). Table 11.3 lists common drugs for osteoporosis.

Hormone replacement therapy (i.e., estrogen alone or estrogen combined with progestin) is generally viewed as the most important intervention for both the prevention and treatment of osteoporosis in postmenopausal women. Hormone replacement therapy can protect bone from rapid demineralization, typical of the early postmenopausal period, and thus decrease fracture rates in postmenopausal women. Women who take estrogen for at least seven years between the onset of menopause and the age of 75 have a 50% reduction in risk of fractures (Levinson and Altkorn 1998). A quantitative review of the evidence from 22 randomized controlled trials of HRT lasting at least 12 months found a cumulative 27% reduction in nonvertebral fractures after HRT (RR = 0.73; 95% CI: 0.56-0.94). The effect was greater (33% reduction in fractures) among women under age 60 (RR = 0.67; 95% CI: 0.46-0.98) than over age 60 (RR = 0.88; 95% CI: 0.71-1.08) (Torgerson and Bell-Syer 2001).

Bone Measurement Techniques

No symptoms accompany bone loss, so it is difficult to diagnose. Bone mass is usually expressed as either bone mineral density (BMD) or bone mineral content (BMC). The two most common measurement techniques used are dual-energy X-ray absorptiometry (DXA), which provides area density (in grams per centimeter squared), and computed tomography (CT), which measures volumetric density (in milligrams per centimeter cubed).

Measuring Bone Mass Density and Bone Mass Content

The DXA method is the most popular technique as it provides precise, fast measurement of BMD with minimal radiation exposure (less than 1/10 of the amount used on a standard chest X ray) and can scan virtually all skeletal sites (Garnero and Delmas 1997). It is the common standard for describing osteoporosis and osteopenia (Kanis et al. 2008).

The anatomic sites most commonly measured by DXA or CT include the proximal femur (i.e., near the hip joint), the spine, and the proximal radius of the arm (near the wrist). The femoral neck and lumbar spine are usually considered optimal for BMD measurement because they are common fracture sites. There is no single site that predicts BMD at

Table 11.3 Common FDA-Approved Drugs for Treating Osteoporosis, Effects on Fracture in Women After Menopause, and Prescription Cost

Drug	Risk reduction		Annual cost
	Spine	Hip or other non-spinal bone	
Estrogens (brand names include Enjuvia, Estrace, Estratab, Estratest, Ogen, Premarin, Prempro/Premplus)	35-40%	35-40%	$165-$900
Alendronate (brand name is Fosamax), 70 mg/week	45%	30-50%	$450 brand name $120 generic
Raloxifene (brand name is Evista), 60 mg/day	35-40%	None	$460-$730 brand name $180-$360 generic
Risedronate (brand name is Actonel), 35 mg/week	40%	30-40%	$400-700
Ibandronate (brand name is Boniva), 150 mg/month	50%	30%	$1400 brand name $300 generic
Teriparatide (brand name is Forteo), 20 microgram injection daily	60-70%	40-70%	$12,600

other skeletal sites, but measurement of the femoral neck currently has the most general application (Sowers 1997).

Blood serum indexes of bone formation and resorption can help detect changes in BMD. Serum bone Gla protein (osteocalcin), the enzyme bone-specific alkaline phosphatase (BAP), and insulin-like growth factor I (IGF-I) are commonly used indicators of bone formation. Another enzyme, tartrate-resistant acid phosphatase (TRACP), and the protein C-terminal cross-linked telopeptide of type I collagen (ICTP) are indicators of bone resorption. Serum levels of 1,25-dihydroxyvitamin D and urinary adenosine 3,5-cyclic monophosphate also have been used as indicators of bone turnover (Menkes et al. 1993). Measurement of bone turnover is a research tool rather than a clinical method for diagnosing or monitoring low bone mass (Sowers 1997).

Measuring Bone Strength

A fracture occurs when an external load exceeds the strength of a bone, depending on the size and mass of bone, its structure (spatial distribution, shape, and microarchitecture), and its material composition (collagen, microdamage, porosity, and mineralization).

Most studies of exercise have used BMD measured by DXA as a proxy measure of bone strength because low BMD is an independent risk factor for predicting fractures in a population (Kanis et al. 2008). However, as many as 80% of fractures occur in individuals who do not have osteoporosis but have osteopenia or even normal BMD as measured by DXA (Järvinen, Kannus, and Sievänen 1999). Other measures such as quantitative computed tomography (QCT), magnetic resonance imaging (MRI), or hip structural analysis (HSA) derived from DXA scans are used to assess the size, shape, and structure of bone. It is now known that even small changes in bone mass distribution and cortical and trabecular structure that increase bone cross section can increase the strength of a bone regardless of overall BMD. Later in the chapter we'll see some evidence that exercise that puts loads on bones in specific sites can increase the cross section and strength of bone by moving trabecular bone to cortical bone. As a result, the bending strength of bone can be increased by exercise even when overall bone density is not changed (Adami et al. 1999; Järvinen et al. 1998).

Physical Activity and Osteoporosis: The Evidence

The scientific advisory committee of the 2008 Physical Activity Guidelines for Americans concluded that a year of exercise training in older adults can increase BMD or slow age-related declines in BMD by 1% to 2% in clinically important regions of the spine and hip. Based on rodent studies it appears that even small improvements in BMD after mechanical loading (i.e., exercise) result in substan-

---

Exercise Recommendations for Bone Health in Adults

Mode: Intermittent weight-loading activities (tennis, stair climbing, jogging, jumping, walking) and resistance exercise (e.g., weightlifting)

Intensity: Bone-loading forces that have moderate-to-high magnitude

Frequency: Three to five days per week for endurance activities and two or three days per week for resistance activities

Duration: 30 to 60 min each session or day consisting of a combination of bone-loading activities that involve major muscle groups

Source: American College of Sports Medicine, 2004

---

tial resistance to fracture (Physical Activity Guidelines Advisory Committee 2008).

There is scientific consensus that physical inactivity is associated with decreased bone mass. Extreme losses of 2% to 10% have been found among young men after four months of bed rest (Buchner and Wagner 1992), but most of that loss is recovered soon after a return to upright posture and normal daily movement. The transience of this bone loss can be attributed to the reduced gravitational load, similar to the loss of bone mass that occurs in microgravity (e.g., during space travel). Nonetheless, there does seem to be a more insidious loss of bone mass among people who live sedentary lifestyles that compounds the natural history of bone loss with increasing age. A recent review of the research literature concluded that physical activity involving high-intensity loading of bone promotes bone density and may help prevent osteoporosis—and that physical activity involving static muscle contractions or slow movements has no effect or smaller effects on bone mass than activities that involve rapidly applied forces (Vuori 2001).

Much of the evidence suggesting the benefits of exercise or sports on bone health initially came from cross-sectional studies that compared athletes or regular exercisers with sedentary people, or from poorly controlled clinical studies of exercise training and bone mass. Cross-sectional studies are reviewed in the next section. Then we discuss population-based studies addressing whether physical activity boosts peak bone mass during adolescence and young adulthood. After that, we discuss clinical trials of the impact of endurance and resistance exercise training on BMD during young adulthood, middle age, and early old age, including comparisons of pre- and postmenopausal women. Finally, we summarize the evidence about whether exercise training retards bone loss as people grow older and whether it reduces the risk of osteoporotic fractures.

Cross-Sectional Studies

Though an early study reported that 41 recreational runners over the age of 50 years had 40% higher BMD than age-matched controls (Lane et al. 1986), bone mass among different types of athletes generally followed the peak weight-bearing activity or localized loading of bone, as in resistance exercise or strength training.

For example, male tennis players 79 years old or older who played tennis for periods ranging from 25 to 72 years showed an increased BMD in their dominant forearms as compared with their age-matched controls (Huddleston et al. 1980). The following are listed from highest to lowest bone mass: weightlifters, weight throwers, gymnasts, tennis players, runners, soccer players, swimmers, and nonathletes (Montoye 1984; Taaffe et al. 1995, 1997). This ranking does not indicate whether high BMD resulted from the particular sport or whether athletes excelled in these sports because of their optimal levels of bone mass. However, a study of college-aged gymnasts found that bone density at relevant sites responded dramatically to high-impact loading, independent of reproductive hormone status and despite high initial BMD values (Taaffe et al. 1997). This provides evidence that mechanical loading, rather than selection bias, underlies the high BMD values characteristic of female gymnasts. Swimming, which imposes smaller peak loads, did not increase BMD in another study (Emslander et al. 1998). Cross-sectional comparisons generally show that, compared with nonathletes, athletes in high-load sports (e.g., weightlifting, gymnastics, basketball, volleyball) have 10% to 15% higher bone mass in the lumbar spine, femoral neck, pelvis, and arm, but that bone mass of athletes who perform repetitive weight-bearing activities (e.g., distance running and Nordic skiing) that don't involve a lot of peak loading is only about 3% to 8% higher.

Greater muscle strength is positively associated with BMD; increased BMD possibly results from stimulation of bone modeling by the transfer of force from muscle to bone. For example, bone mass was positively associated with grip strength and peak torques at the hip and knee joints independently of body weight (Bauer et al. 1993). Among 709 men and 1080 women over age 60 years in the Dubbo Osteoporosis Epidemiology cohort, quadriceps muscle strength predicted bone density at the proximal femur in the men but not the women. After adjustment for age and body weight, BMD at the femoral neck among men and women was about 5% higher in those who had high quadriceps strength and high calcium intake compared with those with low quadriceps strength and low calcium intake (Nguyen et al. 1994).

Several other studies have shown a positive association between activity level and BMD in nonathletes:

• In a population-based cohort of 1254 older Scottish women (mean age 70 years), there were interactions between dietary calcium and self-reported participation in habitual physical activities that loaded bone on BMD at the lumbar spine and hip, independent of other risk factors. At low or medium calcium intakes, BMD was 8% higher among the 33% most active women (Mavroeidi et al. 2009).

• In a nationally representative sample of 4254 U.S. men aged 20 to 59 years from the third National Health and Nutrition Examination Survey (NHANES III), jogging was associated with higher BMD of the total femur (Mussolino, Looker, and Orwoll 2001). A total of 954 men (22.3%) reported jogging in the past month. Bone mineral density was 5% higher among joggers than among nonjoggers and was 8% higher than in 577 nonjoggers who also reported no other leisure activities. Those differences were 3% and 6.5% after adjustment for age at interview, race-ethnicity, body mass index (BMI), dietary protein, calcium, total calorie intake, smoking, alcohol consumption, chronic health conditions, and weight change. Joggers were more likely to report also doing other weight-bearing activities, but their BMD was still higher than that of nonjoggers after further adjustment for total number of leisure physical activities.

• The prevalence of reported osteoporosis in 8073 women 20 years of age or older who participated in NHANES during 1999 to 2004 was 8.9% (95% CI: 7.7-10.1) in sedentary women but 6.2% (95% CI: 4.4-8.5) in women who said they spent at least 30 MET-hours each week doing physical activity (Robitaille et al. 2008).

• Among healthy, reproductive-age (16-33 years) women, non-Hispanic white (n = 247) women who said they spent more than 120 min each week doing weight-bearing physical activities had higher BMD at the femoral neck than those who did less than that. No association between physical activity and BMD was seen in non-Hispanic black (n = 204) or Hispanic women (n = 257) (Berenson, Rahman, and Wilkinson 2009).

Prospective Cohort Studies

There have not been many prospective cohort studies of the effect of physical activity or fitness on bone mass or risk of osteoporosis. Most prospective studies included small samples of about 25 to 200 youths or young adults and lasted only five to 12 months. Despite the short time periods of the studies, most showed a 3% to 10% increase in BMD. Many of those studies did an incomplete job of controlling for diet and other potential confounders that influence bone mass. Nonetheless, the cumulative evidence is encouraging that vigorous physical activity, especially the types that involve high peak loads (e.g., resistance exercise or power sports), might promote higher peak bone mass (Modlesky and Lewis 2002). Some key studies are summarized next.

Nebraska Women

The effects of leisure-time physical activity, diet, and use of oral contraceptives on bone mass measured by DXA were observed for about 3.5 years among 156 healthy, college-aged (mean age 21 years at the beginning of the study) white women (Recker et al. 1992). Estimates of nutrient intake were obtained from repeated seven-day diet diaries. Physical activity was assessed using the Caltrac accelerometer for four days prior to each six-month visit to the clinic. The average gain in BMD in the lumbar spine was 6.8%, and the gain in bone density of the spine was related to both calcium intake and physical activity independently; the least-active women gained an average of 0.3%, and the most active women gained 8.4%.

Framingham Osteoporosis Study

Risk factors for four-year change in BMD at the hip, radius, and spine were examined in nearly 800 elderly women and men aged 67 to 90 years (Hannan et al. 2000). Average four-year BMD loss for women (range, 3.4-4.8%) was greater than the loss for men (range, 0.2-3.6%) at all sites. For women, lower baseline weight, weight loss in interim, and greater alcohol use were associated with BMD loss. For women, current estrogen users had less bone loss than nonusers; at the femoral neck, nonusers lost up to 2.7% more BMD. For men, lower baseline weight and weight loss also were associated with BMD loss. Men who smoked cigarettes at baseline lost more BMD at the trochanter site. Bone loss was not affected by caffeine, serum 25-hydroxyvitamin D, calcium intake, or physical activity. However, a single measure of physical activity taken at the baseline may have imprecisely estimated frequency of exposure in the relatively small groups of men and women.

Rancho Bernardo, California, Men

The BMD of 507 ambulatory community-dwelling men 45 to 92 years old was assessed at the hip by DXA between 1988 and 1992 and again four years later (Bakhireva et al. 2004). Loss of BMD averaged 0.47% at the total hip and 0.34% at the femoral neck each year. The main predictors of BMD loss were an age of 75 years or older, baseline BMI <24 kg/m^2, four-year weight loss of 5% or more, current smoking, and physical inactivity. A high proportion of the men reported regular exercise (30.6% exercised often, and 48.9% exercised sometimes) three or more times per week.

Nord-Trøndelag Health Study (HUNT)

The Nord-Trøndelag Health Study (HUNT) is an ongoing population-based study in North Trøndelag, one of Norway's 19 counties. More than 20,000 women completed an initial health survey during 1984-1986 (HUNT 1), and a follow-up survey was conducted during 1995 through 1997 (HUNT 2). Approximately 8000 women had a measure of BMD at the distal and ultradistal regions of the nondominant forearm at HUNT 2. There were 1396 premenopausal women 31 to 44 years of age after exclusion of those who reported diabetes,

stroke, cancer, epilepsy, severe physical disability, rheumatoid arthritis, hyperthyroidism, perceived very poor health, severe disability, bilateral ovariectomy, or pregnancy. After further exclusion of women who also had osteoporosis or prior fractures, used calcium or vitamin D supplementation, or used asthma medication, there were 2924 postmenopausal women aged 55 to 98 years.

Premenopausal women who said they participated in high-intensity leisure-time physical activity and also did heavy physical occupational work in both 1984 and 1995 had about a 55% reduction in odds of low BMD (less than the lowest 20%) at the ultradistal radius at HUNT 2, with or without adjustments for age, smoking, amenorrhea, BMI, and daily milk consumption (Augested et al. 2004). Among postmenopausal women, odds (adjusted for age, BMI, age at menarche, years since menopause, smoking, milk consumption, and HRT) of having low BMD 10 years later at HUNT 2 at either forearm site were 30% lower in those who at HUNT 1 said they participated in high-intensity recreational physical activity.

Finnish Youths

Bone mass was associated with exercise, smoking, and dietary calcium in a prospective cohort study of 153 females and 111 males ages 9 to 18 who were observed for 11 years; their BMD was assessed by DXA when they were 20 to 29 years old (Valimaki et al. 1994). After adjustment for age and body weight, femoral neck BMD was nearly 8% higher in the women and 10% higher in the men who were the most physically active than in the least-active women and men. Similarly, BMD in the lumbar spine was 8% higher in the most active men than in the least-active men. Exercise predicted BMD in the femoral neck and the lumbar spine of the men independently of smoking.

The University of Saskatchewan Bone Mineral Study

The influence of physical activity on gains in bone mass during adolescence was observed for six years among 53 girls and 60 boys who ranged from 8 to 14 years old at the start of the study (Bailey et al. 1999). Measures of physical activity, diet, height, weight, and bone mineral content (BMC) by DXA were taken every six months. Peak rates of gain in BMC were computed for the total body, lumbar spine, and proximal femur. After adjustment for height and weight gains, the peak rate of gain in BMC in the femoral neck, lumbar spine, and total body was higher for both males and females who were more physically active than in the less active subjects. The BMC in the femoral neck measured one year after the peak rate of gain was 7% higher in boys and 9% in girls in the most active quartile compared with the least-active quartile; total-body gains were 9% and 17% higher in the most active boys and girls, respectively.

Amsterdam Growth and Health Longitudinal Study

Daily physical activity and fitness were monitored from age 13 to 29 years in a cohort of 182 males and females (Kemper et al. 2000). At a mean age of 28 years, BMD was measured by DXA at the lumbar spine, the femoral neck, and the distal radius. Physical activity during the previous three months was determined by interview when participants were between 13 and 16 years old and again between ages 21 and 27. Physical activity was expressed as energy expended (in MET-hours) per week or as peak intensity (in multiples of body mass), independently of the frequency and duration of activity. Physical fitness was measured with a neuromotor fitness test (a composite of six strength, flexibility, and speed tests) and as cardiopulmonary fitness (maximal oxygen uptake). After adjustment for sex, age, body composition, and dietary calcium, both measurements of physical activity and neuromotor fitness during adolescence and in young adulthood were positively related with the bone mass in the lumbar spine and femoral neck measured at a mean age of 28 years. Cardiorespiratory fitness was unrelated to bone mass.

Penn State Young Women's Health Study

The associations of cumulative teenage sport participation and calcium intake with gains in whole-body BMD, measured using DXA between ages 12 and 18 years, and with peak bone mass in the femoral neck at age 18 were studied in a small cohort of 81 females (Lloyd et al. 2000). Diets were assessed from 33 days of food records collected at regular intervals between ages 12 and 18 years. Calcium intake ranged from 500 to 1500 mg per day and was unrelated to femoral bone mass and whole-body gains in bone mass at age 18. The cumulative amount of sport and exercise participation was correlated with peak femoral BMD at age 18 ($r = 0.42$) but not with gains in whole-body BMD.

Swedish Youth

A school-based intervention examined BMD measured by DXA in 40 boys and 40 girls who increased their physical education classes to four times each week for three to four years from age 12 to age 16, compared with a control group of 82 boys and 66 girls of the same age who had two days of physical education each week during the same time period (Sundberg et al. 2001). Bone mineral content, BMD, and volumetric BMD were 8% to 9% higher among the boys who increased the frequency of their physical education classes compared with the control boys. The differences remained after adjustment for possible confounders, including body weight and height, milk consumption, and physical activity after school.

Clinical Studies: Endurance Exercise Training

A quantitative review of 23 randomized and nonrandomized controlled trials of endurance exercise training conducted between 1966 and 1997 concluded that exercise training led to the prevention or reversal of about 1% of the annual loss of BMD or BMC in the lumbar spine and the femoral neck in both pre- and postmenopausal women in randomized controlled trials (Wolff et al. 1999). Effects were about twice that big in the nonrandomized controlled trials; however, they were probably confounded by other factors that affect bone mass but were not controlled for because participants were not randomly assigned to the exercise intervention.

▶ **CUMULATIVE EVIDENCE** from 23 randomized and nonrandomized controlled trials indicates that endurance exercise training prevented or reversed about 1% of annual bone loss in the lumbar spine and the femoral neck.

Kohrt, Ehsani, and Birge (1997) demonstrated larger increases in BMD, especially in the femur, after a program of walking, jogging, and stair climbing up to 70% to 85% of maximal heart rate in women ages 60 to 74 years. Bone mineral density increases for the total body were 2.0% ± 0.8%; in the lumbar spine, 1.8% ± 0.8%; in the proximal femur, 6.1% ± 1.5%; and in the femoral neck, 3.5% ± 0.8%. Although those results were encouraging, they probably overestimated the independent effect of aerobic training because some of the subjects were also receiving estrogen replacement therapy. On balance, it appears that vigorous, repetitive, weight-bearing aerobic training can result in a small net increase in bone mass of 1% to 2% per year among women regardless of age.

Walking interventions in past trials probably were not frequent or lengthy enough to sufficiently load bones in the back and hips more than people's usual daily physical activity. Other evidence indicates that exercise programs that mix age-appropriate impact activities with resistance exercise can increase BMD in young women and retard bone loss in aging women, especially when the activities are unusual. Six randomized and three nonrandomized exercise trials lasting six months or longer included a total of 521 premenopausal women who did unusual or high-impact activity (e.g., vertical jumping or skipping; group exercises such as stamping, bench stepping, and hurdling), often combined with heavy resistance training or the use of weighted vests usually two or three times per week (Martyn-St James and Carroll 2010). Less than half the studies found a significant effect of exercise on BMD, often because not enough women were studied to allow detection of small effects. However, when results were averaged across the studies, BMD was increased at the lumbar

Meta-Analyses of Randomized and Nonrandomized Controlled Trials of Exercise and BMD

POSTMENOPAUSAL WOMEN

Aggregation of results from 13 trials of walking, aerobic dance, leg cycling, or resistance exercise in 700 postmenopausal women yielded a 1% increase (0.005 g/cm^2; 95% CI: 0.001 to 0.009) in BMD in the lumbar spine of 355 exercisers and a decrease of 1% (0.007 g/cm^2; 95% CI: −0.002 to 0.012) in the control group of 344 nonexercisers (±SD = −0.007 ± 0.045 g/cm^2, t = −3.051, p =0.002; 95% CI: −0.012 to 0.002) (Kelley, Kelley, and Tran 2002).

Averaged across eight randomized or nonrandomized trials of walking lasting six to 24 months, the increase in BMD at the lumbar spine was too small to reach statistical significance (0.007 g/cm^2; 95% CI: −0.001 to 0.016) (Martyn-St James and Carroll 2008). Averaged across five trials, there was an increase in BMD at the femoral neck (0.014 g/cm^2; 95% CI: 0.000-0.028). Ten randomized controlled and nonrandomized trials of aerobic and resistance hip loading exercises, lasting 32 to 104 weeks and including 595 postmenopausal women 42 to 92 years old, showed an average increase in BMD at the femoral neck of 0.73%, which was not different from the value in control participants who did not exercise (Kelley and Kelley 2006).

Fourteen groups from randomized controlled trials of high-intensity resistance exercise in postmenopausal women showed an average increase in BMD of 0.006 g/cm^2 (95% CI: 0.002-0.011) at the lumbar spine, and 11 groups from randomized controlled trial studies showed an increase of 0.010 g/cm^2 (95% CI: −0.002 to 0.021) at the femoral neck (Martyn-St James and Carroll 2006a).

A recent meta-analysis of 43 randomized but usually poorly controlled trials of 4320 post-menopausal women concluded that high force, progressive resistance exercise was more effective than weight-bearing exercises such as walking for increasing BMD at about the neck of the femur, whereas programs that combined different types of exercise were more effective for increasing BMD in the spine (Howe et al. 2011).

PREMENOPAUSAL WOMEN

High-intensity progressive resistance training increased BMD at the lumbar spine 1% (0.014 g/cm^2; 95% CI: 0.009-0.019) but not at the femoral neck (0.001 g/cm^2; 95% CI: −0.006 to 0.008) (Martyn-St James and Carroll 2006b).

MEN

Averaged across eight studies including 225 men, increases of about 2.6% (2.1% in the exercisers vs. −0.5% in the controls) were found at the femur and lumbar spine after exercises that put loads on the bone sites assessed. Effects were statistically significant only for men older than 31 years (0.21 SD) (Kelley, Kelley, and Tran 2000).

---

spine (0.009 g/cm^2; 95% CI: 0.002-0.015) and the femoral neck (0.007 g/cm^2; 95% CI: 0.001-0.013). High-impact exercise alone was effective only at the femoral neck (0.024 g/cm^2; 95% CI: 0.002-0.027).

When results were averaged across 15 randomized and nonrandomized trials of nearly 700 postmenopausal women, exercise programs that mixed jogging with other low-impact loading activities such as walking or stair climbing, or that mixed impact activities (e.g., rope skipping or jumping) with resistance training, increased BMD by a range of 0.016 g/cm^2 (95% CI: 0.005-0.027) to 0.025 g/cm^2 (95% CI: 0.004-0.046) at the lumbar spine and from 0.005 g/cm^2 (95% CI: 0.001-0.010) to 0.022 g/cm^2 (95% CI: 0.014-0.030) at the femoral neck (Martyn-St James and Carroll 2009). Exercises that were only high impact or only unusual impact did not increase BMD at either site.

Clinical Studies: Resistance Exercise Training

Consensus has emerged that exercises producing high peak forces that overload bone are effective for increasing and maintaining bone mass, regardless of age (Layne and Nelson 1999; Vuori 2001).

Postmenopausal Women

Several resistance training studies have found that high-intensity (e.g., 80% of maximal strength) training can increase bone mass at specific sites among postmenopausal women without estrogen replacement. Bone mineral density in the lumbar spine was increased (mean ± SE) by 1.6% ± 1.2% after nine months of weight training among

17 postmenopausal women, compared with a 3.6% ± 1.5% loss in BMD in a control group of nine women who did not weight train. Resistance exercise had no effect, though, on BMD at the femoral neck or distal radius at the wrist (Pruitt et al. 1992).

A randomized controlled trial examined whether a high-load, low-repetition program (three sets of 8RM; RM = repetition maximum) designed to maximize strength gains or a low-load, high-repetition program (three sets of 20RM) designed to maximize gains in muscular endurance would have the greater effect on bone mass in 56 postmenopausal women (Kerr et al. 1996). Bone mineral density gains measured by DXA after a year of thrice-weekly progressive resistance training of the forearms and hips on one side of the body were compared between the two types of training and with the other side of the body, which provided a nonexercise control. Strength (1RM) was increased for 10 exercises in both training groups; but with the exception of a single midradial site, the endurance program did not change bone mass. The high-load strength program led to increases of about 1.5% to 2% at the hip sites and 2.4% at the distal radius, whereas the control sites had reductions in BMD of 0.1% to 1.4%.

A subsequent randomized controlled trial conducted by the same investigators compared the effects of a two-year exercise intervention and calcium supplementation (600 mg) on BMD in 126 postmenopausal women (mean age, 60 ± 5 years), who were assigned to either progressive strength training or strength plus leg cycling exercise at a minimal load (Kerr et al. 2001). The two exercise groups completed three sets of the same nine exercises three times a week. Bone mineral density was measured by DXA at the hip, lumbar spine, and forearm sites every six months. Both groups had a 0.9% increase in total-body BMD and a 1.1% increase in hip BMD.

Site-Specific Loading

Some studies have focused on the site-specific principles of mechanical loading. One study compared 12 men who engaged in strength training for at least one year with 50 age-matched controls (Colletti et al. 1989). The exercise group increased BMD compared with the control group in the weight-bearing sites of the lumbar spine, trochanter, and femoral neck, but no increase was seen in the non-weight-bearing site of the midradius. The effects of resistance training and bone density have been seen in older populations.

A program of dynamic loading exercises of the distal forearm was performed three times a week for five months by 14 postmenopausal osteoporotic women; 26 osteoporotic women served as controls (Simkin, Ayalon, and Leichter 1987). After the five-month period, the exercise group had an increase in BMD of 3.8% in the radius, while the control group had a decrease of 1.9%.

Eccentric muscle training may be even more effective in bone formation than concentric training. Eccentric muscle contraction generates more force per muscle area. Twelve

women ages 20 to 23 years at the University of Southern California participated in an 18-week strength training program that involved training one leg using eccentric knee extension and flexion and the opposite leg using concentric extension and flexion (Hawkins et al. 1999). Eight similar women served as controls. There were no significant differences between exercise and control subjects in total BMD or hip BMD at the beginning or end of the study. The eccentric exercise significantly increased BMD in the midfemur by 3.9%; concentric exercise produced a nonsignificant increase of 1.1%; and the control group had a 0.6% increase. These findings suggest that the greater force produced by eccentric exercise was responsible for the greater increase in bone mass.

Other evidence suggests that BMD in young premenopausal women does not benefit from lower body resistance exercise. Aggregated results from 74 exercisers and 69 controls (women who didn't exercise) indicated no change in BMD in the lumbar spine or femoral neck (Kelley and Kelley 2004). However, it is unlikely that the type of exercise maneuvers used in the studies produced peak loads on the low back or hip sufficient to increase bone mineral in normal young bones.

Resistance exercise training also can be effective against glucocorticoid-induced bone loss, which can occur after antirejection drug therapy among heart transplant patients. In a prospective randomized controlled program, eight male transplant recipients participated in a resistance training program and restored almost all of their preoperation total-body, femoral neck, and lumbar spine bone mass, while eight transplant patients in the control group lost bone mass (Braith et al. 1996).

Researchers in Italy reported the first clinical evidence in humans that bones can adapt themselves to increased loading by transferring bone mineral from the trabecular bone compartment to the cortical shell (Adami et al. 1999). Postmenopausal women aged 52 to 72 years either participated in a six-month exercise program ($n = 118$) that specifically loaded the wrist or did not exercise ($n = 116$). The exercisers spent 70 min each session doing exercises that included push-ups and playing volleyball either sitting or standing. Ten minutes were spent in intermittent bouts (3 min every 15 min) of partly supinated forearm curls of a 500 g weight. Frequency of lifts per minute increased progressively from 10 to 25 over the months. Sessions were held twice each week, and the women were asked to do the exercises at home for 30 min or more each day. There was no effect of exercise on BMD measured by DXA at the femoral neck, the lumbar spine, or the radius. However, measures of bone area, BMC, and volumetric density using quantitative computed tomography of the ultradistal radius showed 3% increases both in the cross-sectional area of the cortical bone and in cortical BMC. Because of a greater than 3% decrease in trabecular BMC, there was no net change in total BMC. Thus, the ultradistal radial bone apparently adapted to loading by increasing both the cross-sectional area and density of its cortical component at the expense of its trabecular component. See figure 11.7.

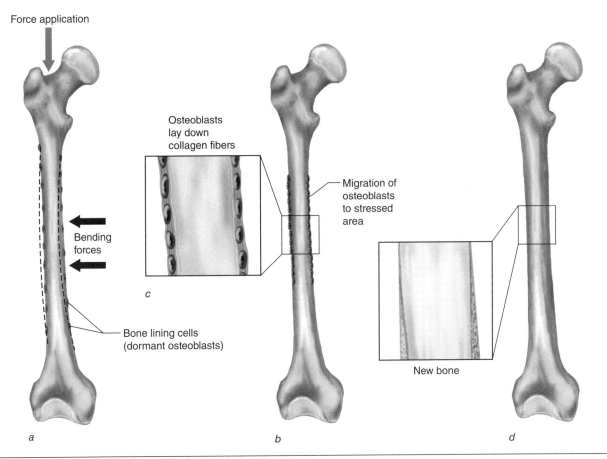

Figure 11.7 Mechanical loads that bend bone will increase periosteal cortical bone.

Reprinted, by permission, from N.R. Ratamess, 2008, Adaptations to anaerobic training programs. In *Essentials of strength training and conditioning*, 3rd ed., by National Strength and Conditioning Association, edited by T.R. Baechle and R.W. Earle (Champaign, IL: Human Kinetics), 103.

This should increase its bending strength. Research on rats has shown that sudden-impact loading on bone does not change its BMC or size as measured by DXA but can increase the load at which the bone will fracture by as much as 14% (Järvinen et al. 1998).

Randomized controlled trials conducted since those early studies have found that exercise enhances whole bone strength at loaded sites in children but not in adults. Aggregated findings from 10 trials lasting six or more months, using quantitative computed tomography (QCT), magnetic resonance imaging (MRI), or DXA-based hip structural analysis (HSA), indicated small effects of 1% to 8% in children and adolescents and 0.5% to 2.5% in premenopausal women who exercised the most (Nikander et al. 2010). There were no effects in postmenopausal women. Only the effect (about 0.20 SD) for boys in prepuberty or early puberty was statistically significant (see figure 11.8). Puberty may affect bone responses to exercise differently in girls and boys. Some evidence suggests that estrogens in girls contribute more to BMD while androgens in boys contribute more to cortical bone growth. However, the types and amounts of exercise varied widely, and many of the studies were too small to detect small or moderate changes.

Canadian Boys

A seven-month jumping program (10 min, three times per week) led to a 1.6% gain in total BMC and a 1% gain in BMD in the femur of 61 prepubertal 10-year-old Asian and white boys from 14 schools in Canada compared to a randomized control group of 60 boys (MacKelvie et al. 2002).

Exercise Plus Hormone Replacement Therapy in Postmenopausal Women

Although estrogen-deficient women can benefit from weight-bearing exercise, exercise alone cannot substitute for HRT during the early postmenopausal phase of rapid bone loss. During the first five years after menopause, women who do not take estrogen can lose up to 35% of their bone mass. The combination of HRT and exercise may yield the greatest effect on bone because estrogen may enhance the osteogenic effect of mechanical loading. Several studies have examined whether estrogen plus weight training is more effective than just weight training or estrogen replacement alone. Notelovitz and colleagues (1991) showed that weight training enhanced the bone-conserving effect of estrogen in

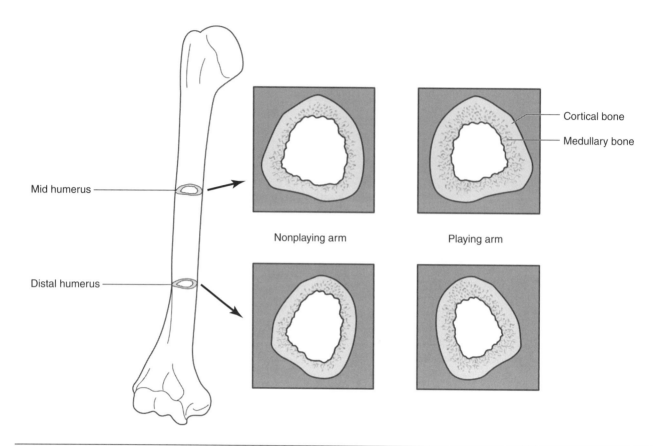

Figure 11.8   Changes in cortical bone in female tennis players. Magnetic resonance imaging of cortical bone (outer layer) and medullary bone (inner layer) of the nondominant and dominant arms of postpubertal tennis players. Bone mineral content strength was about 10% to 15% greater in the playing arm because of increases in periosteal bone that occurred during prepubertal years of playing and remained stable during continued playing after puberty.

Reprinted, by permission, from S.L. Bass et al., 2002, "The effect of mechanical loading on the size and shape of bone in pre-, peri-, and postpubertal girls: A study in tennis players," *Journal Bone Mineral Research* 17: 2274-2280.

surgically postmenopausal women. After one year of weight training plus estrogen therapy, spine BMD significantly increased by 8.3% ± 5.3% while an estrogen-only group merely maintained BMD, with a slight increase of only 1.5% ± 12.4%. Kohrt and colleagues (1995) described a one-year intervention trial that compared the combined and separate effects of HRT and weight-bearing exercises in 32 women with an average age of 66. The combination of HRT and high-intensity exercise had additive and synergistic effects on BMD, depending on the site measured. These findings suggest that each treatment acts via an independent mechanism; thus, exercise can have an additional beneficial effect on bone when used in conjunction with estrogen.

Prince and colleagues (1991) performed the first large prospective study. This two-year study compared four groups: sedentary controls, exercise subjects, an exercise plus calcium group, and an exercise plus HRT group. Each group consisted of 40 postmenopausal women, all with BMD at the distal radius 1 standard deviation below the fracture threshold as determined by CT scan. The mean age of the subjects was 56. Calcium supplementation slowed bone loss, and HRT increased bone mass, but the rate of bone loss was

similar for the exercise-only group and the sedentary controls. However, the exercise stimulus was inadequate in this study. It consisted of 1 h of supervised low-impact aerobics each week, and exercise compliance was less than 50%. Moreover, the wrist would not be expected to respond to low-impact weight-bearing exercise.

In contrast, a randomized controlled trial evaluated the effect of one month or three months of combination estrogen and progesterone therapy on menopausal symptoms, bone density, muscle strength, and lipid metabolism in 78 postmenopausal women ages 49 to 55 years (Heikkinen et al. 1997). Hormone replacement therapy and placebo groups were further randomized to exercise or no-exercise subgroups. Hormone replacement therapy was effective for slowing loss of BMD in the lumbar spine and proximal femur. In addition, exercise slowed bone loss in the placebo group, but exercise provided no additional benefit beyond the effects of HRT in the HRT plus exercise group.

In another study, 167 sedentary, postmenopausal women who received calcium supplements (about 700 to 900 mg/ day) were randomized to a program of progressive, heavy resistance exercise or to control and were followed for four years (Cussler et al. 2005). Half the women were also getting HRT. Exercisers were instructed to complete two sets of six to eight repetitions of exercises at 70% to 80% of 1RM three times weekly. Actual compliance with the frequency ranged from about 25% to 50% of prescribed frequency, on average. The frequency of actual exercise was positively related to BMD increases in the trochanter and neck of the femur, the lumbar spine, and total body. Among hormone therapy users, BMD increased 1.5% in the trochanter and 1.2% in both the femur neck and lumbar spine BMD for every day of weekly exercise. The increases were 1.9% and 2.3%, respectively, among women who were not on hormone therapy. These findings support the long-term effectiveness of strength training exercise for reducing bone loss in postmenopausal women, including those who are using HRT.

Physical Activity and Risks of Falls or Fractures

The scientific advisory committee of the 2008 Physical Activity Guidelines for Americans concluded that a greater amount of physical activity (i.e., frequency, duration, or intensity or more than one of these) has an inverse dose–response relation with the risk of fractures of the hip (i.e., proximal femur) (Physical Activity Guidelines Advisory Committee 2008).

A few studies have suggested that neuromuscular effects of resistance exercise training can aid in the prevention of falls and subsequent fractures in older people (Nelson et al. 1994). However, an early review concluded that observational population-based studies and randomized controlled trials of the effectiveness of physical activity programs to prevent falls had been inconclusive, in part because many studies did not include enough people to show that the modest effects were statistically significant or did not focus on types of exercise training most likely to reduce the risks of falling (Gregg, Pereira, and Caspersen 2000). The reviewers concluded that more recent clinical trials had suggested that exercise training specifically using exercises designed to improve balance and leg strength can reduce the risk of falling, which could reduce the risk of hip and wrist fractures. Finally, they concluded that there was consistent evidence from retrospective case–control and prospective cohort studies of an association between leisure-time physical activity and a 20% to 40% reduced risk of hip fracture but not for an association between physical activity and risks of wrist or spine fractures. Similarly, a meta-analysis concluded that exercise alone does not reduce fall risk in elderly women and men (Gillespie et al. 2001). However, many early studies included frail nursing home residents, who had risk factors for falling besides low strength or poor balance (such as poor eyesight) that would not be helped by exercise; many also used exercise intensities too low to increase strength (American College of Sports Medicine 2004).

A review of 34 randomized controlled trials or nonrandomized trials involving mostly women around the age of 75 years found small improvements in the ability to stand on one leg, reach forward without overbalancing, and walk, especially when mixed types of exercise—balancing, functional movements, and muscle strengthening—were used to target gait (Howe et al. 2007).

British Women and Men

The associations of low dietary calcium intake and physical inactivity measured by interview and medical exam in 1973 to 1974 with 15-year risk of hip fractures were evaluated in a case–control study of 441 women and 542 men 65 years old or older who lived in five areas in England, two areas in Scotland, and an area in Wales (Wickham et al. 1989). Incidence of hip fracture increased with age and was higher in women than in men but was unrelated to a seven-day recall of calcium intake. After adjustment for smoking and BMI, the odds ratio of hip fractures in the lowest tertile for outdoor physical activity compared with the highest tertile was 4.3 (95% CI: 0.7-26.8) and was 3.9 (95% CI: 0.7-23.0) in the lowest tertile for grip strength.

Study of Osteoporotic Fractures

Potential risk factors for osteoporotic fractures, including low bone mass, were studied in 9516 white women 65 years or older living in Baltimore, Minneapolis, or Portland (Oregon) or around Pittsburgh who were able to walk and had no previous hip fracture. The women were examined every four months to determine incidence of hip fracture, which was verified by X ray (Cummings et al. 1995). During an average of 4.1 years of observation, 192 women had a first hip fracture. The incidence ranged from a low of 1.1 fractures per 1000 woman-years among women who had two or fewer risk factors and normal bone density for their age to a high of 27 fractures per 1000 woman-years among those who had five or more risk factors and bone density in the lowest third for their age. Maternal history of hip fracture and current use of anticonvulsant drugs each doubled the risk of hip fracture, while walking for exercise and a resting pulse rate below 80 beats/min reduced risk by 30% and 40%, respectively, regardless of whether the women had lower or higher bone density of the heel or otherwise spent at least 4 h a day on their feet.

Framingham Osteoporosis Study

Seven hundred women and men from the Framingham cohort who had radiographic examinations at baseline in 1967-1969, when they were mostly in their late 40s or mid 50s, were evaluated again in 1992 or 1993 (Samelson et al. 2006). Incident crush fractures of vertebrae were defined as at least mildly deformed (20-25% reduction or more in any vertebral height) at follow-up. Age, height, weight, grip strength, metacarpal cortical area, estrogen use (in women), and physical activity measured at baseline had little or no influence on cumulative incidence of vertebral fracture. However, this is partly explainable by the limited measures of exposure and the small groups of men and women. Odds of fracture were lower in moderately active (middle tertile) men

(OR = 0.44; 95% CI: 0.16-1.18) and women (OR = 0.82; 95% CI: 0.52-1.30) compared to the least active (lowest tertile); but the confidence intervals of the odd ratios included 1.0, partly because of the small numbers of people.

Finnish Men

The association between leisure physical activity measured in 1975 and future risk of osteoporotic hip fracture was studied prospectively for about 21 years in a cohort of 3262 men who were 44 years old or older and did not have any diseases that limited their participation in physical activity (Kujala et al. 2000). After adjustment for the potential confounders height, BMI, baseline diseases, smoking, use of alcohol, work-related physical activity, and occupational group, the relative risk of osteoporotic hip fracture among men participating in vigorous physical activity was 0.38 (95% CI: 0.16-0.91) compared with sedentary men.

Copenhagen, Denmark

Risk of first hip fracture (1121 incident cases) was aggregated from findings from three population studies of 13,183 women and 17,045 men (Høidrup et al. 2001). People who initially were highly or moderately active in their leisure time but became sedentary had about double the risk of hip fracture compared with those who remained moderately physically active. A decline in the physical activity over time was risky, but an increase in physical activity was not protective.

The Nurses' Health Study

Risk of hip fracture in more than 61,000 postmenopausal women was reduced by about 6% for every 3 MET-hours of weekly physical activity (about 1 h of walking per week) (Feskanich, Willett, and Colditz 2002). Women who reported walking at least 4 h each week had a 41% lower risk compared with sedentary women who walked less an hour per week. The protective effect of walking against hip fracture was seen even though those amounts of walking are known to have only a small impact on BMD.

Uppsala Longitudinal Study of Adult Men

A cohort of 2205 men, 49 to 51 years of age, living in Uppsala, Sweden, was followed for 35 years. Leisure physical activity and other lifestyle habits were established at baseline and at ages 60, 70, 77, and 82 years (Michaëlsson et al. 2007). During follow-up, 482 men had at least one fracture, including 134 hip fractures. Sedentary men had about 60% higher risk of any fracture compared to the most active men who said they regularly participated in recreational sport or did heavy gardening for 3 or more hours each week. Compared to the lowest rates of hip fracture in the most active men (about 8%), rates were elevated in men who walked or bicycled only for pleasure (13%; RR = 1.6; 95% CI: 1.1-2.4)

and in men who were sedentary in their leisure time (20%; RR= 2.6; 95% CI: 1.6-4.2). About one-third of hip fractures were potentially preventable by participation in regular sports or heavy gardening activities.

Women's Health Initiative (WHI)

During an average of about eight years of observation, 1132 hip fractures occurred in 93,676 women (0.16% per year) who initially were 50 to 79 years old (Robbins et al. 2007). Eleven factors were independent predictors of hip fracture within five years: age, self-reported health, weight, height, race-ethnicity, history of fracture after age 54 years, parental hip fracture, current smoking, current corticosteroid use, treated diabetes, and low physical activity. An index based on those risk factors had about 70% accuracy for predicting hip fracture compared to 80% prediction accuracy based on DXA bone scanning. Women who said they got 12 or more MET-hours of physical activity each week had 25% lower risk of fracture than women who got between 5 and 12 MET-hours and 40% lower risk than women who were sedentary.

Erlangen-Nuremberg, Germany

About 250 women aged 65 years or older who were living independently were randomized to an 18-month trial of a multipurpose exercise program that emphasized intensity or to a control group that did low-intensity activities less frequently (Kemmler et al. 2010). The exercise group had increases in BMD in the lumbar spine (1.77%) and femoral neck (1%) and a 60% reduction in falls (one fall per exercising woman compared to 1.6 falls per woman in the control group) during the 18 months.

Strength of the Evidence

Randomized controlled studies provide the most valid evaluation of treatment effects by minimizing the effects of confounders that can influence bone outcomes, thus isolating the effects of physical activity. The cumulative, average effect in randomized trials of resistance training on BMD in the lumbar spine and the femoral neck in both pre- and postmenopausal women was about a 0.9% per year when compared with women who did not exercise (Wolff et al. 1999). The effects of exercise reported by nonrandomized trials were nearly twice that size, but these studies probably overestimate the true effects as a result of poor control of confounders such as selection bias introduced by volunteers, who may be more likely to benefit than randomly selected subjects.

A few observational retrospective and prospective cohort studies and case–control studies have suggested that physical activity reduces the risk of falls and osteoporotic fractures. However, there are few well-controlled epidemiologic studies linking physical activity with risk of developing osteoporosis or fractures in a large population base. Analogously to what we acknowledged in previous chapters on other chronic diseases, it is unlikely that a randomized, double-blind, placebo-controlled trial will ever be funded to demonstrate whether physical activity or vigorous exercise carried out during youth, adulthood, or old age reduces osteoporosis-related fractures in old age (Karlsson, Bass, and Seeman 2001). Nonetheless, a circumstantial body of evidence has accumulated that is encouraging. Specifically, studies collectively suggest that resistance exercise is associated with (1) an increase in peak bone mass and (2) a slowing of osteopenia during middle age. A few studies also suggest that resistance exercise training has potential to promote (1) a reversal of bone mass loss in old age, (2) a reduction in risk factors for falls and the incidence of falls, and (3) a reduction in fractures resulting from falls among the elderly.

Modification and Confounders

Though increased bone mass after exercise training has been reported in both premenopausal and postmenopausal women, other age-related factors may modify the osteogenic effects of exercise. Several studies that failed to show a significant increase in bone density after strength training apparently did not impose the high strains, high strain rates, or strain distribution required to induce bone remodeling. Programs that fulfill all of these requirements may not be the most desirable ones for elderly people. For the frail elderly, they may even involve risks.

Beyond meeting the requirements of necessary strains on the bone, there are large differences among training programs in type, duration, frequency, and intensity. Comparing intensities in different programs may be the most difficult aspect because of insufficient and nonstandardized descriptions of intensity. Other important sources of heterogeneity among studies are the use of vitamin D, calcium supplementation, and HRT. All are known to have a positive influence on BMD (Prince et al. 1991).

Bone mass differences at baseline can also explain various treatment effects. Individuals with low bone mass at the beginning of a training program are likely to show a greater increase in bone mass than those who start out with higher bone mass. Bone mass is positively related to body weight (Khosla et al. 1996; Alekel et al. 1995); therefore, weight loss in exercise groups can be a confounder in long-term interventions. Weight loss as a result of the training study might lead to underestimation of the effect of the program (Wolff et al. 1999).

Temporal Sequence

Though more cross-sectional studies of physical activity and bone mass have been reported, several prospective cohort studies had follow-up periods ranging from about three months to 12 years, and randomized controlled trials typically lasted five to 12 months and as long as two years.

Strength of Association

The cumulative evidence from cross-sectional studies suggests that participants in repetitive weight-bearing activities have about 5% higher bone mass than sedentary controls; participants in resistance exercise training or sports that have high peak loads have 10% to 15% higher bone mass than sedentary controls. The few prospective cohort studies suggest a 3% to 10% increase in BMD and an average reduction in risk of fractures of the hip of 20% to 40% among physically active people. The aggregate effect of randomized controlled trials on middle-aged or older women is a reduction or reversal in the loss of bone mass with age of about 1% per year. Even a 1% to 2% change in BMD, coupled with increased strength and better balance, might lower fracture risk as much as 50% (Kemmler et al. 2010).

Consistency

Most prospective observational studies and randomized controlled trials have involved white women, who are at greatest risk of osteoporosis. Nonetheless, the overall evidence for a favorable effect of physical activity on bone health seems to occur in prepubertal youths, adult men, and both pre- and postmenopausal women regardless of race, ethnicity, or age.

However, the way bone adapts to exercise seems to vary by age, skeletal site, and sex. Before and during puberty, increases in the size of the shaft of long bones mainly result from new periosteal bone (i.e., the outer surface), especially in boys. In contrast, at distal skeletal sites that are composed mostly of trabecular bone, exercise increases the density of bone by increasing either the thickness of trabecular bone or new endocortical bone (i.e., the inner surface) (Daly 2007). In adults, the limited data from intervention trials suggest that any increase in bone strength is due largely to increased bone mineral, reduced endocortical bone loss, or both, rather than an increase in bone size (Nikander et al. 2010).

Dose Response

There is no evidence regarding whether the effects of physical activity on peak bone mass in youth and young adulthood depend on the type or intensity of physical activity. Similarly, there is no direct evidence to indicate whether the effect of physical activity on maintaining bone mass in premenopausal women and retarding or reversing bone loss in postmenopausal women is dose dependent. Nonetheless, it appears that site-specific effects on bone mineral content and density are greater for resistance exercise and sporting activities that place high peak loads on bone than for low-impact, repetitive, weight-bearing activities (Vuori 2001). Most studies that show favorable effects of exercise on bone health in children before puberty or in early puberty involved 10 to 60 min durations of moderate to high-strain activity (impact, weight bearing) for two or three or more days per week (Strong et al. 2005).

Minimum levels of physical activity associated with reduced fracture risk in adults are at least 9 to 14.9 MET-hours per week of physical activity, more than 4 h per week of walking, at least 1290 kcal per week of physical activity, and more than 1 h per week of physical activity (Physical Activity Guidelines Advisory Committee 2008).

Biological Plausibility

The skeleton has two main extrinsic forces acting on it during exercise: (1) gravity and (2) the pull of the muscle–tendon unit during muscular contraction, locomotion, and maintenance of posture. These torsion, shearing, bending, and compression forces during exercise can provide the mechanical stress necessary to stimulate bone remodeling and increased bone mass (Khosla et al. 1996).

Research has indicated that the magnitude of loading stress on bone has a greater influence on bone density than the number of cycles of bone loading. Daily activities may provide several loading cycles but usually fail to provide sufficient loading magnitudes (Whalon, Carter, and Steele 1988). Generating the high inertial forces that increase bone mass requires greater muscular exertion and velocities than most people achieve during the physical activities of daily living; consequently most people do not attain the bone densities observed among athletes whose sports require high ground reaction and joint reaction forces.

Although the geometric properties of bone are determined genetically, the internal architecture, BMD, and internal and external bone diameter respond to environmental forces, which influence the balance of bone resorption and bone formation. Bone adapts to mechanical needs by atrophy and hypertrophy. The mechanical laws that regulate the structural architecture of bone tissue are not fully understood (Martin and McCulloch 1987). However, several theories provide plausible ways in which exercise could positively influence bone mass.

Proposed over 100 years ago, Wolff's law posits that mechanical loading applied to the bone causes change or remodeling of the bone's microstructural architecture (Wolff 1892). When bone is bent or is under a mechanical load, it modifies its structure by building layers of new cells on its concave side and by resorption of old cells on its convex side. Long bones tend to align along the axis of force by hypertrophy in the areas that are compressed (Chamay and Tschantz 1972). The biochemical mechanisms that explain how mechanical strain is translated into an increase in BMD are still not fully understood. Several mechanisms have been proposed, including piezoelectric potentials; release of prostaglandins; increased bone blood flow and hormonal response; and a cascade of prostaglandins, nitric oxide, and growth factors in response to load imbalances communicated among bone cells. Most likely, a combination of the following proposed mechanisms is involved in bone formation.

Piezoelectric Effects

An early hypothesis of bone remodeling is that bone acts as a piezoelectric crystal (Bassett and Becker 1962; Brighton et al. 1985; Lanyon and Hartman 1977). Strains that are placed on the bone cause it to bend or vibrate. These strains are translated into biochemical signals that appear to be mediated by electric fields. Loads cause transient electrical potential differences across the bone, which act as pulsed electric fields that stimulate deposits of positively charged calcium ions on the negatively charged side of the bone cell. Conversely, positively charged calcium ions are resorbed from the positively charged side of the bone cell. This is believed to result in an increased ratio of bone osteoblast activity to bone osteoclast activity at the points of stress, yielding formation of new bone. Early studies showed that application of electrical stimulation caused an increase in bone formation in animals (Bassett 1965), and applied electromagnetic fields have more recently been proposed as a clinically useful approach to the prevention of osteoporosis in people who are at high risk of developing osteoporosis (Bassett 1995; Tabrah et al. 1990).

Prostaglandins

Electrical stimulation of bone also increases the production of adenosine 3,5-cyclic monophosphate (cAMP) and prostaglandin E2 (PGE2) by osteoblasts. Prostaglandin is a necessary part of bone formation under loading conditions. The synthesis of PGE2 results from the stretching of bone cell membranes, which exposes cell membrane phospholipids to phospholipase A2 (Chamay and Tschantz 1972). The synthesis of PGE2 increases intracellular levels of cAMP, which acts to increase DNA and RNA synthesis of new bone proteins.

Blood Flow and Hormonal Response

Bone formation may also be stimulated by increased blood flow to the bones as a response to the metabolic demands of exercise, which can increase the diffusion surface area of bone cells and deliver more nutrients to osteocytes, perhaps increasing their production of bone growth factors (Chilibeck, Sale, and Webber 1995). Also, hormonal responses during exercise may stimulate the activity of osteoblasts. For example, osteoblasts have receptors for dihydrotestosterone, which can increase the gene expression of bone DNA by osteoblasts. Muscle contraction can result in spikes of increased testosterone in the blood, and weight training has reportedly led to increased production of endogenous testosterone (Kraemer, Marchitelli, and Gordon 1990). However, because it appears that bone formation is localized, as is seen in the dominant arm of tennis players or carpenters (Huddleston et al. 1980), the influence of general factors such as blood flow and hormonal action on bone changes after exercise seems very limited.

The Error-Strain Distribution Theory of Bone Remodeling

The error-strain distribution theory by Lanyon (1996) proposed that cells derived from osteoblasts and distributed on the surface of bone and in the bone matrix can sense mechanical strain, or load imbalances, and communicate with one another via gap junctions. The feedback about these load imbalances within bone tissue results in an influx of calcium ions, prostaglandins, nitric oxide, and growth hormones to the area of strain. This error-strain mechanism can explain bone remodeling, protection against fatigue cracks, mineral exchange, and repair of microdamage (Rawlinson, Pitsillides, and Lanyon 1996; Lanyon 1993). These feedback responses are determined not only by the magnitude of the load placed on the bone but also by the frequency of the application of these loads (Rubin and Lanyon 1984). High loads and low frequencies, similar to typical resistance exercise, appear to be optimal for inducing bone hypertrophy.

Bone Turnover After Exercise

Cross-sectional studies have shown that strength training is associated with high BMD or with bone metabolism that favors a high BMD (Block et al. 1989). Bell and colleagues (1988) found higher levels of osteocalcin, serum 1,25-dihydroxyvitamin D, and urinary cAMP, indicative of elevated bone turnover, among people who strength trained than among inactive control subjects. In one longitudinal study, serum concentrations of osteocalcin, bone-specific alkaline phosphatase (BAP, an enzyme marker of bone formation), and tartrate-resistant acid phosphatase (TRACP, an enzyme marker of bone resorption) were measured before, during, and after a 16-week strength training program (Menkes et al. 1993). Serum concentrations of osteocalcin

---

Error-Strain Distribution Hypothesis of Mechanical Osteogenesis

1. Bone cells sense mechanical strain from weight-bearing or resistance exercises.

2. Load imbalances are communicated among cells locally, leading to an influx of calcium ions.

3. The calcium ions are followed by prostaglandins, nitric oxide, and growth hormones, leading to bone remodeling.

Adapted from Lanyon 1996.

---

increased by 19% ± 6% after 12 weeks of training and remained significantly elevated after 16 weeks of training compared with those in the control group. Blood levels of BAP increased by 26% ± 11% after 16 weeks of training. Blood levels of TRACP increased at each measured time point, but the differences were not statistically significant. When bone turnover was expressed as a ratio of bone formation to bone resorption (i.e., BAP/TRACP), the exercise training group had a significant increase of 16% ± 9% in bone remodeling after four months.

A more recent study suggests that increased bone density in older people after exercise training depends on bone turnover. Markers of bone turnover were assessed in 62 men and women ages 60 to 83 years after six months of progressive resistance exercise, either 13 repetitions at 50% of 1RM or eight repetitions at 80% of 1RM, three times a week. Serum levels of BAP, osteocalcin, and pyridinoline cross-links were measured (Vincent and Braith 2002). The percentage increase in total strength was about 17% for both exercise intensities. Bone mineral density of the femoral neck increased by 2% in the high-intensity group only. The increase in osteocalcin was 25% after low-intensity training but 39% after high-intensity training. BAP increased by 7% only after high-intensity training.

The effects on bone mass and serum levels of insulin-like growth factor I (IGF-I) of six months of a moderate-intensity, seated resistance training program were compared with those of a high-intensity, standing, free-weight exercise program in healthy older men (mean age about 55 years) and postmenopausal women without estrogen replacement (Maddalozzo and Snow 2000). The high-intensity training resulted in a gain in BMD in the spine and hip in men but not in women, whereas moderate-intensity training produced no changes in either sex at these sites. Despite a nearly 38% increase in strength, the bone mass changes were unrelated to blood levels of IGF-I.

Another study examined the effects of four months of a progressive resistance training program on blood markers of bone turnover, including osteocalcin, BAP, IGF-I, and C-terminal cross-linked telopeptide of type I collagen (ICTP; Sartorio et al. 2001). Thirty men ages 65 to 81 years were randomly assigned to a control group that sustained their usual physical activity or to a group that performed 10 repetitions each of six different sets of exercises using the major muscle groups (two for the lower limb and four for the upper limb) three times a week. The men warmed up each time with 15 min of cycling exercise at 50% of maximal oxygen uptake and 15 repetitions of each exercise at 20% of 1RM. Lower limb training graduated from 50% to 80% of 1RM during the first month. Upper limb exercises graduated from 40% to 65% of 1RM. Resistance exercise did not change osteocalcin or IGF-I levels, but BAP levels increased by 25%, and ICTP levels decreased by 5%. Bone turnover, expressed as the ratio of bone formation to bone resorption

Principles of Exercise to Optimize Bone Health

- Dynamic, not static
- High peak loads that are frequent and intermittent
- Imposition of an unusual loading pattern on the bones
- Support with unlimited nutrient energy
- Adequate calcium and vitamin D3 (cholecalciferol)

Adapted from Borer 2005

(i.e., BAP/ICTP), increased by 34% after the resistance exercise training, whereas no changes in the markers of bone turnover were seen in the control group.

In a large cohort (n = 530) of healthy premenopausal Italian women, BMD levels in the spine and several bone formation markers (osteocalcin and N-terminal propeptide of type 1 procollagen [P1NP]), but not serum C-telopeptide of type I collagen (sCTX), were positively associated with the level of physical activity, even after adjustment for age and BMI. Twenty-four of the women who participated in a month-long community exercise program had a 25% increase in osteocalcin and P1NP but no change in sCTX, regardless of changes in body weight, when compared to 18 age-matched controls who didn't exercise (Adami et al. 2008).

Summary

The two main tactics for reducing risks of bone fracture from low trauma are first to maximize peak bone mineral during childhood and young adulthood and second to minimize the drop in bone mineral after the age of 40 that is partly explainable by aging, including endocrine changes and declining physical activity. Physical activity can increase peak bone mass in children, can mechanically stimulate bone formation and the accumulation of bone mineral, and can help preserve bone mass during aging. Resistance and agility exercises can also strengthen muscles and improve balance, which reduce the risk of falls and fractures in people who are elderly. The adaptation by bone to loads is apparently optimized when the load results in unusually high peak strain applied at a high rate for short intervals (Lanyon 1996). Hence, exercise sessions designed to promote increases in bone mass should hypothetically involve intermittent load-bearing cycles repeated daily or every other day.

Resistance exercise training and endurance exercises that produce high ground reaction forces can increase peak bone mass in young adults by 5% to 10% and retard or reverse bone mass loss by about 1% per year in both pre- and post-menopausal women. Other studies show that estrogen and androgens help potentiate the osteogenic effects of bone loading and suggest that dietary intake of calcium needs to be within the range of 1000 mg to 1300 mg per day in order for the exercise stimulus to promote bone mass. Hence, the prevention and treatment of osteoporosis and osteoporotic fractures should be directed at maximizing peak bone mass by optimizing dietary calcium and vitamin D, normal menstruation, or sex hormone replacement and using vigorous physical activity that involves high peak forces, such as resistance exercise (Layne and Nelson 1999). However, recent evidence from the Women's Health Initiative study showing that estrogen plus progestin HRT increases cardiovascular and breast cancer risks warrants careful consultation by women with their personal physician before the decision is made to use HRT to promote bone health after menopause. Though exercise with or without calcium supplementation is a potentially useful adjuvant for increasing or maintaining bone mass after menopause, maximal benefits for bone health may also require osteogenic drugs when medically indicated.

Notwithstanding the encouraging results of clinical studies of exercise and bone mass, more population-based epidemiologic studies that do a better job of controlling for diet and adjusting for other potential confounders, as well as more randomized controlled trials, are needed to establish the generalizability of results to population segments at risk for developing osteoporosis and to establish the effect of physical activity on risk of osteoporotic fractures. Nonetheless, the cumulative evidence is encouraging that vigorous physical activity, especially the types that involve high peak loads (e.g., sports and games that involve jumping and quick changes in direction or resistance exercise), might promote higher peak bone mass and might retard bone loss with aging. Even without changes in overall bone mass or density, bones can adapt to external loads by reshaping or expanding their cross-sectional area and by redistribution of mineral from trabecular bone to cortical bone, resulting in increased bending and twisting strength.

Gains in BMD from sports during youth are mostly lost in adults who become sedentary (Nordstrom et al. 2005). However, some structural changes (e.g., size of cortical bone) that are more important for bone strength may be mostly retained and might reduce risks of fragility fractures in old age (Karlsson 2007). In order to maximize the goals of public health most effectively, individually adapted, intense, high-impact exercise programs are needed. However, these may be complicated to communicate and difficult to get people to adhere to at the level of the population. Thus, exercise programs that have the highest efficacy for increasing bone health in a laboratory or clinical setting must be judged against popular programs (e.g. aerobic classes, tai chi, and walking) that have less efficacy but may ultimately have better effectiveness because they can be feasibly and safely promoted to reduce risk of osteoporotic fracture in older or more frail men or postmenopausal women (Schmitt, Schmitt, and Dören 2009).

· BIBLIOGRAPHY ·

Adami, S., D. Gatti, V. Braga, D. Bianchini, and M. Rossini. 1999. Site-specific effects of strength training on bone structure and geometry of ultradistal radius in postmenopausal women. *Journal of Bone and Mineral Research* 14: 120-124.

Adami, S., D. Gatti, O. Viapiana, C.E. Fiore, R. Nuti, G. Luisetto, M. Ponte, M. Rossini; BONTURNO Study Group. 2008. Physical activity and bone turnover markers: A cross-sectional and a longitudinal study. *Calcified Tissue International* 83: 388-392.

Alaimo, K., M.A. McDowell, R.R. Briefel, A.M. Bischof, C.R. Caughman, C.M. Loria, and C.L. Johnson. 1994. Dietary intake of vitamins, minerals, and fiber of persons ages 2 months and over in the United States: Third National Health and Nutrition Examination Survey, phase 1, 1988–91. *Advance Data* 14 (258): 1-28.

Alekel, L., J.L. Clasey, P.C. Fehling, R.M. Weigel, R.A. Boileau, J.W. Erdman, and R. Stiliman. 1995. Contributions of exercise, body composition, and age to bone mineral density in premenopausal women. *Medicine and Science in Sports and Exercise* 27: 1477-1485.

Alfredson, H., P. Nordstrom, and R. Lorentzon. 1997. Bone mass in female volleyball players: A comparison of total and regional bone mass in female volleyball players and nonactive females. *Calcified Tissue International* 60: 338-342.

American College of Sports Medicine. 1995. American College of Sports Medicine position stand: Osteoporosis and exercise [review]. *Medicine and Science in Sports and Exercise* 27 (4): I-VII.

American College of Sports Medicine position stand: Physical activity and bone health. 2004. W.M. Kohrt, S.A. Bloomfield, K.D. Little, M.E. Nelson, V.R. Yingling. *Medicine and Science in Sports and Exercise* 36 (11): 1985-1996.

Anderson, J.C., and C. Eriksson. 1970. Piezoelectric properties of dry and wet bone. *Nature* 227: 491-492.

Augestad, L.B., B. Schei, S. Forsmo, A. Langhammer, and W.D. Flanders. 2004. The association between physical activity and forearm bone mineral density in healthy premenopausal women. *Journal of Women's Health (Larchmt)* 13 (3, April): 301-313.

Augestad, L.B., B. Schei, S. Forsmo, A. Langhammer, and W.D. Flanders. 2006. Healthy postmenopausal women - physical activity and forearm bone mineral density: The Nord-Trøndelag health survey. *Journal of Women and Aging* 18 (1): 21-40.

Bailey, D.A., H.A. McKay, R.L. Mirwald, P.R. Crocker, and R.A. Faulkner. 1999. A six-year longitudinal study of the relationship of physical activity to bone mineral accrual in growing children: The University of Saskatchewan bone mineral accrual study. *Journal of Bone and Mineral Research* 14 (10): 1672-1679.

Bakhireva, L.N., E. Barrett-Connor, D. Kritz-Silverstein, and D.J. Morton. 2004. Modifiable predictors of bone loss in older men: A prospective study. *American Journal of Preventive Medicine* 26 (5): 436-442.

Bass, S.L., L. Saxon, R.M. Daly, C.H. Turner, A.G. Robling, E. Seeman, and S. Stuckey. 2002. The effect of mechanical loading on the size and shape of bone in pre-, peri-, and postpubertal girls: A study in tennis players. *Journal of Bone and Mineral Research* 17: 2274-2280.

Bassett, C.A. 1965. Electrical effects in bone. *Scientific American* 213: 18-25.

Bassett, C.A. 1995. Why are the principles of physics and anatomy important in treating osteoporosis? *Calcified Tissue International* 56 (6): 515-516.

Bassett, C.A., and R.O. Becker. 1962. Generation of electric potentials by bone in response to mechanical stress. *Science* 137: 1063-1064.

Bauer, D.C., W.S. Browner, J.A. Cauler, E.S. Orwoll, J.C. Scott, D.M. Black, J.L. Tao, and S.R. Cummings. 1993. Factors associated with appendicular bone mass in older women. *Annals of Internal Medicine* 18 (9): 657-665.

Bell, N.H., R.N. Godsen, D.P. Henry, J. Shary, and S. Epstein. 1988. The effects of muscle-building exercise on vitamin D and mineral metabolism. *Journal of Bone and Mineral Research* 3: 369-373.

Bemben, D.A. 1999. Exercise interventions for osteoporosis prevention in postmenopausal women. *Journal of the Oklahoma State Medical Association* 92 (2): 66-70.

Ben-Noun, L. 2002. What was the disease of the bones that affected King David? *Journals of Gerontology Series A: Biological Sciences and Medical Sciences* 57A: M152-M154.

Berenson, A.B., M. Rahman, and G. Wilkinson. 2009. Racial difference in the correlates of bone mineral content/density and age at peak among reproductive-aged women. *Osteoporosis International* 20: 1439-1449.

Blimkie, C.J.R., S. Rice, C.E. Wegger, J. Martin, D. Levy, and C.L. Gordon. 1996. Effects of resistance training on bone mineral content (BMC) and density in adolescent females. *Canadian Journal of Physiology and Pharmacology* 74: 1025-1033.

Block, J.E., A.L. Friedlander, J.S. Brooks, and P. Steiger. 1989. Determinants of bone density among athletes engaged in weight-bearing and non-weight-bearing activity. *Journal of Applied Physiology* 67: 1100-1105.

Blumenthal, J.A., C.F. Emery, D.J. Madden, R. Schniebok, M.W. Riddle, M. Cobb, M. Higginbotham, and R.W. Coleman. 1991. Effects of exercise training on bone density in older men and women. *Journal of the American Geriatrics Society* 39 (11): 1065-1070.

Borer, K.T. 2005. Physical activity in the prevention and amelioration of osteoporosis in women: Interaction of mechanical, hormonal and dietary factors. *Sports Medicine* 35: 779-830.

Bradney, M., G. Pearce, G. Naughton, C. Sullivan, S. Bass, T. Beck, J. Carlson, and E. Seeman. 1998. Moderate exercise during growth in prepubertal boys: Changes in bone mass, size, volumetric density and bone strength: A controlled prospective study. *Journal of Bone and Mineral Research* 13: 1814-1821.

Braith, R.W., R.M. Mills, M.A. Welsch, J.W. Keller, and M.L. Pollock. 1996. Resistance exercise training restores bone mineral density in heart transplant recipients. *Journal of the American College of Cardiology* 28: 1471-1477.

Brighton, C.T., M.J. Katz, S.R. Goll, C.E. Nichols, and S.R. Pollack. 1985. Prevention and treatment of sciatic denervation disuse osteoporosis in the rat tibia with capacitatively coupled electric stimulation. *Bone* 6: 87-97.

Buchner, D.M., and E.H. Wagner. 1992. Preventing frail health. *Clinics in Geriatric Medicine* 8: 1-17.

Burge, R.T., B. Dawson-Hughes, D. Solomon, J.B. Wong, A.B. King, and A.N.A. Tosteson. 2007. Incidence and economic burden of osteoporotic fractures in the United States, 2005-2025. *J Bone Min Res* 22 (3): 465-475.

Chamay, A., and P. Tschantz. 1972. Mechanical influences on bone remodeling: Experimental research on Wolff's law. *Journal of Biomechanics* 5: 173-180.

Chilibeck, P.D., D.G. Sale, and C.E. Webber. 1995. Exercise and bone mineral density. *Sports Medicine* 19 (2): 103-122.

Clinical practice guidelines for the diagnosis and management of osteoporosis [special supplement]. 1996. *Canadian Medical Association Journal* 155 (8): 1113-1129.

Colletti, L.A., J. Edwards, L. Gordon, J. Shary, and N.H. Bell. 1989. The effects of muscle-building exercise on bone mineral density of the radius, spine, and hip in young men. *Calcified Tissue International* 45: 12-14.

Colón-Emeric, C., M. Kuchibhatla, C. Pieper, W. Hawkes, L. Fredman, J. Magaziner, S. Zimmerman, and K.W. Lyles. 2003. The contribution of hip fracture to risk of subsequent fractures: Data from two longitudinal studies. *Osteoporosis International* 14: 879-883.

Courteix, D., E. Lespessailles, S.L. Peres, P. Obert, P. Germain, and C.L. Benhamou. 1998. Effect of physical training on BMD in prepubertal girls: A comparative study between impact-loading and non-impact-loading sports. *Osteoporosis International* 8: 152-159.

Cummings, S.R. 2006. A 55-year-old woman with osteopenia. *Journal of the American Medical Association* 296 (21, December 6): 2601-2610.

Cummings, S.R., and L.J. Melton. 2002. Epidemiology and outcomes of osteoporotic fractures. *Lancet* 359 (9319, May 18): 1761-1767.

Cummings, S.R., M.C. Nevitt, W.S. Browner, K. Stone, K.M. Fox, K.E. Ensrud, J. Cauley, D. Black, and T.M. Vogt. 1995. Risk factors for hip fracture in white women. Study of Osteoporotic Fractures Research Group. *New England Journal of Medicine* 332 (12, March 23): 767-773.

Cussler, E.C., S.B. Going, L.B. Houtkooper, V.A. Stanford, R.M. Blew, H.G. Flint-Wagner, L.L. Metcalfe, J.E. Choi, and T.G. Lohman. 2005. Exercise frequency and calcium intake predict 4-year bone changes in postmenopausal women. *Osteoporosis International* 16: 2129-2141.

Dalsky, G.P., K.S. Stocke, A.A. Ehsani, E. Slatopolsky, W.C. Lee, and S.J. Birge. 1988. Weight-bearing exercise training and lumbar bone mineral content in postmenopausal women. *Annals of Internal Medicine* 108: 824-828.

Daly, R.M. 2007. The effect of exercise on bone mass and structural geometry during growth. In *Optimizing bone mass and strength. The role of physical activity and nutrition during growth,* edited by R. Daly and M. Petit. *Medicine and Sport Science, Basel, Karger, 51, 33-49.*

Dawson-Hughes, B., S. Harris, E. Krall, and G. Dallal. 1997. Effect of calcium and vitamin D supplementation on bone density in men and women 65 years of age and older. *New England Journal of Medicine* 337: 670-676.

Dequeker, J., D.J. Ortner, A.I. Stix, X.G. Cheng, P. Brys, and S. Boonen. 1997. Hip fracture and osteoporosis in a XIIth dynasty female skeleton from Lisht, upper Egypt. *Journal of Bone and Mineral Research* 12 (6): 881-888.

Emslander, H.C., M. Sinaki, J.M. Muhs, E.Y. Chao, H.W. Wahner, S.C. Bryant, B.L. Riggs, and R. Eastell. 1998. Bone mass and muscle strength in female college athletes (runners and swimmers). *Mayo Clinic Proceedings* 73: 1151-1160.

Feskanich, D., W. Willett, and G. Colditz. 2002. Walking and leisure-time activity and risk of hip fracture in postmenopausal women. *Journal of the American Medical Association* 288: 2300-2306.

Fiatarone, M.A., E.F. O'Neill, N.D. Ryan, K.M. Clements, G.R. Solares, M.E. Nelson, S.B. Roberts, and W.J. Evans. 1994. Exercise training and nutritional supplementation for physical frailty in very elderly people. *New England Journal of Medicine* 330 (25): 1769-1775.

Foldes, A.J., and M.M. Popovtzer. 1996. Osteoporosis 4000 years ago. *New England Journal of Medicine* 334: 735.

Friedlander, A.L., H.K. Genant, S. Sadowsky, N.N. Byl, and C.-C. Gluer. 1995. A two-year program of aerobics and weight training enhances BMD of young women. *Journal of Bone and Mineral Research* 10: 574-585.

Frigo, P., and C. Lang. 1995. Osteoporosis in a woman of the early Bronze Age. *New England Journal of Medicine* 333: 1468.

Garnero, P., and P.D. Delmas. 1997. Osteoporosis. *Endocrinology and Metabolism Clinics of North America* 26: 913-936.

Gillespie, L.D., W.J. Gillespie, M.C. Robertson, S.E. Lamb, R.G. Cumming, and B.H. Rowe. 2001. Interventions for preventing falls in elderly people. *Cochrane Database of Systematic Reviews* (3): CD000340.

Gourlay, M.L., J.P. Fine, J.S. Preisser, R.C. May, C. Li, L.Y. Lui, D.F. Ransohoff, J.A. Cauley, K.E. Ensrud; Study of Osteoporotic Fractures Research Group. 2012. Bone-density testing interval and transition to osteoporosis in older women. *New England Journal of Medicine* 366: 225-233.

Gregg, E.W., M.A. Pereira, and C.J. Caspersen. 2000. Physical activity, falls, and fractures among older adults: A review of the epidemiologic evidence. *Journal of the American Geriatrics Society* 48 (8): 883-893.

Gross, D., and W.S. Williams. 1982. Streaming potential and the electromechanical response of physiologically moist bone. *Journal of Biomechanics* 15: 277-295.

Grove, K.A., and B.R. Londeree. 1992. Bone density in postmenopausal women: High impact vs. low impact exercise. *Medicine and Science in Sports and Exercise* 24: 1190-1194.

Hakkinen, A., T. Sokka, A. Kotaniemi, and P. Hannonen. 2001. A randomized two-year study of the effects of dynamic strength training on muscle strength, disease activity, functional capacity, and bone mineral density in early rheumatoid arthritis. *Arthritis and Rheumatism* 44: 515-522.

Hannan, M.T., D.T. Felson, B. Dawson-Hughes, K.L. Tucker, L.A. Cupples, P.W. Wilson, and D.P. Kiel. 2000. Risk factors for longitudinal bone loss in elderly men and women: The Framingham Osteoporosis Study. *Journal of Bone and Mineral Research* 15: 710-720.

Hatori, M., A. Hasegawa, H. Adachi, A. Shinozaki, R. Hayashi, H. Okano, H. Mizunuma, and K. Murata. 1993. The effects of walking at the anaerobic threshold level on vertebral bone loss in postmenopausal women. *Calcified Tissue International* 52: 411-414.

Hawkins, S.A., E.T. Schroeder, R.A. Wiswell, S.V. Jaque, T.J. Marcell, and K. Costa. 1999. Eccentric muscle action increases site-specific osteogenic response. *Medicine and Science in Sports and Exercise* 31: 1287-1292.

Heikkinen, J., E. Kyllonen, E. Kurttila-Matero, G. Wilen-Rosenqvist, K.S. Lankinen, H. Rita, and H.K. Vaananen. 1997. HRT and exercise: Effects on bone density, muscle strength and lipid metabolism. A placebo controlled 2-year prospective trial on two estrogen-progestin regimens in healthy postmenopausal women. *Maturitas* 26 (2): 139-149.

Heinonen, A., P. Oja, P. Kannus, H. Sievanen, H. Haapasalo, A. Manttari, and I. Vuori. 1995. BMD in female athletes representing sports with different loading characteristics of the skeleton. *Bone* 17: 197-203.

Heinonen, A., P. Oja, P. Kannus, H. Sievanen, A. Manttari, and I. Vuori. 1993. BMD in female athletes of different sports. *Bone and Mineral* 23: 1-14.

Heinonen, A., P. Oja, H. Sievanen, M. Pasanen, and I. Vuori. 1998. Effect of two training regimens on bone mineral density in healthy perimenopausal women: A randomized control trial. *Journal of Bone and Mineral Research* 13: 483-490.

Heinonen, A., H. Sievanen, P. Kannus, P. Oja, M. Pasanen, and I. Vuori. 2000. High-impact exercise and bones of growing girls: A 9-month controlled trial. *Osteoporosis International* 11 (12): 1010-1017.

Høidrup, S., T.I. Sørensen, U. Strøger, J.B. Lauritzen, M. Schroll, and M. Grønbaek. 2001. Leisure-time physical activity levels and changes in relation to risk of hip fracture in men and women. *American Journal of Epidemiology* 154 (1, July 1): 60-68.

Hourigan, S.R., J.C. Nitz, S.G. Brauer, S. O'Neill, J. Wong, and C.A. Richardson. 2008. Positive effects of exercise on falls and fracture risk in osteopenic women. *Osteoporosis* 19 (7): 1077-1086. [Epub, January 11, 2008]

Howe, T.E., L. Rochester, A. Jackson, P.M.H. Banks, and V.A. Blair. 2007. Exercise for improving balance in older people. *Cochrane Database of Systematic Reviews* (4): CD004963.

Howe, T.E., B. Shea, L.J. Dawson, F. Downie, A. Murray, C. Ross, R.T. Harbour, L.M. Caldwell, and G. Creed. 2011. Exercise for preventing and treating osteoporosis in postmenopausal women. *Cochrane Database and Systematic Reviews* Jul 6;(7): CD000333.

Huddleston, A.L., D. Rockwell, D.N. Kulund, and R.B. Harrison. 1980. Bone mass in lifetime tennis athletes. *Journal of the American Medical Association* 244: 1107-1109.

Hui, S.L., C.W. Slemenda, and C.C. Johnston Jr. 1989. Baseline measurement of bone mass predicts fracture in white women. *Annals of Internal Medicine* 111: 355-361.

Järvinen, T.L., P. Kannus, and H. Sievänen. 1999. Have the DXA-based exercise studies seriously underestimated the effects of mechanical loading on bone? *Journal of Bone and Mineral Research* 14: 1634-1635.

Järvinen, T.L.N., P. Kannus, H. Sievänen, P. Jolma, A. Heinonen, and M. Järvinen. 1998. Randomized controlled study of effects of sudden impact loading on rat femur. *Journal of Bone and Mineral Research* 13: 1475-1482.

Johnell, O., and J. Kanis. 2005. Epidemiology of osteoporotic fractures. *Osteoporosis International* 16 (Suppl. 2, March): S3-7.

Johnston, C.C. Jr., and C.W. Slemenda. 1995. Pathogenesis of osteoporosis. *Bone* 17 (Suppl. 2): 19S-22S.

Kanis, J.A., E.V. McCloskey, H. Johansson, A. Oden, L.J. Melton, and N. Khaltaev. 2008. A reference standard for the description of osteoporosis. *Bone* 42: 467-475.

Karlsson, M.K. 2007. Does exercise during growth prevent fractures in later life? *Medicine and Sport Science* 51: 121-136.

Karlsson, M., S. Bass, and E. Seeman. 2001. The evidence that exercise during growth or adulthood reduces the risk of fragility fractures is weak. *Best Practice and Research: Clinical Rheumatology* 15 (3): 429-450.

Katz, W.A., and C. Sherman. 1998. Osteoporosis: The role of exercise in optimal management. *Physician and Sportsmedicine* 26 (2): 33-43.

Kelley, G.A., and K.S. Kelley. 2004. Efficacy of resistance exercise on lumbar spine and femoral neck bone mineral density in premenopausal women: A meta-analysis of individual patient data. *Journal of Women's Health (Larchmt)* 13 (3, April): 293-300.

Kelley, G.A., and K.S. Kelley. 2006. Exercise and bone mineral density at the femoral neck in postmenopausal women: A meta-analysis of controlled clinical trials with individual patient data. *American Journal of Obstetrics and Gynecology* 194 (3): 760-767.

Kelley, G.A., K.S. Kelley, and Z.V. Tran. 2000. Exercise and bone mineral density in men: A meta-analysis. *Journal of Applied Physiology* 88 (5): 1730-1736.

Kelley, G.A., K.S. Kelley, and Z.V. Tran. 2002. Exercise and lumbar spine bone mineral density in postmenopausal women: A meta-analysis of individual patient data. *Journals of Gerontology Series A: Biological Sciences and Medical Sciences* 57 (9): M599-604.

Kemmler, W., S. von Stengel, K. Engelke, L. Haberle, and W.A. Kalender. 2010. Exercise effects on bone mineral density, falls, coronary risk factors, and health care costs in older women: The randomized controlled senior fitness and prevention (SEFIP) study. *Archives of Internal Medicine* 170: 179-185.

Kemper, H.C., J.W. Twisk, W. van Mechelen, G.B. Post, J.C. Roos, and P. Lips. 2000. A fifteen-year longitudinal study in young adults on the relation of physical activity and fitness with the development of the bone mass: The Amsterdam Growth and Health Longitudinal Study. *Bone* 27 (6): 847-853.

Kerr, D., T. Ackland, B. Maslen, A. Morton, and R. Prince. 2001. Resistance training over 2 years increases bone mass in calcium-replete postmenopausal women. *Journal of Bone and Mineral Research* 16 (1): 175-181.

Kerr, D., A. Morton, I. Dick, and R. Prince. 1996. Exercise effects on bone mass in postmenopausal women are site specific and load dependent. *Journal of Bone and Mineral Research* 11: 218-225.

Khosla, S., E.J. Atkinson, B.L. Riggs, and L.J. Melton. 1996. Relationship between body composition and bone mass in women. *Journal of Bone and Mineral Research* 11: 857-863.

Kirk, R., C.F. Sharp, N. Elbaum, D.B. Endres, S.M. Simons, J.G. Mohler, and R.K. Rude. 1989. Effect of long-distance running on bone mass in women. *Journal of Bone and Mineral Research* 4 (4): 515-522.

Kohrt, W.M., A.A. Ehsani, and S.J. Birge. 1997. Effects of exercise involving predominantly either joint reaction or ground reaction forces on bone mineral density in older women. *Journal of Bone and Mineral Research* 12: 1253-1261.

Kohrt, W.M., D.B. Snead, E. Slatopolsky, and S.J. Birge Jr. 1995. Additive effects of weight-bearing exercise and estrogen on BMD in older women. *Journal of Bone and Mineral Research* 10: 1303-1311.

Kohrt, W.M., K.E. Yarasheski, and J.O. Holloszy. 1998. Effects of exercise training on bone mass in elderly women and men with physical frailty. *Bone* 23: S499.

Kraemer, W.J., L. Marchitelli, and S. Gordon. 1990. Hormonal and growth factor responses to heavy resistance exercise protocols. *Journal of Applied Physiology* 69: 1442-1450.

Kujala, U.M., J. Kaprio, P. Kannus, S. Sarna, and M. Koskenvuo. 2000. Physical activity and osteoporotic hip fracture risk in men. *Archives of Internal Medicine* 160 (5): 705-708.

Lane, J.M., and M. Nydick. 1999. Osteoporosis: Current modes of prevention and treatment. *Journal of the American Academy of Orthopaedic Surgeons* 7 (1): 19-31.

Lane, N.E., D.A. Bloch, H.H. Jones, W.H. Marshall Jr., P.D. Wood, and J.F. Fries. 1986. Long-distance running, bone density, and osteoarthritis. *Journal of the American Medical Association* 255: 1147-1151.

Lanyon, L.E. 1993. Osteocytes, strain detection, bone modeling and remodeling. *Calcified Tissue International* 53: 5102-5106.

Lanyon, L.E. 1996. Using functional loading to influence bone mass and architecture: Objectives, mechanisms, and relationship with estrogen of the mechanically adaptive process in bone. *Bone* 18 (Suppl. 1): 37S-43S.

Lanyon, L.E., and W. Hartman. 1977. Strain related electrical potentials recorded in vitro and in vivo. *Calcified Tissue International* 22: 315-327.

Layne, J.E., and M.E. Nelson. 1999. The effects of progressive resistance training on bone density: A review. *Medicine and Science in Sports and Exercise* 31 (1): 25-30.

Lees, B., T. Molleson, T.R. Arnett, and J.C. Stevenson. 1993. Differences in proximal femur bone density over two centuries. *Lancet* 341 (8846): 673-675.

Levinson, W., and D. Altkorn. 1998. Primary prevention of postmenopausal osteoporosis. *Journal of the American Medical Association* 280 (21): 1821-1822.

Lloyd, T., V.M. Chinchilli, N. Johnson-Rollings, K. Kieselhorst, D.F. Eggli, and R. Marcus. 2000. Adult female hip bone density reflects teenage sports-exercise patterns but not teenage calcium intake. *Pediatrics* 106 (1 Pt 1): 40-44.

Lohman, T., S. Going, R. Pamenter, M. Hall, T. Boyden, L. Houtkooper, C. Ritenbaugh, L. Bare, A. Hill, and M. Aickin. 1995. Effects of resistance training on regional and total bone mineral density in premenopausal women: A randomized prospective study. *Journal of Bone and Mineral Research* 10 (7): 1015-1024.

Looker, A.C., L.J. Melton 3rd, T.B. Harris, L.G. Borrud, and J.A. Shepherd. 2010. Prevalence and trends in low femur bone density among older US adults: NHANES 2005-2006 compared with NHANES III. *Journal of Bone and Mineral Research* 25: 64-71.

Looker, A.C., L.J. Melton 3rd, T. Harris, L. Borrud, J. Shepherd, and J. McGowan. 2009. Age, gender, and race/ethnic differences in total body and subregional bone density. *Osteoporosis International* 20 (7): 1141-1149.

Looker, A.C., H.W. Wahner, W.L. Dunn, M.S. Calvo, T.B. Harris, S.P. Heyse, C.C. Johnston Jr., and R. Lindsay. 1998. Updated data on proximal femur bone mineral levels of US adults. *Osteoporosis International* 8 (5): 468-489.

MacKelvie, K.J., H.A. McKay, M.A. Petit, O. Moran, and K.M. Khan. 2002. Bone mineral response to a 7-month randomized controlled, school-based jumping intervention in 121 prepubertal boys: Associations with ethnicity and body mass index. *Journal of Bone and Mineral Research* 17 (5): 834-844.

Maddalozzo, G.F., and C.M. Snow. 2000. High intensity resistance training: Effects on bone in older men and women. *Calcified Tissue International* 66 (6): 399-404.

Marshall, D., O. Johnell, and H. Wedel. 1996. Meta-analysis of how well measures of bone mineral density predict occurrence of osteoporotic fractures. *British Medical Journal* 312: 1254-1259.

Martin, A.D., and R.G. McCulloch. 1987. Bone dynamics: Stress, strain, and fracture. *Journal of Sports Sciences* 5: 155-163.

Martin, D., and M. Notelovitz. 1993. Effects of aerobic training on bone mineral density of postmenopausal women. *Journal of Bone and Mineral Research* 8 (8): 931-936.

Martyn-St James, M., and S. Carroll. 2006a. High-intensity resistance training and postmenopausal bone loss: A meta-analysis. *Osteoporosis International* 17 (8): 1225-1240. [Epub, June 1, 2006]

Martyn-St James, M., and S. Carroll. 2006b. Progressive high-intensity resistance training and bone mineral density changes among premenopausal women: Evidence of discordant site-specific skeletal effects. *Sports Medicine* 36 (8): 683-704.

Martyn-St James, M., and S. Carroll. 2008. Meta-analysis of walking for preservation of bone mineral density in postmenopausal women. *Bone* 43: 521-531.

Martyn-St James, M., and S. Carroll. 2009. A meta-analysis of impact exercise on postmenopausal bone loss: The case for mixed loading exercise programmes. British Journal of Sports Medicine 43: 898-908.

Martyn-St James, M., and S. Carroll. 2010. Effects of different impact exercise modalities on bone mineral density in premenopausal women: A meta-analysis. *Journal of Bone and Mineral Metabolism* 28 (3, May): 251-267.

Mavroeidi, A., A.D. Stewart, D.M. Reid, and H.M. Macdonald. 2009. Physical activity and dietary calcium interactions in bone mass in Scottish postmenopausal women. Osteoporosis International 20 (3): 409-416.

Menkes, A., S. Mazel, R.A. Redmond, K. Koffler, C.R. Libanati, C.M. Gundberg, T.M. Zizic, J.M. Hagberg, R.E. Pratley, and B.F. Hurley. 1993. Strength training increases regional bone mineral density and bone remodeling in middle-aged and older men. *Journal of Applied Physiology* 74: 2478-2484.

Michaëlsson, K., H. Olofsson, K. Jensevik, S. Larsson, H. Mallmin, L. Berglund, B. Vessby, and H. Melhus. 2007. Leisure physical activity and the risk of fracture in men. *PLoS Medicine* 4 (6): e199.

Modlesky, C.M., and R.D. Lewis. 2002. Does exercise during growth have a long-term effect on bone health? *Exercise and Sport Sciences Reviews* 30: 171-176.

Montoye, H.J. 1984. Exercise and osteoporosis. *American Academy of Physical Education Papers* 17: 59-75.

Morris, F.L., G.A. Naughton, J.L. Gibbs, J.S. Carlson, and J.D. Wark. 1997. Prospective ten-month exercise intervention in pre-menarcheal girls: Positive effects on bone and lean mass. *Journal of Bone and Mineral Research* 12: 1453-1462.

Mosca, L. 2000. The role of hormone replacement therapy in the prevention of postmenopausal heart disease. *Archives of Internal Medicine* 160: 2263-2272.

Mussolino, M.E., A.C. Looker, and E.S. Orwoll. 2001. Jogging and bone mineral density in men: Results from NHANES III. *American Journal of Public Health* 91: 1056-1059.

National Institutes of Health. 1994. NIH Consensus Conference. Optimal calcium intake. NIH Consensus Development Panel on optimal calcium intake. *Journal of the American Medical Association* 272: 1942-1948.

National Osteoporosis Foundation. 2002. *America's bone health: The state of osteoporosis and low bone mass.* Washington, DC: National Osteoporosis Foundation.

National Osteoporosis Foundation. 2010. *Clinician's guide to prevention and treatment of osteoporosis.* Washington, DC: National Osteoporosis Foundation.

Nelson, M.E., M.A. Fiatarone, C.M. Morganti, I. Trice, R.A. Greenberg, and W.J. Evans. 1994. Effects of high intensity strength training on multiple risk factors for osteoporotic fractures. *Journal of the American Medical Association* 272: 1909-1914.

Nelson, M.E., E.C. Fisher, F.A. Kilmanian, G.E. Dallal, and W.J. Evans. 1991. A 1-y walking program and increased dietary calcium in postmenopausal women: Effects on bone. *American Journal of Clinical Nutrition* 53: 1304-1311.

Nguyen, T.V., P.J. Kelly, P.N. Sambrook, C. Gilbert, N.A. Pocock, and J.A. Eisman. 1994. Lifestyle factors and bone density in elderly: Implications for osteoporosis prevention. *Journal of Bone and Mineral Research* 9 (9): 1339-1346.

Nichols, D.L., C.F. Sanborn, S.L. Bonnick, B. Gench, and N. DiMarco. 1995. Relationship of regional body composition to BMD in college females. *Medicine and Science in Sports and Exercise* 27: 178-182.

Nichols, D.L., C.F. Sanborn, and A.M. Love. 2001. Resistance training and bone mineral density in adolescent females. *Journal of Pediatrics* 139 (4): 494-500.

Nikander, R., H. Sievänen, A. Heinonen, R.M. Daly, K. Uusi-Rasi, and P. Kannus. 2010. Targeted exercise against osteoporosis: A systematic review and meta-analysis for optimising bone strength throughout life. *BMC Medicine* (8, July 21): 47.

Nordstrom, A., C. Karlsson, F. Nyquist, T. Olsson, P. Nordstrom, et al. 2005. Bone loss and fracture risk after reduced physical activity. *Journal of Bone and Mineral Research* 20: 202-207.

Notelovitz, M., D. Martin, R. Tesar, F.Y. Khan, C. Probart, C. Fields, and L. McKenzie. 1991. Estrogen therapy and variable resistance weight training increases bone mineral in surgically menopausal women. *Journal of Bone and Mineral Research* 6: 583-590.

Olszynski, W.P., K. Shawn Davison, J.D. Adachi, J.P. Brown, S.R. Cummings, D.A. Hanley, S.P. Harris, A.B. Hodsman, D. Kendler, M.R. McClung, P.D. Miller, and C.K. Yuen. 2004. Osteoporosis in men: Epidemiology, diagnosis, prevention, and treatment. *Clinical Therapeutics* 26 (1): 15-28.

Pettersson, U., H. Alfredson, P. Nordstrom, K. Henriksson-Larsen, and R. Lorentzon. 2000. Bone mass in female cross-country skiers: Relationship between muscle strength and different BMD sites. *Calcified Tissue International* 67: 199-206.

Physical Activity Guidelines Advisory Committee. 2008. *Physical Activity Guidelines Advisory Committee report.* Washington, DC: U.S. Department of Health and Human Services.

Prince, R.L., M. Smith, I.M. Dick, R.I. Price, P.G. Webb, N.K. Henderson, and M.M. Harris. 1991. Prevention of postmenopausal osteoporosis: A comparative study of exercise, calcium supplementation, and hormone replacement therapy. *New England Journal of Medicine* 325: 1189-1195.

Pruitt, L.A., R.D. Jackson, R.L. Bartels, and H.J. Lehnard. 1992. Weight training effects on bone mineral density in early postmenopausal women. *Journal of Bone and Mineral Research* 7: 179-185.

Pruitt, L.A., D.R. Taaffe, and R. Marcus. 1995. Effects of a one-year high-intensity versus low-intensity resistance training program on BMD in older women. *Journal of Bone and Mineral Research* 10: 1788-1795.

Ralston, S.H., and A.G. Uitterlinden. 2010. Genetics of osteoporosis. *Endocrine Reviews.* [Epub ahead of print, April 29]

Rawlinson, S.C., A.A. Pitsillides, and L.E. Lanyon. 1996. Involvement of different ion channels in osteoblasts' and osteocytes' early responses to mechanical strain. *Bone* 19: 609-614.

Recker, R.R., K.M. Davies, S.M. Hinders, R.P. Heaney, M.R. Stegman, and D.B. Kimmel. 1992. Bone gain in young adult women. *Journal of the American Medical Association* 268 (17): 2403-2408.

Riggs, B.L., and L.J. Melton. 1986. Involutional osteoporosis. *New England Journal of Medicine* 314: 1676-1686.

Riggs, B.L., and L.J. Melton. 1995. The worldwide problem of osteoporosis: Insights afforded by epidemiology. *Bone* 17 (5 Suppl.): 505S-511S.

Robbins, J., A.K. Aragaki, C. Kooperberg, N. Watts, J. Wactawski-Wende, R.D. Jackson, M.S. LeBoff, C.E. Lewis, Z. Chen, M.L. Stefanick, and J. Cauley. 2007. Factors associated with 5-year risk of hip fracture in postmenopausal women. *Journal of the American Medical Association* 298: 2389-2398.

Robitaille, J., P.W. Yoon, C.A. Moore, T. Liu, M. Irizarry-Delacruz, A.C. Looker, and M.J. Khoury. 2008. Prevalence, family history, and prevention of reported osteoporosis in U.S. women. *American Journal of Preventive Medicine* 35 (1, July): 47-54.

Rossouw, J.E., G.L. Anderson, R.L. Prentice, A.Z. LaCroix, C. Kooperberg, M.L. Stefanick, R.D. Jackson, S.A. Beresford, B.V. Howard, K.C. Johnson, et al. 2002. Risks and benefits of estrogen plus progestin in healthy postmenopausal women:

Principal results from the Women's Health Initiative randomized controlled trial. *Journal of the American Medical Association* 288: 321-333.

Rubin, C.T., and L.E. Lanyon. 1984. Regulation of bone formation by applied dynamic loads. *Journal of Bone and Mineral Research* 66: 397-402.

Samelson, E.J., M.T. Hannan, Y. Zhang, H.K. Genant, D.T. Felson, and D.P. Kiel. 2006. Incidence and risk factors for vertebral fracture in women and men: 25-year follow-up results from the population-based Framingham study. *Journal of Bone and Mineral Research* 21 (8): 1207-1214.

Sartorio, A., C. Lafortuna, P. Capodaglio, V. Vangeli, M.V. Narici, and G. Faglia. 2001. Effects of a 16-week progressive high-intensity strength training (HIST) on indexes of bone turnover in men over 65 years: A randomized controlled study. *Journal of Endocrinological Investigation* 24 (11): 882-886.

Schmitt, N.M., J. Schmitt, and M. Dören. 2009. The role of physical activity in the prevention of osteoporosis in postmenopausal women-An update. *Maturitas* 20: 63 (1, May): 34-38.

Shamos, M.H., and L.S. Lavine. 1964. Physical bases for bioelectric effects in mineralized tissues. *Clinical Orthopaedics and Related Research* 35: 177-188.

Sheth, P. 1999. Osteoporosis and exercise: A review. *Mount Sinai Journal of Medicine* 66 (3): 197-200.

Simkin, A., J. Ayalon, and I. Leichter. 1987. Increased trabecular bone density due to bone-loading exercises in postmenopausal osteoporotic women. *Calcified Tissue International* 40: 59-63.

Sinaki, M., L.A. Fitzpatrick, C.K. Richie, A. Montesano, and W. Wahner. 1998. Site-specificity of bone mineral density and muscle strength in women: Job related physical activity. *American Journal of Physical Medicine and Rehabilitation* 6: 470-476.

Sinaki, M., H.W. Wahner, K.P. Offord, and S.F. Hodgson. 1989. Efficacy of nonloading exercises in prevention of vertebral bone loss in postmenopausal women: A controlled trial. *Mayo Clinic Proceedings* 64: 762-769.

Siris, E.S., S. Baim, and A. Nattiv. 2010. Primary care use of FRAX: Absolute fracture risk assessment in postmenopausal women and older men. *Postgraduate Medicine* 122 (1): 82-90.

Slemenda, C.W., C.H. Turner, M. Peacock, J.C. Christian, J. Sorbel, S.L. Hui, and C.C. Johnston. 1996. The genetics of proximal femur geometry, distribution of bone mass and bone mineral density. *Osteoporosis International* 6 (2): 178-182.

Smith, E., C. Gilligan, M. McAdam, C.P. Ensign, and P.E. Smith. 1989. Deterring bone loss by exercise intervention in premenopausal and postmenopausal women. *Calcified Tissue International* 44: 312-321.

Snow-Harter, C., M.L. Bouxsein, B.T. Lewis, D.R. Carter, and R. Marcus. 1992. Effects of resistance and endurance exercise on bone mineral status of young women: A randomized exercise intervention trial. *Journal of Bone and Mineral Research* 7: 761-769.

Sowers, M.F. 1997. Clinical epidemiology and osteoporosis: Measures and their interpretation. *Endocrinology and Metabolism Clinics of North America* 26: 219-231.

Sowers, M.F., G. Corton, and B. Shapiro. 1993. Bone density and bone turnover with long-term lactation. *Journal of the American Medical Association* 269: 3130-3135.

Speroff, L., R.H. Glass, and N.G. Case. 1994. *Clinical gynecologic endocrinology and infertility.* Baltimore: Williams and Wilkins.

Steinberg, K.I.K., S.B. Thacker, S.J. Smith, S.F. Stroup, M. Sack, D. Flanders, and R.L. Berkelman. 1991. A meta-analysis of the effect of estrogen replacement therapy on the risk of breast cancer. *Journal of the American Medical Association* 265 (15): 1985-1990.

Strong, W.B., R.M. Malina, C.J. Blimkie, S.R. Daniels, R.K. Dishman, B. Gutin, A.C. Hergenroeder, A. Must, P.A. Nixon, J.M. Pivarnik, T. Rowland, S. Trost, and F. Trudeau. 2005. Evidence based physical activity for school-age youth. *Journal of Pediatrics* 146 (6): 732-737.

Sundberg, M., P. Gardsell, O. Johnell, M.K. Karlsson, E. Ornstein, B. Sandstedt, and I. Sernbo. 2001. Peripubertal moderate exercise increases bone mass in boys but not in girls: A population-based intervention study. *Osteoporosis International* 12 (3): 230-238.

Szulc, P., and P.D. Delmas. 2007. Bone loss in elderly men: Increased endosteal bone loss and stable periosteal apposition. The prospective MINOS study. *Osteoporosis International* 18: 495-503.

Taaffe, D.R., T.L. Robinson, C.M. Snow, and R. Marcus. 1997. High-impact exercise promotes bone gain in well-trained female athletes. *Journal of Bone and Mineral Research* 12: 255-260.

Taaffe, D.R., C. Snow-Harter, D.A. Connolly, T.L. Robinson, M.D. Brown, and R. Marcus. 1995. Differential effects of swimming versus weight-bearing activity on bone mineral status of eumenorrheic athletes. *Journal of Bone Mineral Research* 10 (4): 586-593.

Tabrah, F., M. Hoffmeier, F. Gilbert Jr., S. Batkin, and C.A. Bassett. 1990. Bone density changes in osteoporosis-prone women exposed to pulsed electromagnetic fields (PEMFs). *Journal of Bone and Mineral Research* 5 (5): 437-442.

Torgerson, D.J., and S.E.M. Bell-Syer. 2001. Hormone replacement therapy and prevention of nonvertebral fractures: A meta-analysis of randomized trials. *Journal of the American Medical Association* 285: 2891-2897.

Turner, C.H., and A.G. Robling. 2003. Designing exercise regimens to increase bone strength. *Exercise and Sport Sciences Reviews* 31: 45-50.

U.S. Department of Health and Human Services. 2004. *Bone health and osteoporosis: A report of the Surgeon General.* Rockville, MD: U.S. Department of Health and Human Services, Office of the Surgeon General.

Valimaki, M.J., M. Karkkainen, C. Lamberg-Allardt, K. Laitinen, E. Alhava, J. Heikkinen, O. Impivaara, P. Makela, J. Palmgren, R. Seppanen, et al. 1994. Exercise, smoking, and calcium intake during adolescence and early adulthood as determinants of peak bone mass: Cardiovascular risk in young Finns study group. *British Medical Journal* 309 (6949): 230-235.

Vincent, K.R., and R.W. Braith. 2002. Resistance exercise and bone turnover in elderly men and women. *Medicine and Science in Sports and Exercise* 34 (1): 17-23.

Vuori, I.M. 2001. Dose-response of physical activity and low back pain, osteoarthritis, and osteoporosis. *Medicine and Science in Sports and Exercise* 33 (Suppl. 6): S551-S586.

Wallach, J., and M. Lan. 1994. *Rare earths: Forbidden cures.* California: Double Happiness.

Welsh, L., and O.M. Rutherford. 1996. Hip bone mineral density is improved by high-impact aerobic exercise in postmenopausal women and men over 50 years. *European Journal of Applied Physiology* 74: 511-517.

Whalon, R.T., D.R. Carter, and C.R. Steele. 1988. Influence of physical activity on the regulation of bone density. *Journal of Biomechanics* 21: 825-837.

Whitfield, J.F., and P. Morley. 1998. *Anabolic treatments for osteoporosis.* Boca Raton, FL: CRC Press.

Wickham, C.A., K. Walsh, C. Cooper, D.J. Barker, B.M. Margetts, J. Morris, and S.A. Bruce. 1989. Dietary calcium, physical activity, and risk of hip fracture: A prospective study. *British Medical Journal* 299 (6704): 889-892.

Wolff, I., J.J. van Croonenborg, H.C.G. Kemper, P.J. Kostense, and J.W.R. Twisk. 1999. The effect of exercise training programs on bone mass: A meta-analysis of published controlled trials in pre- and postmenopausal women. *Osteoporosis International* 9: 1-12.

Wolff, J. 1892. *Das Gesetz der Transformation der Knochen [The law of bone transformation].* Berlin: Hirschwald.

World Health Organization Study Group. 1994. Assessment of fracture risk and its application to screening for postmenopausal osteoporosis. *WHO Technical Report Service* 843: 1-129.

· PART FIVE ·

Physical Activity, Cancer, and Immunity

In the United States, cancer was predicted to kill about 570,000 people in 2010, second only to cardiovascular disease. Groups such as the International Agency for Research on Cancer and the American Cancer Society have estimated that approximately a third of cancer deaths occurring each year are attributable to poor diet and physical inactivity. Estimates from 15 nations of the European Union suggest that between 165,000 and 330,000 cases of the six major cancers (breast, colon, lung, prostate, endometrial, and ovarian) in 2008 were attributable to insufficient levels of physical activity (Friedenreich, Neilson, and Lynch 2010). The chapters in this section describe the evidence that physical activity is associated with reduced risks of certain cancers, particularly cancers of the colon and breast, two of the most prevalent and deadly cancers in the United States.

Surgical treatment of breast cancer was documented as early as 1600 BC in Egyptian papyrus records; and in the fourth century BC, Hippocrates coined the term *carcinoma*. However, he and Greco-Roman physicians such as Galen and Celsus believed that cancer was not curable. We now know that is not the case. We also have learned that behaviors, including physical activity, can influence the risk of developing cancer. The first chapter in this part of the book describes the contemporary epidemiologic evidence that physical activity indeed reduces the risk of developing cancers of the colon and breast. The second chapter in this part focuses on the emerging evidence that moderate physical activity influences certain aspects of the immune system in ways that might help protect against tumor growth and some inflammatory diseases.

CHAPTER 12

Physical Activity and Cancer

Certain morbid affections come . . . from other causes,
some particular posture of the limbs or unnatural movements of the body.
We must advise men employed in standing trades to interrupt . . . that too prolonged
posture by . . . walking about or exercising the body.

· Bernardino Ramazzini ·
The Diseases of Workers, 1713

CHAPTER OBJECTIVES

▸ Describe the public health burden of cancer, review its pathophysiology, and identify general risk factors

▸ Review and evaluate the strength of epidemiologic evidence that physical activity reduces the risk of colon cancer

▸ Review and evaluate the strength of epidemiologic evidence that physical activity reduces the risk of breast cancer

▸ Review epidemiologic evidence of the association of physical activity and reduced risk of other site-specific cancers

▸ Describe preliminary epidemiologic evidence on the association of physical activity and survival in patients with cancer

Cancer is a family of related diseases that result from uncontrolled growth and spread of abnormal cells, which usually become a tumor (from the Latin word meaning "swelling"; tumors can be benign or malignant, and malignant tumors are called cancers). Some of the oldest evidence of cancer is bone tumors (**osteosarcoma**) found in Egyptian mummies. Papyrus writings dated to about 1600 BC described the surgical treatment of eight cases of breast tumors, but the Greek physician Hippocrates is credited with coining a term for cancer in the fourth century BC. He used the Greek word for crab, *carcinoma,* to describe ulcer-forming tumors, presumably because tumor projections resembled the shape of a crab's body and legs.

The epidemiologic study of cancer was catalyzed by the Italian physician Bernardino Ramazzini (1633-1714) when he reported, first in 1700 and later in 1713, that nuns seldom had uterine cervical cancer but had a high incidence rate of breast cancer. He speculated that the paradox might be explained somehow by their celibacy. Today, nulliparity (i.e., not having given birth) is recognized as a risk factor for breast cancer, and modern-day research on the hormonal effects of pregnancy on cancer risk can be traced in part to Ramazzini's views. He also believed that cancer risk was influenced by physical activity (Ramazzini 1983). Ramazzini is considered the father of occupational medicine (Franco 1999). He chronicled the risk factors associated with infectious diseases and cancer present in the workplace for 55 occupations, including runners and athletes, in his 1713 book *De Morbis Artificum Diatriba* (*The Diseases of Workers,* Ramazzini 1983). He observed that diseases among workers, including cancer, mainly were associated with the toxic materials that they handled and were exacerbated by "violent or irregular motions and unnatural postures of the body." He especially recommended exercise for sedentary workers such as cobblers and tailors (Ramazzini 1983). After a description of cancer and its public health impact, this chapter discusses whether the evidence supports Ramazzini's ideas about physical activity.

▷ **BERNARDINO RAMAZZINI,** the father of occupational medicine and an early cancer epidemiologist, observed in the early 1700s that sedentary workers had elevated risks of chronic disease, including cancer.

Magnitude of the Problem

Cancer is a leading cause of morbidity and mortality in high-income countries. In the United States, cancer was predicted to kill about 569,000 people in 2010 (American Cancer Society 2010), second only to cardiovascular disease (CVD); nearly a third of cancer deaths occurring each year are attributable to poor diet and physical inactivity (Byers et al. 2002; International Agency for Research on Cancer [IARC] 2002). The financial burden of cancer is great. Estimated costs for 2010 were $263 billion from medical costs ($103 billion), lost productivity ($21 billion), and premature mortality ($140 billion) (American Cancer Society 2010). Though the annual incidence of death from cancer is roughly half that of CVD in the United States, cancer deaths rose during the 1980s before leveling off or declining starting in the 1990s. During that time, death rates from CVD steadily declined. Since the 1930s, the death rates from most cancers have generally stayed about the same or decreased. The exception is lung cancer deaths, which steadily increased until 1990 in men and 1999 in women (figure 12.1, *a* & *b*).

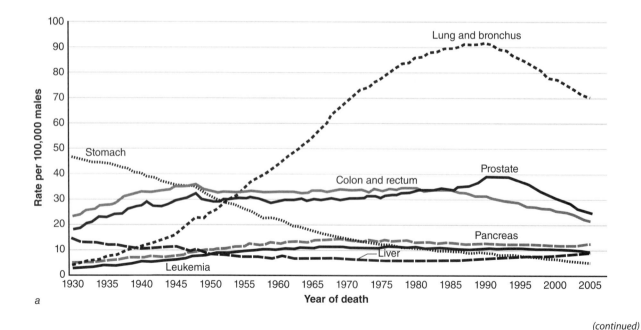

a

(continued)

Figure 12.1 Age-adjusted cancer death rates for *(a)* males and *(b)* females by site. United States: 1930–2005.

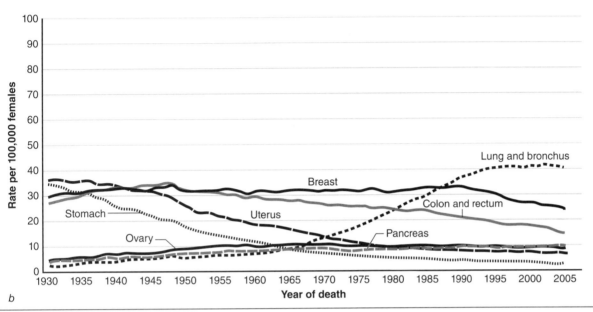

b

Figure 12.1 *(continued).*

American Cancer Society, *Cancer Facts and Figures 2012.* Atlanta: American Cancer Society, Inc.

About 1.53 million new cases of cancer were expected in the United States in 2010. That represented a 25% increase over the past decade, from an estimated incidence of 1.22 million new cases in 1999. Almost half of men (44%) and over a third of women (38%) in the United States will develop some form of cancer during their lifetimes. While all cancers involve the malfunction of genes that control cell growth and division, only about 5% of cancer is strongly hereditary (American Cancer Society 2010), so the primary and secondary prevention of cancer are top priorities for public health.

▷ **ALMOST HALF** of men and over a third of women in the United States will develop some form of cancer during their lifetimes. Only 5% of cancer is strongly hereditary, so the primary and secondary prevention of cancer are top priorities for public health.

Cancers differ in their numbers of new cases each year and annual death rates (tables 12.1 and 12.2). Though prostate cancer in men and breast cancer in women are most commonly diagnosed in the United States, lung cancer is the most deadly in both men and women. Colorectal cancers rank third in both incidence and mortality, regardless of sex.

Etiology of Cancer

Hippocrates believed that the body contained four humors (i.e., fluids), including blood, phlegm, yellow bile, and black bile. Health depended on maintaining a proper balance of these fluids. Hippocrates' idea that an excess of black bile in organs was the cause of cancer was disseminated by the Greco-Roman physician Galen and remained the popular view in medicine until the European Renaissance, around the 14th century. The humoral theory of cancer was then supplanted by a theory that cancer was caused by the fermentation of lymph fluids. John Hunter, an 18th-century Scottish surgeon credited as the first modern physician to suggest that cancers could be cured by surgery, agreed that tumors grew from lymph filtered out of the blood. Around 1840, however, German pathologist Johannes Muller showed that cancer is composed of cells, not lymph. But he thought that cancer cells stemmed from buds (or blastema) extending between normal cells. Later, Muller's student Rudolph Virchow demonstrated that cancer cells, like all cells, result from the reproduction of existing cells (Diamandopoulos 1996; Gallucci 1985).

Cancer originates in two phases: initiation and promotion. In initiation, normal cells are changed into potentially cancerous cells by damage from mutational factors. In the second phase, promotion, tumor growth is stimulated by other

Table 12.1   2010 Estimated U.S. New Cancer Cases

Type	Cases (thousands)	Percent of total
Men		
Prostate	218	28%
Lung	117	15%
Colon and rectum	72	9%
Urinary bladder	53	7%
Melanoma of skin	39	5%
Non-Hodgkin lymphoma	35	4%
Kidney	35	4%
Oral cavity	25	3%
Leukemia	25	3%
Pancreas	21	3%
Total cases	789,620	
Women		
Breast	207	28%
Lung	106	14%
Colon and rectum	70	10%
Uterine corpus	43	6%
Thyroid	34	5%
Non-Hodgkin lymphoma	30	4%
Melanoma of skin	29	4%
Kidney	23	3%
Ovary	22	3%
Pancreas	22	3%
Total cases	739,940	

Table 12.2   2010 Estimated U.S. Cancer Deaths

Type	Deaths (thousands)	Percent of total
Men		
Lung	86	29%
Prostate	32	11%
Colon and rectum	27	9%
Pancreas	19	6%
Liver	13	4%
Leukemia	13	4%
Esophagus	12	4%
Non-Hodgkin lymphoma	11	4%
Urinary bladder	10	3%
Kidney	8	3%
Total deaths	299,200	
Women		
Lung	71	26%
Breast	40	15%
Colon and rectum	25	9%
Pancreas	18	7%
Ovary	14	5%
Non-Hodgkin lymphoma	10	4%
Leukemia	9	3%
Uterine corpus	8	3%
Liver	6	2%
Brain and nerves	6	2%
Total deaths	270,290	

agents, including naturally circulating endogenous hormones. Genes located on chromosomes control the growth, division, and death of cells. Normally, body cells grow, divide, and die according to a systematic schedule. After a person reaches maturity, cell division occurs to replace injured or dying cells. In a normally aging cell, structures located at the end of chromosomes, called **telomeres,** shrink each time the cell divides until they reach a critical length that inhibits the cell from dividing further. Then the cell dies. Research has determined that 80% to 90% of cancer cells produce an enzyme called **telomerase,** which blocks the shrinking of telomeres, thus resulting in uncontrolled division of a cell to form a tumor (Holland et al. 2000).

Certain genes that promote cell division are called **oncogenes.** Others that slow down cell division, or cause cells to die at the right time, are called **tumor suppressor genes.** Cancers can be caused by DNA mutations that activate oncogenes or inactivate tumor suppressor genes. Inherited DNA changes can cause certain cancers to occur very frequently and are responsible for the cancers that run in some families. Most cancer-causing agents (i.e., **carcinogens**) produce DNA mutations that lead to abnormal clones, which progressively

become malignant clones that continue to reproduce (Holland and Frei 1993).

When cells break away from a tumor, they can **metastasize,** that is, migrate through the blood or lymph circulatory systems to other body issues, where they build "colony" tumors at a new site and continue growing, a process first described by English surgeon Stephen Paget in 1889 after he had performed autopsies on 735 women who had died of breast cancer (Paget 1889). Cancers vary in their rates of growth, patterns of spread, and responses to different types of treatment. Benign (noncancerous) tumors do not metastasize and seldom kill people. Cancers are named by their site of origin, even if they spread to another part of the body. In general, those arising from epithelial cells are called **carcinoma.** Those arising from connective tissue are known as **sarcoma.** Cancers are generally categorized according to four stages or as recurrent. Stage I cancers are small, localized tumors that usually are curable. Stage II and III cancers are advanced, localized tumors or have spread to local lymph nodes. Stage IV cancers usually are inoperable or have metastasized. These stages are defined more precisely and differently for each type of cancer and cannot be used to compare the progression of disease among different types of cancer. Staging systems that are specific to the type of cancer are described later in this chapter for cancers of the colon and breast.

▷ CANCERS ARE named by their site of origin, even if they spread to another part of the body. In general, those arising from epithelial cells are called carcinoma. Those arising from connective tissue are known as sarcoma.

Radiation and chemicals can alter a cell's DNA, causing mutations that result in cancer. One of the first practical uses of the X ray—discovered in 1896 by Wilhelm Conrad Roentgen, the first Nobel Prize winner for physics in 1901—was to treat cancer. It was subsequently determined that low daily doses of radiation can shrink tumors but that the wrong dose of radiation, including ultraviolet rays from the sun, can cause cancer growth. The idea that chemicals can cause cancer probably had its origin in the writings of London physician John Hill, who popularized the idea that tobacco is a carcinogen. In 1761, he wrote a book titled *Cautions Against the Immoderate Use of Snuff.*

Viruses also are believed to contribute to cancer by injecting new DNA sequences into cells. For example, chronic hepatitis B infection can turn into liver cancer. A type of herpes virus, Epstein-Barr, which causes mononucleosis, is believed to contribute to non-Hodgkin's lymphoma and to cancer of the nose and throat. Human immunodeficiency virus (HIV) increases the probability of developing non-Hodgkin's lymphoma, while human papilloma virus (HPV) increases the risk of cervical cancer.

The discovery of two tumor suppressor genes, BRCA1 and BRCA2, whose harmful variants greatly increase the risk of breast cancer, allows genetic screening of people at exaggerated risk of developing breast cancer, thus permitting attempts at early primary and secondary prevention (Weber 1996). Other genes have been discovered that are associated with some cancers that run in families, such as cancers of the colon, rectum, kidney, ovary, esophagus, lymph nodes, skin, and pancreas.

Risk Factors

Different cancers have different risk factors, though some risk factors are associated with several cancers. For example, smoking is a risk factor for cancers of the lung, mouth, throat, larynx, esophagus, pancreas, kidney, bladder, and cervix. In 2010, 171,000 cancer deaths (30% of all cancer deaths) were attributed to tobacco use (American Cancer Society 2010). Though several factors like this are associated with higher rates of cancer, how they contribute to the pathophysiology that leads to specific-site cancers is less well understood than for some other chronic diseases such as CVD and type 2 diabetes. For example, excessive sun exposure (especially in fair-skinned people and children and when the skin peels) increases the risk of basal cell and squamous cell carcinomas,

which are diagnosed in about 2 million people each year. Ultraviolet radiation, whether from the sun or tanning lamps and beds, also increases the risk of the most serious form of skin cancer, melanoma, which had an incidence of about 68,000 new cases in 2010 and accounted for 8700 (74%) of the estimated 12,000 deaths from all skin (excluding basal and squamous cell) cancers (American Cancer Society 2010). However, melanomas also occur on parts of the body that do not receive exposure to the sun.

▷ THE ANNUAL rate of cancer death among blacks in the United States is 18% to 35% higher than in whites, and one-third to more than twice as high as in Hispanics, American Indians, and Asian/Pacific Islanders. This discrepancy among races can be attributed to differences in exposure to risk factors, access to regular screening, and timely diagnosis and treatment (Jemal et al. 2009).

In its guidelines for cancer prevention, the American Cancer Society includes a role of regular physical activity (Kushi et al. 2006). The number of studies that have examined the association of physical activity with the rates of various cancers has increased markedly in the past decade, yielding increasing evidence that physical activity does play an important role in the prevention of some cancers. In this chapter, we examine the evidence that physical inactivity is an independent, and plausibly causal, risk factor for some cancers.

Population Studies of Physical Activity: Specificity of Protection?

Two of the earliest epidemiologic studies postulating that physical activity may reduce the risk of developing cancer were published in 1922 (Cherry 1922; Sivertsen and Dahlstrom 1922). In these studies, investigators observed that men who worked in physically demanding occupations had lower cancer mortality rates than men in less demanding ones. Subsequently, there was little research interest in this topic until the 1980s; and especially beginning in the 1990s, a large body of evidence has since accumulated on this topic. This collective body of data led to the conclusion in the Surgeon General's report on physical activity and health that physical activity decreases the risk of colon cancer and possibly other cancers (U.S. Department of Health and Human Services 1996). And, in 2007, an international panel of experts convened by the World Cancer Research Fund and the American Institute for Cancer Research found convincing evidence that physical activity protects against colon cancer, probable evidence of protection against breast cancer (particularly in postmenopausal women) and endometrial cancer, and possible evidence of protection against some other cancers. Most recently, an expert panel charged by the U.S. federal government to comprehensively examine the scientific base for making physical activity recommendations agreed with the main conclusions of the international expert panel, stating that the evidence was clear that physical activity reduces the risks of developing colon and breast cancers (Physical Activity Guidelines Advisory Committee 2008). The U.S. expert panel also found that the evidence was suggestive for lower risks of lung, endometrial, and ovarian cancers associated with physical activity. The experts further stated that the overall data did not support associations with prostate cancer or rectal cancer, while too few data existed for cancers of other sites to allow any conclusions.

The following sections summarize the evidence about the relationship of physical activity and cancer. Only cancers of the colon and breast, for which the evidence is strongest and most consistent, are discussed fully. These also are two of the most commonly occurring and fatal cancers in the United States, on which many physical activity studies have been conducted. Lung cancer, the most commonly fatal and the second most commonly occurring cancer in both men and women, and endometrial cancer, the fourth most commonly occurring cancer in women, are discussed briefly since the data on associations with physical activity for these two cancers are more limited.

The available evidence suggests that the benefits of physical activity appear to be site specific, which is logical because the risk factors for different cancers also are different. Nonetheless, we briefly describe next the early findings from two well-regarded prospective studies of large cohorts that found both physical activity and physical fitness to be associated with reduced risk of all-site cancer deaths. These results likely reflect the combined findings for some cancer sites, where physical activity or fitness does reduce mortality, and other cancer sites, where no relation exists, leading to an overall lower death rate from all cancers.

Harvard Alumni Health Study

Among 17,000 Harvard alumni who were observed for 12 to 16 years, a third of the deaths were attributed to cancer. After adjustment for age, smoking, and body mass index, the men who expended fewer than 500 kcal each week in physical activity—this was estimated from reported walking, stair climbing, and sports and recreational activities—had a 50% higher risk of cancer death than did men who expended 500 kcal or more each week (figure 12.2) (Paffenbarger, Hyde, and Wing 1987).

Aerobics Center Longitudinal Study (ACLS)

In the ACLS cohort, over 10,000 men and 3000 women were observed for about eight years after a clinic fitness test and health exam. The low-fit men and women were nearly three and two times, respectively, more likely to die of cancer than those who had an average level of fitness. Figure 12.3

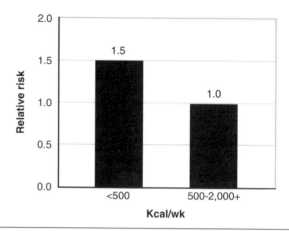

Figure 12.2   Harvard Alumni Health Study examining kilocalories burned per week and relative risk for cancer death.

Data from Paffenbarger, Hyde, and Wing 1987.

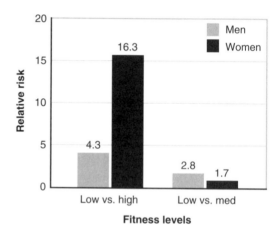

Figure 12.3   Aerobics Center Longitudinal Study comparing fitness levels to relative risk for cancer.

Data from Blair et al. 1989.

illustrates that the lower risk associated with fitness was dose dependent. The low-fit men and women had relative risks of 4.3 and 16.3, respectively, compared with those who had a high fitness level (Blair et al. 1989). The high risk among low-fit women might not be reliable, though, because there were only 18 cancer deaths among women in the ACLS cohort.

Colon and Rectal Cancer

According to the American Cancer Society (2010), about 103,000 new cases of colon cancer (50,000 men and 53,000 women) and 40,000 new cases of rectal cancer (23,000 men and 17,000 women) were predicted to occur in 2010. Colon and rectal cancers were expected to account for more than 51,000 deaths (26,000 in men and 25,000 in women) during 2010. Colon cancer and rectal cancer have common features and often are referred to jointly as colorectal cancer. The death rate from colorectal cancers has been declining during the past 20 years, probably because of fewer new cases, early detection, and improved treatment. The five-year survival rate is 90% for people whose colorectal cancer is found and treated in an early stage, but only about 40% of colorectal cancers are detected before metastasis. After regional metastasis, the five-year survival rate goes down to 70%, and it is merely 11% after metastasis to distant sites. The overall five-year survival rate for colon cancer in the United States is about 67% for whites and 56% for blacks (American Cancer Society 2010).

The remainder of this section focuses only on colon cancer, since as already noted, the totality of evidence does not support a relation between physical activity and rectal cancer incidence (Physical Activity Guidelines Advisory Committee 2008).

Types of Colon Cancer

The colon is a smooth-muscle vessel about 5 ft (1.5 m) long that absorbs water and minerals from fecal matter received from the small intestine. Fecal matter is then passed to the rectum for excretion from the body. The colon has four sections (figure 12.4). (1) The ascending colon (also known as the right colon) extends upward on the right side of the abdomen. (2) The transverse colon crosses the body to the left side, where it connects to (3) the descending colon (also known as the left colon), which continues

downward on the left side. (4) The sigmoid colon, named for its S-like shape, connects to the rectum. Cancer can develop in any of the four sections of the colon or in the rectum and can cause different symptoms in each area (National Cancer Institute 1999).

Stages of Colon Cancer

Once cancer is detected, it is important that its severity be judged in order to plan treatment. Severity is graded in stages based on how far a tumor has spread within the rectum and colon, to nearby tissues, and to other organs as determined by palpation, sigmoidoscopy or colonoscopy, X rays, blood tests, and biopsy. The most common staging systems are the TNM and the Dukes/Modified Astler-Coller equivalents systems, provided in tables 12.3 and 12.4 along with average survival rates. The TNM system is the one used most often. The T staging refers to the invasiveness of the tumor. N describes how far the cancer has spread to nearby lymph

Table 12.3 TNM Staging Table

T Stage		N Stage		M Stage	
T1	Invades submucosa	N0	No nodes involved	M0	No metastases
T2	Invades muscularis propria	N1	One to three local lymph nodes involved	M1	Metastases present
T3	Invades through muscularis into subserosa	N2	Four or more pericolic lymph nodes involved		
T4	Invades other organs or perforates the visceral peritoneum	N3	Any lymph nodes along a named vascular trunk involved		

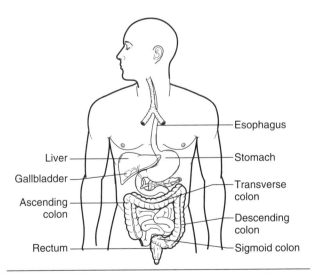

Figure 12.4 Diagram illustrating the four sections of the colon.

Table 12.4 TNM Group Staging and Dukes/Modified Astler-Coller Equivalents

T, N, M grouping	T, N, M stage	Dukes/MAC equivalent	Five-year survival
T1, N0, M0	I	A	90%
T2, N0, M0		B1	75%
T3, N0, M0	II	B2	60%
T4, N0, M0		B3	50%
Any T, N1, M0	III	C1	45%
Any T, N2, M0		C2	40%
Any T, N3, M0		C3	30%
Any T, Any N, M1	IV	D	10%

nodes. M indicates whether the cancer has metastasized to other organs of the body. The information from the T, N, and M categories can be combined into Stages 0 through IV to describe increasing severity of the cancer (table 12.4).

Etiology of Colon Cancer

Like atherosclerosis and type 2 diabetes, colorectal cancers develop over a period of several decades. Before a true cancer develops, there usually are precancerous changes in the lining of the colon or rectum. These changes might be dysplasia (abnormal tissue formation) or adenomatous **polyps** (masses of tissue that bulge, usually on a stalk, from the interior lining of the colon). Polyps grow inward toward the center of the colon or rectum. In contrast, a cancer can grow either inward or outward through the walls of the colon or rectum and can metastasize if not treated. More than 95% of colorectal cancers are adenocarcinomas, gland-like cancers of epithelial cells in the lining of the colon and rectum.

Risk Factors and Screening

Major risk factors for colorectal cancer include a personal or immediate family history of colorectal cancer or polyps, inflammatory bowel disease, age (about 90% of cases occur after age 50), a diet high in red meat and low in fiber, high alcohol intake, obesity, and physical inactivity (Giovan-nucci and Wu 2006).

The progression from normal colorectal mucosa to adenomatous polyp to invasive carcinoma occurs over a decade or longer and is associated with an accumulation of genetic and epigenetic alterations that are either inherited or caused by environmental factors (e.g., obesity, lack of physical activity) (Fearon and Vogelstein 1990). Measures can be taken to reduce mortality rates from colorectal cancer via screening, which can detect this disease in its early stages, when treatment is much more effective. Several tests designed to detect colorectal cancer in its early stages are available. These include a stool blood test that checks for hidden blood in the stool. More invasive screening tests that are recommended include a flexible sigmoidoscopy (inspection of the rectum and lower colon by a camera attached to the end of a flexible tube) or a colonoscopy (inspection of the rectum and entire colon by a camera attached to the end of a flexible tube) (U.S. Preventive Services Task Force 2008).

The more invasive screening procedures can detect the presence of a polyp. An adenomatous polyp is one that is derived from glandular epithelial cells. The most common treatment for polyp removal is surgery ("polypectomy"). Colorectal cancer has hallmark symptoms that include a change in usual bowel habits ranging from diarrhea to con-stipation; blood in the stool or narrower stool than usual;

stomach discomfort such as gas pain, bloating, or cramps; a feeling that a bowel movement is not complete; weight loss without a reason; and persistent fatigue. Surgery is the primary treatment for most patients with colorectal cancer, and this may be combined with chemotherapy and radiation therapy, depending on the stage of the disease.

Physical Activity and Colon Cancer: The Evidence

A recent meta-analysis examined the available evidence relating physical activity to reduced risk of colon cancer (Wolin et al. 2009). A total of 52 studies, 24 case–control and 28 cohort studies, were included. These studies were conducted in many countries, including the United States, Canada, China, Denmark, Finland, Italy, Japan, Korea, New Zealand, Norway, Sweden, Switzerland, Taiwan, and Turkey. Overall, the studies consistently observed an inverse association between physical activity and the risk of develop-ing colon cancer. When the most active versus least-active individuals across all studies are compared, the relative risk was 0.76 (95% CI: 0.72-0.81). The effect was similar in men and women (relative risks of 0.76 and 0.79, respectively), and the results from case–control studies tended to be stronger than those from cohort studies (relative risks of 0.69 and 0.83, respectively). This protective effect of physical activity appears independent of other risk factors for colon cancer (Physical Activity Guidelines Advisory Committee 2008; Harriss et al. 2009).

Many of the studies relating physical activity levels to colon cancer risk categorized subjects according to at least three levels of physical activity, allowing assessment of dose–response relations. In general, the evidence supports an inverse dose–response relation; however, due to the multiple and variable methods used to assess and catego-rize physical activity, it is difficult to determine the shape of the dose–response curve (Physical Activity Guidelines Advisory Committee 2008). With regard to the amount of physical activity required to lower the risk of colon cancer, again, the different methods of physical activity assessment in the different studies make it difficult to provide a detailed answer. Overall, it appears that some 30 to 60 min per day of moderate- to vigorous-intensity physical activity may be necessary to significantly reduce the risk of developing colon cancer.

With regard to whether the association of physical activity and colon cancer risk differs by subgroups of individuals, several studies have separately examined subgroups based on use of menopausal hormone therapy in women, various aspects of diet, or body mass index. Overall, the findings have been largely inconsistent, but they suggest that higher levels of physical activity may ameliorate the adverse impact of high body weight on colon cancer risk (Physical Activity

Guidelines Advisory Committee 2008). Several studies also have examined whether physical activity has different associations with colon cancers occurring at different subsites of the colon. Again, these data have been equivocal (Physical Activity Guidelines Advisory Committee 2008).

▷ **A RECENT REVIEW** of 52 epidemiological studies of physical activity and colon cancer incidence showed a reduction in risk with increasing levels of physical activity (Wolin et al. 2009). This was true for both men and women. On average, physical activity was associated with a 24% reduction in the risk of developing colon cancer. Some 30 to 60 min per day of moderate-to vigorous-intensity physical activity appears necessary to reduce the risk.

Case–Control Studies

Because the body of literature is large, it is not possible to comprehensively discuss each study. Here we provide findings from exemplar case–control studies that have investigated the relation between physical activity and colon cancer risk.

Sweden

This was one of the earliest case–control studies to examine whether physical activity is associated with lower risk of developing colon cancer. Nearly 1200 men and women were studied from 1986 to 1988 (352 cases of colon cancer, 217 cases of rectal cancer; 624 controls) (Gerhardsson de Verdier et al. 1990). Both occupational and recreational physical activity levels were determined by self-reports. Compared with the most active men and women, sedentary men and women had an odds ratio of 3.2 (95% CI: 1.5-7.0) for developing cancer in the left colon; further, this association showed an inverse dose–response relation. There was no association of physical activity with the right colon or rectum. Controlling for year of birth, sex, body mass, and dietary factors (intakes of total energy, protein, total fat, and dietary fiber) did not change the results.

Seattle

In this case–control study, investigators were interested in the associations of different domains of physical activity—specifically leisure-time and occupational activity—with colon cancer risk. Two hundred fifty men and 190 women ages 30 to 62 years who were diagnosed with colon cancer from 1985 to 1989 in three counties of the Seattle metropolitan area were matched by age, sex, and county of residence with 233 male and 193 female control subjects (White, Jacobs, and Daling 1996). Physical activity was assessed by questions about the frequency and duration of various recreational and occupational activities performed at least twice

a month during the 10-year period ending two years before diagnosis (or reference date for controls). Activities were classified as low intensity (<4.5 METs [metabolic equivalents]) or moderate to high intensity (>4.5 METs). Among men and women combined, participation in moderate- or high-intensity leisure-time physical activity two or more times each week was associated with a relative risk of 0.70 (95% CI: 0.45-1.00) compared with that for people reporting no physical activity. The association was stronger for men than women. Paradoxically, the lowest risk was observed in people who said they exercised in their leisure time two or three times a week rather than more often. Occupational activity was not associated with colon cancer overall, but a 70% reduction was found in men 55 years and younger who performed more than 14.5 h/week of moderate activity at work compared with those who had sedentary jobs. Findings were independent of age, body mass index, dietary factors, alcohol use, some other health behaviors, and region of the colon affected by cancer.

California, Utah, and Minnesota

In this case–control study, investigators wanted to examine the details of physical activity required for lower colon cancer risk in order to provide information useful for public health recommendations (Slattery et al. 1997). Study participants came from Northern California, Utah, and the Minneapolis–Saint Paul metropolitan area in Minnesota; there were approximately 2000 men and women with colon cancer and 2400 control subjects matched on sex and age. Long-term involvement (20 years) in high levels of physical activity prior to the onset of colon cancer, equivalent to 60 min or more of vigorous activity each session, was associated with about a 30% reduction in risk of colon cancer (RR = 0.68; 95% CI: 0.52-0.87). The amount of time involved in physical activity had a greater impact than the number of days per week on which activities were performed. Those reporting the highest level of activity, as defined by both duration and intensity, had a 40% reduction in risk compared with those who were sedentary. Associations did not differ by age at diagnosis, site of the tumor within the colon, or sex. The protective effect of physical activity was slightly stronger among those without a family history of colorectal cancer. In the populations studied, 13% of colon cancers could be attributed to lack of vigorous leisure-time activity (i.e., 4.3 cases of colon cancer per 100,000 population could be prevented each year by participation in vigorous leisure-time physical activity).

China

In this large, population-based case–control study, the relation between physical activity conducted during transportation (commuting physical activity) and colon cancer risk was of interest. A total of 931 incident colon cancer cases (462 men and 469 women) diagnosed between 1990 and 1993 in

Shanghai and 1552 randomly selected controls, frequency matched to the age and sex distribution of the cases, were studied (Hou et al. 2004). Subjects reported their means of commuting and the time spent on the round trip to and from work at in-person interviews. There was a significant inverse dose–response relation between commuting physical activity and risk of colon cancer in both men and women: When >94.3 MET-hours/week of commuting was compared with <48.3 MET-hours, the odds ratios were 0.52 (95% CI: 0.27-0.87) in men and 0.56 (0.21-0.91) in women after adjustment for age, education, family income, marital status, and diet, and also number of children and menopausal status in women.

Prospective Cohort Studies

As with the case–control studies, we provide findings here from exemplar cohort studies that have investigated the relation between physical activity and colon cancer risk.

Los Angeles

The protective effect of physical activity against the development of colon cancer was first suggested by an observational study of new colon cancer cases among men ages 20 to 64 years who lived in Los Angeles County from 1972 to 1981 (Garabrant et al. 1984). Physical activity levels were categorized as sedentary, moderately active, and highly active based on job titles. The age-adjusted colon cancer incidence rates per 100,000 men declined linearly, from 24.6 to 21.6 to 13.4, with each increasing physical activity level. The relative risk for those in sedentary occupations was 1.8 times that in the highly active jobs, but the higher rate of cancer among the sedentary men might have been influenced by differences in diet, which was not controlled in the study.

Harvard Alumni Health Study

Prior to the Harvard Alumni Health Study, investigations addressing the influence of physical activity on colon cancer risk generally used a single assessment of physical activity, thus failing to account for changes over time. Additionally, few previous studies had provided information on the amount of physical activity associated with lower colon cancer risk. Thus, investigators from the Harvard Alumni Health Study sought to address these gaps in knowledge. Self-reported stair climbing, walking, and sports play were assessed between 1962 and 1966 and again in 1977 among approximately 17,000 Harvard alumni ages 30 to 79 years who were followed prospectively for the occurrence of colon cancer (n = 220) and rectal cancer (n = 44) from 1965 through 1988 (Lee, Paffenbarger, and Hsieh 1991). Men who consistently expended 1000 to 2500 kcal per week had about half the risk of colon cancer compared with men who were less active in age-adjusted analyses (RR = 0.50; 95% CI: 0.27-0.93). There was no further risk reduction with >2500 kcal per week. Further adjustment for body mass index did not change findings, but diet was not controlled for. Physical activity was unrelated to rectal cancer risk.

In an updated analysis that also controlled for body mass index and parental history of cancer, the inverse relation between physical activity and colon cancer risk was no longer observed among all men, although an inverse relation of borderline significance still existed for heavier men with body mass index of at least 26 kg/m² (Lee and Paffenbarger 1994). It is unclear why the inverse association was no longer observed among all men; one possible reason is that with longer follow-up but no additional updating of physical activity information in the later study, physical activity levels may have changed, leading to random misclassification and biasing observed findings toward no association.

The generalizability of these findings may be limited, since Harvard alumni are unlikely to be representative of the general population. Nonetheless, the observation of an inverse relation between physical activity and colon cancer risk in Harvard alumni is consistent with findings from many other studies conducted in diverse countries and among diverse populations.

Health Professionals Follow-Up Study

In this prospective cohort study, investigators (Giovannucci et al. 1995) examined whether physical inactivity and obesity increase the risk for colon cancer and adenomas. A cohort of nearly 48,000 male health professionals 40 to 75 years of age responded in 1986 to a health survey that included questions about physical activity; questions were similar to those from the Harvard Alumni Health Study although restricted to only eight groups of the most common leisure-time activities, as well as weight and height. Participants were grouped into quintiles based on estimated energy expenditure from leisure-time activities. By 1992, 203 colon cancer cases and 586 adenoma cases were reported and confirmed on medical record review. The rate of left colon cancer was about 50% lower in the highest quintile compared with the lowest quintile of energy expenditure (RR = 0.53; 95% CI: 0.32-0.88) after adjustment for age, history of colorectal polyps, previous endoscopy, parental history of colorectal cancer, smoking, body mass index, use of aspirin, diet, and alcohol. Modest levels of activity (11 MET-hours per week) substantially reduced the risk of colon cancer, with an inverse dose–response relationship existing, up to 46.8 MET-hours per week. The level of physical activity associated with substantially reduced colon cancer risk—11 MET-hours per week—is approximately equivalent to 1000 kcal per week, the amount of activity associated with lower colon cancer risk in the earlier Harvard Alumni Health Study investigation already described. This translates to the approximate equivalent of about 1 h of running, 2 h of tennis, or 3 h of walking a week. Weak inverse associations were observed between physical activity and colon polyps, particularly large polyps of the distal colon.

Nonetheless, the findings were limited to male health professionals, who might be more likely to engage in other healthful behaviors not controlled in the study. Also, only eight groups of the most common leisure-time activities were assessed, which might lead to an underestimation of the amount of physical activity needed for protection against colon cancer.

Nurses' Health Study

None of the prospective studies discussed so far included women. The Nurses' Health Study, which began in 1976, is a prospective cohort study of women's health in 122,000 female registered nurses who were ages 30 to 55 years at baseline. Women provide information about health and behavior on questionnaires that are updated every two years. In a 1997 study that included about 68,000 eligible women followed from 1986 onward, when detailed physical activity information was available (Martinez et al. 1997), investigators examined whether leisure-time physical activity significantly influences the risk of colon cancer in women. Physical activity in this study was self-reported, using a questionnaire similar to that in the Health Professionals Follow-Up Study just discussed; follow-up for ascertainment of colon cancer also used similar procedures. During six years of follow-up, 212 women developed colon cancer. After controlling for age, smoking, family history of colorectal cancer, body mass index, postmenopausal hormone use, use of aspirin, red meat intake, and alcohol, women who expended more than 21 MET-hours per week in leisure-time physical activities had a relative risk of colon cancer of 0.54 (95% CI: 0.33-0.90) compared with women who expended less than 2 MET-hours per week, consistent with observations in men. As in the male health professionals investigation, only eight groups of leisure-time physical activities were assessed, so the amount of activity needed for protection may have been underestimated.

An updated analysis of this study continued to show an inverse, but less marked, association between physical activity and colon cancer risk (Wolin et al. 2007). Women expending at least 21.5 MET-hours per week now had a relative risk of colon cancer of 0.77 compared with women expending <2 MET-hours per week. This updated analysis also sought to examine the kinds of activities needed to reduce risk and found that moderate-to-vigorous leisure-time activities were more strongly related to lower risk than was walking.

California Teachers Study

This is another prospective cohort study of women that examined the relation between physical activity and colon cancer risk (Mai et al. 2007). The California Teachers Study is a study of approximately 133,000 current, recent, and retired female public school teachers and administrators, ages 22 to 84 years, in the California State Teachers Retirement System at the time the study began in 1995. For this particular analysis, about 120,000 women were included. Women reported on questionnaires the average amount of time per week spent in moderate leisure-time activities, and the average months per year, for several time periods in their lives. Parallel questions were asked for vigorous activities.

Between 1996 and 2002, 395 women developed invasive colon cancer. After age and race were controlled for, lifetime moderate and vigorous leisure-time activities were modestly associated with reduced colon cancer risk; the relative risk was 0.75 (95% CI: 0.57-1.00) for women with 4 or more hours per week of such activities versus 0.5 or fewer hours per week. Further adjustments for body mass index, smoking, use of postmenopausal hormone therapy, use of nonsteroidal anti-inflammatory drugs, and diet did not change the findings. The association was stronger among postmenopausal women who had never taken hormone therapy.

Strength of the Evidence

As discussed earlier in this book, cause-and-effect relations can be inferred only from well-designed and well-conducted randomized controlled trials. Epidemiologic studies that have examined the relation between physical activity and cancer risk all have been observational in study design—either case–control or cohort studies. Thus, the available data cannot prove causality of the relation. However, with use of Mill's cannons (see chapter 2) as discussed later, the totality of evidence does support a cause-and-effect relation between physical activity and lower colon cancer rates.

A particular concern for observational studies is the potential for confounding—persons who are physically active also may have other healthy habits or characteristics (e.g., less alcohol intake, better diet, healthier body weight) that may lower colon cancer risk. Thus, it is unclear whether it is the physical activity that is responsible for the lower risk or whether this is a consequence of the other healthy habits. Many of the studies, particularly the more recent studies, have controlled for these other health habits in their analyses and have continued to observe lower colon cancer rates among physically active persons (Physical Activity Guidelines Advisory Committee 2008). For example, in the Health Professionals Follow-Up Study (Giovannucci et al. 1995) discussed earlier, investigators controlled for many other factors (age; prior endoscopy; parental history of colorectal cancer; smoking; intakes of aspirin, animal fat, dietary fiber, folate, methionine, and alcohol) and still found an inverse association between physical activity and risk of colon cancer in men. The Nurses' Health Study (Martinez et al. 1997; Wolin et al. 2007) similarly controlled for many of the same variables and continued to observe lower colon cancer rates among physically active women. On balance, the association between physical activity and lower incidence of colon cancer appears to be independent of other health factors.

Further questions of interest, particularly for public health recommendations, relate to the details of physical activity required. While most studies have examined leisure-time physical activity, the studies described up to this point suggest that occupational and commuting activity also do count. With regard to the amount of physical activity required, few studies have provided sufficient details to be able to answer this question. Some of these studies have been described here; on the whole, the available data suggest that 30 to 60 min a day of moderate-to-vigorous physical activity is required (Physical Activity Guidelines Advisory Committee 2008).

Temporal Sequence

In general, this criterion is well satisfied. In the case–control studies, while the actual investigation took place after exposure (physical activity) and disease (colon cancer) had already occurred, most of the studies asked subjects to recall physical activity at a time in the past, often decades in the past, before the onset of colon cancer (e.g., see case–control study from California, Utah, and Minnesota discussed previously). For the prospective cohort studies, investigators ascertained physical activity at baseline, then followed subjects forward in time, in some cases for decades, for the onset of colon cancer (e.g., see Harvard Alumni Health Study discussed earlier).

Strength of Association

Most studies have reported a moderately strong, inverse association between physical activity and risk of colon cancer, with the relative risks ranging from 1.2 to 3.9 for those who are most sedentary compared with those who are most active (Lee and Oguma 2006; Wolin et al. 2009). A 2009 meta-analysis estimated that the most active individuals have a 24% reduction in the risk of developing colon cancer compared with the least active, and that the magnitude of risk reduction is similar in men and women (Wolin et al. 2009). It has been estimated that colon cancer rates in the United States could be lowered by 7% if the roughly 25% of the U.S. adult population reporting no leisure-time physical activity were to increase energy expenditure by 10 MET-hours (about 3 h of moderate-intensity physical activity) each week (Colditz, Cannuscio, and Frazier 1997). If the overall risk for colon cancer attributable to physical inactivity is 30%, about 15,000 deaths could be prevented if all sedentary Americans became vigorously active.

▶ **IT HAS** been estimated that colon cancer rates in the United States could be lowered by 7% if the 25% of the U.S. adult population with no leisure-time activity were to increase energy expenditure by 10 MET-hours (about 3 h of moderate-intensity physical activity) each week (Colditz, Cannuscio, and Frazier 1997).

Consistency

Overall, the data have been consistent (figure 12.5, *a* & *b*), with studies of physical activity showing significant inverse associations with colon cancer risk in both men and women in different ethnic groups and nations, including the United

States, Canada, China, Japan, Sweden, Denmark, Italy, New Zealand, Switzerland, Taiwan, and Turkey (Lee and Oguma 2006; Wolin et al. 2009). A 2009 meta-analysis estimated that risk reductions were similar in men (RR = 0.76; 95% CI: 0.71-0.82) and women (RR = 0.79; 95% CI: 0.71-0.88) (Wolin et al. 2009).

Dose Response

In a recent review of 23 publications on physical activity and colon cancer risk since the 1996 Surgeon General's report, almost all studies classified subjects according to at least three levels of physical activity, allowing investigators to assess dose response (Physical Activity Guidelines Advisory Committee 2008). About half the case–control studies and two-thirds of the cohort studies reported significant, inverse trends between physical activity and colon cancer risk. Previous reviews that included studies published prior to 1996 also concluded that an inverse dose–response relation is likely (Friedenreich and Orenstein 2002; Lee and Oguma 2006). As discussed earlier, because of the many different methods used to assess and classify physical activity in these studies, it is difficult to ascertain the shape of the dose–response curve; one can note only that a dose–response relation appears likely.

With regard to the amount and intensity of physical activity required, an expert panel charged by the U.S. federal government to comprehensively examine the scientific base for making physical activity recommendations concluded that some 30 to 60 min per day of moderate- to vigorous-intensity physical activity may be necessary to significantly reduce the risk of developing colon cancer (Physical Activity Guidelines Advisory Committee 2008).

Biological Plausibility

While the exact mechanisms underlying a protective effect of physical activity on colon cancer risk have not been identified, several plausible mechanisms have been suggested. As described previously, adenomatous polyps (adenomas) are precursors to most colorectal cancers, and several studies have reported lower risk of adenomas among physically active people. For example, in a colonoscopy study of 200 adenoma cases and 384 adenoma-free controls, women in the top three quartiles of leisure physical activity had half the incidence of colorectal adenomas of those in the least-active quartile (Sandler, Pritchard, and Bangdiwala 1995). There was no protective effect of occupational physical activity among men or women, while men who did not participate in sports had a 70% increase in risk for adenomas. However, in a prospective study of about 1900 men and women, no associations between adenoma recurrence and moderate, vigorous, or total physical activity were found during a three-year follow-up period after colonoscopy (Colbert et al. 2002). One possible explanation for this apparent

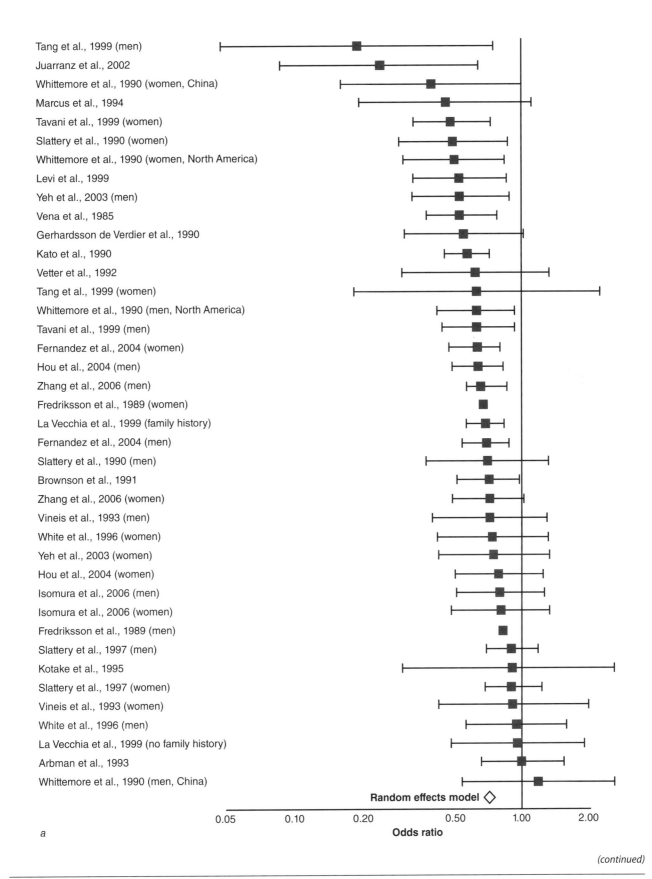

Tang et al., 1999 (men)
Juarranz et al., 2002
Whittemore et al., 1990 (women, China)
Marcus et al., 1994
Tavani et al., 1999 (women)
Slattery et al., 1990 (women)
Whittemore et al., 1990 (women, North America)
Levi et al., 1999
Yeh et al., 2003 (men)
Vena et al., 1985
Gerhardsson de Verdier et al., 1990
Kato et al., 1990
Vetter et al., 1992
Tang et al., 1999 (women)
Whittemore et al., 1990 (men, North America)
Tavani et al., 1999 (men)
Fernandez et al., 2004 (women)
Hou et al., 2004 (men)
Zhang et al., 2006 (men)
Fredriksson et al., 1989 (women)
La Vecchia et al., 1999 (family history)
Fernandez et al., 2004 (men)
Slattery et al., 1990 (men)
Brownson et al., 1991
Zhang et al., 2006 (women)
Vineis et al., 1993 (men)
White et al., 1996 (women)
Yeh et al., 2003 (women)
Hou et al., 2004 (women)
Isomura et al., 2006 (men)
Isomura et al., 2006 (women)
Fredriksson et al., 1989 (men)
Slattery et al., 1997 (men)
Kotake et al., 1995
Slattery et al., 1997 (women)
Vineis et al., 1993 (women)
White et al., 1996 (men)
La Vecchia et al., 1999 (no family history)
Arbman et al., 1993
Whittemore et al., 1990 (men, China)

Random effects model ◇

0.05   0.10   0.20   0.50   1.00   2.00

a

Odds ratio

(continued)

Figure 12.5 Meta-analysis of physical activity and colon cancer: *(a)* case–control studies, and *(b)* cohort studies.

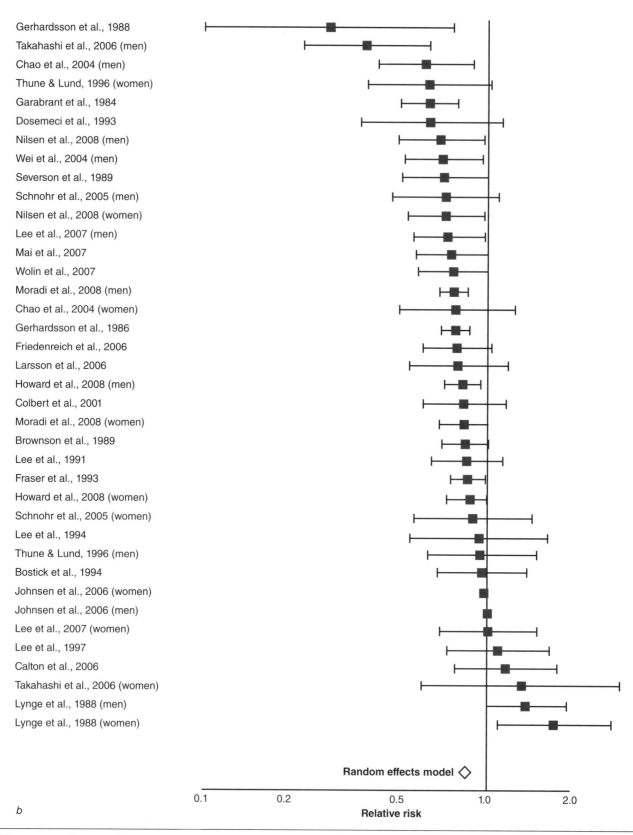

Figure 12.5 *(continued).*

Adapted, by permission, from K.Y. Wolin, Y. Yan, G.A. Colditz, and I.M. Lee, 2009, "Physical activity and colon cancer prevention: A meta-analysis," *British Journal of Cancer* 100: 611-616.

discrepancy is that the types of polyps in these two studies may have differed. Physical activity appears to influence the later stages of disease progression, since stronger inverse associations with physical activity have been noted for large polyps (Giovannucci et al. 1995) and advanced neoplastic polyps (Wallace et al. 2005).

Bowel Transit Time

An initial popular explanation for reduced colon cancer rates among physically active people was that exercise results in a shortened gastrointestinal transit time (e.g., by increasing peristalsis and decreasing fecal segmentation), hence reducing the contact of potential carcinogens with the mucosal lining of the colon (Shephard 1995). However, studies examining gastrointestinal transit time with exercise have presented inconsistent findings (Bingham and Cummings 1989; Coenen et al. 1992; Cordain, Latin, and Behnke 1986; Koffler et al. 1992; Robertson et al. 1993). Additionally, one study reported that four weeks of exercise training had no effect on patients with idiopathic constipation (Meshkinpour et al. 1998), and some population-based studies have found that cancer risk was not related to overall gastrointestinal transit time (Shephard 1996).

Insulin Resistance and Obesity

Currently, there is strong belief that insulin resistance represents an important pathway in the physical activity–colon cancer relation. People diagnosed with colon cancer have a higher than average rate of the metabolic syndrome, which includes features of hyperinsulinemia, hyperglycemia, hypertriglyceridemia, low high-density lipoprotein cholesterol levels, high blood pressure, and central obesity. Physical inactivity is a strong determinant of hyperinsulinemia, which could mediate the effect of inactivity on colon cancer risk because insulin is an important growth factor for colon cancer cells (Giovannucci 2001). Higher colon cancer incidence and mortality also have been noted in those with type 2 diabetes or impaired glucose tolerance, and insulin can enhance tumor development by stimulating cell proliferation or inhibiting apoptosis (Physical Activity Guidelines Advisory Committee 2008). Acute bouts of physical activity improve insulin sensitivity and increase glucose uptake by skeletal muscle for up to 12 h, and chronic exercise training results in prolonged improvements in insulin sensitivity (Physical Activity Guidelines Advisory Committee 2008). Although adiposity is strongly associated with insulin sensitivity, exercise-induced changes in insulin sensitivity can occur from physical activity, independent of the changes in weight or body composition (Physical Activity Guidelines Advisory Committee 2008). And, congruent with this observation is the finding from epidemiologic studies that the inverse relation between physical activity and colon cancer risk is observed among persons of different body mass index (Physical Activity Guidelines Advisory Committee 2008).

▷ **CURRENTLY, THERE** is strong belief that insulin resistance represents an important pathway in the physical activity–colon cancer relation. Physical inactivity is a strong determinant of hyperinsulinemia, which could mediate the effect of inactivity on colon cancer risk because insulin is an important growth factor for colon cancer cells (Giovannucci 2001).

Inflammation

Inflammation may play a role as well; elevated levels of inflammatory markers, such as C-reactive protein (CRP), interleukin (IL)-6, and tumor necrosis factor-alpha (TNF-α) and decreased levels of anti-inflammatory markers such as adiponectin have been linked with increased cancer risk (Schottenfeld and Beebe-Dimmer 2006). Physical activity may reduce systemic inflammation alone or in combination with improved body weight, composition, or both (Physical Activity Guidelines Advisory Committee 2008).

Immune Function

The immune system is thought to play a role in reducing cancer risk by recognizing and eliminating abnormal cells or through immune system components—acquired, innate, or both. Physical activity may enhance the immune system: An exercise session can temporarily elevate levels of some immune cells in the blood (e.g., natural killer cells, cytoxic T lymphocytes, monocytes), which might inhibit colon tumor growth (Shephard 1996).

Other Mechanisms

Other postulated mechanisms for the link between higher physical activity levels and lower colon cancer rates include changes in prostaglandin levels with exercise (Shephard 1996). Prostaglandin F increases gut motility and inhibits the division and spread of colon cancer cells. In contrast, prostaglandin E2, which is elevated in people with colorectal cancer or polyps, decreases gut motility and increases colonic cell proliferation.

Finally, while the findings from animal experiments should be cautiously extrapolated to humans, they do support a protective effect of physical activity on cancer. Most experimental studies used mice or rats that ran in an activity wheel or were forced to swim in order to examine whether physical activity affects tumor growth or survival after tumor implants (Shephard 1996). It is difficult to extrapolate age, duration of training, and rate of body fat accumulation from rats or mice to humans (Shephard 1996). Nevertheless, experimental studies of rodents indicate that prior or concurrent exercise reduces the incidence of chemically induced tumors and produces a 25% to 100% slowing of tumor growth (Shephard 1995, 1996).

Summary and Conclusions

About 50 case–control and cohort studies of physical activity and risk of developing colon cancer have been reported. Overall, the studies showed a protective effect of physical activity. This has been observed in different ethnic groups and many nations, including the United States, Canada, China, Japan, Sweden, Denmark, Italy, New Zealand, Switzerland, Taiwan, and Turkey, indicating high consistency (Physical Activity Guidelines Advisory Committee 2008; Lee and Oguma 2006; Wolin et al. 2009). The reduction in rates of colon cancers among physically active people on average is 24%, similar in men and women (Wolin et al. 2009). Occupational, leisure-time, and commuting physical activity appear to "count" for protection (Physical Activity Guidelines Advisory Committee 2008). Some 30 to 60 min a day of moderate- to vigorous-intensity physical activity appears required for reduced risk (Physical Activity Guidelines Advisory Committee 2008). Generally, study findings have satisfied the criteria of strength of association, consistency between sexes, temporal sequence, dose response, and biological plausibility. Because of cost and feasibility constraints, randomized controlled trials of physical activity and the development of colon cancer among persons at average risk will likely never be conducted. Thus, while there have been no studies of cancer risk in humans after experimental manipulations of physical activity and no studies showing that naturally occurring alterations in physical activity levels are associated with changes in colon cancer rates, the available data do strongly support a protective role of physical activity in preventing colon cancer development.

▷ **ABOUT 50** case–control and cohort studies of physical activity and colon cancer have been reported worldwide. Overall, these studies showed a protective effect of physical activity. The reduction in rates of colon cancers among physically active people on average is 24%, similar in men and women (Wolin et al. 2009).

Breast Cancer

Next to skin cancers, breast cancer is the most prevalent cancer among women, accounting for one of every three cancer diagnoses in the United States. About 207,000 new cases of invasive breast cancer were expected among women in 2010; this is a rare cancer in men, with only 2000 new cases expected among men in 2010 (American Cancer Society 2010). Thus this section focuses on female breast cancers. In the United States, about 40,000 women (and 400 men) were predicted to die from breast cancer in the year 2010; breast cancer mortality is second only to lung cancer mortality. The chance of developing invasive breast cancer at some time in a woman's life is about 1 in 8 (12%),

while the chance that breast cancer will be responsible for a woman's death is about 1 in 35 (3%) (American Cancer Society 2009). Worldwide, the incidence of breast cancer is about 1 million cases per year. Incidence and mortality are highest in western Europe and North America and lowest in Asia and Africa (Brinton and Devesa 1996). Differences in incidence and mortality are greater among countries than within countries and are associated with variations in body weight; diet; reproductive hormone levels; and reproductive history, including menstrual cycle length, **parity**, and lactation (Kelsey and Horn-Ross 1993). Environmental factors, rather than genetic factors, are responsible for most of the variation in breast cancer rates among countries. Studies of migrants to the United States have shown that the incidence rate of migrants and their offspring approaches the level in the native-born population (Ewertz 1995).

▷ **IN THE** United States, about 40,000 women were predicted to die from breast cancer in the year 2010; breast cancer mortality is second only to lung cancer mortality.

According to the American Cancer Society (2010), the overall five-year survival rate for breast cancer has increased from 63% in the early 1940s to the present level of 90%; today, if the breast cancer is local, the survival rate is 98%. However, once the cancer has spread regionally, the survival rate decreases to 84%. For people with distant metastases, the five-year survival rate is only 23%. In the United States, five-year survival rates are higher for white women than black women (91% vs. 79% across all ages) (American Cancer Society 2010), and Asian American women have higher five-year survival rates than white American women (Kelsey and Horn-Ross 1993). Some cancer researchers have proposed that American blacks have poorer survival rates because of less aggressive treatment, lower incidence of estrogen receptor–positive tumors, a higher proportion of poorly differentiated tumors, poorer nutritional status, and higher body mass index. In contrast, women of Asian descent have lower body weight and fewer lymph node metastases than whites (Kelsey and Horn-Ross 1993). A cumulative review of studies involving 189,877 white and 32,004 black patients that controlled for deaths from causes other than cancer concluded that blacks were at a significantly higher risk of death from breast cancer but that the higher mortality rate among blacks was better explained by more advanced stages of cancer at the time of diagnosis than by differences in cancer biology among racial groups (Bach et al. 2002).

Although the incidence rates have been increasing, possibly due to increased mammography utilization, with a peak around 1999 before beginning to decline, mortality rates have remained virtually stable over the past 50 years and have been declining since 1990, probably as a result of earlier detection and better treatment. In the United States, the mortality rate in women less than 65 years old has fallen, but the rates have increased for older white women and black women of all ages.

Types of Breast Cancer

Most breast lumps are benign (not cancerous) and result from fibrocystic changes in breast tissue. Fibrosis refers to excessive scar-like connective tissue. Cysts are fluid-filled sacs. Fibrocystic lumps usually cause breast swelling and pain. The nipple might discharge a clear or cloudy liquid. Benign breast lumps such as fibroadenomas or papillomas are common growths. They cannot spread outside of the breast to other organs. Mammographic abnormalities indicative of breast cancer include pointed, star-like lesions; small, asymmetric lumps; microcalcifications; and any distortion or asymmetry of the breast's shape (Henderson 1995). The most important physical sign of breast cancer is a painless lump in the breast. However, about 10% of patients have breast pain and no mass. Less common symptoms include persistent changes to the breast, such as thickening, swelling, skin irritation, or distortion, and nipple symptoms including spontaneous discharge, erosion, inversion, or tenderness.

Carcinoma in Situ

When a cancer is confined to breast lobules (milk glands) or ducts (milk passages) (figure 12.6) and has not spread to surrounding fat cells in the breast or to other organs, it is called **breast carcinoma in situ.** There are two types of in situ breast cancer: Lobular carcinoma in situ (LCIS) originates in the lobules and does not penetrate through the lobule walls. It usually does not become an invasive cancer, but it is a risk factor for developing invasive cancer. Ductal carcinoma in situ (DCIS) involves cancer cells inside the milk ducts that do not infiltrate the surrounding fat cells in the breast. It is the most common noninvasive breast cancer (National Cancer Institute 2000).

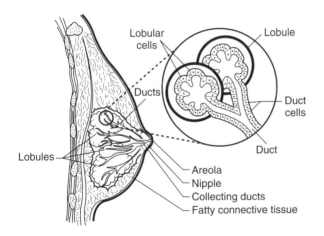

Figure 12.6 Diagram of breast structure.

Invasive Carcinoma

Invasive breast carcinoma spreads in the breast and to other parts of the body. Invasive ductal carcinoma (IDC) originates in a milk duct but breaks through the wall of the duct and invades the fatty tissue of the breast. It can pass into the lymph and blood circulatory systems and spread to other organs. About 70% of breast cancers are IDC. Another 5% to 10% of invasive breast cancers are lobular carcinomas (ILC), which originate in the milk-producing glands. About 5% of breast cancers are medullary carcinomas, which have a distinct border between the tumor cells and normal breast tissue. Other rare forms of invasive breast cancer include colloid carcinoma, which produces mucus; tubular carcinoma; and adenoid cystic carcinoma, which usually develops in the salivary glands, not the breast. Each of these rare types of invasive cancer has a better prognosis than invasive lobular cancer, invasive ductal cancer, or inflammatory breast cancer (IBC), in which the skin is red, feels warm, and may thicken like an orange peel. Though called inflammatory, IBC results from the spread of cancer cells within the lymph circuits in the skin, not from inflammation. It is classified as stage IIIB (breast cancers of any size that have spread to the skin, chest wall, or internal mammary lymph nodes) until it metastasizes (National Cancer Institute 2000).

Etiology of Breast Cancer

The etiology of breast cancer is not well understood. Between 5% to 10% and 27% of breast cancer cases are hereditary, and about half of hereditary cases are believed to result from mutations of the BRCA1 and BRCA2 genes, which normally express proteins that inhibit abnormal cell reproduction (National Human Genome Research Institute 2009). About 35% to 84% of women with inherited BRCA1 or BRCA2 mutations will develop breast cancer by the age of 70, and they also are at elevated risk for ovarian cancer (Nelson et al. 2005). Inherited mutations of the p53 tumor suppressor gene can also increase a woman's risk of developing breast cancer, as well as leukemia, brain tumors, and sarcomas of bone or connective tissue. Most DNA mutations related to breast cancer, however, occur during a woman's life rather than having been inherited. Acquired mutations of oncogenes or tumor suppressor genes may result from radiation or cancer-causing chemicals. So far, however, studies have not been able to identify any chemical in the environment or in our diets that is likely to cause these mutations or a subsequent breast cancer. The cause of most acquired mutations remains unknown.

▷ **BETWEEN 5%** to 10% and 27% of breast cancer cases are hereditary, and about half of hereditary cases are believed to result from mutations of the BRCA1 and BRCA2 genes, which normally express proteins that inhibit abnormal cell reproduction. About 35% to 84% of women with inherited BRCA1 or BRCA2 mutations will develop breast cancer by the age of 70.

Breast Cancer Stages

Stages indicate whether or how far a breast cancer has spread within the breast, to nearby tissues, and to other organs as determined by palpation, diagnostic blood tests, and X rays (Mayo Clinic 2009).

Stage 0 (Noninvasive or In Situ Breast Cancer)

Includes lobular carcinoma in situ and ductal carcinoma in situ.

Stage I

Tumor is smaller than 2 cm (0.8 in.) in diameter and does not appear to have spread beyond the breast.

Stage II

Tumor is less than 2 cm (0.8 in.) but has spread to lymph nodes under the arm, or no tumor is found in the breast, but breast cancer cells are found in lymph nodes under the arm, or tumor is 2-5 cm (0.8-2 in.) and may or may not have spread to lymph nodes under the arm, or tumor is larger than 5 cm (2 in.) but hasn't spread to any lymph nodes.

Stage III

Stage III breast cancers are subdivided into three categories—IIIA, IIIB, and IIIC—based on a number of criteria. By definition, stage III cancers haven't spread to distant sites.

Stage IV

The cancer, regardless of its size, has metastasized to distant sites, such as bones, lungs, or lymph nodes not near the breast.

Tests to identify other acquired changes in oncogenes or tumor suppressor genes (such as p53) may help doctors more accurately predict the prognosis of some women with breast cancer. But, with the exception of the HER2 oncogene, these tests have not yet been shown to be useful for making decisions about treatment and are used only for research purposes. A monoclonal antibody therapy called trastuzumab (Herceptin) has been developed that specifically interrupts the growth-promoting action of the HER2 oncogene.

The female hormone estrogen has been implicated in breast tumor growth since a Scot named Thomas Beatson discovered in 1878 that rabbits stopped producing milk after he removed the ovaries. He then tested whether breast cancer could be treated by oophorectomy (removal of the ovaries) and concluded from his sometimes-successful results that the ovaries might be the cause of breast cancer. The incidence rate of breast cancer in women increases rapidly with age during the childbearing years, until around age 50; the slope rises at a slower pace after **menopause.** This changing rate is not apparent in men, for whom breast cancer incidence continues to increase linearly with age. This has been interpreted as evidence for the involvement of reproductive hormones in the etiology of breast cancer (Ewertz 1995). During menopause, the exposure to estrogen and progesterone decreases. Although these hormones are not carcinogenic themselves, they may act to promote the growth of cells that have already undergone malignant transformation.

Some women with genetic risk choose to take the medication tamoxifen, a drug that blocks the effects of estrogen on breast cells, in an attempt to reduce the likelihood of developing breast cancer. Results from the Breast Cancer Prevention Trial showed that women at high risk for breast cancer are less likely to develop the disease if they take tamoxifen (Fisher et al. 2005). After five years of tamoxifen and seven years of follow-up, these women had 43% fewer breast cancers than women with the same risk factors who did not take tamoxifen. Whether tamoxifen prevents new breast cancer from developing or retards small, initially undetectable cancers has not been determined.

A woman's age increases her exposure to initiators and promoters of cancer. A woman's breast age differs according to the rate of cell divisions in breast tissue. Breast epithelial cell division begins at **menarche** and continues until menopause. The last menstrual cycle ends the division of breast epithelial cells. Physical activity has been proposed as a way to alter this exposure to estrogen (see further discussion later on) and therefore may have a drastic effect on reducing risk by decreasing breast aging.

Estradiol is an endogenous estrogenic hormone that is not toxic to breast epithelial cells but stimulates cell proliferation in the body. Sometimes this proliferation can be excessively rapid and cause a mutation in the DNA. A DNA mutation could cause the production of defective repair enzymes or defective tumor suppressor genes. The defective enzymes might not allow the body to protect itself against excessively rapid proliferation of cells in the tissue, leading to cancer. Breast cancer has been hypothesized to form from excessive exposure to estradiol. Women have a higher risk of DNA mutations and breast cancer because of their increased lifetime exposure to estrogens. Factors such as age, age at menarche, age at menopause, obesity, postmenopausal hormone therapy, and menstrual cycle length can increase hormone exposure in various ways.

▷ **ESTRADIOL CAN** speed the rate of breast cell division. Coupled with gene mutations that inhibit tumor suppressor factors and enzymes that repair cells, this can promote tumor growth. Factors such as age, age at menarche, age at menopause, obesity, postmenopausal hormone therapy, and menstrual cycle length can increase lifetime estradiol exposure.

▷ **HIGHER ESTRADIOL** levels are associated with a doubling of breast cancer risk and have been found in girls whose menarche occurred before the age of 12. These girls were also found to be at higher risk for adiposity and fluctuating testosterone levels during their menstrual cycles, both of which also contribute to breast cancer risk. A delayed menarche may induce irregular menstrual cycles for up to 30 years and thus also lower lifetime estradiol exposure. Irregular cycles alone are associated with a reduction in risk of around 50%.

The risk of breast cancer increases more slowly after menopause as female reproductive hormone levels decline. Nonetheless, postmenopausal women remain at greater risk in part because after menopause their levels of sex hormone–binding globulin (SHBG) decreases. SHBG regulates the amount of active sex hormones circulating throughout the body since it binds to sex hormones, making them inactive. When SHBG decreases, the amount of free—and active—sex hormones circulating increases. Physical activity may help control this problem, mostly by preventing it from getting worse. Obesity in postmenopausal women further decreases the amount of SHBG; physical activity can fight obesity and thus counter further decreases in SHBG.

Risk Factors

Risk factors for breast cancer include older age, high socioeconomic class, having family members with the disease, starting menstruation at an early age or menopause at a late age, and late first pregnancy or **nulliparity.** High fat intake or high overall calorie consumption is also associated with higher risk of breast cancer.

• *Age.* The incidence and mortality of breast cancer increase with age (table 12.5). Each year more than 75% of women newly diagnosed with breast cancer are over the age of 50. Breast cancer is rare in younger women, with an incidence rate of only 1 case per 100,000 for women ages 20 to 24. However, the rate climbs to about 25 cases per 100,000 for ages 30 to 34, to 122 cases for ages 40 to 44, and to 245 cases for ages 50 to 54. Breast cancer is the leading cause of cancer death in women between the ages of 15 and 54.

• *Race.* For all ages combined, white American women are more likely to develop breast cancer than African Ameri-

Table 12.5 Likelihood of Developing Invasive Breast Cancer Among Women According to Age Interval, 2003-2005

Age interval, years	Likelihood (probability)
Birth to 39	1 in 208 (0.48%)
40 to 59	1 in 26 (3.79%)
60 to 69	1 in 29 (3.41%)
70 and older	1 in 16 (6.44%)
Birth to death	1 in 8 (12.03%)

Data from the American Cancer Society, 2009

can women. Between 2001 and 2005, the incidence rate for white women in the United States was 131 cases per 100,000; it was 118 per 100,000 for African American women, 90 per 100,000 for Hispanic/Latino as well as Asian American/Pacific Islander women, and 75 per 100,000 for American Indian/Alaska Native women (American Cancer Society 2009). However, African American women were more likely to die of breast cancer (34 per 100,000) than white women (24 per 100,000). Mortality rates from breast cancer in the other three race–ethnic groups all were lower than for white women, ranging from 13 to 17 per 100,000.

• *Sex.* Although breast cancer is a disease that affects primarily women, about 2000 new cases of breast cancer and 400 deaths occur in men each year. Male breast cancer accounts for less than 1% of the overall incidence and mortality of this disease. Even though men are at low risk of developing breast cancer, they should be aware of risk factors, especially family history, and report any change in their breasts to a physician.

• *Family history of breast cancer.* Having one first-degree relative (mother, sister, or daughter) with breast cancer doubles a woman's risk, and having two first-degree relatives increases her risk fivefold. The first breast cancer susceptibility gene, BRCA1, was identified on chromosome 17 in 1994, and the second gene associated with breast cancer was identified on chromosome 13 a year later. Deleterious mutations of the BRCA1 and BRCA2 genes increase a woman's lifetime risk of breast cancer to 60% to 85% (Nelson et al. 2005), compared with about 12% among all women (table 12.5).

• *Previous proliferative breast disease.* Women who have been diagnosed with proliferative breast disease with usual hyperplasia from an earlier breast biopsy have 1.5 to 2 times higher risk of breast cancer than other women. A previous biopsy result of atypical hyperplasia increases a woman's breast cancer risk four to five times. However, a biopsy diagnosed as fibrocystic changes without proliferative breast disease carries no added risk of breast cancer. A woman with cancer in one breast has a three- to fourfold risk of developing a new cancer in the other breast.

• *Previous breast irradiation.* Women who have had chest-area radiation therapy as children or young women to treat another cancer (such as Hodgkin's disease or non-Hodgkin's lymphoma) are at significantly increased risk for breast cancer.

- *Menstrual history.* Women who started menstruating before age 12 have a 50% greater breast cancer risk than those who started at age 15 or later. Also, women who reached natural menopause at or after age 55 have twice the risk of women who experience menopause before age 45 (Brinton and Devesa 1996). Long-term, repetitive proliferation of breast endothelial cells during the childbearing years can promote the development of malignant cells.

- *High socioeconomic status.* Social class can be regarded as an indicator of a high-risk lifestyle, not necessarily as a direct risk factor of breast cancer. Women of higher socioeconomic status are more likely to have their first child at a later age, to have fewer children, and to use hormone therapy during menopause, all of which may increase the risk of breast cancer (Ewertz 1995).

- *Oral contraceptive use.* It is still not clear what part oral contraceptives (birth control pills) might play in breast cancer risk. In 2005, the International Agency for Research on Cancer classified oral contraceptives containing estrogen and progesterone as a group I carcinogen (the highest rating), increasing the risks of breast, cervical, and liver cancers. However, the increased risk of breast cancer was primarily observed in older studies; the doses of estrogen and progesterone were higher than those in current formulations (Casey, Cerhan, and Pruthi 2008). Moreover, the increased risk was small (24%) among current users and was weaker in recent users, and no risk was observed after discontinuation of use for 10 years or more (Collaborative Group 1996). More recent studies of women using lower-dose formulations do not appear to observe any increased risk for breast cancer (Collaborative Group 1996).

- *Nulliparity.* As first reported in 1713 by Bernardo Ramazzini, nuns had a high rate of breast cancer compared with married women; Ramazzini speculated that this was due to their nulliparous state. Women who have not given birth to children have about a 30% increase in risk compared with women who have (Ewertz et al. 1990). Protection against cancer-inducing factors may be one of the benefits of an early pregnancy. During pregnancy, a differentiation of breast tissue occurs that changes the tissue's sensitivity to endogenous sex hormones. Some evidence indicates that women who give birth before age 20 have about half the risk of developing breast cancer of nulliparous women (Stoll 1995). The increased risk with late pregnancy may be associated with the aging process, or involution, of the breasts.

- *Hormone therapy.* Most studies suggest that long-term use (10 years or more) of hormone therapy (HT) after menopause may increase the risk of breast cancer. Results of the large Women's Health Initiative randomized **clinical trial** showed a 24% increased risk of breast cancer after about five years of hormone therapy that combined estrogen and pro-

gestin treatment (Chlebowski et al. 2003). However, women in this trial who were assigned estrogen-only therapy did not experience any increase in breast cancer risk (Anderson et al. 2004).

- *Alcohol consumption.* Compared with nondrinkers, women who consume alcoholic drinks have an increased risk of breast cancer. A meta-analysis estimated an increase in risk of 22% overall associated with drinking alcohol and indicated that each additional 10 g ethanol per day was associated with a 10% increase in risk (an average drink contains about 12 g of ethanol) (Key et al. 2006). Alcohol is also known to increase the risk of developing cancers of the mouth, throat, and esophagus.

- *Obesity and high-fat diets.* The relation between obesity and breast cancer risk differs for pre- and postmenopausal breast cancers. Obesity increases the risk of postmenopausal breast cancer (Renehan et al. 2008) and weight gain since adolescence also increases risk (World Cancer Research Fund/American Institute for Cancer Research 2007). Also, the effect of obesity on risk is more prominent among women not taking postmenopausal hormone therapy than among those who do. The reason is that endogenous estrogen levels are low in postmenopausal women. Adipose tissue converts estrogen precursors to estrogen, so obese postmenopausal women have higher levels of estrogen compared with lean postmenopausal women. Additionally, SHBG levels tend to be lower in obese women, leading to more free, or active, estrogen circulating in the body. In women taking postmenopausal hormone therapy, the dose of exogenous estrogen is much higher than circulating endogenous estrogen, so any effect of obesity is swamped. In contrast to the increased risk of postmenopausal breast cancer with obesity, higher body weights are instead associated with lower risk of premenopausal breast cancer except in Asia-Pacific populations, where the association is reversed (Renehan et al. 2008). This is likely a consequence of abnormal estrogen and progesterone levels among obese premenopausal women.

Most ecologic studies have found that breast cancer is less common in countries where the typical diet is low in total fat, low in polyunsaturated fat, and low in saturated fat. On the other hand, many studies of women in the United States have not found breast cancer risk to be related to dietary fat intake after controlling for other risk factors for breast cancer such as physical activity level and intake of other nutrients that might also alter breast cancer risk. In the Women's Health Initiative randomized clinical trial, after about eight years of follow-up, 0.42% of women assigned to the low-fat diet group and 0.45% of women in the regular diet group were diagnosed with breast cancer, showing little effect (Prentice et al. 2006). However, it was difficult for women in the study to achieve the goal of 20% of calories from fat; only 14% continued to meet the goal after six years. The American Cancer Society recommends maintaining a healthy weight and limiting the intake of high-fat foods, particularly those from animal sources.

• *Environmental toxins.* Currently, research does not clearly show a link between breast cancer risk and exposure to environmental pollutants, such as the pesticide DDE (chemically related to DDT) or polychlorinated biphenyls (PCBs). Studies on other environmental toxins are under way.

• *Physical inactivity.* Physical activity has been hypothesized to reduce breast cancer, and it is one of the few modifiable behaviors that affect breast cancer risk. Plausible explanations for a protective effect of physical activity include fewer lifetime ovulatory cycles and reduced body fat. The association between physical inactivity and breast cancer risk is discussed more fully in the next section.

Physical Activity and Breast Cancer: The Evidence

A recent review of the results of more than 60 observational, epidemiological studies of physical activity and breast cancer concluded that physically active women have a lower risk of developing breast cancer than sedentary women (Physical Activity Guidelines Advisory Committee 2008). As with the investigations of colon cancer, inverse associations between physical activity and breast cancer have been seen in studies conducted in North America, Europe, Asia, and Australia. Comparison of physically active women with sedentary women showed a median risk reduction of 20% (Lee and Oguma 2006).

Approximately three-quarters of these studies classified women according to three or more levels of physical activity, allowing assessment of a dose–response relation (Lee and Oguma 2006). There appears to be an inverse dose response, with about three-fifths of these studies reporting either a significant inverse trend across levels of physical activity, or relative risks consistent with an inverse dose response that was not tested for statistical significance (Lee and Oguma 2006). A systematic review of case–control studies of recreational activity and breast cancer risk estimated that each additional hour of physical activity per week reduced risk of postmenopausal breast cancer by 6% (95% CI: 3-8%) (Monninkhof et al. 2007).

Whether the association of physical activity with breast cancer risk differs among subgroups of women (e.g., with and without family history, nulliparous vs. parous, lean and overweight women) or by breast tumor characteristics is unclear (Physical Activity Guidelines Advisory Committee 2008). With regard to menopausal status, the inverse relation appears stronger in postmenopausal compared with premenopausal women (Physical Activity Guidelines Advisory Committee 2008; Lee and Oguma 2006). The periods of life that may be the most relevant for the protective effects of physical activity on breast cancer risk have not been established. Several studies have observed that lifetime physical activity is needed to significantly reduce risk (e.g., Bernstein et al. 1994); others

have also noted that physical activity during adolescence (e.g., Maruti et al. 2008) or at various times in life (e.g., Carpenter et al. 1999) is more strongly associated with reduced risk than physical activity carried out at other times.

▷ **MORE THAN** 60 epidemiological studies of physical activity and breast cancer incidence show a reduction in risk with higher levels of physical activity (Physical Activity Guidelines Advisory Committee 2008). On average, physical activity was associated with about a 20% reduction in risk, with the effect stronger for postmenopausal than for premenopausal breast cancer. Each additional hour of physical activity per week reduced risk of postmenopausal breast cancer by 6% (95% CI: 3-8%) (Monninkhof et al. 2007).

Case–Control Studies

More than three dozen population-based case–control studies have examined the relation between physical activity and risk of developing breast cancer (Physical Activity Guidelines Advisory Committee 2008). The majority have assessed the role of recreational or leisure-time physical activity; and overall, most studies indicate that physically active women have a lower risk of developing breast cancer than sedentary women. Risk reductions ranging from 20% to 70% have been noted, with a median of 30% across all studies (Lee and Oguma 2006). Here we describe several exemplar case–control studies that have investigated the association of physical activity with breast cancer risk.

Los Angeles County

In one of the early case–control studies on this topic, Bernstein and colleagues (1994) matched 545 women (ages 40 and younger at diagnosis) who had been newly diagnosed with in situ or invasive breast cancer between 1983 and 1989 with 545 control subjects by date of birth, race, parity, and neighborhood of residence. Lifetime histories of participation in regular exercise activities were obtained during an interview. After adjustment for age at first pregnancy, age at menarche, birth date, family history, months of lactation, number of full-term pregnancies, parity, race, and oral contraceptive use, the average number of hours spent in exercise activities per week from menarche to one year prior to diagnosis was independently associated with reduced breast cancer risk. Overall, the odds ratio of breast cancer among women who participated for 3.8 h or more per week in exercise activities was 58% lower (odds ratio, 0.42; 95% CI: 0.27-0.64) than in inactive women. The inverse association appeared stronger in women with at least one full-term pregnancy.

Shanghai, China

This study showed an inverse association in Chinese women (Matthews et al. 2001) similar to that seen among U.S.

women in the Los Angeles County study. Subjects for this population-based case–control study were 1459 women newly diagnosed with breast cancer and 1556 age-matched controls in urban Shanghai. Interviewers obtained information on physical activity from exercise and sports, household activities, and walking and cycling for transportation during adolescence (age 13-19 years) and adulthood (last 10 years); lifetime occupational activity also was ascertained. After the investigators controlled for age, education, income, family history of breast cancer, history of breast fibroadenoma, age at menarche, age at first live birth, and age at menopause, the risk of developing breast cancer was reduced with exercise only in adolescence (odds ratio, 0.84; 95% CI: 0.70-1.00), exercise only in adulthood (0.68; 0.53-0.88), and exercise at both times (0.47; 0.36-0.62). Household and transportation activities did not show any significant associations with breast cancer risk, while lifetime occupational activity involving more standing and walking was inversely related to risk.

Women's Contraceptive and Reproductive Experiences Study

This was a multicenter, population-based case–control study designed to investigate the predictors of breast cancer (including physical inactivity) among white and black women in Atlanta, Detroit, Los Angeles, Philadelphia, and Seattle (Bernstein et al. 2005). Detailed histories of lifetime recreational physical activity were obtained by interviews with 1605 black and 2933 white women aged 35 to 64 years, with newly diagnosed invasive breast cancer, and 1646 black and 3033 white control women who were frequency matched to cases on age, race, and study site. Among all women, increased levels of lifetime physical activity were associated with decreased breast cancer risk. After controlling for age, study site, race, family history of breast cancer, age at menarche, menopausal status, age at first full-term pregnancy, body mass index, and months of lactation, the most active black women, expending ≥3.0 h/week on average, had an odds ratio for breast cancer of 0.75 (95% CI: 0.61-0.93) compared with inactive women. For white women, the corresponding results were similar (odds ratio, 0.83; 0.70-0.98). For both races, there were significant inverse dose–response trends. Unlike what was seen in the case–control study from Los Angeles County described earlier, the association in this study did not differ between nulliparous and parous women.

Retrospective Cohort Studies

Several retrospective cohort studies also have examined whether physical activity is related to reduced breast cancer risk. We describe two such studies below.

College Alumnae Study

Frisch and colleagues (1985) conducted one of the first major studies to examine the potential protective effects of exercise against breast cancer. This study used a retrospec-

tive cohort study design to evaluate the relation between exercise and the prevalence of female reproductive cancers in a cohort of 5398 living (as of 1981) alumnae from the classes of 1925 to 1981 from 10 U.S. colleges. A total of 69 prevalent breast cancers were reported by the women. Alumnae were classified as athletes (defined as being on at least one varsity team, house team, or other intramural team for one or more years) or nonathletes. After adjustment for age, family history of cancer, age of menarche, number of pregnancies, use of oral contraceptives, use of hormones during menopause, smoking, and leanness, the relative risk of prevalent breast cancer for the athletes, compared with nonathletes, was 0.54 (95% CI: 0.29-1.00). Questionnaires reflected that a larger percentage of the former athletes than of the former nonathletes were physically active after college (74% vs. 57%). The authors concluded that long-term athletic training establishes a lifestyle that lowers the risk of breast cancer. While this early study provided useful information, its limitations included the small number of breast cancers and the investigation only of college exercise in relation to breast cancer risk. Given that nearly 60% of the college nonathletes were currently active at the time of the study, this may have diluted an association with breast cancer. In addition, since the study included only women who were alive in 1981, a selection bias may have occurred since only prevalent cases were included and mortality from breast cancer was not evaluated. If former athletes were likely to live longer than former nonathletes, the prevalence of nonfatal breast cancer would be higher in the athletes; thus, the observed inverse association likely would have been more marked if this bias had been removed.

Washington State

This retrospective cohort study took advantage of occupational information recorded on death certificates in the state of Washington to investigate the association of physical activity with breast cancer mortality (Vena et al. 1987). Vena and colleagues made use of published data from the death certificates of 25,000 white females (excluding women who were housewives) who died in that state from 1974 to 1979. Occupation titles were recorded from the death certificates related to "usual occupation during most of working life, even if retired." Based on their job title, women were classified into five categories of occupational physical activity. Standardized proportionate mortality ratios of specific cause of death were calculated for each category of occupational physical activity through comparison of the observed number of deaths against the expected number of deaths across all occupations, based on sex and calendar year, for that specific cause of death. Women in the most sedentary category of occupation had a standardized mortality ratio for breast cancer of 115 (i.e., 15% higher than expected), while women in the three most active categories of occupational activity, combined, had a standardized mortality ratio of 85% (i.e., 15% lower than expected).

While this study made efficient use of information already collected, it also had several limitations. No adjustments were made for known risk factors of breast cancer that could be related to occupational activity. For example, it was likely that sedentary jobs were held by women with higher socio-economic status and a history of late first pregnancy, both of which are associated with increased risk for breast cancer. In addition, occupational physical activity was based only on the job title listed on the death certificate; lifetime occupational history could not be assessed.

Prospective Cohort Studies

More than two dozen prospective cohort studies have investigated whether physical activity reduces the risk of developing breast cancer (Physical Activity Guidelines Advisory Committee 2008). As with the case–control studies, most of these examined recreational or leisure-time physical activity. The totality of evidence suggests that physically active women have a lower risk of developing breast cancer than sedentary women, with risk reductions ranging from 20% to 80%. Across all studies, the median risk reduction was 10%, a smaller magnitude than that observed in the case–control studies (Lee and Oguma 2006). Here we describe several exemplar prospective cohort studies on this topic.

Norway

This study represents one of the first detailed prospective cohort studies of physical activity and risk of developing breast cancer. Between 1974 and 1978 and again between 1977 and 1983, a total of 25,624 women, 20 to 54 years of age, answered questionnaires about leisure-time and occupational physical activity (Thune et al. 1997). Over nearly 14 years of follow-up, 351 cases of invasive breast cancer were detected. Regular leisure-time physical activity was associated with about a one-third reduction in the risk of breast cancer after adjustment for age, body mass index, height, parity, and county of residence (RR = 0.63; 95% CI: 0.42-0.95). The reduction in risk was greater in premenopausal women than in postmenopausal women, greater in younger women (<45 years at study entry) than in older women (≥45 years), and greater in lean women (body mass index <22.8 kg/m²) than in heavier women. Higher levels of occupational physical activity were associated with lower breast cancer risk as well, and that effect also was stronger among premenopausal women.

University of Pennsylvania Alumnae

Investigators in this study wanted to assess the association of physical activity and breast cancer risk, as well as to determine whether the association differed according to postmenopausal status and body mass index as suggested by the study from Norway just described. Approximately 1600 University of Pennsylvania alumnae who had matriculated between 1916 and 1950 (average age 45.5 years) and who

were initially free of breast cancer, in 1962, were observed until 1993 for breast cancer occurrence (Sesso, Paffenbarger, and Lee 1998). At baseline, women reported their stair climbing, walking, and sport participation and were classified into three levels (<500 kcal/week, 500-999 kcal/week, or ≥1000 kcal/week). During 35,365 person-years of observation, 109 cases of breast cancer cases were detected. After adjustment for age and body mass index, postmenopausal women who expended ≥1000 kcal or more each week had about half the risk of developing breast cancer than women who expended <500 kcal per week (RR = 0.49; 95% CI: 0.28-0.86). There was no significant association for premenopausal women. These analyses updated an earlier retrospective cohort study of women who were from the same cohort but were followed only through 1978 (Paffenbarger, Hyde, and Wing 1987). Physical activity, based on participation in college athletics, was not related to breast cancer risk; however, pre- and postmenopausal breast cancers were not differentiated.

Nurses' Health Study I and II

These two studies are among the few prospective cohort studies that updated information on physical activity over time. The earlier investigation enrolled subjects from Nurses' Health Study II, a prospective cohort study of women's health among approximately 117,000 women who were 25 to 42 years old in 1989 (Rockhill et al. 1998). At the baseline survey, women were asked, "While in high school and between the ages 18 and 22 years, how often did you participate in strenuous physical activity at least twice a week?" Responses to the two time periods were averaged to estimate physical activity in late adolescence. Women were also asked how many hours each week they currently spent in several leisure physical activities using questions similar to those in Nurses' Health Study I, described earlier in the context of physical activity and colon cancer (at that time, the study was referred to as the Nurses' Health Study). During six years of observation, 372 cases of invasive breast cancer were detected. Among these women, who were primarily premenopausal, after adjustment for age, age at menarche, age at first birth, parity, oral contraceptive use, height, alcohol intake, history of benign breast disease, and family history of breast cancer, neither physical activity in adolescence nor contemporary leisure activity was associated with the risk of breast cancer (relative risk for either time period, comparing high with low activity level, was 1.1); this finding was congruent with those seen in the University of Pennsylvania alumnae just discussed.

The second study was based on women from Nurses' Health Study I, a cohort of older women aged 30 to 55 years at baseline in 1976 (Rockhill et al. 1999). For this analysis of physical activity and breast cancer risk, follow-up started in 1980, when women were asked about the average number of hours per week they spent in various moderate and vigorous recreational physical activities during the past year. Physical activity information was updated every two years; and starting in 1986, more detailed questions on eight different groups of recreational activities were asked. During 16 years of observation, 3137 cases of invasive breast cancer (1036 premenopausal and 2101 postmenopausal women) were detected. Women who reported participation in moderate or vigorous physical activity for 7 h or more per week had nearly 20% lower risk of breast cancer than those who averaged less than 1 h per week (RR = 0.82; 95% CI: 0.70-0.97) after adjustment for age, age at menarche, age at first birth, menopausal status, use of postmenopausal hormones, family history of breast cancer, history of benign breast disease, body mass index, and height. There also was a significant, inverse dose response across categories of physical activity. One possible explanation for the different results across these two studies might have been the higher preponderance of postmenopausal breast cancers in the latter study; the overall body of evidence suggests stronger associations for postmenopausal than for premenopausal breast cancer (Physical Activity Guidelines Advisory Committee 2008; Lee and Oguma 2006).

Women's Health Initiative Cohort Study

All of the prospective cohort studies discussed in the preceding sections comprised primarily Caucasian women. In the Women's Health Initiative Cohort Study, the association of physical activity with breast cancer risk was examined among approximately 74,000 women aged 50 to 70 years, 15% of whom were from race–ethnic minority groups, throughout the United States (McTiernan et al. 2003). At baseline between 1993 and 1998, women reported on their walking and on the frequency and duration spent on light-, moderate-, and vigorous-intensity physical activity. During an average follow-up of 4.7 years, 1780 women developed breast cancer. After adjustment for age, race, geographic region, income, education, body mass index, use of postmenopausal hormones, breastfeeding, hysterectomy status, family history of breast cancer, smoking, parity, age at first birth, age at menarche, age at menopause, mammography, and alcohol use, women who expended no, ≤5, 5.1 to 10, 10.1 to 20, 20.1 to 40, and >40 MET-hours/week in physical activity had relative risks (95% CI) for breast cancer of 1.00 (referent), 0.90 (0.77-1.07), 0.82 (0.68-0.97), 0.89 (0.76-1.00), 0.83 (0.70-0.98), and 0.78 (0.62-1.00), respectively; p for trend = 0.03.

Strength of the Evidence

All of the studies examining whether physical activity can reduce the risk of developing breast cancer have been observational epidemiologic studies, a situation similar to that for studies of physical activity and colon cancer risk. Thus, we use Mill's cannons (see chapter 2) here to assess whether the observed inverse association between physical activity and breast cancer risk is likely to be causal.

As with the studies of colon cancer, confounding by other risk factors for breast cancer needs to be evaluated. It is unlikely that confounding completely explains the observation from many studies that physically active women have lower rates of breast cancer. While early studies on this topic generally did not have information to allow comprehensive control of confounding, many later studies, including some of those described here, continued to observe significantly lower rates of breast cancer in active women after adjusting for several potential confounders (Lee and Oguma 2006). For example, in the Women's Health Initiative Cohort Study, a significant inverse relation remained after investigators took into account differences in age, race, geographic region, income, education, body mass index, smoking, alcohol use, ages at menarche and menopause, age at first birth, parity, breastfeeding, use of postmenopausal hormones, hysterectomy status, screening mammography, and family history of breast cancer (McTiernan et al. 2003).

Temporal Sequence

As with the studies of colon cancer, the criterion for temporal sequence is well satisfied, with investigators in case–control studies asking cases to recall physical activity that occurred prior to the onset of breast cancer and those in cohort studies ascertaining, in real time, physical activity prior to the onset of breast cancer. Some degree of recall bias is likely to exist in the case–control studies, since the average magnitude of risk reduction is larger in these studies than in the cohort studies—30% vs. 10%, respectively (Lee and Oguma 2006).

Separate aspects related to the temporal association between physical activity and breast cancer development include, When must exercise begin and for what period of time must it be maintained? Does exercise in adolescence provide protection against premenopausal and postmenopausal risk of breast cancer? Is there a protective benefit from beginning an exercise program after menopause? It is unclear when in the tumor development process exercise may have a protective effect, and studies to date do not provide clear answers (Physical Activity Guidelines Advisory Committee 2008).

Strength of Association

Overall, the strength of association for breast cancer, as reflected by the magnitude of risk reduction, is less strong than for colon cancer. The median relative risk across studies suggests that physical activity reduced the risk of breast cancer by about 20% among all women, with a larger magnitude for postmenopausal compared with premenopausal breast cancer (30% vs. 20% risk reduction, respectively) (Lee and Oguma 2006).

Figure 12.7, *a* and *b*, summarizes the results from case–control and cohort studies of physical activity and breast

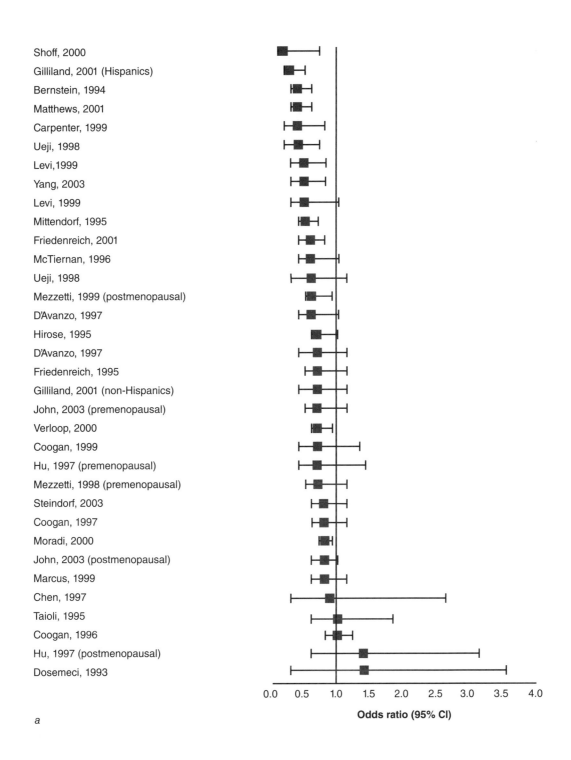

Shoff, 2000
Gilliland, 2001 (Hispanics)
Bernstein, 1994
Matthews, 2001
Carpenter, 1999
Ueji, 1998
Levi,1999
Yang, 2003
Levi, 1999
Mittendorf, 1995
Friedenreich, 2001
McTiernan, 1996
Ueji, 1998
Mezzetti, 1999 (postmenopausal)
D'Avanzo, 1997
Hirose, 1995
D'Avanzo, 1997
Friedenreich, 1995
Gilliland, 2001 (non-Hispanics)
John, 2003 (premenopausal)
Verloop, 2000
Coogan, 1999
Hu, 1997 (premenopausal)
Mezzetti, 1998 (premenopausal)
Steindorf, 2003
Coogan, 1997
Moradi, 2000
John, 2003 (postmenopausal)
Marcus, 1999
Chen, 1997
Taioli, 1995
Coogan, 1996
Hu, 1997 (postmenopausal)
Dosemeci, 1993

0.0   0.5   1.0   1.5   2.0   2.5   3.0   3.5   4.0

Odds ratio (95% CI)

a

(continued)

Figure 12.7   Summary of results from *(a)* case–control studies and *(b)* cohort studies of physical activity and breast cancer.

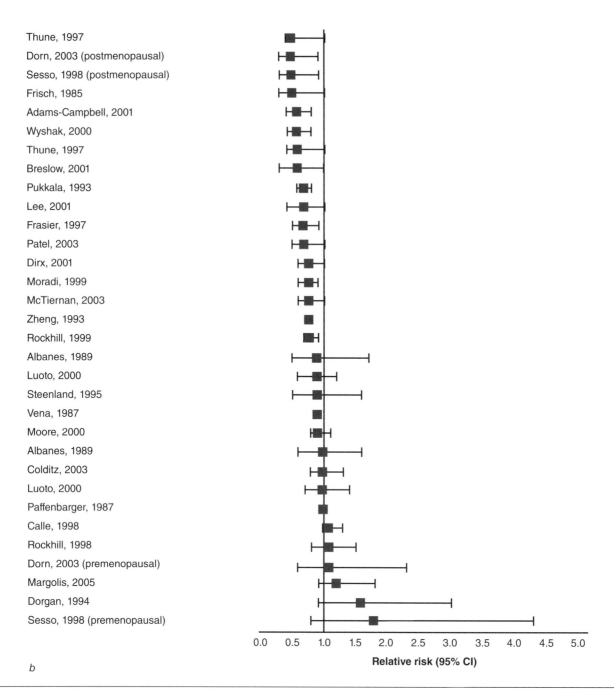

b

Figure 12.7 *(continued).*

Adapted, by permission, from B. Steinfeld and I. Lee, 2009, Physical activity and cancer: The evidence, the issues, and the changes. In *Epidemiologic methods in physical activity studies,* edited by I-M. Lee (New York, NY: Oxford University Press), 184-185.

cancer risk. It shows that while most studies found a decreased risk as indicated by the point estimate of the odds ratio or relative risk, several of the results had 95% confidence intervals (the vertical lines through the point estimates) that included an odds ratio or relative risk of 1.0, indicating nonsignificant results. Those results are too weak to be considered statistically significant, either because not enough women were studied to ensure a sufficient sample of breast cancers, or because the difference in rates between the active and inactive groups was too small to be detected

with certainty given the sample size of the particular study, or for both reasons. Moreover, imprecise physical activity measures can add to variation, further decreasing statistical power.

Consistency

The overall association between physical activity and breast cancer risk among women appears consistent across studies involving different races and ethnicities. However, as discussed already, there appears to be an effect modification by menopausal status, with a stronger association seen for postmenopausal breast cancer. Evidence is insufficient to show whether differences exist in the relation between physical activity and breast cancer risk by subgroups of women according to body mass index, parity, or other characteristics (Physical Activity Guidelines Advisory Committee 2008).

Dose Response

The measures of exercise in studies of physical activity and breast cancer risk have varied, from college athletic status to job classification to commuting physical activity to adult recreational activities and fitness levels. Thus, the type, intensity, or duration of exercise involved in the dose response is difficult to assess. As discussed previously, the available evidence supports an inverse dose–response relation (Physical Activity Guidelines Advisory Committee 2008; Lee and Oguma 2006). A systematic review of recreational activity and breast cancer risk from case–control studies estimated that each additional hour of physical activity per week reduced risk of postmenopausal breast cancer by 6% (95% CI: 3-8%) (Monninkhof et al. 2007). With regard to the minimum amount of activity associated with reduced breast cancer incidence, an expert panel charged by the U.S. federal government to comprehensively examine the scientific base for making physical activity recommendations concluded that some 30 to 60 min per day of moderate- to vigorous-intensity physical activity may be necessary to significantly reduce the risk of developing breast cancer (Physical Activity Guidelines Advisory Committee 2008).

Biological Plausibility

As with colon cancer, the exact mechanisms have not been identified, but several plausible, as yet unproven, biological mechanisms have been suggested (Physical Activity Guidelines Advisory Committee 2008). In addition to enhancing the immune system, which is discussed in chapter 13, the key possible mechanisms for the protective effect of physical activity may include its influence on menstrual function and sex steroid hormones, reduction in blood levels of insulin-like growth factor as a result of negative energy balance, or indirect associations with lower body weight (e.g., higher levels of SHBG and hence lower levels of free estrogen, less inflammation).

Sex Hormones

A popular hypothesis for explaining how physical activity might protect against breast cancer is that it reduces the cumulative lifetime exposure to circulating ovarian hormones, especially estrogen, since higher levels of estrogen are associated with increased breast cancer risk. Physical activity has been found to decrease risk by delaying the age of menarche, decreasing adiposity, and helping to maintain hormonal balance in the body. Thus, physical activity

during early adolescence could have protective benefits on a woman's risk later in life.

Menstrual Function

Strenuous physical activity during adolescence may increase the age at menarche (Gammon and John 1993) and is also associated with longer menstrual cycles (Hoffman-Goetz et al. 1998). In general, a 20% reduction in breast cancer risk is observed for every year that menarche is delayed (Henderson and Bernstein 1996). Conversely, women with relatively frequent, short, and regular ovulatory cycles are at increased risk for breast cancer. These women spend more of their time in the luteal phase of the menstrual cycle, when both estrogen and progesterone are high. Susceptibility to breast cancer increases because peak mitotic activity in breast epithelium occurs during the luteal phase (Henderson and Bernstein 1996). Therefore, if exercise delays menarche and lengthens regular menstrual cycles, cumulative exposure to estrogen and progesterone would be reduced, thus decreasing the risk of breast cancer. For menarche to occur, a girl must attain a critical ratio of body mass relative to height. Height is determined genetically, while weight is determined mostly by caloric intake. Once the critical mass-to-height ratio has been met, the critical mass must be maintained to maintain menstruation. Those who lose weight from vigorous activity and cease menstruating might gain protection against breast cancer. Irregular menstrual cycles and amenorrhea, with associated low levels of estrogen, have been reported among some competitive female athletes who train at very high levels of exertion. However, exercising to such extremes for potential protection against breast cancer is not recommended.

Vigorous training in sports such as swimming, running, gymnastics, and dance has been associated with delayed menarche in young girls. Whether the delayed menarche results from the exercise or from the smaller body mass of girls who naturally select such sports has not been established (Malina 1983). Nonetheless, one study found that even a moderate amount of physical activity, 600 kcal/week, increased the odds of irregular menstrual cycles compared with less activity (Cooper et al. 1996). Thus, even moderate physical activity might have a protective effect against breast cancer by reducing lifetime exposure to endogenous steroid hormones.

Onset of Menopause

It is also plausible that physical activity could be associated with an earlier age at menopause. Women who experience natural menopause before age 45 are estimated to have half the risk of breast cancer of women whose natural menopause occurs after age 55 (Brinton and Devesa 1996). Physically active women tend to be leaner than inactive women, and obesity is associated with a late age at menopause (Friedenreich and Rohan 1995). Frisch and colleagues (1985) also observed that athletes had an earlier age of natural menopause than nonathletes. It is worth noting, however, that many epidemiologic studies that did control for differences in age at menopause continued to find lower breast cancer rates among active women.

Energy Balance, Body Weight, and Endogenous Sex Hormones

Obesity also independently influences breast cancer risk, increasing the risk of postmenopausal breast cancer. Overall obesity, as well as abdominal obesity, is related to higher circulatory estrogen levels and increased conversion of androgens to estrogen (World Cancer Research Fund/American Institute for Cancer Research 2007). After menopause, estrogen is primarily produced from sources other than the ovaries, such as adipose cells that aid the conversion of androgens to estrogen.

Low body fat has also been associated with increased metabolism of estradiol to its less potent metabolite, 2-hydroxyestrone. Former female college athletes have been found to have lower body mass, higher 2-hydroxyestrone levels, and lower risk for breast cancer than nonathletes. Thus, physical activity could protect both pre- and postmenopausal women by converting excess estradiol to 2-hydroxyestrone.

Exercise influences body composition by increasing energy expenditure, retarding loss of muscle mass, and increasing metabolic rate. Caloric availability is reduced by physical activity, and caloric restriction is proposed to be of benefit in reducing breast cancer risk. Exercise may also promote other health behaviors, including dietary changes in the type and amount of fat consumed. However, as discussed earlier in the chapter, a recent randomized clinical trial of low-fat diet did not show any effect on breast cancer rates, but few women managed to achieve the low-fat target of 20% of calories from fat (Prentice et al. 2006). Given the range of influences of physical activity, it is thus difficult to assess whether the relationships among exercise, estrogen, and breast cancer risk are related to a direct effect of activity on ovulatory cycles; an indirect effect through diet, body composition, and caloric expenditure; or some combination of these.

Experimental studies have used chemically induced mammary tumors in rodents as a model for human breast cancer, though it remains unclear whether the carcinogens used and the dose and duration of exposure in the animal studies would induce malignant tumor growth in humans. In any case, a summary of these studies indicates that mammary tumor incidence was decreased by exercise performed during the time of tumor initiation and promotion (Friedenreich and Rohan 1995). However, the effects of diet and energy balance were not well controlled in those studies, so the independent effect of exercise was not clearly shown (Hoffman-Goetz et al. 1998). Additionally, no dose–response relationship has been established for exercise and mammary tumors. Other research has shown increased tumor development and worse survival rates after chronic exercise in mice with a gene mutation that causes mammary tumors (Colbert et al. 2009). Thus,

the experimental studies also proved inconclusive regarding the protective effects of exercise (vs. diet) on breast tumor growth.

▷ **THE CUMULATIVE** evidence from more than 60 studies shows that physical activity is associated with reduced risk of breast cancer (Physical Activity Guidelines Advisory Committee 2008). On average, physically active women have about a 20% reduction in risk compared with sedentary women.

Summary and Conclusions

A recent review from an expert panel, convened by the U.S. federal government to examine the literature to provide a scientific base for physical activity recommendations, included more than 60 studies of physical activity and breast cancer risk conducted in many countries throughout the world (Physical Activity Guidelines Advisory Committee 2008). The panel concluded that there are clear data showing that higher levels of physical activity are associated with lower breast cancer rates, particularly in postmenopausal women, and that this inverse association is supported by several plausible biologic mechanisms. On average, active women have about a 20% reduction in risk compared with inactive women (Lee and Oguma 2006). There also appears to be an inverse dose response.

Aside from a more marked effect of physical activity on postmenopausal breast cancer, whether specific subgroups of the population (e.g., by body mass index, parity) may experience a greater decrease in breast cancer with increased levels of physical activity remains unclear. While several plausible mechanisms have been suggested, the precise underlying biological mechanisms are unknown. Additional questions related to the features of physical activity that affect the risk, such as the type (occupational, recreational, or household), frequency, intensity, and duration, as well as the times of life associated with risk reduction, remain. Investigations that examine the effect of physical activity at different stages of breast cancer are needed. As is also the case for colon cancer, there have been no randomized controlled trials of physical activity and breast cancer risk. Also, no studies have shown that naturally occurring alterations in physical activity levels are associated with a change in breast cancer rates. However, randomized controlled trials of physical activity and breast cancer in a population at average risk will likely never be completed because of cost and feasibility constraints. Randomized controlled trials of physical activity and factors related to breast cancer risk, such as decreased adiposity, support the hypothesis that physical activity can lower breast cancer rates. Thus, while no randomized controlled trials of breast cancer occurrence exist, the totality of evidence does strongly support a protective role of physical activity in preventing breast cancer development.

Other Cancers

Epidemiologic studies investigating the association of physical activity with other site-specific cancers also have been conducted. Below, we summarize the evidence on lung and endometrial cancers, for which the data suggest inverse relations with physical activity, and rectal and prostate cancers, for which the data indicate no associations with physical activity.

Lung Cancer

Lung cancer is the second most commonly occurring cancer in the United States and the leading cause of cancer deaths for both men and women, accounting in 2010 for an estimated 15% and 14% of all new cancer cases in men and women, respectively (American Cancer Society 2010). It also is the leading cause of cancer deaths worldwide (Herbst, Haymach, and Lippman 2008). According to the American Cancer Society, in 2010 approximately 222,520 persons (116,750 men and 105,770 women) were expected to develop lung cancer, and 157,300 persons (86,220 men and 71,080 women) were expected to die from this disease (American Cancer Society 2010). In men, lung cancer mortality rates peaked around 1990 and have been declining about 2% each year since; in women, lung cancer mortality rates continued to rise in the 1990s, leveling off in the late 1990s and staying about the same since 2003 (American Cancer Society 2010). African American men have higher lung cancer incidence rates and mortality rates than white men; but in women, the rates in the two races are similar (American Cancer Society 2009). Lung cancer has a poorer prognosis than the other two cancers we have discussed, with overall five-year survival rates of 16% (American Cancer Society 2010).

The two major forms of lung cancer are non–small-cell lung cancer (about 85% of all lung cancers) and small-cell lung cancer (about 15%). Non–small-cell lung cancer can be further divided into three major histologic subtypes: squamous cell carcinoma, adenocarcinoma, and large-cell lung cancer (Herbst, Haymach, and Lippman 2008). Smoking is a strong risk factor for all types of lung cancer, particularly small-cell lung cancer and squamous cell carcinoma, while adenocarcinoma is the most common type in patients who have never smoked (Herbst, Haymach, and Lippman 2008). Passive smoking (secondhand smoke) also increases the risk of lung cancer (Molina et al. 2008). Other factors associated with increased lung cancer risk include occupational exposures (especially to asbestos), air pollution, alcohol intake, and possibly low intakes of antioxidants in the diet (Molina et al. 2008). There also is a hereditary component to lung cancer; several lung cancer susceptibility genes have been reported in recent years (Molina et al. 2008).

Of interest in this textbook is the observation from several epidemiologic studies that higher levels of physical activ-ity may be associated with lower lung cancer risk. A 2006 review based on six case–control and 15 cohort studies found a median of 20% risk reduction for lung cancer in the most versus the least-active subjects (Lee and Oguma 2006). And a 2008 review by a federal expert panel, focusing on studies published between 1996 and 2006, reported similar findings (Physical Activity Guidelines Advisory Committee 2008). The two reviews showed similar findings in men and women and stronger results from case–control than from cohort studies, possibly reflecting some degree of recall bias in the case–control design. There also appears to be an inverse dose response relation; a 2005 meta-analysis of 11 studies of leisure-time physical activity and lung cancer risk reported relative risks of 1.00 (referent), 0.87 (95% CI: 0.79-0.95), and 0.70 (0.62-0.79), respectively, for low, moderate, and high levels of leisure-time activity (p trend <0.01) (Tardon et al. 2005).

A concern regarding these observational epidemiologic studies is the potential for confounding by smoking, a powerful risk factor for lung cancer. Most of the studies on the association of physical activity and lung cancer did adjust for cigarette smoking, but the potential for residual confounding exists. One way to prevent confounding is to examine the association of physical activity with lung cancer risk among never smokers; however, this is a rare cancer among never smokers, so power is limited. More consistent inverse associations have been observed in former or current smokers than in never smokers (Kubik et al. 2004; Lee, Sesso, and Paffenbarger 1999; Mao et al. 2003; Sinner et al. 2006). Another strategy to examine whether the inverse relation between physical activity and lung cancer risk is due to residual confounding is to examine the relation separately for different histological types of lung cancer, some of which are more weakly related to smoking (in particular adenocarcinoma). The findings from such studies have been unclear, in part because of the limited sample sizes (Mao et al. 2003; Steindorf et al. 2006; Thune and Lund 1997).

Possible mechanisms for an inverse relation between physical activity and lung cancer risk include enhancement of the immune system by physical activity, antioxidant effects of exercise, and decreased inflammation associated with physical activity and reduced body weight (Friedenreich 2001; Puntoni et al. 2008).

Endometrial Cancer

Endometrial cancer is the most common gynecologic cancer and the fourth most commonly occurring cancer in women (American Cancer Society 2010). In 2010, the American Cancer Society estimated that about 43,470 new cases would occur and that 7950 women would die from this cancer (American Cancer Society 2010). Incidence and mortality rates have remained relatively stable in the past one to two decades (American Cancer Society 2009). The incidence of endometrial cancer in white women is twice that in African American women; but when matched stage for stage, African American women have a less favorable prognosis (Sorosky 2008)—about 8% worse survival at all stages of diagnosis (American Cancer Society 2010). The five-year survival rate in white women is 86%; in African American women, it is 61% (American Cancer Society 2009).

Endometrial cancer is commonly classified into three types (Sorosky 2008). Type I cancers represent the vast majority of endometrial cancers. These are estrogen related and are usually low grade; the most common histology is endometrioid. Type II cancers are high grade, and the final type of endometrial cancer is hereditary or genetic. Risk factors are best known for Type 1 cancers; high levels of estrogen, whether from an endogenous or exogenous source, are a strong risk factor. Continuous estrogen stimulation from reproductive or menstrual factors or comorbidities increases the risk of endometrial cancer. As described previously, adipose tissue represents a significant source of estrogen in postmenopausal women; thus obesity is strongly related to endometrial cancer (IARC 2002). Obese women have some two- to fourfold increased risk compared with lean women (Conroy et al. 2009; Schouten, Goldbohm, and van den Brandt 2004). Extreme levels of obesity also are associated with worse survival from this cancer (Sorosky 2008). Post-menopausal hormone therapy, particularly estrogen-alone regimens, increases risk of endometrial cancer. Tamoxifen, a selective estrogen receptor modulator used in the chemo-prevention of breast cancer, also increases risk (Sorosky 2008). Other conditions such as estrogen-producing tumors and cirrhosis (a condition associated with increased estrogen production) can result in excess estrogen stimulation to the endometrium and hence increased risk of endometrial cancer (Sorosky 2008).

Several epidemiologic studies also suggest a relation between physical activity and endometrial cancer risk, although the data are not entirely consistent. A recent meta-analysis estimated a summary odds ratio of 0.71 (95% CI: 0.63-0.80) in active compared to inactive women in 13 case–control studies and a corresponding relative risk of 0.77 (0.70-0.85) in seven cohort studies (Voskuil et al. 2007). However, results varied across studies, with studies of better quality supporting an inverse relation. More research is needed to clarify the association, since a recent large prospective cohort study with good measures of physical activity did not find any relation between physical activity and risk. In the Women's Health Study, after adjusting for age, body mass index, smoking status, alcohol use, saturated fat intake, fiber intake, fruit/vegetable intake, parity, use and type of postmenopausal hormone therapy, and menopausal status, investigators did not find any association between physical activity—whether total leisure-time activity, walking, or vigorous-intensity activity—and risk of endometrial cancer (Conroy et al. 2009).

One explanation for an inverse relation between physical activity and endometrial cancer risk is that physical activity is associated with leaner body weight, and obesity increases risk of this cancer. However, several studies that did control for difference in body mass index or other measures of adiposity have continued to report lower rates of endometrial cancer among active women (Physical Activity Guidelines Advisory Committee 2008; Sternfeld and Lee 2009). Other mechanisms, including beneficial effects of physical activity on the immune system (Physical Activity Guidelines Advisory Committee 2008) and inflammation, may play a role (Modugno et al. 2005).

Rectal Cancer

At least 30 studies, conducted in North America, Europe, Asia, and Australia, have examined whether physical activity is related to rectal cancer risk (Physical Activity Guidelines Advisory Committee 2008; Lee and Oguma 2006; Sternfeld and Lee 2009). Overall, there is little support for any effect of physical activity; when active and inactive persons are compared, the median relative risk is 1.00, and results differ little between men and women (Lee and Oguma 2006).

Prostate Cancer

There also is a large body of evidence on the relation between physical activity and prostate cancer risk (Physical Activity Guidelines Advisory Committee 2008; Lee and Oguma 2006; Sternfeld and Lee 2009). In the approximately 40 studies, the overall findings have been inconsistent: While some individual studies have reported significantly lower rates of prostate cancer among active men, others have not. A recent expert panel concluded that the data on the whole do not support an association of physical activity with prostate cancer risk (Physical Activity Guidelines Advisory Committee 2008).

Cancers of Other Sites

There are too few studies of other cancers to permit firm conclusions regarding their associations with physical activity (Friedenreich, Neilson, and Lynch 2010). It is possible that physical activity also decreases the risk of other cancers, including ovarian (Cust 2011) and pancreatic cancers (Physical Activity Guidelines Advisory Committee 2008; Carnide, Kreiger, and Coterchio 2009; Lee and Oguma 2006; Olsen et al. 2007; Rossing et al. 2010; Sternfeld and Lee 2009), but the accumulated evidence so far is against a role of physical activity in reducing pancreatic cancer risk (Bao and Michaud 2008; O'Rorke et al. 2010).

Physical Activity and Cancer Survivors

The term "cancer survivor" refers to all living persons who have ever received a diagnosis of cancer. There are more than 10 million cancer survivors in the United States today

(Anonymous 2004). This represents a remarkable increase over the past three decades—in 1971, there were an estimated 3.0 million cancer survivors. The large increase in the number of cancer survivors has likely been the consequence of several factors, including earlier detection of cancers and improved treatments for the initial and recurrent disease, as well as the aging of the U.S. population (since cancer rates increase exponentially with age). After a diagnosis of cancer, many cancer survivors are highly motivated to seek health information about whether lifestyle changes beyond standard therapies, such as physical activity, can improve their response to treatment, quality of life, and survival (Brown et al. 2003).

In recent years, several studies have examined whether physical activity can improve various health outcomes in cancer survivors. Among cancer survivors, physical activity improves cardiorespiratory fitness; a smaller body of evidence suggests that it may also improve muscular strength and endurance, as well as flexibility (Physical Activity Guidelines Advisory Committee 2008). Additionally, physical activity improves quality of life and cancer-related fatigue and may ameliorate weight gain that can occur after a diagnosis of breast cancer (Physical Activity Guidelines Advisory Committee 2008; Speck et al. 2010). For breast cancer patients, surgical removal or irradiation of axillary lymph nodes as part of treatment for the cancer can damage the lymphatic system and cause swelling and pain in the affected arm. Lymphedema, considered a chronic condition, occurs in 6% to 70% of breast cancer survivors. Breast cancer survivors with lymphedema may limit the use of their affected arm out of fear of worsening the lymphedema. However, none of the five studies of aerobic or resistance exercise in breast cancer survivors reported negative effects on limb swelling; instead, symptoms may be reduced (Physical Activity Guidelines Advisory Committee 2008; Schmitz et al. 2009).

While there have been many studies on physical activity and the *prevention* of cancer, as discussed previously in this chapter, very few have addressed whether physical activity improves prognosis in cancer patients. Among women with breast cancer, 9 to 14.9 MET-hours/week of physical activity was associated with half the breast cancer mortality rate, compared with <3 MET-hours/week (Holmes et al. 2005). At higher levels of physical activity, beyond 14.9 MET-hours/week, there was no additional reduction in breast cancer deaths (risk reductions of 40-44%). For total mortality, the reduction was 41% among women exercising 9 to 14.9 MET-hours/week; again there was no additional reduction with higher levels of activity (risk reductions of 35-44%). In two other studies of men and women with colorectal cancer, physical activity was associated with decreased mortality from the cancer and also decreased overall mortality (Meyerhardt et al. 2006a, 2006b). The amount of physical activity associated with significantly better survival, however, was at least 18 MET-hours/week, substantially higher than that observed for women with breast cancer. Physical activity also appears to be associated with better survival among men with prostate cancer (Kenfield et al. 2011).

Summary

Cancer is a major cause of morbidity and mortality in the United States and worldwide. A modifiable factor that can reduce the risk of developing cancer is physical activity. A large body of epidemiologic evidence clearly indicates that active men and women have lower rates of colon cancer and that active women have lower rates of breast cancer compared with inactive individuals. The magnitude of risk reduction is on the order of 20% to 30% for both types of cancer. Approximately 30 to 60 min per day of moderate- to vigorous-intensity physical activity appears necessary to reduce the risk of both types of cancer. Several plausible biological mechanisms support the data from the epidemiologic studies.

With regard to other cancers, the accumulated evidence does not support a role of physical activity in preventing rectal or prostate cancers. For other cancer sites, the data are more limited: Physical activity may lower the risks of lung and endometrial cancers and possibly other cancers. Among cancer survivors, emerging literature suggests that physical activity may improve survival.

· BIBLIOGRAPHY ·

American Cancer Society. 2009. *Cancer facts and figures 2009.* Atlanta: American Cancer Society.

American Cancer Society. 2010. *Cancer facts and figures 2010.* Atlanta: American Cancer Society.

Anderson, G.L., M. Limacher, A.R. Assaf, T. Bassford, S.A. Beresford, et al. 2004. Effects of conjugated equine estrogen in postmenopausal women with hysterectomy: The Women's Health Initiative randomized controlled trial. *Journal of the American Medical Association* 291: 1701-1712.

Anonymous. 2004. Cancer survivorship—United States, 1971-2001. *MMWR Morb Mortal Wkly Rep* 53: 526-9.

Bach, P.B., D. Schrag, O.W. Brawley, A. Galaznik, S. Yakren, and C.B. Begg. 2002. Survival of blacks and whites after a cancer diagnosis. *Journal of the American Medical Association* 287: 2106-2113.

Bao, Y., and D.S. Michaud. 2008. Physical activity and pancreatic cancer risk: A systematic review. *Cancer Epidemiology, Biomarkers and Prevention* 17 (10): 2671-2682.

Bernstein, L., B.E. Henderson, R. Hanisch, J. Sullivan-Halley, and R.K. Ross. 1994. Physical exercise and reduced risk of breast cancer in young women. *Journal of the National Cancer Institute* 86: 1403-1408.

Bernstein, L., A.V. Patel, G. Ursin, J. Sullivan-Halley, M.F. Press, et al. 2005. Lifetime recreational exercise activity and breast cancer risk among black women and white women. *Journal of the National Cancer Institute* 97: 1671-1679.

Bingham, S.A., and J.H. Cummings. 1989. Effect of exercise and physical fitness on large intestinal function. *Gastroenterology* 97: 1389-1399.

Blair, S.N., H.W. Kohl 3rd, R.S. Paffenbarger Jr., D.G. Clark, K.H. Cooper, and L.W. Gibbons. 1989. Physical fitness and all-cause mortality. A prospective study of healthy men and women. *Journal of the American Medical Association* 262: 2395-2401.

Brinton, L.A., and S.S. Devesa. 1996. Etiology and pathogenesis of breast cancer: Incidence, demographics, and environmental factors. In *Diseases of the breast,* edited by J.R. Harris, M.E. Lippman, M. Morrow, and S. Hellman, pp. 159-168. Philadelphia: Lippincott-Raven.

Brown, J.K., T. Byers, C. Doyle, K.S. Courneya, W. Demark-Wahnefried, et al. 2003. Nutrition and physical activity during and after cancer treatment: An American Cancer Society guide for informed choices. *CA: A Cancer Journal for Clinicians* 53: 268-291.

Byers, T., M. Nestle, A. McTiernan, C. Doyle, A. Currie-Williams, et al. 2002. American Cancer Society guidelines on nutrition and physical activity for cancer prevention: Reducing the risk of cancer with healthy food choices and physical activity. *CA: A Cancer Journal for Clinicians* 52: 92-119.

Cancer survivorship—United States, 1971-2001. 2004. *Morbidity and Mortality Weekly Report* 53: 526-529.

Carnide, N., N. Kreiger, and M. Cotterchio. 2009. Association between frequency and intensity of recreational physical activity and epithelial ovarian cancer risk by age period. *European Journal of Cancer Prevention* 18 (4): 322-330.

Carpenter, C.L., P.K. Ross, A. Paganini-Hill, and L. Bernstein. 1999. Lifetime exercise activity and breast cancer risk among postmenopausal women. *British Journal of Cancer* 80: 1852-1858.

Casey, P.M., J.R. Cerhan, and S. Pruthi. 2008. Oral contraceptive use and risk of breast cancer. *Mayo Clinic Proceedings* 83: 86-90; quiz 90-1.

Cherry, T. 1922. A theory of cancer. *Medical Journal of Australia* 1: 425-438.

Chlebowski, R.T., S.L. Hendrix, R.D. Langer, M.L. Stefanick, M. Gass, et al. 2003. Influence of estrogen plus progestin on breast cancer and mammography in healthy postmenopausal women: The Women's Health Initiative Randomized Trial. *Journal of the American Medical Association* 289: 3243-3253.

Coenen, C., M. Wegener, B. Wedmann, G. Schmidt, and S. Hoffmann. 1992. Does physical exercise influence bowel transit time in healthy young men? *American Journal of Gastroenterology* 87: 292-295.

Colbert, L.H., E. Lanza, R. Ballard-Barbash, M.L. Slattery, J.A. Tangrea, et al. 2002. Adenomatous polyp recurrence and physical activity in the Polyp Prevention Trial (United States). *Cancer Causes and Control* 13: 445-453.

Colbert, L.H., K.C. Westerlind, S.N. Perkins, D.C. Haines, D. Berrigan, L.A. Donehower, R. Fuchs-Young, and S.D. Hursting. 2009. Exercise effects on tumorigenesis in a p53-deficient mouse model of breast cancer. *Medicine and Science in Sports and Exercise* 41 (8): 1597-1605.

Colditz, G.A., C.C. Cannuscio, and A.L. Frazier. 1997. Physical activity and reduced risk of colon cancer: Implications for prevention. *Cancer Causes and Control* 8: 649-667.

Collaborative Group on Hormonal Factors in Breast Cancer. 1996. Breast cancer and hormonal contraceptives: Collaborative reanalysis of individual data on 53 297 women with breast cancer and 100 239 women without breast cancer from 54 epidemiological studies. *Lancet* 347: 1713-1727.

Conroy, M.B., J.R. Sattelmair, N.R. Cook, J.E. Manson, J.E. Buring, and I.M. Lee. 2009. Physical activity, adiposity, and risk of endometrial cancer. *Cancer Causes and Control* 20: 1107-1115.

Cooper, G.S., D.P. Sandler, E.A. Whelan, and K.R. Smith. 1996. Association of physical and behavioral characteristics with menstrual cycle patterns in women age 29-31 years. *Epidemiology* 7: 624-628.

Cordain, L., R.W. Latin, and J.J. Behnke. 1986. The effects of an aerobic running program on bowel transit time. *Journal of Sports Medicine and Physical Fitness* 26: 101-104.

Cust, A.E. 2011. Physical activity and gynecologic cancer prevention. *Recent Results in Cancer Research* 186: 159-185.

Diamandopoulos, G.T. 1996. Cancer: An historical perspective. *Anticancer Research* 16: 1595-1602.

Ewertz, M. 1995. Risk from age, race, and social class. In *Reducing breast cancer risk in women,* edited by B.A. Stoll, pp. 41-45. Dordrecht, The Netherlands: Kluwer Academic.

Ewertz, M., S.W. Duffy, H.O. Adami, G. Kvale, E. Lund, et al. 1990. Age at first birth, parity and risk of breast cancer: A meta-analysis of 8 studies from the Nordic countries. *International Journal of Cancer* 46: 597-603.

Fearon, E.R., and B. Vogelstein. 1990. A genetic model for colorectal tumorigenesis. *Cell* 61: 759-767.

Fisher, B., J.P. Costantino, D.L. Wickerham, R.S. Cecchini, W.M. Cronin, et al. 2005. Tamoxifen for the prevention of breast cancer: Current status of the National Surgical Adjuvant Breast and Bowel Project P-1 study. *Journal of the National Cancer Institute* 97: 1652-1662.

Franco, G. 1999. Ramazzini and workers' health. *Lancet* 354: 858-861.

Friedenreich, C.M. 2001. Physical activity and cancer prevention: From observational to intervention research. *Cancer Epidemiology, Biomarkers and Prevention* 10 (4): 287-301.

Friedenreich, C.M., H.K. Neilson, and B.M. Lynch. 2010. State of the epidemiological evidence on physical activity and cancer prevention. *European Journal of Cancer* 46 (14): 2593-2604.

Friedenreich, C.M., and M.R. Orenstein. 2002. Physical activity and cancer prevention: Etiologic evidence and biological mechanisms. *Journal of Nutrition* 132: 3456S-3464S.

Friedenreich, C.M., and T.E. Rohan. 1995. A review of physical activity and breast cancer. *Epidemiology* 6: 311-317.

Frisch, R.E., G. Wyshak, N.L. Albright, T.E. Albright, I. Schiff, et al. 1985. Lower prevalence of breast cancer and cancers of the reproductive system among former college athletes compared to non-athletes. *British Journal of Cancer* 52: 885-891.

Gallucci, B.B. 1985. Selected concepts of cancer as a disease: From the Greeks to 1900. *Oncology Nursing Forum* 12: 67-71.

Gammon, M.D., and E.M. John. 1993. Recent etiologic hypotheses concerning breast cancer. *Epidemiologic Reviews* 15: 163-168.

Garabrant, D.H., J.M. Peters, T.M. Mack, and L. Bernstein. 1984. Job activity and colon cancer risk. *American Journal of Epidemiology* 119: 1005-1014.

Gerhardsson de Verdier, M., G. Steineck, U. Hagman, A. Rieger, and S.E. Norell. 1990. Physical activity and colon cancer: A case-referent study in Stockholm. *International Journal of Cancer* 46: 985-989.

Giovannucci, E. 2001. Insulin, insulin-like growth factors and colon cancer: A review of the evidence. *Journal of Nutrition* 131: 3109S-3120S.

Giovannucci, E., A. Ascherio, E.B. Rimm, G.A. Colditz, M.J. Stampfer, and W.C. Willett. 1995. Physical activity, obesity, and risk for colon cancer and adenoma in men. *Annals of Internal Medicine* 122: 327-334.

Giovannucci, E., and K. Wu. 2006. Cancers of the colon and rectum. In *Cancer epidemiology and prevention,* edited by D. Schottenfeld and J.F. Fraumeni Jr., pp. 809-829. New York: Oxford University Press.

Harriss, D.J., G. Atkinson, A. Batterham, K. George, N.T. Cable, T. Reilly, N. Haboubi, A.G. Renehan; Colorectal Cancer, Lifestyle, Exercise and Research Group. 2009. Lifestyle factors and colorectal cancer risk (2): A systematic review and meta-analysis of associations with leisure-time physical activity. *Colorectal Disease* 11 (7): 689-701.

Henderson, B.E., and L. Bernstein. 1996. Etiology and pathogenesis of breast cancer: Endogenous and exogenous hormonal factors. In *Diseases of the breast,* edited by J.R. Harris, M.E. Lippman, M. Morrow, and S. Hellman, pp. 185-200. Philadelphia: Lippincott-Raven.

Henderson, I.C. 1995. Breast cancer. In *Clinical oncology,* edited by G.P. Murphy, W.L. Lawrence, and R.E. Lenhard. Atlanta: American Cancer Society.

Herbst, R.S., J.V. Heymach, and S.M. Lippman. 2008. Lung cancer. *New England Journal of Medicine* 359: 1367-1380.

Hoffman-Goetz, L., D. Apter, W. Demark-Wahnefried, M.I. Goran, A. McTiernan, and M.E. Reichman. 1998. Possible mechanisms mediating an association between physical activity and breast cancer. *Cancer* 83: 621-628.

Holland, J.F., and E. Frei, eds. 1993. *Cancer medicine.* 3rd edition. Philadelphia: Lea & Febiger.

Holland, J.F., D.W. Kufe, R.E. Pollock, R.R. Weichselbaum, E.I. Frei, and R.C. Bast Jr., eds. 2000. *Holland-Frei cancer medicine.* 5th edition. Hamilton, ON: Decker.

Holmes, M.D., W.Y. Chen, D. Feskanich, C.H. Kroenke, and G.A. Colditz. 2005. Physical activity and survival after breast cancer diagnosis. *Journal of the American Medical Association* 293: 2479-2486.

Hou, L., B.T. Ji, A. Blair, Q. Dai, Y.T. Gao, and W.H. Chow. 2004. Commuting physical activity and risk of colon cancer in Shanghai, China. *American Journal of Epidemiology* 160: 860-867.

International Agency for Research on Cancer. 2002. *Weight control and physical activity.* Lyon: International Agency for Research on Cancer.

Jemal, A., R. Siegel, E. Ward, Y. Hao, J. Xu, and M.J. Thun. 2009. Cancer statistics, 2009. *CA: A Cancer Journal for Clinicians* 59: 225-249.

Kelsey, J.L., and P.L. Horn-Ross. 1993. Breast cancer: Magnitude of the problem and descriptive epidemiology. *Epidemiologic Reviews* 15: 7-16.

Kenfield, S.A., M.J. Stampfer, E. Giovannucci, and J.M. Chan. 2011. Physical activity and survival after prostate cancer diagnosis in the health professionals follow-up study. *Journal of Clinical Oncology* 29: 726-732.

Key, J., S. Hodgson, R.Z. Omar, T.K. Jensen, S.G. Thompson, et al. 2006. Meta-analysis of studies of alcohol and breast cancer with consideration of the methodological issues. *Cancer Causes and Control* 17: 759-770.

Koffler, K.H., A. Menkes, R.A. Redmond, W.E. Whitehead, R.E. Pratley, and B.F. Hurley. 1992. Strength training accelerates gastrointestinal transit in middle-aged and older men. *Medicine and Science in Sports and Exercise* 24: 415-419.

Kubik, A.K., P. Zatloukal, L. Tomasek, N. Pauk, L. Havel, et al. 2004. Dietary habits and lung cancer risk among non-smoking women. *European Journal of Cancer Prevention* 13: 471-480.

Kushi, L.H., T. Byers, C. Doyle, E.V. Bandera, M. McCullough, et al. 2006. American Cancer Society Guidelines on Nutrition and Physical Activity for cancer prevention: Reducing the risk of cancer with healthy food choices and physical activity. *CA: A Cancer Journal for Clinicians* 56: 254-281; quiz 313-4.

Lee, I-M., and Y. Oguma. 2006. Physical activity. In *Cancer epidemiology and prevention,* edited by D. Schottenfeld and J.F. Fraumeni Jr., pp. 449-467. New York: Oxford University Press.

Lee, I.M., and R.S. Paffenbarger Jr. 1994. Physical activity and its relation to cancer risk: A prospective study of college alumni. *Medicine and Science in Sports and Exercise* 26: 831-837.

Lee, I.M., R.S. Paffenbarger Jr., and C. Hsieh. 1991. Physical activity and risk of developing colorectal cancer among college alumni. *Journal of the National Cancer Institute* 83: 1324-1329.

Lee, I.M., H.D. Sesso, and R.S. Paffenbarger Jr. 1999. Physical activity and risk of lung cancer. *International Journal of Epidemiology* 28: 620-625.

Mai, P.L., J. Sullivan-Halley, G. Ursin, D.O. Stram, D. Deapen, et al. 2007. Physical activity and colon cancer risk among women in the California Teachers Study. *Cancer Epidemiology, Biomarkers and Prevention* 16: 517-525.

Malina, R.M. 1983. Menarche in athletes: A synthesis and hypothesis. *Annals of Human Biology* 10: 1-24.

Mao, Y., S. Pan, S.W. Wen, and K.C. Johnson. 2003. Physical activity and the risk of lung cancer in Canada. *American Journal of Epidemiology* 158: 564-575.

Martinez, M.E., E. Giovannucci, D. Spiegelman, D.J. Hunter, W.C. Willett, and G.A. Colditz. 1997. Leisure-time physical activity, body size, and colon cancer in women. *Journal of the National Cancer Institute* 89: 948-955.

Maruti, S.S., W.C. Willett, D. Feskanich, B. Rosner, and G.A. Colditz. 2008. A prospective study of age-specific physical activity and premenopausal breast cancer. *Journal of the National Cancer Institute* 100: 728-737.

Matthews, C.E., X.O. Shu, F. Jin, Q. Dai, J.R. Hebert, et al. 2001. Lifetime physical activity and breast cancer risk in the Shanghai Breast Cancer Study. *British Journal of Cancer* 84: 994-1001.

Mayo Clinic. 2009. Breast cancer. www.mayoclinic.com/health/stage-of-breast-cancer/BR00011 (Accessed 1/10/12).

McTiernan, A., C. Kooperberg, E. White, S. Wilcox, R. Coates, et al. 2003. Recreational physical activity and the risk of breast cancer in postmenopausal women: The Women's Health Initiative Cohort Study. *Journal of the American Medical Association* 290: 1331-1336.

Meshkinpour, H., S. Selod, H. Movahedi, N. Nami, N. James, and A. Wilson. 1998. Effects of regular exercise in management of chronic idiopathic constipation. *Digestive Diseases and Sciences* 43: 2379-2383.

Meyerhardt, J.A., E.L. Giovannucci, M.D. Holmes, A.T. Chan, J.A. Chan, et al. 2006a. Physical activity and survival after colorectal cancer diagnosis. *Journal of Clinical Oncology* 24: 3527-3534.

Meyerhardt, J.A., D. Heseltine, D. Niedzwiecki, D. Hollis, L.B. Saltz, et al. 2006b. Impact of physical activity on cancer recurrence and survival in patients with stage III colon cancer: Findings from CALGB 89803. *Journal of Clinical Oncology* 24: 3535-3541.

Modugno, F., R.B. Ness, C. Chen, and N.S. Weiss. 2005. Inflammation and endometrial cancer: A hypothesis. *Cancer Epidemiology, Biomarkers and Prevention* 14: 2840-2847.

Molina, J.R., P. Yang, S.D. Cassivi, S.E. Schild, and A.A. Adjei. 2008. Non-small cell lung cancer: Epidemiology, risk factors, treatment, and survivorship. *Mayo Clinic Proceedings* 83: 584-594.

Monninkhof, E.M., S.G. Elias, F.A. Vlems, I. van der Tweel, A.J. Schuit, et al. 2007. Physical activity and breast cancer: A systematic review. *Epidemiology* 18: 137-157.

National Cancer Institute. n.d. Cancer survivorship research. http://dccps.nci.nih.gov/ocs/index.html.

National Cancer Institute. 1999. *Information about detection, symptoms, diagnosis, and treatment of colon and rectal cancer.* Publication No. 99-1552. Bethesda, MD: National Institutes of Health.

National Cancer Institute. 2000. *Information about detection, symptoms, diagnosis, and treatment of breast cancer.* Publication No. 00-1556. Bethesda, MD: National Institutes of Health.

National Human Genome Research Institute. 2009. Learning about breast cancer. http://genome.gov/10000507.

Nelson, H.D., L.H. Huffman, R. Fu, and E.L. Harris. 2005. Genetic risk assessment and BRCA mutation testing for breast and ovarian cancer susceptibility: Systematic evidence review for the U.S. Preventive Services Task Force. *Annals of Internal Medicine* 143: 362-379.

Olsen, C.M., C.J. Bain, S.J. Jordan, C.M. Nagle, A.C. Green, D.C. Whiteman, P.M. Webb; Australian Ovarian Cancer Study Group. 2007. Recreational physical activity and epithelial ovarian cancer: A case-control study, systematic review, and meta-analysis. *Cancer Epidemiology, Biomarkers and Prevention* 16 (11): 2321-2330.

O'Rorke, M.A., M.M. Cantwell, C.R. Cardwell, H.G. Mulholland, and L.J. Murray. 2010. Can physical activity modulate pancreatic cancer risk? A systematic review and meta-analysis. *International Journal of Cancer* 126: 2957-2968.

Paffenbarger, R.S. Jr., R.T. Hyde, and A.L. Wing. 1987. Physical activity and incidence of cancer in diverse populations: A preliminary report. *American Journal of Clinical Nutrition* 45: 312-317.

Paget, S. 1889. The distribution of secondary growths in cancer of the breast. *Lancet* 1: 571-573.

Physical Activity Guidelines Advisory Committee. 2008. *Physical Activity Guidelines Advisory Committee report.* Washington, DC: U.S. Department of Health and Human Services.

Prentice, R.L., B. Caan, R.T. Chlebowski, R. Patterson, L.H. Kuller, et al. 2006. Low-fat dietary pattern and risk of invasive breast cancer: The Women's Health Initiative Randomized Controlled Dietary Modification Trial. *Journal of the American Medical Association* 295: 629-642.

Puntoni, M., D. Marra, S. Zanardi, and A. Decensi. 2008. Inflammation and cancer prevention. *Annals of Oncology* 19 (Suppl. 7): vii225-229.

Ramazzini, B. 1983. *Diseases of workers.* Latin text of 1713 revised with translation and notes by Wilmer Cave Wright. New York: Classics of Medicine Library, Division of Gryphon Editions.

Renehan, A.G., M. Tyson, M. Egger, R.F. Heller, and M. Zwahlen. 2008. Body-mass index and incidence of cancer: A systematic review and meta-analysis of prospective observational studies. *Lancet* 371 (9612): 569-578.

Robertson, G., H. Meshkinpour, K. Vandenberg, N. James, A. Cohen, and A. Wilson. 1993. Effects of exercise on total and segmental colon transit. *Journal of Clinical Gastroenterology* 16: 300-303.

Rockhill, B., W.C. Willett, D.J. Hunter, J.E. Manson, S.E. Hankinson, and G.A. Colditz. 1999. A prospective study of recreational physical activity and breast cancer risk. *Archives of Internal Medicine* 159: 2290-2296.

Rockhill, B., W.C. Willett, D.J. Hunter, J.E. Manson, S.E. Hankinson, D. Spiegelman, and G.A. Colditz. 1998. Physical activity and breast cancer risk in a cohort of young women. *Journal of the National Cancer Institute* 90: 1155-1160.

Rossing, M.A., K.L. Cushing-Haugen, K.G. Wicklund, J.A. Doherty, and N.S. Weiss. 2010. Recreational physical activity and risk of epithelial ovarian cancer. *Cancer Causes and Control* 21 (4): 485-491.

Sandler, R.S., M.L. Pritchard, and S.I. Bangdiwala. 1995. Physical activity and the risk of colorectal adenomas. *Epidemiology* 6: 602-606.

Schmitz, K.H., R.L. Ahmed, A. Troxel, A. Cheville, R. Smith, et al. 2009. Weight lifting in women with breast-cancer-related lymphedema. *New England Journal of Medicine* 361: 664-673.

Schottenfeld, D., and J. Beebe-Dimmer. 2006. Chronic inflammation: A common and important factor in the pathogenesis of neoplasia. *CA: A Cancer Journal for Clinicians* 56: 69-83.

Schouten, L.J., R.A. Goldbohm, and P.A. van den Brandt. 2004. Anthropometry, physical activity, and endometrial cancer risk: Results from the Netherlands Cohort Study. *Journal of the National Cancer Institute* 96: 1635-1638.

Sesso, H.D., R.S. Paffenbarger Jr., and I.M. Lee. 1998. Physical activity and breast cancer risk in the College Alumni Health Study (United States). *Cancer Causes and Control* 9: 433-439.

Shephard, R.J. 1995. Exercise and cancer: Linkages with obesity? *International Journal of Obesity and Related Metabolic Disorders* 19 (Suppl. 4): S62-68.

Shephard, R.J. 1996. Exercise and cancer: Linkages with obesity? *Critical Reviews in Food Science and Nutrition* 36: 321-339.

Sinner, P., A.R. Folsom, L. Harnack, L.E. Eberly, and K.H. Schmitz. 2006. The association of physical activity with lung cancer incidence in a cohort of older women: The Iowa Women's Health Study. *Cancer Epidemiology, Biomarkers and Prevention* 15: 2359-2363.

Sivertsen, I., and A.W. Dahlstrom. 1922. The relation of muscular activity to carcinoma: A preliminary report. *Journal of Cancer Research* 6: 365-378.

Slattery, M.L., S.L. Edwards, K.N. Ma, G.D. Friedman, and J.D. Potter. 1997. Physical activity and colon cancer: A public health perspective. *Annals of Epidemiology* 7: 137-145.

Sorosky, J.I. 2008. Endometrial cancer. *Obstetrics and Gynecology* 111: 436-447.

Speck, R.M., K.S. Courneya, L.C. Mâsse, S. Duval, and K.H. Schmitz. 2010. An update of controlled physical activity trials in cancer survivors: A systematic review and meta-analysis. *Journal of Cancer Survivorship: Research and Practice* 4 (2): 87-100.

Steindorf, K., C. Friedenreich, J. Linseisen, S. Rohrmann, A. Rundle, et al. 2006. Physical activity and lung cancer risk in the European Prospective Investigation into Cancer and Nutrition Cohort. *International Journal of Cancer* 119: 2389-2397.

Sternfeld, B., and I.M. Lee. 2009. Physical activity and cancer: The evidence, the issues, and the challenges. In *Epidemiologic methods in physical activity studies,* edited by I.M. Lee. New York: Oxford University Press.

Stoll, B.A. 1995. Childbearing and related risk factors In *Reducing breast cancer risk in women,* edited by B.A. Stoll, pp. 19-28. Dordrecht, The Netherlands: Kluwer Academic.

Tardon, A., W.J. Lee, M. Delgado-Rodriguez, M. Dosemeci, D. Albanes, et al. 2005. Leisure-time physical activity and lung cancer: A meta-analysis. *Cancer Causes and Control* 16: 389-397.

Thune, I., T. Brenn, E. Lund, and M. Gaard. 1997. Physical activity and the risk of breast cancer. *New England Journal of Medicine* 336: 1269-1275.

Thune, I., and E. Lund. 1997. The influence of physical activity on lung-cancer risk: A prospective study of 81,516 men and women. *International Journal of Cancer* 70: 57-62.

U.S. Department of Health and Human Services. 1996. *Physical activity and health: A report of the Surgeon General.* Atlanta: U.S. Department of Health and Human Services, Centers for Disease Control and Prevention, National Center for Disease Control and Prevention and Health Promotion.

U.S. Preventive Services Task Force. 2008. Screening for colorectal cancer: U.S. Preventive Services Task Force recommendation statement. *Annals of Internal Medicine* 149: 627-637.

Vena, J.E., S. Graham, M. Zielezny, J. Brasure, and M.K. Swanson. 1987. Occupational exercise and risk of cancer. *American Journal of Clinical Nutrition* 45: 318-327.

Voskuil, D.W., E.M. Monninkhof, S.G. Elias, F.A. Vlems, and F.E. van Leeuwen. 2007. Physical activity and endometrial cancer risk, a systematic review of current evidence. *Cancer Epidemiology, Biomarkers and Prevention* 16: 639-648.

Wallace, K., J.A. Baron, M.R. Karagas, B.F. Cole, T. Byers, et al. 2005. The association of physical activity and body mass index with the risk of large bowel polyps. *Cancer Epidemiology, Biomarkers and Prevention* 14: 2082-2086.

Weber, B.L. 1996. Genetic testing for breast cancer. *Scientific American Science and Medicine* 3: 12-21.

White, E., E.J. Jacobs, and J.R. Daling. 1996. Physical activity in relation to colon cancer in middle-aged men and women. *American Journal of Epidemiology* 144: 42-50.

Wolin, K.Y., I.M. Lee, G.A. Colditz, R.J. Glynn, C. Fuchs, and E. Giovannucci. 2007. Leisure-time physical activity patterns and risk of colon cancer in women. *International Journal of Cancer* 121: 2776-2781.

Wolin, K.Y., Y. Yan, G.A. Colditz, and I.M. Lee. 2009. Physical activity and colon cancer prevention: A meta-analysis. *British Journal of Cancer* 100: 611-616.

World Cancer Research Fund/American Institute for Cancer Research. 2007. *Food, nutrition, physical activity, and the prevention of cancer: A global perspective.* Washington, DC: American Institute for Cancer Research.

Physical Activity
and the Immune System

Violent, prolonged, exhausting work produces a leucocytosis . . . made up
principally by an increase in the polymorphonuclear . . . neutrophiles. . . . More than one
cause acts to produce the leucocytosis—probably a temporary, mechanical cause, and a toxic
cause, more slow to develop, but lasting as long as the exercise continues.

• Ralph C. Larrabee •
"Leucocytosis After Violent Exercise," 1902

CHAPTER OBJECTIVES

▸ Discuss the role of the immune system in cancers and patients with inflammatory diseases including HIV-AIDS, multiple sclerosis, and cancer survivors

▸ Provide a brief history of immunology as it applies to public health and clinical medicine

▸ Identify and describe the origin and function of key cells of the immune system

▸ Identify and describe the major lymphokines and how they regulate cells of the immune system

▸ Describe how the autonomic nervous system and the endocrine system are believed to alter immune function

▸ Describe the known and hypothesized effects of physical activity on the immune system, including circulating levels of lymphokines, neutrophils, monocytes and macrophages, lymphocytes, and natural killer cells

▸ Describe and evaluate the strength of evidence that physical activity and exercise training alters immune responses in people with inflammatory diseases

Though the site-specific mechanisms that explain the reduced risks for colon, breast, lung, and endometrial cancers are not yet understood clearly, the possibility that moderate levels of physical activity may have a positive influence on the immune system remains a likely explanation for general benefits that might extend to several different types of cancers. It is believed that persistent inflammation is part of the pathogenesis in tumor growth but also in the development of atherosclerosis, insulin resistance, and neurodegenerative diseases of the central nervous system. Hence, regular physical activity and exercise could exert part of their protective effects against cardiovascular diseases, type 2 diabetes, dementia, and depression through anti-inflammatory effects, either by reduction in abdominal fat that secretes inflammatory **cytokines** or by the release of anti-inflammatory myokines during skeletal muscle contraction (Pedersen 2006, 2009, 2011). See figure 13.1. It is also possible that favorable effects of exercise on aspects of innate (i.e., natural) and adaptive or acquired (i.e., learned) immunity help protect tissues and organs from damage by viruses, bacteria, and other microbes.

Regular exercise may also promote health in people with several of the chronic diseases discussed in earlier chapters

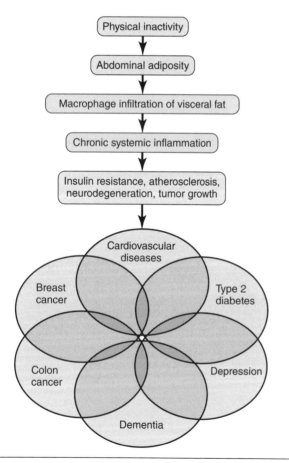

Figure 13.1 Hypothesized inflammatory effects and contributions to disease risk of physical inactivity.

Reprinted, by permission, from B.K. Pedersen, 2011, "Muscles and their myokines," *Journal of Experimental Biology* 214(2): 337-346.

that often feature low-grade inflammation (e.g., cardiovascular disease, obesity, type 2 diabetes, and cancer) and immune disorders, such as HIV/AIDS and multiple sclerosis (MS), that increase mortality risk and impair quality of life. Multiple sclerosis (*disseminated sclerosis* or *encephalomyelitis disseminata*) is an autoimmune disease that results in chronic inflammation and demyelination of the brain and spinal cord. It has an estimated prevalence between 2 and 150 people per 100,000 people worldwide (about 2.1 to 2.5 million people) (National Institute of Medicine 2001; Rosati et al. 2001), including up to 400,000 in the United States (Noonan et al. 2010), with varying severity of symptoms and disability. Neurological symptoms include loss of sensitivity; tingling; pricking or numbness; muscle weakness; muscle spasms; difficulties with moving, coordination, and balance; problems in speech or swallowing; vision problems; fatigue; chronic pain; and bladder and bowel difficulties. Cognitive impairment and depression are also common. Life expectancy is five to 10 years shorter in people with MS. The causes of MS are not known, but people with MS are more likely to have mutations in genes for tumor necrosis factor (TNF) and interferon (IFN) signaling (De Jager et al. 2009). Emerging evidence shows that physical activity can help manage symptoms, and possibly delay the onset, of MS (Motl and Gosney 2008; Snook and Motl 2009; White et al. 2004).

In 2008, AIDS accounted for 2.0 million deaths worldwide (1.4 million in sub-Saharan Africa), while 2.7 million people were newly infected with the HIV-1 virus. According to the Joint United Nations Program on HIV/AIDS, approximately 33.4 million people are living with HIV disease (UNAIDS 2009). In the United States, HIV/AIDS was a major cause of death, with the death rate increasing every year, between 1987 and 1994. However, mortality slowed dramatically after the introduction of new antiretroviral drugs, highly active antiretroviral therapy (HAART), especially protease inhibitors. See figure 13.2. As the number of people living in the United States with HIV disease has grown to more than 1 million (about 500,000 have AIDS) (Centers for Disease Control and Prevention [CDC] 2009), deaths in HIV outpatients from non-AIDS diseases have increased disproportionately, especially from non-AIDS cancers, liver disease, and cardiovascular and pulmonary disease (Palella et al. 2006; Quinn 2008). A substantial body of evidence accumulated during the past 20 years confirms that regular exercise improves fitness and cardiometabolic risk factors in people with HIV disease, with little risk of adverse events (Fillipas et al. 2010; O'Brien et al. 2010).

The acute effects of exercise on the immune system were first reported over 100 years ago, when German physiologist G. Schulz (1893) noted that muscle contractions produced an increase in the number of leukocytes circulating in the blood. Rohde and Wachholder (1953) later reported that the leukocyte increase peaked within the first minute of exercise.

Physical activity may also influence the risk of infections. A modern-day belief among athletes and coaches is that intense, strenuous exercise temporarily increases

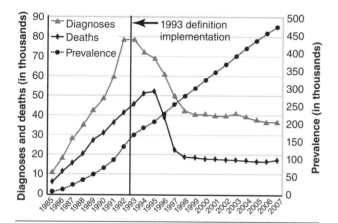

Figure 13.2 Trends from 1985 through 2007 in the estimated numbers of AIDS diagnoses, deaths of persons with AIDS, and persons living with an AIDS diagnosis in the 50 states, the District of Columbia, and the U.S. dependent areas. In 1993, the CDC expanded the AIDS surveillance case definition to include all HIV-infected persons who have less than 200 CD4+ T lymphocytes per cubic centimeter, or a CD4+ T lymphocyte percentage of total lymphocytes of less than 14.

Reprinted from Centers for Disease Control. Available: http://www.cdc.gov/hiv/topics/surveillance/resources/slides/index.htm

susceptibility to infection, especially upper respiratory infection (URI). A few studies seem to confirm that view for some sports and activities, such as marathon running and training for cross-country skiing. In contrast, an equally common belief among the public is that regular physical activity of a moderate intensity and duration increases resistance to URI or days of sickness with a common cold (Nieman 2003). Neither of these views is as yet well documented by experimental evidence, but each remains plausible.

Whether physical activity affects the immune system in a way that meaningfully reduces the risk of developing cancer or other chronic diseases is even less well established. No studies have shown such benefits among humans. However, experimental studies using rats and mice have shown that moderate physical activity seems to slow the growth of experimentally induced tumors (Cohen et al. 1992, 1993).

Thus, there remains good reason to continue to study the effects of physical activity on the immune system. This chapter describes the immune system and its function and then discusses the scientific evidence about the effects of physical activity on the immune system and inflammatory diseases.

An Abridged History of Immunology

The Greek historian Thucydides is credited with the first description of the concept of acquired immunity (from the Greek word *immunus,* meaning "exemption") in his 430 BC account of the plague of smallpox that swept Greece after the Peloponnesian War: "It was with those who had recovered from the disease that the sick and the dying found most compassion. These knew what it was from experience, and had now no fear for themselves; for the same man was never attacked twice—never at least fatally" (Sprat 1667). Later, Chinese physicians around AD 1000 and the Circassians in Turkey during the 1600s practiced variolation, whereby people were inoculated via scratching of the skin with smallpox taken from pustules of infected people.

▷ **IMMUNOLOGY IN** Western medicine has its roots in the 1796 finding by British physician Edward Jenner that injection of cowpox virus into humans resulted in protection against human smallpox.

However, **immunology** as a field of study in Western medicine has its roots in the 1796 observation by British physician Edward Jenner that injection of cowpox virus into humans resulted in inoculation against human smallpox, hence the term *vaccination,* from the Latin root *vaccinnus,* meaning "relating to a cow." Jenner reportedly got the idea when, while serving as an apprentice to an apothecary, he overheard a farm girl tell her doctor that she could not contract smallpox because she had once had cowpox. That actually was a common observation among English milkmaids, who

Early Immunology Milestones

Cowpox

A farmer named Benjamin Jesty can be credited with the first cowpox inoculation after noticing that his milkmaid was seemingly protected from smallpox. However, when Jesty's children and wife became violently ill after a botched attempt at variolation (probably because of unsterile procedures in a barnyard), he was scorned by neighbors who felt his attempts were immoral.

Early Discoveries

Milestones in the history of immunology include the discovery in the mid-to-late 1800s by the French biochemist Louis Pasteur that most infectious diseases are caused by germs, including the discoveries of staphylococcus, streptococcus, and pneumococcus bacteria. Pasteur also discovered that weakened

forms of a microbe could be used as an immunization against more virulent forms of the microbe and that rabies was transmitted by submicroscopic agents, thus discovering viruses and contributing to the development of vaccination against viruses. Around the same time, German physician Emil Adolph von Behring discovered antibodies through his pioneering research on immunization against diphtheria and tetanus by injecting what he termed "antitoxins." For that work, he received the first Nobel Prize in physiology and medicine in 1901. During the same era, the Russian biologist Ilya Mechnikov introduced the theory of **phagocytosis,** that is, that certain white blood cells can engulf bacteria. He won the 1908 Nobel Prize in physiology and medicine for using the concept of antibodies to treat diphtheria.

had reduced risk of contracting smallpox because of their exposure to cowpox. After 1770, Jenner was inspired by his mentor, famous London surgeon and anatomist John Hunter, to continue experiments with cowpox. Jenner found that there were two forms of cowpox but that only one provided immunity against smallpox. On May 14, 1796, Jenner tested his hypothesis by inoculating a healthy 8-year-old boy, James Phipps, with cowpox. Two months later, he exposed the boy to smallpox virus from the dairymaid Sarah Nelmes, but the boy did not get the disease. Jenner submitted a manuscript describing his findings to the Royal Society of Medicine, but it was rejected. He then published a book about his studies in 1798 (figure 13.3), but it was largely ignored by physicians at the time. Later, an influential physician named William Woodville, who was director of London Smallpox and Inoculation Hospital, conducted extensive trials of successful vaccination on several thousand patients. Those studies led to the acceptance of Jenner's ideas by the Royal Society and set the stage for the modern study of immunology.

HIV and AIDS

The initial or index case of human immunodeficiency virus (HIV) disease/acquired immune deficiency syndrome (AIDS), treated in Los Angeles during 1981 by Michael S. Gottlieb, MD, had fewer than 50 CD4+ cells and Pneumocystis carinii pneumonia, a rare form of pneumonia that is usually found only in patients with severe immune suppression. Together with Gottlieb and other local physicians, Wayne Shandera, MD, the Epidemic Intelligence Service officer stationed at the Los Angeles County Department of Public Health,

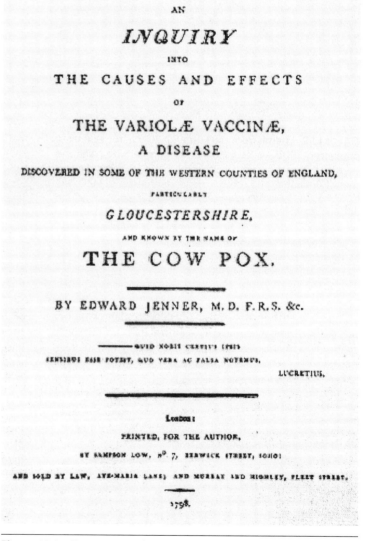

Figure 13.3 Frontispiece of British physician Edward Jenner's book on his studies of smallpox, published in 1798.

Reprinted from E. Jenner 1798.

prepared a report on five cases of Pneumocystis carinii pneumonia among previously healthy young men in Los Angeles and submitted it for publication by CDC in *Morbidity and Mortality Weekly Report* in early May 1981 (CDC 1981). The CDC now defines AIDS in adults or teenagers as a CD4⁺ T cell count less than 200 cells per cubic millimeter (mm³) of blood or the presence of one of 25 AIDS-related clinical conditions that mainly represent opportunistic infections (such as pneumocystis pneumonia, candidiasis, cytomegalovirus, herpes symplex with chronic ulcerations, mycobacterium, histoplasmosis, lymphoma, multifocal leukoencephalopathy, toxoplasmosis of brain, encephalopathy due to HIV, wasting syndrome due to HIV, Kaposi's sarcoma, and some other pneumonias) (CDC 1987). The case definition in adults and adolescents was expanded in 1993 to include HIV infection in an individual (CDC 1992).

The virus responsible for AIDS was initially termed human T lymphotropic virus type III/lymphadenopathy-associated virus (HTLV-III/LAV). French researchers Francoise Barre-Sinoussi and Luc Montagnier won the 2008 Nobel Prize in medicine for their discovery in 1983 of human immunodeficiency virus, or HIV-1. HIV is a retrovirus that uses the enzyme reverse transcriptase to replicate DNA from its single-stranded RNA in a host cell. Mutated DNA is then incorporated into the host's DNA by an integrase enzyme. Then, HIV-1 protease cleaves a newly synthesized HIV protein to create an active, infectious protein. HIV-1 specifically targets CD4⁺ cells (i.e., helper T cells), which are killed by the mutation or by cytotoxic CD8⁺ cells, thereby severely suppressing adaptive or acquired immunity. Hence, HIV disease progresses to AIDS.

Since the introduction of HAART in 1996, the progression of HIV disease has dropped markedly in regions that have access to antiretrovirals (Cohen et al. 2008). Currently, there are over 20 antiretroviral drugs in five distinct pharmacological classes: nucleoside/nucleotide reverse transcriptase inhibitors (NRTIs), non-nucleoside reverse transcriptase inhibitors (NNRTIs), protease inhibitors (PIs), entry inhibitors, and, most recently, integrase inhibitors (Quinn 2008). In 1995-1996, 58% of HIV patients treated with HAART achieved a clinical goal of reduced viral load (i.e., 500 copies/ml or less of HIV-1 RNA) by six months compared with 83% in 2002-2003 (May et al. 2006). However, despite retardation of the expansion of viral load in HIV patients and an increase in survival time in AIDS patients, there has not been a corresponding drop in overall AIDS mortality (May et al. 2006), in part because of disproportionate increases in rates of chronic diseases, especially non-AIDS-related cancers and cardiovascular disease in HIV patients undergoing HAART (Gill et al. 2010). Figure 13.4 shows a common progression of declining CD4⁺ counts and increasing viral load after HIV-1 infection. Most clinical symptoms of AIDS start appearing when CD4⁺ cells fall below 400. A count below 200 cells/mm³ is a criterion for AIDS.

The Immune System

The **immune system** is an integrated network of molecules, cells, tissues, and organs that defends an organism against infection by foreign substances (e.g., bacteria and viruses) and against mutated native cells (i.e., tumors). It also helps to repair damaged tissues and to clean up the debris of dead cells (e.g., after muscle injury). Historically, the immune system has been regarded as self-regulating, independent of other regulatory mechanisms. However, it is now known that, in mammals at least, it interacts with the nervous and

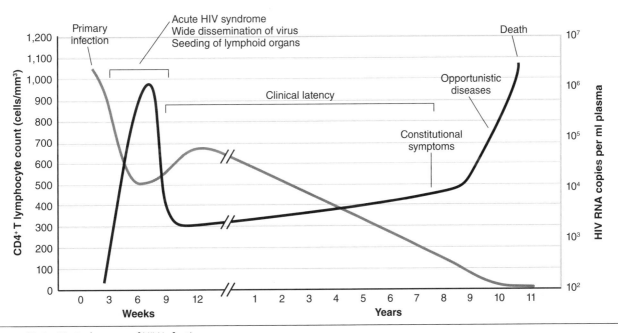

Figure 13.4 Typical course of HIV infection.

Adapted from National Institute of Allergy and Infectious Diseases 2011.

endocrine systems in ways that could plausibly be altered by exercise. There are two main types of immunities: innate (i.e., natural) and adaptive (i.e., acquired) immunity. They differ mainly in whether prior exposure is required for an immune response to occur. **Innate immunity** means that immune cells can recognize a foreign substance (an antigen) without prior exposure; **adaptive immunity** refers to immune cells' memory whereby they recognize a pathogen from a prior encounter, permitting a quicker and larger immune response upon a subsequent exposure (figure 13.5).

▷ **THE IMMUNE** system is a network of molecules, cells, tissues, and organs that defend an organism against infection by foreign substances and against mutated native cells. It also helps repair damaged tissues by cleaning up the debris of dead cells.

Innate Immunity

Innate, or natural, immunity provides the initial defense against various infectious agents and cancer. It can be activated by pathogens to which an organism is exposed through contact with skin, inhalation, or ingestion in food or water. Innate immunity can also be activated by tissue necrosis (e.g., muscle damage from exercise) or release of heat shock or oxidative stress proteins from the liver, heart, and skeletal muscle (Whitham and Forte 2008) and acute-phase proteins from the liver (e.g., C-reactive protein). Heat shock proteins, especially Hsp70, are involved in binding antigens and presenting them to the immune system. C-reactive protein is an acute-phase protein that is also activated by adipokines secreted by fat cells. Natural immunity is accomplished by **phagocytic cells** such as macrophages, **neutrophils,** and **natural killer (NK) cells.** It includes physical and chemical barriers such as the

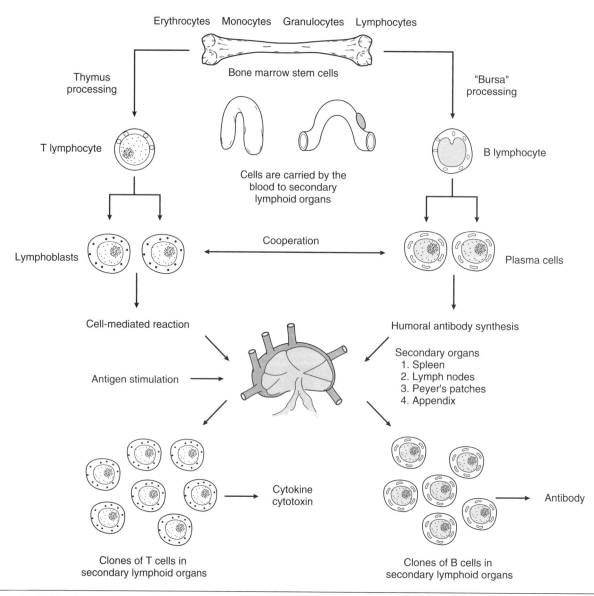

Figure 13.5   The immune system.

epidermis and epithelia. Even human sweat contains an anti-bacterial peptide that helps regulate microbes on the surface of the skin (Schittek et al. 2001). Innate immune cells are also activated by Toll-like receptor (TLR) proteins found in mast cells and intestinal epithelium that recognize the presence of microbes (e.g., bacteria, fungi, amoebas, and protozoa) that have penetrated the skin or intestinal tract mucosa. TLRs are also expressed by dendritic cells, monocytes/macrophages, and B lymphocytes. They participate in the acute-phase and inflammatory responses to infection by stimulating the production of cytokines such as interleukin-1 (IL-1), tumor necrosis factor-alpha (TNF-α), interleukin-8 (IL-8), and interleukin-12 (IL-12). The innate immune system also is composed of factors that cause **inflammation,** which is a localized response of increased blood flow, increased capillary permeability, influx of neutrophils and macrophages, and secretion of cytokines (nonantibody proteins secreted by inflammatory leukocytes, and some other cells including skeletal muscle, that act as intercellular mediators).

Innate immunity also involves blood proteins that are components of the **complement system,** which is capable of lysing bacteria and viruses coated with antibodies. The complement system is composed of about 25 proteins produced mainly by macrophages, the liver, and the intestine, which function in a cascade leading to cell lysis. Innate immunity is not very able to recognize specific antigens but provides general response against most infectious agents.

Inflammation is commonly an acute, transitory response to infection or injury. However, people can have persistent low-grade inflammation, which is usually characterized by small increases in neutrophils and NK cells in the blood and levels of inflammatory and anti-inflammatory cytokines and acute-phase proteins (e.g., C-reactive protein) that are two to four times higher than normal.

Adaptive Immunity

Adaptive or acquired immunity is able to recognize highly specific antigens as a result of previous exposure and offers different responses to different types of microbes. Memory enables a rapid and strong response to the same microbes when an organism is exposed to them again. Lymphocytes, such as T and B cells, and the products of plasma cells, **antibodies,** provide adaptive immunity. The molecules of the innate and adaptive immune systems function cooperatively as an integrated defense mechanism.

Cells of the Immune System

The immune system consists of different cell populations and molecules that migrate into and out of the blood and **lymph** circulations and are distributed in lymph organs and other tissues except in the central nervous system. **Leukocytes** (white blood cells) include lymphocytes, monocytes, and granulocytes (figure 13.6).

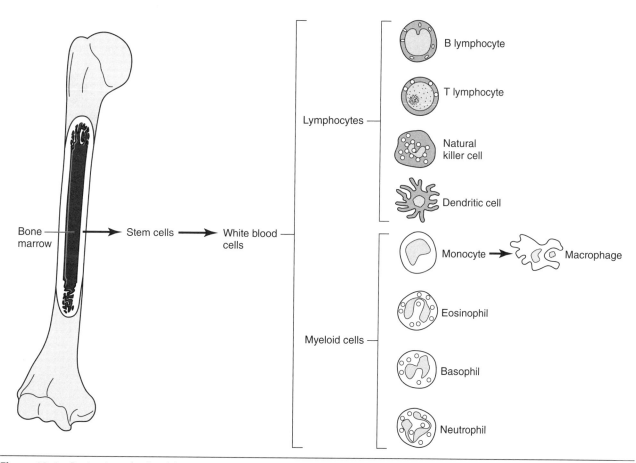

Figure 13.6 Derivation of cells of the immune system.

Lymphocytes are the major cells of adaptive immunity. **B lymphocytes** mature in bone marrow in mammals and differentiate into plasma cells, which produce antibodies after exposure to an antigen. B lymphocytes provide humoral (i.e., of the blood) immunity. They do not require mediating cell-to-cell contact in order to kill foreign cells during a primary (i.e., initial) infection by an antigen, but they require activation by helper T cells during a secondary (i.e., recurrent) infection by an antigen. Each B cell displays an antibody that has binding sites specific to a particular antigen. Antibodies are classified by five main types of **immunoglobulin (Ig)** that differ in their relative amounts in the blood: IgG, 80%; IgA, 10% to 15%; IgM, 5% to 10%; and IgE, 1%. Antibodies can coat antigens with opsonin (a process termed **opsonization**), a substance that makes it easier for antigens to be engulfed by a phagocyte. Binding of a B lymphocyte to an antigen presented by an **antigen-presenting cell** (APC) (cells that engulf antigens and present them to B or T lymphocytes in a recognizable form [e.g., in a major histocompatibilty complex class II molecule], such as a macrophage or a dendritic cell) results in activation and **clonal expansion** of the B lymphocyte (figure 13.7). Other B lymphocytes are memory B cells, which mainly reside in the lymph nodes and spleen. Some memory B cells circulate in the blood as sentinels, ready to respond quickly and forcefully if they encounter the same antigen again. B cells can also serve as APCs for T lymphocytes. Macrophages and dendritic cells are termed "professional" APCs because they are effective at inducing a second-messenger signal needed for T and B cell activation.

T lymphocytes, derived from bone marrow, differentiate in the thymus. T lymphocytes are classified by the surface molecules, called the cluster of differentiation (CD), as CD4+ or CD8+ cells, which are also known by their functional names, helper T (T_H) cells and suppressor/cytotoxic T ($T_{S/C}$) cells, respectively. T cells participate in cell-mediated immunity, which means that they require cell-to-cell contact in order to generate cytotoxic cells and to activate macrophages. Helper T cells are differentiated into T_{H-1} and T_{H-2} (see figure 13.8). T_{H-1} cells activate macrophages and cytotoxic T cells (figures 13.9 and 13.10). T_{H-2} cells activate B lymphocytes (figure 13.7).

The specificity of T cells against antigens results from their ability to recognize peptide structures associated with the major histocompatibility complex (MHC) expressed on the surface of an APC. Cytotoxic T cells recognize MHC I proteins, while helper T cells recognize MHC II proteins. For example, when an APC first internalizes the antigen, it decomposes it into smaller peptides (epitopes) by digestion with lysosyme and then displays a fragment of the antigen on the APC's MHC class II molecule so that the helper T cell recognizes the antigen and is activated. The main function of cytotoxic T cells is **lysis** of tumor cells and virus-infected cells. When activated, helper T cells secrete cytokines that promote the growth and differentiation of T cells and other lymphocytes and activate inflammatory cells such as mononuclear phagocytes, neutrophils, and **eosinophils.**

Natural killer cells represent a distinct class of lymphocytes found in blood and **lymphoid** organs, especially the spleen. They have a shape similar to that of other lymphocytes but are granular, so they are also called large granular lymphocytes (LGL). Natural killer cells are an important part of innate immunity that do not require prior exposure to

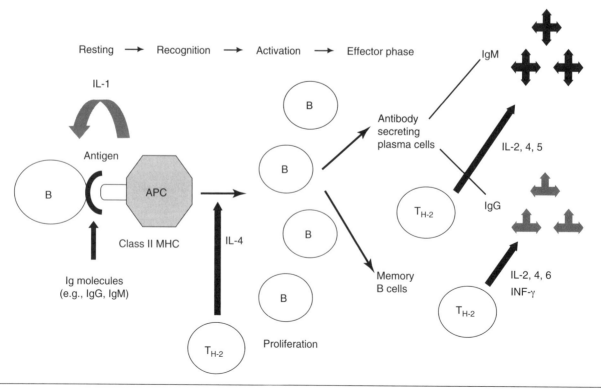

Figure 13.7   Activation of B cells and antibody secretion after presentation of an antigen.

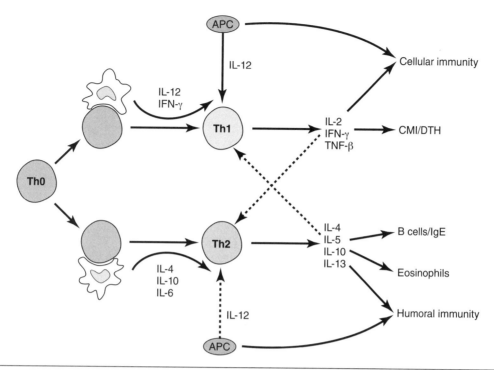

Figure 13.8 Differentiation of T_{H-1} and T_{H-2} cells.

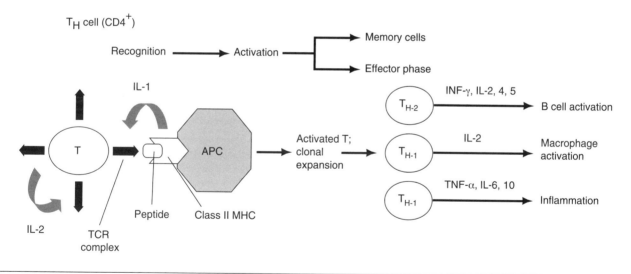

Figure 13.9 The presentation of an antigen to a helper T cell and the cascade of immune responses, including cloning of the activated helper T and subsequent activation of B cells, macrophages, granulocytes, and cytotoxic T cells, assisted by secretion of cytokines from other helper T cells.

recognize an antigen. Thus, NK cells play an important role in early defense against microbes by producing cell membrane damage (e.g., osmotically lysing) or inducing apoptosis (the process of genetically programmed cell death characterized by cell shrinkage and DNA fragmentation) in virus-infected cells and tumor cells. Natural killer cells can also secrete cytotoxic cytokines, including TNF-α and IFN-γ.

▷ **NATURAL KILLER** cells are a class of large, granular lymphocytes found in blood and lymphoid organs, especially the spleen. They do not require prior exposure to recognize an antigen and thus play an important role in innate immunity. Acute exercise increases the numbers and possibly the activity of NK cells in the blood.

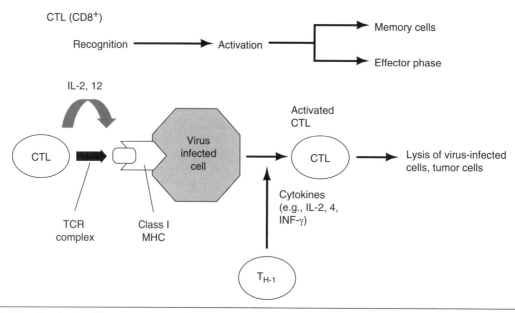

Figure 13.10   T cell activation. The presentation of an antigen directly to a cytotoxic T cell.

Monocytes are produced in bone marrow and are released into the bloodstream, where they act as phagocytes, cytokine producers, regulators of blood clotting, and APCs for about a week while they travel to fixed sites in body tissues or special vessels. There they mature to become fully functioning macrophages, which are major phagocytes and APCs that produce cytokines during localized tissue infections. IL-1 secreted by macrophages is the key activator of helper T cells and stimulates the cascade of defense during an adaptive immune response to infection.

Macrophages classically activated by IFN-γ or lipopolysaccharides (LPS) on bacteria secrete pro-inflammatory cytokines such as IL-1, IL-6, IL-12, and TNF-α (Mosser and Edwards 2008). LPS are cell wall constituents of Gram-negative bacteria that bind to LPS-binding proteins (LBP) in plasma to activate macrophages. Macrophages are alternatively activated by IL-4, IL-13, and transforming growth factor-beta (TGF-β) to scavenge injured or dead tissue, secrete anti-inflammatory cytokines IL-10 and IL-1 receptor antagonist (IL-1ra), and release TGF-β and vascular endothelial growth factor (VGEF), which promote tissue repair and healing. Hence, macrophages have three main functions (figure 13.11): host defense, wound healing, and regulation of other immune cells (Mosser and Edwards 2008).

Dendritic cells are the most efficient APCs, but they are present in low numbers in the body, mainly in the skin (Langerhans cells) and in the inner lining of the nose, lungs, stomach, and intestines.

Granulocytes, which originate in bone marrow, include neutrophils, eosinophils, **basophils,** and **mast cells.** Neutrophils make up about 80% to 90% of granulocytes and are major phagocytes of bacteria. They are abundant in the blood circulation but not in tissues. Neutrophils are chemically attracted and rapidly migrate from the blood to the site of an inflammation (a process called chemotaxis), especially a bacterial infection, where they ingest the bacteria. Neutrophils kill ingested bacteria by releasing lysosomal enzymes (e.g., proteases) or by an oxidative burst, using oxygen free radicals, nitric oxide, and hydrogen peroxide, which are toxic to microbes. Dead neutrophils compose part of the pus that forms at the site of infection.

▶ **NEUTROPHILS ARE** the main type of granulocytes that digest bacteria at the site of infection. They increase in number during and immediately after acute exercise.

Cytokines differ from classical hormones because they are produced by several types of cells rather than by specialized glands. There are more than 60 cytokines, which are usually named according to their function or the cells that release them. Some cytokines that communicate between leukocytes are called **interleukins (IL).** Cytokines produced by lymphocytes are often termed lymphokines. Monocytes and macrophages secrete monokines.

Chemokines are a class of pro-inflammatory cytokines that are released by phagocytes, endothelial cells, fibroblasts, and smooth muscle cells in response to bacteria, viruses, and cell damage at the site of infection. Chemokines chemically attract and activate leukocytes in infected tissue by (1) binding with leukocytes and stabilizing the binding of integrin molecules with the endothelium, (2) providing a chemokine gradient across the endothelium that chemically attracts leukocytes across the vessel wall, and (3) activating phagocytic lysis. Chemokines are classified into two main types according to variations in shared cysteine molecules. C-X-C or α

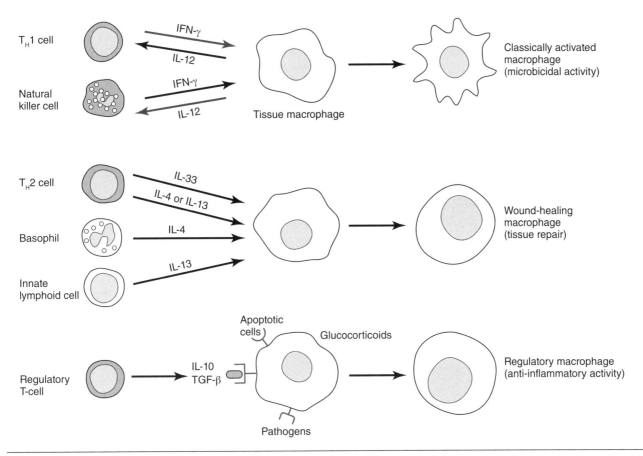

Figure 13.11   Functions of macrophages.
Adapted from Mosser and Edwards 2008.

chemokines (e.g., IL-8) have paired cysteines separated by a different amino acid; they act as chemoattractants for neutrophils and fibroblasts involved with healing wounds. C-C or β chemokines (e.g., monocyte chemoattractant protein-1 [MCP-1]) have paired cysteines; they act as chemoattractants for monocytes, lymphocytes, eosinophils, and basophils.

Interferons boost resistance against viruses, inhibit proliferation of normal and malignant cells, impede multiplication of intracellular parasites, enhance macrophage and granulocyte phagocytosis, and augment NK cell activity. Interferon-gamma (IFN-γ) is the main interferon produced by stimulated lymphocytes. Cytokines mediate both innate (e.g., TNF-α, IL-1, IL-6, IL-10, IL-12, and IL-15) and adaptive immune responses (e.g., IFN-γ, TGF-β, IL-2, IL-4, and IL-5). Cytokines released by resident phagocytes at the site of infection have local effects, including leukocyte adhesion to the vascular endothelium, expression of class I MHC molecules, and augmentation of activity of phagocytes.

Cytokines also have general effects when they are released into the blood circulation. For example, pro-inflammatory cytokines such as IL-1β and TNF-α contribute to increased body temperature, which can inhibit the growth of some bacteria and enhance some immune reactions. They also induce the **acute-phase response,** which can result in fever, fatigue, loss of appetite, and nausea, as well as output by the liver of proteins that function like antibodies and boost innate immunity. A key acute-phase protein is C-reactive protein (discussed in chapter 5 in the context of inflammation and coronary heart disease), which binds to some bacteria and fungi, serving as both an opsonin and a complement catalyst. Another general effect of pro-inflammatory cytokines during initial infection is **leukocytosis,** which is an increase in the number of leukocytes circulating in the blood coming from bone marrow and, to a much lesser extent, the marginal pool.

Adipokines are cytokines secreted by adipocytes (i.e., fat cells). As discussed in chapter 9 on obesity, they include proteins that act locally or as hormones to regulate energy intake and expenditure (e.g., adiponectin [glucose and fatty acid oxidation], leptin [appetite suppression by inhibition of neuropeptide Y in the hypothalamus], resistin [promotion of insulin resistance], and chemerin [stimulation of lipolysis]). Adiponectin is inversely related to inflammatory cytokines associated with obesity, but is elevated in autoimmune disorders such as rheumatoid arthritis, systemic lupus erythematosus, inflammatory bowel disease, type 1 diabetes, and cystic fibrosis (Fantuzzi 2008).

Types of Adipokines

- Tumor necrosis factor-alpha (TNF-α)
- Interleukin-6 (IL-6)
- Plasminogen activator inhibitor-1 (PAI-1) (promotes fibrosis)
- Visfatin (mimics effects of insulin and also inhibits apoptosis (i.e., programmed cell death) of neutrophils

Myokines are peptides released by contracting skeletal muscle that have cell signaling effects on fat oxidation and glucose uptake within the muscle, but also have local paracrine (act on receptors on nearby cells) and systemic endocrine (carried by blood and lymph fluids to cells they act upon) effects outside the muscle to mediate anti-inflammatory responses (Pedersen 2006). See figure 13.12. The first proposed myokine, IL-6, acts as an anti-inflammatory cytokine by its inhibitory effects on TNF-α and IL-1, as well as activation of the IL-1 receptor and the

Key Cytokines of the Immune System

- **Interleukin-1 (IL-1),** produced mainly by macrophages, activates acute-phase responses during the first few hours of infection or tissue damage. Such responses include fever, redistribution of amino acids, and increased liver production of antimicrobial plasma proteins. IL-1 also activates the cascade of humoral and cellular immune responses against infection by activating helper T cells and the clonal expansion of B cells, and by inducing the expression of adhesion molecules to aid emigration of leukocytes from the blood to infected tissue (Cannon et al. 1986).

- **Interleukin-2 (IL-2)** is produced mainly by activated T_H lymphocytes. Its main functions are self-priming (i.e., it upregulates its own activity), activation of cytotoxic T cells and NK cells, increased expression of IL-2 receptors on other lymphocytes, and stimulation for the release of other cytokines such as IFN.

- **Interleukin-6 (IL-6)** is produced primarily by activated T_{H-2} lymphocytes, monocytes, and macrophages (Mackinnon 1999). Its main functions are to stimulate B cells to form plasma cells and secrete antibodies and to induce acute-phase protein synthesis by the liver in response to inflammation (Sprenger et al. 1992). Hence, it is an anti-inflammatory cytokine. IL-6 is secreted by skeletal muscle during violent exercise that induces muscle injury and also during moderate exercise. The IL-6 response to moderate exercise is a putative regulator of fuel metabolism of fat and glucose during exercise (Febbraio and Pedersen 2002), but it also has potentially positive immunological effects. It promotes an anti-inflammatory cascade characterized by increased levels of cytokine inhibitors, IL-1 receptor antagonist (IL-1ra), TNF receptors (TNF-R), and the anti-inflammatory cytokine IL-10; and it inhibits the production of the pro-inflammatory cytokine TNF-α (Pedersen 2006, 2011).

- **Interleukin-8 (IL-8)** is a chemokine released mainly by resident macrophages and epithelial cells in damaged tissue. It acts as a chemoattractant for neutrophils and fibroblasts involved with healing wounds.

- **Interleukin-10 (IL-10)** is an anti-inflammatory cytokine produced by T_{H-2} lymphocytes. It was initially termed cytokine synthesis inhibitory factor because it inhibits cytokine production by macrophages in order to downregulate T_{H-1} cells. IL-10 also downregulates MHC II expression on antigen-presenting cells and acts in concert with IL-4 to decrease macrophage inflammatory activity.

- **Interleukin-12 (IL-12)** is secreted by macrophages and B cells. It activates T_{H-1} lymphocytes and NK cells. In combination with IL-2, IL-12 also activates cytotoxic T cells.

- **Interleukin-15 (IL-15)** is structurally and functionally similar to IL-2. It is secreted by monocytes and macrophages after viral infection. It modulates T and B lymphocytes and induces proliferation of NK cells.

- **Tumor necrosis factor-alpha (TNF-α)** is primarily produced by macrophages. It activates the killing of tumor cells and plays a role in antiviral activity (Mackinnon 1999). It also is an anti-inflammatory mediator of the acute-phase response (Rivier et al. 1994). Paradoxically, high levels of TNF-α have harmful effects, including chronic inflammation and muscle wasting (Mackinnon 1999).

- **Tumor necrosis factor-beta (TNF-β)** is produced by T lymphocytes. It activates tumor lysis, enhances phagocytic activity by macrophages, and is involved with mediating inflammation.

- **Interferon-gamma (IFN-γ)** is produced by activated T_{H-1} and cytotoxic lymphocytes and NK cells. It plays a major role in antimicrobial and antitumor responses as well as antiviral effects and inhibition of antigen proliferation and differentiation (Sprenger et al. 1992). IFN-γ activates macrophages so that they are more phagocytic and increases their expression of class II MHC so that they have increased capacity as APCs.

- **Transforming growth factor-beta (TGF-β)** is released by platelets, macrophages, and lymphocytes. It increases IL-1 production by activated macrophages, converts proliferating B cells to IgA, and is a chemoattractant for monocytes and macrophages. It also inhibits lymphocyte proliferation during inflammation, thus facilitating wound healing by restraining inflammation after cell injury.

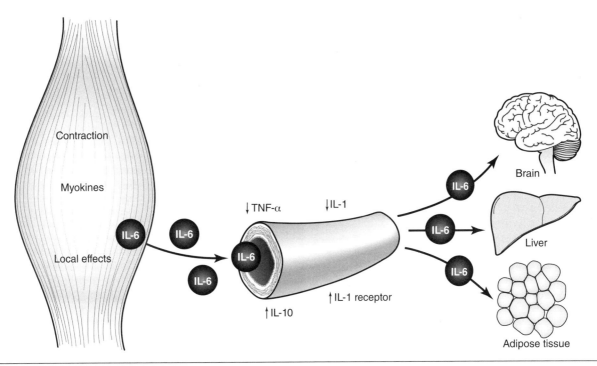

Figure 13.12 Contracting skeletal muscle releases myokines into the circulation.
Data from Pedersen 2011.

anti-inflammatory cytokine IL-10 (Febbraio and Pedersen 2005). Myokines may ultimately help explain molecular (i.e., cell signaling) mechanisms by which skeletal muscle communicates with adipose tissue, the liver, the pancreas, and the brain to counteract inflammatory responses that can contribute to chronic diseases (Pedersen 2009).

Colony-Stimulating Factors

Leukocytosis from bone marrow is regulated by colony-stimulating factors (CSF), which are glycoproteins (conjugated protein–carbohydrate compounds) found in the blood that stimulate the proliferation of bone marrow cells and the formation of colonies of granulocytes or macrophages. They include granuloctye–macrophage colony-stimulating factor (GM-CSF), granulocyte colony-stimulating factor (G-CSF), macrophage colony-stimulating factor (M-CSF), and IL-3. GM-CSF is produced in response to several inflammatory factors in blood and at the site of infection. It stimulates the production of neutrophils, macrophages, and mixed granulocyte–macrophage colonies from bone marrow cells. It can also stimulate the formation of eosinophil colonies and stimulate activities in mature granulocytes and macrophages. G-CSF induces the survival, proliferation, and differentiation of neutrophilic granulocyte precursor cells and functionally activates mature blood neutrophils. M-CSF stimulates the survival, proliferation, and differentiation of monocyte-macrophages. IL-3, also termed multi-CSF because it is secreted by lymphocytes, epithelial cells, and astrocytes, stimulates clonal proliferation and differentiation of various types of blood and tissue cells.

Organs of the Immune System

Immune cells migrate to and are concentrated in the primary and secondary lymphoid organs. See figure 13.13. The primary lymphoid organs include bone marrow, where hematopoiesis (generation of blood cells) occurs, and the thymus, where thymocytes mature to become T lymphocytes. The secondary lymphoid organs, where the contact between lymphocytes and antigens occurs, consist of lymph nodes, the spleen, the mucosal-associated lymphoid tissue (MALT) (e.g., **Peyer's patches** in the small intestine and the tonsils), and the cutaneous immune system (e.g., epidermic or dermic lymphocytes). Foreign antigens in the lymph are collected and transported to lymph nodes, which are located throughout the lymphatic vessels, and other lymphoid tissues, where they can be recognized by lymphocytes. The spleen removes foreign substances from the blood, stores immune cells, and provides another site for immune responses to blood-borne antigens. Migration and recirculation of monocytes, neutrophils, and lymphocytes to the different sites in the body where antigens can be localized are critical in immune responses.

Responses to Infection

Host responses to an infection have three main phases: (1) innate, nonadaptive defense involving epithelial cell surfaces, resident phagocytes, and complement activation; (2) early induced responses, including inflammation, activation of phagocytes and NK cells, and cytokine release; and (3) the adaptive immune response involving the clonal expansion

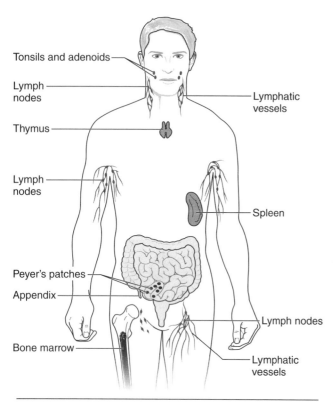

Figure 13.13 Organs of the immune system.

of cytoxic T cells and B cells (Abbas, Lightman, and Pober 1997).

The first phase occurs within a few hours after infection. If the complement system and resident phagocytes (e.g., macrophages) do not sufficiently limit the infection, the second phase of early nonadaptive responses is induced. Key aspects of this phase are inflammation and the migration of leukocytes (e.g., monocytes and granulocytes) to the site of infection. Inflammation and migration are regulated by cytokines (e.g., IL-6 and IL-8) and other inflammatory factors such as prostaglandins and leukotrienes released by phagocytes during the initial, innate response, as well as by complement proteins C5a, C3a, and C4a. Localized actions of these inflammatory factors culminate in local dilation of postcapillary venules, a reduced rate of blood flow, and increased permeability of vessel walls leading to edema (i.e., swelling), heat, and pain. The vascular changes also result in **margination** of leukocytes to the slower, peripheral area of the bloodstream, thereby increasing contact between circulating leukocytes and the endothelial cells that line the vessels and facilitating the transmigration of leukocytes that circulate in the blood across the vessel walls into infected tissues. This margination and emigration from the blood of leukocytes is a three-step process termed **extravasation**, which is regulated by **adhesion molecules** expressed by both the leukocyte and the endothelium (Collins 1995) (figure 13.14). Expression

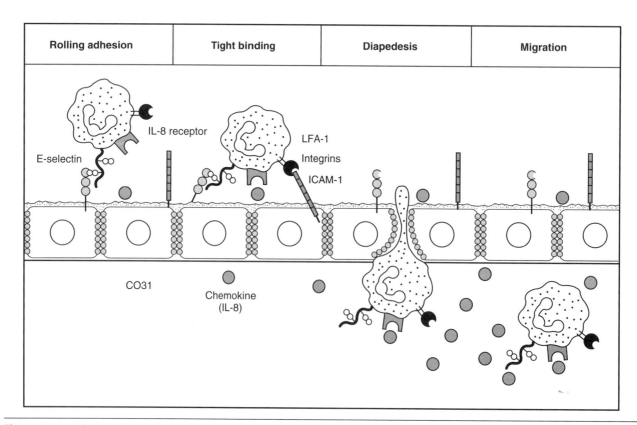

Figure 13.14 Extravasation and transmigration of a leukocyte to the site of an infection, regulated by adhesion molecules and chemokines.

of adhesion molecules by endothelial cells is regulated by inflammatory cytokines including IL-1 and TNF-α.

The first step of extravasation is mediated by **selectin molecules** (e.g., L-selectin, P-selectin, E-selectin) expressed by the endothelium of venules, which bind with glycoproteins on leukocytes and cause leukocytes to roll along a "sticky" endothelial surface of the blood vessel. This is a rapid process. For example, E-selectin is activated by TNA-α in about 1 h. The second step involves binding of **integrin molecules** (e.g., lymphocyte function–associated antigen-1 [LFA-1], leukocyte adhesion receptor [Mac-1], very late antigen-4 [VLA-4], and murine mucosal homing receptor-1 [LPAM-1]) on leukocytes with adhesion molecules on the endothelial surface (e.g., intercellular adhesion molecule-1 [ICAM-1] binds with LFA-1 integrin; vascular cell adhesion molecule-1 [VCAM-1] binds with integrin VLA-4 and LPAM-1; and mucosal addressin cell adhesion molecule-1 [MAdCAM-1] assists homing of lymphocytes to specific lymphoid sites) so that leukocytes stop rolling and become loosely attached to the endothelium, where they form the **marginal pool.** This is a slower process. For example, activation of VCAM-1 by IL-4 and other pro-inflammatory cytokines and ICAM-1 by IFN-γ takes 5 or more hours. The last step is transmigration of the leukocyte through the vascular wall into the infected tissue. This step, termed **diapedesis,** depends on the binding of leukocyte integrins with platelet endothelial cell adhesion molecule-1 (PECAM-1), an adhesion molecule expressed by platelets and on the junctions between endothelial cells, and erosion of the endothelial basement membrane by proteases (enzymes that decompose proteins) released by the leukocyte. After an infection is contained, lymphocytes return to the bloodstream via the thoracic duct; and some recirculate in the lymph and blood through the same tissue, acting as antigen sentinels based on memory of past antigen exposure (this is called "homing"). Monocytes and granulocytes do not reenter the lymph and blood circulation from infected tissue.

Immunomodulation by the Nervous and Endocrine Systems

Activation of the sympathetic nervous system and the **hypothalamic-pituitary-adrenocortical axis (HPA axis)** helps regulate the immune response during heavy exercise and other types of stress (figure 13.15).

Sympathetic Innervation and Immunomodulation

The autonomic nervous system (ANS) includes the parasympathetic nervous system (PNS) and the sympathetic nervous system (SNS), which regulate the organism's internal

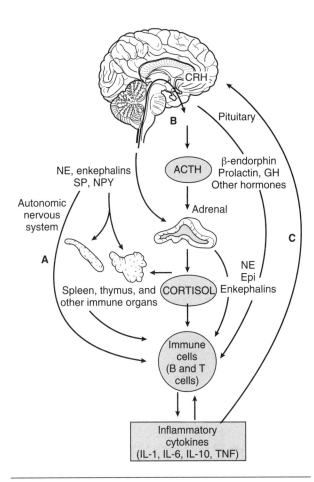

Figure 13.15 Schematic of the interaction between the autonomic nervous and hypothalamic-pituitary-adrenal cortical systems and the immune system.

Adapted, by permission, from S.F. Maier and L.R. Watkins, 1998, "Cytokines for psychologists: Implications of bi-directional immune-to-brain communication for understanding behavior, mood, and cognition," *Psychological Review* 105(1): 83-107.

environment. The SNS controls the flight-or-fight reaction to **stressors,** whereas the PNS governs rest and, along with the **enteric nervous system,** digestion. In a stressful situation, the SNS is activated by the **hypothalamus,** resulting in increased sympathetic nerve traffic to target organs such as the heart and immune tissues. Immune organs are stimulated by catecholamines (norepinephrine and epinephrine) released from the sympathetic nerve terminals and are modulated by the hormonal effects of these catecholamines after they are secreted into the blood from the adrenal medulla (Maier and Watkins 1998). Figure 13.16 illustrates the influence of catecholamines on leukocytosis, the migration of leukocytes from lymphoid organs into the blood.

Noradrenergic nerves to the spleen and noradrenergic nerve ends in the spleen have been found in rats. In humans, β-adrenergic receptors have been identified on lymphocytes, including NK cells. Infusion of epinephrine results in increased numbers of NK cells activated by lymphokines such

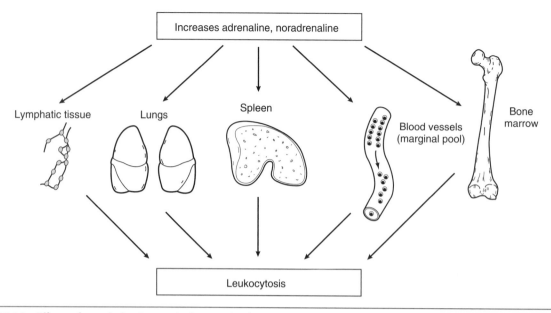

Figure 13.16 Effects of catecholamines on leukocyte circulation.

Adapted from *Brain, Behavior, and Immunity,* Vol. 10, R.J. Benschop, M. Rodriguez-Feuerhahn, and M. Schedlowski, "Catecholamine-induced leukocytosis: Early observation, current research, and future directions," pgs. 77-91, Copyright 1996, with permission from Elsevier.

as IL-2 (Kappel et al. 1998) and an immediate but short-lived increase in the **cytolytic** (i.e., cell killing) activity of NK cells (Tonnesen, Christensen, and Brinklov 1987). It is now known that epinephrine increases the number of lymphocytes, especially NK cells, that leave the spleen or other lymphoid organs by activating β_2-adrenoreceptors. The influence of catecholamines on the trafficking of granulocytes from the spleen to the blood is regulated by α-adrenoreceptors (Ernstrom and Sandberg 1973). Prior to those findings, it was thought that epinephrine caused the spleen to contract, spilling its store of lymphocytes by mechanical action. This view was abandoned, though, when studies showed that epinephrine still induced lymphocytosis in animals after the spleen had been removed. In the 1990s it was found that emotional stress or an injection of norepinephrine increased blood levels of NK cells in people without a spleen as much as or more than in people with spleens. The most likely explanation for this observation is that catecholamines cause NK cells to leave the marginal pool, apparently by inhibiting adhesion molecules on NK cells.

The shearing force of increased blood flow can also contribute to the exit of leukocytes from the marginal pool. The additional circulating granulocytes induced by catecholamines come both from the marginal pool and from bone marrow. In contrast, the increased NK cells appear to come mainly from the marginal pool rather than bone marrow. Natural killer cells do not follow the same recirculation pathway between lymph and blood (i.e., via lymph nodes and the thoracic duct) as do other lymphocytes.

▷ **LEUKOCYTOSIS FROM** the marginal pool is mainly explained by inhibition of adhesion molecules by catecholamines and by shearing forces of increased blood flow during exercise.

Activation of the HPA Axis and Immunomodulation

Neuroendocrine responses to stressors include increased levels of **glucocorticoids,** such as **cortisol** and corticosterone, in circulating blood as a result of activation of the HPA axis. Synthesis and secretion of releasing factors such as **corticotropin-releasing hormone (CRH)** by the hypothalamus activate the pituitary gland to secrete hormones such as **adrenocorticotropic hormone (ACTH),** which in turn leads to the release of glucocorticoids from the **adrenal cortex.** Increased levels of circulating glucocorticoids regulate organs and cells of the immune system that possess receptors for these hormones (Maier and Watkins 1998). The effects of cortisol on immunity are inconsistent in humans, but many studies show that short-term increases in blood levels of cortisol contribute to the migration of granulocytes and lymphocytes from the blood circulation back to lymph organs as a stress response ends. However, long-term exposure of lymphocytes to cortisol, as during periods of repeated severe stress, can contribute to suppression of the immune system's ability to fight an infection.

▷ **SHORT-TERM INCREASES** in blood levels of cortisol help regulate the migration of granulocytes and lymphocytes from the blood circulation back to lymph organs after a stress response ends. Long-term exposure of lymphocytes to cortisol during repeated stress can suppress the immune system's ability to fight an infection.

Other Mechanisms

In addition to the SNS stimulation of immune tissues and increased level of adrenal hormones, opiates and **endogenous** opioid peptides appear to play a role in the regulation of immunity during stress. Opioid receptors have been found on large, granular lymphocytes, which include NK cells. Intermittent stress can activate the opioid system and suppress NK cell activity. That suppression is blunted by opioid antagonists.

Physical Activity and Immunity: The Evidence

After the German physiologist G. Schulz (1893) reported that muscle activity produced an increase in the number of leukocytes in the blood, severalfold increases in blood leukocytes were reported in four men after they ran the Boston Athletic Association's marathon of 1901 (Larrabee 1902) and in another group of men after a 400 m race (Garrey and Butler 1929). Lymphocytes increased in number within the first 10 min of exercise, and this was followed by an increase in neutrophils—the same pattern seen after an injection of epinephrine. Hence, it was hypothesized that an increase in epinephrine levels during exercise was responsible for leukocytosis during exercise (Martin 1932). Modern studies have generally confirmed those early observations of leukocytosis in response to exercise (Pedersen and Hoffman-Goetz 2000; Woods et al. 1999a; Woods, Lowder, and Keylock 2002).

Acute Exercise

Among normal, healthy people, the numbers of several types of immune cells, especially NK cells and neutrophils, are usually elevated during and immediately after a session of moderate- to high-intensity exercise (50-85% $\dot{V}O_2$max; Fiatarone et al. 1988; Lewicki et al. 1988; Moyna et al. 1996; Murray et al. 1992; Palmo et al. 1995; Rhind et al. 1999). Neutrophils remain elevated for several hours, and lymphocytes return to normal levels within 2 h (Lewicki et al. 1988) to 24 h after the exercise (Espersen et al. 1996). However, after heavy, prolonged exercise, numbers of lymphocytes and NK cells can be depressed below normal levels for up to 6 h (Espersen et al. 1996). One view is that this period of immunosuppression after heavy exercise provides a window of susceptibility to infection if exposure to a pathogen occurs while the number of cytotoxic cells is below normal (Hoffman-Goetz and Pedersen 1994).

▷ **A TEMPORARY SUPPRESSION** of the immune system after heavy exercise may provide a window of susceptibility to infection if exposure to a pathogen occurs while the number of cytotoxic cells is below normal.

Macrophages

Acute exercise increases the number of monocytes circulating in the blood. This increase in monocytes (as for other leukocytes) is best explained by an influx of cells from the marginal pool. Exceptions to this increase are the migration of monocytes from the blood during prolonged exercise of several hours and a likely increase in the region of an infection after exhaustive exercise. The latter exception makes sense, as a localized infection would logically have higher biological priority than would circulatory adjustments during exercise. Exercise also has stimulatory effects on phagocytosis, antitumor activity, reactive oxygen and nitrogen metabolism, and chemotaxis of macrophages; but most of the studies that investigated these effects used mice rather than humans as subjects (Woods et al. 1999b). Studies of mice also have shown that exercise training can increase macrophage antitumor activity, regardless of age. However, not all macrophage functions are enhanced by exercise. Reductions in the expression of MHC II by macrophages and in their antigen-presenting capacity have been reported. Hence, it has been suggested that exercise temporarily increases the phagocytic function of macrophages while inhibiting their accessory cell functions (Woods et al. 2000).

Lymphocytes

Many studies have suggested that the ability of T and B lymphocytes to proliferate (i.e., to grow and to reproduce by cloning) is increased when they are exposed to some mitogenic factors (factors that induce clonal expansion by lymphocytes, e.g., IL-2 and pokeweed) and inhibited when they are exposed to other mitogenic factors (e.g., phytohemagglutinin and concanavalin A). However, it appears that those changes mainly reflect the number of lymphocytes circulating in the blood during and immediately after exercise, not a real change in the growth and division of individual lymphocytes (Pedersen and Hoffman-Goetz 2000) (table 13.1). Entry of lymphocytes into the blood (i.e., lymphocytosis) during acute exercise seems to mainly depend on the release of catecholamines (i.e., norepinephrine from sympathetic nerves and epinephrine from the adrenal gland). Cytotoxic

Table 13.1 Effects of Strenuous Exercise on the Immune System

Measure	During exercise	After exercise
Neutrophil count	↑	↑↑
Monocyte count		↑
Lymphocyte count	↑	↓
CD4+ count	↑	↓
CD8+ count	↑	↓
CD19+ count	↑	↓
CD16+56+ count	↑	↓
Lymphocyte apoptosis	↑	↑
Proliferative response to mitogens	↓	↓
Antibody response in vitro	↓	↓
Saliva IgA	↓	↓
Delayed-type hypersensitivity response (skin test)		↓
NK cell activity	↑	↓
Lymphokine-activated killer cell activity	↑	↓
C-reactive protein		↑

↑, increase; ↓, decrease; ↑↑, marked increase

Reprinted from B.K. Pedersen and L. Hoffman-Goetz, 2000, "Exercise and the immune system: Regulation, integration, and adaptation," *Physiological Reviews* 80: 1055-1081. Used with permission.

T (CD8+) lymphocytes, especially effector-memory T cells (Simpson et al 2007), are more responsive to exercise than helper T (CD4+) or B lymphocytes, probably because they have more β_2-adrenoreceptors and adhesion molecules on their surface that respond to catecholamines and aid their removal from the marginal pool.

Within an hour or so of the end of an exercise session, lymphocyte numbers in the blood, especially NK cells, paradoxically fall below their preexercise levels (lymphocytopenia), possibly because of increased levels of cortisol from the adrenal cortex. Several hours later, but within 24 h, blood lymphocyte counts return to normal. A decrease in mitogen-stimulated T cell proliferation and T cell release of IL-2 and IFN-γ has been reported immediately after intense exercise (Gleeson and Bishop 2005).

Natural Killer Cells

A quantitative review of 27 published studies conducted on a total of 390 people indicated that the cumulative effect of acute exercise was an increase in NK cytotoxicity (i.e., the killing of tumor cells **in vivo** by NK cells) of 1.2 standard deviations (95% confidence interval [CI]: 0.37-2.1; Hong and Dishman 2004). Results changed distinctly over time, with a marked increase in cytotoxicity during and soon after exercise, a decrease below preexercise basal levels 1 to 3 h after exercise, and a return to the basal level within 24 h. Changes did not differ according to the mode or intensity

of the exercise but were larger for exercise that lasted between 20 min and 2 h than for exercise longer than 2 h (e.g., Espersen et al. 1996; Nielsen et al. 1998; Rhind et al. 1999). Changes were larger among people who were either sedentary or physically active in their leisure but had not undergone exercise training designed to increase their physical fitness. The changes in NK cytotoxicity after exercise are probably more the result of changes in the number of NK cells in the blood than of changes in the ability of individual NK cells to lyse tumor cells. For example, most studies have found that when cytolytic activity of NK cells in the blood is appropriately expressed relative to NK cell number, it is not changed by exercise (Moyna et al. 1996; Nieman et al. 1995b; Palmo et al. 1995), except when intense, unusual, and prolonged exercise can depress the cytolytic activity of NK cells for several hours (Gleeson and Bishop 2005).

Levels of prostaglandins (e.g., PGE2), β-endorphin, and catecholamines have been investigated as possible mechanisms or mediators of altered NK cell activity after acute exercise (Fiatarone et al. 1988; Moyna et al. 1996; Murray et al. 1992; Rhind et al. 1999), but there are too few studies using uniform methods to allow drawing conclusions. Some evidence indicates that the activity of neutrophils, including chemotaxis, phagocytosis, and the oxidative burst, is enhanced after moderate-intensity exercise, especially in the upper airways.

▷ **THE INCREASED** killing of tumor cells by NK cells after acute exercise is probably the result of an increased number of NK cells in the blood rather than an increase in the ability of individual NK cells to kill tumor cells.

Eccentric Muscle Contraction

Eccentric resistance exercise involving smaller muscle groups has been found both to increase (Palmo et al. 1995) and to decrease (Malm, Lenkei, and Sjodin 1999) NK cell numbers in the blood circulation during exercise. In addition, the number of NK cells increases after a heavy exercise bout (80% $\dot{V}O_2$max) but not after light exercise (40% $\dot{V}O_2$max) (Strasner et al. 1997). Other studies have shown that prolonged endurance exercise (e.g., 2-3 h) and shorter-term, heavy eccentric exercise can induce an inflammation-like response resulting in increased secretion of inflammatory cytokines (e.g., IL-1, IL-6, and TNF-α) by stimulating the liver's biosynthesis of acute-phase proteins. Also, neutrophils and macrophages migrate to the area of muscle damage to remove the debris of dead cells.

Natural Killer Cells After Exercise Training

Too few studies of the effects of chronic exercise on macrophages, neutrophils, and T- and B lymphocytes have been conducted to allow conclusions about the adaptations of these immune cells to repeated physical activity (Woods et al. 1999b). Results are somewhat clearer for NK cells, which are perhaps the most responsive immune cell to acute exercise in humans. A half-dozen exercise training studies and another handful of cross-sectional comparisons between exercise-trained and untrained people showed a cumulative mean increase in numbers of NK cells of 0.6 standard deviations (95% CI: 0.3-0.9) and 1.0 standard deviation (95% CI: 0.7-1.4), respectively (Hong and Dishman 2004).

Results of individual studies have not consistently shown significant changes in NK cell activity, however (Shephard and Shek 1999). No change in NK cell activity or in blood mononuclear cell numbers or proliferation was found in 18 rheumatoid arthritis patients after eight weeks of progressive cycle exercise training (Baslund et al. 1993). Neither 12 to 15 weeks of a walking exercise program (45 min at 60-75% maximal heart rate, five days per week; Nieman et al. 1990b) nor eight weeks of a combination of aerobic and resistance training (Scanga et al. 1998) influenced NK cell activity or circulating levels. Six months of aerobic exercise by elderly men and women did not significantly affect NK cell activity or leukocyte counts (Woods et al. 1999b). In contrast, a cross-sectional study by Rhind and colleagues (1994) showed that physically trained individuals (with $\dot{V}O_2$max of 57 ml · kg^{-1} · min^{-1}) had higher levels of circulating total leukocytes, granulocytes, and NK cells than previously untrained control individuals ($\dot{V}O_2$max of 39 ml · kg^{-1} · min^{-1}).

Compared with the evidence from human studies, evidence of the effect of exercise training on NK cell cytotoxicity in mice has been more consistent. An hour and a half of daily, moderate-intensity swimming for 20 days increased NK cell activity in mice (Ferrandez and De la Fuente 1996). Hoffman-Goetz, Arumugam, and Sweeny (1994) conducted a series of studies on NK cell activity and tumor metastasis following exercise training in mice. After nine weeks of wheel running and treadmill training exercise, male C3H mice were injected with tumor cells. After three weeks of tumor development and no exercise, the mice were killed. Trained mice demonstrated enhanced splenic NK cell activity and lower tumor cell retention in the lungs (MacNeil and Hoffman-Goetz 1993b). Treadmill training for 10 weeks enhanced NK cytotoxicity in mice measured **in vitro** (Simpson and Hoffman-Goetz 1990), and nine weeks of both voluntary wheel running and treadmill training resulted in increased cytotoxicity both in vivo and in vitro (MacNeil and Hoffman-Goetz 1993a). A dissociation between NK cytotoxicity and tumor metastasis was found in female mice that received an injection of tumor cells; mice with previously elevated LAK cell (NK cells activated by lymphokines) activity measured in vitro showed higher tumor multiplicity after eight weeks of voluntary wheel running (Hoffman-Goetz, Arumugam, and Sweeny 1994).

In contrast to findings from studies of mice, basal splenic NK cell activity in rats did not change after six weeks of voluntary wheel running (Dishman et al. 1995), six weeks of treadmill running (Dishman et al. 2000b), or 15 weeks of treadmill running (Nasrullah and Mazzeo 1992). Conversely, reduced immune functions including NK cell activity in obese Zucker rats were restored after treadmill exercise five days per week for 40 weeks (Moriguchi et al. 1998).

The balance of the evidence in humans and in rodents is that chronic physical activity does not alter basal NK activity, despite a temporary enhancement of NK cytotoxicity right after an exercise session. However, other studies in rats indicate that chronic physical activity, independently of any fitness changes, protects against the suppression of NK cell activity after stress (Dishman et al. 1995; Dishman et al. 2000a, 2000b).

> ▶ **DESPITE STRONG** evidence that acute exercise temporarily increases the number of NK cells in the blood, the effects of exercise training on basal NK activity have been inconsistent in studies of both humans and rodents.

Investigators have not always clearly described the use of force in studies of swimming and treadmill running and have used various strains of rats and mice that differ in their inherent running behavior. Hence, it remains important to determine the effects of chronic exercise independently of the co-occurring stress of forced, rather than voluntary, exercise. Although exercise training has been found to augment NK cell activity in rats and mice, it has not been shown whether exercise training enhances peripheral blood NK cytotoxicity in humans. The insignificant effect of exercise training on resting NK cell activity observed in human studies raises questions regarding the nature of the exercise program (its intensity, duration, etc.) as it might affect different adaptations in NK cell activity. Also, there are at least two distinct subsets of human NK cells based on the expression intensity of CD56: CD56(bright) and CD56(dim) cells. During exercise, CD56(dim) cells are more responsive, but up to 1 h of recovery after exercise, CD56(bright) cells are more responsive, which may have implications for the use of exercise as an adjuvant in the treatment of inflammatory diseases such as MS (Timmons and Cieslak 2008).

Table 13.2 summarizes the effects of acute and chronic exercise training on the immune system.

Table 13.2　Effects of Exercise on the Immune System

Type of exercise	Increases	Decreases
Acute	• Blood levels of granulocytes (mainly neutrophils) • Blood levels of monocytes • Phagocytic activity of macrophages • Blood levels of NK cells	• Blood levels of T lymphocytes • NK cell cytotoxicity (strenuous exercise)
Chronic	• NK cell cytotoxicity? • Risk of upper respiratory infection (strenuous exercise)	• Risk of upper respiratory infection (moderate exercise) • Tumor growth

Data from Pedersen and Hoffman-Goetz 2000

Physical Activity, Exercise, and Low-Grade Systemic Inflammation

Production of C-reactive protein in the liver is part of an acute-phase response to infection that is stimulated by cytokines such as IL-6, IL-1, and TNF-α. All those inflammatory markers can be elevated in people who are obese or have any of several other chronic health conditions, such as diabetes, cystic fibrosis, chronic obstructive pulmonary disease, MS, cancer (including cancer cachexia—i.e., wasting syndrome), and immunosenescence associated with old age. Increased physical activity could plausibly counter low-grade systemic inflammation by secreting anti-inflammatory cytokines during muscle contraction (Pedersen 2006; Lira et al. 2009; Senchina and Kohut 2007). Or, physical activity can contribute to fat loss and thus reduce inflammation indirectly by reducing inflammatory adipokines and macrophages that reside in adipose tissue (Woods, Vieira, and Keylock 2009).

An early review of published studies of exercise and C-reactive protein concluded that strenuous exercise (e.g., marathons and road races, triathlon) induced a transitory, acute-phase inflammatory response but that exercise training seemed to result in a persistent anti-inflammatory adaptation. With just a handful of exceptions, nearly 20 cross-sectional studies showed that endurance athletes or physically active men and women of varying ages had lower levels of C-reactive protein measured at rest compared to less active or sedentary people. Also, two of three small exercise trials reported a reduction in C-reactive protein after endurance exercise training (Kasapis and Thompson 2005). Although a number of exercise studies adjusted for body mass index (BMI), most studies have not demonstrated that the association between physical activity and inflammatory markers is independent of fatness, which is a risk factor for low-grade inflammation (Wärnberg et al. 2010). Additionally, most of the investigations showing physical activity to be associated with lower levels of inflammation are cross-sectional studies.

Thus, it is unclear whether physical activity leads to decreased inflammation, or whether a reduced state of inflammation serves as a marker for healthier persons who may be more able and likely to be physically active. Subsequent evaluations of randomized controlled trials concluded that exercise training sufficient to increase fitness in people who are overweight or obese does not reliably lower C-reactive protein unless there is substantial weight loss (Kelley and Kelley 2006; Stewart et al. 2010).

The INFLAME Study

This was randomized controlled trial of the effects of four months of supervised aerobic exercise training (16 kcal/kg body weight per week) at a vigorous intensity on elevated C-reactive protein concentrations (≥ 2.0 mg/L; median = 4.0 mg/L) in 162 initially sedentary, obese women and men who were mostly between ages 40 and 60 years (Thompson et al. 2008). There was no effect of exercise on C-reactive protein levels regardless of gender or baseline body weight. However, change in weight was associated with change in C-reactive protein. Only women who lost an average of about 6.5 lb (2.9 kg) or more ($\geq 3\%$) had a significant reduction in C-reactive protein (about 1 mg/L) (Church et al. 2010).

The Dose Response to Exercise in Women (DREW) Study

More than 400 sedentary, overweight or obese postmenopausal women were randomized into one of four groups: a nonexercise control or one of three aerobic exercise groups. The exercise groups expended an exercise energy of 4, 8, or 12 kcal · kg^{-1} · week^{-1} for six months at a training intensity of 50% of peak $\dot{V}O_2$ (Stewart et al. 2010). Median levels of C-reactive protein ranged from 3.4 to 4.9. There was no effect of exercise on blood levels of C-reactive protein or on IL-6 and TNF-α or adiponectin (Arsenault et al. 2009) regardless of energy expenditure. Even though increases in peak $\dot{V}O_2$ were dose related, the decreases in waist circumference were similar in all the exercise groups. Only women who lost about 5.75 lb (2.6 kg) or more ($\geq 3\%$) had a reduction in C-reactive protein (about 1 mg/L), regardless of control or exercise group.

Seattle, Washington

A similar 12-month randomized controlled trial of exercise in sedentary, overweight men and women, only some of whom had elevated initial levels, also found no effect on C-reactive protein levels despite a 2% reduction in body fat (Campbell et al. 2008). However, in a subsequent analysis of results from postmenopausal women who were obese, abdominally obese, or both, exercise reduced C-reactive protein by more than 10%, even though weight loss was modest and IL-6 was not affected by the exercise (Campbell et al. 2009).

▷ **REDUCING BODY** fatness seems to be the key to reducing elevated C-reactive protein with an exercise program in people who are obese and who have elevated levels.

The Lifestyle Interventions and Independence for Elders (LIFE) Trial

This was a long-term intervention that examined the effect of exercise on biomarkers of inflammation (C-reactive protein and IL-6) in 424 elderly (aged 70-89), nondisabled, community-dwelling men and women at risk for physical disability. Participants were randomly assigned to a 12-month moderate-intensity physical activity (PA) intervention or a successful aging (SA) health education intervention at sites in Dallas, Texas; Stanford, California; Pittsburgh, Pennsylvania; and Winston-Salem, North Carolina (Nicklas et al. 2008). After adjustment for baseline IL-6, sex, clinic site, and diabetes, the exercise group had 8.5% lower IL-6 levels than the heath education group, but exercise did not affect C-reactive protein. An ancillary analysis of 368 participants showed no effects of exercise on blood levels of adiponectin, TNF-α, or IL-15, or on receptors for IL-1, IL-1 inhibitor, IL-2, IL-6, and TNF. IL-8 levels were 10% lower after exercise training, but that could have been a chance finding (Beavers et al. 2010). Overall, there was no evidence of an anti-inflammatory effect of exercise training.

Youths

The few studies of physical activity and inflammatory markers in adolescents have yielded results similar to those found in adults (Rubin and Hackney 2010). Several cross-sectional comparisons of physically active boys and girls and a few exercise training studies lasting two to three months showed 25% to 35% higher levels of adiponectin, 25% to 50% lower levels of IL-6, 30% reductions in C-reactive protein, and lower or unchanged TNF-α than in less active or sedentary boys and girls. However, body fatness was not well controlled in most of those studies, and randomized controlled trials with obese youths suggest that the effects of exercise on adipokines and inflammatory cytokines in obese youths, as in adults, depend on weight loss (Balagopal et al. 2005; Kelly et al. 2007).

Patients With Inflammatory Disease

A review of 19 studies examined whether acute exercise (seven studies in children and eight in adults) and chronic exercise training (five studies in adults) elicit an abnormal inflammatory response in patients with an inflammatory disease (e.g., MS, chronic fatigue, McArdle disease, chronic obstructive pulmonary disease [COPD], congestive heart failure, type 2 diabetes, and rheumatoid arthritis) (Ploeger et al. 2009). The authors concluded that single sessions of exercise might elicit an aggravated inflammatory response in patients with type 1 diabetes mellitus, cystic fibrosis, or COPD. Levels of IL-6, T lymphocytes, and total leukocytes remained elevated longer into the recovery period following an acute bout of exercise in patients compared with healthy controls. In contrast, chronic endurance exercise training programs typically reduced or did not change those markers in patients with chronic heart failure and type 2 diabetes mellitus.

People With Multiple Sclerosis

In a pilot study, 11 MS patients and 11 control participants (eight women and three men in each group), matched in age, height, body mass, body fat, and peak $\dot{V}O_2$, completed 30 min of cycling exercise at 60% of peak O_2 uptake three days a week for eight weeks (Castellano, Patel, and White 2008). Plasma cytokine concentrations were determined before and after exercise at the beginning of the study and after four and eight weeks. The response of plasma IL-6, TNF-α, and IFN-γ after a single session of exercise was similar in MS and control participants. After exercise training, resting levels of IL-6 tended to decrease in both groups, whereas levels of plasma TNF-α and IFN-γ were elevated in MS patients but unchanged in control participants.

Men With Congestive Heart Failure

Twenty middle-aged male patients with stable congestive heart failure were randomized to a control group or to aerobic training that increased peak $\dot{V}O_2$ by 29% after six months. Blood levels of TNF-α, IL-6, and IL-1β were not affected by exercise, but reductions of 38% to 48% in skeletal muscle were accompanied by reductions in their gene expression The authors proposed that the local anti-inflammatory effects of exercise might mitigate the catabolic wasting process associated with the progression of congestive heart failure (Gielen et al. 2003).

People With HIV/AIDS

Several groups have examined whether men diagnosed as positive for HIV-1 respond favorably to chronic exercise. Though long-term morbidity and mortality studies with large numbers of men have not been conducted, small clinical studies generally have found that the prudent use of aerobic and resistance exercise training within professionally accepted guidelines for healthy adults (e.g., Pollock et al. 1998) leads to increased cardiorespiratory and muscular fitness without adverse effects on the numbers of blood lymphocytes or health (LaPerriere et al. 1990; Rigsby et al. 1992). The first randomized controlled trial of exercise to measure T lymphocytes in men seropositive for the HIV-1 virus and also diagnosed with AIDS-related complex showed that 13 men assigned to 20 min of cycling exercise and 35 min of strength and flexibility training three days a week for 12 weeks had increased aerobic fitness, strength, and body weight and decreased skinfold thickness, but no improvement in clinical health status, when compared to 11 men assigned to a counseling control group that met 1 to 2 h twice each week (Rigsby et al. 1992). There were no extra adverse outcomes of exercise, and there was a small increase of CD4+ (helper T lymphocytes) cells from about 335 cells to 395 cells/ mm³. That increase was about 1/3 SD when compared to the number in the counseling group, which did not change from 310 cells. If the sample size had been doubled, the effect would have reached statistical significance. In AIDS patients with CD+ cell counts below 200, a change of 50 cells is commonly viewed as clinically important. The study included only three men diagnosed with AIDS, but most of the men had immunosuppression. Their range in cell counts was from 9 to 804 cells/mm³. Normal ranges are from about 400 to 1500.

One meta-analysis summarized 10 randomized controlled trials, including 87 female and 245 male HIV-1 adults 18 to 66 years of age with CD4+ cell counts less than 100 to more than 1000 cells/mm³, that compared resistance exercise training or resistance exercise plus aerobic exercise training at least three times a week for at least four weeks with no exercise or another intervention (O'Brien et al. 2008). There were nonsignificant changes in CD4+ count (weighted mean difference: 39 cells/mm³; 95% CI: −8 to 85; 106 people) and viral load (weighted mean difference: 0.31 log$_{10}$ copies; 95% CI: −0.13 to 0.74; 63 people), increases in body weight for resistance exercise alone (4.2 kg; 95% CI: 1.8-6.7; 46 people) or resistance plus aerobic exercise (2.7 kg; 95% CI: 1.8-6.7; 106 people), and increased arm and thigh girth (7.9 cm; 95% CI: 2.2-13.7%; 46 people). Nine of the 10 studies reported increases in strength.

A companion meta-analysis included 14 randomized trials of 454 HIV-positive adults 18 to 58 years of age (70% males) at varying stages of HIV-1 infection and AIDS progression, with CD4+ cell counts ranging from less 100 to more than 1000 cells/mm³, who performed aerobic exercise or aerobic exercise plus resistance exercise for at least 20 min at least three times per week for at least five weeks (O'Brien et al. 2010). Aerobic exercise was associated with small nonsignificant changes in CD4+ count (weighted mean difference: 18 cells/mm³; 95% CI: −12 to 48; 306 people), viral load (weighted mean difference: 0.40 log$_{10}$copies; 95% CI: −0.28 to 1.07; 63 people), and V̇O$_2$max (weighted mean difference: 2.6 ml · kg^{-1} · min^{-1}; 95% CI: 1.2-4.1; 276 people). The studies showed no change in body weight or BMI but a decrease in estimated body fatness (−1.1%, 95% CI: −0.07% to −2.2%; 119 people).

Another meta-analysis of nine RCTs of 469 people living with HIV (41% females) concluded that aerobic exercise

HIV/AIDS-Related Metabolic Syndrome

A common side effect of highly active antiretroviral therapy (HAART) is lipodystrophy syndrome, which features HIV/AIDS-related metabolic syndrome. Main characteristics are a reduction of subcutaneous fat (lipoatrophy) in the face and limbs, especially with reverse transcriptase inhibiting drugs, and an increase (lipohypertrophy) in abdominal, intra-abdominal, and dorsocervical fat that is accompanied by dyslipidemia and insulin resistance, especially in HAART with protease inhibitors (Anuurad, Bremer, and Berglund 2010). The pathogenesis of HAART-associated metabolic syndrome and atherogenesis involves direct effects of the drugs on lipid metabolism, endothelial and adipocyte cell function (e.g., leptin deficiency and hypoadiponectinemia), activation of pro-inflammatory cytokines, and mitochondrial dysfunction (Barbaro and Iacobellis 2009; Tsiodras et al. 2010; Villarroya, Domingo, and Giralt 2010).

Among 30 otherwise healthy people treated for HIV-1 with protease inhibitors, non-nucleoside reverse transcriptase inhibitors, or both, 12 weeks of aerobic exercise plus a recommended low-fat diet increased V̇O$_2$peak by 25% more than the diet plus weekly stretching and relaxation (Terry et al. 2006). However, reductions in body weight, body fat, and waist-to-hip ratio were similar in the two groups, and neither condition altered immune variables or blood levels of triglycerides, total cholesterol, or high-density lipoprotein (HDL) cholesterol levels.

In another study, 20 sedentary HIV-infected men with lipodystrophy were randomly assigned to supervised strength or endurance training three times a week for 16 weeks (Lindegaard et al. 2008). Insulin-dependent glucose uptake increased by about 15% in each group. Only strength training increased total fat-free mass (about 2 kg) and decreased total fat mass (about 3 kg), trunk fat (2.5 kg), and limb fat (0.75 kg). Endurance training reduced total cholesterol, low-density lipoprotein (LDL) cholesterol, free fatty acids, C-reactive protein, IL-6, IL-18, and TNF-α and increased HDL cholesterol. Strength training decreased triglycerides, free fatty acids, and IL-18 and increased HDL cholesterol.

compared to control decreased BMI (-1.3 kg/m^2; 95% CI: -2.59 to -0.03; $n = 186$), triceps skinfold thickness of subcutaneous fat (-1.83 mm; 95% CI: -2.36 to -1.30; $n = 144$), total body fat (%) (-0.37; 95% CI: -0.74 to -0.01; $n = 118$), and waist circumference (-0.74 mm, 95% CI: -1.08 to -0.39; $n = 142$). Progressive resistive exercise increased body weight (5.09 kg; 95% CI: 2.13-8.05; $n = 46$) and arm and thigh girth (1.08 cm; 95% CI: 0.35-1.82; $n = 46$) (Fillipas et al. 2010).

These reviews confirmed that exercise training positively affects fitness and body composition of people with HIV/AIDS without further compromising their immune system. However, long-term health outcomes of exercise still have not been determined.

The introduction of antiretroviral drugs and HAART has resulted in a significant reduction in AIDS-related mortality and improved survival rates but a disproportionate increase in deaths from chronic diseases not directly attributable to AIDS. In 13 HIV cohort studies in Europe and North America, 792 deaths were AIDS related (49.5% of all deaths attributable to a specific cause), but substantial proportions were attributable to non-AIDS cancers (189; 11.8%), non-AIDS infections (131; 8.2%), liver disease (113; 7.0%), and cardiovascular disease (103; 6.5%) (Gill et al. 2010). The proportion of deaths classified as AIDS related decreased with increasing duration of antiretroviral therapy. As HAART becomes more accessible in sub-Saharan Africa, metabolic syndromes, body fat redistribution (BFR), and cardiovascular disease may eventually become more prevalent. A six-month randomized controlled trial of aerobic exercise training that increased cardiorespiratory fitness among HAART-treated HIV(+) Africans living in Rwanda also reduced waist circumference (-7.13 cm), sum skinfold thickness (-6.15 mm), and percent body fat mass (-1.5 kg) (Mutimura et al. 2008).

Cancer Survivors

There have been at least a dozen studies on whether regular exercise can positively influence the immune system of cancer survivors. A comprehensive review of those published between 1994 and 2000 reported that four of the six studies showed statistically significant improvements in a number of cancer-related immune system components associated with exercise (Fairey et al. 2002). A meta-analysis of seven controlled trials of exercise training in cancer survivors found a small, nonsignificant overall effect (-0.73; CI: -1.93 to 0.47), but there were too few effects for each outcome (e.g., neutrophil counts, NK cell cytolytic activity, and C-reactive protein) to allow estimation of specific effects of exercise training (Speck et al. 2010).

Another review of 10 randomized controlled trials and four nonrandomized controlled clinical trials, mostly combining progressive resistance exercise and aerobic training, concluded that there were no favorable or adverse effects of training on body composition or endocrine and immune function, despite overall training effects of 39% to 65% for aerobic fitness and 11% to 110% for strength (De Backer et al. 2009). Methodological problems of small samples, weak research designs that incompletely controlled for confounders, poorly standardized prescriptions of the exercise dose, or limited measures of physical fitness and immune responses were noted by the authors of the review as limitations that prevent a clear interpretation of the results. Nonetheless, the preliminary findings are sufficiently encouraging to show the need for controlled clinical trials to determine whether exercise can independently reduce the risk of cancer recurrence and secondary malignancies and increase survival times among cancer survivors.

Breast Cancer

An investigation by Nieman and colleagues (1995) showed no effects of eight weeks of aerobic and resistance exercise for an hour three days each week on blood levels of neutrophils, T lymphocytes and NK cells, or NK cytolytic activity in six female breast cancer survivors compared to six controls (Nieman et al. 1995a). Fifty-three postmenopausal breast cancer survivors were randomly assigned to an exercise ($n = 25$) or control group ($n = 28$). The exercise group trained on cycle ergometers three times per week for 15 weeks. Exercise training increased NK cell cytolytic activity and unstimulated [3H]thymidine uptake by peripheral blood lymphocytes, but had no effects on whole blood neutrophil function or the production of pro-inflammatory (IL-1α, TNF-α, IL-6) or anti-inflammatory (IL-4, IL-10, TNF-1β) cytokines (Fairey et al. 2005b). However, the exercise group had a reduction in C-reactive protein levels (Fairey et al. 2005a).

Breast cancer patients ($n = 28$) who had undergone chemotherapy and then participated three days a week in a six-month program of moderate-intensity aerobic and resistance exercise had similar blood levels of NK cells, T and B lymphocytes, IL-6, and IFN-γ, but a greater percentage of CD4$^+$ T cells that were activated by mitogen stimulation, than patients ($n = 21$) who did not exercise (Hutnick et al. 2005). Another study showed no effects of six months of aerobic and resistance exercise on C-reactive protein, interleukin-1β, and tumor necrosis factor receptor in 30 premenopausal patients with breast cancer on adjuvant chemotherapy (Demark-Wahnefried et al. 2008).

Colorectal Cancer

In 13 patients with curatively treated colorectal cancer, two weeks of moderate-intensity exercise 30 to 40 min daily had no effect on blood levels of IL-1, IL-6, TNF, and anti-inflammatory cytokines (IL-1ra, TNF receptors I and II) (Allgayer, Nicolaus, and Schreiber 2004). However, The LPS-stimulated IL-1ra response to lipopolysaccharides (LPS) was decreased. Lipopolysaccharides are cell wall constituents of Gram-negative bacteria that bind to LPS-binding proteins (LBP) in plasma to activate macrophages.

Stomach Cancer

Stomach cancer patients who had undergone surgery were randomly divided into an exercise group ($n = 17$) and a control group ($n = 18$) (Na et al. 2000). After two weeks of moderate-intensity arm and leg cycling twice a day, five days a week, NK cytolytic activity was increased in the exercise group compared to the control group.

Prostate Cancer

Effects of 20 weeks of twice per week high-intensity upper and lower body resistance training on blood levels of hormones and inflammatory markers at rest, and following acute bouts of exercise, were examined in 10 prostate cancer patients undergoing androgen deprivation by luteinizing hormone–releasing hormone agonist (LHRHa), or antiandrogen medications that block the androgen receptors, or both (Galvão et al. 2008). Androgen deprivation therapy can have several adverse effects, including reduced muscle strength, reduced lean and bone mass, increased fat mass and fracture risk, and low-grade systemic inflammation. Neither testosterone nor prostate-specific antigen changed at rest or following an acute bout of exercise. Acute resistance exercise combining concentric and eccentric contractions led to normal increases in total leukocytes, neutrophils, monocytes, lymphocytes, IL-6, and TNF-α. Resting level of IL-8 increased during the study, but levels of IL-6, IL-1ra, TNF-α, and C-reactive protein did not change during the 20 weeks of training.

Stem Cell Transplants

In a randomized study, 33 cancer patients receiving high-dose chemotherapy followed by autologous peripheral blood stem cell transplantation performed an exercise program consisting of biking on an ergometer in the supine position after an interval training pattern for 30 min daily during hospitalization. Durations of neutropenia (low neutrophil counts) and thrombopenia (low platelet counts) were reduced in the training group (Dimeo et al. 1997).

After peripheral blood stem cell transplant, six cancer patients with immunosuppression underwent three months of aerobic (three days a week) and resistance exercise training (two days a week) at moderate intensities. Exercise had no effect on white blood cell counts or CD4+ and CD8+ T lymphocyte counts or their proliferative response to mitogen stimulation when compared to results for six patients who did not exercise (Hays et al. 2003).

Overtraining and Immune Suppression in Athletes

A few population-based surveys suggested that heavy, prolonged exercise can have a negative impact on immunity. Among 2300 runners in the 1987 Los Angeles Marathon, the incidence of self-reported infection during the week after the

race was six times higher (13%) than among similar runners who did not run the marathon (Nieman et al. 1990a). In a cohort of over 500 runners, those who trained more than 17 miles (27 km) a week for a year had twice the rate of URI of those who ran less than 10 miles (16 km) a week (Heath et al. 1991). Some small clinical studies have reported decreased levels of neutrophils and increased rates of URI among endurance athletes undergoing heavy training, but, to date, no clear association between those two responses has been shown (Davis and Colbert 1997).

In cross-country skiing, the chronic stress of strenuous training may combine with the drying effect of breathing cold, dry air to both suppress immunoglobulin responses in the airways and reduce the mucus barrier against bacteria and viruses. Also, some studies suggest that temporary immune suppression or an "open window" for infection between 3 to 72 h after heavy, prolonged exertion (e.g., a marathon race) may lower resistance to URI (Nieman and Pedersen 1999), especially when people are exposed to novel pathogens during travel or they lose sleep, experience mental stress, consume a poor diet, or lose a lot of weight (Nieman 2003). Figure 13.17 shows that survival rates in mice infected with influenza virus were improved by 20 to 30 min of moderate exercise but were dramatically worsened by 2.5 h of prolonged exercise. A common clinical recommendation by physicians is to avoid exercise when the symptoms of an infection extend below the neck, as is the case during a bout of flu or high fever. When symptoms are localized about the neck, exercise does not appear to worsen symptoms.

Nonetheless, there are unanswered questions about exercise training and mucosal immunity, including whether

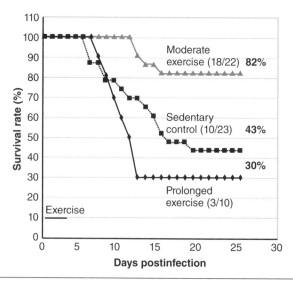

Figure 13.17 Survival rates in exercising mice after influenza infection. The mice began exercising four days after infection. A total of 55 mice were divided into three groups for the experiment.

Reprinted from Brain Behavior & Immunity, Vol. 19 (2), T. Lowder, D.A. Padgett, and J.A. Woods, "Moderate exercise protects mice from death due to influenza virus," pgs. 377-380, copyright 2005, with permission of Elsevier.

athletes are really more prone to illness; whether illness affects athletic performance; what are characteristics of people or features of the training exposure that modify the mucosal immune responses to exercise; what are the mechanisms by which exercise influences the acute mucosal immune response; and whether moderate exercise directly affects mucosal immune status (Gleeson, Pyne, and Callister 2004). In overtrained athletes, heavy exercise can elevate cortisol and anti-inflammatory cytokines (e.g. IL-6, IL-10, IL-Ira), causing temporary inhibition of type 1 T cell cytokine production with a relative dampening of the type 1 (cell mediated) response (Gleeson and Bishop 2005).

Mechanisms of Alterations in Monocytes, Granulocytes, and Natural Killer Cells After Acute Exercise

Acute exercise induces leukocytosis, but the mechanisms have yet to be clearly elucidated. The major catalysts of leukocytosis during infection are colony-stimulating factors. If exercise induces an acute-phase-like response, as several researchers believe, it is plausible that increases in circulating granulocytes and monocytes in response to exercise are mainly the result of increases in colony-stimulating factors, independently of epinephrine. A recent study found that increases in blood levels of IL-6 and G-CSF after a maximal treadmill exercise test were each correlated with the increase in circulating neutrophils measured 1 to 2 h after the exercise ended (Yamada et al. 2002). Another study of vigorous, prolonged exercise (running at 75% of $\dot{V}O_2$max for 2.5 h) showed a nearly 30-fold increase in circulating IL-6 and a threefold increase in circulating neutrophils (Steensberg et al. 2001). Epinephrine infusion resulted in just a sixfold increase in IL-6 and no increase in neutrophils. In contrast, exercise and epinephrine infusion increased the numbers of circulating lymphocytes to a similar level (Steensberg et al. 2001).

Likewise, the mechanisms underlying the marked increase in NK cell percentage after exercise are not fully known. The role of the spleen in leukocyte redistribution during or after acute exercise was investigated in individuals who had undergone splenectomy (Baum, Geitner, and Liesen 1996). Marked leukocytosis occurred after exhaustive cycling exercise but did not differ between splenectomized and control individuals. Markedly increased blood pressure and cardiac output during acute exercise might contribute to leukocytosis by freeing cells that are loosely attached to the vessel walls. It has been hypothesized that acute exercise results in a shedding of adhesion molecules on lymphocytes, resulting in lymphocytes' detaching from the vascular endothelium and surging into the circulation.

Increased levels of neutrophils and lymphocytes have been observed after intense resistance exercise (six sets of

10RM [repetition maximum] leg squats) in women, but the percentages of T, B, and NK cells that expressed the adhesion molecule L-selectin decreased in peripheral blood (Miles et al. 1998). That finding suggests a shedding of L-selectin. Adrenergic mechanisms have been hypothesized to influence shedding of adhesion molecules on lymphocytes, including NK cells, which affects lymphocytes' migration and homing to circulation and lymphoid tissues (Benschop, Rodriguez-Feuerhahn, and Schedlowski 1996; Benschop et al. 1997b; Carlson, Fox, and Abell 1997). Treadmill running to exhaustion led to increased levels of circulating adhesion factors, which were diminished by administration of a β-adrenoreceptor-blocking drug treatment (Rehman et al. 1997).

Whether these results indicate an exercise-induced decrease in the capacity of NK cells to adhere to adjacent tissues and cells or whether they indicate altered NK cell cytotoxicity during or after acute exercise is not established. However, it is possible that the molecular signaling that results in shedding of the adhesion molecules during exercise might also affect adhesion of NK cells to target cells, which could influence NK cell cytotoxicity.

Exercise and Cytokines

Only a few of the more than 60 known cytokines are likely to be influenced by exercise (Pedersen et al. 2001). Table 13.3 shows the effects of acute exercise on specific cytokines, such as IL-1, IL-2, IL-6, IL-7, interferons, and TNF, as determined by experimental studies (Moldoveanu, Shephard, and Shek 2001). Those known as inflammatory cytokines (e.g., IL-1, IL-6, IL-8, IL-10, and TNF) are part of the acute-phase response to infection or injury. Some researchers believe that acute exercise produces an acute-phase-like response. It is also likely that very heavy exercise, especially novel eccentric exercise that damages muscle cells, evokes an inflammation-like response to clean up the debris of dead muscle cells.

Table 13.3 Plasma Levels of Lymphokines During and After Vigorous Exercise

Lymphokines	During exercise	After exercise
Interleukin-1	↑	↑
Interleukin-6	↑↑	↑
Interleukin-8	↑	↑
Interleukin-10	↑	↑
Tumor necrosis factor-α	↑	↑
Tumor necrosis factor receptors	↑	↑
Interferon	↔	↔

↑, increase; ↑↑, marked increase; ↔, no change.

Data from Pedersen and Hoffman-Goetz 2000.

Interleukin-1 (IL-1)

Blood levels of IL-1 are unchanged from resting levels immediately after exercise but are elevated 2 to 3 h after exercise (Cannon et al. 1986; Evans et al. 1986; Haahr et al. 1991; Lewicki et al. 1988). Most studies did not use a control group that did not exercise, however, so some of the increases in IL-1 after exercise might be explainable by natural circadian variations in IL-1 levels during the day (e.g., Smith et al. 1992). Other possible explanations include a delay in the synthesis of new cytokines that requires some time after exercise ends or altered migration of cytokines between lymph tissues and the blood.

IL-1 levels in muscles are elevated immediately after heavy eccentric resistance exercise of the type that damages muscle cells (Fielding et al. 1993). Levels remained elevated five days postexercise, in spite of decreasing muscle damage. This is consistent with the concept that IL-1 contributes to prolonged metabolic alterations following eccentric exercise.

Interleukin-2 (IL-2)

IL-2 levels in blood are lowered during exercise (Espersen et al. 1990; Lewicki et al. 1988; Tvede et al. 1993) and 2 h after exercise (Lewicki et al. 1988; Tvede et al. 1993). That decrease in IL-2 is followed by a compensatory increase in the numbers of IL-2 receptors observed after exercise (Espersen et al. 1990; Sprenger et al. 1992). The changes in IL-2 numbers after exercise probably reflect the initial exit and subsequent return to the blood circulation of T lymphocytes, which produce IL-2. An increase in IL-2 levels has been found 24 h after strenuous exercise sufficient to cause muscle damage and inflammation (Espersen et al. 1990).

Interleukin-6 (IL-6)

Contracting skeletal muscle synthesizes and releases IL-6 into extracellular fluids, especially during eccentric contractions, and accounts for most of the increased IL-6 in the blood during and soon after acute exercise. The response is dose dependent regardless of mode (e.g., during leg extensions and curls, cycling, running, and rowing) (Fischer 2006).

Blood levels of IL-6 are increased by as much as 100 times basal levels after acute exercise, depending upon the intensity, duration, and type of exercise (Febbraio and Pedersen 2002). The timing of peak levels of IL-6 in the blood also depends on the type of muscle contraction. IL-6 levels increased during a graded cycling or treadmill test to exhaustion and remained elevated between about 20 min and 1 h after the tests ended (Rivier et al. 1994; Yamada et al. 2002). A 20 km run lasting about 2 h resulted in increased levels of IL-6 in both blood and urine during, 1 h after, and 5 h after the run (Sprenger et al. 1992).

Treadmill running at 75% of $\dot{V}O_2$max for 2.5 h led to a 29-fold increase in blood levels of IL-6 during exercise (Steensberg et al. 2001). Though the main sources of IL-6 are activated monocytes, macrophages, fibroblasts, and vascular endothelial cells, increased levels of IL-6 in the blood after exercise appear to come from contracting skeletal muscle. Because IL-6 has effects in the liver, adipose tissue, and the HPA axis, it is plausible that increases in IL-6 with exercise promote muscle energy metabolism (e.g., glycogenolysis and lipolysis) and enhance insulin sensitivity by inhibiting TNF-α (which has an insulin resistance effect). Because IL-6 affects leukocytes (e.g., monocytes and macrophages), it also is likely that IL-6 is indicative of an inflammatory response to muscle damage, depending upon the nature of the muscle contraction. IL-6 increases resulting from muscle damage are smaller and occur later than increases resulting directly from muscle contraction (Febbraio and Pedersen 2002); they seem to be independent of epinephrine and lactate responses to exercise but are blocked by indomethacin, a nonsteroidal anti-inflammatory drug (Rhind et al. 2002). Increases in IL-6 after prolonged, intense exercise are followed by smaller increases in the anti-inflammatory cytokine IL-10 (Febbraio and Pedersen 2002), suggesting a compensatory, homeostatic response.

Changes in calcium use, impaired glucose availability, and increased formation of reactive oxygen species (ROS) are all capable of activating transcription factors that regulate IL-6 synthesis. However, marked increases in blood levels of IL-6 require prolonged exercise involving a significant amount of contracting muscle. A common adaptation to chronic exercise training is a reduction in basal IL-6 production and the IL-6 response to acute exercise, possibly by blunting the factors that stimulate IL-6 release from muscle during exercise (Fischer 2006).

Studies using rodents have found that a single session of exercise results in activation of stress response genes in the liver (including those activated by IL-6 cell signaling) that are threefold higher than seen in contracting skeletal muscle (Hoene and Weigert 2010). This is plausible because nonexhaustive exercise energy depletion occurs more in the liver than in skeletal muscle and because the liver is exposed to altered concentrations of insulin and glucagon in the portal vein.

Tumor Necrosis Factor-Alpha

Studies generally agree that plasma TNF-α levels are unchanged during exercise (Espersen et al. 1990; Haahr et al. 1991; Rivier et al. 1994; Smith et al. 1992), 20 min after exercise (Rivier et al. 1994), and 2 to 24 h after exercise (Haahr et al. 1991; Smith et al. 1992). One study reported increased levels of TNF-α in urine during and 1 h after exercise (Sprenger et al. 1992), suggesting that TNF-α is rapidly removed from circulation. Quick excretion of TNF-α is plausible as a protection against the toxic effects of the accumulation of high levels of TNF-α in blood and other tissues. The response by TNF-α to exercise may depend on the duration or intensity of exercise, as strenuous, prolonged exercise such as marathon running is accompanied by a small increase in blood levels of TNF-α near the end of the run and afterward (Febbraio and Pedersen 2002).

Interferon-Gamma

Early studies of IFN-γ in response to exercise have shown no effects. Haahr and colleagues (1991) reported no change in plasma levels of IFN-γ during exercise and 2 and 24 h following exercise. Sprenger and colleagues (1992) reported elevated urine levels of IFN-γ during exercise but a return to baseline levels within 1 h. Most studies since have shown no effect of acute exercise on blood levels of IFN (Pedersen and Hoffman-Goetz 2000).

Chronic Effects of Exercise in Trained Versus Untrained People

Though a single session of vigorous exercise appears to be accompanied by a temporary activation of the immune system that is similar to the acute phases of inflammation and response to infection, it is not clear that chronic exercise has a meaningful effect on cytokines. In one study, basal levels of IL-1 in the blood at rest were higher among exercise-trained men than in untrained men (Evans et al. 1986). Also, all the untrained men, but only one of the trained men, had an increase in IL-1 blood levels 3 h after exercise. That finding could be plausibly explained by more muscle cell damage in the untrained men than in the trained men. In another study (Smith et al. 1992), exercise-trained and untrained men had the same blood levels of IL-1, IL-6, and TNF-α measured at rest and after exercise. The discrepant findings might be explainable by the extent or type of exercise training.

Possible Mechanisms

One plausible mechanism to explain the effects of strenuous, intense exercise on cytokine levels is that it elicits a response similar to the acute-phase response to infection. However, the elevation in blood IL-1 levels induced by exercise is smaller than that found during infection (Cannon et al. 1986; Evans et al. 1986). A popular hypothesis is that cytokine release in response to exercise occurs most reliably in response to localized muscle damage, especially IL-1 increases after eccentric resistance exercise (Fielding et al. 1993), in order to activate phagocytic removal of dead or injured cells as part of the healing process.

A second plausible mechanism is a hormone-induced elevation of cytokine levels. Elevated blood levels of stress hormones, especially epinephrine and norepinephrine, during exercise cause changes in lymphocyte number, which suggests that increased IL-1 and IL-6 levels after exercise may be the result of increased blood levels of catecholamines (Cannon et al. 1986; Haahr et al. 1991) or other neuropeptides (Jonsdottir 2000). Another possible explanation is that increased blood flow during exercise results in synthesis and release of cytokines in order to regulate a greater flux and mixing of leukocytes caused by the increased blood flow. One study concluded that prolonged (3 h) cycling and inclined walking was accompanied by leukocytosis and elevated blood concentrations of IL-1, IL-6, and TNF-α but no changes in **messenger RNA** for those cytokines, suggesting that acute upregulation of gene expression does not explain the increased levels of cytokines (Moldoveanu, Shephard, and Shek 2000).

Problems With the Research

Several problems with the methods used limit conclusions about whether exercise has an independent effect on cytokines. Few studies of acute effects of a single session of exercise used an appropriate control group to show that the changes after exercise were not just normal fluctuations that would also have been seen at rest during the same amount of time. Also, the intensity, duration, and type of exercise were dissimilar among many studies, making it impossible to compare dose responses across studies. Studies of whether exercise training affects cytokines typically compare a group of people who are already trained with a group who are regarded as untrained. Randomized clinical trials have not been reported, and mostly men have been studied. Few of the cross-sectional studies controlled for medication intake, alcohol intake, diet, activity level prior to the experiment, or existing illnesses. The methods used to assay cytokines also differed widely among studies, introducing unknown sources of error in the measurements.

Nonetheless, exercise appears to enhance the release of cytokines in plasma, urine, and muscle. IL-1 and IL-6 levels appear to increase after exercise. IL-2 levels decrease, with a concomitant increase in IL-2 receptor expression. TNF and IFN remained constant during exercise in the few studies that examined these particular cytokines. Trained individuals have higher cytokine levels than untrained individuals. Extremely intense activity has been shown to reduce immune function, presumably by reducing the production of glutamine in skeletal muscles and increasing oxidative stress. Glutamine metabolism has been found to provide essential fuel to immune cells, and decreased production leads to slower immune response and recovery. The oxidative stress that physical activity may cause may also increase the body's vulnerability to cell and tissue damage by free radicals. Free radicals have been hypothesized to be initiators of cancer; therefore, people should avoid overtraining in order to experience the protective benefits of physical activity without the negative effects.

Summary

Acute exercise results in a temporary increase in the numbers of white blood cells circulating in the blood, mainly neutrophils, NK cells, and monocytes. This leukocytosis is plausibly explained by increases in pro-inflammatory cytokines that induce an inflammatory-like, acute-phase response that activates colony-stimulating factors to induce the proliferation of neutrophils and monocytes from bone marrow. The influx of NK cells into the blood probably comes mainly from the marginal pool, resulting from shearing forces of increased blood flow and inhibition of adhesion molecules that help lymphocytes adhere briefly to the endothelial cells of blood vessels. The general pattern of the leukocytosis is a marked increase during and shortly after moderate-intensity to vigorous exercise that lasts from 20 min up to 2 h, followed by a reduction below preexercise basal levels that lasts for 1 to 3 h but returns to basal levels within 24 h. The clinical meaning of this pattern of leukocytosis has not yet been confirmed in humans, but some experts have proposed that the transient reduction in leukocytes after heavy exercise might open a window of susceptibility to infections. A limited amount of epidemiologic evidence showing increased risk of upper respiratory infections after marathon running has been interpreted by some researchers as being consistent with that idea. Acute exercise also results in elevations of several lymphokines in the blood, suggesting that acute exercise mimics an acute-phase response to infection. However, increases in many of these lymphokines (e.g., interleukins) can be explained simply by the fact that the numbers of the lymphocytes secreting them have increased, so whether exercise simulates an infection-like response remains to be verified.

Adaptations by the immune system to chronic exercise have been harder to document, but the majority of exercise training studies and cross-sectional comparisons of exercise-trained men and women with sedentary people generally suggest an enhancement of innate immunity as evidenced by increased killing of tumor cells by NK cells. A very few studies found increased killing of bacteria by neutrophils and greater phagocytosis by macrophages.

To date, most studies of physical activity and the immune response among humans have understandably been limited to descriptions of cells in the blood. Animal studies using mice and rats have been able to examine the effects of exercise on immune responses in lymph tissues other than blood and have begun to clarify the potential mechanisms and health consequences of immune responses to exercise. Preliminary findings suggest that moderately intense exercise can have a positive influence on cancer survivors, increase fitness among men who have HIV disease without further impairing the immune system, and possibly reduce the risk of upper respiratory infections. In contrast, exhausting exercise and heavy endurance training have been associated with increased risk of infection in a few studies. The anti-inflammatory effects of regular exercise in people with inflammatory disease seem to depend mainly on fat loss, but the cumulative effects of myokines secreted by contracting skeletal muscle on immune function and health are not as yet fully known. Though limited in quantity and scientific quality, the available evidence is encouraging enough to justify more randomized controlled trials and prospective cohort studies to clarify the health implications of short- and long-term physical activity on overall immune function, resistance to infection, low-grade systemic inflammation, and cancer risk.

· BIBLIOGRAPHY ·

Abbas, A.K., A.H. Lightman, and J.S. Pober. 1997. *Cellular and molecular immunology.* 3rd edition. Philadelphia: Saunders.

Allgayer, H., S. Nicolaus, and S. Schreiber. 2004. Decreased interleukin-1 receptor antagonist response following moderate exercise in patients with colorectal carcinoma after primary treatment. *Cancer Detection and Prevention* 28 (3): 208-213.

Anuurad, E., A. Bremer, and L. Berglund. 2010. HIV protease inhibitors and obesity. *Current Opinion in Endocrinology, Diabetes, and Obesity* 17 (5): 478-485.

Arsenault, B.J., M. Côté, A. Cartier, I. Lemieux, J.P. Després, R. Ross, C.P. Earnest, S.N. Blair, and T.S. Church. 2009. Effect of exercise training on cardiometabolic risk markers among sedentary, but metabolically healthy overweight or obese postmenopausal women with elevated blood pressure. *Atherosclerosis* 207 (2): 530-533.

Balagopal, P., D. George, H. Yarandi, V. Funanage, and E. Bayne. 2005. Reversal of obesity-related hypoadiponectinemia by lifestyle intervention: A controlled, randomized study in obese adolescents. *Journal of Clinical Endocrinology and Metabolism* 90 (11): 6192-6197.

Barbaro, G., and G. Iacobellis. 2009. Metabolic syndrome associated with HIV and highly active antiretroviral therapy. *Current Diabetes Reports* 9 (1): 37-42.

Baslund, B., K. Lyngberg, V. Andersen, J. Halkjaer-Kristensen, M. Hansen, M. Klokker, and B.K. Pedersen. 1993. Effect of 8 wk of bicycle training on the immune system of patients with rheumatoid arthritis. *Journal of Applied Physiology* 75 (4): 1691-1695.

Baum, M., T. Geitner, and H. Liesen. 1996. The role of the spleen in the leukocytosis of exercise: Consequences for physiology and pathophysiology. *International Journal of Sports Medicine* 17: 604-607.

Beavers, K.M., F.C. Hsu, S. Isom, S.B. Kritchevsky, T. Church, B. Goodpaster, M. Pahor, and B.J. Nicklas. 2010. Long-term physical activity and inflammatory biomarkers in older adults. *Medicine and Science in Sports and Exercise* 42 (12): 2189-2196.

Benschop, R.J., R. Geenen, P.J. Mills, B.D. Naliboff, J.K. Kiecolt-Glaser, T.B. Herbert, G. van der Pompe, G.E. Miller, K.A. Matthews, G.L.R. Godaert, et al. 1997a. Cardiovascular and immune responses to acute psychological stress in young and old women: A meta-analysis. *Psychosomatic Medicine* 60: 290-296.

Benschop, R.J., M. Rodriguez-Feuerhahn, and M. Schedlowski. 1996. Catecholamine-induced leukocytosis: Early observations, current research, and future directions. *Brain, Behavior, and Immunity* 10: 77-91.

Benschop, R.J., M. Schedlowski, H. Wienecke, R. Jacobs, and R.E. Schmidt. 1997b. Adrenergic control of natural killer cell circulation and adhesion. *Brain, Behavior, and Immunity* 11: 321-332.

Brines, R., L. Hoffman-Goetz, and B.K. Pedersen. 1996. Can you exercise to make your immune system fitter? *Immunology Today* 17 (6): 252-254.

Campbell, K.L., P.T. Campbell, C.M. Ulrich, M. Wener, C.M. Alfano, K. Foster-Schubert, R.E. Rudolph, J.E. Potter, and A. McTiernan. 2008. No reduction in C-reactive protein following a 12-month randomized controlled trial of exercise in men and women. *Cancer Epidemiology, Biomarkers and Prevention* 17 (7): 1714-1718.

Campbell, P.T., K.L. Campbell, M.H. Wener, B.L. Wood, J.D. Potter, A. McTiernan, and C.M. Ulrich. 2009. A yearlong exercise intervention decreases CRP among obese postmenopausal women. *Medicine and Science in Sports and Exercise* 41 (8): 1533-1539.

Cannon, J., W. Evans, V. Hughes, C. Meredith, and C. Dinarello. 1986. Physiological mechanisms contributing to increased interleukin-1 secretion. *Journal of Applied Physiology* 61 (5): 1869-1874.

Carlson, S.L., S. Fox, and K.M. Abell. 1997. Catecholamine modulation of lymphocyte homing to lymphoid tissues. *Brain, Behavior, and Immunity* 11: 307-320.

Castellano, V., D.I. Patel, and L.J. White. 2008. Cytokine responses to acute and chronic exercise in multiple sclerosis. *Journal of Applied Physiology* 104 (6): 1697-1702.

Centers for Disease Control (CDC). 1981. Pneumocystis pneumonia—Los Angeles. *Morbidity and Mortality Weekly Report* 30: 250-252.

Centers for Disease Control. 1987. Classification for human immunodeficiency virus (HIV) infection in children under 13 years of age. *Morbidity and Mortality Weekly Report* 35: 224-235.

Centers for Disease Control. 1992. 1993 revised classification system for HIV infection and expanded surveillance case definition for AIDS among adolescents and adults. *Morbidity and Mortality Weekly Report* 41: 1-19.

Centers for Disease Control and Prevention (CDC). 2009. *HIV/AIDS Surveillance Report, 2009.* Vol. 21. Atlanta: U.S. Department of Health and Human Services. www.cdc.gov/hiv/surveillance/resources/reports/2009report/index.htm

Church, T.S., C.P. Earnest, A.M. Thompson, E.L. Priest, R.Q. Rodarte, T. Saunders, R. Ross, and S.N. Blair. 2010. Exercise without weight loss does not reduce C-reactive protein: The INFLAME study. *Medicine and Science in Sports and Exercise* 42 (4): 708-716.

Cohen, L.A., E. Boylan, M. Epstein, and E. Zang. 1992. Voluntary exercise and experimental mammary cancer. *Advances in Experimental and Medical Biology* 322: 41-59.

Cohen, L.A., M.E. Kendall, C. Meschter, M.A. Epstein, J. Reinhardt, and E. Zang. 1993. Inhibition of rat mammary tumorigenesis by voluntary exercise. *In Vivo* 2: 151-158.

Cohen, M.S., N. Hellmann, J.A. Levy, K. DeCock, and J. Lange. 2008. The spread, treatment, and prevention of HIV-1: Evolution of a global pandemic. *Journal of Clinical Investigation* 118 (4): 1244-1254.

Collins, T. 1995. Adhesion molecules in leukocyte emigration. *Scientific American Science and Medicine* 2 (6): 29-37.

Compston, A., and A. Coles. 2008. Multiple sclerosis. *Lancet* 372 (9648): 1502-1517.

Davis, J.M., and L.H. Colbert. 1997. The athlete's immune system, intense exercise, and overtraining. In *Perspectives in exercise science and sports medicine,* edited by D.R. Lamb and R. Murray, Vol. 10, *Optimizing sport performance,* pp. 269-311. Carmel, IN: Cooper.

De Backer, I.C., G. Schep, F.J. Backx, G. Vreugdenhil, and H. Kuipers. 2009. Resistance training in cancer survivors: A systematic review. *International Journal of Sports Medicine* 30 (10): 703-712.

De Jager, P.L., X. Jia, J. Wang, P.I. de Bakker, L. Ottoboni, N.T. Aggarwal, L.E. Piccio, S. Raychaudhuri, D. Tran, C. Aubin, R. Briskin, S. Romano; International MS Genetics Consortium, S.E. Baranzini, J.L. McCauley, M.A. Pericak-Vance, J.L. Haines, R.A. Gibson, Y. Naeglin, B. Uitdehaag, P.M. Matthews, L. Kappos, C. Polman, W.L. McArdle, D.P. Strachan, D. Evans, A.H. Cross, M.J. Daly, A. Compston, S.J. Sawcer, H.L. Weiner, S.L. Hauser, D.A. Hafler, and J.R. Oksenberg. 2009. Meta-analysis of genome scans and replication identify CD6, IRF8 and TNFRSF1A as new multiple sclerosis susceptibility loci. *Nature Genetics* 41 (7): 776-782.

Demark-Wahnefried, W., L.D. Case, K. Blackwell, P.K. Marcom, W. Kraus, N. Aziz, D.C. Snyder, J.K. Giguere, and E. Shaw. 2008. Results of a diet/exercise feasibility trial to prevent adverse body composition change in breast cancer patients on adjuvant chemotherapy. *Clinical Breast Cancer* 8 (1): 70-79.

Dimeo, F., S. Fetscher, W. Lange, R. Mertelsmann, and J. Keul. 1997. Effects of aerobic exercise on the physical performance and incidence of treatment-related complications after high-dose chemotherapy. *Blood* 90 (9, November 1): 3390-3394.

Dishman, R.K., S. Hong, J. Soares, G.L. Edwards, B.N. Bunnell, L. Jaso-Friedmann, and D.L. Evans. 2000a. Activity wheel running blunts suppression of natural killer cell cytotoxicity after sympathectomy and footshock. *Physiology and Behavior* 71: 297-304.

Dishman, R.K., J.M. Warren, S. Hong, B.N. Bunnell, E.H. Mougey, J.L. Meyerhoff, L. Jaso-Friedmann, and D.L. Evans. 2000b. Treadmill exercise training blunts suppression of splenic natural killer cell cytolysis after footshock. *Journal of Applied Physiology* 88: 2176-2182.

Dishman, R.K., J.M. Warren, S.D. Youngstedt, H. Yoo, B.N. Bunnell, E.H. Mougey, J.L. Meyerhoff, L. Jaso-Friedmann, and D.L. Evans. 1995. Activity-wheel running attenuates suppression of natural killer cell activity after foot shock. *Journal of Applied Physiology* 78 (4): 1547-1554.

Ernstrom, U., and G. Sandberg. 1973. Effects of adrenergic alpha- and beta-receptor stimulation on the release of lymphocytes and granulocytes from the spleen. *Scandinavian Journal of Haematology* 11: 275-286.

Espersen, G., A. Elbaek, E. Ernst, E. Toft, S. Kaalund, C. Jersild, and N. Grunnet. 1990. Effect of physical exercise on cytokines and lymphocyte subpopulations in human peripheral blood. *Acta Pathologica, Microbiologica, et Immunologica Scandinavica* 98: 395-400.

Espersen, G.T., A. Elbaek, S. Schmidt-Olsen, E. Ejlersen, K. Varming, and N. Grunnet. 1996. Short-term changes in the immune system of elite swimmers under competition conditions: Different immunomodulation induced by various types of sport. *Scandinavian Journal of Medicine and Science in Sports* 6 (3): 156-163.

Evans, W., C. Meredith, J. Cannon, C. Dinarello, W. Frontera, V. Hughes, B. Jones, and H. Knuttgen. 1986. Metabolic changes following eccentric exercise in trained and untrained men. *Journal of Applied Physiology* 61: 1864-1868.

Fairey, A.S., K.S. Courneya, C.J. Field, G.J. Bell, L.W. Jones, B.S. Martin, and J.R. Mackey. 2005a. Effect of exercise training on C-reactive protein in postmenopausal breast cancer survivors: A randomized controlled trial. *Brain, Behavior, and Immunity* 19 (5): 381-388.

Fairey, A.S., K.S. Courneya, C.J. Field, G.J. Bell, L.W. Jones, and J.R. Mackey. 2005b. Randomized controlled trial of exercise and blood immune function in postmenopausal breast cancer survivors. *Journal of Applied Physiology* 98 (4): 1534-1540.

Fairey, A.S., K.S. Courneya, C.J. Field, and J.R. Mackey. 2002. Physical exercise and immune system function in cancer survivors: A comprehensive review and future directions. *Cancer* 94 (2): 539-551.

Fantuzzi, G. 2008. Adiponectin and inflammation: Consensus and controversy. *Journal of Allergy and Clinical Immunology* 121 (2): 326-330.

Febbraio, M.A., and B.K. Pedersen. 2002. Muscle-derived interleukin-6: Mechanisms for activation and possible biological roles. *Journal of the Federation of American Societies for Experimental Biology* 16: 1335-1347.

Febbraio, M.A., and B.K. Pedersen. 2005. Contraction-induced myokine production and release: Is skeletal muscle an endocrine organ? *Exercise and Sport Sciences Reviews* 33 (3): 114-119.

Felten, D.L., S.Y. Felten, D.L. Bellinger, S.L. Carlson, K.D. Ackerman, K.S. Madden, J.A. Olschowka, and S. Livnat. 1987. Noradrenergic sympathetic neural interactions with the immune system: Structure and function. *Immunological Review* 100: 225-260.

Felten, D.L., and J. Olschowka. 1987. Noradrenergic sympathetic innervation of the spleen: II. Tyrosine hydroxylase (TH)–positive nerve terminals form synaptic-like contacts on lymphocytes in the splenic white pulp. *Journal of Neuroscience Research* 18: 37-48.

Ferrandez, M.D., and M. De la Fuente. 1996. Changes with aging, sex and physical exercise in murine natural killer activity and antibody-dependent cellular cytotoxicity. *Mechanisms of Ageing and Development* 86 (2): 83-94.

Fiatarone, M.A., J.E. Morley, E.T. Bloom, D. Benton, T. Makinodan, and G.F. Solomon. 1988. Endogenous opioids and the exercise-induced augmentation of natural killer cell activity. *Journal of Laboratory and Clinical Medicine* 112 (5): 544-552.

Fielding, R., T. Manfredi, W. Ding, M. Fiatarone, W. Evans, and J. Cannon. 1993. Acute phase response in exercise: III. Neutrophil and IL-1 beta accumulation in skeletal muscle. *American Journal of Physiology* 265: R166-R172.

Fillipas, S., C.L. Cherry, F. Cicuttini, L. Smirneos, and A.E. Holland. 2010. The effects of exercise training on metabolic and morphological outcomes for people living with HIV: A systematic review of randomised controlled trials. *HIV Clinical Trials* 11 (5, September-October): 270-282.

Fischer, C.P. 2006. Interleukin-6 in acute exercise and training: What is the biological relevance? *Exercise Immunology Review* 12: 6-33.

Gahmberg, C.G., L. Valmu, S. Fagerholm, P. Kotovuori, E. Ihanus, L. Tian, and T. Pessa-Morikawa. 1998. Leukocyte integrins and inflammation. *Cellular and Molecular Life Sciences* 54: 549-555.

Galvão, D.A., K. Nosaka, D.R. Taaffe, J. Peake, N. Spry, K. Suzuki, K. Yamaya, M.R. McGuigan, L.J. Kristjanson, and R.U. Newton. 2008. Endocrine and immune responses to resistance training in prostate cancer patients. *Prostate Cancer and Prostatic Disease* 11 (2): 160-165.

Garrey, W.E., and V. Butler. 1929. Physiological leucocytosis. *American Journal of Physiology* 90: 355-356.

Gielen, S., V. Adams, S. Möbius-Winkler, A. Linke, S. Erbs, J. Yu, W. Kempf, A. Schubert, G. Schuler, and R. Hambrecht. 2003. Anti-inflammatory effects of exercise training in the skeletal muscle of patients with chronic heart failure. *Journal of the American College of Cardiology* 42 (5): 861-868.

Gill, J., M. May, C. Lewden, M. Saag, M. Mugavero, P. Reiss, et al.; Antiretroviral Therapy Cohort Collaboration. 2010. Causes of death in HIV-1-infected patients treated with antiretroviral therapy, 1996-2006: Collaborative analysis of 13 HIV cohort studies. *Clinical Infectious Diseases* 50 (10): 1387-1396.

Gleeson, M. 2005. Assessing immune function changes in exercise and diet intervention studies. *Current Opinion in Clinical Nutrition and Metabolic Care* 8 (5, September): 511-515.

Gleeson, M., and N.C. Bishop. 2005. The T cell and NK cell immune response to exercise. *Annals of Transplantation* 10 (4): 43-48.

Gleeson, M., D.B. Pyne, and R. Callister. 2004. The missing links in exercise effects on mucosal immunity. *Exercise Immunology Review* 10: 107-128.

Haahr, P., B. Pedersen, A. Fomsgaard, N. Tvede, M. Diamant, K. Karlund, J. Halkjaer-Kristensen, and K. Bendtzen. 1991. Effect of physical exercise on in vitro production of interleukin-1, interleukin-6, tumor necrosis factor-α, interleukin-2 and interferon-γ. *International Journal of Sports Medicine* 12: 223-227.

Hayes, S.C., D. Rowbottom, P.S. Davies, T.W. Parker, and J. Bashford. 2003. Immunological changes after cancer treatment and participation in an exercise program. *Medicine and Science in Sports and Exercise* 35 (1): 2-9.

Heath, G.W., E.S. Ford, T.E. Craven, C.A. Macera, K.L. Jackson, and R.R. Pate. 1991. Exercise and the incidence of upper respiratory tract infections. *Medicine and Science in Sports and Exercise* 23: 152-157.

Hoene, M., and C. Weigert. 2010. The stress response of the liver to physical exercise. *Exercise Immunology Review* 16: 163-183.

Hoffman-Goetz, L., ed. 1996. *Exercise and immune function.* Boca Raton, FL: CRC Press.

Hoffman-Goetz, L., D. Apter, W. Denmark-Wahnefried, M.I. Goran, A. McTiernan, and M.E. Reichman. 1998. Possible mechanisms mediating an association between physical activity and breast cancer. *Cancer* 83 (3 Suppl.): 621-628.

Hoffman-Goetz, L., Y. Arumugam, and L. Sweeny. 1994. Lymphokine activated killer cell activity following voluntary physical activity in mice. *Journal of Sports and Medicine in Physical Fitness* 34 (1): 83-90.

Hoffman-Goetz, L., and B.K. Pedersen. 1994. Exercise and the immune system: A model of the stress response? *Immunology Today* 15: 382-387.

Hong, S., and R.K. Dishman. 2004. The effect of exercise on natural killer cell activity: A quantitative synthesis. Unpublished manuscript, University of Georgia, Athens.

Hutnick, N.A., N.I. Williams, W.J. Kraemer, E. Orsega-Smith, R.H. Dixon, A.D. Bleznak, and A.M. Mastro. 2005. Exercise and lymphocyte activation following chemotherapy for breast cancer. *Medicine and Science in Sports and Exercise* 37 (11): 1827-1835.

Irwin, M., R.L. Hauger, and M. Brown. 1992. Central corticotropin releasing hormone activates the sympathetic nervous system and reduces immune function: Increased responsivity of the aged rat. *Endocrinology* 131: 1047-1053.

Irwin, M., R.L. Hauger, M. Brown, and L. Britton. 1988. CRF activates autonomic nervous system and reduces natural killer cytotoxicity. *American Journal of Physiology* 5 (2): R744-R747.

Irwin, M., R.L. Hauger, L. Jones, M. Provencio, and K.T. Britton. 1990. Sympathetic nervous system mediates central corticotropin-releasing factor induced suppression of natural killer cytotoxicity. *Journal of Pharmacology and Experimental Therapeutics* 255: 101-107.

Jonsdottir, I.H. 2000. Neuropeptides and their interaction with exercise and immune function. *Immunology and Cell Biology* 78: 562-570.

Kanter, M.M. 1994. Free radicals, exercise, and antioxidant supplementation. *International Journal of Sport Nutrition* 4: 451-455.

Kappel, M., T.D. Poulsen, H. Galbo, and B.K. Pedersen. 1998. Influence of minor increases in plasma catecholamines on natural killer cell activity. *Hormone Research* 49: 22-26.

Kasapis, C., and P.D. Thompson. 2005. The effects of physical activity on serum C-reactive protein and inflammatory markers: A systematic review. *Journal of the American College of Cardiology* 45 (10): 1563-1569.

Katafuchi, T., S. Take, and T. Hori. 1993. Roles of sympathetic nervous system in the suppression of cytotoxicity of splenic natural killer cells in the rat. *Journal of Physiology (Lond)* 465: 343-357.

Kelley, G.A. and K.S. Kelley. 2006. Effects of aerobic exercise on C-reactive protein, body composition, and maximum oxygen consumption in adults: A meta-analysis of randomized controlled trials. *Metabolism* 55: 1500-1507.

Kelly, A.S., J. Steinberger, T.P. Olson, and D.R. Dengel. 2007. In the absence of weight loss, exercise training does not improve adipokines or oxidative stress in overweight children. *Metabolism* 56 (7): 1005-1009.

LaPerriere, A.R., M.H. Antoni, N. Schneiderman, G. Ironson, N. Klimas, P. Caralis, and M.A. Fletcher. 1990. Exercise intervention attenuates emotional distress and natural killer cell decrements following notification of positive serologic status for HIV-1. *Biofeedback and Self-Regulation* 15: 229-242.

Larrabee, R.C. 1902. Leucocytosis after violent exercise. *Journal of Medical Research* 7: 76-82.

Lee, I.M. 1995. Exercise and physical health: Cancer and immune function. *Research Quarterly for Exercise and Sport* 66: 286-291.

Lewicki, R., H. Tchorzewski, E. Majewska, Z. Nowak, and Z. Baj. 1988. Effect of maximal physical exercise on T-lymphocyte subpopulations and on interleukin-1 (IL-1) and interleukin-2 (IL-2) production in vitro. *International Journal of Sports Medicine* 9 (2): 114-117.

Lindegaard, B., T. Hansen, T. Hvid, G. van Hall, P. Plomgaard, S. Ditlevsen, J. Gerstoft, and B.K. Pedersen. 2008. The effect of strength and endurance training on insulin sensitivity and fat distribution in human immunodeficiency virus-infected patients with lipodystrophy. *Journal of Clinical Endocrinology and Metabolism* 93 (10): 3860-3869.

Lira, F.S., J.C. Rosa, N.E. Zanchi, A.S. Yamashita, R.D. Lopes, A.C. Lopes, M.L. Batista Jr., and M. Seelaender. 2009. Regulation of inflammation in the adipose tissue in cancer cachexia: Effect of exercise. *Cell Biochemistry and Function* 27 (2): 71-75.

Lowder, T., D.A. Padgett, and J.A. Woods. 2005. Moderate exercise protects mice from death due to influenza virus. *Brain, Behavior, and Immunity* 19 (5): 377-380.

Mackinnon, L. 1999. *Advances in exercise immunology.* Champaign, IL: Human Kinetics.

MacNeil, B., and L. Hoffman-Goetz. 1993a. Chronic exercise enhances in vivo and in vitro cytotoxic mechanisms of natural immunity in mice. *Journal of Applied Physiology* 74 (1): 388-395.

MacNeil, B., and L. Hoffman-Goetz. 1993b. Exercise training and tumour metastasis in mice: Influence of time of exercise onset. *Anticancer Research* 13 (6A): 2085-2088.

Madden, K.S., K.D. Ackerman, S. Livnat, S.Y. Felten, and D.L. Felten. 1993. Neonatal sympathetic denervation alters development of natural killer (NK) cell activity in F344 rats. *Brain, Behavior, and Immunity* 7: 344-351.

Maier, S.F., and L.R. Watkins. 1998. Cytokines for psychologists: Implications of bidirectional immune-to-brain communication for understanding behavior, mood, and cognition. *Psychological Review* 105 (1): 83-107.

Maisel, A.S., T. Harris, C.A. Rearden, and M.C. Michel. 1990. β-adrenergic receptors in lymphocyte subsets after exercise: Alterations in normal individuals and patients with congestive heart failure. *Circulation* 82 (6): 2003-2010.

Malm, C., R. Lenkei, and B. Sjodin. 1999. Effects of eccentric exercise on the immune system in men. *Journal of Applied Physiology* 86 (2): 461-468.

Mandler, R.N., W.E. Mandler, and S.A. Serrate. 1986. β-endorphin augment the cytolytic activity and interferon production of natural killer cells. *Journal of Immunology* 136: 934-939.

Martin, H.E. 1932. Physiological leucocytosis. *Journal of Physiology* 75: 113-129.

May, M.T., J.A. Sterne, D. Costagliola, C.A. Sabin, A.N. Phillips, A.C. Justice, F. Dabis, J. Gill, J. Lundgren, R.S. Hogg, F. de Wolf, G. Fätkenheuer, S. Staszewski, A. d'Arminio Monforte, M. Egger; Antiretroviral Therapy (ART) Cohort Collaboration. 2006. HIV treatment response and prognosis in Europe and North America in the first decade of highly active antiretroviral therapy: A collaborative analysis. *Lancet* 368 (9534): 451-458.

Miles, M.P., S.K. Leach, W.J. Kraemer, K. Dohi, J.A. Bush, and A.M. Mastro. 1998. Leukocyte adhesion molecule expression during intense resistance exercise. *Journal of Applied Physiology* 84 (5): 1604-1609.

Moldoveanu, A.I., R.J. Shephard, and P.N. Shek. 2000. Exercise elevates plasma levels but not gene expression of IL-1beta, IL-6, and TNF-alpha in blood mononuclear cells. *Journal of Applied Physiology* 89 (4): 1499-1504.

Moldoveanu, A.I., R.J. Shephard, and P.N. Shek. 2001. The cytokine response to physical activity and training. *Sports Medicine* 31 (2): 115-144.

Moriguchi, S., M. Kato, K. Sakai, S. Yamamoto, and E. Shimizu. 1998. Exercise training restores decreased cellular immune functions in obese Zucker rats. *Journal of Applied Physiology* 84 (1): 311-317.

Morville, R., P.C. Pesquies, and C.Y. Guezennee. 1979. Plasma variations in testicular and adrenal androgens during prolonged physical exercise in man. *Annals in Endocrinology* 40: 501-515.

Mosser, D.M., and J.P. Edwards. 2008. Exploring the full spectrum of macrophage activation. *Nature Reviews Immunology* 8 (12): 958-969.

Motl, R.W., and J.L. Gosney. 2008. Effect of exercise training on quality of life in multiple sclerosis: A meta-analysis. *Multiple Sclerosis* 14 (1): 129-135.

Moyna, N.M., G.R. Acker, K.M. Weber, J.R. Fulton, F.L. Goss, R.J. Robertson, and B.S. Rabin. 1996. The effects of incremental submaximal exercise on circulating leukocytes in physically active and sedentary males and females. *European Journal of Applied Physiology* 74 (3): 211-218.

Murray, D.R., M. Irwin, C.A. Rearden, M. Ziegler, H. Motulsky, and A.S. Maisel. 1992. Sympathetic and immune interactions during dynamic exercise: Mediation via a beta 2-adrenergic-dependent mechanism. *Circulation* 86 (1): 203-213.

Mutimura, E., N.J. Crowther, T.W. Cade, K.E. Yarasheski, and A. Stewart. 2008. Exercise training reduces central adiposity and improves metabolic indices in HAART-treated HIV-positive subjects in Rwanda: A randomized controlled trial. *AIDS Research and Human Retroviruses* 24 (1): 15-23.

Na, Y.M., M.Y. Kim, Y.K. Kim, Y.R. Ha, and D.S. Yoon. 2000. Exercise therapy effect on natural killer cell cytotoxic activity in stomach cancer patients after curative surgery. *Archives of Physical Medicine and Rehabilitation* 81 (6): 777-779.

Nasrullah, I., and R.S. Mazzeo. 1992. Age-related immunosenescence in Fischer 344 rats: Influence of exercise training. *Journal of Applied Physiology* 73: 1932-1938.

National Institute of Medicine. 2001. *Multiple sclerosis: Current status and strategies for the future,* edited by J.E. Joy and R.B. Johnston Jr. Committee on Multiple Sclerosis: Current Status and Strategies for the Future. Board on Neuroscience and Behavioral Health. Institute of Medicine, National Academies. Washington, DC: National Academy Press.

Newsholme, E.A., and M. Parry-Billings. 1994. Effects of exercise on the immune system. In *Physical activity, fitness, and health,* edited by C. Bouchard, R. Shephard, and T. Stephens, pp. 451-455. Champaign, IL: Human Kinetics.

Nicklas, B.J., F.C. Hsu, T.J. Brinkley, T. Church, B.H. Goodpaster, S.B. Kritchevsky, and M. Pahor. 2008. Exercise training and plasma C-reactive protein and interleukin-6 in elderly people. *Journal of the American Geriatrics Society* 56 (11): 2045-2052.

Nielsen, H.B., N.H. Secher, M. Kappel, and B.K. Pedersen. 1998. N-acetylcysteine does not affect the lymphocyte proliferation and natural killer cell activity responses to exercise. *American Journal of Physiology* 275 (4 Pt 2): R1227-R1231.

Nieman, D.C. 2003. Current perspective on exercise immunology. *Current Sports Medicine Reports* 2 (5): 239-242.

Nieman, D.C., V.D. Cook, D.A. Henson, J. Suttles, W.J. Rejeski, P.M. Ribisl, O.R. Fagoaga, and S.L. Nehlsen-Cannarella. 1995a. Moderate exercise training and natural killer cell cytotoxic activity in breast cancer patients. *International Journal of Sports Medicine* 16 (5): 334-337.

Nieman, D.C., D.A. Henson, G. Gusewitch, B.J. Warren, R.C. Dotson, D.E. Butterworth, and S.L. Nehlsen-Cannarella. 1993. Physical activity and immune function in elderly women. *Medicine and Science in Sports and Exercise* 25: 823-831.

Nieman, D.C., D.A. Henson, C.S. Sampson, J.L. Herring, J. Suttles, M. Conley, M.H. Stone, D.E. Butterworth, and J.M. Davis. 1995b. The acute immune response to exhaustive resistance exercise. *International Journal of Sports Medicine* 16 (5): 322-328.

Nieman, D.C., L.M. Johannsen, J.W. Lee, and K. Arabatzis. 1990a. Infectious episodes in runners before and after the Los Angeles Marathon. *Journal of Sports Medicine and Physical Fitness* 30: 316-328.

Nieman, D.C., S.L. Nehlsen-Cannarella, P.A. Markoff, A.J. Balk-Lamberton, H. Yang, D.B. Chritton, J.W. Lee, and K. Arabatzis. 1990b. The effects of moderate exercise training on natural killer cells and acute upper respiratory tract infections. *International Journal of Sports Medicine* 11: 467-473.

Nieman, D.C., and B.K. Pedersen. 1999. Exercise and immune function. *Sports Medicine* 27: 73-80.

Noonan, C.W., D.M. Williamson, J.P. Henry, R. Indian, S.G. Lynch, J.S. Neuberger, et al. 2010. The prevalence of multiple sclerosis in 3 US communities. *Preventing Chronic Disease* 7 (1): A12. www.cdc.gov/pcd/issues/2010/Jan/08_0241.htm

O'Brien, K., S. Nixon, A.M. Tynan, and R. Glazier. 2010. Aerobic exercise interventions for adults living with HIV/AIDS. *Cochrane Database of Systematic Reviews,* August 4 (8): CD001796.

O'Brien, K., A.M. Tynan, S. Nixon, and R.H. Glazier. 2008. Effects of progressive resistive exercise in adults living with HIV/AIDS: Systematic review and meta-analysis of randomized trials. *AIDS Care* 20 (6): 631-653.

Palella, F.J. Jr., R.K. Baker, A.C. Moorman, J.S. Chmiel, K.C. Wood, J.T. Brooks, et al. 2006. Mortality in the highly active antiretroviral therapy era: Changing causes of death and disease in the HIV outpatient study. *Journal of Acquired Immune Deficiency Syndrome* 43: 27-34.

Palmo, J., S. Asp, J.R. Daugaard, E.A. Richter, M. Klokker, and B.K. Pedersen. 1995. Effect of eccentric exercise on natural killer cell activity. *Journal of Applied Physiology* 78 (4): 1442-1446.

Pedersen, B.K. 2006. The anti-inflammatory effect of exercise: Its role in diabetes and cardiovascular disease control. *Essays in Biochemistry* 42: 105-117.

Pedersen, B.K. 2009. Edward F. Adolph distinguished lecture: Muscle as an endocrine organ: IL-6 and other myokines. *Journal of Applied Physiology* 107 (4): 1006-1014.

Pedersen, B.K. 2011. Muscles and their myokines. *Journal of Experimental Biology* 214 (2): 337-346.

Pedersen, B.K., and L. Hoffman-Goetz. 2000. Exercise and the immune system: Regulation, integration, and adaptation. *Physiological Reviews* 80: 1055-1081.

Pedersen, B.K., A. Steensberg, C. Fischer, C. Keller, K. Ostrowski, and P. Schjerling. 2001. Exercise and cytokines with particular focus on muscle-derived IL-6. *Exercise Immunology Review* 7: 18-31.

Ploeger, H.E., T. Takken, M.H. de Greef, and B.W. Timmons. 2009. The effects of acute and chronic exercise on inflammatory markers in children and adults with a chronic inflammatory disease: A systematic review. *Exercise Immunology Review* 5: 6-41.

Pollock, M.L., G.A. Gaesser, J.D. Butcher, J.P. Despres, R.K. Dishman, B.A. Franklin, and C.E. Garber. 1998. Recommended quantity and quality of exercise for developing and maintaining cardiorespiratory and muscular fitness, and flexibility in healthy adults. *Medicine and Science in Sports and Exercise* 30: 975-991.

Quinn, T.C. 2008. HIV epidemiology and the effects of antiviral therapy on long-term consequences. *AIDS* 22 (Suppl. 3): S7-12.

Rehman, J., P.J. Mills, S.M. Carter, J. Chou, J. Thomas, and A.S. Maisel. 1997. Dynamic exercise leads to an increase in circulating ICAM-1: Further evidence for adrenergic modulation of cell adhesion. *Brain, Behavior, and Immunity* 11: 343-351.

Rhind, S.G., G.A. Gannon, R.J. Shephard, and P.N. Shek. 2002. Indomethacin modulates circulating cytokine responses to strenuous exercise in humans. *Cytokine* 19: 153-158.

Rhind, S.G., G.A. Gannon, M. Suzui, R.J. Shephard, and P.N. Shek. 1999. Indomethacin inhibits circulating PGE2 and reverses postexercise suppression of natural killer cell activity. *American Journal of Physiology* 276 (5 Pt 2): R1496-R1505.

Rhind, S.G., P.N. Shek, S. Shinkai, and R.J. Shephard. 1994. Differential expression of interleukin-2 receptor alpha and beta chains in relation to natural killer cell subsets and aerobic fitness. *International Journal of Sports Medicine* 15 (6): 311-318.

Rigsby, L.W., R.K. Dishman, A.W. Jackson, G.S. Maclean, and P.B. Raven. 1992. Effects of exercise training on men seropositive for the human immunodeficiency virus-1. *Medicine and Science in Sports and Exercise* 24: 6-12.

Rivier, A., J. Pene, P. Chanez, F. Anselme, C. Caillaud, C. Prefaut, P. Godard, and J. Bousquet. 1994. Release of cytokines by blood monocytes during strenuous exercise. *International Journal of Sports Medicine* 15 (4): 192-198.

Rohde, C.P., and K. Wachholder. 1953. Weibes blutbid und muskelarbeit. *Arbeitsphysiologie* 15: 165-174.

Romeo, J., J. Wärnberg, T. Pozo, and A. Marcos. 2010. Physical activity, immunity and infection. *Proceedings of the Nutrition Society* 69 (3): 390-399.

Rosati, G. 2001. The prevalence of multiple sclerosis in the world: An update. *Neurological Sciences* 22 (2): 117-139.

Rubin, D.A., and A.C. Hackney. 2010. Inflammatory cytokines and metabolic risk factors during growth and maturation: Influence of physical activity. *Medicine and Sport Science* 55: 43-55.

Scanga, C.B., T.J. Verde, A.M. Paolone, R.E. Andersen, and T.A. Wadden. 1998. Effects of weight loss and exercise training on natural killer cell activity in obese women. *Medicine and Science in Sports and Exercise* 30 (12): 1666-1671.

Schittek, B., R. Hipfel, B. Sauer, J. Bauer, H. Kalbacher, S. Stevanovic, M. Schirle, K. Schroeder, N. Blin, F. Meier, G. Rassner, and C. Garbe. 2001. Dermcidin: A novel human antibiotic peptide secreted by sweat glands. *Nature Immunology* 2: 1133-1137.

Schulz, G. 1893. Experimentelle Untersuchungen über das Vorkommen und die diagnostische Bedeutung der Leukozytose. *Deutsches Archiv für Klinische Medizin* 51: 234.

Senchina, D.S., and M.L. Kohut. 2007. Immunological outcomes of exercise in older adults. *Clinical Interventions in Aging* 2 (1): 3-16.

Shavit, Y., G.W. Terman, J.W. Lewis, et al. 1986. Effects of footshock stress and morphine on natural killer lymphocytes in rats: Studies of tolerance and cross-tolerance. *Brain Research* 372: 382-385.

Shephard, R.J. 2002. Cytokine responses to physical activity, with particular reference to IL-6: Sources, actions, and clinical implications. *Critical Reviews in Immunology* 22: 165-182.

Shephard, R.J., and P.N. Shek. 1995. Cancer, immune function, and physical activity. *Canadian Journal of Applied Physiology* 20: 1-25.

Shephard, R.J., and P.N. Shek. 1999. Effects of exercise and training on natural killer cell counts and cytolytic activity. *Sports Medicine* 28: 177-195.

Simpson, J.R., and L. Hoffman-Goetz. 1990. Exercise stress and murine natural killer cell function. *Proceedings of the Society for Experimental Biology and Medicine* 195 (1): 129-135.

Simpson, R.J., D.G. Florida-James, C. Cosgrove, G.P. Whyte, S. Macrae, H. Pircher, and K. Guy. 2007. High-intensity exercise elicits the mobilization of senescent T lymphocytes into the peripheral blood compartment in human subjects. *Journal of Applied Physiology* 103 (1): 396-401.

Smith, J., R. Telford, R. Baker, A. Hapel, and M. Weidermann. 1992. Cytokine immunoreactivity in plasma does not change after moderate endurance exercise. *Journal of Applied Physiology* 73 (4): 1396-1401.

Snook, E.M., and R.W. Motl. 2009. Effect of exercise training on walking mobility in multiple sclerosis: A meta-analysis. *Neurorehabilitation and Neural Repair* 23 (2): 108-116.

Speck, R.M., K.S. Courneya, L.C. Mâsse, S. Duval, and K.H. Schmitz. 2010. An update of controlled physical activity trials in cancer survivors: A systematic review and meta-analysis. *Journal of Cancer Survivorship* 4 (2): 87-100.

Sprat, T. 1667. The plague of Athens which hapned in the second year of the Peloponnesian Warr / first described in Greek by Thucydides, then in Latin by Lucretius, now attempted in English by Tho. Sprat. London: Printed by E.C. for Henry Brome.

Sprenger, H., C. Jacobs, M. Nain, M. Gressner, H. Prinz, W. Wesemann, and D. Gemsa. 1992. Enhanced release of cytokines, interleukin-2 receptors, and neopterin after long-distance running. *Clinical Immunology and Immunopathology* 63 (2): 188-195.

Steensberg, A., C. Keller, R.L. Starkie, T. Osada, M.A. Febbraio, and B.K. Pedersen. 2002. IL-6 and TNF-alpha expression in, and release from, contracting human skeletal muscle. *American Journal of Physiology: Endocrinology and Metabolism* 283: E1272-E1278.

Steensberg, A., A.D. Toft, P. Schjerling, J. Halkjaer-Kristensin, and B.K. Pedersen. 2001. Plasma interleukin-6 during strenuous exercise: Role of epinephrine. *American Journal of Physiology: Cell Physiology* 281: C1001-C1004.

Stewart, L.K., C.P. Earnest, S.N. Blair, and T.S. Church. 2010. Effects of different doses of physical activity on C-reactive protein among women. *Medicine and Science in Sports and Exercise* 42 (4): 701-707.

Strasner, A., J.M. Davis, M.L. Kohut, R.R. Pate, A. Ghaffar, and E. Mayer. 1997. Effects of exercise intensity on natural killer cell activity in women. *International Journal of Sports Medicine* 18 (1): 56-61.

Terry, L., E. Sprinz, R. Stein, N.B. Medeiros, J. Oliveira, and J.P. Ribeiro. 2006. Exercise training in HIV-1-infected individuals with dyslipidemia and lipodystrophy. *Medicine and Science in Sports and Exercise* 38 (3): 411-417.

Thompson, A.M., C.R. Mikus, R.Q. Rodarte, B. Distefano, E.L. Priest, E. Sinclair, C.P. Earnest, S.N. Blair, and T.S. Church. 2008. Inflammation and exercise (INFLAME): Study rationale, design, and methods. *Contemporary Clinical Trials* 29 (3): 418-427.

Timmons, B.W., and T. Cieslak. 2008. Human natural killer cell subsets and acute exercise: A brief review. *Exercise Immunology Review* 14: 8-23.

Tonnesen, E., N.J. Christensen, and M.M. Brinklov. 1987. Natural killer cell activity during cortisol and adrenaline infusion in healthy volunteers. *European Journal of Clinical Investigation* 17: 497-503.

Tsiodras, S., A. Perelas, C. Wanke, and C.S. Mantzoros. 2010. The HIV-1/HAART associated metabolic syndrome - novel adipokines, molecular associations and therapeutic implications. *Journal of Infection* 61 (2): 101-113.

Tvede, N., M. Kappel, J. Halkjaer-Kristensen, H. Galbo, and B. Pedersen. 1993. The effect of light, moderate and severe bicycle exercise on lymphocyte subsets, natural and lymphokine activated killer cells, lymphocyte proliferative response and interleukin 2 production. *International Journal of Sports Medicine* 14 (5): 275-282.

UNAIDS, Joint United Nations Programme on HIV/AIDS and WHO. 2009. AIDS epidemic update. www.unaids.org/en/data-analysis/epidemiology/2009aidsepidemicupdate/.

Villarroya, F., P. Domingo, and M. Giralt. 2010. Drug-induced lipotoxicity: Lipodystrophy associated with HIV-1 infection and antiretroviral treatment. *Biochimica et Biophysica Acta* 1801 (3): 392-399.

Wärnberg, J., K. Cunningham, J. Romeo, and A. Marcos. 2010. Physical activity, exercise and low-grade systemic inflammation. *Proceedings of the Nutrition Society* 69 (3): 400-406.

White, L.J., S.C. McCoy, V. Castellano, G. Gutierrez, J.E. Stevens, G.A. Walter, and K. Vandenborne. 2004. Resistance training improves strength and functional capacity in persons with multiple sclerosis. *Multiple Sclerosis* 10 (6): 668-674.

Whitham, M., and M.B. Fortes. 2008. Heat shock protein 72: Release and biological significance during exercise. *Frontiers in Bioscience* 13: 1328-1339.

Woods, J.A., M.A. Ceddia, B.W. Wolters, J.K. Evans, Q. Lu, and E. McAuley. 1999a. Effects of 6 months of moderate aerobic exercise training on immune function in the elderly. *Mechanisms of Ageing and Development* 109 (1): 1-19.

Woods, J.A., J.M. Davis, J.A. Smith, and D.C. Nieman. 1999b. Exercise and cellular innate immune function. *Medicine and Science in Sports and Exercise* 31: 57-66.

Woods, J.A., T.W. Lowder, and K.T. Keylock. 2002. Can exercise training improve immune function in the aged? *Annals of the New York Academy of Sciences* 959: 117-127.

Woods, J.A., Q. Lu, M.A. Ceddia, and T. Lowder. 2000. Special feature for the Olympics: Effects of exercise on the immune system: Exercise-induced modulation of macrophage function. *Immunology and Cell Biology* 78: 545-553.

Woods, J.A., V.J. Vieira, and K.T. Keylock. 2009. Exercise, inflammation, and innate immunity. *Immunology and Allergy Clinics of North America* 29 (2): 381-393.

Wu, A.H., A.S. Whittemore, L.N. Kolonel, E.M. John, R.P. Gallagher, D.W. West, J. Hankin, C.Z. Teh, D.M. Dreon, and R.S. Paffenbarger Jr. 1995. Serum androgens and sex hormone–binding globulins in relation to lifestyle factors in older African-American, white, and Asian men in the United States and Canada. *Cancer Epidemiology, Biomarkers and Prevention* 4 (7): 735-741.

Yamada, M., K. Suzuki, S. Kudo, M. Totsuka, S. Nakaji, and K. Sugawara. 2002. Raised plasma G-CSF and IL-6 after exercise may play a role in neutrophil mobilization into the circulation. *Journal of Applied Physiology* 92: 1789-1794.

PART SIX

Physical Activity, and Special Concerns

At the start of new millennium, the American Psychological Association initiated the "Decade of Behavior," an interdisciplinary effort to promote behavioral and social science research. One of the themes of that effort was health. The preceding parts of this book have shown why the promotion of leisure-time physical activity has emerged as an important initiative for public health and quality of living in many economically developed nations and, more recently, in developing nations. The chapters in this part expand the view of public health beyond chronic diseases and premature death. The World Health Organization has already endorsed disability-adjusted life expectancy as an important way to judge healthy living beyond mere life expectancy in years. Moreover, the WHO has projected that depression will be second only to cardiovascular disease as the world's leading cause of death and disability by the year 2020 and will be number one by 2030, ahead of cardiovascular disease, with dementia then ranking third. Chapter 14 describes the accumulated evidence that physical activity protects against depression and anxiety disorders, as well as cognitive decline and dementia associated with aging. Chapter 15 provides a broad overview of progress made in understanding physical activity in disability and other special populations that have health disparities.

Nonetheless, it is important to acknowledge that participation in vigorous physical activity carries with it some risk. Chapter 16 discusses the adverse events and hazards of physical activity. Leisure-time physical activity has remained below recommended levels in nations that keep population statistics about physical activity. The final chapter, chapter 17, deals with the promotion of a safe, physically active lifestyle among all segments of the population.

CHAPTER 14

Physical Activity and Mental Health

Opposite to Exercise is Idleness or want of exercise, the bane of body and minde . . . the chiefe author of all mischiefe, one of the seven deadly sinnes, and the sole cause of melancholy.

• Robert Burton •
Anatomy of Melancholy, 1632

Our muscular vigor will . . . always be needed to furnish the background of sanity, serenity, and cheerfulness to life, to give moral elasticity to our disposition, to round off the wiry edge of fretfulness, and make us good-humored . . .

• William James •
Talks to Teachers on Psychology: And to Students on Some of Life's Ideals, 1899

CHAPTER OBJECTIVES

▸ Describe the public health burden of depression, anxiety disorders, and dementia including their prevalence in population groups, costs, and their roles in the risk of cardiovascular diseases, early mortality, and reduced quality of life

▸ Identify common tests used to diagnose and screen for depression and anxiety in the population

▸ List common drugs used to treat depression and anxiety disorders and their common side effects

▸ Identify the major modifiable and nonmodifiable risk factors for depression and anxiety and common causes of dementia

▸ Identify and describe the function of key brain structures and neural networks that regulate motivation and emotional responses during stress

▸ Discuss the putative social, cognitive, and neurobiological mechanisms that might explain mental health benefits of physical activity and exercise training

▸ Describe and evaluate the strength of evidence that physical activity reduces the risk of developing depression, anxiety disorders, and dementia in population groups and that exercise training reduces symptoms in people diagnosed with these disorders

Although chronic diseases (e.g., cardiovascular disease, diabetes, cancer) and obesity receive most of the attention in public health, mental health problems are a public health burden worldwide, decreasing the quality of life and adding substantially to health care costs. The medical cost of treating depression, schizophrenia, and dementia is 1% to 2% each of total health care costs in many nations (Hu 2006). In the United States, estimated costs of mental disorders are a combined 6.2% of health care expenditures (Mark et al. 2007). Depression and dementia were among the 10 leading risk factors of disability-adjusted life expectancy in high-income nations during 2001 (Lopez et al. 2006), and they are projected to rank first and third worldwide by the year 2030 (Mathers and Loncar 2006). In the United States, dementia and other disorders of the central nervous system are leading causes of death, and mental disorders account for more than 40% of years lost to disability (Michaud et al. 2006). Evidence continues to accumulate to support that physical activity reduces odds of disorders such as depression, anxiety, and cognitive decline associated with aging while promoting better sleep and feelings of energy and well-being. And, those outcomes don't occur just because people expect benefits from exercise. Neuroscience studies show that exercise improves brain health through positive neurogenerative (new cells), neurotrophic (cell growth), neuroprotective (cell survival), neuroplastic (density and complexity of synapses), and vascular (better circulation) changes.

The most comprehensive estimates of mental health problems among U.S. adults come from the National Comorbidity Survey Replication (NCS-R), a nationally representative survey during 2001-2002 of 9282 English-speaking household residents ages 18 years and older in the contiguous United States (Kessler et al. 2004). Twelve-month prevalence estimates (NCS 2007) were 19.1% for anxiety disorders, 9.7% for mood disorders, 10.5% for impulse control disorders, and 13.4% for substance abuse (including 11% for nicotine dependence). See figure 14.1. Schizophrenia and other psychoses unrelated to mood disorders were not assessed. About 26% of people had at least one disorder during the past year, of which 22.3% were serious, 37.3% were moderately severe, and 40.4% were mild. Fifty-five percent of people had only one disorder; 22% had two, and 23% had three or more diagnoses. There were three clusters of people who had very high comorbidities (mainly high rates of phobias, social anxiety, generalized anxiety, and major depressive episode or dysthymia) that represented 7% of the population but 44% of all serious cases (Kessler et al. 2005b).

The combined prevalence rates of anxiety disorders, mood disorders, and substance abuse disorders in people 18 to 54 years of age (30.5%) had not changed since 1990-1992 (29.4%) (with the exception of now including nicotine dependence as a substance abuse disorder), but the rate of treatment had increased. About 12% of the population got treatment for emotional disorders in 1990-1992. That rose to 20% in 2001-2003 (Kessler et al. 2005b). Just half the people treated met diagnostic criteria for mental disorders. Among people diagnosed with a disorder, 32.9% received treatment in 2001-2003 compared to 20.3% in 1990-1992 (Kessler et al. 2005c).

A serious mental illness in the United States costs about $16,000 in annual lost earnings, a total impact of $193.2 billion on the economy (Kessler et al. 2008). The total cost of mental health problems in the United States, including medical costs, mortality, and lost income, is about $300 billion each year (Greenberg et al. 2003; Rice and Miller

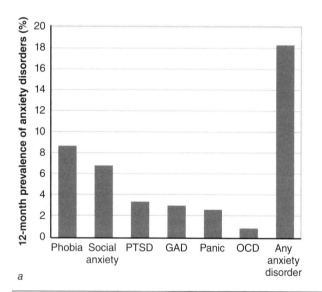

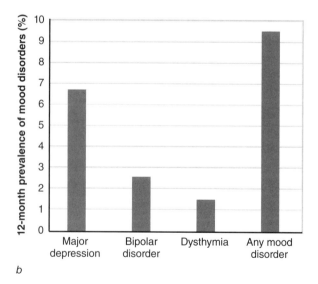

a

b

Figure 14.1 Twelve-month prevalence estimates of *(a)* anxiety disorders and *(b)* mood disorders in U.S. adults.

Data from Kessler et al. 2005, "Prevalence, severity, and comorbidity of 12-month DSM-IV disorders in the National Comorbidity Survey Replication," and National Comorbidity Survey 2007, http://www.hcp.med.harvard.edu/ncs/.

1995; Insel 2008). The most common disorders, anxiety and depression, each cost about $85 billion a year. Estimated costs of depression in the United States for 2000 were $26.1 billion (31%) in direct medical costs, $5.4 billion (7%) in suicide-related mortality costs, and $51.5 billion (62%) in lost productivity at the workplace (Greenberg et al. 2003). Anxiety costs haven't been updated for the United States since an annual estimate of $46.6 billion in 1990, which was 31.5% of total mental health costs at that time (Rice and Miller 1998). However, anxiety costs have surely kept pace with costs of depression.

The total annual cost of depression in Europe was estimated as 118 billion euros in 2004, which corresponds to a cost of 253 euros per capita (Sobocki et al. 2006). Depression was the most costly brain disorder in Europe, accounting for 33% of the total mental health care costs and 1% of the gross domestic product (GDP) or total economy of Europe.

Nearly half of Americans will meet the criteria for at least one DSM-IV disorder sometime in their life, usually first in childhood or adolescence. Lifetime prevalence estimates are about 29.9% for anxiety disorders, 21.4% for mood disorders, 25% for impulse control disorders, and 35.3% for substance use disorders (including 29.6% for nicotine dependence) (Kessler et al. 2005a; NCS 2007). Median age of onset is much earlier for anxiety or impulse control disorders (each 11 years of age) than for substance use (20 years) and mood (30 years) disorders. Half of all lifetime cases start by age 14 years and three-fourths by age 24 years (Kessler et al. 2005a). The World Health Organization (WHO) World Mental Health Surveys on the global burden of mental disorders found that the combined prevalence rates for anxiety, mood, impulse control, and substance use disorders ranged from about 10% to 19% annually and 18% to 36% over a lifetime for the middle 50% of the 17 participating countries (Kessler et al. 2009).

Rates of anxiety, mood, and substance use disorders in the United States differ according to people's sex, age, and race. Women's lifetime odds are 60% higher than men's for any anxiety disorder and 50% higher for any mood disorder. In contrast, men are 2.5 times more likely than women to have a substance use disorder and 40% more likely to have an impulse control disorder during their lifetime (Kessler

et al. 2005a). Figure 14.2 shows that the prevalence of all anxiety disorders, major depressive disorder, and dysthymia increases with age until age 60 years. Alcohol abuse and dependence follows a similar pattern, while drug disorders start to decline after age 45.

These declines in rates in older age groups might seem counterintuitive because we expect that greater lifetime exposure will lead to higher lifetime prevalence. Remember, though, that the estimates come from a cross-sectional survey of age cohorts, not from a longitudinal observation of birth cohorts. The lower lifetime estimates in ages after 60 years can be mainly explained by lower incidence rates after middle age, increasing incidence in more recent birth cohorts, early mortality in people with mental health problems, and perhaps failure to recall early health problems.

Data on 5424 Hispanics, non-Hispanic blacks, and non-Hispanic whites from the National Comorbidity Survey Replication (Breslau et al. 2006) showed that both minority groups had lower risk for depression, generalized anxiety disorder, and social phobia. Also, Hispanics had lower risk for dysthymia, oppositional-defiant disorder, and attention deficit hyperactivity disorder; non-Hispanic blacks had

Suicide Risk in Youth and Young Adults

According to the CDC (2010a, 2010b), suicide is the second leading cause of death among 25- to 34-year-olds and the third leading cause of death among 15- to 24-year-olds.

- Among 15- to 24-year-olds, suicide accounts for 12.2% of all deaths annually.

- 13.8% of students in grades 9 through 12 seriously considered suicide in the previous 12 months (17.4% of females and 10.5% of males).

- 6.3% of students reported making at least one suicide attempt in the previous 12 months (8.1% of females and 4.6% of males).

- Suicide death rates are highest among elderly men.

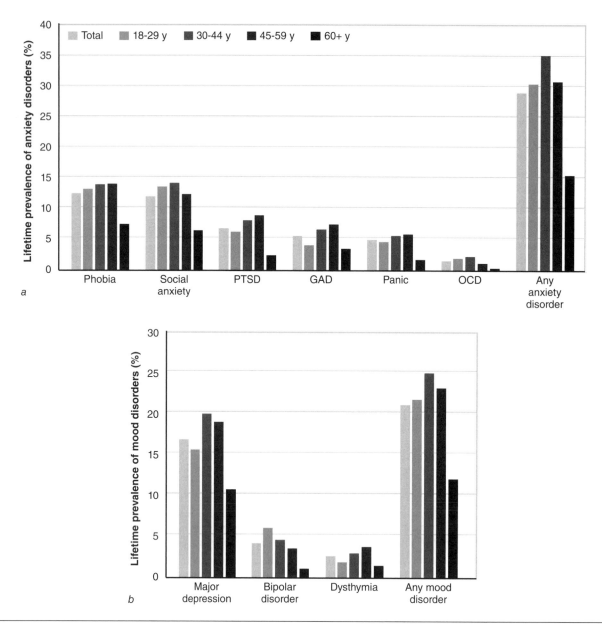

Figure 14.2   Lifetime prevalence estimates of *(a)* anxiety disorders and *(b)* mood disorders in U.S. adults according to age.

Data from Kessler et al. 2005, "Lifetime prevalence and age-of-onset distributions of DSM-IV disorders in the National Comorbidity Survey Replication."

lower risk for panic disorder, substance use disorders, and early-onset impulse control disorders. Lower risk among minorities was more pronounced at lower levels of education. See figure 14.3.

About 80% of people in the United States who attempt suicide have a prior mental disorder (especially mood, anxiety, impulse control, and substance use disorders) (Nock et al. 2010). There are nearly a million suicide deaths each year worldwide. In the United States, more than 30,000 people commit suicide each year, making suicide the 11th leading cause of death. In 2008, suicide was the seventh leading cause of death for males and the 15th leading cause of death for

females. Suicide is the second leading cause of death among American Indians and Alaska Natives ages 15 to 34 years. Almost four times as many males as females die by suicide, but women are two to three times more likely to attempt suicide. For every suicide in the United States, there are 24 nonfatal suicide attempts (Centers for Disease Control and Prevention [CDC] 2010a).

The father of American psychology, William James, recognized the usefulness of exercise for decreasing worry and elevating **mood** at the turn of the 20th century. Hippocrates had prescribed exercise for his patients suffering from depression, which he called *melancholia,* a term still

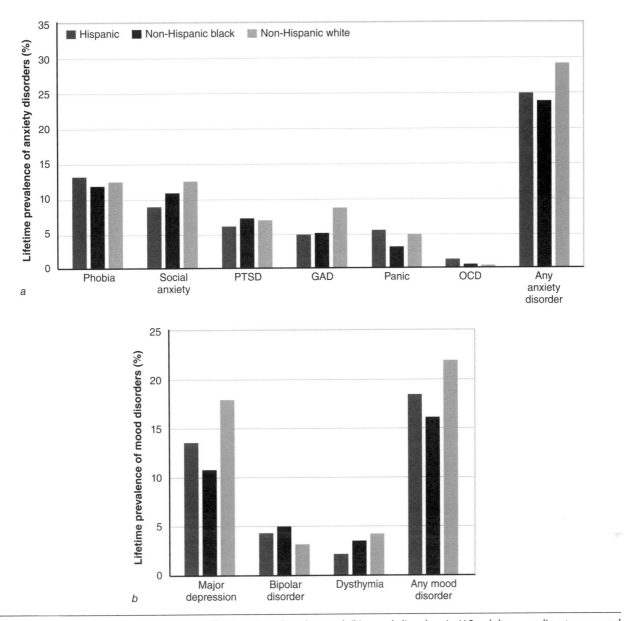

Figure 14.3 Lifetime prevalence estimates of *(a)* anxiety disorders and *(b)* mood disorders in U.S. adults according to race and ethnicity.

Data from Breslau et al. 2006.

used today for severe, somatic depression. As noted by the 17th-century scholar Robert Burton (1632) in *The Anatomy of Melancholy,* sloth or physical inactivity had been regarded as a cause of depression since antiquity. The report of the U.S. Surgeon General on mental health included physical activity as an important part of mental hygiene (U.S. Department of Health and Human Services 1999). This chapter describes the evidence that supports the clinical observations of Hippocrates and James.

A protective effect of physical activity against the primary (i.e., initial incidence) and secondary (i.e., recurrence) risk of developing depression and anxiety disorders would have great potential importance for public health. Not only are anxiety and mood disorders the most prevalent mental health problems in the United States; they are also risk factors for cardiovascular morbidity and mortality.

Depression

The American Psychiatric Association recognizes four types of mood disorders: (1) depression, (2) bipolar or **manic–depressive disorder,** (3) mood disorders due to a medical condition, and (4) substance-induced mood disorders. The first category includes **major depression** and the milder

<table>
<tr><td colspan="2">

Manic–Depressive Disorders

Bipolar I: Major depression alternates with mania, or uncontrollable elation.

Bipolar II: Major depression alternates with hypomania, a milder form of elation.

Cyclothymia: Swings between hypomania and milder depression.
</td></tr>
</table>

chronic form, **dysthymia.** The two principal subtypes of major depression are melancholic and atypical depression, although about half of patients who meet the criteria for major depression do not meet the criteria for either subtype. The second category, bipolar or manic–depressive disorder, is characterized by periods of depression alternating with periods of elevated, expansive, or irritable mood; exaggerated self-confidence; risky or asocial behavior; or even paranoia.

According to the *Diagnostic and Statistical Manual of Mental Disorders,* 4th edition (DSM-IV) (American Psychiatric Association 2000a), people have a major depressive episode when they experience at least five of the following nine symptoms during the same two-week period and these symptoms represent a change from previous functioning. In addition, one of the symptoms must be depressed mood or marked loss of interest or pleasure in activities that were once enjoyable. These are the nine diagnostic symptoms of major depression:

- Depressed mood most of the day, nearly every day
- Marked loss of interest or pleasure in almost all activities most of the day, nearly every day
- Significant weight loss or weight gain when not dieting (e.g., more than 5% of body weight in a month), decrease or increase in appetite nearly every day
- Insomnia or hypersomnia nearly every day
- Psychomotor agitation or retardation nearly every day, observable by others
- Fatigue or loss of energy nearly every day
- Feelings of worthlessness or of excessive and inappropriate guilt nearly every day
- Diminished ability to think or concentrate, or indecisiveness, nearly every day
- Recurrent thoughts of death (not just fear of dying), recurrent ideas of suicide with or without a specific plan, or a suicide attempt

In Europe, the **International Classification of Diseases (ICD-10)** endorsed in 1992 by the WHO in Geneva, Switzerland, defines a depressive episode as depressed mood, loss of interest and enjoyment, and reduced energy leading to increased fatigability (often after only slight effort) and diminished activity (WHO 1992). The depressive episode is classed as mild, moderate, or severe. During a depressive episode, the lowered mood is usually persistent from day to day for at least two weeks, regardless of circumstances, yet tends to improve during the day. A depressive episode may be diagnosed when symptoms have not lasted for two weeks but are very severe and have appeared very rapidly. In some cases, **anxiety** and motor agitation can be more prominent symptoms than depressed mood. Also, mood disturbance can be less apparent than other features such as irritability; abuse of alcohol; and worsening of existing comorbid phobias, obsessions, or preoccupation with physical symptoms.

Some symptoms included in the ICD-10 classification system have special clinical significance for defining typical somatic depression and are similar to those in the American DSM-IV system for the diagnosis of **melancholia.** At least four of the following are required for diagnosis of somatic depression:

- Loss of interest or pleasure in activities that are normally enjoyable
- Lack of emotional reactivity to normally pleasurable surroundings and events
- Waking in the morning 2 h or more before the usual time
- Worse depression in the morning
- Objective evidence of definite psychomotor retardation or agitation (remarked on or reported by other people)
- Marked loss of appetite
- Weight loss (defined as 5% or more of body weight in the past month)
- Marked loss of libido

When a person experiences a major depressive episode, these symptoms cause significant distress and impairment in social and occupational settings as well as in other areas of the person's life. Depression is not considered a major depressive episode if it is caused by drug abuse or medication or a medical condition such as hyperthyroidism, heart disease, diabetes, multiple sclerosis, hepatitis, or rheumatoid arthritis. Also, many people have these symptoms within the first two months after a loved one has died, but this is not considered major depression unless the symptoms are associated with marked functional impairment, a preoccupation with worthlessness, ideas of suicide, psychotic symptoms, or psychomotor retardation.

A DSM-IV diagnosis of dysthymia requires a depressed mood and two or more of the other symptoms of major depression for more days than not, for at least two years, without an interruption of symptoms for more than two

Common Symptoms of a Depressive Episode According to the International Classification of Diseases (ICD-10)

- Reduced concentration and attention
- Reduced self-esteem and self-confidence
- Ideas of guilt and unworthiness (even in a mild type of episode)
- Bleak and pessimistic views of the future
- Ideas or acts of self-harm or suicide
- Disturbed sleep
- Diminished appetite

WHO 1992.

months. In children and adolescents, mood can be irritable, and duration must be at least one year.

Minor depression is not a formal diagnostic category. It is not as severe as major depression and is characterized by at least two symptoms of depression, one of which must be depressed mood or loss of pleasure, most days for at least two weeks.

▷ **THE WHO** has projected that depression will be second only to cardiovascular disease as the world's leading cause of death and disability by the year 2020 and will be first by 2030.

Magnitude of the Problem

Estimates from epidemiologic research in England, Finland, Australia, and the United States suggest that 8% of women and 4% of men have some form of clinical depression at any point in time (Lehtinen and Joukamaa 1994). In the United States, 4.5% to 9.3% of all women and 2.3% to 3.2% of all men have a major depressive disorder. The annual prevalence of major depression in the United States has increased steadily during the past 50 years. African Americans tend to experience less depression than white Americans, while nonwhites of Hispanic ancestry have more depression than whites. The National Comorbidity Survey found a lifetime rate of 17% for major depression (21% for women and 13% for men) and a rate of 5% when people were asked whether they had been depressed in the previous month (Kessler et al. 1994). The replication of that survey 10 years later estimated that the lifetime prevalence of major depression among U.S. adults was 16% (Kessler et al. 2003). Except for manic episodes in bipolar disorder, women have nearly twice the rate of depression as men.

Results From the National Comorbidity Survey

The National Comorbidity Survey Replication in the United States and the WHO World Mental Health Surveys found that people who have had major depression are two to three times more likely than others to attempt suicide. The odds of suicidal thoughts are elevated in people who are depressed, but people who have severe anxiety or agitation (e.g., post-traumatic stress disorder) and poor impulse control (e.g., conduct disorder or substance use disorders) are most likely to then plan or attempt suicide (Nock et al. 2009, 2010).

The onset of increased rates of depression occurs during early adolescence, affecting about 8% to 9% of boys and girls annually (Rushton, Forcier, and Schectman 2002). The annual rate of depression among teenagers and young adults is about twice that of adults 25 to 44 years of age and four times the rate among people over age 65 (Kessler et al. 1994). Worldwide, 12-month prevalence estimates of suicide thoughts, plans, and attempts are about 2.0%, 0.6%, and 0.3% of the populations, respectively, in developed nations and are similar in developing nations (Borges et al. 2010).

Risk Factors for Suicidal Behaviors

- Female sex
- Younger age
- Less education, low income or unemployed
- Unmarried
- Parental psychopathology
- Childhood adversities
- Presence of 12-month DSM-IV mental disorders

Source: Borges et al. 2010

Why Is the Rate of Depression Higher in Women?

Four possible reasons have been proposed:

- They ruminate more about their problems.
- They are more introspective and more likely to seek help.
- In many cultures they have less control over their lives than men, leading to helplessness and despair.
- Flux in reproductive hormones such as estrogen increases risk of depression during menstruation and menopause, while women are taking birth control pills, and after childbirth.

Etiology of Depression

There are many causes of depression, and at least 10 different theoretical models of the etiology of depressive disorders have been proposed, including existential models, based on loss of purpose; social models, based on loss of role status; cognitive models, based on irrational thought; learning modes, based on loss of control and helplessness; and biochemical models, based on malfunction of brain neurotransmission. A modern biological framework, which encompasses social and psychological factors, for the etiology and treatment of depression and other mental disorders is based on the following five principles proposed by Nobel Prize–winning psychiatrist Eric Kandel (1998):

1. Actions at the brain level are responsible for all mental and psychological processes.
2. Brain functioning is controlled by genes.
3. Social, developmental, and environmental factors can produce alterations in gene expression.
4. Alterations in gene expression induce changes in brain functioning.
5. Treatments for mental illness exert their effect by producing alterations in gene expression, resulting in beneficial changes in brain function.

Within this framework, depression is thought to result from disturbances in brain neuronal function; and effective treatments for depression, such as psychotherapy, medication, or exercise, are hypothesized to produce treatment responses in brain function at a genetic level that result in alleviation of depressive symptoms.

The etiology of depression can include catastrophic events such as major physical illness, loss of a loved one through death or separation, loss of **self-esteem** (e.g., feeling unworthy for not meeting academic goals), or chronic anxiety or stress (e.g., worry or a feeling that life is out of one's control). Depression, especially a somatic or melancholic depressive episode, can also occur for no apparent reason. A direct genetic abnormality leading to depression has not been confirmed, but some people are more vulnerable to depression. Regardless of cause, depression is associated with imbalances in **neurotransmitters,** chemicals that influence the activity of brain cells that regulate mood, pleasure, and rational thought.

Studies of neurotransmitter systems involved in depression have focused primarily on **noradrenergic** and **serotonergic** systems mainly because most effective pharmacotherapies modulate either or both of these neurotransmitter systems. The norepinephrine system originates primarily in the **locus coeruleus,** a small region in the brain stem, and projects to numerous brain regions, including areas associated with the regulation of emotion, such as the hippocampus, amygdala, and frontal cortex, as well as a dopamine circuit between the ventral tegmentum and the nucleus accumbens in the ventral striatum. The **serotonin,** or 5-hydroxytryptamine (5-HT), system similarly sends projections to those areas, including the locus coeruleus, from the **raphe nuclei** in the brain stem (figure 14.4).

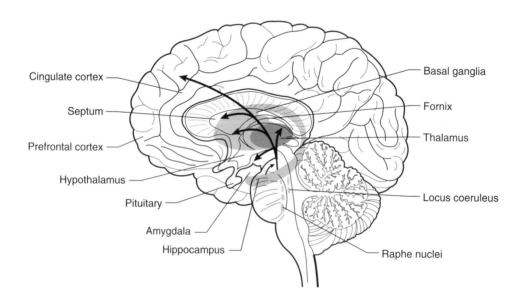

Figure 14.4   Cross section of the central nervous system showing limbic structures (hippocampus, amygdala, cingulate cortex, fornix). Arrows show the pathways from the raphe nuclei to the central structures.

Reprinted, by permission, from J. Buckworth and R.K. Dishman, 2002, *Exercise psychology* (Champaign, IL: Human Kinetics), 48.

Brain Neurobiology in Depression

A neurobiological perspective on depression integrates cognitive and neurological theories. For example, neural circuits involved with depression must involve brain neural circuits that regulate mood, pleasure, pain, memories about reward for behavior, and abstract **cognitions** such as optimism. The effects of these different neural systems are dependent on several neurotransmitters, which have been targets for the pharmacologic treatment of depressive disorders.

The evidence accumulated from neuroscience studies that have used the techniques of brain lesioning, **electrophysiological measures,** and **neuroimaging** has so far identified six key brain regions that seem to be most involved in the expression of human **emotion**, including depression and anxiety (Davidson and Irwin 1999; Drevets 1998). These are (1) the **prefrontal cortex;** (2) the **amygdala,** especially the central portion; (3) the **hippocampus;** (4) the **ventral striatum,** especially the **nucleus accumbens** located below the front of the caudate and putamen; (5) the **cingulate cortex,** a layer of gray matter lying between the cerebrum and the lateral ventricle; and (6) the **insular cortex,** an island of involuted cortex near the temporal lobe. These brain regions function synergistically, but they each appear to have some unique functions:

• The prefrontal cortex stores memories of the consequences of behaviors or experiences that were aversive or pleasurable; this permits an emotion to be sustained long enough to direct behavior toward the goal that is appropriate for that emotion.

• The amygdala plays a key role in integrating overt behavior, autonomic responses, and hormonal responses during stress and emotion. It influences the valence (i.e., pleasantness or unpleasantness of an experience or memory). Also, its tonic level of activity is sensitive to negative mood. For example, activity in the amygdala is elevated among patients diagnosed with depression and anxiety disorders.

• The hippocampus processes memories of the environmental context in which an emotion occurs before those memories are stored in the brain region where they were experienced (e.g., visual, auditory, or gustatory [taste] memories). People who have damage to the hippocampus still experience emotion but often at inappropriate times or places.

• The ventral striatum, especially the nucleus accumbens, is in the pathway of **dopamine** neurons in the midbrain that are key in what is known as reward-motivated behavior. It plays a role in regulating approach behaviors (e.g., drives, urges, and cravings) that result in pleasure.

• The anterior cingulate cortex is part of the primitive cortex common to species other than humans. It helps regulate attention during the processing of pleasure or displeasure during an emotion.

• The insular cortex receives sensory inputs from the autonomic nervous system, especially cardiovascular responses, and sends signals to the central amygdala and the hypothalamus, which each regulate cardiac and endocrine responses during stress.

In addition to these brain regions, the dopaminergic neuronal circuit between the **ventral tegmental area (VTA)** (a group of neural cell bodies in the underside of an area at the top of the brain stem, between the pons and the fourth ventricle of the brain), the nucleus accumbens, and the prefrontal cortex is key in regulating motivation through its involvement in pleasure and the memory of pleasurable events (figure 14.5).

Many antidepressant drugs target the monoamines (i.e., serotonin, norepinephrine, and dopamine). The drugs that are currently most popular target serotonergic systems by blocking serotonin reuptake or acting on serotonergic receptors as agonists or antagonists. In addition, norepinephrine reuptake inhibitors have a long history of **efficacy** in the treatment of depression, and new dopamine agonists are also efficacious as antidepressants.

The synthesis and metabolic pathways for norepinephrine and its receptors in the brain are the same as for peripheral noradrenergic nerves to the heart and blood vessels as described in chapter 7 on hypertension. Drugs that block β-adrenorecptors are sometimes used with anxiety patients to reduce cardiovascular symptoms. Drugs that block the reuptake of norepinephrine by the neuron (selective norepinephrine reuptake inhibitors [SNRIs]) after its release by inhibiting

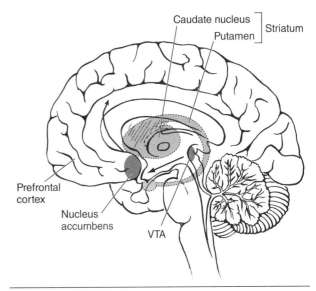

Figure 14.5 The ventral tegmental area (VTA), a major site of brain dopamine, is shown in relation to the basal ganglia (caudate nucleus, putamen, and nucleus accumbens). Reward pathway from the VTA to the nucleus accumbens to the prefrontal cortex.

Reprinted, by permission, from J. Buckworth and R.K. Dishman, 2002, *Exercise psychology* (Champaign, IL: Human Kinetics), 55.

proteins that act as a norepinephrine transporter (NET) are used to treat both anxiety and depressive disorders. Other commonly prescribed antidepressant medications specifically target the serotonin system. For example, selective serotonin reuptake inhibitors (SSRIs) act to block serotonin reuptake by inhibiting a serotonin transporter (SERT), allowing the neurotransmitter to remain in the synapse. The synthesis of serotonin from the amino acid tryptophan, its metabolic pathways, and its receptors are illustrated in figure 14.6.

Although research has focused primarily on the role of norepinephrine and serotonin in depression, more attention has recently been paid to understanding the role of dopamine in the etiology of depression and its symptoms. Because the dopamine system plays a critical role in reward, motivation, and motor functions, **dysregulation** of this system may contribute to the anhedonia (i.e., loss of pleasure) and psychomotor disturbances that are observed in depression. Also, prolonged elevations in cortisol during chronic stress have been accompanied by dysfunction of dopamine neurons (Chrousos 1998), and some antidepressant drugs influence the activity of dopamine neurons by targeting dopamine receptors or altering dopamine metabolism (Willner 1995). Dopamine is the precursor molecule for the synthesis of

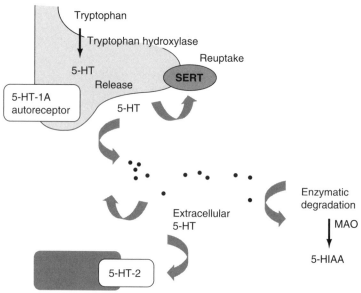

Figure 14.6 Serotonin synthesis, action at the synapse, and metabolism reuptake.

norepinephrine, so the two share the same synthetic and metabolic pathways. Key receptors for dopamine in brain neurons are depicted in figure 14.7. Later in this chapter, we present evidence that exercise could protect against depression by altering brain monoamines and the function of their neurons.

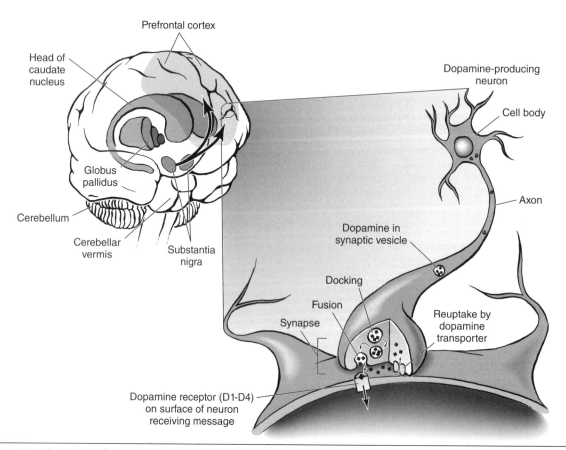

Figure 14.7 Structures of the basal ganglia and the actions of dopamine from production to postsynaptic activation.

Treatment of Depression

Despite their higher prevalence of depression, women respond to treatment as well as or better than men. Most adults who suffer depression can be effectively treated as outpatients with antidepressant medications, psychotherapy, or a combination of the two treatments. People who do not respond to those treatments are switched to another anti-depressant or given augmentation therapy that combines different types of antidepressant drugs. Or, they may be helped by electroconvulsive therapy (ECT), or electroshock treatment, in which small amounts of electric current are passed through the brain. Most depression is called uni-polar, characterized only by depressed mood. A smaller percentage of people have manic–depressive disorder. As already mentioned, they experience periods of depressed mood alternating with periods of elevated, expansive, or irritable mood; exaggerated self-confidence; risky or asocial behavior; or even paranoia. They are often treated with a drug called lithium.

The treatment of depression, by either drugs or psy-chotherapy, involves acute, continuation, and maintenance stages as depicted in figure 14.8. Hospitalization is required for about 5% to 10% of major depressive episodes and for about half of manic episodes, mainly because of debilitating symptoms and risk of suicide or self-harm.

Because of high costs, the average hospital stay is about a week for depression and 10 days to two weeks for mania, but depressive symptoms are seldom reduced within one to two weeks, and patients usually require follow-up out-patient care.

Acute Phase

Acute-phase treatment continues until a clinically meaning-ful treatment response is observed, which is defined as a reduction in symptoms of more than 50%, or long enough that the patient no longer meets diagnostic criteria of a depressive episode (i.e., remission). When pharmacotherapy is indicated, this commonly takes six to eight weeks, during which patients are observed each or every other week in order to monitor symptoms and side effects and to adjust medication dosage. Psychotherapy commonly consists of six to 20 weekly sessions during the acute phase of depression treatment. About 50% to 70% of depressed patients treated as outpatients respond favorably to drug treatment or psy-chotherapy. Drugs are typically changed if a patient does not respond within four to six weeks and are often added to psychotherapy if symptoms have not improved within three to four months. It is acknowledged that acute response to treatment includes the combined effects of placebo expec-tancy, spontaneous remission, and active treatment.

Psychotherapy

The two most effective types of psychotherapy used to treat depression are behavioral therapy and cognitive–behavioral therapy. Behavioral therapy teaches patients how to control their environment in ways that reduce the risk of depression and how to minimize situations that compound symptoms. Cognitive–behavioral therapy builds on the behavioral approach by helping patients better understand faulty thinking that contributes to their feelings of helplessness, hopeless-ness, and despair.

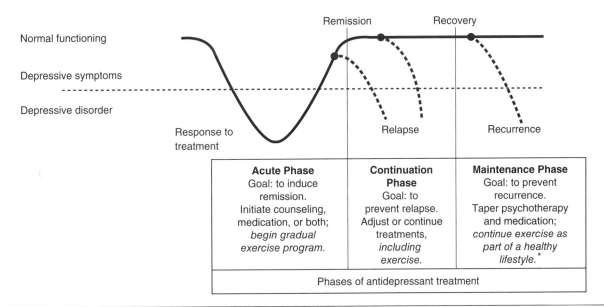

Figure 14.8 Phases of antidepressant treatment. Because depressive episodes often recur, long-term maintenance of remission is an important clinical issue. While pharmacotherapy and psychotherapy are tapered and withdrawn following remission of depres-sion, exercise may be continued and incorporated into the individual's lifestyle. Thus, unlike those of most other traditional treat-ments, the potential antidepressant effects of exercise are not time limited.

Adapted, by permission, from H.A. O'Neal, A.L. Dunn, and E.W. Martinsen, 2000, "Depression and exercise," *International Journal of Sports Psychology* 31: 113.

Pharmacotherapy

More than 30 drugs are being used in the United States and worldwide to treat depression; common ones are listed in the sidebar. In 2005, an estimated 27 million Americans used antidepressant medication, including 2.5% of children ages 6 to 17 years (Olfson and Marcus 2009). Half of the patients used the drugs for back or nerve pain, fatigue, sleep difficulties, or other problems aside from depression.

Among users of antidepressants, the percentage receiving psychotherapy fell from 31.5% in 1996 to less than 20% in 2005. About 80% of patients were treated by doctors other than psychiatrists. In 2009, an estimated 169 million prescriptions were filled for antidepressants in the United States, making them the third most often prescribed class of drugs behind only lipid drugs and codeine-based medicines used mainly for pain (IMS Health 2010).

▶ **IN 2009,** an estimated 169 million prescriptions were filled for antidepressants in the United States, making them the third most prescribed class of drugs behind only lipid drugs and codeine-based medicines.

The most common drugs used to treat depression are tricyclics, introduced in the 1940s, which block the reuptake of monoamines released by brain neurons; monoamine oxidase inhibitors (MAOIs), introduced in the 1950s, which block the deamination (i.e., metabolism) of monoamines after neuronal release; and selective serotonin reuptake inhibitors (SSRIs), introduced in the late 1980s, that block reentry of serotonin into the neuron after release. The SSRIs are currently the most popular, not because they are more effective but because they have fewer side effects (e.g., less sedation, dry mouth, dizziness, faintness, stomach upset, and weight gain) than do the tricyclics.

During the 1990s, selective norepinephrine reuptake inhibitors (SNRIs; e.g., reboxetine), which selectively block the reuptake of norepinephrine, and drugs that simultaneously block the reuptake of both norepinephrine and serotonin (e.g., venlafaxine) or that block reuptake of dopamine (e.g., amineptine and bupropion) more than norepinephrine and serotonin, became popular. Some other tetracyclic antidepressants (also known as noradrenergic and specific serotonin antidepressants (NaSSAs), first introduced in the 1970s, have a different chemical structure from tricyclics and MAOIs. They do not affect the reuptake or metabolism of monoamines; rather, they block receptors (e.g., mianserin blocks 5-HT$_2$ [serotonin] receptors, and mirtazapine blocks α_2 [norepinephrine] autoreceptors). By blocking α_2-adrenergic autoreceptors, as well as α_1 and 5-HT$_3$ receptors, NaSSAs enhance adrenergic and serotonergic neurotransmission, especially 5-HT$_{1A}$-mediated transmission.

Common Antidepressant Drugs

Tricyclics

Anafranil (clomipramine)
Asendin (amoxapine)
Aventyl (nortriptyline)
Elavil (amitriptyline)
Norpramin (desipramine)
Pamelor (nortriptyline)
Sinequan (doxepin)
Surmontil (trimipramine)
Tofranil (imipramine)
Vivactil (protriptyline)

Monoamine Oxidase Inhibitors

Marplan (isocarboxazid)
Nardil (phenelzine sulfate)
Parnate (tranylcypromine sulfate)

Selective Serotonin Reuptake Inhibitors

Celexa (citalopram)
Desyrel (trazodone), now available as generic
Lexapro (escitalopram)
Ludiomil (maprotiline)
Paxil (paroxetine)
Prozac (fluoxetine)
Selfemra (fluoxetine)
Zoloft (sertraline)

Selective Serotonin and Noradrenaline Reuptake Inhibitors

Cymbalta (duloxetine)
Effexor (venlafaxine)
Luvox (fluvoxamine)
Pristiq (sustained-release desvenlafaxine)
Serzone (nefazodone)

Dopamine Agonists

Wellbutrin (bupropion)
Zyban (sustained-release bupropion)

Tetracyclic Noradrenergic and Specific Serotonin Antidepressants

Mianserin (Bolvidon, Norval, Tolvon)
Mirtazapine (Remeron, Avanza, Zispin)
Setiptiline (Tecipul)

Neuronal Effects of Antidepressant Drugs

First Line, Acute

- Blocked reuptake of norepinephrine or serotonin
- Reduced norepinephrine cell firing in brain stem
- Temporary reduction of norepinephrine synthesis and turnover
- Blocked α_1 and α_2 receptors for norepinephrine

Baldessarini 1989.

Second Line, Chronic (10 to 20 Days)

- Sustained blockade of norepinephrine or serotonin reuptake
- Transient **downregulation** of α_2 receptors
- Normalization of norepinephrine cell firing rate and turnover; increased norepinephrine synthesis and release
- Downregulation of β_1 and upregulation of α_1 and serotonin 5-HT receptors

People suffering from bipolar disorder, or manic depression, are usually treated with lithium carbonate (Baldessarini et al. 2002), lithium citrate, or aripiprazole (Abilify), which is an atypical-type antipsychotic drug. Lithium is an alkaline metal like sodium and potassium and forms a salt when combined with carbonate or citrate. The mechanism by which lithium controls manic episodes and reduces severe depression is not fully known, but lithium alters sodium transport and may interfere with ion exchange mechanisms (e.g., preventing reentry of potassium into brain neurons) and nerve conduction. Lithium enhances the reuptake of norepinephrine and serotonin by the brain neurons that release them, reduces the release of norepinephrine from brain neurons, and inhibits production of the neural second messenger cyclic adenosine monophosphate (cAMP). Though lithium can disturb the regulation of body water and electrolytes, which can impair temperature regulation and cardiovascular function, studies have confirmed that exercise does not alter lithium metabolism (Jefferson et al. 1982).

Though many people with depression respond well to prescription drugs or psychological treatments, about half the people who have an episode of clinical depression go undiagnosed or misdiagnosed. Of people who are correctly diagnosed with depression and would be helped by antidepressant drugs, half have never taken them, and less than a third are prescribed the appropriate dose (Kessler et al. 2007). The drugs have varying negative side effects for many people, including somnolence (sleepiness), dry mouth, stomach and intestinal distress, increased appetite, weight gain, dizziness, blurred vision, and sexual impairment, as well as more serious cardiovascular problems such as low blood pressure and irregular heart rate.

About half of depressed patients treated with antidepressant drugs still have residual symptoms after two or more months of treatment. In the Sequenced Treatment Alternatives to Relieve Depression (STAR*D) study, only 47% of nearly 2900 depressed patients had a favorable response (i.e., a 50% drop in symptoms) after six to eight weeks or more of antidepressant treatment with the SSRI citalopram. Only 27% remitted (i.e., no longer had symptoms). Then, nonremitters who still had symptoms were switched to either sertraline (another SSRI), venlafaxine (a combination SSRI and SNRI), or bupropion-SR (a norepinephrine and dopamine reuptake inhibitor). About 25% of those patients subsequently remitted (Rush et al. 2006; Trivedi et al. 2006a). Another group of nonremitters were switched to cognitive therapy and had a similar remission rate (31%) during the second round of treatment. Psychotherapy was better tolerated than drug therapy, but augmentation of citalopram with another drug was quicker acting than augmentation with cognitive therapy (40 days compared with 55 days, on average) (Gaynes et al. 2009).

These facts indicate the potential importance of self-help behaviors, such as exercise, that can enhance mental hygiene (Freeman et al. 2010). Many studies agree that regular physical activity can reduce symptoms after a person becomes depressed and can reduce the odds that a person will experience depression. As discussed later, exercise may have effects on the brain monoamine systems similar to the effects of antidepressant drugs; or the exercise setting may have cognitive effects that are beneficial, such as increasing physical self-esteem. Exercise can also help offset residual symptoms of ineffective drug therapy by increasing feelings of energy and by promoting better sleep and improved sexual function. Exercise training has even been successful as an augmentation therapy among patients who have not responded to pharmacotherapy (Trivedi et al. 2006b).

Physical Activity and Depression: The Evidence

The first reports by psychiatrists using exercise to treat depression in the United States appeared in 1905. The mood and reaction times of two depressed men were improved on days they exercised for about 2 h compared with days they rested (Franz and Hamilton 1905). The use of exercise in psychiatry continued in the United States through the 1950s (Campbell and Davis 1939-1940; Layman 1960) without scientific evaluation.

William P. Morgan and colleagues at the University of Missouri (Morgan et al. 1970) conducted the first experimental study showing that self-ratings of depressive symptoms could be reduced in men after an exercise training program. That finding was extended by Morgan with psychiatrist John Greist in a small, randomized clinical trial of psychiatric outpatients at the University of Wisconsin, which showed that the reduction in depressive symptoms after 12 weeks of running therapy was equivalent to or greater than that with two forms of group psychotherapy (Greist et al. 1978). Moreover, nine of the 10 patients treated with running therapy were still running and not depressed nine months later, while depressive symptoms had returned in the other patients.

In 1984, the National Institute of Mental Health Workshop on Exercise and Mental Health concluded that exercise is associated with a decreased level of mild to moderate depression (Morgan and Goldston 1987). That conclusion was upheld at the Second International Consensus Symposium on Physical Activity, Fitness, and Health held in Toronto in 1992 (Bouchard, Shephard, and Stephens 1994), by the U.S. Surgeon General's report *Physical Activity and Health* (U.S. Department of Health and Human Services 1996), and by the scientific advisory committee of the 2008 Physical Activity Guidelines for Americans (Physical Activity Guidelines Advisory Committee 2008).

The documentation of an association between exercise and the reduction in symptoms of mild to moderate depression has come from population studies, narrative and quantitative (i.e., **meta-analyses**) reviews of research literature, and exercise training studies conducted with clinical and nonclinical populations. About 30 studies qualify as prospective population-based, epidemiologic studies; about 90 studies were randomized controlled trials of patients with chronic medical conditions other than depression; and about 30 studies were randomized controlled trials of people diagnosed as having depression. Most studies of exercise and depression have been conducted in young to middle-aged adults. Among people over age 65, the evidence suggests that the benefits of exercise for reducing symptoms of depression may diminish as people age (O'Connor, Aenchbacher, and Dishman 1993; Physical Activity Guidelines Advisory Committee 2008); however, despite more age-related depression-like symptoms among older people (e.g., sleep and cognitive disorders), older people have a lower prevalence of clinically diagnosed depression than young and middle-aged adults. The benefits of physical activity for helping *prevent* depression and for reducing depression symptoms usually occur regardless of people's age, sex, race, or socioeconomic status.

▷ THE BENEFITS of physical activity for helping prevent depression occur regardless of people's age, sex, race, or socioeconomic status.

Preventing Depression: Observational Studies

More than 150 observational, epidemiological studies have shown an association between physical activity levels and lower odds of depression symptoms. More than three-fourths of these have been published in the past decade. About 85% of the studies have shown lower depression with higher physical activity.

Early Studies

Two early prospective studies followed depression over time and compared people's risk with their physical activity:

• In the Alameda County (California) Study, about 5000 nondepressed adult men and women completed surveys on physical activity and depression in 1965 (Camacho et al. 1991). Those who were not depressed in 1965 were studied again in 1974 and 1983. Participants were classified as low active, medium active, or high active based on self-reported frequency (i.e., never, sometimes, often) and intensity of physical activity in the categories of active sports, swimming, walking, doing exercises, or gardening. Inactive people who were not depressed in 1965 had a 70% increase in risk of depression in 1974 compared with those who were initially highly active. Associations between changes in activity from 1965 to 1983 and symptoms of depression in 1983 suggested that the risk of depression was alterable by increasing exercise, but this association was not independent of the other risk factors for depression.

• In a study of about 10,000 male Harvard University alumni from the mid-1960s through 1977, physical activity was shown to reduce the likelihood of developing physician-diagnosed depression (Paffenbarger, Lee, and Leung 1994). Figure 14.9 illustrates that those who expended 1000 to 2500 kcal per week by walking, climbing stairs, or playing sports had 17% less risk of developing depression compared with their less active peers. Those who expended more than 2500 kcal per week had a 28% lower risk.

Cross-Sectional Studies

An association between leisure-time physical activity and reduced symptoms of depression among adults has been generally supported in more than 100 population-based, cross-sectional observational studies from many countries published since 2000, including nationally representative samples of nearly 200,000 Americans. Active people on average had nearly 45% lower odds of depression symptoms than did inactive people. In the national samples of Americans, active people had approximately 30% lower odds of depression. The studies did not have the temporal sequencing needed to infer that lower depression resulted from more physical activity and often failed to adjust for other risk

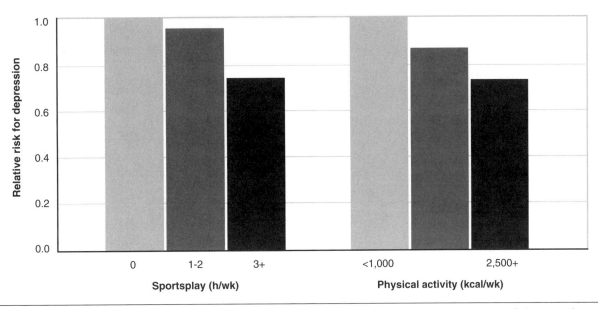

Figure 14.9   Harvard alumni study of 10,201 males. Measured activity habits in 1962 to 1966 and incidence of physician-diagnosed depression during 23- to 27-year follow-up.

Data from Paffenbarger, Lee, and Leung 1994.

factors of depression that might have also been less prevalent among more active people. Nonetheless, these studies provide some evidence for dose–response associations and consistency across population subgroups.

U.S. National Comorbidity Survey

Goodwin (2003) analyzed data from the U.S. National Comorbidity Survey (n = 5877), a nationally representative sample of adults ages 15 to 54 in the United States. People who said they regularly got physical exercise for recreation or at work had 25% lower odds of being diagnosed with major depression during the past year (OR = 0.75; 95% CI: 0.6-0.94) after adjustment for age, gender, race, marital status, education, income, physical illnesses, and other mental disorders. There was a dose–response reduction in the odds of major depression, dysthymia, and bipolar disorder with higher frequency of physical activity. See figure 14.10.

CARDIA

History of elevated depression symptoms was measured by the Center for Epidemiologic Studies Depression Scale (CES-D) (number of times scores were 16 or more from three assessments, years 5, 10, and 15 of follow-up) in black (1157 men and 1480 women) and white (1171 men and 1307 women) Americans enrolled in the Coronary Artery Risk Development in Young Adults Study (Knox et al. 2006). After adjustment for age, education, alcohol use, smoking, and body mass index (BMI), there was an inverse association (about 28 fewer metabolic equivalents [METs] during the past year for each episode of elevated depression symptoms)

between history of depression symptoms and physical activity at year 15 that was consistent across race.

The Medical Expenditure Panel Survey

A nationally representative survey of the U.S. population in 2003 asked 23,283 adults whether they engaged in moderate or vigorous activity for 30 min or more, three times per week (Morrato et al. 2007). Depressive disorder or major depression was diagnosed from survey responses according to the International Classification of Diseases, version 9. Among all adults, odds of depression were 40% lower in people who were physically active (OR = 0.60; 95% CI: 0.55-0.66). Lower odds of depression in active people were attenuated but remained significant after adjustment for sex, age, race and ethnicity, education, income, BMI, cardiovascular disease, hypertension, hyperlipidemia, and physical disability.

The 2006 Behavioral Risk Factor Surveillance Survey

This was a random-digit-dialed telephone survey of 217,379 participants in 38 states, the District of Columbia, Puerto Rico, and the U.S. Virgin Islands (Strine et al. 2008). About 24% of participants in the BRFSS said they had not participated in any leisure-time physical activity or exercise during the past 30 days. Regardless of age, inactive people were three times more likely to have current depression symptoms (OR= 2.9; 95% CI: 2.7-3.2) and 50% more likely to have ever been told they had depression by a physician or health provider (OR = 1.5; 95% CI: 1.5-1.6). Those odds were still elevated after adjustment for age, sex, race and ethnicity, education,

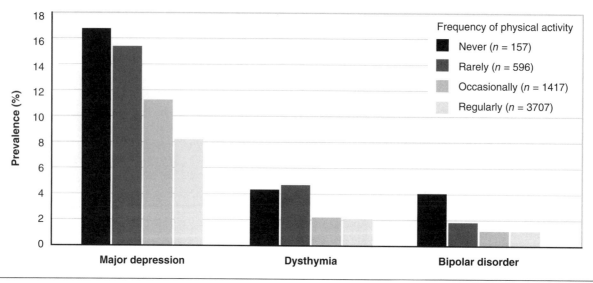

Figure 14.10 Twelve-month prevalence rates of mood disorders according to frequency of physical activity in the U.S. National Comorbidity Survey.

Data from Goodwin 2003.

marital and job status, chronic medical conditions, smoking, obesity, and heavy alcohol use.

The Netherlands Twin Registry

This sample consisted of 12,450 adolescents (at least 10 years old) and adults who participated in a study on lifestyle and health from 1991 to 2002 (De Moor et al. 2006). The prevalence of exercise participation (at least an hour each week in activities rated at 4 METs or more) was 51.4%. After adjustment for gender and age, odds of symptoms of depression were approximately 17% lower among exercisers (OR = 0.83; 95% CI: 0.78-0.89). However, that association was likely confounded by personality because the exercisers also were more extraverted and emotionally stable; these are traits that reduce the risks of anxiety and depression disorders. In fact, among pairs of identical twins (479 male and 943 female) aged 18 to 50 years, the twin who exercised more did not report fewer symptoms of depression than the twin who exercised less (De Moor et al. 2008).

Prospective Cohort Studies

More than 30 population-based prospective studies of exercise and depression have been reported around the world since the first one in 1988. These have included about 50,000 adults from studies from the United States and 11 other countries (Australia, Canada, China, Denmark, England, Finland, Germany, Israel, Italy, Netherlands, and Japan). Nearly all of them showed that symptoms of depression are more likely to appear among people who report little or no leisure-time physical activity; but about half the results did not reach a high level of statistical significance, often because the sample

sizes were too small (a fourth of the comparisons included 500 or fewer people) given the relatively small and varying reductions in risk. Because these studies were prospective and satisfied temporal sequencing, it is less likely that the associations seen were explainable by people's becoming less active after they experienced depression symptoms. The average follow-up was about four years (ranging from nine months to 37 years).

When averaged across the studies, the odds of elevated symptoms were about 33% lower among active compared with inactive people, without adjustments for depression risk factors that might have differed between the active and inactive groups (OR = 0.67; 95% CI: 0.59-0.77). After adjustment for risk factors such as age, sex, race, education, income, smoking, alcohol use, chronic health conditions, and other social and psychological risk factors, the odds remained about 20% lower among active people (OR = 0.82; 95% CI: 0.78-0.86). See figure 14.11.

The apparently protective effect of physical activity against depression is not limited to self-rated symptoms measured by questionnaires. At least 10 studies have reported lower rates of physician-diagnosed incident depression among people who were active at baseline. After adjustment for risk factors such as age, sex, race, education, income, smoking, alcohol use, and medical conditions (but not psychiatric comorbidities), average odds were about 25% lower among active people (OR = 0.74; 95% CI: 0.67-0.81).

Alameda County Study

Participants, 1947 adults aged 50 to 94 years living near Oakland and Berkeley, California, were assessed in 1994 and then followed for five years (Strawbridge et al. 2002). The

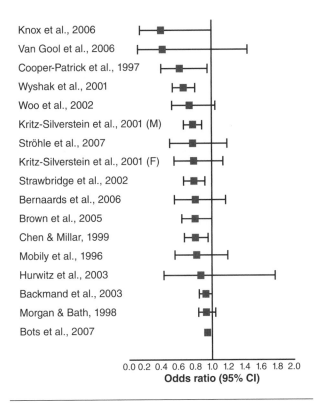

Figures 14.11 Adjusted odds ratios and 95% confidence intervals from prospective cohort studies of physical activity and depression published between 1995 and 2008.

Data from Physical Activity Guidelines Advisory Committee 2008

incident rate of depression measured using DSM-IV diagnostic criteria was 5.4% of the cohort. After adjustment for age, sex, ethnicity, financial strain, chronic health conditions, disability, BMI, alcohol use, smoking, and social relations, there was a 17% reduction in risk of incident depression over five years for each point scored on a physical activity measure in 1994 (OR = 0.83; 95% CI: 0.73-0.96) over five years.

Australian Longitudinal Study on Women's Health

This study examined the dose–response relations between physical activity and depressive symptoms in a population-based cohort of 9207 middle-aged women who completed mailed surveys about physical activity in 1996, 1998, and 2001 (Brown et al. 2005). After adjustment for education, marital status, occupation, smoking, BMI, menopause, health conditions, and scores on another measure of feelings of depression and anxiety, odds ratios for elevated CES-D scores in 1998 and 2001 (a score of 10 or more) in 2001 were 30% to 40% lower among women who reported an hour or more of moderate-intensity physical activity per week currently or in the preceding years, compared with those who reported less than an hour. Women who were in the lowest physical activity category in 1996 (i.e., less than 200 MET-minutes per week),

but who subsequently reported 600 or more MET-minutes per week, had lower odds of elevated scores in 2001 (OR = 0.78; 95% CI: 0.61-1.01) than women who were still in the lowest activity group in 2001 (i.e., < 240 MET-minutes per week).

In another cohort of 6677 young women (22-27 years in 2000), depressive symptoms were reported in 2000 and at follow-up in 2003 (Ball, Burton, and Brown 2008). Figure 14.12 shows that women in each of the low to high levels of physical activity in 2000 had lower odds of elevated symptoms in 2003 compared to women who said they got less then 300 MET-minutes of weekly physical activity. Women who were sedentary in 2000 (none or very low) had a 25% reduction in adjusted odds of elevated depression symptoms in 2003 if they increased their activity to a moderate level and a 50% reduction if they became highly active in 2003.

Northern Rivers Mental Health Study, Australia

A cohort of community residents living in the Richmond Valley of New South Wales was followed for a two-year period in order to identify the factors that were predictive of changes in their mental health status regardless of their past history (Beard et al. 2007). After random telephone screening to recruit a cohort at risk of mental disorders, 1407 invited subjects completed baseline face-to-face interviews using the Mini WHO CIDI diagnostic interview (ICD-10 criteria) (859 [51.4%] likely cases and 548 [56.9%] likely noncases). After two years, 968 adults ages 18 to 85 were reinterviewed. Higher baseline levels of walking more than 105 min per week (OR = 0.47; 95% CI: 0.20-1.12), but not minutes of

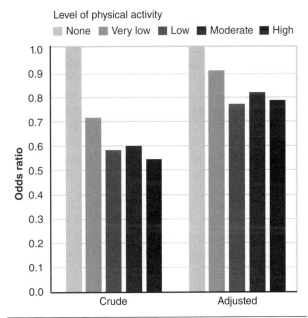

Figure 14.12 Dose response of physical activity and incident reports of depression symptoms in the Australian Longitudinal Study on Women's Health.

Data from Ball, Burton, and Brown 2008.

vigorous physical activity, were protective against incident depression (excluding bipolar disorder and dysthymia). The benefit of walking no longer held after adjustment for age, stressful life events, emotional stability, and symptoms of distress measured at baseline.

U.S. Black Women's Health Study

A total of 35,224 African American women ages 21 to 69 answered mailed questions on past and current exercise levels at baseline (1995) and follow-up (1997) (Wise et al. 2006). The CES-D was used to measure elevated depressive symptoms in 1999. Women who reported a physician-diagnosed depression before 1999 were excluded. After adjustment for age, education, occupation, marital status, BMI, heath conditions, smoking, alcohol use, and child care, odds of elevated depression symptoms were inversely related to weekly vigorous physical activity during adulthood up to 3 to 4 h each week but not more. Women who said they got vigorous exercise both in high school (5 or more hours per week) and adulthood (2 or more hours per week) had the lowest odds of depressive symptoms (OR = 0.76; 95% CI: 0.71-0.82) compared to women who said they were never active.

Copenhagen City Heart Study

Leisure-time physical activity and potential confounders were measured in 18,146 residents of Copenhagen, Denmark, at baseline in 1976-1978 and again in 1981-1983 and 1991-1994 (Mikkelsen et al. 2010). Depression incident cases through 2002 were obtained from two Danish hospital registers according to ICD diagnostic criteria. Depression risk at each of the two follow-up assessments was predicted by physical activity and confounders measured at the preceding assessment (i.e., ~5 to 10 years earlier). Adjustments were made for age, education, and chronic diseases. Compared to women with a high physical activity level, women with a moderate level of physical activity had 7% elevated risk of incident depression (OR = 1.07; 95% CI: 0.80-1.44), while women with a low level of physical activity had an 80% higher risk (OR = 1.80; 95% CI: 1.29-2.51). Compared to men with a high physical activity level, men with a moderate level of physical activity had 11% higher risk of incident depression (OR = 1.11; 95% CI: 0.73-1.68), while men with a low level of physical activity had 39% higher risk (OR = 1.39; 95% CI: 0.83-2.34). See figure 14.13.

Danish National Birth Cohort

More than 100,000 pregnancies were recorded between 1990 and 2002 among 70,866 women who had their medical records linked to the Danish Psychiatric Central Register and the Danish Register for Medicinal Product Statistics to identify clinical cases of depression up to one year postpartum (Strøm et al. 2009). Physical activity was assessed by a telephone interview at week 12 of gestation. Women who said they got no exercise (63%) had 27% higher odds of getting an antidepressant prescription filled than women who said

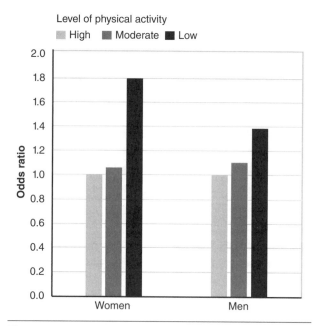

Figure 14.13 Copenhagen City Heart Study of incident depression in inactive women and men.

Data from Mikkelsen et al. 2010.

they exercised (OR = 1.26; 95% CI: 0.98-1.27). There was no dose–response reduction in risk across quartiles of physical activity (MET-hours/week). However, women who said they spent at least 25% of their exercise time during pregnancy in activities with an intensity of 6 METs or higher (13% of the women) had about 20% lower risk of getting an antidepressant prescription (adjusted OR = 0.81; 95% CI: 0.66-0.99) compared to women who said they got no exercise,

Swedish Health Professionals

Cohort data collected in 2004 and 2006 from health care professionals and social insurance workers in western Sweden (2694 women, 420 men) were analyzed (Jonsdottir et al. 2010). Compared to those who were sedentary, people who said they engaged in either light physical activity (gardening, walking, bicycling to work at least 2 h each week) or moderate-to-vigorous physical activity (aerobics, dancing, swimming, soccer, or heavy gardening at least 2 h each week; or 5 h at high intensity) during the past three months in 2004 were less likely than sedentary people to report elevated symptoms of depression at follow-up in 2006 (OR = 0.37; 95% CI: 0.21-0.63 and OR = 0.29; 95% CI: 0.15-0.57, respectively).

The Honolulu-Asia Aging Study

A total of 1282 elderly men 71 to 93 years of age reported their daily walking distance (12 city blocks = 1 mile) in 1991 through 1993 and their symptoms of depression eight years later in 1999-2000 (T.L. Smith et al. 2010). Age-adjusted eight-year incidence rates of depression symptoms (having elevated CES-D scores or taking antidepressant medication) were 13.6%, 7.6%, and 8.5% for low (<0.25 miles/day), moderate (0.25-1.5 miles/day), and high (>1.5 miles/day) walking groups, which approximated tertiles of walking distance at baseline. After adjustment for age, education, marital status, BMI, diabetes, alcohol use, smoking, cancer, Parkinson's disease, cognitive impairment or dementia, and disability, men in the lowest walking group had 60% to 90% higher odds of incident depression symptoms than did the men in moderate and high walking groups, respectively (OR = 1.92; 95% CI: 1.20-3.13 and OR = 1.64; 95% CI: 1.10-2.56).

Taiwan's Health and Living Status of the Elderly Survey

A nationally representative cohort of 3778 adults aged 50 years and older in 1996 were followed in 1999 and 2003 (Ku, Fox, and Chen 2009). There were 420 incident cases of elevated depression symptoms (CES-D after seven years of follow-up). People classified as low active (*n* = 1139) in 1996 (they said they engaged in less than three sessions of physical activity each week in their leisure time) had 34% higher odds than active people (three or more sessions per week) of developing elevated CES-D symptoms in 2003 (OR = 1.43; 95% CI: 1.04-1.95).

Dose Response in Prospective Cohort Studies

Fewer than 10 prospective cohort studies included the three or more levels of physical activity necessary to judge whether the odds of depression symptoms had a dose–gradient reduction with increased levels of exposure to physical activity (Physical Activity Guidelines Advisory Committee 2008). After adjustment for age, sex, and other risk factors, the reduction of odds was smaller for the lowest level of physical activity (OR = 0.86; 95% CI: 0.79-0.94) compared to the next two levels, which did not differ (OR = 0.77; 95% CI: 0.72-0.82). Also, about half the prospective cohort studies provided enough information to determine whether active people were meeting public health recommendations for participation in moderate or vigorous physical activity (i.e., moderate-intensity aerobic physical activity for a minimum of 30 min on five days per week, or vigorous-intensity aerobic physical activity for a minimum of 20 min on three days per week). After adjustment for other risk factors, there was a protective benefit for people who performed moderate or vigorous physical activity (OR = 0.77; 95% CI: 0.72-0.82) compared to people who were active but did not reach the recommended levels (OR = 0.84; 95% CI: 0.78-0.90).

Causality in Prospective Cohort Studies

Longitudinal studies satisfy temporal sequence, but they cannot confirm that physical inactivity resulted in incident depression when physical activity exposure is only mea-

sured once at the baseline or beginning of the observation period. Even adjustment for confounders at baseline does not rule out that there could be residual confounding by other traits common to both physical activity and proneness to depression. Results from the Canadian National Population Health Survey showed that major depressive episodes were associated with a 60% increased risk of becoming physically inactive (RR = 1.6; 95% CI: 1.2-1.9) (Patten et al. 2009).

Findings from a cohort of 424 adults diagnosed with major or minor depressive disorder using Research Diagnostic Criteria showed that physical activity counteracted the effects of medical conditions and negative life events on depression, but physical activity was not associated with subsequent depression (Harris, Cronkite, and Moos 2006). Measures of physical activity during the past month (swimming, tennis, and long hikes or walks), depression, and other demographic and psychosocial constructs were measured at baseline and one year, four years, and 10 years later. More physical activity was associated with less concurrent depression, even after gender, age, medical problems, and negative life events were controlled for.

▶ **PHYSICAL ACTIVITY** and depression may influence each other. Annual assessments of 496 adolescent girls for six years showed that physical activity reduced depression symptoms and the risk of meeting diagnostic criteria for major or minor depression. Conversely, depressive symptoms and a diagnosis of either major or minor depression subsequently reduced future physical activity (Jerstad et al. 2010).

With few exceptions, cohort studies have been limited to just one or two estimates of physical activity exposure, despite follow-up periods lasting many years. Depression incidence rates were often not related to the dose of physical activity. However, most studies relied on poorly validated self-reports of physical activity and used various criteria and methods to classify people into activity groups that were not equivalent across studies. Thus, their ability to detect a dose-response was limited by weak methods. Moreover, none of the studies assessed change in physical activity exposure or sequential measures of outcome. This is necessary for estimating trajectories of change and judging misclassification errors that result when people over- or underreport their physical activity. It is also necessary for discounting residual confounding by fluctuating traits common to physical inactivity and depression risk, including psychiatric comorbidities of depression such as anxiety and alcohol abuse or sleep disorders, which were not assessed. Cardiorespiratory fitness (CRF) provides an objective, surrogate measure of physical activity exposure. The decline in CRF seen in healthy adults during ages 40 to 60 is best explained by reduced moderate-to-vigorous physical activity, after age, BMI, and smoking have been accounted for (Jackson et al. 2009).

The Aerobics Center Longitudinal Study is one study that included measures of cardiorespiratory fitness and depression. Cardiorespiratory fitness was assessed at four clinic visits, each separated by two to three years, to objectively measure cumulative physical activity exposure in 7936 men and 1261 women from the Aerobics Center Longitudinal Study who had not complained of depression at their first clinic visit (Dishman et al. 2012). Across subsequent visits, there were 446 incident cases of depression in men and 153 cases in women. After adjustment for age, time between visits, BMI, and fitness at visit 1, each minute decline in treadmill endurance (i.e., a decline in fitness of one-half MET) between ages 51 and 55 in men and ages 53 and 56 in women increased the odds of incident depression by approximately 2% and 9.5%, respectively. The increased odds remained significant but were attenuated to 1.3% and 5.4% after further adjustment for smoking, alcohol use, medical conditions, anxiety, and sleep problems. See figure 14.14. The results support that maintenance of cardiorespiratory fitness during late middle age, when decline in fitness typically accelerates, helps protect against the onset of depression complaints made to a physician.

▷ **MODERATE AND** high levels of physical activity similarly reduce the odds of developing depression symptoms compared to low levels of physical activity exposure, which is nonetheless more protective than inactivity or very low levels of physical activity. An increase in physical fitness is not required to reduce symptoms, but maintaining fitness during middle age helps reduce risk of developing depression.

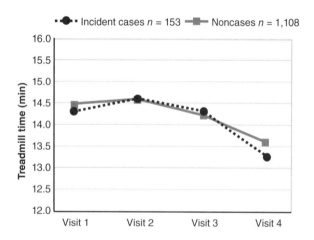

- • - Incident cases *n* = 153   ■— Noncases *n* = 1,108

Figure 14.14 Decline in cardiorespiratory fitness and incident depression in women adjusted for age, time between visits, BMI, smoking, alcohol use, number of medical conditions, and complaints of anxiety or sleep problems.

Reprinted from *American Journal of Preventive Medicine*, R.K. Dishman et al., issue 10, "Decline in cardiorespiratory fitness and odds of incident depression," copyright 2012, with permission from Elsevier.

Other Risk Factors for Depression Often Controlled Statistically in Population Studies of Physical Activity

Age

Education

Chronic health conditions

Perceived health

Physical disability

Physical symptoms

Feelings of autonomy

Social isolation

Stressful life events: moving, job loss, separation or divorce, death of spouse, and financial difficulties

Confounders in Prospective Cohort Studies

To build a case that physical activity causes reduced risk of depression, it must be demonstrated that the effect of physical activity is independent of other factors, such as age, overall health, and psychosocial variables, that might be associated with physical activity levels and also influence depression. Nearly all prospective cohort studies measured confounding factors only at baseline, yet they assessed prevalence or incidence of depression after many years of follow-up. This makes it hard to discount residual confounding by fluctuating traits in people that may be common to physical inactivity and depression risk, including psychiatric comorbidities of depression such as anxiety and alcohol abuse or sleep disorders, which have been ignored in many studies. Thus, there is limited evidence that physical inactivity is an independent risk factor for depression. However, stronger evidence for causality comes from randomized controlled trials.

Treating Depression: Experimental Studies

Most of the experimental research showing that exercise improves self-ratings of depressive mood has been done with people who had normal mental and physical health, but about 30 randomized controlled trials involving people diagnosed with mild to moderate unipolar depression have shown improvements in mood after several weeks of moderately intense exercise.

Though exercise appears comparable to psychotherapy and drug therapy for treating mild to moderate depression, its clinical effects on reducing symptoms occur later than those of drug therapy. The minimal or optimal type or amount of exercise for reducing depression is not yet known, but it appears that an increase in physical fitness is not required, and resistance exercise has been effective in a few studies.

Reviews and Meta-Analyses

Several subjective reviews and quantitative meta-analyses of exercise and depression research indicate that exercise reduces depression symptoms among people diagnosed with depression by about 1 standard deviation (SD) and among chronically ill patients without diagnosed depression by about 1/3 SD (Herring et al. 2012; Lawlor and Hopker 2001; Mead et al. 2009). Those changes represent reductions of about 5 to 10 points on standard self-rating scales of symptoms. An effect of 1 SD is statistically large, comparable to increasing a grade from a C to a B in a course graded using a normal or bell-shaped curve.

Most studies of chronic exercise and depression have used an aerobic exercise intervention such as walking or jogging. However, the types of people studied, the severity of initial depression, the use of appropriate comparison groups, and the type and amount of exercise varied among studies. Nonetheless, it appears that aerobic endurance exercise and resistance exercise each have potential to reduce depression symptoms.

▷ **BOTH AEROBIC** and resistance exercise training have a positive effect on patients diagnosed as having mild to moderate depression.

Early studies of the effects of exercise training on symptoms among hospitalized psychiatric patients diagnosed with major depression were conducted by Norwegian psychiatrist Egil Martinsen and his colleagues at the Modum Bads Nervesanatorium (Martinsen, Hoffart, and Solberg 1989b; Martinsen, Medhus, and Sandvik 1985). In the first study, 43 patients were randomly assigned to either exercise or an occupational therapy control group in addition to their standard treatment, which included psychotherapy and medication. After nine weeks of training, patients in the exercise group had significantly larger reductions in self-reported symptoms of depression than the control group. In the second study, 99 patients diagnosed with unipolar depressive disorders (major depression, dysthymic disorder, and atypical depression) were randomly assigned to either aerobic or nonaerobic exercise. After eight weeks of training, both groups had significant reductions in depression scores. The change in depression scores did not differ between the two conditions, but the aerobic group had significant increases in fitness, defined as maximal oxygen uptake ($\dot{V}O_2$max), while the fitness of the nonaerobic group did not change.

Meta-Analysis of Randomized Controlled Trials

A meta-analysis of 14 trials of chronic exercise among people diagnosed with depression (Lawlor and Hopker 2001) showed that exercisers had a 1.1 SD (95% CI: −1.5 to −0.60) reduction in depression symptoms measured using the Beck Depression Inventory compared with people who were not treated, equivalent to a 7-point reduction in symptoms (95% CI: −10.0 to −4.6) on a scale that ranges up to 61. People who score at least 10 are judged to be mildly depressed; higher scores indicate increasingly severe depression. The effects of exercise were similar to the effects of cognitive psychotherapy. Collectively, the studies had several scientific weaknesses that made it hard to conclude that the reduced depression symptoms were the independent result of exercise:

- Use of volunteers
- Use of symptom ratings rather than clinical diagnoses as the measure of treatment response
- Failure to conceal group assignment
- Exclusion of dropouts from the treatment response tally

An update of that review located 23 randomized controlled trials of 907 adult patients diagnosed with depression, excluding women with postpartum depression, and showed that on average, exercise reduced symptoms −0.82 SD (95% CI: −1.12 to −0.51) (Mead et al. 2009). The effect was half that size, though, in the three trials judged by the authors to have the best quality control (e.g., treatments were concealed from the patients, and dropouts were included in outcome assessments).

Another review identified eight of 13 trials that adequately concealed which group patients had been assigned to, six that blinded raters of symptoms from those group assignments, and five that used intention-to-treat analyses (i.e., included dropouts in the average effect of exercise and control conditions) (Krogh et al. 2010). The mean effect of exercise was a −0.40 SD reduction in symptoms (95% CI: −0.66 to −0.14). Effects varied across studies and were inversely related to the length of the intervention, which ranged from four to 16 weeks. However, adherence ranged from 100% to 42%, and some of the longest trials had the lowest adherence and smallest effect on depression (e.g., Krogh et al. 2009). The three studies judged to have the best research design (adequately concealed random assignment to groups, blinded outcome assessment, and intention-to-treat analysis) had a smaller effect that was not statistically significant (−0.19 SD; 95% CI: −0.70 to 0.31). Each of those three studies compared an exercise group to a group that might have undergone active treatment without exercise (e.g., stretching or relaxation exercises or biweekly visits with a psychiatrist) rather than to a control that received no treatment (e.g., a group that was untreated but was offered the exercise program after the control period passed). Those "placebo" comparisons judge whether exercise is better than some other minimally effective treatment, but they underestimate the efficacy of exercise alone, which is also important to know given the high rates of people who have depression but do not seek treatment from a health professional.

A clinical response in a treatment for depression is usually judged as favorable when the symptom reduction is 50% or more of the initial number or strength of symptoms. However, about half of patients who respond to treatment do not have remission of their symptoms, which is the desired end point of treatment. Remission is generally defined as a score of 7 or less on the 17-item HAM-D (HAM-D[17]) physician rating scale; minimal or no symptoms of depression; loss of the diagnosis, that is, the patient no longer meets the criteria for major depressive disorder listed in the DSM-IV; and the return of normal psychosocial and occupational function (Zajecka 2003). With few exceptions (e.g., Dunn et al. 2005; Singh et al. 2005) exercise trials have not reported whether the reduction in symptoms was sufficient to indicate a favorable response or remission.

The first experimental report comparing the effectiveness of resistance exercise with aerobic exercise for reducing depression symptoms was reported by Doyne and colleagues (1987). Forty women ages 18 to 35 years who were diagnosed with depression were assigned to an aerobic exercise (running) or a weightlifting group. After eight weeks of exercise training, both exercise groups exhibited significant reductions in depression scores, while a control group showed no changes. The reduction in depression scores was similar for the two forms of exercise. Singh, Clements, and Fiatarone (1997b) conducted a 10-week, progressive resistance exercise training study among elderly subjects who met DSM-IV criteria for depression or dysthymia. Compared with a control group that received health education only, the

resistance exercise group had larger reductions (about 4 to 5 SDs) in depressive symptoms on both Beck self-ratings and diagnostic interview ratings by clinicians. Results from these studies and those by Martinsen in Norway show that changes in aerobic capacity are not necessary to confer the antidepressant effects of physical activity.

The cumulative evidence shows that exercise can be as effective as psychotherapy. Whether the effects of exercise operate through a different mechanism from psychotherapy and thus are additive to the treatment response of psychotherapy alone is not yet known. For example, Fremont and Craighead (1987) compared aerobic exercise to traditional psychotherapy for depression in a sample of 49 men and women 19 to 62 years of age with self-reported symptoms of mild to moderate depression (figure 14.15). Participants were randomly assigned to supervised running, individual cognitive psychotherapy, or combined running and psychotherapy. After 10 weeks of treatment, all groups exhibited significant reductions in depression scores, but no differences were found among the groups. Thus, exercise was found to be as effective as a traditional psychotherapy, but there was no additional benefit when exercise was added to psychotherapy.

Research has also shown that exercise can be generally as effective as drug therapy for reducing depression symptoms. Aerobic exercise was compared with standard medication in a training study of 156 older men and women who were

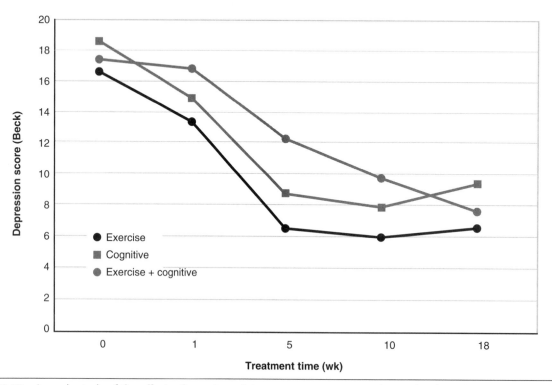

Figure 14.15 An early study of the effects of exercise training on symptoms among hospitalized psychiatric patients diagnosed with major depression showed that after eight weeks of training, running and psychotherapy groups each exhibited significant reductions in depression scores.

Data from Fremont and Craighead 1987.

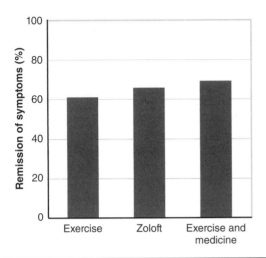

Figure 14.16 Changes in depression remission rates across treatments.

Data from Blumenthal et al., 1999.

clinically diagnosed with major depressive disorder (Blumenthal et al. 1999). Participants were randomly assigned to an aerobic exercise, antidepressant, or combined exercise and medication group. Figure 14.16 illustrates that after the 16-week program, the three groups demonstrated similar decreases in depression that were statistically and clinically significant. The medication-only group exhibited the fastest initial response; but by the end of the program, the exercise treatment was equally effective in reducing depression in this older sample. Also, the exercise group was more likely to have fully recovered and less likely to have relapsed into depression six months after treatment than the drug treatment patients (Babyak et al. 2000). A later study of 37 adults 65 years of age or older who had minor depression showed that symptoms were similarly reduced after 16 weeks of supervised aerobic and resistance exercise (about an hour, three times each week) and drug treatment with the SSRI sertraline when compared to usual medical care (Brenes et al. 2007).

Dose Response in Randomized Controlled Trials

About three-fourths of the randomized controlled trials (RCTs) of healthy adults and nonpsychiatric medical patients used a moderate-to-vigorous exercise intensity of 60% to 80% of people's aerobic capacity or maximum strength three days per week. Intensity was lower or the frequency was two days per week in the other studies. The average duration of each session was about 35 min, but it was less than 30 min in a fourth of the studies and more than 1 h in another fourth. However, fewer than half the studies were clear about how the time was partitioned into warm-up, exercise, and cool-down. Nonetheless, reductions in depression symptoms have not consistently differed across these varying features of exercise. However, these studies did not experimentally

examine whether the apparently antidepressant effects of physical activity depend on the type or amount of physical activity. Two of three well-executed studies of depressed patients have shown a dose–response effect on symptom reduction.

Aerobic Exercise Dose Study

The DOSE study was the first RCT designed to test the dose–response relation of aerobic exercise with reduction in depression symptoms in patients (Dunn et al. 2005). Eighty adults diagnosed with mild to moderate major depressive disorder were assigned to either a placebo control (three days a week of flexibility exercise) or to one of four solitary aerobic exercise treatments conducted in a supervised laboratory, which varied by energy expenditure each session and weekly frequency: low dose (7.0 kcal $\cdot$ kg^{-1} $\cdot$ week^{-1} [about 100-150 calories each session]) or high dose (17.5 kcal $\cdot$ kg^{-1} $\cdot$ week^{-1} [about 250-400 calories each session]) and a weekly frequency of either three days or five days. The primary outcome was the score on a physician diagnostic rating scale of depression symptoms. Depression scores at 12 weeks were reduced by 47% from baseline in the high-dose group, compared with 30% and 29% for the low-dose and control groups. There was no main effect of exercise frequency at 12 weeks, but figure 14.17 shows that people in the high-dose group who exercised five days a week were about twice as likely to have a favorable response (i.e., a 50% or more reduction in their entry symptoms) and a remission in symptoms (i.e., no longer enough symptoms to be judged as depressed; ≥7 on HAM-D).

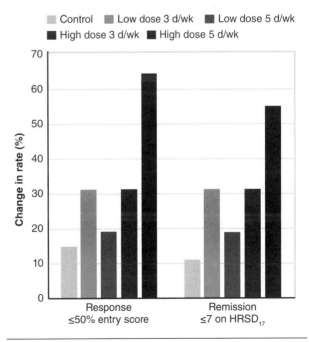

Figure 14.17 Changes in depression response and remission rates across two doses of exercise treatment.

Data from Dunn et al. 2005.

Experimental Evidence of Improved Depression Symptoms

About a dozen experiments have found that patients recovering from a heart attack report a moderate reduction in self-rated depression (about 1/2 SD) when they participate in a cardiac rehabilitation exercise program (Kugler, Seelbach, and Kruskemper 1994). Improvements in symptoms of depression have also been reported among breast cancer survivors who exercised (Segar et al. 1998).

Resistance Exercise Dose Study

Sixty community-dwelling adults ages 60 years or older who had major or minor depression were randomized to usual care by a physician or to supervised progressive resistance exercise of high intensity (80% maximum load) or low intensity (20% maximum load) three days per week for eight weeks (Singh et al. 2005). The rate of favorable response (i.e., 50% reduction in physician-rated symptoms) in the high-intensity group (61% of those patients) was twice as high as in the low-intensity group (29%) and the standard care group (21%).

DEMO Trial

This was a randomized pragmatic trial for patients with unipolar depression conducted from January 2005 through July 2007. Patients were referred from general practitioners or psychiatrists and were eligible if they fulfilled ICD-10 criteria for unipolar depression and were between 18 and 55 years of age. Patients ($n = 165$) were allocated to two weekly sessions of supervised strength, aerobic, or relaxation training during a four-month period (Krogh et al. 2009). The primary outcome measure was the 17-item Hamilton Rating Scale for Depression (HAM-D[17]). Despite an increase in strength in the resistance group and maximal oxygen uptake in the aerobic group, changes in depression symptoms after four months were not different from those in the relaxation group. However, 40% of the participants left the study, and those who remained averaged just one day of supervised exercise each week, so the exposure to exercise may have been insufficient to affect symptoms. Exercise outside the program wasn't verified, so the fitness scores, which were based on performance rather than objective physiological criteria, might have improved because of motivation to perform better by the exercisers the second time they were tested.

Physical Activity and Depression in Youth

No RCTs of children or adolescents diagnosed with depression have been reported. A meta-analysis located five poorly controlled trials including healthy youths aged 11 to 19 years

that compared exercise training with a no-exercise condition (Larun et al. 2006). On average, there was a moderately large reduction in depression scores after exercise (−0.66 SD; 95% CI: −1.25 to −0.08) regardless of exercise intensity. Two small trials of children who were being treated for depression found a small, statistically nonsignificant effect of exercise for reducing symptoms (−0.31 SD; 95% CI: −0.78 to 0.16). Whether those effects are generalizable to a reduction in the primary risk of developing depression among adolescents is not yet established.

A prospective cohort study examined naturally occurring changes in physical activity, and changes in depressive symptoms were studied during early adolescence, when depression risk begins to increase markedly (Motl et al. 2004). Nearly 4600 boys and girls in Minnesota reported their frequency of physical activity outside of school and completed the CES-D in the fall of 1998 (beginning of 7th grade; baseline data), spring of 1999 (end of 7th grade; interim data), and spring of 2000 (end of 8th grade; follow-up data). Results indicated that a 1 SD change in the frequency of leisure-time physical activity was inversely related to a 1/3 SD in depressive symptoms in both boys and girls. This effect was attenuated but remained statistically significant after adjustment for any confounding effects of smoking and alcohol consumption; socioeconomic status; and the value students placed on their health, appearance, and achievement. Thus, physical activity was independently and inversely related to depressive symptoms, providing evidence that physical activity indeed represents a feasible target of population-based interventions designed to reduce depression risk among adolescent boys and girls in the United States.

In a four-year longitudinal study of 2548 adolescents and young adults aged 14 to 24 years in Munich, Germany, incident rates were 8% for major depression and 2% for dysthymia. Those who said they regularly exercised or played sports at baseline had a lower incidence of dysthymia (OR = 0.34; 95% CI: 0.16-0.74), but lower risk of major depression was weak (OR = 0.73; 95% CI: 0.50-1.04) (Ströhle et al. 2007).

A recent British study of 2789 7th- and 9th-grade students in East London found that after adjustment for confounders, both boys and girls who were more physically active at baseline had 8% lower odds of elevated depression symptoms for each hour of exercise each week. However, there was no association between a change in physical activity from baseline and depressive symptoms in cohort ($n = 2093$) follow-up two years later (Rothon et al. 2010).

Strength of the Evidence

The case for a protective effect of leisure-time physical activity on the primary and secondary prevention of depression is encouraging but as yet incomplete. Most of the population-based studies of physical activity and depression show lower risk of depression among people who say they are physically active in their leisure time, but only about half of the studies found effects large enough to be statistically significant, often because of relatively small population samples (e.g., less than 500 people). About half the studies did an incomplete job of controlling confounders, and they used imprecise measures of physical activity or depression.

Many clinical studies have found that both acute and chronic exercise are followed by lower scores on self-report questionnaires designed to measure depressed mood. This has been seen in about 30 RCTs of depressed adults, but most of the studies did not report whether the reduction in symptoms was enough to judge a favorable response to treatment (i.e., a 50% reduction in symptoms) or result in a diagnosis of remission. Also, exercising patients commonly received treatment by psychotherapy or drug therapy, so it wasn't possible to determine the sole, independent effect of exercise on their symptoms.

Many exercise programs with depressed patients were conducted in groups outdoors during daylight, so it was hard to determine whether the benefits attributed to exercise could be explained by social effects or light exposure; each could have antidepressant effects regardless of the physical exertion. Reduced scores on depression scales have also been reported after exercise by people who have normal fluctuations in mood but have not been diagnosed with depression. However, it has not been determined whether this mood-elevating response reduces the risk of future development of depression.

Temporal Sequence

The mean follow-up of 30 or prospective cohort studies is about four years, ranging from nine months to 37 years. However, physical activity and depression can influence each other, so it is challenging to demonstrate temporal causality in observational studies.

Also, the cohort studies have mainly been limited to just one or two estimates of physical activity exposure, despite follow-up periods lasting many years. This makes it hard to estimate trajectories of change and judge misclassification errors resulting from people who over- or underreport their physical activity—and makes it impossible to judge how other risk factors of depression that change over time may confound the prospective association of physical activity with depression symptoms. Future exercise interventions in experimental studies should be of sufficient length to allow observation of whether reductions in depression occur in a manner consistent with theoretical biological explanations and should incorporate follow-up assessments to evaluate whether antidepressant effects are maintained over time.

Strength of Association

Averaged across prospective cohort studies, the odds of elevated symptoms are about one-third lower among active compared with inactive people. After adjustment for depression risk factors that might have differed between active and inactive groups, the odds of developing symptoms of depression stayed about 20% lower among active people.

Quantitative reviews of RCTs using people with normal mood and people diagnosed with mild to moderate depression have found a moderately large reduction in symptoms of depression, ranging from about 1/3 SD in patients with medical conditions other than depression to about 1 SD in patients diagnosed with depression, an effect comparable to the benefits of psychotherapy. Most exercise studies did not show that the reduction in symptoms was large enough for a diagnosis of remission or maintenance of remission, though a recent study encouraged the view that exercise might be more effective for maintenance than drug treatment is (Babyak et al. 2000). And, exercise has been successfully used as an augmentation treatment for depressed patients who did not respond to drug therapy (Trivedi et al. 2006b).

Consistency

It is important to consider whether the effects of exercise are the same for women and men and among races or ethnicities and ages to establish the scientific consistency of the effects, as well as for the practical reason of implementing optimal physical activity interventions within segments of the population. Observational population studies have come from Australia, Canada, China, England, Finland, Germany, Israel, Italy, Netherlands, and Japan, as well as the United States. In general, physical activity has been associated with decreased risk for depression in both males and females, across age groups, and in multiple cultures. However, few studies were designed to compare population subgroups on their depression responses to exercise.

One prospective study showed that lower levels of depression symptoms were associated with more physical activity in both men and women (Kritz-Silverstein et al. 2001). Only a third of cohort studies specified the proportions of racial and ethnic groups included, and only four studies in the United States had evidence of good representation of African Americans, Hispanics/Latinos, or both. One study reported that the odds of depression symptoms were similarly lower among white and African American adults who were active (Knox et al. 2006). Other studies had poor or no representation of other minority groups. Race and ethnicity were poorly represented or not described in most RCTs.

There have been few observational or controlled studies of children and adolescents, and most studies of people over age 65 measured symptoms of depression but did not demonstrate clinically meaningful remission of symptoms among people diagnosed with a depressive disorder.

Dose Response

On balance, it appears that being sedentary increases risk of depression; moderate and high levels of physical activity similarly reduce the odds of developing depression symptoms compared to low levels of physical activity exposure, which is nonetheless more protective than inactivity or very low levels of physical activity. About half the prospective cohort studies provided enough information to determine whether active people were meeting public health recommendations for participation in moderate or vigorous physical activity (i.e., moderate-intensity aerobic physical activity for a minimum of 30 min on five days per week, or vigorous-intensity aerobic physical activity for a minimum of 20 min on three days per week). After adjustment for other risk factors, these studies showed that people who engaged in moderate or vigorous physical activity benefited from a protective effect compared to people who were active but did not reach the recommended levels. An increase in physical fitness does not appear to be necessary for antidepressant effects of exercise. However, two RCTs of depressed patients found that symptom reductions were greater after a higher dose of aerobic or resistance exercise.

Plausibility

The second-century Greek physician Galen recognized the importance of exercise for stimulating the four humors of Hippocrates (blood, black bile, yellow bile, and phlegm), which Galen extended to help explain mood. Sanguine, melancholic, choleric, and phlegmatic are adjectives derived from those humors to describe people's temperament. In more modern times, it was proposed that exercise was beneficial to people who were depressed because it stimulated nerves and increased glandular secretions (Vaux 1926). The following paragraphs discuss the evidence that supports a biological explanation of activity's effect on mood. However, unlike the situation with the other chronic diseases discussed in this book, biological mechanisms are not the only plausible explanations for the mental health effects of physical activity. Cognitive explanations, especially increased self-esteem, and social support are also popular hypotheses to explain physical activity's antidepressant effect. It is important to remember, though, that regardless of whether the pivotal mechanism whereby physical activity reduces depression is viewed as cognitive or social, it ultimately can be explained in biochemical and physiological terms as the regulation of neurons by genes (e.g., Kandel 1998).

Cognitive and Social Factors

Cognitive changes, such as enhancement of self-esteem, and social support have been proposed as explanations for the effects of physical activity on depression. However, there's little evidence to permit conclusions about the roles these factors play. Observational population studies have not included measures of self-esteem and social support to determine whether they confound or mediate the lower rates of depressive symptoms observed among physically active people. Also, most RCTs did not examine whether reduced depression after exercise training was mediated by enhanced self-esteem (Motl et al. 2005), nor did they use the proper comparison groups to demonstrate that reduced depression after exercise was independent of social support. Nonetheless, cognitive and social factors deserve further study, especially self-esteem.

Self-esteem is a cornerstone of mental health and behavior, and depression is often associated with low self-esteem. Because body image is related to general **self-concept,** an improvement in body image or physical skills can contribute to general self-esteem in people who place high value on physical attributes relative to the other aspects of self-concept (Sonstroem 1998) and might reduce the primary or secondary risk of depression.

• *Self-esteem.* Self-esteem is the value people place on their conception or view of themselves. It reflects a person's feelings about and evaluations of specific personal features, including physical attributes—such as appearance, endurance, strength, and sport skills—and social, academic or professional, emotional, and spiritual attributes (Sonstroem and Morgan 1989). Positive comments from others about one's fitness or physique, or merely expectations of increased fitness, can improve self-esteem even when actual fitness has not improved. A sense of achievement is key. Participants' self-esteem tends to improve more after fitness training than after participating in competitive sports, in which success and feelings of accomplishment are less assured (Fox 2000; Spence, McGannon, and Poon 2005). A few poorly controlled randomized trials have shown a moderately large effect (0.49 SD; 95% CI: 0.16-0.81) of mainly aerobic exercise or sports training on self-esteem in children and youths (Ekeland, Heian, and Hagen 2005). Correlational evidence suggests that physical activity and sport participation might reduce depression risk among adolescent girls through positive influences on physical self-concept that operate to increase self-esteem independently of girls' fitness; BMI; and perceptions of sport competence, body fatness, and appearance (Dishman et al. 2006b). The biggest gains in self-esteem usually occur for people who value physical fitness or appearance and are not satisfied with their current status in these areas. Believing that you are doing something positive for yourself may be enough to improve self-esteem. Supporting this idea is a study by Desharnais and colleagues (1993) in which college students' self-esteem improved after participation in an exercise program whose stated goal was to improve psychological well-being. Students in the same study who were not told of the goal did not report improvements in self-esteem even though they showed similar fitness improvements. People who improve their fitness can gain an increased sense of mastery over physical tasks. Some evidence suggests that this confidence can extend beyond physical activity settings to enhance overall self-concept and life adjustment and therefore help reduce depression.

• *Social support.* In one RCT of 30 depressed elderly men and women, participants either walked outdoors for 20 min twice weekly for six weeks with a young companion or spent the same amount of time with another young companion. Compared with control, both conditions resulted in reductions in self-ratings of depression; but the condition that combined walking with social contact was not more effective than the condition of social contact alone (McNeil, LeBlanc, and Joyner 1991). Hence, walking added no benefit beyond social contact.

Although enhanced self-esteem remains a plausible explanation for the antidepressant effects of exercise, it has not been empirically tested as a mediator of depression reduction after exercise in well-designed studies. Moreover, if self-esteem was the only mechanism underlying the treatment responses observed in exercise programs, this mechanism would not be unique to exercise and would not support an independent, causal effect of exercise for reducing depression symptoms because self-esteem can exert its influence in many settings that do not involve physical activity. Likewise, social influences that contribute to reductions in depression after exercise would be part of the setting in which exercise takes place, not exercise itself, that might be no different from other therapeutic settings.

Biological Plausibility

Several neurobiological mechanisms represent potential avenues by which exercise could influence physiological mediators of depression. The following discussion provides an overview of the primary biological hypotheses regarding exercise and depression.

• *Endorphin hypothesis.* One proposed mechanism for the antidepressant effect of exercise is that elevations in **endorphin** levels following exercise produce improvements in mood (referred to as the **endorphin hypothesis**). Endorphins such as **enkephalins** are opioids, proteins with analgesic properties that occur naturally in the brain and spinal cord, but also in the adrenal gland, gut, and sympathetic nerves. They help modulate body temperature and the cardiovascular system during stress, including exercise; they can elevate mood and reduce pain, with effects similar to those of the powerful opiates like morphine (e.g., enkephalins, β-endorphin, and morphine each bind to μ-opioid receptors). β-Endorphin, though found in the brain, is released from the pituitary into the blood during stress. Although blood levels of β-endorphin have been shown to be elevated following intense exercise, it has not been shown that β-endorphin crosses the blood–brain barrier during or after exercise. For β-endorphin to be a plausible mechanism for the antidepressant effects of exercise, it must induce changes in brain regions that regulate mood. Endorphins modulate the actions of monoamines throughout brain regions involved with emotions and increase in the brain after exercise in rats and mice (Hoffman 1997). However, those studies were not designed to show changes in depression-like behaviors. In addition, several studies of humans using drugs to block the action of opioids did not prevent changes in depressive mood following exercise. Thus, the available experimental evidence in humans has failed to support the endorphin hypothesis of mood change after exercise (Dishman 1998; Dishman and

O'Connor 2009). Nonetheless, one action of β-endorphin in the brain is to inhibit the tonic inhibition of dopamine, the key neurotransmitter in brain regions involved with pleasure (e.g., the ventral tegmental area) and motivation (e.g., the nucleus accumbens). So, it is plausible that β-endorphin could indirectly influence positive moods through its role in regulating dopamine. Peripheral opioid responses also could indirectly influence mood by reducing pain, but this has not been confirmed. A recent uncontrolled study reported a correlation between self-reports of euphoria and brain opioid binding measured by positron emission tomography in 10 experienced distance runners (Boecker et al. 2008). This is the first and only evidence that brain opioids are influenced by exercise in humans in a way that may help explain mood changes associated with running. Whether an endorphin response during exercise affects dopamine and symptoms of depression is not known.

• *Brain blood flow hypothesis.* Research has demonstrated that cerebral blood flow is increased during moderately intense cycling exercise (Ogoh and Ainslie 2009), including to areas of the brain involved in motor control (J.C. Smith et al. 2010) and the control of cardiovascular responses (Williamson, Fadel, and Mitchell 2006). Some of those areas can be involved with emotional and cognitive processes (e.g., the cingulate and insular cortexes). Blood flow and oxygen levels are also increased in the frontal cortex during moderate-to-hard cycling, rowing, or treadmill running, though they decline at maximal, exhaustive exercise (Rooks et al. 2010). Because an increase in blood flow is associated with elevated cellular metabolism, enhanced blood flow to brain regions involved in the regulation of emotion could mediate changes in mood with exercise. However, alterations in blood flow or oxygen levels during exercise to brain areas that are involved with the regulation of mood have not been shown during exercise, so there is currently little evidence to support the role of brain blood flow in mediating the effects of exercise on depression.

• *HPA hypothesis.* Disruption of the hypothalamic-pituitary-adrenocortical (HPA) axis, the system that regulates much of the body's endocrine response to stress, has also been implicated in the etiology of depression. In response to a physical or psychological stressor, the hypothalamus produces corticotropin-releasing hormone (CRH), which acts on the pituitary to signal the release of adrenocorticotropic hormone (ACTH). ACTH then exerts its effect on the adrenal gland to stimulate the release of cortisol. The integrated function of this system is to prepare the body for fight or flight in response to a real or perceived threat. Although activation of this system is critical for an appropriate stress response, excess activation of the HPA axis may play a role in the development of depression. Depressed individuals frequently exhibit a blunted ACTH response to CRH, and hyperactivation of the HPA axis and hypercortisolism are also commonly seen in patients with depression. Because CRH and glucocorticoids such as cortisol influence brain regions important in emotional responses, including the nucleus accumbens, amygdala, and hippocampus, elevated levels of CRH and cortisol under conditions of chronic stress may disrupt functioning in brain regions that regulate mood and may lead to depression (Gold and Chrousos 1998). Both acute and chronic exercise can influence functioning of the HPA axis. Acute bouts of exercise result in activation of this system, whereas exercise training attenuates the effect of acute exercise at a given absolute workload. However, the effect of exercise training on this system in relation to depression is unclear. For example, when rats with access to activity wheels were compared with sedentary animals following a foot-shock stressor, responses in plasma levels of ACTH and corticosterone did not differ between the groups (Dishman et al. 1995, 1997). In contrast, increased levels of ACTH have been observed in treadmill-trained rats after immobilization stress (White-Welkley et al. 1995). Further investigation is needed to clarify the effects of exercise on the HPA axis and to determine how these effects may influence depression.

• *Improved sleep.* Chronic insomnia increases mortality and psychiatric problems and decreases work productivity. About one-third of all adults will experience insomnia sometime in their lives, and people suffering from depression or an anxiety disorder commonly have disturbed sleep. Exercise is frequently included as a component of good sleep hygiene and could plausibly reduce other depression symptoms by improving sleep (Youngstedt 2000). Moderately large reductions (nearly 1/2 SD) in rapid eye movement (REM) sleep (about 7-10 min) and increased **latency** for REM sleep (about 12-15 min) have been reported (Kubitz et al. 1996; Youngstedt, O'Connor, and Dishman 1997). The changes in REM sleep after exercise could help explain the antidepressant effects of exercise, as REM sleep deprivation has been shown to be an effective treatment for some depressed patients. Resistance exercise training led to improved sleep and reduced depression symptoms in older depressed adults who reported sleep problems (Singh, Clements, and Fiatarone 1997a, 1997b).

• *Monoamine hypothesis.* Much of the physiological research on exercise and depression has focused on the brain monoaminergic systems, which include the neurotransmitters dopamine, norepinephrine, and serotonin (Chaouloff 1997a, 1997b; Dishman 1997b; Meeusen and De Meirleir 1995), primarily because most effective pharmacotherapies modulate one or more of these neurotransmitter systems. Animal research has provided evidence of a mediating effect of exercise on the monoaminergic systems implicated in depression. Studies using rats have demonstrated that acute exercise results in increased release of norepinephrine, dopamine, and serotonin in the brain (Meeusen, Piacentini, and De Meirleir 2001; Wilson and Marsden 1996) and that repeated treadmill training attenuates norepinephrine release during exercise (Pagliari and Peyrin 1995b).

Subsequent studies on rats conducted at the University of Georgia showed that brain noradrenergic adaptations to chronic exercise are related to antidepressant-like effects. First, Dunn and colleagues (1996) found that both treadmill exercise training and activity-wheel running led to increased levels of norepinephrine in regions of the brain stem that contain norepinephrine cell bodies. Next, it was shown that such increases in brain norepinephrine in the locus coeruleus and raphe nuclei were accompanied by protection against depletion of brain norepinephrine (Dishman et al. 1997). That was the first study to experimentally test a neurobiological mechanism for the antidepressant effects of exercise. Next, a pharmacologic model of depression was used to compare exercise and antidepressant treatment in animals treated neonatally with clomipramine, a serotonin reuptake inhibitor (Yoo et al. 2000b). Treadmill exercise training and activity-wheel running each increased brain levels of norepinephrine and decreased the number of β-adrenoreceptors in the brain frontal cortex, effects that are similar to those obtained with chronic administration of the antidepressant imipramine. Chronic activity-wheel runners also had attenuated release of norepinephrine in the frontal cortex during uncontrollable electric foot shock compared with sedentary animals but no change in gene expression for the synthetic enzyme tyrosine hydroxylase (Soares et al. 1999). Those findings suggest a downregulation in activity by the locus coeruleus that could preserve brain norepinephrine during stress. Subsequent research suggested that this attenuated stress response after wheel running can be partly explained by increased gene expression for **galanin,** a neuropeptide that appears to inhibit neuronal discharge by the locus coeruleus (O'Neal et al. 2001). In addition, both acute and chronic exercise in animals have been shown to influence dopaminergic activity, and changes in the density and affinity of dopamine receptors have been observed following chronic training in animals (for reviews, see Chaouloff 1989; Mazzeo 1991; Meeusen and De Meirleir 1995; Tantillo et al. 2002). Dishman and colleagues (1997) found that sedentary animals had 50% higher dopamine concentrations in the hypothalamus than animals with access to activity wheels following uncontrollable foot shock; this brain region is important in the regulation of hormone release from the pituitary. Moreover, sedentary animals exhibited 30% more serotonin in the amygdala following foot shock. Thus, exercise training appears to influence monoamine systems, and these adaptations may help explain the biological effects of exercise as a treatment for depression.

• *Depression-like behavior.* In rats, the escape-deficit model after uncontrollable stress, first reported by McCulloch and Bruner (1939), was the first animal model of depression. The hallmark response to uncontrollable, inescapable foot shock is increased latency to escape from controllable shock administered 24 to 72 h later, presumably resulting from depletion of norepinephrine in the locus coeruleus and a subsequent upregulation of β-adrenoreceptors in the brain cortex. The escape-deficit model is an attempt to simulate the so-called learned helplessness or behavioral despair common in human depression. The model is mostly **isomorphic** with human depression, featuring weight loss, reduced sexual behavior, sleep disturbances (decreased REM sleep latency), and anhedonia. Though self-reward tasks such as feeding choices between water and water with added sucrose and intracranial self-stimulation are used as surrogate measures in the rat for the phenomenological **construct** of pleasure experienced by humans, it is not possible to determine whether a rat feels helpless or hopeless.

Some types of depression and anxiety in humans appear to be endogenous; they cannot be attributed to an uncontrollable stressor. One model of endogenous depression in the rat involves injecting neonatal pups with clomipramine, leading to decreased REM sleep latency and other key behavioral signs of depression upon reaching adulthood. Another endogenous model disturbs brain neurotransmitter systems, including norepinephrine and serotonin, by surgically removing the olfactory bulbs located below the brain frontal cortex (Kelly, Wrynn, and Leonard 1997). These models each are responsive to pharmacotherapy. Studies conducted at the University of Georgia showed that chronic activity-wheel running protects against depression-like behavioral abnormalities in all of the rat models mentioned. Female wheel runners were protected from learned helplessness when exposed to electrical shock (Dishman et al. 1997), and male wheel runners were protected against impaired sexual behavior after neonatal clomipramine injections (Yoo et al. 2000b) and after olfactory bulbectomy, which elicits brain monoamine abnormalities and depression-like behaviors in rats (Van Hoomissen et al. 2001). Not only were behavioral signs of depression reduced among wheel runners, but responses by the brain noradrenergic and serotonergic systems, as well as enhanced neuron growth factors, were comparable to those with antidepressant drug treatment (Dishman et al. 1997; O'Neal et al. 2001; Van Hoomissen et al. 2003; Yoo et al. 2000b).

New areas of research implicate other potential biological mechanisms for antidepressant effects of exercise. For example, neurotrophic peptides such as brain-derived neurotrophic factor (BDNF), VGF, and neuropeptide Y enhance the growth and maintenance of several neuronal systems and might have an important role in the neuropathology and treatment of depression, similar to their suspected roles in mediating the effects of antidepressant drugs (Bjørnebekk, Mathé, and Brené 2006, 2010; Greenwood and Fleshner 2008; Hunsberger et al. 2007; Russo-Neustadt 2003).

Because the procedures used to study the monoaminergic systems directly are extremely invasive, much of the research has been limited to animal models of depression, with obviously limited application to human depression. However, refinement of neurobiological diagnostic procedures in humans, including brain imaging techniques such as **functional magnetic resonance imaging (FMRI)** and **positron emission tomography (PET),** should allow researchers and clinicians to gain a better understanding of the effects of exercise on neuronal activity in brain systems and their role in the etiology of depression (Davidson et al. 2003; Kalin et al. 1997; Nemeroff 1998; Nemeroff, Kilts, and Berns 1999). It is likely that future studies of exercise and depression that include brain imaging assessments will greatly enhance our understanding of the neurobiological adaptations associated with exercise. For the time being, however, although there is evidence that neurobiological mechanisms underlying depression may be responsive to exercise stimuli, current evidence is inadequate to conclusively determine a biologically plausible explanation for physical activity's effect on depression.

Summary and Conclusions

A limitation of the exercise and depression research literature has been the failure to fully characterize the mental status of subjects. There are several types of depressive disorders, and symptoms exhibited by individuals with depression can vary widely depending on the nature of their illness. Furthermore, depressed individuals often suffer from anxiety or other mental disorders (Kessler et al. 2005b), yet most studies do not assess comorbidity or analyze data to investigate whether effects are dependent on the nature of the depressive disorder. The substantial number of prospective cohort studies with sufficient follow-up periods generally agree that regular participation in leisure-time physical activity is associated with lowered risk of developing depression symptoms. However, only about half the studies adjusted for other risk factors that might confound that association. Although studies have come from several nations, population subgroups were usually underrepresented or not specifically evaluated. Well-controlled studies that encompass a range of demographic groups and fully consider subject characteristics are needed to determine whether the relationship between exercise and depression is consistent across sexes, ages, races, ethnicities, levels of education, socioeconomic levels, and mental status. In addition, better descriptions of the exercise exposure are needed to determine whether the effects are consistent for all modes, intensities, frequencies, and durations of physical activity.

Numerous studies have demonstrated that exercise programs are associated with a reduction in depression symptoms. However, most studies had methodological limitations that may have obscured the actual effect of exercise training. For example, most RCTs have not fully discounted that favorable outcomes are at least partly influenced by people's expectation of benefits. Few studies have been conducted using a blinded design to protect against experimenter bias, and it is difficult to protect against bias due to participant expectancies. The failure to use appropriate comparison groups is another common design limitation in this area of research. Studies that compare an exercise group to a no-treatment control group reveal little about the clinical meaningfulness of the results, since the only conclusion that can be made is that exercise is better than no treatment and thus might merely be a placebo effect. Because standard therapies have been shown to be effective in treating depression, a placebo group or minimal-intervention control group is needed to adequately evaluate the effectiveness of exercise in alleviating depression. Medication is the best-documented treatment for depression, but only one published study has compared exercise and medication in the treatment of depression—with promising results, however (Blumenthal et al. 1999). Research design must also provide rigorous control of other features of physical activity settings that could influence mood and depression, such as increased social contact and increased light exposure, so that the direct effect of the exercise exposure can be established.

The use of valid measures of physical activity and depression is also an important research consideration. Physical activity should be adequately described, and physiological status before and after training should be measured using appropriate methods. Level of depression should be assessed with valid inventories that have good psychometric properties. Therapist interviews as well as self-report questionnaires should be employed, because both methods are needed to confirm that a clinically meaningful remission of symptoms occurs after exercise.

▶ **ALTHOUGH MODERATE** exercise during leisure time is associated with reduced risk of depression and with reduced depression symptoms, excessive exercise training (i.e., over-training), especially in endurance sports, can result in depression in some athletes (Morgan et al. 1987). Most youths and adults are sedentary, though, so depression resulting from overtraining is not a concern for the general population.

Few studies used resistance or flexibility exercise; most used jogging as the mode of activity, and a few used cycling. Exercise training usually was prescribed based on the guidelines of the American College of Sports Medicine for the types and amounts of exercise recommended for cardiorespiratory fitness in otherwise healthy people (Pollock et al. 1998). Because no adverse effects were reported in these studies, the following exercise guidelines should be appropriate for people with depression who are otherwise healthy:

- Three to five days a week
- 20 to 60 min each session
- 55% to 90% of maximal heart rate

Though beginners should always increase the intensity and length of their workouts gradually, gradual progress is especially important for someone who is depressed. Gradual progress helps to maximize feelings of success and control and to minimize potential feelings of failure if the person cannot sustain the exercise program due to overly rapid progression. It is important to remember that continued participation is more important for reducing depression than is increasing fitness.

▶ **BEING SEDENTARY** increases the risk for depression, but very high levels of physical activity may not be any more protective than moderate levels.

Anxiety Disorders

Anxiety is characterized by apprehension or worry and is typically accompanied by agitation, feelings of tension, and bodily arousal. Other signs and symptoms of **anxiety disorders** vary in number and severity. They include excessive alertness, confusion, muscle tension, tremors, high heart rate, palpitations, flushing, sweating, dry mouth, and urinary and gastrointestinal problems. Though anxiety often occurs with depression, and chronic anxiety can contribute to the risk of depression, people most often experience anxiety apart from depression.

Anxiety is a common human experience during imagined or real threatening circumstances. The term **state anxiety** can be used to refer to this condition if the feelings of anxiety are temporary and fluctuate from moment to moment ("How do I feel right now?"); the term **trait anxiety** is used if these feelings and symptoms are constant and persistent ("How have I been feeling generally?"). Anxiety disorders, however, are illnesses that cause people to feel frightened, distressed, and uneasy for extended periods of time for no apparent reason. Left untreated, these disorders can reduce productivity and diminish the quality of life.

Though apprehension, agitation, and activation of the autonomic nervous system are core signs and symptoms present to varying degrees in all anxiety states, there are several recognized types of anxiety disorders. According to the American Psychiatric Association (2000a), the major types include the following:

- *Phobias.* A **phobia** is an intense fear of an object, place, or situation. A person with a specific phobia experiences extreme fear of something that poses little or no actual danger; the fear causes people with phobias to avoid these objects or situations and most likely limits their lives unnecessarily.

- *Social phobia.* People with social phobia (i.e., social anxiety disorder) have an overwhelming fear of scrutiny and embarrassment in social situations, which causes them to avoid many potentially enjoyable activities. Social phobias are equally common in men and women. They may be discrete (e.g., restricted to eating in public, to public speaking, or to encounters with the opposite sex) or diffuse, involving almost all social situations outside the family circle. A fear of vomiting in public may be important. Direct eye-to-eye confrontation may be particularly stressful in some cultures. Social phobias are usually associated with low self-esteem

Diagnostic Guidelines

Social Phobias

All the following criteria should be fulfilled for a diagnosis of social phobia:

- The psychological, behavioral, or autonomic symptoms must be primarily manifestations of anxiety and not secondary to other symptoms such as delusions or obsessional thoughts.
- The anxiety must be restricted to or must predominate in particular social situations.
- Avoidance of the phobic situations must be a prominent feature.

Panic Disorder (Episodic Paroxysmal Anxiety)

Panic disorder should be the main diagnosis only in the absence of any of the phobias. For a definite diagnosis, several severe attacks of autonomic anxiety should have occurred within a period of about one month

- in circumstances where there is no objective danger,
- without being confined to known or predictable situations, and
- with comparative freedom from anxiety symptoms between attacks (although anticipatory anxiety is common).

Obsessive–Compulsive Disorder

Obsessional symptoms or compulsive acts, or both, must be present on most days for at least two successive weeks and must be a source of distress or interference with activities. The obsessional symptoms should have the following characteristics:

- They must be recognized as the individual's own thoughts or impulses.
- There must be at least one thought or act that is still resisted unsuccessfully, even though others may be present that the sufferer no longer resists.

WHO 1992.

- The thought of carrying out the act must not in itself be pleasurable (simple relief of tension or anxiety is not regarded as pleasure in this sense).
- The thoughts, images, or impulses must be unpleasantly repetitive.

Posttraumatic Stress Disorder

This disorder should not generally be diagnosed unless there is evidence that it arose within six months of a traumatic event of exceptional severity. In addition to evidence of trauma, there must be a repetitive, intrusive recollection or reenactment of the event in memories, daytime imagery, or dreams. Conspicuous emotional detachment, numbing of feeling, and avoidance of stimuli that might arouse recollection of the trauma are often present but are not essential for the diagnosis. Autonomic disturbances, mood disorder (e.g., depression, dramatic bursts of fear or panic), and behavioral abnormalities (aggression disorder, alcohol abuse) all contribute to the diagnosis but are not key.

Generalized Anxiety Disorder

Primary symptoms of anxiety must be present most days for at least several weeks at a time and usually for several months. These symptoms should usually involve elements of

- apprehension (worries about future misfortunes, feeling "on edge," difficulty concentrating, etc.);
- motor tension (restless fidgeting, tension headaches, trembling, inability to relax); and
- autonomic overactivity (light-headedness, sweating, tachycardia or tachypnea, epigastric discomfort, dizziness, dry mouth, etc.).

In children, frequent need for reassurance and recurrent somatic complaints may be prominent.

and fear of criticism. Symptoms often involve flushing, hand tremor, nausea, or urgent need to urinate; a person with social phobia is sometimes sure that one of these secondary symptoms of anxiety is the primary problem. Symptoms may progress to panic attacks. Agoraphobia, which is fear of open spaces, and depressive disorders are often prominent, and both may contribute to the person's becoming housebound.

• *Panic disorder.* Panic disorder involves repeated episodes of intense fear that strike without warning and without an obvious source. Physical symptoms include chest pain;

heart palpitations; choking sensations or shortness of breath; dizziness; abdominal distress; feelings of unreality; and fear of dying, losing control, or going crazy. A panic attack usually lasts for minutes, during which a crescendo of fear and autonomic symptoms builds and leads the person to flee and subsequently avoid the situation in which the attack occurred, often producing fear of being alone or going into public places and persistent fear of another attack.

• *Obsessive–compulsive disorder (OCD).* This disorder is characterized by repeated, unwanted thoughts or compulsive behaviors that seem impossible to stop and is typified by repetitive acts or rituals to relieve anxiety.

• *Posttraumatic stress disorder.* This manifests as a delayed or prolonged response to a stressful event or situation (either short or long lasting) that was especially threatening or catastrophic (e.g., natural disaster; combat; serious accident; witnessing the violent death of others; or being the victim of torture, terrorism, rape, or other crime). Symptoms of **posttraumatic stress disorder** commonly include flashbacks or dreams of the original trauma, a state of autonomic hyperarousal with hypervigilance, an enhanced startle reaction, and insomnia.

• *Generalized anxiety disorder (GAD).* **Generalized anxiety disorder (GAD)** comprises recurrent or persistent excessive, uncontrollable worry about everyday, routine life events and activities, on more days than not for at least six months. Freud called this "free-floating" anxiety. It is accompanied by at least three of six symptoms of tension and vigilance and causes significant distress or impairment. The diagnostic criteria for GAD are still being refined. It is still controversial whether excessive worry is a necessary criterion (e.g., excessive worry is not required by the International Classification of Diseases-10) (Weisberg 2009). These are the symptoms of GAD, as defined by the American Psychiatric Association (2000a):

- Restlessness or feeling keyed up or on edge
- Being easily fatigued
- Difficulty concentrating or mind going blank
- Irritability
- Muscle tension
- Sleep disturbance (difficulty falling or staying asleep, or restless unsatisfying sleep)

Magnitude of the Problem

Anxiety disorders are the most common mental illnesses in the United States, affecting about 23 million people (4% of women and 2% of men) each year. As is the case with depression, young people tend to have more anxiety than do older people. People in the age group of 15 to 24 years experience episodes of anxiety about 40% more often than people 25 to 54 years old, regardless of race.

Social phobia is the most common anxiety disorder, with reported prevalence rates of up to 18.7%. The onset of social phobia typically occurs in childhood or adolescence; and the clinical course, if it is left untreated, is usually chronic, unremitting, and associated with significant functional impairment. Social phobia exhibits a high degree of comorbidity with other psychiatric disorders, including mood disorders, anxiety disorders, and substance abuse or dependence. Few people with social phobia seek professional help despite the existence of beneficial treatment approaches (Van Ameringen et al. 2003).

One of the most commonly encountered anxiety disorders in the primary care setting, panic disorder is a chronic and debilitating illness. Patients with panic disorder have medically unexplained symptoms that lead to overutilization of health care services (Pollack et al. 2003). Panic disorder is often comorbid with agoraphobia and major depression, and patients may be at increased risk of cardiovascular disease and, possibly, suicide.

Generalized anxiety disorder is a common disorder with a lifetime prevalence of 4% to 7% in the general population. Onset of GAD symptoms usually occurs during an individual's early 20s; however, high rates of GAD have also been seen in children and adolescents. The clinical course of GAD is often chronic, with 40% of patients reporting illness lasting more than five years. Generalized anxiety disorder is associated with pronounced functional impairment, resulting in decreased vocational function and reduced quality of life. Patients with GAD tend to be high users of outpatient medical care, which contributes significantly to health care costs (Allgulander et al. 2003).

Etiology of Anxiety Disorders

Just as people can have a depressive **temperament,** people can also, through genetics and early experiences, have an anxious temperament. Fluctuations in anxiety are a major part of most people's emotional lives, even those who do not have an anxiety disorder. Anxiety, like depression, is a stress emotion. Uncertainties about important events can lead to worry and apprehension, especially when a person feels a lack of control over how the event is going to turn out. Life events and desires such as romance, divorce, paying bills, making good grades, making a good impression on others, and getting a good job contribute to anxieties that affect the quality of life. Smaller hassles of daily living, such as catching the bus on time, making it to class on time, and dealing with a noisy neighbor or a nagging friend or relative, can add to stress emotions, including anxiety.

Anxiety can also be more subconscious, leading to tension, digestion problems, headaches, high blood pressure, and sleep problems, even when people do not report feeling worried. Feelings of helplessness or loss of control can lead to anxiety, as they do to depression.

Brain Neurobiology in Anxiety Disorders

A neurobiological perspective of anxiety integrates cognitive and neurological theories. For example, neural circuits involved in the experience of anxiety must include **afferent nerves** that allow potentially threatening stimuli to be sensed so that they can be interpreted as threatening by higher brain areas. These brain areas must appraise the input and integrate it with relevant memories. If the stimuli are then interpreted as representing a threat, the response depends on **efferent nerves** that generate a coordinated endocrine, autonomic, and muscular response. The effects of these different neural systems depend on several neurotransmitters, which have been targets for the pharmacologic treatment of anxiety disorders.

As is the case for depression, evidence from human and animal research indicates that the amygdala, locus coeruleus, midbrain, **thalamus,** right hippocampus, anterior cingulate cortex, insular cortex, and right prefrontal cortex (shown previously in figure 14.4) are involved in the genesis and expression of anxiety (Goddard and Charney 1997; Reiman 1997). The amygdala seems to be the critical central neural structure involved in the psychophysiological components of fear and anxiety responses (Goddard and Charney 1997; LeDoux 1998). The amygdala receives input from the thalamus and locus coeruleus and from sensations that have been integrated in higher cortical areas. Other key brain regions involved in anxiety include the hypothalamus and the **periaqueductal gray area,** which is a doughnut-shaped region that surrounds the cerebrospinal fluid channel between the third and fourth ventricles of the brain. The periaqueductal gray processes neuronal signals associated with pain and aversive behavior.

Each of those brain regions is modulated by the actions of serotonin (mainly originating from the dorsal raphe nuclei), norepinephrine (mainly originating from the locus coeruleus), and the inhibitory neurotransmitter **gamma-aminobutyric acid (GABA).** Several **anxiolytic** drugs affect serotonergic systems by blocking serotonin reuptake or by acting on serotonergic receptors as agonists or antagonists. The brain noradrenergic system is also involved in anxiety (O'Connor, Raglin, and Martinsen 2000). Inhibiting the effects of norepinephrine with β-adrenergic blockers, which downregulate the norepinephrine receptor–effector system, has been shown to be efficacious in the treatment of social phobia (Gorman and Gorman 1987). However, GABA is the major neural inhibitory brain neurotransmitter involved in anxiety disorders. GABA neurons and receptors are widely distributed in brain areas thought to be important for the expression of anxiety (Menard and Treit 1999).

Treatment of Anxiety Disorders

Anxiety disorders can be treated with psychotherapy or medications. Among antianxiety drugs, benzodiazepines are most commonly used to treat short-term symptoms, although SSRIs are also used to treat certain anxiety disorders.

Psychotherapy

The two most effective forms of psychotherapy used to treat anxiety disorders are behavioral and cognitive–behavioral therapy. Behavioral therapy helps patients change their actions through breathing techniques or through gradual exposure to what is frightening them. Cognitive–behavioral

therapy, in addition to these techniques, teaches patients to understand their thinking patterns so that they can react differently to the situations that cause them anxiety.

Pharmacotherapy

Although nearly two of three anxiety patients in the United States were treated with antidepressant drugs in 2005 (Olfson and Marcus 2005), a classification of drugs called the benzodiazepines (BDZs) provides the most effective short-term treatment of several anxiety disorders, especially generalized anxiety (Ballenger 2001). Across 12 years of observation in the National Population Health Survey of Canada, the prevalence of use of BDZs or similar sedatives was 2% to 3% of the population (Patton et al. 2010). In the Netherlands, anxiety patients who had other psychiatric conditions got twice as many antidepressant prescriptions and twice as many BDZ prescriptions during the year after diagnosis as did patients diagnosed only with anxiety (Smolders et al. 2007).

Benzodiazepines bind to the $GABA_A$ receptor and inhibit neuron activity by opening a chloride channel that raises the discharge threshold. Benzodiazepines are central nervous system depressants that are in a class of drugs known as sedative-hypnotics. Sedative drugs reduce anxiety (anxiolytic) and have a calming effect. Hypnotic drugs produce a state of drowsiness that helps people go to sleep and stay asleep. Other sedative–hypnotic drugs are barbiturates; alcohol; meprobamate (Miltown); and newer drugs like zolpidem (Ambien), eszopiclone (Lunesta), and zaleplon (Sonata) that are used to treat insomnia.

Fourteen BDZs are available in the United States, including alprazolam (Xanax), clonazepam (Klonopin), chlorazepate (Tranzene), diazepam (Valium), estazolam (ProSom), flurazepam (Dalmane), halazapam (Paxipam), lorazepam (Ativan), midazolam (Versed), oxazepam (Serax), prazepam (Centrax), quazepam (Doral), temazepam (Restoril), and triazolam (Halcion). Many other BDZs are available in Europe, Central and South America, and Asia that are not legally available in the United States. One notable example is flunitrazepam (Rohypnol), illegally imported into the United States, which has been used in conjunction with alcohol as a "date rape" drug due to its hypnotic and amnesic properties.

In 2009, an estimated 88 million prescriptions were filled in the United States for BDZs, making them the 10th most prescribed class of drugs (IMS Health 2010). Xanax (alprazolam) is by far the most prescribed BDZ in the United States (44.4 million prescriptions filled in 2009), followed by Klonopin (clonazepam), Ativan (lorazepam), Valium (diazepam), and then Restoril (temazepam) (IMS Health 2010). Benzodiazepines inhibit activity of neurons in the brain by opening a chloride channel and hyperpolarizing the cell. Benzodiazepines vary in the strength of their central nervous system depressant and muscle-relaxing effects, but they all are less sedating and hypnotic than barbiturates, which were commonly used to treat anxiety before BDZs. The BDZs are effective in treating GAD. Benzodiazepines are only weakly effective in the treatment of OCD and posttraumatic stress disorder, which are more effectively treated by SSRI antidepressants.

Excessive responses by nerves that manufacture and release noradrenaline contribute to signs and symptoms of anxiety, especially panic. Drugs that block receptors for noradrenaline, called beta-blockers (e.g., propranolol), help reduce panic symptoms, especially rapid heartbeat and palpitations. In contrast, inadequate responses by brain neurons that manufacture and release serotonin also play a role in anxiety disorders, especially OCD. SSRI antidepressants are clinically effective in treating anxiety. The tricyclic SSRI clomipramine is especially effective in treating OCD because it has antiobsessional effects (March et al. 1997).

Buspirone (BuSpar) is an atypical antianxiety drug that does not block the neuronal reuptake of monoamines. Rather, it binds with brain D2 dopamine receptors, where it acts as an antagonist and agonist, and with 5-HT_{1A} receptors, where it acts as an agonist (Stahl 1996). Like tricyclic and SSRI antidepressants, buspirone takes about a month to be effective in treating GAD, especially when combined with SSRIs; but it is not effective alone for the treatment of panic, OCD, or posttraumatic stress disorder (Stahl 1996).

High-potency BDZs (e.g., alprazolam, clonazepam, and lorazepam) are effective in treating panic disorder and panic attacks with or without agoraphobia and as add-on therapy to SSRIs in the treatment of OCD and panic disorders (Chouinard 2004). SSRIs are frontline treatments for social anxiety and panic disorder. Treatment of social phobia may need to be continued for several months to consolidate response and achieve full remission (Van Ameringen et al. 2003). An integrated treatment approach that combines pharmacotherapy with cognitive–behavioral therapy may provide the best treatment for panic disorder. Long-term efficacy and ease of use are important considerations in treatment selection, as maintenance treatment is recommended for at least 12 to 24 months, and in some cases, indefinitely (Pollack et al. 2003). Currently, BDZs and buspirone are prescribed frequently to treat GAD. Benzodiazepines are not recommended for long-term treatment of GAD due to associated development of tolerance, psychomotor impairment, cognitive and memory changes, physical dependence, and a withdrawal reaction on discontinuation. SSRIs (e.g., Paroxetine) and serotonin and noradrenaline reuptake inhibitors (e.g., extended-release Venlafaxine) appear to be effective in treating GAD. Of the psychological therapies, cognitive–behavioral therapy (CBT) shows the greatest benefit in treating GAD patients. Treatment gains after a 12-week course of CBT may be maintained for up to one year. Currently, no guidelines exist for the long-term treatment of GAD (Allgulander et al. 2003).

Common Drugs Used to Treat Anxiety

Benzodiazepines

Ativan (lorazepam)

Centrax (prazepam)

Halcion (triazolam)

Klonopin (clonazepam)

Paxipam (halazepam)

Restoril (temazepam)

Serax (oxazepam)

Valium (diazepam)

Versed (midazolam), intravenous injection in hospital only

Xanax (alprazolam)

Barbiturates

Librium (chlordiazepoxide)

Tranxene (clorazepate)

Tricyclic

Surmontil (trimipramine), panic disorder and OCD

Serotonin Antagonist

BuSpar (buspirone)

Selective Serotonin Reuptake Inhibitors

Celexa (citalopram)

Luvox (fluvoxamine)

Paxil (paroxetine)

Selfemra (fluoxetine), panic attacks, OCD

Zoloft (sertraline)

Selective Serotonin and Noradrenaline Reuptake Inhibitors

Cymbalta (duloxetine), generalized anxiety disorder

Effexor (venlafaxine), generalized anxiety disorder

Luvox (fluvoxamine), OCD, social anxiety, panic disorder, posttraumatic stress disorder, GAD

Dopamine Agonist

Wellbutrin (bupropion), panic disorder

Side effects include sedation, low muscle tone, and anticonvulsant effects; tolerance or dependence and withdrawal may develop.

Physical Activity and Anxiety: The Evidence

The 1996 U.S. Surgeon General's report on physical activity and health (U.S. Department of Health and Human Services 1996) concluded that regular physical activity reduces feelings of anxiety. However, the scientific advisory committee for the 2008 Physical Activity Guidelines for Americans concluded that the evidence to support that physical activity or exercise reduces symptoms in anxiety patients or protects against developing an anxiety disorder was minimal (Physical Activity Guidelines Advisory Committee 2008).

In contrast to the work on physical activity and depression, very few prospective epidemiologic studies have examined whether regular physical activity protects against developing an anxiety disorder, and even fewer RCTs have tested whether an exercise program can reduce anxiety symptoms in people diagnosed with an anxiety disorder. Most studies have been experimental studies of the effects of acute exercise on state anxiety or of chronic exercise on trait anxiety among people without anxiety disorders, or in patients with medical conditions other than anxiety who were enrolled in RCTs of exercise mainly to improve their primary medical condition or fitness level.

Preventing Anxiety: Observational Studies

An early cross-sectional population study suggested that active people had lower anxiety symptoms than inactive people (Stephens 1988). The Canada Health Survey asked nearly 11,000 Canadians aged 15 years and older questions about anxiety and their physical activity during the past two weeks. Women over 40 years of age and men (both under and over 40) who said they expended the equivalent of 5 or more kcal/kg of their body weight each day in leisure-time physical activity reported fewer anxiety-like symptoms than those who expended less than 2 kcal/kg of body weight each day. Since that first survey, several population-based studies using cross-sectional or prospective cohort designs have further examined the association between physical activity levels and risk of elevated anxiety symptoms.

Cross-Sectional Studies

At least five large population-based cross-sectional studies published during the past decade, including data from nationally representative samples of nearly 350,000 Americans, show that regular physical activity is associated with lower odds of anxiety symptoms.

U.S. National Comorbidity Survey

Goodwin (2003) analyzed data from the U.S. National Comorbidity Survey (n = 5877), a nationally representative sample of adults ages 15 to 54 in the United States. After adjustment for age, gender, race, marital status, education, income, physical illnesses, and other mental disorders, people who said they regularly got physical exercise for recreation or at work had 25% to 35% lower odds of being diagnosed with anxiety disorders during the past year, namely, agoraphobia (OR = 0.64; 95% CI: 0.43-0.94), social anxiety (OR = 0.65; 95% CI: 0.53-0.80), specific phobias (OR = 0.78; 95% CI: 0.63-0.97), and panic attacks (OR = 0.73; 95% CI: 0.56-0.96). A nearly 40% reduction in the odds of GAD (OR = 0.61; 95% CI: 0.42-0.88) was no longer significant after adjustment for other mental disorders (OR = 0.76; 95% CI: 0.52-1.11), likely reflecting the high comorbidity between GAD with depression and other anxiety disorders. There was a dose–response reduction in the odds of each anxiety disorder with higher frequency of physical activity. See figure 14.18.

The 2006 Behavioral Risk Factor Surveillance Survey

This was a random-digit-dialed telephone survey of 217,379 participants in 38 states, the District of Columbia, Puerto Rico, and the U.S. Virgin Islands (Strine et al. 2008). About 11% of people (14.3% of women and 8.2% of men) said they had at least once been told by a physician or health provider that they had an anxiety disorder (including acute stress disorder, anxiety, GAD, OCD, panic attacks, panic disorder, phobia, posttraumatic stress disorder, or social anxiety disorder). About 24% of participants said they had not participated in any leisure-time physical activity or exercise during the past 30 days. Regardless of age, inactive people were 40% more likely to have a lifetime anxiety disorder (OR = 1.4; 95% CI: 1.3-1.5). After adjustment for age, sex, race and ethnicity, education, marital and job status, chronic medical

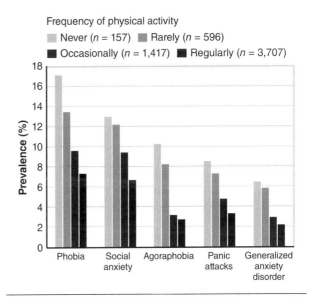

Figure 14.18 Twelve-month prevalence rates of anxiety disorders according to frequency of physical activity in the U.S. National Comorbidity Survey.

Data from Goodwin 2003.

conditions (cardiovascular disease, diabetes, asthma), smoking, obesity (BMI ≥30 kg/m²), and alcohol use (drinks per day: more than two for men, more than one for women), that risk remained elevated by 10%.

Health Study of North Trøndelag County, Norway

A total of 1260 survivors of testicular cancer and 20,207 men from the general population completed a mailed questionnaire that assessed leisure-time physical activity (including walking to work) and symptoms of anxiety (Thorsen et al. 2005). People who said they had spent less than 1 h each week during the past year in low-intensity physical activity (i.e., not hard enough to produce sweating or breathlessness) or no time in high-intensity physical activity were classified as physically inactive (18% of the people). The prevalence of elevated anxiety symptoms was higher among those who were physically inactive (17%) than among those who were active (13%), regardless of cancer diagnosis (OR = 1.36; 95% CI: 1.23-1.51). After adjustment for age, BMI, education, living alone, smoking, and elevated depression symptoms, odds of elevated anxiety symptoms were no longer higher among physically inactive people.

The Netherlands Twin Registry

The sample consisted of 12,450 adolescents (at least 10 years old) and adults who participated in a study on lifestyle and health from 1991 to 2002 (De Moor et al. 2006). The prevalence of exercise participation (at least an hour each week in activities rated at 4 METs or more) was 51.4%. After adjustment for gender and age, odds of general feelings of anxiety were approximately 16% lower among exercisers (OR = 0.84; 95% CI: 0.81-0.87). However, that association was likely confounded by personality because the exercisers also were more extraverted and emotionally stable; these are traits that reduce the risks of anxiety disorders. Among pairs of identical twins (479 male and 943 female) aged 18 to 50 years, the twin who exercised more did not report less anxiety than the twin who exercised less (De Moor et al. 2008). Also longitudinal analysis (follow-up ranged from two to 11 years) showed that increases in exercise participation did not predict decreases in anxiety.

Prospective Cohort Studies

At least three population-based studies that used a prospective cohort design have shown that physical activity is associated with 25% to 40% reductions in the risk of an anxiety disorder.

Northern Rivers Mental Health Study, Australia

A cohort of community residents living in the Richmond Valley of New South Wales was followed for a two-year period in order to identify the factors that were predictive of changes in their mental health status regardless of their past history (Beard et al. 2007). After random telephone screening to recruit a cohort at risk of mental disorders, 1407 invited subjects completed baseline face-to-face interviews using the Mini WHO Composite International Diagnostic Interview (ICD-10 criteria) (859 [51.4%] likely cases and 548 [56.9%] likely noncases). After two years, 968 adults ages 18 to 85 were reinterviewed. Those who reported more than 3 h per week of vigorous physical activity at baseline had 43% lower odds of developing any anxiety disorder compared to those who said they got no activity (OR = 0.57; 95% CI: 0.31-1.05), but the odds reduction was extinguished after adjustment for sex, stressful life events, emotional stability, and symptoms of distress measured at baseline.

SUN (Sequimiento Universidad de Navarra) Study

A reduction in the incidence of anxiety was observed in a cohort of 10,381 graduates (mean age about 43 ± 12 years) of the University of Navarra, Spain, who were followed up for four to six years (Sanchez-Villegas et al. 2008). There were 731 incident cases of anxiety disorder defined as self-reported physician-diagnosed anxiety or habitual tranquilizer use. After adjustment for age, gender, calorie intake, smoking, marital status, arthritis, ulcers, and cancer at baseline, odds of incident anxiety were reduced by one-third in the 20% of the people who expended at least 19 but less than 33 MET-hours per week in leisure-time physical activity (OR = 0.67; 95% CI: 0.52-0.85) and by 25% in the 20% who expended 33 MET-hours per week or more (OR = 0.74; 95% CI: 0.58-0.94) compared to the 20% least-active people.

Swedish Health Professionals

Cohort data collected in 2004 and 2006 from health care professionals and social insurance workers in western Sweden (2694 women, 420 men) were analyzed (Jonsdottir et al. 2010). Compared to those who were sedentary, people who said they engaged in either light physical activity (gardening, walking, or bicycling to work at least 2 h each week) or moderate-to-vigorous physical activity (aerobics, dancing, swimming, soccer, or heavy gardening at least 2 h each week; or 5 h at high intensity) during the past three months in 2004 were less likely than sedentary people to report elevated symptoms of anxiety at follow-up in 2006 (OR = 0.64; 95% CI: 0.42-1.02 and OR = 0.56; 95% CI: 0.34-0.94, respectively).

State Anxiety

The first modern-day controlled study of exercise and state anxiety was reported by William P. Morgan (1973) of the University of Wisconsin. He measured state anxiety in 40 men before, shortly after, and 20 to 30 min after 45 min of vigorous exercise. There was a slight increase in anxiety immediately after exercise but a significant decrease below preexercise anxiety 20 to 30 min later. In a subsequent study, the reduction in state anxiety after 20 min of exercise at 70% of aerobic capacity was comparable to reductions after meditation or quiet rest in a group of 75 middle-aged men (Bahrke and Morgan 1978). That study was especially important because it generated the **distraction hypothesis,** the hypothesis that the key feature common to each of the conditions was time out, or diversion, from the source or symptoms of anxiety and that distraction might be a plausible explanation for anxiety reduction after exercise. This hypothesis recently has found support (Breus and O'Connor 1998).

Since Morgan's seminal studies, a large body of research has shown about a 1/2 SD reduction in self-rated anxiety after aerobic exercise in adults without anxiety disorders (e.g., Landers and Petruzzello 1994), with larger changes typically occurring 5 to 30 min after exercise that lasted about 20 to 30 min. Although vigorous, acute exercise can temporarily increase state anxiety (O'Connor et al. 1995), confirming Morgan's seminal finding, moderate intensities of exercise lasting at least 30 min are generally associated with the largest reductions in self-rated state anxiety. Several studies suggested that acute exercise is as effective as meditation (Bahrke and Morgan 1978) and biofeedback and drugs (Broocks et al. 1998) but no more effective than quiet rest or distraction in decreasing state anxiety (Bahrke and Morgan 1978; Breus and O'Connor 1998). However, the anxiolytic effects of exercise apparently last longer than those of rest or distraction, and short periods of exercise have been associated with decreases in state anxiety that have persisted up to several hours. For example, Raglin and Wilson (1996) reported that state anxiety remained decreased up to 2 h after 20 min of cycling at either 40%, 60%, or 70% of $\dot{V}O_2$max.

Trait Anxiety

Landers and Petruzzello (1994) concluded from a meta-analysis of exercise and anxiety research that the typical reduction in trait anxiety after exercise training was nearly 1/2 SD, a change of about 5 points on the most common rating scale used in the studies, Spielberger's state–trait anxiety inventory, which ranges from 20 (almost never anxious) to 80 (almost always anxious). Despite the fact that virtually none of the people who were studied had diagnosed anxiety disorders, greater reductions were seen among people who had higher trait anxiety. Effects for exercise were as good as for other active treatments and better than for control conditions.

Long and van Stavel (1995) subsequently reported a mean effect of 0.40 SD for decreases in trait anxiety after exercise training averaged across 40 quasi-experimental and experimental studies of healthy adults. Since 1995, about 50 RCTs of exercise training have been reported. A recent meta-analysis of 40 RCTs including 2914 patients with chronic medical conditions other than anxiety disorders found that exercise training significantly reduced anxiety symptoms by a small amount (0.29 SD; 95% CI: 0.23-0.36) when compared to results for control groups that did not exercise (Herring, O'Connor, and Dishman 2010). See figure 14.19. Anxiety reductions were greatest in trials lasting no more than three

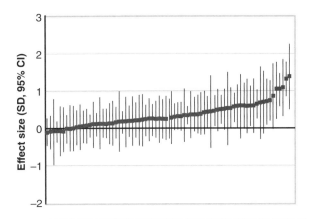

Figure 14.19 Randomized controlled trials of exercise training and anxiety symptoms among patients with medical conditions other than anxiety.

Data from Herring, O'Connor, and Dishman 2010.

months, when sessions lasted at least 30 min, and when people reported their experience of anxiety symptoms for more than the past week.

Treating Anxiety: Exercise Training by Patients With Anxiety Disorders

Few training studies have been conducted with people diagnosed with anxiety disorders, but generally there are reductions in anxiety regardless of training intensity or changes in aerobic capacity. Early RCTs with anxiety patients were conducted by Norwegian psychiatrist Egil Martinsen at the Modum Bads Nervesanatorium in the mid-1980s. Martinsen, Hoffart, and Solberg (1989a) examined the effects of aerobic (walking, jogging) and nonaerobic (strength, flexibility, relaxation) exercise on 79 inpatients with various anxiety disorders.

Patients randomly assigned to the groups exercised for 1 h three days per week. After eight weeks of training, patients in the two groups showed similar and significant reductions in anxiety regardless of changes in aerobic capacity. Benefits of exercise training were also documented in another study of 44 inpatients with a variety of anxiety disorders (Martinsen, Sandvik, and Kolbjørnsrud 1989). Patients performed 1 h of aerobic exercise five times a week for eight weeks. All exhibited improvements in anxiety symptoms during the study except those diagnosed with social phobia. Patients with GAD and agoraphobia without panic attacks had maintained their improvements at follow-up one year later. Sexton, Mære, and Dahl (1989) also reported persistence in anxiety reduction six months after hospitalized patients had participated in eight weeks of moderate- or low-intensity aerobic exercise training. In addition, improvements in psychological symptoms were similar for the two intensities.

Most of the clinical research on anxiety and exercise has focused on panic disorders, in part because of a concern in psychiatry since the 1960s that vigorous exercise poses a risk of inducing panic attacks in patients diagnosed with panic disorder, presumably resulting from hypersensitivity to bodily symptoms induced from blood lactate (O'Connor, Raglin, and Martinsen 2000). Contrary to that concern, empirical evidence from 15 studies conducted since 1987 refutes the association between exercise and panic attacks; only five panic attacks were reported during exercise involving 444 exercise bouts performed by 420 panic disorder patients (O'Connor, Smith, and Morgan 2000). Research has also shown that lactate accumulation resulting from exercise is not related to increased risk of panic attacks among patients with panic disorder (Martinsen et al. 1998) or to postexercise anxiety in normal individuals (e.g., Garvin, Koltyn, and Morgan 1997). A half hour of moderate-to-vigorous treadmill exercise reduces the intensity of experimentally induced panic attacks among panic patients (Ströhle et al. 2009).

At least three RCTs have shown a reduction in anxiety after exercise training among people who have an anxiety disorder (e.g., Broocks et al. 1998; Herring et al. 2012; Merom et al. 2008).

Aerobic Exercise Versus SSRIs for Panic Disorder and Agoraphobia

A randomized clinical trial showed that 10 weeks of aerobic exercise training was effective in reducing symptoms of anxiety among patients with panic disorder and agoraphobia, though not as effective as drug therapy (Broocks et al. 1998). In that study, 46 outpatients suffering from moderate to severe panic disorder with agoraphobia (four did not have agoraphobia) were randomly assigned to a 10-week treatment consisting of regular aerobic exercise (running), the serotonin reuptake inhibitor clomipramine (112.5 mg/day), or placebo pills. The dropout rate was 31% for the exercise group, 27% for the placebo group, and 0% for the clomipramine treatment group. Compared with placebo, both exercise and clomipramine were accompanied by a significant decrease in symptoms, but clomipramine treatment improved anxiety symptoms sooner and more effectively. See figure 14.20. Though some evidence has suggested that individuals with panic disorders are physically inactive and actually avoid exercise (Broocks et al. 1997), there is no scientific consensus that patients diagnosed with panic disorder avoid physical activity because of fear (O'Connor, Smith, and Morgan 2000).

Walking Plus Group Cognitive–Behavioral Therapy

A group randomized trial in an outpatient clinic for people diagnosed with panic disorder, GAD, or social phobia compared a home-based walking program added to group

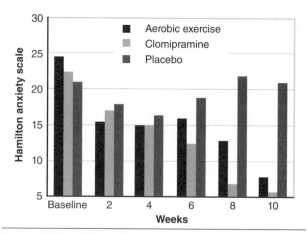

Figure 14.20 Effects of aerobic exercise or drug therapy on panic disorder.

Data from Broocks et al. 1998.

cognitive–behavioral therapy (GCBT + walking) (21 people) with GCBT and educational sessions (GCBT + education) (20 people) (Merom et al. 2008). After adjustment for self-ratings of depression, anxiety, and stress at study outset and type of anxiety disorder, the GCBT + walking group reported fewer symptoms of depression, anxiety, and stress than did the GCBT + education group.

Generalized Anxiety Disorder

Thirty sedentary women 18 to 37 years of age at the University of Georgia who had a primary DSM-IV diagnosis of GAD were randomly assigned to six weeks of resistance exercise training or aerobic exercise training or to a wait list control group who had the opportunity to participate in an exercise program after the trial ended (Herring et al. 2012). About 70% of the women had a comorbidity with another anxiety or mood disorder, and one-third of them were being treated with antidepressants (mainly a SSRI or a NSRI). Women exercised two times a week under supervision, performing either lower body weightlifting or leg cycling matched between conditions by body region, positive work, load progression, and time actively engaged in exercise. There were no adverse events. Remission rates were 60%, 40%, and 30% for resistance exercise, aerobic exercise, and the control condition. Worry symptoms were reduced by the exercise conditions compared to the control condition. Most research on anxiety and exercise has examined the effects of aerobic, low-resistance exercises such as swimming, cycling, or running at moderate or high intensities. Anxiety reductions following high-resistance exercise such as weightlifting have been examined less frequently.

In 1993, Raglin, Turner, and Eksten found no decrease in state anxiety after weight training but significant decreases after leg cycle exercise. Focht and Koltyn (1999) found a reduction in state anxiety after resistance exercise at 50% but not 80% of 1-repetition maximum (1RM), although this effect was delayed by more than 60 min after exercise. In another study, anxiety reductions after resistance exercise were delayed until 1.5 to 2 h after exercise (O'Connor et al. 1993). Bartholomew and Linder (1998) found decreased state anxiety after 20 min of resistance exercise at 40% to 50% of 1RM, and this effect occurred 15 and 30 min after exercise. They also found that anxiety was increased 5 and 15 min after 20 min of high-intensity resistance exercise (75-85% of 1RM).

Dose Response in Studies of Physical Activity and Anxiety

No exercise training studies have manipulated exercise program length or exercise type to see whether the size of anxiety reductions differs. About half the studies used aerobic exercise alone (walking, jogging, or cycling), and one-fourth used resistance exercise alone or combined aerobics with resistance training, usually low-intensity strength training. The magnitude of anxiety reduction has been similar regardless of type of exercise or duration (usually 25 min up to an hour) or regardless of whether it was continuous or intermittent (i.e., with rest breaks). However, most studies were imprecise in describing how much time was actually spent in active exercise compared to warming up, resting, and cooling down.

It is not known whether intensity of aerobic or resistance exercise affects anxiety reduction in clinical trials. More than half the trials used moderate-to-vigorous exercise intensity (i.e., 60-80% of aerobic capacity or maximum strength) with a weekly frequency of three or more days per week. Reductions in anxiety symptoms were similar across those variations in exercise intensity.

Physical Activity and Anxiety in Youth

No RCTs of children or adolescents diagnosed with anxiety disorders have been reported. A meta-analysis located six poorly controlled trials including youths aged 11 to 19 years from the general population that compared exercise training with a no-treatment condition or with an intervention other than drugs or psychotherapy (Larun et al. 2006). The exercise group showed a moderately large but statistically nonsignificant effect of exercise in reducing anxiety scores (−0.48 SD; 95% CI: −0.97 to 0.01) regardless of exercise intensity. Whether that apparent effect is generalizable to a reduction in the primary risk of developing depression among adolescents is not yet established. A four-year longitudinal study of 2548 adolescents and young adults aged 14 to 24 years in Munich, Germany, showed that those who said they regularly exercised or played sports at baseline had a lower overall incidence of any mental disorder and anxiety (Ströhle et al. 2007).

Strength of the Evidence

There is no compelling evidence that increased physical activity or fitness changes a person's temperament from anxious to calm and relaxed. However, studies have shown that a single session of physical activity can reduce state anxiety and that regular exercise can reduce trait anxiety. Because there is no evidence that physical activity causes the underlying sources of anxiety to disappear or causes people to perceive events as less threatening, how can these reductions in anxiety be explained?

Temporal Sequence

Controlled prospective cohort studies of the association between physical activity and anxiety symptoms or the risk of developing anxiety disorders have yet to be reported. About 100 experimental studies, which have the proper temporal sequence to establish cause and effect, of the effects of acute exercise on state anxiety and of chronic exercise on trait anxiety in people without anxiety disorders have generally agreed that exercise decreases self-rated symptoms of anxiety to a small to moderate degree.

Strength of Association

More than 250 small-sample studies cumulatively have shown a small to moderate reduction either in self-rated state anxiety after acute exercise (about 0.50 SD) or in trait anxiety after chronic exercise in healthy adults (about 0.40 SD) or patients with medical conditions other than anxiety disorders (about 0.30 SD). A handful of studies show reductions in symptoms among patients diagnosed with panic disorders, social phobia, or GAD, even suggesting better remission rates after aerobic or resistance exercise. However, there is not yet enough evidence to allow judgment on the clinical benefits of exercise training as a first-line or adjuvant treatment for anxiety disorders.

Consistency

As is the case for studies of depression, most studies of anxiety and exercise were not designed to compare demographic groups on their anxiety responses to exercise and were limited to ages younger than 55 years; or they arbitrarily used middle age (e.g., 40 or 45 years) as a criterion for aging effects. There have been very few controlled studies of children and of people over age 65. Quantitative reviews concluded that age did not moderate reductions in self-ratings of state anxiety and trait anxiety (e.g., Landers and Petruzzello 1994). Neither men nor women had reduced state anxiety in one review (Schlict 1994); but the small number of studies reviewed led to low statistical power, and it appears that sampling errors prevented powerful tests of age in both analyses. Another quantitative review found that state anxiety was reduced after exercise among men but not women. Reductions in physiological variables under nonstress conditions were significant for subjects under 45 years but not over 45 years. Although it is likely that sociocultural factors differently influence the ways in which women and men of different ages, education levels, races, or ethnicities perceive exercise, its outcomes, and its context, the current evidence does not permit conclusions about whether the association of exercise with anxiety is consistent across demographic groups.

Dose Response

There are biological reasons to expect that the effects of physical activity on anxiety would vary according to exercise intensity (e.g., increases in body temperature, whose relevance for anxiety is explained later in this chapter, and endocrine and metabolic responses during exercise). However, available data do not show dose-dependent reductions in anxiety with increasing exercise intensity. Changes in state anxiety after exercise reported in studies published before 1993 did not differ significantly among exercise intensities expressed as percentages of $\dot{V}O_2$peak (Landers and Petruzzello 1994; Petruzzello et al. 1991), but most of those studies did not quantify relative exercise intensity according to different levels of cardiorespiratory fitness or compare intensities within the same participants.

Often, aerobic capacity was estimated based on submaximal fitness tests or heart rate, which can be up to 20% off from actual aerobic capacity. Accurate assessment of exercise intensity is critical for determining the necessary or optimal exercise intensity for reducing anxiety for prescribing a training program. Studies published since 1993 typically have used standard methods for quantifying exercise intensity. The researchers reported decreased or unchanged anxiety after intensities ranging from 40% to 70% $\dot{V}O_2$peak (Breus and O'Connor 1998; Dishman, Farquhar, and Cureton 1994; Garvin, Koltyn, and Morgan 1997; Koltyn and Morgan 1992; O'Connor and Davis 1992; Raglin and Wilson 1996) and increased, decreased, or unchanged anxiety after maximal exercise testing with different samples of participants (Koltyn, Lynch, and Hill 1998; O'Connor et al. 1995).

Also, too few studies have been conducted to permit a statistically powerful quantitative analysis of the concomitant effects of intensity and duration. It appears that moderate intensities of exercise lasting up to about 30 min generally are associated with the largest reductions, but there have been few studies of short durations (e.g., 5-10 min) or intermittent sessions. A few studies have specifically contrasted the effects of different intensities or durations of exercise on anxiety, but they confounded intensity and duration and used only slightly different intensities or used intensities too high and durations too short for clinical applications.

With the exception of two reports (Herring et al. 2012; Pronk et al. 1994), studies examining dose–response effects of acute or chronic exercise on state or trait anxiety have not attempted to equate the total energy expenditure of exercise conditions of varying intensity and duration. Thus, the effects of different total energy expenditures may be falsely attributed to variations in the intensity or duration of the activity.

Plausibility

As with depression, biological plausibility is not the only concept that can explain mental health outcomes of physical activity. Next is a discussion of several of the most popular cognitive and social explanations, followed by a traditional examination of biological plausibility.

Cognitive and Social Factors

It is important to determine whether reduced anxiety after acute exercise or an exercise training program can be explained by a direct effect of exercise or merely by other aspects of the exercise setting. It is unlikely that exercise would directly decrease the occurrence of some forms of anxiety. For example, there is no reason to expect that exercise would reduce simple phobias. A person afraid of spiders will experience anxiety when exposed to one whether he or she is active and fit or sedentary. However, physical activity might help people cope with the experience of anxiety, distract them from worry, or reduce some symptoms.

Physiological sensations from exercise might help redefine the subjective meaning of arousal and could thus compete with the perception of anxiety symptoms. This has been proposed as a way in which exercise could help panic patients who are very sensitive to somatic symptoms of arousal. Repeated exercise might help people with panic disorder learn to perceive arousal as less threatening. Sensations of the heart pounding during exercise can be reinterpreted as a sign of a good workout rather than a symptom of anxiety.

Exercise can also distract attention from anxiety-provoking thoughts and provides a time-out from cares and worries (Bahrke and Morgan 1978). Breus and O'Connor (1998) tested this distraction hypothesis by measuring state anxiety in 18 highly trait-anxious college women before and after exercise at moderate intensity (40% of aerobic capacity), exercise during studying, studying only, and quiet rest. There was no change in anxiety after exercise during studying, studying only, or quiet rest. There was a significant decrease in anxiety after the exercise-only condition, which indicates that the anxiolytic effect of exercise (exercise as a distraction from worries and concerns) was blocked by studying.

Herring and colleagues found that women diagnosed with GAD reported less worry after six weeks of resistance or aerobic exercise training (Herring et al. 2012).

▷ **THE DISTRACTION** hypothesis states that exercise distracts attention from anxiety-provoking thoughts and provides a time-out from cares and worries.

Biological Plausibility

Physical activity is unique among behavioral treatments for mental health. The increased metabolism of physical exertion produces several acute responses during exercise and more long-lasting adaptations to chronic exercise that appear to improve mental health. Possible explanations for reduced anxiety after exercise include body warming, alterations in endorphins, reduced arousal, altered brain electrocortical activity, changes in the brain noradrenaline and serotonin systems, and influences on the brain GABA/benzodiazepine system.

• *Body warming.* Increases in body temperature in the range that occurs with moderate to intense exercise (about 1-1.5 °C) at normal environmental temperatures have been associated with reduced muscle tension. The speculation that reduced anxiety after exercise depends on increased body temperature is biologically plausible, but the dozen or so studies that tested the idea did not support it (Koltyn 1997). Changes in anxiety after acute exercise have not corresponded with manipulations of body temperature before or during exercise. However, the studies that simulated natural exercise (e.g., underwater finning exercise with or without a wet suit) did an incomplete job of controlling temperature or used inadequate nonexercise control conditions. A study that effectively controlled temperature during exercise did so in an unnatural exercise setting: Subjects cycled in shoulder-deep water (Youngstedt et al. 1993). It remains plausible that increased temperature during typical exercise contributes to reduced anxiety, but body warming probably is not the sole or direct cause of the reduced anxiety or improved mood.

• *Endorphins.* For the same reasons discussed earlier regarding depression, brain opioids could plausibly be involved with anxiety reduction after acute exercise, but there currently is no compelling evidence to support that idea (Dishman and O'Connor 2009). Studies in humans that used opioid-blocking drugs during exercise still found that people reported reduced state anxiety or feelings of tension (e.g., Farrell et al. 1982). Other research has shown that men who had the largest increases in blood levels of β-endorphin during cycling exercise also had the largest increase in state anxiety, exactly the converse of the endorphin hypothesis.

• *Physiological arousal.* A few early studies reviewed by de Vries (1981) and a more recent study (Smith et al. 2002) have shown that acute and chronic exercise can reduce muscle reflexes and tension. It is not yet clear, though, whether reduced muscle tension after exercise is part of anxiety reduction or is a biological response to exercise that is independent of anxiety. Recent research on the **Hoffmann reflex,** which has been presumed to be an objective index of relaxation after acute exercise (Bulbulian and Darabos 1986; de Vries et al. 1981; Petruzzello et al. 1991), showed that reductions in the Hoffman reflex after mild or vigorous cycling exercise were not related to reductions in self-rated state anxiety (Motl, O'Connor, and Dishman 2004). Likewise, reductions in blood pressure after exercise have been interpreted by some investigators as indirect evidence of an anxiolytic effect of exercise (e.g., Petruzzello et al. 1991;

Raglin, Turner, and Eksten 1993). However, postexercise hypotension (i.e., lowered blood pressure for up to 2 h after exercise) is a well-known physiological phenomenon that occurs even when anxiety is not lowered after exercise (e.g., Youngstedt et al. 1993). In contrast, one modern theory proposes that an **electromyogram (EMG)** measure of the startle response provides an index of people's predisposition to interpret environmental events as negative or threatening (Lang, Bradley, and Cuthbert 1998). A recent study showed that a reduction in startle response was related to reduced self-ratings of state anxiety after both quiet rest and moderate-intensity cycling exercise (Smith et al. 2002).

• *Brain electroencephalographic activity.* Another contemporary theory of emotional response proposes that **electroencephalograms (EEGs)** of **hemispheric asymmetry** in brain oscillatory activity (i.e., brain waves) provide another index of a predisposition to interpret environmental events as negative or threatening (R.J. Davidson 1998). Recently, EEG asymmetry in the alpha frequency band has been shown to be related to self-ratings of anxiety after moderately intense treadmill and cycling exercise (Crabbe, Smith, and Dishman 2007; Petruzzello and Landers 1994; Petruzzello and Tate 1997). However, moderate to large increases in the frequency band of **alpha wave activity** measured by EEG are common during and after exercise (Crabbe and Dishman 2004; Kubitz and Mott 1996; Petruzzello et al. 1991; figure 14.21). Increased alpha activity is traditionally viewed as an index of relaxed wakefulness, but this view is not universally held by EEG experts, and the exercise studies did not show that the increased alpha activity was caused by the exercise or related to reduced anxiety; other brain wave frequencies also increase after exercise (Crabbe and Dishman 2004).

• *Brain neurotransmitters: serotonin, norepinephrine, and GABA.* Animal studies have found increased activity of serotonin neurons in the raphe nucleus during treadmill running (Jacobs and Fornal 1999), increased brain release of serotonin during treadmill running (Wilson and Marsden 1996), and increased release of serotonin and increased levels of serotonin in several brain regions after exercise

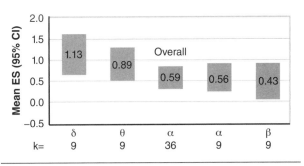

Figure 14.21 Effects of acute exercise on brain oscillatory activity.

Data from Crabbe and Dishman 2004.

training (Dunn and Dishman 1991; Meeusen and De Meirleir 1995). There is also indirect evidence of effects of exercise on central serotonergic systems based on measures of tryptophan disposition in the blood and concentrations of 5-HIAA (a serotonin metabolite) in cerebrospinal fluid (Chaouloff 1997a). One mechanism for increased brain levels of serotonin with exercise is the effect of exercise on increasing the transport of the amino acid tryptophan from the bloodstream into the brain. Exercise induces increased lipolysis, or the breakdown of triglycerides into free fatty acids, which are used to fuel increased levels of muscular contraction. Increased serum levels of free fatty acids compete with tryptophan for binding with albumin, leading to increases in free tryptophan. This increase in free tryptophan stimulates an influx of tryptophan into the brain and thus the potential for increased synthesis of serotonin.

Chronic activity-wheel running and treadmill exercise training increase levels of norepinephrine in the locus coeruleus, amygdala, hippocampus, and hypothalamus (Dishman et al. 2000b) and decrease the number of β-adrenoreceptors in the frontal cortex (Yoo et al. 2000b). Chronic activity-wheel running also reduces the release of norepinephrine in the frontal cortex during stress (Soares et al. 1999), possibly by upregulating the expression of genes for neuropeptides such as galanin and **neuropeptide Y** that inhibit locus coeruleus activity (O'Neal et al. 2001). All those changes are similar to some of the actions of antidepressant drugs that presumably underlie their therapeutic effects. Chronic activity-wheel running also increases levels of GABA and decreases the number of GABA$_A$ receptors in the corpus striatum, consistent with an anxiolytic effect (Dishman et al. 1996). The explanation for the anxiolytic effect of exercise based on GABA may be the effects of exercise on central cholinergic function, which is inhibited by BDZ receptor agonists.

An increase in locomotion usually reflects an adaptive motivational state in rats, indicating reduced behavioral inhibition (e.g., less freezing; Dishman 1997a). An increase in open-field locomotion has been reported in rats following forced exercise swimming and after motorized treadmill running. Locomotion by the rat in an open field is associated inversely with observer ratings of anxiety when the locomotion appears purposeful and the animal exhibits other exploratory behaviors such as rearing or approaching the center of the open field. In contrast, low levels of locomotion, few approaches to the center of the open field, freezing, defecation, urination, and shivering are conventionally regarded as isomorphic with the hypervigilance, hesitancy, fear, and autonomic activation common in human anxiety. Under certain circumstances of threat, increased locomotion seems to indicate panic (e.g., the flight response to a predator). A study conducted at the University of Georgia found that chronic activity-wheel running led to increased open-field locomotion and changes in GABA receptor binding, consistent with an anxiety-reducing effect (Dishman et al. 1996).

Cognitive Function and Dementia

Cognition involves selection, manipulation, storage, and retrieval of information and the use of that information to guide behavior. Cognitive functions generally develop in childhood, reach a peak during young adulthood, and then decline after middle age. Normal function can become impaired with age or after trauma. Further deterioration can lead to dementia.

In 1906, German psychiatrist and pathologist Aloysius Alzheimer described the dementia that bears his name after he observed amyloid plaques, neurofibril tangles, and arteriosclerotic pathologies during autopsy of the brain of a 51-year-old woman who had a five-year history of progressive cognitive and social impairments in functioning before her death (Möller and Graeber 1998). One hundred years later, there are an estimated 24.3 million people worldwide with dementia (Ferri et al. 2005). Dementia is projected to be the world's third leading cause of death and disability by the year 2030 (Mathers and Loncar 2006). Based on an expected 4.6 million new cases of dementia each year since 2001, the number of cases is expected to double every 20 years to 81.1 million by 2040 (Ferri et al. 2005). Most people (60% in 2001) with dementia live in developing countries. That rate is predicted to be 71% by 2040. In contrast, projected average increases in developed nations are expected to double during that time but to increase by 300% in India, China, south Asia, and the western Pacific.

According to the nationally representative Aging, Demographics, and Memory Study conducted in the United States, the estimated prevalence of any dementia among people ages 71 and older was 13.9% in 2002, about 3.4 million people. The prevalence of Alzheimer's dementia was 9.7% (2.4 million people), accounting for approximately 69.9% of all dementia. Vascular dementia, the next most common form, accounted for 17.4%. Dementia rates have been shown to increase with age, from 5.0% of those aged 71 to 79 years to 37.4% of those aged 90 and older (Plassman et al. 2007). In the United States, the annual cost of informal care was $18 billion per year in 1998 (Langa et al. 2001).

Only about 5% of people with Alzheimer's disease have the early-onset, or familial, form, which develops in peoples ages 30 to 60 years. Some of those cases are caused by gene mutations on chromosomes 21, 14, and 1, which result in abnormal proteins. Mutations on chromosome 21 cause the formation of abnormal amyloid precursor protein, which forms plaques outside brain cells. Those plaques make brain cells more vulnerable to the subsequent accumulation of a lethal protein named tau which spreads through neural memory circuits after starting mainly in the entorhinal cortex of the hippocampus. A mutation on chromosome 14 causes abnormal presenilin 1 to be made, and a mutation on chromosome 1 leads to abnormal presenilin 2. Mutations in prese-

---

Causes of Dementia

Degenerative Disorders

- Alzheimer's disease
- Frontotemporal dementias
- Dementia with Lewy bodies (abnormal aggregates of protein that develop inside nerve cells)
- Parkinson's disease dementia
- Huntington's disease
- Progressive supranuclear palsy

Vascular Causes

- Multi-infarct dementia
- Lacunar infarcts
- Binswanger's disease
- Cerebral autosomal dominant arteriopathy with subcortical infarcts and leukoencephalopathy
- Vasculitis (e.g., lupus erythematosus)

---

nilins impair their ability to recycle normal proteins and to catabolize damaged proteins and cell organelles that are toxic to neurons. Most cases of Alzheimer's, though, are late onset, after age 60. In early 1993, one of the four variant alleles of the apo E gene on chromosome 19, apo E-ε4, was identified as a genetic risk factor for late-onset Alzheimer's disease. As discussed in chapter 8 in the context of lipoproteins, apo E is a protein that regulates cholesterol and fat metabolism. Apo E-ε4 occurs in about 40% of all people who develop late-onset Alzheimer's disease and is present in about 25% to 30% of the population (Alzheimer's Disease Genetics Fact Sheet 2008). Middle-aged adult carriers of the apo E-ε4 mutation who have normal cognitive function nonetheless have abnormally low rates of brain glucose metabolism in the medial parietal, the posterior cingulate, parietotemporal, and the frontal cortexes, which may signal early pathology (Reiman et al. 2005).

Like the other constructs discussed in this chapter, cognition is not an objective thing. Rather, it is inferred from performance on tests. There are more than 400 tests designed to assess specific types of mental processing (Lezak, Howieson, and Loring 2004). They include those designed to assess specific processes such as working memory, information-processing speed, and inhibition and those that assess global mental functioning involving multiple processes, such as intelligence and abstract reasoning. They also include tests for evaluating the effects of traumatic head injury or degenerative diseases and those that measure how healthy people normally differ from each other. Exercise studies during the past decade have focused mainly on executive control processes, which

include response inhibition, attentional control, working memory, and rule discovery; these are mainly regulated by neural activity in the prefrontal cortexes of the brain, areas that are further modulated by activity in the temporal and parietal cortexes, the hippocampus, and several other brain areas involved with motivated behavior (Royall et al. 2002).

Physical Activity and Cognitive Function: The Evidence

The scientific advisory committee of the Physical Activity Guidelines for Americans concluded that the weight of the available evidence from prospective cohort studies supports the conclusion that physical activity delays the incidence of dementia and the onset of cognitive decline associated with aging. The committee also concluded that evidence from RCTs of healthy older adults and people with Alzheimer's disease or other dementias support that regular participation in physical activity improves aspects of cognitive function or reduces symptoms of dementia (Physical Activity Guidelines Advisory Committee 2008).

Early studies yielded mixed evidence about the benefits of regular exercise or cardiorespiratory fitness on cognitive functioning (e.g., Tomporowski and Ellis 1986). Reevaluation of that evidence and more recent research suggest some positive effects of both acute and chronic exercise on some aspects of cognitive function in healthy, older adults (McAuley, Kramer, and Colcombe 2004) and children (Davis et al. 2011; Tomporowski 2003). First, the influence of fitness on cognitive performance among older adults seems to depend on features of the cognitive tasks. Studies show that cardiorespiratory fitness and chronic aerobic exercise training facilitate executive control functions of cognition among older adults (Colcombe et al. 2004). The cumulative evidence has shown small to moderately large positive effects of 1/3 to 1/2 SD on several types of cognitive performance after either acute and chronic exercise (Etnier et al. 1997; Lambourne

Cognitive Skills Affected by Dementia

- Decision making, judgment
- Memory
- Spatial orientation
- Thinking, reasoning
- Verbal communication

and Tomporowski 2011; Sibley and Etnier 2003). Whether those effects depend directly upon physical fitness remains unclear, however (Etnier et al. 2007).

A meta-analysis of 18 RCTs of aerobic exercise training in middle-aged adults (ages 55 years and older), mainly people living in the community without cognitive impairment (Colcombe and Kramer 2003), found a benefit of nearly 1/3 SD averaged across all tasks studied. However, the largest effect of exercise, about 0.60 SD, was for executive control tasks that measured goal-oriented decision-making behavior. In a subsequent meta-analysis of RCTs comparing aerobic physical activity programs with any other intervention or no intervention, eight out of 11 studies reported an average increase in maximal oxygen uptake of 14% and also improvements in cognitive function, especially for motor function (1.17 SD) and auditory attention (0.50 SD). There were also small effects (1/4 SD) for information-processing speed and visual attention (Angevaren et al. 2008).

Numerous prospective population-based cohort studies have assessed the relation between people's level of physical activity and the onset of age-related decline in cognitive functioning or incident cases of dementia. Odds ratios from 11 prospective, observational studies of ~23,000 people in the United States (four studies) and Australia, Canada, France, Japan, and Sweden showed that physically active people had an average reduction of nearly 40% in the risk of developing dementia. See figure 14.22.

In a subsequent meta-analysis of those 11 cohort studies plus two others, including 2731 incident cases of Alzheimer's disease or other dementia at follow-up, people classified as being in the highest physical activity level in each study had an average 45% lower risk of Alzheimer's disease (RR = 0.55; 95% CI: 0.36-0.84) and 28% lower risk of all dementia (RR = 0.72; 95% CI: 0.60-0.86) compared to the least-active groups (Hamer and Chida 2009).

Other prospective cohort studies of elderly women in Canada (Middleton, Kirkland, and Rockwood 2008) and the United States (Yaffe et al. 2001), including nearly 19,000 women 70 to 81 years of age from the Nurses' Health Study (Weuve et al. 2004), have reported that those who were the most active during their leisure time, performing either walking or other moderate-to-vigorous activities, had 20% to 40% lower risk of cognitive decline, without dementia, across periods of two to eight years, even after adjustment for education, alcohol use, smoking, aspirin use, and vascular risk factors (e.g., heart disease, stroke, high blood pressure, and diabetes). In a retrospective study of 9000 U.S. women, those who reported being physically active at any point over the life course, especially as teenagers, had a 20% to 35% lower likelihood of cognitive impairment in late life. Also, women who said they were physically inactive as teenagers but became active in later life had lower risk than those who remained inactive (Middleton et al. 2010).

No RCT has shown that regular physical activity prevents dementia, but a few show improvement in some aspects of cognitive functioning in people with dementia, including Alzheimer's disease (Heyn, Abreu, and Ottenbacher 2004; Rolland, Abellan van Kan, and Vellas 2010). For example, a 12-month exercise program (1 h, twice each week, of walking and strength, balance, and flexibility training) led to slower decline in an index of activities of daily living (0.40 SD) compared to usual medical care, but no change in behavioral disturbance or depression, in 134 ambulatory patients with mild to severe Alzheimer's disease living in five nursing homes (Rolland et al. 2007).

▷ **PROSPECTIVE COHORT** studies support the conclusion that physical activity delays the incidence of dementia and the onset of cognitive decline associated with aging.

A recent RCT of 17 women and 16 men ages 55 to 85 years who had mild cognitive impairment (partial loss of memory) compared the effects of high-intensity aerobic exercise to those of stretching for six months (45 to 60 min/day, four days per week) (Baker et al. 2010). In women, aerobic exercise improved glucose metabolism, reduced insulin and BDNF levels in the plasma, and improved performance on several tests of executive function. In men, aerobic exercise increased plasma levels of insulin-like growth factor I and improved performance on only one of the cognitive function tests.

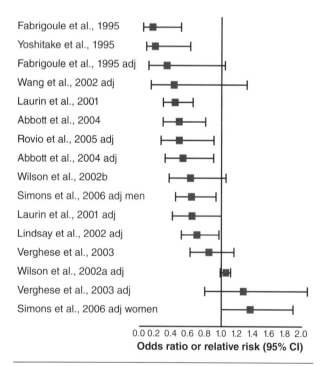

Figure 14.22 Prospective cohort studies of physical activity and dementia risk.

Data from Physical Activity Guidelines Advisory Committee 2008.

Effect Modification of Dementia Risk—Apo E-ε4 Mutation

After adjustment for age, education, alcohol consumption, smoking, and cognitive functioning at baseline, more than an hour of physical activity favorably modified the risk of cognitive decline among carriers of the apo E-ε4 mutation in one Dutch study (Schuit et al. 2001). See figure 14.23. After adjustment for age, gender, and education in a subsequent study, people judged as physically active had faster reaction times during a working memory test if they were apo E-ε4 carriers (Deeny et al. 2008). Among 90 older women who had normal cognitive function, aerobic fitness was associated with significantly better performance on executive function tests that measured working memory in the women who inherited the ε4 allele from both parents (Etnier et al. 2007). Brain imaging showed that sedentary ε4 carriers had less activation of the right temporal lobe during testing than physically active ε4 carriers. A recent cross-sectional study used functional brain imaging to test the modifying effect of physical activity level and apo E-ε4 on brain activation during memory processing of famous names in 68 older (ages 65-85) adults without dementia (Smith et al. 2011). Participants with the apo E-ε4 risk factor for dementia who were high in physical activity showed greater memory activation in nine of 15 brain regions than people who were low risk, low active, or both.

Cognitive Performance in Children

A meta-analysis of 44 studies found a small, cumulative effect of 1/3 SD on improved cognitive function after exercise training among children, regardless of whether the exercise was in physical education classes or was special training for the purpose of trying to improve motor skills, muscular strength, or aerobic fitness (Sibley and Etnier 2003). Effects were a little larger than average for children in early elementary grades and middle school. Also, the size of the effects differed according to type of cognitive task, with effects larger for tests of perceptual skills (ES = 0.49), followed by IQ (ES = 0.34), achievement (ES = 0.30), and then math tests (ES = 0.20) and verbal tests (ES = 0.17).

However, the studies generally weren't well controlled, so the strength of the evidence was weak for several reasons as discussed by Tomporowski and colleagues (2008). First, it's not as yet clear why short-term exercise interventions would change global measures of intellectual functioning and academic achievement, which are formed by learning experiences or motivation to perform. Process-specific tests designed to measure specific components of mental functioning might be more likely to change after exercise. Second, specific types of exercise training may facilitate cognitive functioning more than others. For example, children who are involved in play and structured games that entail learning and group cooperation may adapt differently than children involved in individual physical activities that are performed in relative isolation for the purpose of aerobic fitness (e.g., treadmill running or stationary cycling). Third, different types of children may respond to exercises in different ways. For example, environmental and social contexts in which physical activity occurs may have different effects on children depending upon their gender or cultural background and interests. Fourth, the effect of an exercise intervention may depend on a child's developmental maturity. For example, impulse control (i.e., the ability to inhibit one's actions) may develop mainly during the preschool years whereas other aspects, such as planning and working memory, may continue to develop through the middle school years. Hence an exercise intervention might improve inhibition in preschoolers but not in school-age children.

Acute Exercise

A few studies that examined cognition during moderately intense or exhaustive exercise reported an enhancement of performance on decision-making tasks (e.g., Davranche and Audiffren 2004; Paas and Adam 1991) or an impairment of performance on perceptual (Paas and Adam 1991) and executive control (Dietrich and Sparling 2004) tasks. The cumulative evidence indicates that performance on most cognitive tasks is impaired during exercise of short duration (i.e., 20 min or less), but performance during exercise is enhanced on tasks that involve rapid decisions and automatic behaviors. A meta-analysis of the effects of acute exercise on cognitive function in adults ages 18 to 30 years evaluated 21 studies (292 people) of cognitive performance during an exercise session and 29 studies (545 people) of cognitive performance after an exercise session ended (Lambourne and Tomporowski 2010). During exercise, cognitive task performance was impaired over the first 20 min; but after

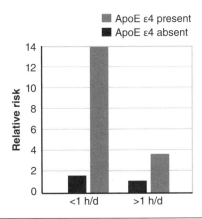

Figure 14.23 Physical activity modifies risk of apo E-ε4 for dementia onset.

Data from Schuit et al. 2001

that, performance on tasks that involved rapid decisions and automated behaviors were improved during the exercise. After exercise ended, cognitive task performance improved by a small amount (0.20 SD; 95% CI: 0.14-0.25), especially for speeded mental processes and memory storage and retrieval. Finally, cognitive performance was affected differently depending on the mode of exercise. Cycling was associated with enhanced performance during and after exercise, whereas treadmill running led to impaired performance during exercise and a small improvement in performance following exercise.

The findings regarding steady-state exercise confirm predictions made by several researchers that metabolic recovery occurs gradually and that the heightened level of arousal during this period facilitates cognitive function (Tomporowski 2003). The mean effects of exercise were larger for tests of memory than for tests of executive function or information-processing time. A subsequent study also showed that acute exercise transiently improves sensory processing without altering executive processing (Lambourne, Audiffren, and Tomporowski 2010).

Strength of the Evidence

Numerous observational studies, including a few prospective cohort studies, and RCTs show that physically active or physically fit people perform better on some types of cognitive function and have lowered odds of cognitive decline or dementia after middle-age when compared with inactive or unfit people.

Temporal Sequence

Follow-up periods in the observational studies of dementia or cognitive decline in middle-age and older adults ranged from two to 21 years and averaged about five years. A few years of observation are unlikely to reveal measurable or marked decline in healthy, middle-aged people, but function can deteriorate rapidly in people with early onset dementia and older people, especially if they have vascular disease.

Strength of Association

Odds ratios from prospective, observational studies show 30% to 40% lower risk of cognitive decline or dementia. This is a meaningful reduction. However, less than half the studies controlled for other risk factors that might confound the association. Hence, the real size of risk reduction remains unclear.

Consistency

More than two-thirds of 20 or so prospective studies from the United States, Australia, Canada, China, France, Japan, Finland, and Sweden showed that physically active people, especially older women, had lower risk of developing dementia or cognitive decline. Early-life, midlife, and current levels of physical activity all appear to postpone symptoms of dementia or cognitive decline.

Dose Response

About half the prospective cohort studies of the risk of cognitive decline or dementia with aging in healthy people examined more than two levels of physical activity exposure. About half of those studies, including the Nurses' Health Study, reported a dose-dependent decrease in risk at higher levels of physical activity participation. The use of self-report measures of physical activity is a unique limitation of prospective studies of cognitive function when the measures of physical activity include leisure activities involving social and cognitive activities but light physical exertion (e.g., crossword puzzles, card games). A RCT designed specifically to assess the dose–effect relation between resistance training and information processing in healthy older adults reported that similar benefits were derived from interventions that involved weight loads of either 50% or 80% of maximal strength (Cassilhas et al. 2007). The number of different physical activities in which older adults engage may be more important than their frequency, intensity, or duration for reducing the odds of dementia (Podewils et al. 2005). The dose of physical activity has not been manipulated in most RCTs. Cognitive function and some measures of brain health have been associated with levels of and gains in cardiorespiratory fitness among healthy, older adults; but the cumulative evidence does not provide clear support that cardiorespiratory fitness results in improved cognitive performance.

Plausibility

Plausible mechanisms that might explain enhanced cognitive function in response to exercise include (1) plasticity and survival of brain neurons; (2) increased brain blood flow; and (3) enhanced neural circuits that support attention, learning, or memory (Dishman et al. 2006a; van Praag 2008).

Plasticity and Survival of Brain Neurons

Voluntary activity-wheel running induces gene expression for brain neurotrophins such as VGF, galanin, and BDNF in the hippocampus, which is involved with contextual memories (e.g., Adlard and Cotman 2004; van Praag 2008). Chronic wheel running also reduces extracellular amyloid-β plaques in the frontal cortex and hippocampus that are found in humans with Alzheimer's disease, probably by changing the processing of the amyloid precursor protein (Adlard et al. 2005). In a study of older adults without dementia, people who had higher fitness levels also had enhanced spatial memory. This association was partly explained (i.e., mediated) by the observation that people who were fit and those who had better memory also tended to have a larger hippocampus (Erickson et al. 2009). Exercise training that increased cardiorespiratory fitness led to increases in hippocampal volume and better short-term memory in healthy and schizophrenic adults (Pajonk et al. 2010). In a study of patients who had early-stage Alzheimer's disease, those who had higher fitness were also more likely to have larger volumes of brain cortex in the parietal and medial temporal regions when compared to older adults without dementia (Honea et al. 2009).

Neurotrophins such as brain-derived neurotrophic factor (BDNF) and nerve growth factor (NGF), vascular endothelial growth factor (VEGF), and galanin play key roles in regulating survival, growth, and maintenance of neurons (van Praag 2008; Reiss et al. 2009). Hippocampal samples from Alzheimer's donors show decreased BDNF expression, but blood levels of BDNF have been reported to be both lower and higher than normal in people with impaired memory or Alzheimer's disease (Angelucci et al. 2010). Three months of endurance training (an hour daily at 65% of $\dot{V}O_2$max or until 600 kcal had been expended) led to an estimated threefold elevation in blood BDNF from the brain at rest but did not alter the amount of BDNF released from the brain during exercise (Seifert et al. 2010). It is not known, however, whether the apparent release of BDNF into the blood after prolonged exercise or after exercise training has an effect on cognitive function or mood.

Brain Blood Flow

Recent studies indicate that aerobic exercise training increases vascular density in the primary motor cortex and the rate of learning in monkeys (Rhyu et al. 2010) and cerebral blood volume and short-term memory in humans (Pereira et al. 2007). Exercise may also affect neural plasticity and function in other brain regions involved with cognition. In one study of fitness training, older adults had lower blood flow in the anterior cingulate cortex and better performance during an error-detection executive function task (Colcombe et al. 2004). Neuroimaging research suggests that cerebral white matter is decreased in older adults, especially in the prefrontal regions, and mediates age-related differences in cognitive function (Madden et al. 2009). A recent cross-sectional study found that aerobic fitness was related to greater white matter integrity in the cingulum (which projects from the cingulate cortex to the entorhinal cortex, the main neural input to the hippocampus), but not the prefrontal brain regions, in both young and old adults who had no neurological impairment (Marks et al. 2007). Aerobically active older adults also have more small vessels and less twisting of vessels in the brain than do less active people, which might contribute to cerebral white matter integrity (Bullitt et al. 2009).

Most studies of brain blood flow during acute exercise have been conducted to enhance understanding of limits to performance and central fatigue rather than cognitive function (Nybo and Secher 2004; Rooks et al. 2010).

Enhanced Neural Circuits

A recent brain imaging study reported that overweight children who participated in a 13-week RCT of daily after-school aerobic exercise known to improve an executive function called planning (i.e., strategy generation and application, self-regulation, intentionality, and use of knowledge) had a bilateral elevation in brain activation of the prefrontal cortex and lowered activation in the posterior parietal cortex during a visual fixation-inhibition task when they were compared to peers not in the program (Davis et al. 2011). In addition, research has shown that attention and executive cognitive functions such as working memory are influenced by changes in alpha and theta oscillatory EEG frequencies that can uncouple, especially in anterior and posterior neural circuits on the brain cortex that receive input from the thalamus (Hughes and Crunelli 2005; Klimesch et al. 2008). Activation of neural input from carotid and cardiopulmonary baroreceptors into cardiovascular centers in the brain stem is alerting and increases indices of arousal, including hippocampal theta activity and activity in the insular cortex. It is plausible that brain cortical systems are altered generally in response to the increased metabolic arousal of physical exertion and the regulation of physical fatigue by the brain to modulate cognitive performance during or soon after an exercise session (Crabbe and Dishman 2004; Magnie et al. 2000; Nybo and Nielsen 2001; Nybo and Secher 2004; Pfaff 2006).

Summary

Despite imperfect methods, there are enough population-based prospective cohort studies to allow the conclusion that physical inactivity is associated with a small to moderate increase in the risk of depression symptoms among adults. Similarly, there are enough RCTs to conclude that regular exercise can reduce symptoms among patients who are chronically ill or who are diagnosed with mild to moderate unipolar depression. Some studies have shown that the effects of exercise are similar, but not additive, to the effects of psychotherapy and drug therapy. However, it has not yet been possible to conclude that the reduction in symptoms is reliably large enough for an improved clinical diagnosis of remission. Also, studies have not yet completely shown that exercise alone is responsible for the effects, independently of increased social contact or placebo effects. Many studies have shown that acute exercise reduces self-rated anxiety and that regular exercise reduces trait anxiety in young to middle-aged adults without anxiety disorders, including patients with chronic medical conditions; but only a small amount of population-based evidence indicates that such effects prevent future anxiety disorders. Only a few RCTs have been conducted to show that regular exercise reduces symptoms among anxiety patients. Contrary to popular clinical opinion, exercise does not appear to pose a risk for panic patients. Enough observational population studies and RCTs exist to permit a conclusion that regular physical activity is associated with reduced odds of dementia or cognitive decline in later years.

At this point, more prospective, large cohort studies are needed that include enough people of varying ages and races or ethnicities to permit comparisons of the effects of physical activity on the risk of depression and anxiety disorders, insomnia, and dementia among subgroups of the population. Ideally, such studies would include measures across several time periods to permit an examination of whether naturally occurring changes in physical activity precede changes in mental health outcomes. Also, more RCTs that include diverse ethnic groups of all ages are needed to clarify the true role of physical activity in mental health. In addition to that type of evidence, many advances are needed in understanding the biological mechanisms of the mental health outcomes associated with exercise and physical activity.

A recent body of evidence clearly showed that chronic activity-wheel running in rats increased gene expression for brain neurotrophins, especially brain-derived neurotrophic factor (BDNF) in the hippocampus (Cotman and Engesser-Cesar 2002), similar to the effects of the tricyclic antidepressant drug imipramine (Russo-Neustadt, Beard, and Cotman 1999; Russo-Neustadt et al. 2001). Though neurotrophins are cell growth factors that help protect brain neurons from damage, their potential role in helping to explain the antidepressant and cognitive-enhancing effects of exercise has not yet been confirmed using valid animal models (Dishman et al. 2006a; Russo-Neustadt et al. 2001; Van Hoomissen et al. 2003; van Praag 2008; Yoo et al. 2000a). BDNF is also expressed outside the central nervous system, including in skeletal muscle (Gómez-Pinilla et al. 2001), where it may aid fat oxidation (Matthews et al. 2009). By measuring the difference between the concentration of BDNF in arterial blood and blood from the internal jugular vein (cerebrospinal fluid drains into the superior sagittal sinus atop and behind the brain, which then empties into the internal jugular veins), investigators have estimated that about 75% of the nearly threefold increase in BDNF that appears in peripheral blood circulation after prolonged, moderate-intensity exercise comes from the brain in very fit people (Rasmussen et al. 2009). However, it took 4 h (even 2 h wasn't enough) of rowing to show the increase, so it is still not clear whether usual exercise increases BDNF in human brains.

A study that reported increased levels of **endocannabinoids** in the blood after acute running (Sparling et al. 2003) has been interpreted as a possible explanation for elevated mood after exercise (Dietrich and McDaniel 2004). Endocannabinoids are endogenous physiological ligands that bind to the same cannabinoid receptors that mediate the psychoactive effects of Cannabis (i.e., marijuana), including reduction of anxiety and pain, elevation of mood, and impairment of short-term memory. However, as is the case for endorphins and BDNF in the blood, that conclusion is not yet valid for several reasons. First, the origin and function of endocannaboids during exercise are unknown. Second, a link between blood levels of endocannabinoids and psychological responses to exercise has not yet been established. Third, endocannabinoids are also found outside the brain (e.g., in the gastrointestinal tract, pancreas, uterus, liver, adipose tissue, and skeletal muscle, as well as in the spleen and tonsils); and they have many functions that are not psychoactive, including anti-inflammatory effects, dilation of blood vessels and airways, and modulation of the HPA axis during stress (Hill and McEwen 2010). Long-term, endocannabinoids promote storage of body fat by increasing appetite and reducing the metabolic rate in brain, adipose tissue, liver, and skeletal muscle (Ginsberg and Woods 2009).

Only recently have human studies shown that brain changes after exercise training are accompanied by improved mental functions (e.g., short-term, working memory). Technological advances in brain neuroimaging, including spatially and time-resolved near-infrared spectroscopy (Wolf, Ferrari, and Quaresima 2007), functional magnetic resonance imaging (J.C. Smith et al. 2010), and transcranial ultrasound (Willie et al. 2011), will permit more objective evidence that physical activity improves brain health, including functional changes in brain plasticity, metabolism, and neurotransmission that can be compared to changes in symptoms of anxiety and depression (Nemeroff, Kilts, and Berns 1999), as well as feelings of energy, well-being, and cognitive function after exercise.

· BIBLIOGRAPHY ·

Adlard, P.A., and C.W. Cotman. 2004. Voluntary exercise protects against stress-induced decreases in brain-derived neurotrophic factor protein expression. *Neuroscience* 124: 985-992.

Adlard, P.A., V.M. Perreau, V. Pop, and C.W. Cotman. 2005. Voluntary exercise decreases amyloid load in a transgenic model of Alzheimer's disease. *Journal of Neuroscience* 25 (17): 4217-4221.

Aksiskal, H.S., and W.T. McKinney. 1975. Overview of recent research in depression: Integration of ten conceptual models into a comprehensive clinical frame. *Archives of General Psychiatry* 32: 285-305.

Allgulander, C., B. Bandelow, E. Hollander, S.A. Montgomery, D.J. Nutt, A. Okasha, M.H. Pollack, D.J. Stein, R.P. Swinson; World Council of Anxiety. 2003. WCA recommendations for the long-term treatment of generalized anxiety disorder. *CNS Spectrums* 8 (Suppl. 1): 53-61.

Alzheimer's disease genetics fact sheet. 2008. Alzheimer's Disease Education and Referral (ADEAR) Center. A service of the National Institute on Aging, National Institutes of Health, U.S. Department of Health and Human Services. NIH Publication No. 08-6424, November.

American Psychiatric Association. 1998. Practice guidelines for the treatment of patients with panic disorder. *American Journal of Psychiatry* 155 (Suppl. 12): 1-34.

American Psychiatric Association. 2000a. *Diagnostic and statistical manual of mental disorders.* 4th edition, text revision. Washington, DC: American Psychiatric Association.

American Psychiatric Association. 2000b. Practice guidelines for the treatment of patients with major depressive disorder (revision). *American Journal of Psychiatry* 157 (4): 1-45.

Angelucci, F., G. Spalletta, F. di Iulio, A. Ciaramella, F. Salani, L. Colantoni, A.E. Varsi, W. Gianni, G. Sancesario, C. Caltagirone, and P. Bossù. 2010. Alzheimer's disease (AD) and mild cognitive impairment (MCI) patients are characterized by increased BDNF serum levels. *Current Alzheimer Research* 7 (1, February): 15-20.

Angevaren, M., G. Aufdemkampe, H.J. Verhaar, A. Aleman, and L. Vanhees. 2008. Physical activity and enhanced fitness to improve cognitive function in older people without known cognitive impairment. *Cochrane Database of Systematic Reviews,* July 16 (3): CD005381.

Babyak, M., J.A. Blumenthal, S. Herman, P. Khatri, M. Doraiswamy, K. Moore, W.E. Craighead, T.T. Baldewicz, and K.R. Krishnan. 2000. Exercise treatment for major depression: Maintenance of therapeutic benefit at 10 months. *Psychosomatic Medicine* 62: 633-638.

Bahrke, M.S., and W.P. Morgan. 1978. Anxiety reduction following exercise and meditation. *Cognitive Therapy and Research* 2 (4): 323-333.

Baker, L.D., L.L. Frank, K. Foster-Schubert, P.S. Green, C.W. Wilkinson, A. McTiernan, S.R. Plymate, M.A. Fishel, G.S. Watson, B.A. Cholerton, G.E. Duncan, P.D. Mehta, and S. Craft. 2010. Effects of aerobic exercise on mild cognitive impairment: A controlled trial. *Archives of Neurology* 67 (1): 71-79.

Baldessarini, R.J. 1989. Current status of antidepressants: Clinical pharmacology and therapy. *Journal of Clinical Psychiatry* 50 (4): 117-126.

Baldessarini, R.J., L. Tondo, J. Hennen, and A.C. Viguera. 2002. Is lithium still worth using? An update of selected recent research. *Harvard Review of Psychiatry* 10 (2): 59-75.

Ball, K., N.W. Burton, and W.J. Brown. 2008. A prospective study of overweight, physical activity, and depressive symptoms in young women. *Obesity (Silver Spring)* 17 (1): 66-71.

Ballenger, J.C. 2001. Overview of different pharmacotherapies for attaining remission in generalized anxiety disorder. *Journal of Clinical Psychiatry* 62 (Suppl. 19): 11-19.

Ballenger, J.C., J.R. Davidson, Y. Lecrubier, D.J. Nutt, J. Bobes, D.C. Beidel, Y. Ono, and H.G. Westenberg. 1998. Consensus statement on social anxiety disorder from the International Consensus Group on Depression and Anxiety. *Journal of Clinical Psychiatry* 59 (Suppl. 17): 54-60.

Barlow, D.H., and C.L. Lehman. 1996. Advances in the psychosocial treatment of anxiety disorders. *Archives of General Psychiatry* 53: 727-735.

Bartholomew, J.B., and D.E. Linder. 1998. State anxiety following resistance exercise: The role of gender and exercise intensity. *Journal of Behavioral Medicine* 21 (2): 205-219.

Beard, J.R., K. Heathcote, R. Brooks, A. Earnest, and B. Kelly. 2007. Predictors of mental disorders and their outcome in a community based cohort. *Social Psychiatry and Psychiatric Epidemiology* 42 (8): 623-630.

Beck, A.T. 1976. *Cognitive therapy and the emotional disorders.* New York: International Universities Press.

Beck, A.T., A.J. Rush, and B.F. Shaw. 1979. *Cognitive therapy of depression.* New York: Guilford Press.

Bjørnebekk, A., A.A. Mathé, and S. Brené. 2006. Running has differential effects on NPY, opiates, and cell proliferation in an animal model of depression and controls. *Neuropsychopharmacology* 31 (2): 256-264.

Bjørnebekk, A., A.A. Mathé, and S. Brené. 2010. The antidepressant effects of running and escitalopram are associated with levels of hippocampal NPY and Y1 receptor but not cell proliferation in a rat model of depression. *Hippocampus* 20 (7): 820-828.

Blumenthal, J.A., M.A. Babyak, K.A. Moore, W.E. Craighead, S. Herman, P. Khatri, R. Waugh, M.A. Napolitano, L.M. Forman, M. Appelbaum, et al. 1999. Effects of exercise training on older patients with major depression. *Archives of Internal Medicine* 159: 2349-2356.

Boecker, H., T. Sprenger, M.E. Spilker, G. Henriksen, M. Koppenhoefer, K.J. Wagner, M. Valet, A. Berthele, and T.R. Tolle. 2008. The runner's high: Opioidergic mechanisms in the human brain. *Cerebral Cortex* 18 (11, February 21): 2523-2531.

Borges, G., M.K. Nock, J.M. Haro Abad, I. Hwang, N.A. Sampson, J. Alonso, L.H. Andrade, M.C. Angermeyer, A. Beautrais, E. Bromet, R. Bruffaerts, G. de Girolamo, S. Florescu, O. Gureje, C. Hu, E.G. Karam, V. Kovess-Masfety, S. Lee, D. Levinson, M.E. Medina-Mora, J. Ormel, J. Posada-Villa, R. Sagar, T. Tomov, H. Uda, D.R. Williams, and R.C. Kessler. 2010. Twelve-month prevalence of and risk factors for suicide attempts in the World Health Organization world mental health surveys. *Journal of Clinical Psychiatry,* August 24. [Epub ahead of print]

Bouchard, C., R. Shephard, and T. Stephens, eds. 1994. *Physical activity, fitness, and health: International proceedings and consensus statement.* Champaign, IL: Human Kinetics.

Brenes, G.A., J.D. Williamson, S.P. Messier, W.J. Rejeski, M. Pahor, E. Ip, and B.W. Penninx. 2007. Treatment of minor depression in older adults: A pilot study comparing sertraline and exercise. *Aging and Mental Health* 11 (1): 61-68.

Breslau, J., S. Aguilar-Gaxiola, K.S. Kendler, M. Su, D. Williams, and R.C. Kessler. 2006. Specifying race-ethnic differences in risk for psychiatric disorder in a US national sample. *Psychological Medicine* 36 (1): 57-68.

Breus, M.J., and P.J. O'Connor. 1998. Exercise-induced anxiolysis: A test of the "time out" hypothesis in high anxious females. *Medicine and Science in Sports and Exercise* 30 (7): 1107-1112.

Broocks, A., B. Bandelow, G. Pekrun, A. George, T. Meyer, U. Bartmann, U. Hillmer-Vogel, and E. Rüther. 1998. Comparison of aerobic exercise, clomipramine, and placebo in the treatment of panic disorder. *American Journal of Psychiatry* 155: 603-609.

Broocks, A., T.F. Meyer, B. Bandelow, U. Bartmann, E. Rüther, and U. Hillmer-Vogel. 1997. Exercise avoidance and impaired endurance capacity in patients with panic disorder. *Neuropsychobiology* 36: 182-187.

Broocks, A., T. Meyer, A. George, U. Hillmer-Vogel, D. Meyer, B. Bandelow, G. Hajak, U. Bartmann, C.H. Gleiter, and E. Rüther. 1999. Decreased neuroendocrine responses to meta-chlorophenylpiperazine (m-CPP) but normal responses to ipsapirone in marathon runners. *Neuropsychopharmacology* 20 (2): 150-161.

Brown, D., D. Galuska, J. Zhang, D. Eaton, J. Fulton, R. Lowry, and L.M. Maynard. 2007. Physical activity, sport participation, and suicidal behavior: US high school students. *Medicine and Science in Sports and Exercise* 39: 2248-2257.

Brown, W.J., J.H. Ford, N.W. Burton, A.L. Marshall, and A.J. Dobson. 2005. Prospective study of physical activity and depressive symptoms in middle-aged women. *American Journal of Preventive Medicine* 29 (4): 265-272.

Buckworth, J.B., and R.K. Dishman. 2002. *Exercise psychology.* Champaign, IL: Human Kinetics.

Bulbulian, R., and B.L. Darabos. 1986. Motor neuron excitability: The Hoffmann reflex following exercise of low and high intensity. *Medicine and Science in Sports and Exercise* 18: 697-702.

Bullitt, E., F.N. Rahman, J.K. Smith, E. Kim, D. Zeng, L. Katz, and B.L. Marks. 2009. The effect of exercise on the cerebral vasculature of healthy aged subjects as visualized by MR angiography. *American Journal of Neuroradiology* 30: 1857-1863.

Bunney, W.E. Jr., and J.M. Davis. 1965. Norepinephrine in depressive reactions: A review. *Archives of General Psychiatry* 13: 483-494.

Burton, R. 1632. *The anatomy of melancholy.* Oxford: Printed by Ion Lichfield for Henry Cripps.

Calfas, K.J., and W.C. Taylor. 1994. Effects of physical activity on psychological variables in adolescents. *Pediatric Exercise Science* 6: 406-423.

Camacho, T.C., R.E. Roberts, N.B. Lazarus, G.A. Kaplan, and R.D. Cohen. 1991. Physical activity and depression: Evidence from the Alameda County Study. *American Journal of Epidemiology* 134: 220-231.

Campbell, D.D., and J.E. Davis. 1939-1940. Report of research and experimentation in exercise and recreational therapy. *American Journal of Psychiatry* 96: 915-933.

Cassilhas, R.C., V.A. Viana, V. Grassmann, R.T. Santos, R.F. Santos, S. Tufik, and M.T. Mello. 2007. The impact of resistance exercise on the cognitive function of the elderly. *Medicine and Science in Sports and Exercise* 39 (8): 1401-1407.

Centers for Disease Control and Prevention. 2010a. Web-based Injury Statistics Query and Reporting System (WISQARS) [online]. National Center for Injury Prevention and Control, CDC, producer. www.cdc.gov/injury/wisqars/index.html.

Centers for Disease Control and Prevention. 2010b. Youth Risk Behavior Surveillance—United States, 2009. Surveillance Summaries, June 4. *Morbidity and Mortality Weekly Report* 59 (SS-5): 117-126.

Chambliss, H.O., and R.K. Dishman. 2004. Physical activity and depression: A quantitative synthesis. Unpublished manuscript. University of Georgia, Athens.

Chaouloff, F. 1989. Physical exercise and brain monoamines: A review. *Acta Physiologica Scandinavica* 137: 1-13.

Chaouloff, F. 1994. Influence of physical exercise on 5-HT1A receptor- and anxiety-related behaviours. *Neuroscience Letters* 176 (2): 226-230.

Chaouloff, F. 1997a. Effects of acute physical exercise on central serotonergic systems. *Medicine and Science in Sports and Exercise* 29: 58-62.

Chaouloff, F. 1997b. The serotonin hypothesis. In *Physical activity and mental health,* edited by W.P. Morgan, pp. 179-198. Washington, DC: Hemisphere.

Charney, D.S. 1998. Monoamine dysfunction and the pathophysiology and treatment of depression. *Journal of Clinical Psychiatry* 59 (Suppl. 14): 11-14.

Charney, D.S., S.W. Woods, W.K. Goodman, and G.R. Heninger. 1987. Serotonin function in anxiety: II. Effects of the serotonin agonist MCPP in panic disorder patients and healthy subjects. *Psychopharmacology* 92 (1): 14-24.

Charney, D.S., S.W. Woods, J.H. Krystal, L.M. Nagy, and G.R. Heninger. 1992. Noradrenergic neuronal dysregulation in panic disorder: The effects of intravenous yohimbine and clonidine in panic disorder patients. *Acta Psychiatrica Scandinavica* 86 (4): 273-282.

Charron, S., and E. Koechlin. 2010. Divided representation of concurrent goals in the human frontal lobes. *Science* 328: 360-363.

Chouinard, G. 2004. Issues in the clinical use of benzodiazepines: Potency, withdrawal, and rebound. *Journal of Clinical Psychiatry* (Suppl. 5): 7-12.

Chrousos, G.P. 1998. Stressors, stress, and neuroendocrine integration of the adaptive response. *Annals of the New York Academy of Sciences* 851: 311-335.

Colcombe, S.J., K.I. Erickson, P.E. Scalf, J.S. Kim, R. Prakash, E. McAuley, S. Elavsky, D.X. Marquez, L. Hu, and A.F. Kramer. 2006. Aerobic exercise training increases brain volume in aging humans. *Journals of Gerontology Series A: Biological Sciences and Medical Sciences* 61 (11): 1166-1170.

Colcombe, S., and A.F. Kramer. 2003. Fitness effects on the cognitive function of older adults: A meta-analytic study. *Psychological Science* 14 (2): 125-130.

Colcombe, S.J., A.F. Kramer, K.I. Erickson, P. Scalf, E. McAuley, N.J. Cohen, A. Webb, G.J. Jerome, D.X. Marquez, and S. Elavsky. 2004. Cardiovascular fitness, cortical plasticity, and aging. *Proceedings of the National Academy of Sciences U.S.A.* 101 (9): 3316-3321.

Cooper-Patrick, L., D.E. Ford, L.A. Mead, P.P. Chang, and M.J. Klag. 1997. Exercise and depression in midlife: A prospective study. *American Journal of Public Health* 87: 670-673.

Cotman, C.W., and C. Engesser-Cesar. 2002. Exercise enhances and protects brain function. *Exercise and Sport Sciences Reviews* 30 (2): 75-79.

Crabbe, J.B., and R.K. Dishman. 2004. Brain electrocortical activity during and after exercise: A quantitative synthesis. *Psychophysiology* 41 (4): 563-574.

Crabbe, J.B., J.C. Smith, and R.K. Dishman. 2007. Emotional & electroencephalographic responses during affective picture viewing after exercise. *Physiology and Behavior* 90 (2-3): 394-404.

Craft, L.L., and D.M. Landers. 1998. The effect of exercise on clinical depression and depression resulting from mental illness: A meta-analysis. *Journal of Sport and Exercise Psychology* 20: 339-357.

Davidson, J.R. 1998. Pharmacotherapy of social anxiety disorder. *Journal of Clinical Psychiatry* 59 (Suppl. 17): 47-53.

Davidson, R.J. 1998. Anterior electrophysiological asymmetries, emotion, and depression: Conceptual and methodological conundrums. *Psychophysiology* 35: 607-614.

Davidson, R.J., and W. Irwin. 1999. The functional neuroanatomy of emotion and affective style. *Trends in Cognitive Sciences* 3 (1): 11-21.

Davidson, R.J., W. Irwin, M.J. Anderle, and N.H. Kalin. 2003. The neural substrates of affective processing in depressed patients treated with venlafaxine. *American Journal of Psychiatry* 160: 64-75.

Davis, C.L., P.D. Tomporowski, J.E. McDowell, B.P. Austin, P.H. Miller, N.E. Yanasak, J.D. Allison, and J.A. Nagliere. 2011. Exercise improves executive function and achievement and alters brain activation in overweight children: A randomized, controlled trial. *Health Psychology* 30: 91-98.

Davranche, K., and M. Audiffren. 2004. Facilitating effects of exercise on information processing. *Journal of Sport Sciences* 22: 419-428.

Deeny, S.P., D. Poeppel, J.B. Zimmerman, S.M. Roth, J. Brandauer, S. Witkowski, J.W. Hearn, A.T. Ludlow, J.L. Contreras-Vidal, J. Brandt, and B.D. Hatfield. 2008. Exercise, APOE, and working memory: MEG and behavioral evidence for benefit of exercise in epsilon4 carriers. *Biological Psychology* 78 (2): 179-187.

De Moor, M.H., A.L. Beem, J.H. Stubbe, D.I. Boomsma, and E.J. De Geus. 2006. Regular exercise, anxiety, depression and personality: A population-based study. *Preventive Medicine* 42 (4): 273-279.

De Moor, M.H., D.I. Boomsma, J.H. Stubbe, G. Willemsen, and E.J. de Geus. 2008. Testing causality in the association between regular exercise and symptoms of anxiety and depression. *Archives of General Psychiatry* 65 (8): 897-905.

Desharnais, R., J. Jobin, C. Cote, L. Levesque, and G. Godin. 1993. Aerobic exercise and the placebo effect: A controlled study. *Psychosomatic Medicine* 55: 149-154.

DeVane, C.L. 2000. Pharmacologic characteristics of ideal antidepressants in the 21st century. *Journal of Clinical Psychiatry* 61 (Suppl. 11): 4-8.

de Vries, H.A. 1981. Tranquilizer effect of exercise: A critical review. *Physician and Sportsmedicine* 9: 47-55.

de Vries, H.A., R.A. Wiswell, R. Bulbulian, and T. Moritani. 1981. Tranquilizer effect of exercise. Acute effects of moderate aerobic exercise on spinal reflex activation level. *American Journal of Physical Medicine* 60: 57-66.

Dietrich, A. 2003. Functional neuroanatomy of altered states of consciousness: The transient hypofrontality hypothesis. *Consciousness and Cognition* 12: 231-256.

Dietrich, A., and W.F. McDaniel. 2004. Endocannabinoids and exercise. *British Journal of Sports Medicine* 38 (5): 536-541.

Dietrich, A., and P. Sparling. 2004. Endurance exercise selectively impairs prefrontal-dependent cognition. *Brain and Cognition* 55: 9.

Dishman, R.K. 1997a. Brain monoamines, exercise, and behavior stress: Animal models. *Medicine and Science in Sports and Exercise* 29 (1): 63-74.

Dishman, R.K. 1997b. The norepinephrine hypothesis. In *Physical activity and mental health,* edited by W.P. Morgan, pp. 199-212. Washington, DC: Hemisphere.

Dishman, R.K. 1998. Physical activity and mental health. In *Encyclopedia of mental health,* edited by H.S. Friedman, Vol. 3, pp. 171-188. San Diego: Academic Press.

Dishman, R.K., H.R. Berthoud, F.W. Booth, C.W. Cotman, V.R. Edgerton, M.R. Fleshner, S.C. Gandevia, F. Gomez-Pinilla, B.N. Greenwood, C.H. Hillman, A.F. Kramer, B.E. Levin, T.H. Moran, A.A. Russo-Neustadt, J.D. Salamone, J.D. Van Hoomissen, C.E. Wade, D.A. York, and M.J. Zigmond. 2006a. Neurobiology of exercise. *Obesity (Silver Spring)* 14: 345-356.

Dishman, R.K., A. Dunn, S. Youngstedt, J.M. Davis, M.L. Burgess, S.P. Wilson, and M.A. Wilson. 1996. Increased open-field locomotion and decreased striatal GABAA binding after activity wheel running. *Physiology and Behavior* 60: 699-705.

Dishman, R.K., R. Farquhar, and K.J. Cureton. 1994. Responses to preferred intensities of exertion in men differing in activity levels. *Medicine and Science in Sports and Exercise* 26: 783-790.

Dishman, R.K., D.P. Hales, K.A. Pfeiffer, G.A. Felton, R. Saunders, D.S. Ward, M. Dowda, and R.R. Pate. 2006b. Physical self-concept and self-esteem mediate cross-sectional relations of physical activity and sport participation with depression symptoms among adolescent girls. *Health Psychology* 25 (3): 396-407.

Dishman, R.K., S. Hong, J.M. Warren, S.D. Youngstedt, H. Yoo, B.N. Bunnell, E.H. Mougey, J.L. Meyerhoff, L. Jaso-Friedmann, and D.L. Evans. 2000a. Treadmill exercise training blunts suppression of natural killer cell activity after footshock. *Journal of Applied Physiology* 83: 1547-1554.

Dishman, R.K., and P.J. O'Connor. 2009. Lessons in exercise neurobiology: The case of endorphins. *Mental Health and Physical Activity* 2: 4-9.

Dishman, R.K., K.J. Renner, J.E. White-Welkley, and B.N. Bunnell. 2000b. Treadmill exercise training augments brain norepinephrine response to familiar and novel stress. *Brain Research Bulletin* 52: 337-342.

Dishman, R.K., K.J. Renner, S.D. Youngstedt, T.G. Reigle, B.N. Bunnell, K.A. Burke, H.S. Yoo, E.H. Mougey, and J.L. Meyerhoff. 1997. Activity wheel running reduces escape latency and alters brain monoamine levels after footshock. *Brain Research Bulletin* 42 (5): 399-406.

Dishman, R.K., M. Sui, T.S. Church, G.A. Hand, M.H. Trivedi, and S.N. Blair. 2012. Decline in Cardiorespiratory Fitness and Odds of Incident Depression. *American Journal of Preventive Medicine,* October issue (number 10).

Dishman, R.K., J.M. Warren, S.D. Youngstedt, H. Yoo, B.N. Bunnell, E.H. Mougey, J.L. Meyerhoff, L. Jaso-Friedmann, and D.L. Evans. 1995. Activity wheel running attenuates suppression of natural killer cell activity after footshock. *Journal of Applied Physiology* 78: 1547-1554.

Doyne, E.J., D.J. Ossip-Klein, E.D. Bowman, K.M. Osborn, I.B. McDougall-Wilson, and R.A. Neimeyer. 1987. Running versus weight lifting in the treatment of depression. *Journal of Consulting and Clinical Psychology* 55 (5): 748-754.

Drevets, W.C. 1998. Functional neuroimaging studies of depression: The anatomy of melancholia. *Annual Review of Medicine* 49: 341-361.

Dunn, A.L., and R.K. Dishman. 1991. Exercise and the neurobiology of depression. *Exercise and Sport Sciences Reviews* 19: 41-98.

Dunn, A.L., T.G. Reigle, S.D. Youngstedt, R.B. Armstrong, and R.K. Dishman. 1996. Brain norepinephrine and metabolites after treadmill training and wheel running in rats. *Medicine and Science in Sports and Exercise* 28: 204-209.

Dunn, A.L., M.H. Trivedi, J.B. Kampert, C.G. Clark, and H.O. Chambliss. 2005. Exercise treatment for depression: Efficacy and dose response. *American Journal of Preventive Medicine* 28 (1): 1-8.

DuPont, R.L., D.P. Rice, L.S. Miller, S.S. Shiraki, C.R. Rowland, and H.J. Harwood. 1996. Economic cost of anxiety disorders. *Anxiety* 2: 167-172.

Ekeland, E., F. Heian, and K.B. Hagen. 2005. Can exercise improve self esteem in children and young people? A systematic review of randomised controlled trials. *British Journal of Sports Medicine* 39 (11): 792-798.

Erickson, K.I., R.S. Prakash, M.W. Voss, L. Chaddock, L. Hu, K.S. Morris, S.M. White, T.R. Wojcicki, E. McAuley, and A.F. Kramer. 2009. Aerobic fitness is associated with hippocampal volume in elderly humans. *Hippocampus* 19: 1030-1039.

Ernst, E., J.I. Rand, and C. Stevinson. 1998. Complementary therapies for depression: An overview. *Archives of General Psychiatry* 55: 1026-1032.

Etnier, J.L., R.J. Caselli, E.M. Reiman, G.E. Alexander, B.A. Sibley, D. Tessier, and E.C. McLemore. 2007. Cognitive performance in older women relative to ApoE-epsilon4 genotype and aerobic fitness. *Medicine and Science in Sports and Exercise* 39 (1): 199-207.

Etnier, J.L., P.M. Nowell, D.M. Landers, and B.A. Sibley. 2006. A meta-regression to examine the relationship between aerobic fitness and cognitive performance. *Brain Research Reviews* 52 (1): 119-130.

Etnier, J.L., W. Salazar, D.M. Landers, S.J. Petruzzello, M. Han, and P. Nowell. 1997. The influence of physical fitness and exercise upon cognitive functioning: A meta-analysis. *Journal of Sport and Exercise Psychology* 19: 249-277.

Farrell, P.A., W.K. Gates, M. Maksud, and W.P. Morgan. 1982. Increases in plasma b-endorphin/b-lipotropin immunoreactivity after treadmill running in humans. *Journal of Applied Physiology* 52: 1245-1249.

Ferri, C.P., M. Prince, C. Brayne, H. Brodaty, L. Fratiglioni, M. Ganguli, K. Hall, K. Hasegawa, H. Hendrie, Y. Huang, A. Jorm, C. Mathers, P.R. Menezes, E. Rimmer, M. Scazufca; Alzheimer's Disease International. 2005. Global prevalence of dementia: A Delphi consensus study. *Lancet* 366 (9503): 2112-2117.

Focht, B.C., and K.F. Koltyn. 1999. Influence of resistance exercise of different intensities on state anxiety and blood pressure. *Medicine and Science in Sports and Exercise* 31 (3): 456-463.

Fox, K.E. 2000. Self-esteem, self-perceptions and exercise. *International Journal of Sport Psychology* 31: 228-240.

Franz, S.I., and G.V. Hamilton. 1905. The effects of exercise upon the retardation in conditions of depression. *American Journal of Insanity* 62: 239-256.

Freeman, M.P., M. Fava, J. Lake, M.H. Trivedi, K.L. Wisner, and D. Mischoulon. 2010. Complementary and alternative medicine in major depressive disorder: the American Psychiatric Association Task Force report. *Journal of Clinical Psychiatry* 71: 669-681.

Fremont, J., and L.W. Craighead. 1987. Aerobic exercise and cognitive therapy in the treatment of dysphoric moods. *Cognitive Therapy and Research* 11 (2): 241-251.

Garvin, A.W., K.F. Koltyn, and W.P. Morgan. 1997. Influence of acute physical activity and relaxation on state anxiety and blood lactate in untrained college males. *International Journal of Sports Medicine* 18: 1-7.

Gaynes, B.N., D. Warden, M.H. Trivedi, S.R. Wisniewski, M. Fava, and A.J. Rush. 2009. What did STAR*D teach us? Results from a large-scale, practical, clinical trial for patients with depression. *Psychiatric Services* 60: 1439-1445.

Ginsberg, H.N., and S.C. Woods. 2009. The endocannabinoid system: Potential for reducing cardiometabolic risk. *Obesity (Silver Spring)* 17 (10): 1821-1829. [Epub, April 16]

Goddard, A.W., and D.S. Charney. 1997. Toward an integrated neurobiology of panic disorder. *Journal of Clinical Psychiatry* 58 (Suppl. 2): 4-12.

Goddard, A.W., and D.S. Charney. 1998. SSRIs in the treatment of panic disorder. *Depression and Anxiety* 8 (Suppl. 1): 114-120.

Gold, P.W., and G.P. Chrousos. 1998. The endocrinology of melancholic and atypical depression: Relation to neurocircuitry and somatic consequences. *Proceedings of the Association of American Physicians* 111 (1): 22-34.

Gómez-Pinilla, F., Z. Ying, P. Opazo, R.R. Roy, and V.R. Edgerton. 2001. Differential regulation by exercise of BDNF and NT-3 in rat spinal cord and skeletal muscle. *European Journal of Neuroscience* 13 (6): 1078-1084.

Goodwin, R.D. 2003. Association between physical activity and mental disorders among adults in the United States. *Preventive Medicine* 36: 698-703.

Gorman, J.M., and L.K. Gorman. 1987. Drug treatment of social phobia. *Journal of Affective Disorders* 13 (2): 183-192.

Greenwood, B.N., and M. Fleshner. 2008. Exercise, learned helplessness, and the stress-resistant brain. *Neuromolecular Medicine* 10 (2): 81-98.

Greenberg, P.E., R.C. Kessler, H.G. Birnbaum, S.A. Leong, S.W. Lowe, P.A. Berglund, and P.K. Corey-Lisle. 2003. The economic burden of depression in the United States: How did it change between 1990 and 2000? *Journal of Clinical Psychiatry* 64 (12): 1465-1475.

Greenberg, P.E., L.E. Stiglin, S.N. Finkelstein, and E.R. Berndt. 1993. The economic burden of depression in 1990. *Journal of Clinical Psychiatry* 54 (11): 405-418.

Greist, J.H., M.H. Klein, R.R. Eischens, J. Faris, A.S. Gurman, and W.P. Morgan. 1978. Running through your mind. *Journal of Psychosomatic Research* 22: 259-294.

Gruber, J. 1986. Physical activity and self-esteem development in children: A meta-analysis. In *Effects of physical activity on children: Papers of the American Academy of Physical Education,* edited by G.A. Stull and H.M. Eckhardt, Vol. 19, pp. 30-48. Champaign, IL: Human Kinetics.

Hamer, M., and Y. Chida. 2009. Physical activity and risk of neurodegenerative disease: A systematic review of prospective evidence. *Psychological Medicine* 39: 3-11.

Harris, A.H., R. Cronkite, and R. Moos. 2006. Physical activity, exercise coping, and depression in a 10-year cohort study of depressed patients. *Journal of Affective Disorders* 93 (1-3): 79-85.

Herring, M.P., M.L. Jacob, C. Suveg, R.K. Dishman, and P.J. O'Connor. 2012. Feasibility of exercise training for the short-term treatment of generalized anxiety disorder: A randomized controlled trial. *Psychotherapy and Psychosomatics* 81: 21-28.

Herring, M.P., P.J. O'Connor, and R.K. Dishman. 2010. The effect of exercise training on anxiety symptoms among patients: A systematic review. *Archives of Internal Medicine* 170 (4): 321-331.

Herring, M.P., T.W. Puetz, P.J. O'Connor, and R.K. Dishman. 2012. The effect of exercise training on depression symptoms among patients: A systematic review. *Archives of Internal Medicine* 172 (2): 101-111.

Heyn, P., B.C. Abreu, and K.J. Ottenbacher. 2004. The effects of exercise training on elderly persons with cognitive impairment and dementia: A meta-analysis. *Archives of Physical Medicine and Rehabilitation* 85 (10): 1694-1704.

Hill, M.N., and B.S. McEwen. 2010. Involvement of the endocannabinoid system in the neurobehavioural effects of stress and glucocorticoids. *Progress in Neuropsychopharmacology and Biological Psychiatry* 34 (5): 791-797.

Hirschfeld, R.M.A., M.B. Keller, S. Panico, B.S. Arons, D. Barlow, F. Davidoff, J. Endicott, J. Froom, M. Goldstein, J.M. Gorman, et al. 1997. The National Depressive and Manic-Depressive Association consensus statement on the undertreatment of depression. *Journal of the American Medical Association* 277: 333-340.

Hoffman, P. 1997. The endorphin hypothesis. In *Physical activity and mental health,* edited by W.P. Morgan, pp. 163-177. Washington, DC: Hemisphere.

Honea, R.A., G.P. Thomas, A. Harsha, H.S. Anderson, J.E. Donnelly, W.M. Brooks, and J.M. Burns. 2009. Cardiorespiratory fitness and preserved medial temporal lobe volume in Alzheimer disease. *Alzheimer Disease and Associated Disorders* 23: 188-197.

Hu, T.W. 2006. Perspectives: An international review of the national cost estimates of mental illness, 1990-2003. *Journal of Mental Health Policy and Economics* 9 (1): 3-13.

Hughes, S.W., and V. Crunelli. 2005. Thalamic mechanisms of EEG alpha rhythms and their pathological implications. *Neuroscientist* 11: 357-372.

Hunsberger, J.G., S.S. Newton, A.H. Bennett, C.H. Duman, D.S. Russell, S.R. Salton, and R.S. Duman. 2007. Antidepressant actions of the exercise-regulated gene VGF. *Nature Medicine* 13 (12): 1476-1482.

Ide, K., and N.H. Secher. 2000. Cerebral blood flow and metabolism during exercise. *Progress in Neurobiology* 61: 397-414.

Insel, T.R. 2008. Assessing the economic costs of serious mental illness. *American Journal of Psychiatry* 165: 663-665.

Jackson, A.S., X. Sui, J.R. Hébert, T.S. Church, and S.N. Blair. 2009. Role of lifestyle and aging on the longitudinal change in cardiorespiratory fitness. *Archives of Internal Medicine* 169 (19): 1781-1787.

Jacobs, B.L., and C.A. Fornal. 1999. Activity of serotonergic neurons in behaving animals. *Neuropsychopharmacology* 21 (Suppl. 2): 9-15.

James, H. 1926. *The letters of William James.* Boston: Little, Brown.

James, W. 1899. *Talks to teachers on psychology: And to students on some of life's ideals.* New York: Holt.

Jefferson, J.W., J.H. Greist, P.J. Clagnze, R.R. Eischens, W.C. Marten, and M.A. Evenson. 1982. Effects of strenuous exercise on lithium level in man. *American Journal of Psychiatry* 139: 1593-1595.

Jerstad, S.J., K.N. Boutelle, K.K. Ness, and E. Stice. 2010. Prospective reciprocal relations between physical activity and depression in female adolescents. *Journal of Consulting and Clinical Psychology* 78 (2): 268-272.

Jonsdottir, I.H., L. Rödjer, E. Hadzibajramovic, M. Börjesson, and G. Ahlborg Jr. 2010. A prospective study of leisure-time physical activity and mental health in Swedish health care workers and social insurance officers. *Preventive Medicine* 51 (5): 373-377.

Kalin, N.H., R.J. Davidson, W. Irwin, G. Warner, J.L. Orendi, S.K. Sutton, B.J. Mock, J.A. Sorenson, M. Lowe, and P.A. Turski. 1997. Functional magnetic resonance imaging studies of emotional processing in normal and depressed patients: Effects of venlafaxine. *Journal of Clinical Psychiatry* 58 (Suppl. 16): 32-39.

Kandel, E.R. 1998. A new intellectual framework for psychiatry. *American Journal of Psychiatry* 155 (4): 457-469.

Kelly, J.P., A.S. Wrynn, and B.E. Leonard. 1997. The olfactory bulbectomized rat as a model of depression: An update. *Pharmacology and Therapeutics* 74 (3): 299-316.

Kent, J.M., J.D. Coplan, and J.M. Gorman. 1998. Clinical utility of the selective serotonin reuptake inhibitors in the spectrum of anxiety. *Biological Psychiatry* 44: 812-824.

Kessler, R.C., S. Aguilar-Gaxiola, J. Alonso, S. Chatterji, S. Lee, J. Ormel, T.B. Üstün, and P.S. Wang. 2009. The global burden of mental disorders: An update from the WHO World Mental Health (WMH) surveys. *Epidemiologia e Psichiatria Sociale* 18 (1, January-March): 23-33.

Kessler, R.C., P. Berglund, W.T. Chiu, O. Demler, S. Heeringa, E. Hiripi, R. Jin, B.E. Pennell, E.E. Walters, A. Zaslavsky, and H. Zheng. 2004. The US National Comorbidity Survey Replication (NCSR): Design and field procedures. *International Journal of Methods in Psychiatric Research* 13: 69-92.

Kessler, R.C., P. Berglund, O. Demler, R. Jin, D. Koretz, K.R. Merikangas, A.J. Rush, E.E. Walters, and P.S. Wang. 2003. The epidemiology of major depressive disorder: Results from the National Comorbidity Survey Replication (NCSR). *Journal of the American Medical Association* 289: 3095-3105.

Kessler, R.C., P. Berglund, O. Demler, R. Jin, K.R. Merikangas, and E.E. Walters. 2005a. Lifetime prevalence and age-of-onset distributions of DSM-IV disorders in the National Comorbidity Survey Replication. *Archives of General Psychiatry* 62: 593-602.

Kessler, R.C., W.T. Chiu, O. Demler, K.R. Merikangas, and E.E. Walters. 2005b. Prevalence, severity, and comorbidity of 12-month DSM-IV disorders in the National Comorbidity Survey Replication. *Archives of General Psychiatry* 62 (6): 617-627.

Kessler, R.C., O. Demler, R.G. Frank, M. Olfson, H.A. Pincus, E.E. Walters, P. Wang, K.B. Wells, and A.M. Zaslavsky. 2005c. Prevalence and treatment of mental disorders, 1990 to 2003. *New England Journal of Medicine* 352 (24): 2515-2523.

Kessler, R.C., S. Heeringa, M.D. Lakoma, M. Petukhova, A.E. Rupp, M. Schoenbaum, P.S. Wang, and A.M. Zaslavsky. 2008. Individual and societal effects of mental disorders on earnings in the United States: Results from the national comorbidity survey replication. *American Journal of Psychiatry* 165 (6): 703-711.

Kessler, R.C., K.A. McGonagle, S. Zhao, C.B. Nelson, M. Hughes, S. Eshleman, H.U. Wittchen, and K.S. Kendler. 1994. Lifetime and 12-month prevalence of DSM-III-R psychiatric disorders in the United States: Results from the National Comorbidity Survey. *Archives of General Psychiatry* 51 (1): 8-19.

Kessler, R.C., K.R. Merikangas, and P.S. Wang. 2007. Prevalence, comorbidity, and service utilization for mood disorders in the United States at the beginning of the twenty-first century. *Annual Review of Clinical Psychology* 3: 137-158.

Knox, S., A. Barnes, C. Kiefe, C.E. Lewis, C. Iribarren, K.A. Matthews, N.D. Wong, and M. Whooley. 2006. History of depression, race, and cardiovascular risk in CARDIA. *International Journal of Behavioral Medicine* 13: 44-50.

Koechlin, E., and A. Hyafil. 2007. Anterior prefrontal function and the limits of human decision-making. *Science* 318: 594-598.

Koloski, N.A., N. Smith, N.A. Pachana, and A. Dobson. 2008. Performance of the Goldberg Anxiety and Depression Scale in older women. *Age and Ageing* 37 (4): 464-467.

Koltyn, K. 1997. The thermogenic hypothesis. In *Physical activity and mental health,* edited by W.P. Morgan, pp. 213-226. Washington, DC: Hemisphere.

Koltyn, K., N.A. Lynch, and D.W. Hill. 1998. Psychological responses to brief exhaustive cycling exercise in the morning and evening. *International Journal of Sport Psychology* 29: 145-156.

Koltyn, K.F., and W.P. Morgan. 1992. Influence of underwater exercise on anxiety and body temperature. *Scandinavian Journal of Medicine and Science in Sports* 2: 249-253.

Krause, N., L. Goldenhar, J. Liang, G. Jay, and D. Maeda. 1993. Stress and exercise among the Japanese elderly. *Social Science Medicine* 36: 1429-1441.

Kritz-Silverstein, D., E. Barrett-Connor, and C. Corbeau. 2001. Cross-sectional and prospective study of exercise and depressed mood in the elderly: The Rancho Bernardo study. *American Journal of Epidemiology* 153: 596-603.

Krogh, J., M. Nordentoft, J.A. Sterne, and D.A. Lawlor. 2010. The effect of exercise in clinically depressed adults: A systematic review and meta-analysis of randomized controlled trials. *Journal of Clinical Psychiatry,* October 19. [Epub ahead of print]

Krogh, J., B. Saltin, C. Gluud, and M. Nordentoft. 2009. The DEMO trial: A randomized, parallel-group, observer-blinded clinical trial of strength versus aerobic versus relaxation training for patients with mild to moderate depression. *Journal of Clinical Psychiatry* 70 (6): 790-800.

Ku, P.W., K.R. Fox, and L.J. Chen. 2009. Physical activity and depressive symptoms in Taiwanese older adults: A seven-year follow-up study. *Preventive Medicine* 48 (3): 250-255.

Kubitz, K.A., D.M. Landers, S.J. Petruzzello, and M. Han. 1996. The effects of acute and chronic exercise on sleep: A meta-analytic review. *Sports Medicine* 21: 277-291.

Kubitz, K.A., and A.A. Mott. 1996. EEG power spectral densities during and after cycle ergometer exercise. *Research Quarterly for Exercise and Sport* 67: 91-96.

Kugler, J., H. Seelbach, and G.M. Kruskemper. 1994. Effects of rehabilitation exercise programmes on anxiety and depression in coronary patients: A meta-analysis. *British Journal of Clinical Psychology* 33: 401-410.

Kupfer, D.J. 1991. Long-term treatment of depression. *Journal of Clinical Psychiatry* 52 (Suppl. 5): 28-34.

Lambourne, K., M. Audiffren, and P.D. Tomporowski. 2010. Effects of acute exercise on sensory and executive processing tasks. *Medicine and Science in Sports and Exercise* 42 (7): 1396-1402.

Lambourne, K., and P. Tomporowski. 2011. The effect of exercise-induced arousal on cognitive task performance: A meta-regression analysis. *Brain Research* 1341: 12-24.

Landers, D.M., and S.J. Petruzzello. 1994. Physical activity, fitness, and anxiety. In *Physical activity, fitness, and health: International proceedings and consensus statement,* edited by C. Bouchard, R.J. Shephard, and T. Stephens, pp. 868-882. Champaign, IL: Human Kinetics.

Lang, P.J., M.M. Bradley, and B.N. Cuthbert. 1998. Emotion, motivation, and anxiety: Brain mechanisms and psychophysiology. *Biological Psychiatry* 44: 1248-1263.

Langa, K.M., M.E. Chernew, M.U. Kabeto, et al. 2001. National estimates of the quantity and cost of informal caregiving for the elderly with dementia. *Journal of General Internal Medicine* 16: 770-778.

Larun, L., L.V. Nordheim, E. Ekeland, K.B. Hagen, and F. Heian. 2006. Exercise in prevention and treatment of anxiety and depression among children and young people. *Cochrane Database of Systematic Reviews* (3): doi:10.1002/14651858.

Lawlor, D.A., and S.W. Hopker. 2001. The effectiveness of exercise as an intervention in the management of depression: Systematic review and meta-regression analysis of randomised controlled trials. *British Medical Journal* 322: 1-8.

Layman, E.M. 1960. Contributions of exercise and sports to mental health and social adjustment. In *Science and medicine of exercise and sports,* edited by W.R. Johnson. New York: Harper.

LeDoux, J.E. 1998. Fear and the brain: Where have we been, and where are we going? *Biological Psychiatry* 44 (12): 1229-1238.

Lehtinen, V., and M. Joukamaa. 1994. Epidemiology of depression: Prevalence, risk factors and treatment situation. *Acta Psychiatrica Scandinavica* 377 (Suppl.): 7-10.

Levinson, D., M.D. Lakoma, M. Petukhova, M. Schoenbaum, A.M. Zaslavsky, M. Angermeyer, G. Borges, R. Bruffaerts, G. de Girolamo, R. de Graaf, O. Gureje, J.M. Haro, C. Hu, A.N. Karam, N. Kawakami, S. Lee, J.P. Lepine, M.O. Browne, M. Okoliyski, J. Posada-Villa, R. Sagar, M.C. Viana, D.R. Williams, and R.C. Kessler. 2010. Associations of serious mental illness with earnings: Results from the WHO World Mental Health surveys. *British Journal of Psychiatry* 197: 114-121.

Lezak, M.D., D.B. Howieson, and D.W. Loring. 2004. *Neuropsychological assessment.* 4th edition. Oxford and New York: Oxford University Press.

Long, B.C., and R. van Stavel. 1995. Effects of exercise training on anxiety: A meta-analysis. *Journal of Applied Sport Psychology* 7: 167-189.

Lopez, A.D., C.D. Mathers, M. Ezzati, D.T. Jamison, and C.J. Murray. 2006. Global and regional burden of disease and risk factors, 2001: Systematic analysis of population health data. *Lancet* 367 (9524): 1747-1757.

Lydiard, R.B., O. Brawman-Mintzer, and J.C. Ballenger. 1996. Recent developments in the psychopharmacology of anxiety disorders. *Journal of Consulting and Clinical Psychology* 64: 660-668.

Maas, J.W. 1979. Neurotransmitters and depression: Too much, too little, or unstable? *Trends in the Neurosciences* 2: 306-308.

Madden, D.J., J. Spaniol, M.C. Costello, B. Bucur, L.E. White, R. Cabeza, S.W. Davis, N.A. Dennis, J.M. Provenzale, and S.A. Huettel. 2009. Cerebral white matter integrity mediates adult age differences in cognitive performance. *Journal of Cognitive Neuroscience* 21: 289-302.

Magnie, M.N., S. Bermon, F. Martin, M. Madany-Lounis, G. Suisse, W. Muhammad, and C. Dolisi. 2000. P300, N400, aerobic fitness, and maximal aerobic exercise. *Psychophysiology* 37: 369-377.

Manger, T.A., and R.W. Motta. 2005. The impact of an exercise program on posttraumatic stress disorder, anxiety, and depression. *International Journal of Emergency Mental Health* 7: 49-57.

March, J.S., A. Frances, D. Carpenter, and D.A. Kahn. 1997. Treatment of obsessive-compulsive disorder: The expert consensus panel for obsessive-compulsive disorder. *Journal of Clinical Psychiatry* 58: 2-72.

Mark, T.L., K.R. Levit, R.M. Coffey, D.R. McKusick, H.J. Harwood, E.C. King, E. Bouchery, J.S. Genuardi, R. Vandivort-Warren, J.A. Buck, and K. Ryan. 2007. *National expenditures for mental health services and substance abuse treatment, 1993–2003.* SAMHSA Publication SMA 07-4227. Rockville, MD: Substance Abuse and Mental Health Services Administration.

Marks, B.L., D.J. Madden, B. Bucur, J.M. Provenzale, L.E. White, R. Cabeza, and S.A. Huettel. 2007. Role of aerobic fitness and aging on cerebral white matter integrity. *Annals of the New York Academy of Sciences* 1097: 171-174.

Martinsen, E.W. 1994. Physical activity and depression: Clinical experience. *Acta Psychiatrica Scandinavica* 377 (Suppl.): 23-27.

Martinsen, E.W., S. Friis, and A. Hoffart. 1995. Assessment of depression: A comparison between Beck Depression Inventory and Comprehensive Psychopathological Rating Scale. *Acta Psychiatrica Scandinavica* 92: 460-463.

Martinsen, E.W., A. Hoffart, and Ø.Y. Solberg. 1989a. Aerobic and non-aerobic forms of exercise in the treatment of anxiety disorders. *Stress Medicine* 5: 115-120.

Martinsen, E.W., A. Hoffart, and Ø.Y. Solberg. 1989b. Comparing aerobic with nonaerobic forms of exercise in the treatment of clinical depression: A randomized trial. *Comprehensive Psychiatry* 30 (4): 324-331.

Martinsen, E.W., and A. Medhus. 1989. Adherence to exercise and patients' evaluation of physical exercise in a comprehensive treatment programme for depression. *Nordisk Psykiatrisk Tidsskrift* 43: 411-415.

Martinsen, E.W., A. Medhus, and L. Sandvik. 1985. Effects of aerobic exercise on depression: A controlled study. *British Medical Journal* 291: 109.

Martinsen, E.W., J.S. Raglin, A. Hoffart, and S. Friis. 1998. Tolerance to intensive exercise and high levels of lactate in panic disorder. *Journal of Anxiety Disorders* 12 (4): 333-342.

Martinsen, E.W., L. Sandvik, and O.B. Kolbjørnsrud. 1989. Aerobic exercise in the treatment of nonpsychotic mental disorders: An exploratory study. *Nordisk Psykiatrisk Tidsskrift* 43: 521-529.

Mathers, C.D., and D. Loncar. 2006. Projections of global mortality and burden of disease from 2002 to 2030. *PLoS Medicine* 3 (11): e442.

Matthews, V.B., M.-B. Åström, M.H.S. Chan, C.R. Bruce, O. Prelovsek, T. Åkerström, C. Yfanti, C. Broholm, O.H. Mortensen, M. Penkowa, P. Hojman, A. Zankari, M.J. Watt, B.K. Pedersen, and M.A. Febbraio. 2009. Brain derived neurotrophic factor is produced by skeletal muscle cells in response to contraction and enhances fat oxidation via activation of AMPK. *Diabetologia* 52: 1409-1418.

Mazzeo, R.S. 1991. Catecholamine responses to acute and chronic exercise. *Medicine and Science in Sports and Exercise* 23 (7): 839-845.

McAuley, E., A.F. Kramer, and S.J. Colcombe. 2004. Cardiovascular fitness and neurocognitive function in older adults: A brief review. *Brain Behavior and Immunity* 18 (3): 214-220.

McCloskey, D.P., D.S. Adamo, and B.J. Anderson. 2001. Exercise increases metabolic capacity in the motor cortex and striatum, but not in the hippocampus. *Brain Research* 891: 168-175.

McCulloch, T.L., and J.S. Bruner. 1939. The effect of electric shock upon subsequent learning in the rat. *Journal of Psychology* 7: 333-336.

McNeil, J.K., E.M. LeBlanc, and M. Joyner. 1991. The effect of exercise on depressive symptoms in the moderately depressed elderly. *Psychology and Aging* 6: 487-488.

Mead, G.E., W. Morley, P. Campbell, C.A. Greig, M. McMurdo, and D.A. Lawlor. 2009. Exercise for depression. *Cochrane Database of Systematic Reviews,* July 8 (3): CD004366.

Meeusen, R., and K. De Meirleir. 1995. Exercise and brain neurotransmission. *Sports Medicine* 20 (3): 160-188.

Meeusen, R., M.F. Piacentini, and K. De Meirleir. 2001. Brain microdialysis in exercise research. *Sports Medicine* 31 (14): 965-983.

Meeusen, R., I. Smolders, S. Sarre, K. De Meirleir, H. Keizer, M. Serneels, G. Ebinger, and Y. Michotte. 1997. Endurance training effects on neurotransmitter release in rat striatum: An in vivo microdialysis study. *Acta Physiologica Scandinavica* 159 (4): 335-341.

Menard, J., and D. Treit. 1999. Effects of centrally administered anxiolytic compounds in animal models of anxiety. *Neuroscience and Biobehavioral Review* 23 (4): 591-613.

Merom, D., P. Phongsavan, R. Wagner, T. Chey, C. Marnane, Z. Steel, D. Silove, and A. Bauman. 2008. Promoting walking as an adjunct intervention to group cognitive behavioral therapy for anxiety disorders—a pilot group randomized trial. *Journal of Anxiety Disorders* 22 (6): 959-968.

Micallef, J., and O. Blin. 2001. Neurobiology and clinical pharmacology of obsessive-compulsive disorder. *Clinical Neuropharmacology* 24 (4): 191-207.

Michaud, C.M., M.T. McKenna, S. Begg, N. Tomijima, M. Majmudar, M.T. Bulzacchelli, S. Ebrahim, M. Ezzati, J.A. Salomon, J.G. Kreiser, M. Hogan, and C.J. Murray. 2006. The burden of disease and injury in the United States 1996. *Population Health Metrics* 4: 11.

Middleton, L.E., D.E. Barnes, L.Y. Lui, and K. Yaffe. 2010. Physical activity over the life course and its association with cognitive performance and impairment in old age. *Journal of the American Geriatrics Society* 58 (7): 1322-1326.

Middleton, L., S. Kirkland, and K. Rockwood. 2008. Prevention of CIND by physical activity: Different impact on VCI-ND compared with MCI. *Journal of the Neurological Sciences* 269 (1-2): 80-84.

Mikkelsen, S.S., J.S. Tolstrup, E.M. Flachs, E.L. Mortensen, P. Schnohr, and T. Flensborg-Madsen. 2010. A cohort study of leisure time physical activity and depression. *Preventive Medicine* 51 (6): 471-475.

Möller, H.J., and M.B. Graeber. 1998. The case described by Alois Alzheimer in 1911. Historical and conceptual perspectives based on the clinical record and neurohistological sections. *European Archives of Psychiatry and Clinical Neuroscience* 248 (3): 111-122.

Morgan, W.P. 1973. Influence of acute physical activity on state anxiety. In *Proceedings, annual meeting of the College Physical Education Association for Men,* edited by C.E. Mueller, pp. 113-121. Minneapolis: University of Minnesota.

Morgan, W.P. 1979. Anxiety reduction following acute physical activity. *Psychiatric Annals* 9 (3): 36-41.

Morgan, W.P. 1994. Physical activity, fitness, and depression. In *Physical activity, fitness and health,* edited by C. Bouchard, R.J. Shephard, and T. Stephens, pp. 851-867. Champaign, IL: Human Kinetics.

Morgan, W.P., ed. 1997. *Physical activity and mental health.* Washington, DC: Taylor & Francis.

Morgan, W.P., D.R. Brown, J.S. Raglin, P.J. O'Connor, and K.A. Ellickson. 1987. Psychological monitoring of overtraining and staleness. *British Journal of Sports Medicine* 21: 107-114.

Morgan, W.P., and S.E. Goldston. 1987. *Exercise and mental health.* Washington, DC: Hemisphere.

Morgan, W.P., J.A. Roberts, F.R. Brand, and A.D. Feinerman. 1970. Psychological effect of chronic physical activity. *Medicine and Science in Sports* 2: 213-217.

Morrato, E.H., J.O. Hill, H.R. Wyatt, V. Ghushchyan, and P.W. Sullivan. 2007. Physical activity in U.S. adults with diabetes and at risk for developing diabetes, 2003. *Diabetes Care* 30 (2): 203-209.

Motl, R.W., A.S. Birnbaum, M.Y. Kubik, and R.K. Dishman. 2004. Naturally occurring changes in physical activity are inversely related to depressive symptoms during early adolescence. *Psychosomatic Medicine* 66 (3): 336-342.

Motl, R.W., J.F. Konopack, E. McAuley, S. Elavsky, G.J. Jerome, and D.X. Marquez. 2005. Depressive symptoms among older adults: Long-term reduction after a physical activity intervention. *Journal of Behavioral Medicine* 28 (4): 385-394.

Motl, R.W., and E. McAuley. 2010. Physical activity, disability, and quality of life in older adults. *Physical Medicine and Rehabilitation Clinics of North America* 21 (2): 299-308.

Motl, R.W., P.J. O'Connor, and R.K. Dishman. 2004. Effects of cycling exercise on state anxiety and the soleus H-reflex among males with low or high trait anxiety. *Psychophysiology* 41 (1): 96-105.

Murray, C.J., and A.D. Lopez. 1997. Alternative projections of mortality and disability by cause 1990–2020: Global Burden of Disease Study. *Lancet* 349 (9064): 1498-1504.

NCS (National Comorbidity Survey). 2007. National Comorbidity Survey (NCS) and National Comorbidity Survey Replication (NCS-R). Harvard School of Medicine. Available: http://www.hcp.med.harvard.edu/ncs/.

Nemeroff, C.B. 1998. Psychopharmacology of affective disorders in the 21st century. *Biological Psychiatry* 44: 517-525.

Nemeroff, C.B., C.D. Kilts, and G.S. Berns. 1999. Functional brain imaging: Twenty-first century phrenology or psychobiological advance for the millennium? *American Journal of Psychiatry* 156: 671-673.

Nock, M.K., I. Hwang, N.A. Sampson, and R.C. Kessler. 2010. Mental disorders, comorbidity and suicidal behavior: Results from the National Comorbidity Survey Replication. *Molecular Psychiatry* 15 (8): 868-876.

Nock, M.K., I. Hwang, N. Sampson, R.C. Kessler, M. Angermeyer, A. Beautrais, G. Borges, E. Bromet, R. Bruffaerts, G. de Girolamo, R. de Graaf, S. Florescu, O. Gureje, J.M. Haro, C. Hu, Y. Huang, E.G. Karam, N. Kawakami, V. Kovess, D. Levinson, J. Posada-Villa, R. Sagar, T. Tomov, M.C. Viana, and D.R. Williams. 2009. Cross-national analysis of the associations among mental disorders and suicidal behavior: Findings from the WHO World Mental Health surveys. *PLoS Medicine* 6 (8): e1000123.

Nybo, L., and B. Nielsen. 2001. Perceived exertion is associated with an altered brain activity during exercise with progressive hyperthermia. *Journal of Applied Physiology* 91: 2017-2023.

Nybo, L., and N.H. Secher. 2004. Cerebral perturbations provoked by prolonged exercise. *Progress in Neurobiology* 72: 223-261.

O'Connor, P.J., L.E. Aenchbacher, and R.K. Dishman. 1993. Physical activity and depression in the elderly. *Journal of Aging and Physical Activity* 1: 34-58.

O'Connor, P.J., C.X. Bryant, J.P. Veltri, and S.M. Gebhardt. 1993. State anxiety and ambulatory blood pressure following resistance exercise in females. *Medicine and Science in Sports and Exercise* 25: 516-521.

O'Connor, P.J., and J.C. Davis. 1992. Psychobiologic responses to exercise at different times of the day. *Medicine and Science in Sports and Exercise* 24: 714-719.

O'Connor, P.J., S.J. Petruzzello, K.A. Kubitz, and T.L. Robinson. 1995. Anxiety responses to maximal exercise testing. *British Journal of Sports Medicine* 29: 97-102.

O'Connor, P.J., J.S. Raglin, and E.W. Martinsen. 2000. Physical activity and anxiety disorders. *International Journal of Sport Psychology* 31: 136-155.

O'Connor, P.J., J.C. Smith, and W.P. Morgan. 2000. Physical activity does not provoke panic attacks in patients with panic disorder: A review of the evidence. *Anxiety, Stress, and Coping* 13: 333-353.

Ogoh, S., and P.N. Ainslie. 2009. Cerebral blood flow during exercise: Mechanisms of regulation. *Journal of Applied Physiology* 107: 1370-1380.

Olfson, M., and S.C. Marcus. 2009. National patterns in antidepressant medication treatment. *Archives of General Psychiatry* 66: 848-856

O'Neal, H.A., A.L. Dunn, and E.W. Martinsen. 2000. Depression and exercise. *International Journal of Sport Psychology* 31: 110-135.

O'Neal, H.A., J.D. Van Hoomissen, P.V. Holmes, and R.K. Dishman. 2001. Prepro-galanin messenger RNA levels are increased in rat locus coeruleus after exercise training. *Neuroscience Letters* 299 (1-2): 69-72.

Orwin, A. 1974. Treatment of a situational phobia: A case for running. *British Journal of Psychiatry* 125: 95-98.

Paas, F.G., and J.J. Adam. 1991. Human information processing during physical exercise. *Ergonomics* 34: 1385-1397.

Paffenbarger, R.S., I.-M. Lee, and R. Leung. 1994. Physical activity and personal characteristics associated with depression and suicide in American college men. *Acta Psychiatrica Scandinavica* 377 (Suppl.): 16-22.

Pagliari, R., and L. Peyrin. 1995a. Norepinephrine release in the rat frontal cortex under treadmill exercise: A study with microdialysis. *Journal of Applied Physiology* 78 (6): 2121-2130.

Pagliari, R., and L. Peyrin. 1995b. Physical conditioning in rats influences the central and peripheral catecholamine responses to sustained exercise. *European Journal of Applied Physiology* 71: 41-52.

Pajonk, F.G., T. Wobrock, O. Gruber, H. Scherk, D. Berner, I. Kaizl, A. Kierer, S. Müller, M. Oest, T. Meyer, M. Backens, T. Schneider-Axmann, A.E. Thornton, W.G. Honer, and P. Falkai. 2010. Hippocampal plasticity in response to exercise in schizophrenia. *Archives of General Psychiatry* 67 (2): 133-143.

Patten, S.B., J.V. Williams, D.H. Lavorato, and M. Eliasziw. 2009. A longitudinal community study of major depression and physical activity. *General Hospital Psychiatry* 31 (6): 571-575.

Patten, S.B., J.V. Williams, D.H. Lavorato, A. Kassam, and C.D. Sabapathy. 2010. Pharmacoepidemiology of benzodiazepine and sedative-hypnotic use in a Canadian general population cohort during 12 years of follow-up. *Canadian Journal of Psychiatry* 55 (12): 792-799.

Pereira, A.C., D.E. Huddleston, A.M. Brickman, A.A. Sosunov, R. Hen, G.M. McKhann, R. Sloan, F.H. Gage, T.R. Brown, and S.A. Small. 2007. An in vivo correlate of exercise-induced neurogenesis in the adult dentate gyrus. *Proceedings of the National Academy of Sciences U.S.A.* 104: 5638-5643.

Perry, P.J., T. Sanger, and C. Beasley. 1997. Olanzapine plasma concentrations and clinical response in acutely ill schizophrenic patients. *Journal of Clinical Psychopharmacology* 17: 472-477.

Petruzzello, S.J., and D.M. Landers. 1994. State anxiety reduction and exercise: Does hemispheric activation reflect such changes? *Medicine and Science in Sports and Exercise* 26 (8): 1028-1035.

Petruzzello, S.J., D.M. Landers, B.D. Hatfield, K.A. Kubitz, and W. Salazar. 1991. A meta-analysis on the anxiety-reducing effects of acute and chronic exercise. Outcomes and mechanisms. *Sports Medicine* 11 (3): 143-182.

Petruzzello, S.J., and A.K. Tate. 1997. Brain activation, affect, and aerobic exercise: An examination of both state-independent and state-dependent relationships. *Psychophysiology* 34: 527-533.

Pfaff, D. 2006. *Brain arousal and information theory: Neural and genetic mechanisms.* Cambridge, MA: Harvard University Press.

Physical Activity Guidelines Advisory Committee. 2008. *Physical Activity Guidelines Advisory Committee report.* Washington, DC: U.S. Department of Health and Human Services, pp. 1-683.

Plassman, B.L., K.M. Langa, G.G. Fisher, S.G. Heeringa, D.R. Weir, M.B. Ofstedal, J.R. Burke, M.D. Hurd, G.G. Potter, W.L. Rodgers, D.C. Steffens, R.J. Willis, and R.B. Wallace. 2007.

Prevalence of dementia in the United States: the aging, demographics, and memory study. *Neuroepidemiology* 29: 125-132.

Podewils, L.J., E. Guallar, L.H. Kuller, L.P. Fried, O.L. Lopez, M. Carlson, and C.G. Lyketsos. 2005. Physical activity, APOE genotype, and dementia risk: Findings from the Cardiovascular Health Cognition Study. *American Journal of Epidemiology* 161 (7): 639-651.

Pollack, M.H., C. Allgulander, B. Bandelow, G.B. Cassano, J.H. Greist, E. Hollander, D.J. Nutt, A. Okasha, R.P. Swinson; World Council of Anxiety. 2003. WCA recommendations for the long-term treatment of panic disorder. *CNS Spectrums* 8 (Suppl. 1): 17-30.

Pollock, M.L., G.A. Glaser, J.D. Butcher, J.P. Despre, R.K. Dishman, B.F. Franklin, and C.E. Garber. 1998. The recommended quantity and quality of exercise for developing and maintaining cardiorespiratory and muscular fitness, and flexibility in healthy adults. *Medicine and Science in Sports and Exercise* 30 (6): 975-991.

Pontifex, M.B., and C.H. Hillman. 2007. Neuroelectric and behavioral indices of interference control during acute cycling. *Clinical Neurophysiology* 118: 570-580.

Prange, A.J. 1964. The pharmacology and biochemistry of depression. *Diseases of the Nervous System* 25: 217-221.

Pronk, N.P., A.F. Jawad, S.F. Crouse, and J.J. Rohack. 1994. Acute effects of walking on mood profiles in women: Preliminary findings in postmenopausal women. *Medicine, Exercise, Nutrition, and Health* 3: 148-153.

Raab, S., and K.H. Plate. 2007. Different networks, common growth factors: Shared growth factors and receptors of the vascular and the nervous system. *Acta Neuropathologica* 113 (6): 607-626.

Raglin, J.S. 1997. Anxiolytic effects of physical activity. In *Physical activity and mental health,* edited by W.P. Morgan, pp. 107-126. Washington, DC: Taylor & Francis.

Raglin, J.S., P.E. Turner, and F. Eksten. 1993. State anxiety and blood pressure following 30 min of leg ergometry or weight training. *Medicine and Science in Sports and Exercise* 25: 1044-1048.

Raglin, J.S., and M. Wilson. 1996. State anxiety following 20 minutes of bicycle ergometer exercise at selected intensities. *International Journal of Sports Medicine* 17: 467-471.

Rajala, U., A. Uusimaki, S. Keinanen-Kiukaanniemi, and S.L. Kivela. 1994. Prevalence of depression in a 55-year-old Finnish population. *Society of Psychiatry and Psychiatric Epidemiology* 29: 126-130.

Rasmussen, K., D.A. Morilak, and B.L. Jacobs. 1986. Single unit activity of locus coeruleus neurons in the freely moving cat: I. During naturalistic behaviors and in response to simple and complex stimuli. *Brain Research* 371: 324-334.

Rasmussen, P., P. Brassard, H. Adser, M.V. Pedersen, L. Leick, E. Hart, N.H. Secher, B.K. Pedersen, and H. Pilegaard. 2009. Evidence for a release of brain-derived neurotrophic factor from the brain during exercise. *Experimental Physiology* 94 (10): 1062-1069.

Regier, D.A., J.H. Boyd, J.D. Burke Jr., D.S. Rae, J.K. Myers, M. Kramer, L.N. Robins, L.K. George, M. Karno, and B.Z. Locke.

1988. One-month prevalence of mental health disorders in the United States. *Archives of General Psychiatry* 45: 977-986.

Regier, D.A., D.S. Rae, W.E. Narrow, C.T. Kaelber, and A.F. Schatzberg. 1998. Prevalence of anxiety disorders and their comorbidity with mood and addictive disorders. *British Journal of Psychiatry* 34 (Suppl.): 24-28.

Reiman, E.M. 1997. The application of positron emission tomography to the study of normal and pathologic emotions. *Journal of Clinical Psychiatry* 58 (Suppl. 16): 4-12.

Reiman, E.M., K. Chen, G.E. Alexander, R.J. Caselli, D. Bandy, D. Osborne, A.M. Saunders, and J. Hardy. 2005. Correlations between apolipoprotein E epsilon4 gene dose and brain-imaging measurements of regional hypometabolism. *Proceedings of the National Academy of Sciences U.S.A.* 102 (23): 8299-8302.

Reiss, J.I., R.K. Dishman, H.E. Boyd, J.K. Robinson, and P.V. Holmes. 2009. Chronic activity wheel running reduces the severity of kainic acid-induced seizures in the rat: Possible role of galanin. *Brain Research* 1266: 54-63.

Rhyu, I.J., J.A. Bytheway, S.J. Kohler, H. Lange, K.J. Lee, J. Boklewski, K.M. McCormick, N.I. Williams, G.B. Stanton, W.T. Greenough, and J.L. Cameron. 2010. Effects of aerobic exercise training on cognitive function and cortical vascularity in monkeys. *Neuroscience,* March 6. [Epub ahead of print]

Rice, D.P., and L.S. Miller. 1995. The economic burden of affective disorders. *British Journal of Psychiatry* 166 (Suppl. 27): 34-42.

Rice, D.P., and L.S. Miller. 1998. Health economics and cost implications of anxiety and other mental disorders in the United States. *British Journal of Psychiatry, Supplement* (34): 4-9.

Rolland, Y., G. Abellan van Kan, and B. Vellas. 2010. Healthy brain aging: Role of exercise and physical activity. *Clinics in Geriatric Medicine* 26 (1, February): 75-87.

Rolland, Y., F. Pillard, A. Klapouszczak, E. Reynish, D. Thomas, S. Andrieu, D. Rivière, and B. Vellas. 2007. Exercise program for nursing home residents with Alzheimer's disease: A 1-year randomized, controlled trial. *Journal of the American Geriatrics Society* 55 (2): 158-165.

Rooks, C.R., N.J. Thom, K.K. McCully, and R.K. Dishman. 2010. Effects of incremental exercise on cerebral oxygenation measured by near-infrared spectroscopy: A systematic review. *Progress in Neurobiology* 92 (2): 134-150.

Rothon, C., P. Edwards, K. Bhui, R.M. Viner, S. Taylor, and S.A. Stansfeld. 2010. Physical activity and depressive symptoms in adolescents: A prospective study. *BMC Medicine* 28 (8): 32. www.biomedcentral.com/1741-7015/8/32.

Roy, C., and C. Sherrington. 1890. On the regulation of the blood supply of the brain. *Journal of Physiology* 11: 85-108.

Royall, D.R., E.C. Lauterbach, J.L. Cummings, A. Reeve, T.A. Rummans, D.I. Kaufer, W.C. LaFrance Jr., and C.E. Coffey. 2002. Executive control function: A review of its promise and challenges for clinical research. A report from the Committee on Research of the American Neuropsychiatric Association. *Journal of Neuropsychiatry and Clinical Neurosciences* 14: 377-405.

Rudorfer, M.V., M.E. Henry, and H.A. Sackheim. 1997. Electroconvulsive therapy. In *Psychiatry,* edited by A. Tasman, J. Kay, and J.A. Lieberman, pp. 1535-1556. Philadelphia: Saunders.

Rush, A.J., M.H. Trivedi, S.R. Wisniewski, et al. 2006. Bupropion-SR, sertraline, or venlafaxine-XR after failure of SSRIs for depression. *New England Journal of Medicine* 354: 1231-1242.

Rushton, J.L., M. Forcier, and R.M. Schectman. 2002. Epidemiology of depressive symptoms in the National Longitudinal Study of Adolescent Health. *Journal of the American Academy of Child and Adolescent Psychiatry* 41: 199-205.

Russo-Neustadt, A. 2003. Brain-derived neurotrophic factor, behavior, and new directions for the treatment of mental disorders. *Seminars in Clinical Neuropsychiatry* 8: 109-118.

Russo-Neustadt, A., R.C. Beard, and C.W. Cotman. 1999. Exercise, antidepressant medications, and enhanced brain derived neurotrophic factor expression. *Neuropsychopharmacology* 21 (5): 679-682.

Russo-Neustadt, A., T. Ha, R. Ramirez, and J.P. Kesslak. 2001. Physical activity–antidepressant treatment combination: Impact on brain-derived neurotrophic factor and behavior in an animal model. *Behavioural Brain Research* 120 (1): 87-95.

Sanchez-Villegas, A., I. Ara, F. Guillén-Grima, M. Bes-Rastrollo, J.J. Varo-Cenarruzabeitia, and M.A. Martínez-González. 2008. Physical activity, sedentary index, and mental disorders in the SUN cohort study. *Medicine and Science in Sports and Exercise* 40 (5): 827-834.

Schildkraut, J.J. 1965. The catecholamine hypothesis of affective disorders: A review of the supporting evidence. *American Journal of Psychiatry* 122: 509-522.

Schlict, W. 1994. Does physical exercise reduce anxious emotions? A meta-analysis. *Anxiety, Stress, and Coping* 6: 275-288.

Schuit, A.J., E.J. Feskens, L.J. Launer, and D. Kromhout. 2001. Physical activity and cognitive decline, the role of the apolipoprotein e4 allele. *Medicine and Science in Sports and Exercise* 33 (5): 772-777.

Secher, N.H., T. Seifert, and J.J. Van Lieshout. 2008. Cerebral blood flow and metabolism during exercise: Implications for fatigue. *Journal of Applied Physiology* 104: 306-314.

Segar, M.L., V.L. Katch, R.S. Roth, A.W. Garcia, T.I. Portner, S.G. Glickman, S. Haslinger, and E.G. Wilkins. 1998. The effect of aerobic exercise on self-esteem and depressive and anxiety symptoms among breast cancer survivors. *Oncology Nursing Forum* 25: 107-113.

Seifert, T., P. Brassard, M. Wissenberg, P. Rasmussen, P. Nordby, B. Stallknecht, H. Adser, A.H. Jakobsen, H. Pilegaard, H.B. Nielsen, and N.H. Secher. 2010. Endurance training enhances BDNF release from the human brain. *American Journal of Physiology: Regulatory, Integrative, and Comparative Physiology* 298 (2): R372-377.

Sexton, H., A. Mære, and N.H. Dahl. 1989. Exercise intensity and reduction in neurotic symptoms. *Acta Psychiatrica Scandinavica* 80: 231-235.

Sheehan, D.V., M.T. Eaddy, M.B. Shah, and R.P. Mauch. 2005. Differences in total medical costs across the SSRIs for the treatment of depression and anxiety. *American Journal of Managed Care* 11 (12 Suppl.): S354-361.

Sibley, B.A., and J.L. Etnier. 2003. The relationship between physical activity and cognition in children: a meta-analysis. *Pediatric Exercise Science* 15: 243–256.

Singh, N.A., K.M. Clements, and M.A. Fiatarone. 1997a. A randomized controlled trial of the effects of exercise on sleep. *Sleep* 20: 40-46.

Singh, N.A., K.M. Clements, and M.A. Fiatarone. 1997b. A randomized controlled trial of progressive resistance training in depressed elders. *Journal of Gerontology* 52A (1): M27-M35.

Singh, N.A., T.M. Stavrinos, Y. Scarbek, G. Galambos, C. Liber, and M.A. Fiatarone Singh. 2005. A randomized controlled trial of high versus low intensity weight training versus general practitioner care for clinical depression in older adults. *Journals of Gerontology Series A: Biological Sciences and Medical Sciences* 60: 768-776.

Smith, J.C., K.A. Nielson, J.L. Woodard, M. Seidenberg, S. Durgerian, P. Antuono, A.M. Butts, N.C. Hantke, M.A. Lancaster, and S.M. Rao. 2011. Interactive effects of physical activity and APOE-ε4 on BOLD semantic memory activation in healthy elders. *Neuroimage* 54 (1): 635-644.

Smith, J.C., P.J. O'Connor, J.B. Crabbe, and R.K. Dishman. 2002. Emotional responsiveness after low- and moderate-intensity exercise and seated rest. *Medicine and Science in Sports and Exercise* 34: 1158-1167.

Smith, J.C., E.S. Paulson, D.B. Cook, M.D. Verber, and Q. Tian. 2010. Detecting changes in human cerebral blood flow after acute exercise using arterial spin labeling: Implications for fMRI. *Journal of Neuroscience Methods* 191 (2): 258-262.

Smith, T.L., K.H. Masaki, K. Fong, R.D. Abbott, G.W. Ross, H. Petrovitch, P.L. Blanchette, and L.R. White. 2010. Effect of walking distance on 8-year incident depressive symptoms in elderly men with and without chronic disease: The Honolulu-Asia Aging Study. *Journal of the American Geriatrics Society* 58 (8): 1447-1452.

Smolders, M., M. Laurant, E. van Rijswijk, J. Mulder, J. Braspenning, P. Verhaak, M. Wensing, and R. Grol. 2007. The impact of co-morbidity on GPs' pharmacological treatment decisions for patients with an anxiety disorder. *Family Practice* 24 (6): 538-546.

Soares, J., P.V. Holmes, K.J. Renner, G.L. Edwards, B.N. Bunnell, and R.K. Dishman. 1999. Brain noradrenergic responses to footshock after chronic activity-wheel running. *Behavioral Neuroscience* 113: 558-566.

Sobocki, P., B. Jönsson, J. Angst, and C. Rehnberg. 2006. Cost of depression in Europe. *Journal of Mental Health Policy and Economics* 9 (2): 87-98.

Sonstroem, R.J. 1998. Physical self-concept: Assessment and external validity. *Exercise and Sport Sciences Reviews* 26: 133-164.

Sonstroem, R.J., and W.P. Morgan. 1989. Exercise and self-esteem: Rationale and model. *Medicine and Science in Sports and Exercise* 21: 329-337.

Sothmann, M.S., J. Buckworth, R.P. Claytor, R.H. Cox, J.E. White-Welkley, and R.K. Dishman. 1996. Exercise training and the cross-stressor adaptation hypothesis. *Exercise and Sport Sciences Reviews* 24: 267-287.

Sparling, P.B., A. Giuffrida, D. Piomelli, L. Rosskopf, and A. Dietrich. 2003. Exercise activates the endocannabinoid system. *Neuroreport* 14 (17, December 2): 2209-2211.

Spence, J.C., K.R. McGannon, and P. Poon. 2005. The effect of exercise on global self-esteem: A quantitative review. *Journal of Sport and Exercise Psychology* 27: 311-334.

Stahl, S.M. 1996. *Essential psychopharmacology: Neuroscientific basis and clinical applications.* New York: Cambridge University Press.

Stephens, T. 1988. Physical activity and mental health in the United States and Canada: Evidence from four population surveys. *Preventive Medicine* 17: 35-47.

Strawbridge, W.J., S. Deleger, R.E. Roberts, and G.A. Kaplan. 2002. Physical activity reduces the risk of subsequent depression for older adults. *American Journal of Epidemiology* 156 (4): 328-334.

Strine, T.W., A.H. Mokdad, L.W. Balluz, O. Gonzalez, R. Crider, J.T. Berry, and K. Kroenke. 2008. Depression and anxiety in the United States: Findings from the 2006 Behavioral Risk Factor Surveillance System. *Psychiatric Services* 59 (12): 1383-1390.

Ströhle, A., B. Graetz, M. Scheel, A. Wittmann, C. Feller, A. Heinz, and F. Dimeo. 2009. The acute antipanic and anxiolytic activity of aerobic exercise in patients with panic disorder and healthy control subjects. *Journal of Psychiatric Research* 43 (12): 1013-1017.

Ströhle, A., M. Höfler, H. Pfister, A-G. Müller, J. Hoyer, H-U. Wittchen, and R. Lieb. 2007. Physical activity and prevalence and incidence of mental disorders in adolescents and young adults. *Psychological Medicine* 37: 1657-1666.

Strøm, M., E.L. Mortensen, T.I. Halldorson, M.L. Osterdal, and S.F. Olsen. 2009. Leisure-time physical activity in pregnancy and risk of postpartum depression: A prospective study in a large national birth cohort. *Journal of Clinical Psychiatry* 70 (12): 1707-1714.

Sui, X., J.N. Laditka, T.S. Church, et al. 2009. Prospective study of cardiorespiratory fitness and depressive symptoms in women and men. *Journal of Psychiatric Research* 43 (5): 546-552.

Tantillo, M., C.M. Kesick, G.W. Hynd, and R.K. Dishman. 2002. The effects of exercise on children with attention-deficit hyperactivity disorder. *Medicine and Science in Sports and Exercise* 34: 203-212.

Thorsen, L., W. Nystad, H. Stigum, O. Dahl, O. Klepp, R.M. Bremnes, E. Wist, and S.D. Fosså. 2005. The association between self-reported physical activity and prevalence of depression and anxiety disorder in long-term survivors of testicular cancer and men in a general population sample. *Supportive Care in Cancer* 13 (8): 637-646.

Tomporowski, P.D. 2003. Effects of acute bouts of exercise on cognition. *Acta Psychologica* 112: 297-324.

Tomporowski, P.D., C.L. Davis, P.H. Miller, and I.A. Naglieri. 2008. Exercise and children's intelligence, cognition, and academic achievement. *Educational Psychology Review* 20 (2): 111-131.

Tomporowski, P.D., and N.R. Ellis. 1986. The effects of exercise on cognitive processes: A review. *Psychological Bulletin* 99: 338-346.

Trivedi, M.H., M. Fava, S.R. Wisniewski, et al. 2006a. Medication augmentation after the failure of SSRIs for depression. *New England Journal of Medicine* 354: 1243-1252.

Trivedi, M.H., T.L. Greer, B.D. Grannemann, H.O. Chambliss, and A.N. Jordan. 2006b. Exercise as an augmentation strategy for treatment of major depression. *Journal of Psychiatric Practice* 12 (4): 205-213.

U.S. Department of Health and Human Services. 1996. *Physical activity and health: A report of the Surgeon General.* DHHS Publication No. (PH5) 017-023-00196-5. Atlanta: U.S. Department of Health and Human Services, Centers for Disease Control and Prevention, National Center for Chronic Disease Prevention and Health Promotion.

U.S. Department of Health and Human Services. 1999. *Mental health: A report of the Surgeon General—executive summary.* Rockville, MD: U.S. Department of Health and Human Services, Substance Abuse and Mental Health Services Administration, Center for Mental Health Services, National Institutes of Health, National Institute of Mental Health.

Van Ameringen, M., C. Allgulander, B. Bandelow, J.H. Greist, E. Hollander, S.A. Montgomery, D.J. Nutt, A. Okasha, M.H. Pollack, D.J. Stein, R.P. Swinson; World Council of Anxiety. 2003. WCA recommendations for the long-term treatment of social phobia. *CNS Spectrums* 8 (Suppl. 1): 40-52.

Van Hoomissen, J.D., H.O. Chambliss, P.V. Holmes, and R.K. Dishman. 2003. The effects of chronic exercise and imipramine on mRNA for BDNF after olfactory bulbectomy in rat. *Brain Research* 974: 228-235.

Van Hoomissen, J.D., H.A. O'Neal, J.E. Dishman, P.V. Holmes, and R.K. Dishman. 2000. Serotonin transporter mRNA in dorsal raphe is unchanged by treadmill running. *Medicine and Science in Sports and Exercise* 32 (Suppl. 5): S42.

Van Hoomissen, J.D., H.A. O'Neal, P.V. Holmes, and R.K. Dishman. 2001. The effects of exercise on masculine sexual behavior and BDNF mRNA after olfactory bulbectomy in rats. Abstracts, Society for Neuroscience 31st Annual Meeting, p. 133. San Diego, November 10-15.

van Praag, H. 2008. Neurogenesis and exercise: Past and future directions. *Neuromolecular Medicine* 10 (2): 128-140.

Vaux, C.L. 1926. A discussion of physical exercise and recreation. *Occupational Therapy and Rehabilitation* 5: 329-333.

Veale, D., K. Le Fevre, C. Pantelis, V. de Souza, A. Mann, and A. Sargeant. 1992. Aerobic exercise in the adjunctive treatment of depression: A randomized controlled trial. *Journal of the Royal Society of Medicine* 85: 541-544.

Vissing, J., M. Andersen, and N.H. Diemer. 1996. Exercise-induced changes in local cerebral glucose utilization in the rat. *Journal of Cerebral Blood Flow and Metabolism* 16: 729-736.

Weisberg, R.B. 2009. Overview of generalized anxiety disorder: Epidemiology, presentation, and course. *Journal of Clinical Psychiatry* 70 (Suppl. 2): 4-9.

Weissman, M.M., R.C. Bland, G.J. Canino, C. Faravelli, S. Greenwald, H.G. Hwu, P.R. Joyce, E.G. Karam, C.K. Lee, J. Lellouch, et al. 1997. The cross-national epidemiology of panic disorder. *Archives of General Psychiatry* 54 (4): 305-309.

Weissman, M.M., J.S. Markowitz, R. Ouellette, S. Greenwald, and J.P. Kahn. 1990. Panic disorder and cardiovascular/cerebrovascular problems: Results from a community survey. *American Journal of Psychiatry* 147: 1504-1508.

Westenberg, H.G. 1996. Developments in the drug treatment of panic disorder: What is the place of the selective serotonin reuptake inhibitors? *Journal of Affective Disorders* 40: 85-93.

Weuve, J., J.H. Kang, J.E. Manson, M.M. Breteler, J.H. Ware, and F. Grodstein. 2004. Physical activity, including walking, and cognitive function in older women. *Journal of the American Medical Association* 292 (12): 1454-1461.

White-Welkley, J.E., B.N. Bunnell, E.H. Mougey, J.L. Meyerhoff, and R.K. Dishman. 1995. Treadmill exercise training and estradiol differentially modulate hypothalamic-pituitary-adrenal cortical responses to acute running and immobilization. *Physiology and Behavior* 57: 533-540.

Williamson, J.W., P.J. Fadel, and J.H. Mitchell. 2006. New insights into central cardiovascular control during exercise in humans: A central command update. *Experimental Physiology* 91: 51-58.

Willner, P. 1995. Animal models of depression: Validity and applications. In *Depression and mania: From neurobiology to treatment,* edited by G. Gessa, W. Fratta, L. Pani, and G. Serra, pp. 19-41. New York: Raven Press.

Wilson, W.M., and C.A. Marsden. 1996. In vivo measurement of extracellular serotonin in the ventral hippocampus during treadmill running. *Behavioural Pharmacology* 7: 101-104.

Wise, L.A., L.L. Adams-Campbell, J.R. Palmer, and L. Rosenberg. 2006. Leisure time physical activity in relation to depressive symptoms in the Black Women's Health Study. *Annals of Behavioral Medicine* 32: 68-76.

Wolf, M., M. Ferrari, and V. Quaresima. 2007. Progress of near-infrared spectroscopy and topography for brain and muscle clinical applications. *Journal of Biomedical Optics* 12: 62-104.

World Health Organization (WHO). 1992. *International Classification of Diseases-10.* Geneva: World Health Organization.

Workman, E.A., and D.D. Short. 1993. Atypical antidepressants versus imipramine in the treatment of major depression: A meta-analysis. *Journal of Clinical Psychiatry* 54: 5-12.

Wyshak, G. 2001. Women's college physical activity and self-reports of physician-diagnosed depression and of current symptoms of psychiatric distress. *Journal of Women's Health and Gender-Based Medicine* 10: 363-370.

Yaffe, K., D. Barnes, M. Nevitt, L.Y. Lui, and K. Covinsky. 2001. A prospective study of physical activity and cognitive decline in elderly women: Women who walk. *Archives of Internal Medicine* 161 (14): 1703-1708.

Yoo, H.S., B.N. Bunnell, J.B. Crabbe, L.R. Kalish, and R.K. Dishman. 2000a. Failure of neonatal clomipramine treatment to alter forced swim immobility: Treadmill or activity wheel running and imipramine. *Physiology and Behavior* 70: 407-411.

Yoo, H.S., R.L. Tackett, B.N. Bunnell, J.B. Crabbe, and R.K. Dishman. 2000b. Antidepressant-like effects of physical activity vs. imipramine: Neonatal clomipramine model. *Psychobiology* 28: 540-549.

Youngstedt, S.D. 2000. The exercise–sleep mystery. *International Journal of Sport Psychology* 35: 242-255.

Youngstedt, S.D. 2005. Effects of exercise on sleep. *Clinical Sports Medicine* 24 (2): 355-365, xi.

Youngstedt, S.D., R.K. Dishman, K.J. Cureton, and L.J. Peacock. 1993. Does body temperature mediate anxiolytic effects of acute exercise? *Journal of Applied Physiology* 74: 825-831.

Youngstedt, S.D., and C.E. Kline. 2006. Epidemiology of exercise and sleep. *Sleep and Biological Rhythms* 4 (3): 215-221.

Youngstedt, S.D., P.J. O'Connor, J.B. Crabbe, and R.K. Dishman. 1998. Acute exercise reduces caffeine-induced anxiogenesis. *Medicine and Science in Sports and Exercise* 30 (5): 740-745.

Youngstedt, S.D., P.J. O'Connor, J.B. Crabbe, and R.K. Dishman. 2000. Effects of acute exercise on caffeine-induced insomnia. *Physiology and Behavior* 68: 563-570.

Youngstedt, S.D., P.J. O'Connor, and R.K. Dishman. 1997. The effects of acute exercise on sleep: A quantitative synthesis. *Sleep* 20: 203-213.

Zajecka, J.M. 2003. Treating depression to remission. *Journal of Clinical Psychiatry* 64 (Suppl. 15): 7-12.

Physical Activity
and Special Populations

*The disparities . . . in men [sic] are superficial . . . Each is incomparably superior
to his companion in some faculty. His want of skill in other directions has added to his fitness
for his own work. Each seems to have some compensation yielded to him by his infirmity,
and every hindrance operates as a concentration of his force.*

· Ralph Waldo Emerson (1844) ·

*We believe that the best way to improve our public health system and ultimately
to improve and protect the health of all Americans is to ask ourselves
why some people are lagging behind in certain areas and what can we do to correct that.*

· David Satcher, MD, PhD ·
Former Surgeon General and Assistant Secretary of Health and Human Services (2000)

*The reality is that for too long we provided lesser care to people with disabilities.
Today, we must redouble our efforts so that people with disabilities achieve full access
to disease prevention and health promotion services.*

· Richard H. Carmona, MD, MPH, FACS ·
Former U.S. Surgeon General (2005)

CHAPTER OBJECTIVES

▸ Describe current disparities for physical activity levels and sedentary behavior among persons by age, race or ethnicity, gender, socioeconomic status, and ability

▸ Recognize and understand the impact of these patterns on the health of diverse populations

▸ Describe the prevalence and types of disability in the United States

▸ Discuss the connections between physical inactivity and the development of disabling conditions, particularly in connection with aging

▸ Discuss the relationship between physical activity or inactivity and long-term health in people with disabilities

▸ Recognize and understand some of the potential barriers to physical activity for diverse populations

In this chapter we review the pattern of physical activity and inactivity among persons who represent diverse racial–ethnic groups, persons of lower socioeconomic status, and persons with disabilities. In particular, the chapter seeks to describe and discuss the physical activity and health disparities that exist among these "special populations" compared with the patterns of physical activity seen among majority groups in the United States (e.g., white, middle to higher income, and without disabilities). The rationale for a chapter devoted to these topics is the need to examine in more detail disparities of physical activity patterns that are clearly associated with discrepancies in health status and disease occurrence. These disparities are important to consider in epidemiologic discussions about the health promoting and disease prevention effects of adequate physical activity and risks of inactivity.

Physical Activity Among Diverse Racial–Ethnic Populations

The risk and burden of premature morbidity and mortality from chronic diseases in the United States are higher among diverse racial–ethnic groups than among non-Hispanic whites (National Center for Health Statistics 2007). Many of these chronic diseases and conditions have been demonstrated to be associated with physical inactivity and low levels of physical activity (Physical Activity Guidelines Advisory Committee 2008). Deaths due to coronary heart disease, cancer of the colon, breast cancer, type 2 diabetes, hypertension, obesity, and stroke have all demonstrated a disparate distribution according to race-ethnicity and lower socioeconomic status (SES) in the United States (National Center for Health Statistics 2007). These disease or condition outcomes also have independent associations with inactivity and low levels of physical activity (Physical Activity Guidelines Advisory Committee 2008). Thus, the examination of physical inactivity and physical activity levels among racial–ethnic groups compared with the majority population may provide key insights into addressing these health disparities.

Magnitude of the Problem

The public health burden imposed by low levels of physical activity appears to be disproportionately high among diverse race–ethnic and lower-SES communities (Eyler et al. 2002; Whitt-Glover et al. 2007; Ham et al. 2007; He and Baker 2005). (See figure 15.1.) African Americans, American Indians/Alaska Natives, Asian Americans, Pacific Islanders, and Latinos have significantly lower levels of regular physical activity and significantly higher levels of inactivity than do whites (Marshall et al. 2007). Currently, public health surveillance systems and national surveys tend to aggregate selected racial–ethnic groups when reporting health-related data. Historically, this has been true for Asian Americans

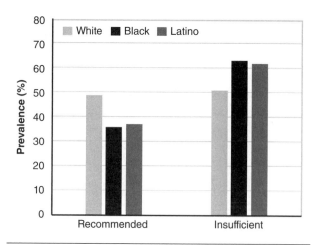

Figure 15.1 Prevalence of physical activity among adults in the United States by race/ethnicity, Behavioral Risk Factor Surveillance System, 2007.

*Recommended level is at least 30 min of moderate physical activity, five days per week, or at least 20 min of vigorous physical activity, three days per week.

Data from Centers for Disease Control 2008.

and Pacific Islanders as well as Latino/Hispanic populations. The disaggregation of these groups into their respective race–ethnic identities (e.g., Asian American, Pacific Islander, Mexican American, Puerto Rican, Central American, and South American) appears prudent because of the variability in such health indicators as body weight, hypertension, and type 2 diabetes mellitus, which are influenced by physical activity. These differences are highlighted by recent data that document low levels of objectively measured moderate-to-vigorous physical activity, as well as high levels of inactivity, across the entire U.S. population, but especially among diverse race–ethnic groups (Matthews et al. 2008; Troiano et al. 2008; Adams and Schoenborn 2006).

That racial–ethnic disparities exist for most physical activity–related chronic diseases and conditions is well accepted (Adams and Schoenborn 2006; Ogden et al. 2006); however, these relationships appear to persist even when studies control for SES (Wang and Beydoun 2007).

Physical Activity and Health in Diverse Populations

Despite the current public health consensus and recent physical activity surveillance data from the National Health Interview Survey (NHIS; Pleis, Lucas, and Ward 2009) (table 15.1) identifying physical inactivity as an important correlate of health disparities across race–ethnic populations, there remains a paucity of studies examining the role of physical activity in association with chronic disease outcomes among racially and ethnically diverse populations. These investigational deficiencies are further confounded by the disproportionate representation of racial–ethnic

www.cdc.gov/nchs/icd/icf.htm. Site of the National Center for Health Statistics, Centers for Disease Control and Prevention, International Classifications of Diseases, International Classification of Function. Provides introduction to international nomenclature in defining and classifying impairments and disabilities.

www.ncpad.org. Website for the National Center for Physical Activity and Disabilities at the University of Illinois, Chicago. Provides resources and links describing physical activity programming and research which addresses the needs of persons with disabilities. Resources include intervention program models, tools for measuring physical activity, and links to condition-specific organizations.

http://minorityhealth.hhs.gov. The Office of Minority Health of the Department of Health and Human Services. Provides specific and general information about the health indices, grant opportunities, and resources for understanding the health challenges of persons associated with specific race or ethnic groups in the United States.

www.healthypeople.gov/2020/topicsobjectives2020/overview.aspx?topicid=9. This site contains physical activity objectives that are specific to persons with disabilities as well as those without disabilities.

www.cdc.gov/omhd/Populations/Disability/Disability.htm. Centers for Disease Control and Prevention website specific to the Office of Minority Health and Disabilities. Provides resources and links within the CDC to resources, data, and tools specific to the public health issues among persons of race or ethnic diversity and persons with disabilities.

www.ihpnet.org. Provides specific information about the health status and links to specific faith-based initiatives and information regarding the health of racial or ethnic minorities within the United States.

www.naphsis.org/NAPHSIS/files/ccLibraryFiles/Filename/000000001003/Race%20and%20Ethnicity.pdf. Provides the current and specific classification of races and ethnicities within the United State from the Office of Management and Budget of the United States.

populations who are classified as lower SES compared with non-Hispanic whites (He and Baker 2005; Ford et al. 1991). Socioeconomic status explains some, but usually not all, racial–ethnic physical activity differences. Some investigators have shown that race-ethnicity is not associated with physical activity levels when multiple sociodemographic variables are used to reflect SES (He and Baker 2005), while others demonstrate the independent effects of race-ethnicity on physical activity despite controlling for SES (Sternfeld et al. 2000). Thus, comparing physical activity and health outcomes within and between racial–ethnic groups is difficult when one considers the effects of SES. This is due in part to the proportional differences in SES among non-Hispanic whites, who characteristically have a smaller proportion of lower-SES people, compared with the racial–ethnic populations of African American, Latino or Hispanic, and American Indian, and interethnic who have greater proportions of lower SES. These observations further complicate understanding the role of physical activity and health outcomes among these diverse groups. As a result, inadequate subsamples of lower-SES non-Hispanic whites or higher-SES diverse racial–ethnic participants hinder analytical disaggregation by race-ethnicity and SES. Therefore, most of the studies reviewed here, focusing on racial–ethnic differences in physical activity and health-related outcomes, recognize that race-ethnicity is, in part, a proxy measure for SES.

All-Cause Mortality

A number of recent studies with nationally representative samples from across population subgroups in the United States have demonstrated that persons representing diverse racial–ethnic populations derive the same health and reduced-mortality benefits as the majority non-Hispanic white population from increased levels of physical activity. The National Health Information Survey (NHIS) is a yearly survey conducted by agencies of the Department of Health and Human Services (DHHS) that provides details on selected health-related data as well as sociodemographic information. These surveys are collected yearly and involve substantial sample sizes. In addition, the NHIS allows for longitudinal follow-up of selected cohorts. Gregg and colleagues (2003), using an NHIS cohort, examined the walking and physical activity behaviors among people with type 2 diabetes mellitus and the association with total and cardiovascular disease (CVD) mortality. The authors demonstrated that for all race–ethnic groups and for both sexes, increased levels of walking and leisure-time physical activity were associated with significant reductions in total and CVD mortality. However, they noted that the proportion of those engaging in increased levels of walking and leisure-time physical activity varied by race-ethnicity, with the lowest frequencies of these behaviors occurring among Latinos and African Americans.

Richardson and colleagues (2004), using data from the Health and Retirement Study (HRS), a large nationally representative cohort of preretirement-aged U.S. adults designed to assess the relationships between health, economic factors, and retirement, examined physical activity and total mortality among people at various levels of risk for CVD. Their results indicate that the protective effect of regular physical activity transcended gender and race-ethnicity, as well as SES. Indeed, the effect of physical activity in preventing premature mortality was strongest among those with the highest CVD risk across all subgroups (Richardson et al. 2004). Ostbye et al. (2002), using the HRS data, examined the relationship of physical activity and total mortality among the oldest old

Table 15.1   Physical Activity Among U.S. Adults by Sex, Age, and Race

Selected characteristic	Leisure-time physical activity status among persons 18 years of age and over				Frequency of vigorous leisure-time physical activity per week among persons 18 years of age and over					
	Total	Inactive	Some leisure-time activity	Regular leisure-time activity	Total	Never	Less than 1	1-2	3-4	5 or more
Total (age-adjusted)	100.0	36.4 (0.61)	31.1 (0.47)	32.5 (0.47)	100.0	58.6 (0.57)	3.0 (0.16)	12.7 (0.33)	14.1 (0.33)	11.6 (0.31)
Total (crude)	100.0	36.5 (0.61)	31.1 (0.47)	32.4 (0.46)	100.0	58.9 (0.57)	3.0 (0.16)	12.6 (0.32)	14.0 (0.32)	11.5 (0.30)
Sex										
Male	100.0	34.1 (0.79)	31.2 (0.67)	34.8 (0.67)	100.0	52.8 (0.77)	3.7 (0.27)	14.7 (0.47)	15.4 (0.49)	13.4 (0.44)
Female	100.0	38.3 (0.66)	31.1 (0.56)	30.6 (0.56)	100.0	63.8 (0.62)	2.4 (0.18)	10.9 (0.39)	12.9 (0.41)	9.9 (0.38)
Age										
18–44 years	100.0	31.1 (0.79)	32.6 (0.65)	36.3 (0.67)	100.0	49.4 (0.81)	3.7 (0.26)	16.3 (0.52)	17.3 (0.50)	13.2 (0.46)
45–64 years	100.0	37.4 (0.88)	30.9 (0.75)	31.7 (0.70)	100.0	62.1 (0.82)	2.9 (0.24)	11.0 (0.47)	12.8 (0.47)	11.3 (0.48)
65–74 years	100.0	46.0 (1.22)	27.9 (1.09)	26.1 (1.05)	100.0	76.5 (0.99)	0.8 (0.21)	5.5 (0.57)	8.3 (0.69)	8.8 (0.70)
75 years and over	100.0	56.0 (1.39)	25.5 (1.24)	18.5 (1.06)	100.0	86.0 (1.02)	*0.9 (0.29)	3.6 (0.51)	4.6 (0.64)	4.9 (0.61)
Race										
One race	100.0	36.4 (0.61)	31.0 (0.47)	32.6 (0.47)	100.0	58.6 (0.57)	3.0 (0.17)	12.7 (0.33)	14.2 (0.33)	11.6 (0.31)
White	100.0	34.8 (0.67)	31.3 (0.53)	33.9 (0.53)	100.0	57.2 (0.64)	3.1 (0.19)	13.0 (0.37)	14.7 (0.38)	12.1 (0.34)
Black or African American	100.0	47.6 (1.21)	27.3 (1.01)	25.0 (0.94)	100.0	66.2 (1.04)	2.6 (0.38)	10.7 (0.72)	11.1 (0.67)	9.4 (0.66)
American Indian or Alaska Native	100.0	48.3 (4.43)	26.3 (3.60)	25.4 (3.01)	100.0	67.5 (3.42)	†	12.9 (2.16)	11.2 (1.96)	7.9 (2.29)
Asian	100.0	33.8 (1.78)	36.0 (1.66)	30.3 (1.71)	100.0	59.9 (1.91)	3.6 (0.69)	13.1 (1.14)	13.4 (1.36)	10.1 (1.07)
Native Hawaiian or Other Pacific Islander	100.0	35.3 (7.45)	*19.4 (7.38)	45.3 (8.49)	100.0	60.5 (9.66)	–	*8.1 (3.87)	*21.9 (10.35)	†
Two or more races	100.0	31.5 (3.10)	38.5 (3.44)	30.0 (2.96)	100.0	59.1 (3.19)	†	17.9 (2.71)	10.8 (1.90)	10.5 (1.97)
Black or African American, white	100.0	54.6 (10.91)	*26.0 (9.93)	19.4 (5.74)	100.0	68.0 (10.42)	–	*21.7 (9.68)	†	†
American Indian or Alaska Native, white	100.0	35.0 (4.91)	37.8 (5.97)	27.2 (5.27)	100.0	63.8 (5.69)	†	*14.5 (5.65)	*8.0 (2.80)	13.2 (3.90)
Hispanic or Latino origin and race										
Hispanic or Latino	100.0	47.5 (1.22)	27.3 (1.02)	25.2 (1.02)	100.0	69.1 (1.06)	2.0 (0.32)	9.7 (0.65)	10.5 (0.65)	8.7 (0.60)
Mexican or Mexican American	100.0	47.3 (1.57)	26.1 (1.22)	26.6 (1.41)	100.0	68.8 (1.38)	2.0 (0.41)	9.4 (0.75)	11.0 (0.86)	8.9 (0.86)
Not Hispanic or Latino	100.0	34.4 (0.64)	31.6 (0.51)	33.9 (0.51)	100.0	56.7 (0.61)	3.2 (0.19)	13.2 (0.36)	14.8 (0.36)	12.1 (0.34)
White, single race	100.0	32.1 (0.71)	32.0 (0.59)	35.9 (0.59)	100.0	54.7 (0.71)	3.3 (0.22)	13.6 (0.41)	15.6 (0.43)	12.8 (0.40)
Black or African American, single race	100.0	47.7 (1.23)	27.5 (1.03)	24.8 (0.96)	100.0	66.2 (1.06)	2.7 (0.38)	10.8 (0.74)	11.0 (0.67)	9.4 (0.67)

Values are percent distribution, with standard error shown in parentheses. Frequency of vigorous leisure-time activity refers to the number of instances of vigorous activity of at least 10 minutes' duration in a given week.

*Relative standard error > 30%.

† Relative standard error > 50%; estimate not shown.

Adapted from Pleis, Lucas, and Ward 2008.

enrolled in the HRS and found a protective effect with regard to premature mortality among the most physically active compared with the least active. These results were similar for each of the race–ethnic subgroups.

Manini and colleagues (2006), using data from the Health, Aging, and Body Composition (Health ABC Study), explored the association between total daily energy expenditure, as measured by doubly labeled water, and total mortality among older (aged 70-79) men and women. The sample included 48.3% African Americans within a total sample size of ~3100 subjects. The uniqueness of this study lay in the methods of energy expenditure assessment, which included daily energy expenditure, and the oversampling of African Americans, which permitted adequate power to test for differences when findings were compared with those for non-Hispanic white subjects. For all race–ethnic and gender groups, there was a strong association of higher levels of free-living energy expenditure with a lower risk of mortality among healthy older adults. Using data from the Puerto Rico Heart Health Program, Crespo and colleagues (2002) demonstrated a positive relationship between increased levels of physical activity and reductions in total mortality in this Latino/Hispanic population. And among Japanese men living on the island of Oahu, Hawaii, Hakim and her colleagues found that those who engaged in regular daily walking had a lower risk of premature mortality compared to men who did not walk or whose walking was irregular (Hakim et al. 1998).

All of these studies showed no apparent racial–ethnic differences when examining the effects of physical activity on all-cause mortality.

Cardiovascular Health

Few studies conducted in the United States have used adequate race–ethnic sample sizes or a sufficient number of clinical outcomes to adequately assess the association between physical activity and CVD outcomes including fatal and nonfatal myocardial infarction, coronary heart disease, angina pectoris, and stroke. Although recent efforts have been made by the DHHS to enroll more women and people representing diverse racial–ethnic populations, only a paucity of longitudinal studies addressing these relationships is currently available. The Women's Health Initiative Observational Study (WHI) is a prospective, racially and ethnically diverse multicenter clinical trial and observational study designed to address the major causes of illness and death in postmenopausal women (Manson et al. 2002). This observational study included 61,574 non-Hispanic white women and 5661 African American women. At the time of Manson's work, the women had been followed since the initiation of the study for a mean of 3.2 years. Physical activity was expressed in MET-hours per week, and subjects were stratified into quintiles of MET-hours per week. Comparing the top two quintiles with the lowest quintile for physical activity revealed a significant association between physical

activity and CVD outcomes for both the non-Hispanic white women and the African American women; a significant protective effect (relative risk) was seen for the highest versus the lowest quintile of activity in white women and African American women (0.56 and 0.48, respectively). In contrast, an earlier report from the Atherosclerosis Risk in Communities (ARIC) study population suggested a measureable inverse relation between activity level and CVD outcomes in white men and women but apparently no such association among African American men or women (Folsom et al. 1997). The authors interpreted these findings as possibly due to an inadequate sample of African Americans who reported engaging in vigorous levels of physical activity (5% of the African American men vs. 15% of the white men).

McGruder and colleagues (2004), using an aggregate of NHIS data for the years 1999, 2000, and 2001, investigated CVD risk levels among 2265 stroke survivors with a racial–ethnic breakdown consisting of 10% Latino/Hispanics, 20% African Americans, and 70% non-Hispanic whites. Their findings clearly identified Latinos and African Americans as more likely than whites to report having had a stroke. In addition, significant disparities in CVD risk levels were apparent in comparisons across the three race–ethnic groups, with whites consistently having a "better" CVD risk profile. Inadequate levels of physical activity (defined as less than 30 min of moderate to vigorous physical activity less than five days per week) were strongly associated with stroke among all race–ethnic groups. However, when the association of CVD risk factors with the outcome of stroke was examined, inadequate physical activity had one of the strongest associations with stroke outcome in African American and Latino stroke survivors compared with non-Hispanic whites (figure 15.2).

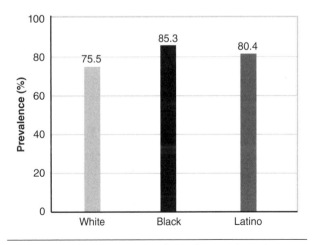

Figure 15.2 The prevalence of insufficient physical activity among U.S. adults reporting a previous stroke, by race/ethnicity, 2000-2001, National Health Interview Survey.

Data from Altman and Bernstein 2008.

Cancer

McTiernan and colleagues (2003) looked at the Women's Health Initiative cohort study population and determined the association between increased levels of physical activity and reduced risk of breast cancer among postmenopausal women. They documented 1780 newly diagnosed cases of breast cancer over a mean follow-up of 4.7 years. Compared with less active women, women who engaged in regular strenuous physical activity at age 35 years had a 14% decreased risk of breast cancer. Similar but attenuated findings were observed for strenuous physical activity at ages 18 years and 50 years. Although there were too few cases to examine racial–ethnic subgroups separately, the investigators attempted to do so with African American women (the largest subgroup apart from non-Hispanic whites) and found the results to be similar to those for the majority white women. Thus, physical activity in this study appeared to be protective against breast cancer across race–ethnic groups.

The Women's Contraceptive and Reproductive Experiences Study (WCRES), a population-based case–control study examining predictors of risk for invasive breast cancer among white and African American women (Bernstein et al. 2005), showed that the lifetime risk of breast cancer was reduced with increasing physical activity levels when these levels were averaged over a woman's lifetime (from age 10 years to the reference age). An annual average of at least 1.3 h of exercise activity per week (or 6.7 MET-hours per week) from age 10 years onward was associated with nearly a 20% reduction in breast cancer risk. Notably in this study, higher levels of lifetime exercise activity were associated with lower breast cancer risk among African American women as well (Bernstein et al. 2005). Similar findings documenting the role of physical activity in reducing the risk of breast cancer among African American women were provided by Adams-Campbell and colleagues (2001) in their study of strenuous physical activity and breast cancer risk among women who were part of the Black Women's Health Study. The authors found that the likelihood for the development of breast cancer was reduced significantly in women who engaged in ~7 h per week of vigorous activity compared to those engaging in vigorous activity less than 1 h per week. Results were specific to the age at which the women were exposed to strenuous physical activity. Women who engaged in strenuous activity at age 21 had a reduced odds for breast cancer overall and for premenopausal breast cancer; women who performed these levels of activity at age 30 had only a reduced odds for breast cancer overall; and women engaging in such activity at age 40 were protected from postmenopausal breast cancer. Similar findings came from the New Mexico Women's Health Study, in which Gilliland and coworkers (2001) showed that both pre- and postmenopausal Latino/Hispanic women had decreased risk for breast cancer with increasing levels of activity while physical activity was protective among post-menopausal non-Hispanic white women only. Slattery and colleagues (2007) documented, among non-Hispanic white,

Latino/Hispanic, and American Indian women residing in the southwestern United States, that physical activity is important in reducing risk of breast cancer among women from all three race–ethnic groups.

Yang and colleagues (2003) explored data from the Los Angeles County Cancer Surveillance Program to examine the relationship between lifetime recreational physical activity and breast cancer among Asian American women. The investigators were able to show that increasing years and levels (average MET-hours per week) of lifetime recreational activity, compared with no lifetime recreational physical activity, were significantly associated with a reduced risk of breast cancer after adjustment for demographic factors, migration history, and menstrual and reproductive factors.

In addition to studies showing the strong association of increased levels of physical activity with prevention of breast cancer are studies that have pointed to the relationship between physical activity and the prevention of other cancers such as colon (Wolin et al. 2009) and prostate (Orsini et al. 2009) cancers. However, very few of these studies have included women and men representing diverse racial–ethnic populations. Drawing from the National Institutes of Health (NIH)-AARP Diet and Health Study, Moore and colleagues (2009), after following 160,006 white and 3671 black men ages 51 to 72 years for seven years, identified 9624 white men and 371 black men who developed prostate cancer. Among white men, physical activity had no association with prostate cancer regardless of age period or activity intensity. Among black men, engaging in >4 h of moderate- to vigorous-intensity physical activity versus infrequent activity during ages 19 years to 29 years was related to a 35% lower risk of prostate cancer (relative risk, 0.65; 95% confidence interval [CI]: 0.43-0.99). Similar findings among Mexican American men were obtained by Strom and coauthors (2008). Although a lifetime history of moderate to vigorous physical activity was shown to protect against prostate cancer, this was true only for occupationally related physical activity and not for recreational activity levels.

Although few studies as yet have examined the benefits of physical activity in relation to cancers such as colon and prostate cancer, the benefits among people representing more diverse racial–ethnic populations appear to be similar to those documented among non-Hispanic white populations.

Overweight and Obesity

Sternfeld and colleagues (2004), examining three years of follow-up data from a multiethnic sample of postmenopausal women (non-Hispanic whites, African Americans, Latinas, and Asian Americans), found that in their longitudinal analysis, higher levels of sports or exercise and daily routine physical activity were independently associated with lower weight and waist circumference among all race–ethnic subgroups. Women who engaged in more frequent or more intense levels of activity in both these active living domains also tended to have a lower risk of substantial weight gain. Furthermore, when the authors investigated within-woman changes in weight and waist circumference in relation to a categorical change in activity, women who increased their activity in either or both domains gained the least weight while those who decreased their activity gained the most (Sternberg et al. 2004). Slattery and colleagues (2006) documented among Hispanic and non-Hispanic women that increased levels of physical activity were associated with decreased levels of overweight and obesity. The majority of both Hispanic and non-Hispanic white women did not perform 30 min of activity five days or more per week, although a greater percentage of Hispanic women met that goal if they reported higher levels of language acculturation. However, the types and intensities of activities performed by Hispanic and non-Hispanic women differed; Hispanic women reported more housework, dependent caregiving, dancing, and work activity. In another study, Hornbuckle and colleagues (2005) recruited 75 African American women to investigate measured walking behavior through pedometry in relation to body weight, waist-to-hip ratio (WHR), body composition assessment using the BodPod, and dietary intake. The findings confirmed results that have been seen among non-Hispanic white women. The African American women who accumulated more steps per day had lower body mass index (BMI) values, body fat percentages, waist and hip circumferences, and WHR. The authors found statistically significant differences ($P < 0.05$) for all these variables except WHR when comparing the least-active and most active groups (Hornbuckle, Basset, and Thompson 2005).

Metabolic Syndrome

Historically, metabolic syndrome has been defined by international and national scientific organizations as a cluster of metabolic indicators that include at least three of the following: glucose level at least 110 mg/dl (6.1 mmol/L); high blood pressure (BP) (systolic BP $\geq$130 or diastolic BP $\geq$85 mmHg); waist circumference greater than 88 cm (women) or greater than 102 cm (men); triglyceride level at least 150 mg/dl (1.70 mmol/L); and high-density lipoprotein (HDL) cholesterol level less than 50 mg/dl (1.30 mmol/L) in women or less than 40 mg/dl (1.04 mmol/L) in men (Adult Treatment Panel III 2001). Although few epidemiologic studies to date have looked at the association of physical activity, fitness, or exercise with metabolic syndrome among racially and ethnically diverse populations exclusively, a number of recent studies have been designed to examine multiethnic populations and to gather information about physical activity and metabolic syndrome and other pertinent risk factors for chronic diseases. Carnethon and her colleagues, using 15-year follow-up data from the CARDIA study, explored the relationship between measured cardiorespiratory fitness and the prevalence of metabolic syndrome among ~4500 men and women; approximately 47% of the participants were African American, and the remaining were non-Hispanic white (Carnethon et al. 2003). The investigators observed that cardiorespiratory fitness

in young men and women, estimated by the duration of a maximal treadmill exercise test, was inversely associated with the risk of developing metabolic syndrome in middle age. In addition, they documented an inverse association of fitness with the presence of hypertension, type 2 diabetes, and hypercholesterolemia at follow-up.

The Diabetes Prevention Program study was a randomized clinical trial testing the effectiveness of the drug metformin, compared with a lifestyle program of healthy eating and regular physical activity, in preventing type 2 diabetes among glucose-intolerant adults (Diabetes Prevention Program Research Group 1999) The study afforded investigators the opportunity to explore the role of these two interventions in preventing metabolic syndrome among a multiethnic population of non-Hispanic white, Latino/Hispanic, African American, and American Indian men and women (Orchard et al. 2005). At the time the trial was halted, the investigators identified through use of life-table analyses (log-rank test) that incidence of the metabolic syndrome was reduced by 41% in the lifestyle group ($P < 0.001$) and by 17% in the metformin group ($P < 0.03$) compared with placebo (Orchard et al. 2005). The three-year cumulative incidences of metabolic syndrome were 51%, 45%, and 34% in the placebo, metformin, and lifestyle groups, respectively. There were no significant differences by race–ethnicity across these groups (Orchard et al. 2005).

Although the role of regular physical activity appears to be clearly associated with a reduced risk for metabolic syndrome among men and women across all major race–ethnic groups, most studies discussed here focused on occupational, leisure, and recreational physical activity and did not examine the complete spectrum of activity that includes inactivity and sedentary behavior (e.g., sitting at a work station, commuting in a car, watching TV, playing video or computer games). Sisson and her colleagues, examining an aggregate sample of the National Nutrition and Health Examination Surveys (NHANES), sought to investigate the association of leisure-time sedentary behavior (LTSB) with the prevalence of metabolic syndrome among men and women 20 years and older (Sisson et al. 2009). The data were for a total of 1868 men and 1688 women who were a representative sample of the U.S. population, consisting of respondents representing European Americans, African Americans, and Mexican Americans and another race–ethnic group including all participants not falling into one of these three groups. With race-ethnicity controlled for, men who had higher levels of LTSB were at the greatest odds of having metabolic syndrome regardless of their physical activity status (meeting or not meeting physical activity guidelines). Among women, again with race-ethnicity controlled for, women who did not meet physical activity guidelines and who also had high levels of LTSB were at the greatest odds of having metabolic syndrome; women who met physical activity guidelines even with high levels LTSB apparently were protected from the syndrome (Sisson et al. 2009). In light of the disparate findings for men and women, the authors concluded, "The reason for the discrepancies between genders pertaining to LTSB and metabolic syndrome stratified by physical activity level and LTSB and individual CVD risk factors is not clearly understood. We hypothesize that it could be due to subtle differences in daily patterns of behavior" (Sisson et al. 2009, p. 533).

Type 2 Diabetes

Three large cohort studies in the United States that included only women (Hu et al. 2003, 2001; Weinstein et al. 2004) all demonstrated an association between increased levels of physical activity and a lower risk of type 2 diabetes. However, in a subsequent study carried out by Hsia and colleagues, this association was observed only among non-Hispanic white women and not among African American, Hispanic, or Asian women (Hsia et al. 2005).

Examining the 20-year follow-up data from the CARDIA study, Carnethon and coworkers recently found, among both non-Hispanic white and African American men and women, that participants who developed diabetes over 20 years had experienced significantly larger declines in relative fitness during the 20 years compared to those who did not. Thus the authors concluded, "Low fitness is significantly associated with diabetes incidence and explained in large part by the relationship between fitness and BMI" (Carnethon et al. 2009, p. 1284). Similar findings were recently published by the Diabetes Prevention Program (DPP) (Diabetes Prevention Program Research Group 2009). Reporting on the 10-year follow-up of participants in the DPP study (those randomized to the drug metformin and to the intensive lifestyle intervention [i.e., physical activity programming/counseling, dietary counseling, behavioral weight management strategies]), the investigators revealed that diabetes incidence in the 10 years since the randomization was reduced by 34% (24-42%) in the lifestyle group and 18% (7-28%) in the metformin group compared with placebo (Diabetes Prevention Project Research Group 2009). These results were consistent across genders and the two race–ethnic groups. The authors concluded, "During follow-up after the DPP, incidences in the former placebo and metformin groups fell to equal those in the former lifestyle group, but the cumulative incidence of diabetes remained lowest in the lifestyle group. Prevention or delay of diabetes with lifestyle intervention or metformin can persist for at least 10 years." (Diabetes Prevention Project Research Group 2009, p. 1677).

Summary

Across all studies reviewed here, results indicate that physical activity is related to a number of chronic disease outcomes among diverse racial–ethnic populations. The direction of these associations is similar among all racial–ethnic groups, with physical activity providing a protective effect. Across studies, findings suggest that no minimum threshold of effect exists, especially among low-active and inactive people (i.e., the majority of U.S. adults). In other words, some activity is better than none.

Physical Activity and Disability

Disability traditionally has denoted limitations in ability to perform life activities because of an impairment, including activities of daily living (ADL) and instrumental activities of daily living (IADL) (LaPlante 1991). For example, disability has been characterized by deleterious anatomical or structural changes or the loss of mental or physiological function as a result of active disease, residual losses from formerly active disease, or congenital losses or injury not associated with active disease (LaPlante 1991). The Americans with Disabilities Act (ADA) of 1991 defines someone with a disability as either a person with a physical or mental impairment that substantially limits one or more of the major life activities, or a person with a medical record of such an impairment, or a person regarded as having such an impairment (Public Law 101-336). This definition has been more clearly specified through the recent decisions of the Supreme Court, according to which a **person with a disability** is defined as "someone who struggles to do basic tasks that are 'central to daily life,' not the special tasks that go with a particular job" (National Council on Disability 2002).

Definitions used for surveillance and assessment of disability are more clearly understood if they are linked to a conceptual framework of the consequences of disease and injury. The **International Classification of Functioning, Disability, and Health (ICF)** is such a conceptual framework (World Health Organization [WHO] 2001). In the ICF, the consequences of disease and injury are defined in two parts. Part 1, Functioning and Disability, consists of the Body component, including body functions and structures, and the Activities and Participation component. Part 2, Contextual Factors, consists of the components Environmental Factors and Personal Factors. Each component in Part 1 and Part 2 can be expressed in both positive and negative terms. Within this system, *disability* is an umbrella term for impairments, **activity limitations**, or participation restrictions (Centers for Disease Control and Prevention [CDC] 2001).

Magnitude of the Problem

Using the NHIS findings, the National Center for Health Statistics of the CDC reported that during 2001-2005, almost 30% of the noninstitutionalized adult (18 years and older) U.S. population (approximately 62 million people) had basic actions difficulty, as indicated by reporting of at least some difficulty with basic movement or sensory, cognitive, or emotional difficulties (Altman and Bernstein 2008). More than one-fifth of the noninstitutionalized adult population reported difficulty with basic movement actions such as walking, bending, reaching overhead, or using their fingers to grasp something. About 13% of the adult population reported vision or hearing difficulties (hearing is measured without the use of hearing aids). Only

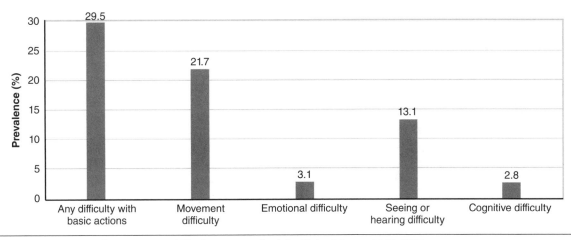

Figure 15.3 Prevalence of basic actions difficulty among all adults, United States, 2001-2005.
Reprinted from Altman and Bernstein 2008.

3% of the population reported emotional difficulties, and 3% reported cognitive difficulties (figure 15.3).

Work limitation was the most commonly reported complex activity limitation (12% of adults), followed by social limitation (7%) and self-care limitation (4%) (figure 15.4). Adults under 65 years of age made up 64% of those with complex activity limitation and 67% of those having difficulty with basic actions (figure 15.5). More than one-half of noninstitutionalized adults with self-care limitations were aged 65 years and over (52%), and approximately one-half of adults with emotional difficulties were under 45 years of age (figures 15.6 and 15.7). Adults without disabilities were more than twice as likely to have a college degree as adults with complex activity limitation and 70% more likely to have a college degree than those with basic actions difficulty (figure 15.8).

Almost one-third of adults with complex activity limitation and 30% of adults with basic actions difficulty were obese (on the basis of self-reported height and weight) during the 2001-2005 period, compared with 19% of adults with no

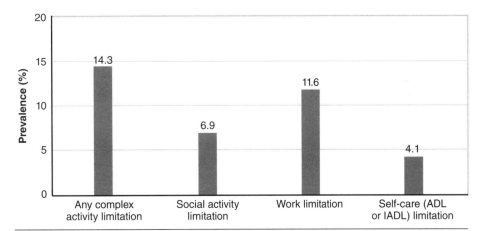

Figure 15.4 Prevalence of complex activity limitation among all adults: United States, 2001-2005.
Reprinted from Altman and Bernstein 2008.

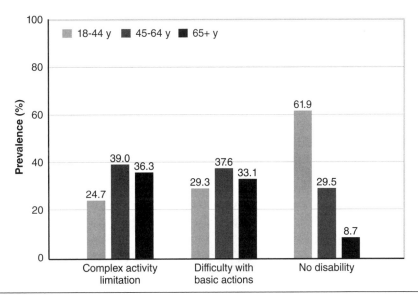

Figure 15.5 Age distribution among adults with and without a disability: United States, 2001-2005.
Reprinted from Altman and Bernstein 2008.

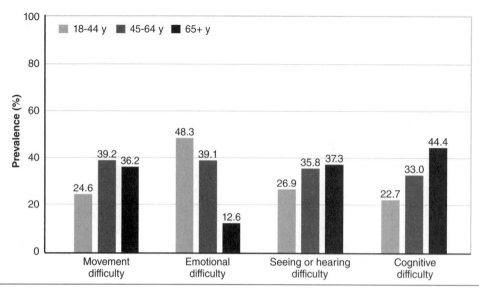

Figure 15.6 Age distribution among adults with basic actions difficulty, by type of difficulty: United States, 2001-2005.
Reprinted from Altman and Bernstein 2008.

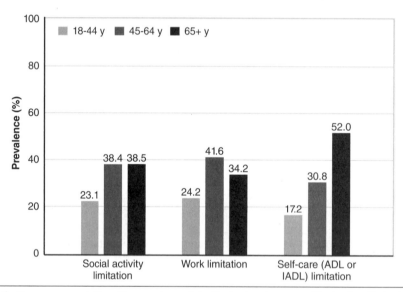

Figure 15.7 Age distribution among adults with complex activity limitation, by type of limitation: United States, 2001-2005.
Reprinted from Altman and Bernstein 2008.

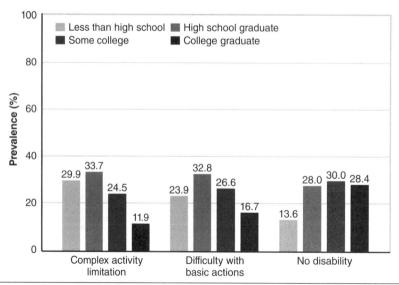

Figure 15.8 Educational attainment distribution among persons with and without disabilities: United States, 2001-2005.
Reprinted from Altman and Bernstein 2008.

reported disability. About 40% of adults aged 18 to 44 years with either complex activity limitation or basic actions difficulty reported currently smoking, compared with 22% of nondisabled adults in this age group (Altman and Bernstein 2008). Only 15% of adults with complex activity limitation reported engaging in regular physical activity, compared with 21% of adults with basic actions difficulties and 35% of adults with no disability (figure 15.9). Among adults 18 to 64 years of age, 19% of those with no disability or with a basic actions difficulty, as well as 17% of those with a complex activity limitation, were uninsured at a point in time (Altman and Bernstein 2008).

The racial and ethnic distribution in the population with disabilities differs from that in the population without disabilities (figure 15.10). Among those without disabilities, 70% were white, compared with adults who had complex activity limitation (76% white) and adults who had basic actions difficulty (77% white). The proportion of the population who were African American/black was similar for those with no disability and for those with basic actions difficulty (11%). However, 13% of those with complex activity limitation were African American/black. The population with complex activity limitation included far fewer people of Latino/Hispanic origin (7.8% compared with 13.2% without disabilities) or Asian American adults (approximately 1% compared with 2.6% among nondisabled people). The prevalence of basic actions difficulty was similar across all race–ethnic groups.

Among adults aged 18 to 64 years, employment was substantially lower among those with basic actions difficulty (42% reported working for pay in the past week) compared with adults with no disability (75% reported working during the past week). One-half of adults with complex activity limitation and almost 40% of those with basic actions difficulty reported family income below 200% of the federal poverty threshold, compared with only about one-quarter of nondisabled adults (Altman and Bernstein 2008). About one-half of adults with a complex activity limitation assessed their overall health as fair or poor, as did about one-third of people with basic actions difficulty but only 3% of adults with no disability. Adults were more likely to report fair or poor health status if they had cognitive difficulty (64%) or self-care limitations (65%) than were adults with other types of basic actions difficulty or complex activity limitation (figures 15.11 and 15.12).

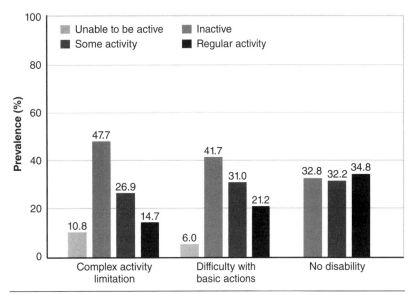

Figure 15.9 Leisure-time physical activity distribution among adults with and without disabilities: United States, 2001-2005.

Reprinted from Altman and Bernstein 2008.

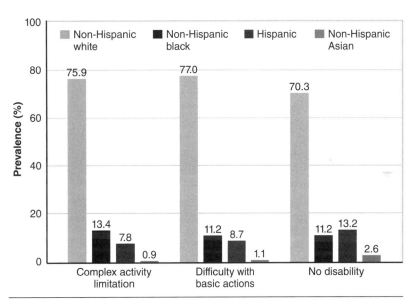

Figure 15.10 Race and ethnicity distribution among adults with and without a disability: United States, 2001-2005.

Reprinted from Altman and Bernstein 2008.

According to results from the more recent 2008 NHIS (Pleis, Lucas, and Ward 2009), 14% of noninstitutionalized U.S. adults (18 years and older), or about 33 million people, reported having difficulty with physical functioning, where functioning included the ability to walk a quarter of a mile; climb 10 steps without resting; stand for 2 h; sit for 2 h; stoop, bend, or kneel; reach over the head; use the fingers to grasp or handle small objects; lift or carry 10 lb; or push or pull large objects.

Using data from the Survey of Income and Program Participation (SIPP) conducted by the Bureau of the Census, the number of persons reported with self-identified disabilities as 21.8% of the population, or more than 47 million noninstitutionalized adults over the age of 18 years who lived in the United States (CDC 2009). On the basis of these survey results, the proportion of people reporting a disability increased with age (18-44 years, 11.0%; 45-64 years, 23.9%; and >65 years, 51.8%) and was significantly higher among women (24.4%; CI: 23.7-25.1) compared with men (19.1%; CI: 18.5-19.7) overall and in all age groups.

A total of 94% of SIPP participants reporting a disability also reported a cause. Arthritis or rheumatism was the most common cause of disability overall (19.0%; estimated population affected = 8.6 million) and for women (24.3%). Back or spine problems were the second most common cause of disability overall (16.8%, estimated population affected = 7.6 million) and the most common cause for men (16.9%). Heart trouble was the third most common cause of disability overall (6.6%, estimated population affected = 3.0 million) and for both sexes (8.4% men, 5.4% women) (table 15.2).

Physical Activity and Disabling Conditions

A consistent finding across national surveys is that the most prevalent chronic conditions and impairments causing disability include orthopedic impairments, arthritis, heart disease, hypertension, visual impairments, diabetes, mental disorders, asthma, intervertebral disc disorders, and nervous disorders. In addition, the proportion of people reporting a disability due to chronic health conditions and impairments appears to have been increasing since the early 1980s (LaPlante and Carlson 1996; CDC 2009). Finally, a disproportionate number of persons above the age of 65 report having a disability (CDC 2009).

Thus trying to understand and describe the patterns of regular physical activity, sport participation, and active recreation among subgroups of the population who report having a disability assumes growing importance. Little information is available on the extent to which a reported disability is a consequence of a chronic condition per se, or self-imposed physical inactivity, or a combination the two. Examining the patterns of regular physical activity among persons with disabilities not only provides some insight into this issue but also helps define the role of physical activity in maintaining function and preventing the progression of the primary

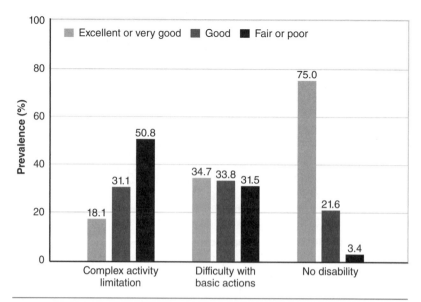

Figure 15.11 Respondent-assessed health status distribution among adults with and without a disability: United States, 2001-2005.

Reprinted from Altman and Bernstein 2008.

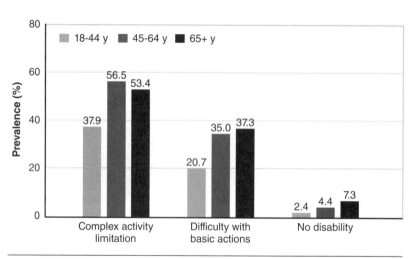

Figure 15.12 Respondent-assessed fair or poor health status among adults with and without a disability, by age: United States, 2001-2005.

Reprinted from Altman and Bernstein 2008.

disabling condition itself, preventing complications of disabilities associated with physical inactivity, and preventing the compounding of disability.

In general, people with disabilities are less active and have a lower work capacity than people without disabilities (Altman and Bernstein 2008; CDC 2009). Figure 15.9 illustrates that Americans who have a disability are less physically active than people without disability when compared on each of the major 2010 Healthy People objectives for the nation established by the U.S. Department of Health and Human Services. An inactive lifestyle compounds the effects of the disability itself and makes this a major public health issue. Poor stamina, reduced muscle strength, and limited flexibility

Table 15.2 Main Cause of Disability Among U.S. Adults 18 Years and Older With Self-Reported Disabilities

Condition	All persons Estimated population†	%	(95% CI)	Men Estimated population	%	(95% CI)	Women Estimated population	%	(95% CI)
Arthritis or rheumatism	8552	19.0	(18.0-20.0)	2154	11.5	(10.3-12.7)	6398	24.3	(22.9-25.7)
Back or spine problems	7589	16.8	(15.9-17.7)	3158	16.9	(15.5-18.3)	4431	16.8	(15.6-18.0)
Heart trouble	2988	6.6	(6.0-7.2)	1570	8.4	(7.3-9.5)	1418	5.4	(4.7-6.1)
Lung or respiratory problem	2224	4.9	(4.4-5.4)	925	4.9	(4.1-5.7)	1299	4.9	(4.2-5.6)
Mental or emotional problem	2203	4.9	(4.4-5.4)	982	5.2	(4.3-6.1)	1222	4.6	(3.9-5.3)
Diabetes	2012	4.5	(4.0-5.0)	907	4.8	(4.0-5.6)	1106	4.2	(3.5-4.9)
Deafness or hearing problem	1908	4.2	(3.7-4.7)	1272	6.8	(5.8-7.8)	635	2.4	(1.9-2.9)
Stiffness or deformity of limbs or extremities	1627	3.6	(3.1-4.1)	664	3.6	(2.9-4.3)	963	3.7	(3.1-4.3)
Blindness or vision problem	1460	3.2	(2.8-3.6)	722	3.9	(3.2-4.6)	738	2.8	(2.3-3.3)
Stroke	1076	2.4	(2.0-2.8)	574	3.1	(2.4-3.8)	503	1.9	(1.5-2.3)
Cancer	1007	2.2	(1.8-2.6)	449	2.4	(1.8-3.0)	558	2.1	(1.6-2.6)
Broken bone or fracture	969	2.1	(1.7-2.5)	358	1.9	(1.4-2.4)	610	2.3	(1.8-2.8)
High blood pressure	857	1.9	(1.6-2.2)	299	1.6	(1.1-2.1)	558	2.1	(1.6-2.6)
Mental retardation	671	1.5	(1.2-1.8)	327	1.7	(1.2-2.2)	344	1.3	(0.9-1.7)
Senility, dementia, or Alzheimer's disease	546	1.2	(0.9-1.5)	195**	1.0	(0.6-1.4)	350	1.3	(0.9-1.7)
Head or spinal cord injury	516	1.1	(0.8-1.4)	287	1.5	(1.0-2.0)	229	0.9	(0.6-1.2)
Learning disability	492	1.1	(0.8-1.4)	298	1.6	(1.1-2.1)	195**	0.7	(0.4-1.0)
Kidney problems	411	0.9	(0.7-1.1)	221	1.2	(0.8-1.6)	190**	0.7	(0.4-1.0)
Stomach or digestive problems	358	0.8	(0.6-1.0)	138**	0.7	(0.4-1.0)	220	0.8	(0.5-1.1)
Paralysis of any kind	257	0.6	(0.4-0.8)	128**	0.7	(0.4-1.0)	129**	0.5	(0.3-0.7)
Epilepsy	256	0.6	(0.4-0.8)	107**	0.6	(0.3-0.9)	149**	0.6	(0.4-0.8)
Hernia or rupture	229	0.5	(0.3-0.7)	109**	0.6	(0.3-0.9)	120**	0.5	(0.3-0.7)
Cerebral palsy	223	0.5	(0.3-0.7)	145**	0.8	(0.5-1.1)	78**	0.3	(0.1-0.5)
Missing limbs or extremities	209	0.5	(0.3-0.7)	159**	0.8	(0.4-1.2)	50**	0.2	(0.1-0.3)
Alcohol or drug problem	201	0.4	(0.2-0.6)	148**	0.8	(0.5-1.1)	53**	0.2	(0.1-0.3)
Tumor, cyst, or growth	123**	0.3	(0.2-0.4)	37**	0.2	(0.0-0.4)	86**	0.3	(0.1-0.5)
Thyroid problems	110**	0.2	(0.1-0.3)	26**	0.1	(0.0-0.2)	84**	0.3	(0.1-0.5)
AIDS or AIDS-related condition	90**	0.2	(0.1-0.3)	45**	0.2	(0.0-0.4)	45**	0.2	(0.1-0.3)
Speech disorder	72**	0.2	(0.1-0.3)	28**	0.1	(0.0-0.2)	44**	0.2	(0.1-0.3)
Other	5830	12.9	(12.1-13.7)	2,268	12.1	(10.8-13.4)	3,562	13.5	(12.4-14.6)
Total*	45,070	100.0		18,701	100.0		26,369	100.0	

* Based on responses from an estimated 45.1 million persons (94% of total) reporting a disability (i.e., difficulty with activities of daily living, instrumental activities of daily living, specific functional limitations [except vision, hearing, or speech], limitation in ability to do housework or work at a job or business) who also reported the main cause of their disability.

† Weighted numbers in 1,000s.

§ Participants reporting disability were asked: "Which condition or conditions cause these difficulties?" and shown this list of conditions. Those who chose more than one condition were asked to identify the main cause of their disability.

CI = Confidence interval.

** Weighted estimates less than 200,000 are based on a small sample size, are likely unreliable, and should be interpreted with caution (4).

Reprinted from Centers of Disease Control 2005.

restrict functional ability and therefore personal independence. This loss of autonomy through inactivity amplifies its importance; but above all else, inactivity deserves attention because it may not be inevitable and may well be, in part, reversible.

The long-term effects of inactivity among people with disabilities should be a legitimate concern for the public health community. Improvements in medical care, assistive technology, and the removal of social and environmental barriers for persons with disabilities have brought the prospect of a longer, more satisfying and productive life for those with chronic disabling conditions. Since an inactive lifestyle increases the risk of CHD, high blood pressure, thrombosis, osteoporosis, obesity, and type 2 diabetes mellitus among the general population and persons with disabilities are often limited in the types and frequency of daily lifestyle activities, the importance of regular physical activity among persons with disabilities may be even more critical to their health and well-being than for persons without disabilities. Persuading people with a disability to adopt a more active lifestyle poses a major challenge, including the need to raise expectations of the people themselves, their caregivers, and the professional groups that support them.

Many people because of their impairment expend more energy participating in normal ADLs. The extra metabolic cost of performing physical tasks may arise because of reduced muscle mass, because of inefficient locomotion and abnormal posture attributable to paralysis, or because of high ventilatory effort due to respiratory impairment. For example, a person with an above-the-knee amputation uses about 50% more energy than a person without this impairment to walk at an average pace (Davis 1993). Although there have been substantial attempts, summarized in current reviews (Physical Activity Guidelines Advisory Committee 2008; Heath and Fentem1997), to document fitness levels among people with disabilities, very little information exists regarding their physical activity levels and patterns. Dearwater and colleagues (1986) recognized the absence of such information and attempted to document the activity levels of people at what they considered the lowest level of the physical activity spectrum, that of patients with spinal cord injury (SCI). Recognizing the difficulty of using conventional physical activity questionnaires, the investigators employed physical activity movement counters to document the physical activity patterns of persons with paraplegia and quadriplegia. In comparisons of college students, blue-collar men, and older women to persons with SCI, the mean counts per hour were 126.7, 33.2, 32.3, and 24.2 (SCI, wrist), and 4.0 (SCI, ankle), respectively. No subsequent studies among people with disabilities have been conducted using this assessment methodology. In addition, the values obtained from these movement measures may not accurately reflect actual energy expenditure. Godin and colleagues (1986) used a questionnaire to assess the physical activity levels of 62 adults with a lower limb disability and found the cause of disability to be a strong predictor of physical activity. Other investigators have attempted to document

the physical activity or exercise behavior of persons with SCI (Noreau et al. 1993), multiple sclerosis (Ponichtera-Mulcare 1993), mental retardation (Rimmer et al. 1999; Rimmer et al. 2004), and arthritis (Minor and Hewett 1995); each of these studies has demonstrated a lower participation rate in physical activity in people with the disability compared to those without. Unfortunately, few studies among people with disabilities have used standardized, valid, and reliable measures to assess physical activity, thus leaving little room for comparison with persons without disabilities.

Historically, Canada and the United States have collected, at the national level, self-reported information about the physical activity and recreational patterns of persons with disabilities. The earliest data from Canada were collected in 1981 as part of the Canada Fitness Survey (Dowler and Jordan-Simpson 1990). The prevalence of people with disabilities in this survey was 13.7%. Respondents were asked about selected leisure-time physical activities. Based on their having participated at least once in the past year, 58% reported walking, 29% gardening, 24% bicycling, 22% home exercises, 22% swimming, 9% dancing, 9% jogging, 8% skating, 9% individual sports, and 8% team sports. The nature and extent of the disability were not explored in any detail. In a subsequent survey, the Canadian Health and Activity Limitations Survey (HALS), 65% of respondents with a disability did not report any physical activities such as walking, swimming, bicycling, or jogging (Hamilton 1989; Dowler and Jordan-Simpson 1990) on a regular basis, that is, at least once per week. Thirty-five percent of people with disabilities reported that they would like to have participated more in walking, swimming, bicycling, or jogging but were prevented by their condition. In the United States, it is estimated from the results of the NHIS that over 30% of persons with disabilities report not doing any leisure-time physical activity compared to 22% of persons without a disability. Twenty-seven percent of persons with a disability compared to 37% of people without a disability engaged in regular moderate physical activity, while 9.6% and 14% of people with and without a disability, respectively, engaged in regular intense or vigorous physical activity (Altman and Bernstein 2008; CDC 2009). These differences in activity patterns between persons with and without disabilities are often confounded by age, SES, and health status, suggesting several potentially effective physical activity intervention points for people with disabilities.

Inactivity and Aging

As mentioned in the previous section, older adults are more likely to experience a disability than younger adults (LaPlante and Carlson 1996; Altman and Bernstein 2008). This is due, in part, to the greater likelihood of older adults having an existing chronic condition or disease that limits their activity (LaPlante and Carlson 1996). Additionally, as people grow older they generally become less physically active.

The reduced activity contributes to a lowering of capacity beyond that induced by a condition or disease or related to age. A negative spiral of deterioration is established, leading to loss of autonomy and reduction in the quality of life. Cross-sectional (Heath et al. 1981; Larsson et al. 1984) and longitudinal studies (Hagberg 1987; Pollock et al. 1987; Kasch et al. 1999) of individuals who have maintained high activity levels over many years provide strong evidence that many of the expected declines in physical capacity with increasing age are not inevitable.

Several long-term studies of people who remained very active have not shown the expected deterioration in stamina with age (Pollock et al. 1987). Athletes aged 50 to 70 years had a maximum work capacity 60% higher than that of untrained middle-aged men. Physiological changes in cardiovascular function with age limit exercise capacity. Older people have lower maximal heart rates than younger people (Heath 1994; Lakatta and Levy 2003), but maximal cardiac output and maximal work rate can, in general, be preserved through increases in stroke volume, provided that health is good and activity is maintained (Hagberg 1987; Pollock et al. 1987; Lakatta and Levy 2003). Athletes who have trained to peak capacity may over the years experience a decline; but for the majority of active people, work capacity can certainly be maintained at levels well above the average (Wang et al. 2002). With good stamina, a wide range of activities, including the occasional demands of extra exertion, may be continued safely and comfortably. Some deterioration is inevitable. The number of muscle cells decreases with increasing age (Grimby et al. 1992); this is thought to be due to loss of the motor neurons. The result is that muscles become weaker and contract more slowly (Davies, Thomas, and White 1986). Regular physical activity appears to moderate this loss. In a five-year study of 70-year-olds, those engaged in moderate physical activity had greater muscle strength and therefore greater reserves of strength than their sedentary peers (Grimby et al. 1992). Reserve muscle strength is vital to independent life. To rise from the toilet or a chair, the average healthy 80-year-old woman uses maximum quadriceps strength (Young 1986; Tseng et al. 1995). If the reserve capacity is already close to such a critical threshold, an illness or other period of inactivity may place the individual below the threshold at which independent function can be resumed.

Impairment of the range of movement of joints and pain on movement are the most frequent health problems among older adults. Thirty-one percent of all people classified as having a disability have some form of arthritis or joint disorder (LaPlante 1991). Joints tend to degenerate with age (Bell and Hoshizaki 1981), and there is an average reduction in joint flexibility of 25% to 30% from young adulthood to older adulthood (Adrian 1981). This results in a decline in the ability to perform many of the normal ADLs. Inability to accomplish such tasks as dressing or climbing onto a bus or entering a vehicle seriously restricts independent life.

Long-term physical activity may reduce the risk of degenerative noninflammatory joint disease, with the resulting severe restrictions on independent life occurring in later years (Burry 1987). A sedentary occupation and low leisure activity were both shown to be associated with greater joint disability in later life (Bergström et al. 1985).

Improvements in stamina, as measured by maximum work capacity (Seals et al. 1984), have been documented in older people when they engage in regular physical activity. Greater functional strength, attributable to either better neural recruitment or to intrinsic changes in the exercised muscle cells, is common (Agre et al. 1988; Frontera et al. 1988). Improvements in flexibility resulted from physical activity programs in both older women (Raab et al. 1988) and men (Chapman, de Vries, and Swezey 1972). These improvements have been documented to some extent among the frail elderly as well, leading to the conclusion that frailty itself can possibly be prevented by instituting early remedial programs of physical activity among older adults (Fiatarone et al. 1994).

Most intervention studies involving physical activity exclude older people who have physical impairments arising from chronic and degenerative diseases, but some studies have been conducted exclusively with people in this subgroup. While the results of one study did not demonstrate any significant changes in maximal capacity after 16 weeks of intervention, there were favorable changes in many of the measured parameters, including workload, strength, blood pressure, and plasma lipids (Thompson et al. 1988). In another study of older men, which did not exclude those with disabilities, a four-month-long physical activity program led to significant favorable changes. Although the dropout rate was high, 76% of those who completed the program had one or more chronic diseases. Those who completed the program showed increases in treadmill time, abdominal strength, and hip flexibility; decreases in both resting and submaximal heart rate; and a reduction in body fat (Morey et al. 1989). There were no adverse reactions to the program in either study, and participants reported subjective improvements and were enthusiastic about continuing to be physically active (Thompson et al. 1988). Walking for most older people is equivalent to jogging in younger people in terms of relative effort. Improvements in stamina are possible with a modest walking program or some physical activity equivalent for those who cannot use their legs to get about. Walking or its equivalent is also beneficial for maintaining or improving bone density. A prospective study concluded that walking at least 1 mile three times per week reduced risk of suffering a fracture among older women by a third (Sorock et al. 1988). A program can be devised based on sitting and standing exercises that load the bones adequately when walking is impossible (Smith 1981). Swimming is also beneficial in that it maintains both range of motion and strength of a large number of joints and muscles (Suominen, Heikkinen, and Parkatti 1977) without loading damaged joint surfaces. Since swimming appears to be ineffective for maintaining bone density (Jacobson et al. 1984), some other exercise should also be performed regularly.

Physical Activity and Long-Term Health Among People With Disabilities

Prolonged physical inactivity is associated with long-term risks of disease in persons with and without a disability. To date, no studies have been conducted to determine whether the long-term benefits of physical activity seen among persons without disabilities, such as lower risks of CHD (Powell et al. 1987), osteoporosis (Chow et al. 1986), and obesity (Bouchard, Despres, and Trembley 1993), also apply to people with disabilities. It is reasonable to argue that the greater life expectancy of those with even the most severe disabilities now places them at risk from these diseases in later life. Thus it makes sense if people who have a disability seek to protect themselves from inactivity-determined conditions that may either exacerbate existing disabilities or contribute to a premature death.

Cardiovascular Health

It has been argued that, for the general population, physical inactivity is as great a risk factor for CHD as hypertension, hypercholesterolemia, or smoking (Powell et al. 1987). With greater longevity, CHD has become a significant cause of death in people who are paraplegic or who have bilateral lower limb amputations due to trauma. Physical activity appears to lower risk through its favorable effect on blood lipid levels (Wood et al. 1983), arterial blood pressure (Blair et al. 1984), blood clotting factors (Williams et al. 1980), and glucose tolerance and insulin sensitivity among people without disabilities.

A recent review (Physical Activity Guidelines Advisory Committee 2008) provided evidence that cardiorespiratory fitness can be improved among people with physical and cognitive disabilities. The review demonstrated positive cardiorespiratory fitness changes in response to increased levels of physical activity or exercise among persons with lower limb loss, multiple sclerosis, SCI, stroke, mental illness, traumatic brain injury, intellectual disability, cerebral palsy, muscular dystrophy, Alzheimer's disease, and Parkinson's disease. The reviewers outlined 21 randomized clinical trials that targeted improvements in cardiorespiratory fitness in persons with physical and cognitive disabilities. Among these studies, 18 (86%) reported significant favorable cardiorespiratory fitness outcomes. Twenty-one of an additional 25 studies that were not randomized clinical trials reported significant favorable cardiorespiratory fitness outcomes (Physical Activity Guidelines Advisory Committee 2008).

Lipid Metabolism

There is strong evidence that high concentrations of HDL in the blood are inversely related to the incidence of CHD (Castelli et al. 1986). Evidence is also strong that a positive relationship exists between levels of physical activity and plasma levels of HDL (Wood et al. 1983). Levels of HDL are generally lower among people who use manual or electric wheelchairs than among persons who do not use wheelchairs (Brenes et al. 1986). Brenes and colleagues (1986) showed this to be associated with inactivity. The authors estimated that among people with SCI, men face a 60% and women a 90% greater than average risk of suffering a myocardial infarction. Increased levels of physical activity appear to lead to higher HDL levels among people with SCI (Brenes et al. 1986). This same finding has been obtained among other people with disabilities, including those with rheumatoid arthritis (Minor 1995) and those with visual impairments (Shindo, Komagai, and Tanaka 1987). Brenes and colleagues (1986) showed that athletes who trained and competed using manual wheelchairs had higher levels of HDL and lower levels of total cholesterol than control subjects who did not participate in regular wheelchair physical activity. The levels of HDL of the wheelchair athletes were similar to those found among active people without disabilities.

The evidence presented by Physical Activity Guidelines Advisory Committee (2008) on the use of physical activity and its effects on lipid levels among persons with disabilities included just four intervention studies that reported significant reductions in total cholesterol and triglycerides. Two studies showed no differences in cholesterol reduction after an exercise intervention. Lipid outcomes targeted in these studies included triglycerides and total cholesterol. In people with physical disabilities, three of four studies showed reductions in cholesterol (SCI) and triglycerides (multiple sclerosis). In people with cognitive disability, one of two studies reported a reduction in triglycerides (mental illness). In three of the four studies, subjects had high cholesterol and triglycerides at baseline.

Hypertension

Hypertension is the most common manifestation of CVD among persons with SCI (Cowell, Squires, and Raven 1986). Physical activity has been shown to reduce arterial blood pressure in people without disabilities who have mild or moderate hypertension (Cade et al. 1984; Hagberg et al. 1983). While no reports were found regarding the effect of regular physical activity on arterial blood pressure among persons with disabilities, it seems plausible to suppose that the effect is similar. Although it seems likely that chronic physical inactivity in people with disabilities contributes to an increased risk of CHD and that increased levels of physical activity could reduce this risk, the role of multiple risk factors for CHD should be acknowledged. As with the population of people without disabilities, moderate- to vigorous-intensity physical activity is no absolute guarantee against developing CHD.

Deep Vein Thrombosis

As prolonged physical inactivity is associated with the development of lower limb deep vein thrombosis, this is an important potential complication of prolonged immobility (Housley 1988). Regular physical activity has been shown to reduce this risk and consequently that of pulmonary embolus, the more serious related complication.

Metabolic Health: Overweight and Obesity

Physical activity is important in preventing weight gain and in managing weight reduction in people who become overweight. Because persons with disabilities are often less active, their risk of gaining weight is greater. Excess body weight may itself have a disabling effect, further restricting mobility, particularly when leg muscles may be weak already. Severe obesity, that is, weight more than 30% above desirable weight for height, exacerbates the effects of other conditions and increases the risk of death before age 65 (Bouchard, Despres, and Trembley 1993). Regular physical activity can reduce weight. This has been established among people with and without a disability (Findlay et al. 1987; Leon et al. 1979).

There is evidence that physical activity or exercise can improve body composition in persons with stroke, intellectual disability, mental illness, traumatic brain injury, and a combined group of individuals with different types of physical disabilities (DHHS 2008). As to metabolic factors, evidence exists for improvements in fasting glucose and insulin sensitivity in the two disability subgroups of stroke (Ivey et al. 2007) and mental illness (Beebe et al. 2005). Three physical activity intervention studies targeted improvements in metabolic factors (e.g., fasting glucose, insulin sensitivity, fasting insulin, and insulin-like growth factor-binding protein-3) among people with stroke (Ivey et al. 2007) and schizophrenia (Wu et al. 2007), while one study reported nonsignificant findings among people with SCI (de Groot et al. 2003).

Musculoskeletal Health

Additional benefits of physical activity among persons with disabilities have been documented beyond the cardiovascular and metabolic health benefits. These include the health-related components of muscular strength, flexibility and reduced joint pain, and improved bone density and prevention of osteoporosis.

Muscular Strength

When muscle strength is decreased and the mass of functional muscle is reduced by paralysis or disease, it is beneficial to increase the strength of the remaining muscle. Indeed, it is vital that residual capacities be both strengthened and maintained. Evidence from studies with both older adults and people with disabilities demonstrate that brief contractions of the muscles, repeated at frequent intervals (Einarsson 1991), lead to an increase in the size of the muscle cells (Gaffney et al. 1981; Kristensen, Hansen, and Saltin 1980) and the

strength of the muscles used (Gehlsen, Grigsby, and Winant 1984; Nilsson, Staff, and Pruett1975). Improvements in muscle strength protect against damage to joints, ligaments, and the muscles themselves by stabilizing the joints and by minimizing the damaging effects of sudden movements and unexpected strain. Evidence indicates that resistance exercise, aerobic exercise, or a combination of the two increases muscle strength in various subgroups with physical and cognitive disabilities.

The Physical Activity Guidelines Advisory Committee Report cited 37 physical activity and exercise interventions among people with disabilities that examined improvements in muscle strength (Physical Activity Guidelines Advisory Committee 2008). Among 14 studies that employed better designs and exposure and outcome measures, investigators reported significant improvements in muscle strength in persons with cerebral palsy (Dodd et al. 2003; Andersson et al. 2003), multiple sclerosis (Petajan et al. 1996; White et al. 2004), muscular dystrophy (van der Kooi et al. 2004), SCI (Tordi et al. 2001; Nash et al. 2007), and stroke (Pang et al. 2005; Ouellette et al. 2004). Even among studies using the least-desirable designs (e.g., cross-sectional), significant improvement in strength among persons with selected disabilities was noted in 95% of trials reported (Physical Activity Guidelines Advisory Committee 2008).

Joint Pain and Flexibility

It appears that long-term regular use of a joint has a beneficial effect. Rather than wearing out joint surfaces, regular movement increases joint nutrition and lubrication, protecting the surfaces and so preventing degenerative joint disease (Ahlqvist 1985; Burry 1987). Gentle motion, by lubricating the joint, makes movement less painful, which is particularly beneficial to those with joint disease (Nordemar et al. 1981; Van Deusen 1987). Suppleness or range of joint movement becomes reduced with inactivity due to joint diseases, paralysis, or aging per se. Muscles and tendons shorten if the full range of joint movement is not regularly used. Simple daily stretching exercises help to avoid this. Habitual sitting leads to flexion contractures, which make an individual rigid. Rigidity leads to problems in changing position and makes personal hygiene and transfer from bed to chair or similar movements difficult. Walking—or stretching exercises when walking is impossible—appears helpful in avoiding joint contractures (Hardy 1986). Children with paralysis due to spina bifida who were able to walk and did so had virtually no joint contractures, while for those consistently using a wheelchair, contractures were a severe problem (Agre et al. 1988). Improvements in stamina, strength, and flexibility widen the range of activities an individual can undertake. The importance of being able to walk a bit farther, transfer into and out of a chair, or brush one's own hair cannot be overestimated. Recent evidence has accrued to suggest improvements in flexibility among individuals with Parkinson's disease (Schenkman et al. 1998), stroke (Rimmer,

Rubin, and Braddock 2000; Jeong and Kim . 2007), traumatic brain injury (Driver et al. 2004), SCI (Rodgers et al. 2001), and combined cognitive and physical disabilities (Podgorski et al. 2004).

Bone Density and Osteoporosis

There is strong evidence that bone density and bone mass are partially determined by habitual levels of physical activity among people with disabilities (Cowell, Squires, and Raven 1986) as in persons without (Chow et al. 1986). Bone is lost rapidly during bed rest or immobility. The rate of loss can be as high as 5% of mass per month on average (Schneider and McDonald 1984). Studies have shown that moderate physical activity can reverse this loss. Two factors regarding maintenance of bone emerge from studies among persons without disabilities: (1) The effect appears to be specific to the bones that are load bearing during the particular physical activity; (2) gravity and the impact of weight bearing appear to be important (Jacobson et al. 1984; Schneider and McDonald 1984). No reports were found concerning the effects of physical activity on bone density with weight-bearing physical activity among persons with disabilities, but it is reasonable to hypothesize that the effect would be the same as observed in older adults (Smith 1981). Walking appears to be an ideal form of physical activity for the purpose of maintaining bone mass. Walking provides a gravity-dependent stimulus to the bones of the back and lower limbs, and these bones are most at risk for osteoporotic fracture. According to what is known of the mechanisms (Yeh and Rodan 1984), the impact of walking with crutches, braces, or orthoses, even for brief periods, should trigger the osteogenic activity of the bone-building cells and maintain density. Maintaining bone density presents a particular problem for people who cannot stand. Paralyzed limbs are most at risk for osteoporotic fracture. Bone can become so fragile that fractures occur with little or no trauma (Cowell, Squires, and Raven 1986). These problems are not, however, insurmountable. The ingenious use of a tilt board for people with tetraplegia (quadriplegia) to gain the effects of weight bearing and gravity during strengthening exercises resulted in a significant reduction in calcium loss (Kaplan 1981). The same strengthening exercises performed without the tilt board resulted in no reduction (Kaplan 1981).

Reducing calcium loss may also decrease the incidence of kidney stones common among people with SCI (Cowell, Squires, and Raven 1986). Evidence also exists on the use of exercise for improving bone density among people with physical and cognitive disabilities. At least two studies have used physical activity interventions to improve bone density among people with a disability. One involved youth with cerebral palsy (Chad et al. 1999), and the other involved adults with stroke (Pang et al. 2005). In the cerebral palsy study, following exposure to 24 weeks of progressive large muscle activity, the investigators showed significant improvement in bone density compared to that in controls (Chad et al. 1999).

In the study among adults following a unilateral stroke who were exposed to six weeks of regular aerobic physical activity, the researchers concluded that physical activity appeared to slow the decline in bone mineral loss in the affected femoral neck (Pang et al. 2005).

Role of Physical Activity in the Prevention of Secondary Complications

Individuals with disabilities are likely to be at increased risk for a number of preventable health problems referred to as *secondary conditions*. According to *Healthy People 2020* (DHHS 2010), secondary conditions are "physical, medical, cognitive, emotional, or psychosocial consequences to which persons with disabilities are more susceptible by virtue of an underlying impairment, including adverse outcomes in health, wellness, participation and quality of life." Several secondary conditions are prominent among people with disabilities, and pain and fatigue are reported to be two of the most common secondary conditions observed in people with physical and cognitive disabilities (Iezzoni and Freedman 2008).

Regular physical activity and exercise training will never completely restore the capacity lost through damage or disease, but some improvement is possible and within the reach of many people with a disability (Nilsson, Staff, and Pruett 1975) and older adults (Seals et al. 1984). The high levels of "fitness" of participants in the Paralympics and similar competitions (Madorsky 1983; Shephard 1991)

Physical Activity and Secondary Conditions

Fatigue. A number of physical activity intervention studies among persons with disabilities have examined fatigue as an outcome. Studies in people with multiple sclerosis (Surakka et al. 2004) and muscular dystrophy (van der Kooi et al. 2007) have demonstrated decreased fatigue.

Pain. Evidence exists that among selected persons with disabilities pain can be reduced with increased levels of physical activity. Significant reductions in musculoskeletal pain among persons with SCI have been demonstrated following an endurance exercise training intervention (Ginis et al. 2003). Other studies have shown site-specific pain reduction following an aerobic and resistance training intervention with reductions in shoulder pain among persons with SCI (Nash et al. 2007).

demonstrate what can be achieved by some people with disabilities. However, even small increases in stamina, strength, and flexibility can lead to large improvements in quality of life. Increases in stamina have been achieved with a modest increase in physical activity by previously inactive older adults who have taken up walking (Frontera et al. 1988). This is equivalent to jogging in younger people in terms of the production of worthwhile improvement in maximal work capacity (deVries 1978; Suominen, Heikkinen, and Parkatti 1977). Given a suitable and interesting physical activity program, such improvements occur among people who have a variety of disabilities, including those that make walking or standing impossible (Hoskins 1975; Nilsson, Staff, and Pruett 1975). Reviews of exercise interventions with frail elderly people concluded that relatively long-lasting and highly intensive multicomponent exercise programs (most using facility-based group exercise performed three times a week for 45-60 min), but not lower extremity strength training by itself, have a positive effect on disability among community-living moderately active frail older persons (Chin et al. 2008; Daniels et al. 2008).

Quality of Life: Psychological Aspects and Mental Health

Success in overcoming physical impairments and psychological and social barriers helps in adjusting to a disability. There are also benefits to self-image. In a society that can devalue individuals for having a disability, they may devalue themselves. Physical achievement can provide an important opportunity for people with disabilities to gain more control over their bodies and lives. In doing so, they may change their perception of their disabilities and abilities. This can provide a tremendous psychological boost (Shephard 1991; Meyer 1981).

The Physical Activity Guidelines Advisory Committee (2008) reviewed more than 20 studies in which physical activity interventions among people with disabilities targeted depression. In the majority of these studies, investigators reported improvement in depression scores. Participants had multiple sclerosis (Petajan et al. 1996; Rasova et al. 2006), SCI (Hicks et al. 2003; Ginis et al. 2003), stroke (Lai et al. 2006), or Alzheimer's disease (Teri et al. 2003). Other studies have documented other mental health benefits from regular physical activity and exercise. Following an exercise intervention, improved self-esteem has been demonstrated among persons with muscular dystrophy (Wenneberg, Bernstein, and Wu 2004), traumatic brain injury (Driver et al. 2005), and intellectual disability (Heller, Hsieh, and Rimmer 2004). Other benefits have included improved quality of sleep in persons with SCI (De Mello et al. 2004) and Alzheimer's disease (McCurry et al. 2005); and people with stroke were shown to manifest enhanced interpersonal relationships (Jeong and Kim 2007).

Functional Health for Daily Living

For persons with disabilities who are not interested in sport or exercise, a physical activity plan may be based on customary activities (Gloag 1985). For example, getting out of a chair with minimal use of arms can maximize quadriceps strength training. Many such activities have been designed for older adults and can be adapted for use among persons with disabilities (Fentem 1992).

In addition to the risk of decline in physical capacities due to a gradual decline in activities, there is risk of deterioration even with relatively brief periods of bed rest (Coyle et al. 1985; Siegel, Blomqvist, and Mitchell 1970). Periods of bed rest must be as short as the impairment or intercurrent illness allows, and subsequent rehabilitation needs to be energetic. Functional health has a broad association with several performance measures related to basic ADLs and IADLs. These include walking speed, walking distance, quality of life, functional independence, and balance. Evidence from a variety of studies supports the use of exercise to improve walking speed and distance and other measures of functional health across a range of disabilities. A recent review examined a total of 74 physical activity interventions that targeted one or more measures of functional health under the categories of walking speed, walking distance, quality of life and well-being, functional independence, and balance (DHHS 2008). This review provided strong evidence for the use of exercise in improving walking speed in persons with multiple sclerosis, stroke, and intellectual disability. While sufficient evidence appears to exist for physical activity interventions among people with Parkinson's disease, Alzheimer's disease, cerebral palsy, and SCI, further evidence is lacking among persons with other types of disabilities (Physical Activity Guidelines Advisory Committee 2008).

The construct Health-Related Quality of Life (HRQOL) is a self-reported measure assessing both physical and mental health functioning (Zahran et al. 2005). A number of studies provide evidence that people with disabilities who are more physically active show improved measures of HRQOL. Such findings have been demonstrated in persons with multiple sclerosis (Schulz et al. 2004; Rampello et al. 2007), SCI (Hicks et al. 2003), stroke (Jeong and Kim 2007), muscular dystrophy (van der Kooi et al. 2007), Alzheimer's disease (Teri et al. 2003), intellectual disability (Heller, Hsieh, and Rimmer 2004), and mental illness (Skrinar et al. 2005).

With regard to balance as an outcome, a limited number of studies provide evidence that exercise interventions improve balance in people with Parkinson's disease (Hirsch et al. 2003) and stroke (Leroux 2005). The body of evidence for improved walking speed among persons with disabilities was identified in over 30 studies in the current literature that reported significant increases in walking speed, walking distance, or both among persons with a variety of mobility impairments or disabilities (Physical Activity Guidelines Advisory Committee 2008).

Physical Work Capacity

Low physical work capacity is reversible. The physiologic and biochemical improvements that occur in the muscles, in the heart, and in vascular function with regular physical activity do not depend on enormous physical effort. Rather they depend on a physical effort greater than that to which the individual is accustomed. While athletes may require work at a high intensity to improve their fitness and performance, sedentary or relatively inactive individuals require little exertion for improvement. Training occurs when the effort of an activity is somewhat greater than what the individual is accustomed to. The degree of improvement depends on the intensity, duration, and frequency of the activity (Hickson et al. 1982). In people with low exercise tolerance, improvements have resulted from rhythmic physical activity of very short duration (i.e., less than 2 min) if it is performed sufficiently frequently (Harkcom et al. 1985). Greater reserve capacity compensates for the increased energy expenditure caused by the impairment. Training can also improve the skill with which a maneuver can be performed and reduce the inefficiency of movements. This also reduces effort. Thus, physical activity training–induced improvements in reserve capacity are especially important.

Summary

Regular physical activity, sport participation, and active recreation are essential behaviors for the prevention of disease, promotion of health, maintenance of functional independence, and reduction in health disparities in special populations. This health behavior is essential for persons with and without disabilities. Population-based surveys have consistently demonstrated that people with disabilities are less likely to be physically active than persons without such limitations. However, these observations are based on relatively few surveys and on physical activity assessment methods that may not be sensitive and specific enough for persons with disabilities.

Studies clearly demonstrate that many persons, representing a variety of disabilities, can adapt to increased levels of physical activity as evidenced by alterations in various components of physical fitness. More importantly, other studies consistently provide evidence that participation in regular physical activity among persons with selected impairments and disabilities results in improved functional status and HRQOL.

Further efforts are critically needed in the area of physical activity assessment methodology for persons with disabilities. These methods need to be developed to provide survey researchers and those in public health surveillance the capacity to measure and monitor the activity patterns of people who have disabilities. This information is important not only for public health officials but also for health policy analysts, service providers, and disability advocacy groups. Further understanding of the role of physical activity in the maintenance of function and independence among persons with disabilities is needed. Finally, environmental and social barriers to physical activity among people with disabilities and the determinants of physical activity require further exploration, including the use of **assistive technology** and maximization of the intrinsic capacity of functional anatomy and physiology.

The lack of participation in recommended amounts of physical activity is a serious public health concern for all, but it is even more important for persons with disabilities, who are demonstrably at much greater risk of developing the types of serious health problems associated with a sedentary lifestyle. *Healthy People 2020* outlines current levels of physical activity and exercise for various subpopulations in the United States based on cross-sectional surveys, as well as goals for the year 2020 (DHHS 2010).

Patterns of low physical activity reported among persons with disabilities should raise serious concerns about their health and well-being, particularly as they reach the later periods of the life cycle when the effects of aging per se are exacerbated by years of inactivity and significant physical deconditioning (Rimmer 2005). Since it is known that persons with disabilities are less physically active than the general population (CDC 2008; Ginis and Hicks 2007), have poorer health status (CDC 2008), and specifically are more likely to experience chronic and secondary conditions such as obesity, pain, fatigue, and depression (CDC 2008), an integrated approach to measuring and promoting physical activity among persons with disabilities should be a high priority as part of a comprehensive approach to population health.

· BIBLIOGRAPHY ·

Adams, P.F., and C.A. Schoenborn. 2006. Health behaviors of adults: United States, 2002-04. *Vital Health Statistics* 10 (230, September): 1-140.

Adams-Campbell, L.L., L. Rosenberg, R.S. Rao, and J.R. Palmer. 2001. Strenuous physical activity and breast cancer risk in African-American women. *Journal of the National Medical Association* 93 (7-8, July): 267-275.

Adrian, M.J. 1981. Flexibility in the aging adult. In *Exercise and aging: The scientific basis,* edited by E.L. Smith and R.C. Serfass, pp. 45-57. Hillside, NJ: Enslow.

Agre, J.C., L.E. Pierce, D.M. Raab, M. McAdams, and E.L. Smith. 1988. Light resistance and stretching exercise in elderly women: Effect upon strength. *Archives of Physical Medicine and Rehabilitation* 69: 273-276.

Ahlqvist, J. 1985. On the structural and physiological basis of the influence of exercise, movement and immobilization in inflammatory joint diseases. *Annales Chirurgiae et Gynaecologiae* 198 (Suppl.): 10-18.

Altman, B., and A. Bernstein. 2008. *Disability and health in the United States, 2001–2005.* Hyattsville, MD: National Center for Health Statistics.

Andersson, C., W. Grooten, M. Hellsten, K. Kaping, and E. Mattsson. 2003. Adults with cerebral palsy: Walking ability after progressive strength training. *Developmental Medicine and Child Neurology* 45 (4): 220-228.

Aniansson, A., L. Sperling, K. Rundgren, and E. Lehnberg. 1983. Muscle function in 75-year-old men and women. A longitudinal study. *Scandinavian Journal of Rehabilitation Medicine* (Suppl. 9): 92-102.

Barcenas, C.H., A.V. Wilkinson, S.S. Strom, Y. Cao, K.C. Saunders, S. Mahabir, M.A. Hernandez-Valero, M.R. Forman, M.R. Spitz, and M.L. Bondy. 2007. Birthplace, years of residence in the United States, and obesity among Mexican-American adults. *Obesity* 15 (4): 1043-1052.

Beebe, L.H., L. Tian, N. Morris, A. Goodwin, S.S. Allen, and J. Kuldau. 2005. Effects of exercise on mental and physical health parameters of persons with schizophrenia. *Issues in Mental Health Nursing* 26 (6): 661-676.

Bell, R.D., and T.B. Hoshizaki. 1981. Relationships of age and sex with range of motion of seventeen joint actions in humans. *Canadian Journal of Applied Sport Sciences* 6: 202-206.

Bergström, G., A. Aniansson, A. Bjelle, G. Grimby, B. Lundgren-Lindquist, and A. Svanborg. 1985. Functional consequences of joint impairment at age 79. *Scandinavian Journal of Rehabilitation Medicine* 17: 183-190.

Bernstein, L., A.V. Patel, G. Ursin, J. Sullivan-Halley, M.F. Press, D. Deapen, J.A. Berlin, J.R. Daling, J.A. McDonald, S.A. Norman, et al. 2005. Lifetime recreational exercise activity and breast cancer risk among black women and white women. *Journal of the National Cancer Institute* 97 (22, November 16): 1671-1679.

Bjarnadottir, O.H., A.D. Konradsdottir, K. Reynisdottir, and E. Olafsson. 2007. Multiple sclerosis and brief moderate exercise. A randomised study. *Multiple Sclerosis* 13 (6): 776-782.

Blair, S.N., N.N. Goodyear, L.W. Gibbons, and K.H. Cooper. 1984. Physical fitness and incidence of hypertension in healthy normotensive men and women. *Journal of the American Medical Association* 252: 487-490.

Booth, F.W., S.H. Weeden, and B.S. Tseng. 1994. Effect of aging on human skeletal muscle and motor function. *Medicine and Science in Sports and Exercise* 26 (5): 556-560.

Bouchard, C., J.P. Despres, and A. Tremblay. 1993. Exercise and obesity. *Obesity Research* 1: 133-147.

Brenes, G.S., S. Dearwater, R. Shapera, R.E. LaPorte, and E. Collins. 1986. High density lipoprotein cholesterol concentrations in physically active and sedentary spinal cord injured patients. *Archives of Physical Medicine and Rehabilitation* 67: 445-450.

Breslow, L., and N. Breslow. 1993. Health practices and disability: Some evidence from Alameda County. *Preventive Medicine* 22: 86-95.

Britton, A., M. McKee, N. Black, K. McPherson, C. Sanderson, and C. Bain. 1999. Threats to applicability of randomised trials: Exclusions and selective participation. *Journal of Health Services and Research Policy* 4 (2, April): 112-121.

Burry, H.C. 1987. Sport, exercise and arthritis. *British Journal of Rheumatology* 26: 386-388.

Byrne, N.M., R.L. Weinsier, G.R. Hunter, R. Desmond, M.A. Patterson, B.E. Darnell, and P.A. Zuckerman. 2003. Influence of distribution of lean body mass on resting metabolic rate after weight loss and weight regain: Comparison of responses in white and black women. *American Journal of Clinical Nutrition* 7 (6): 1368-1373.

Cade, R., D. Mars, H. Wagemaker, C. Zauner, D. Packer, M. Privette, M. Cade, J. Peterson, and D. Hood-Lewis. 1984. Effect of aerobic exercise training on patients with systemic arterial hypertension. *American Journal of Medicine* 77: 785-790.

Carnethon, M.R., S.S. Gidding, R. Nehgme, S. Sidney, D.R. Jacobs Jr., and K. Liu. 2003. Cardiorespiratory fitness in young adulthood and the development of cardiovascular disease risk factors. *Journal of the American Medical Association* 290 (23, December 17): 3092-3100.

Carnethon, M.R., B. Sternfeld, P.J. Schreiner, D.R. Jacobs Jr., C.E. Lewis, K. Liu, and S. Sidney. 2009. Association of 20-year changes in cardiorespiratory fitness with incident type 2 diabetes: The Coronary Artery Risk Development in Young Adults (CARDIA) fitness study. *Diabetes Care* 32: 1284-1288.

Castelli, W.P., R.J. Garrison, P.W.F. Wilson, R.D. Abbott, S. Kalousdian, and W.B. Kannel. 1986. Incidence of coronary heart disease and lipoprotein cholesterol levels: The Framingham Study. *Journal of the American Medical Association* 256: 2835-2838.

Centers for Disease Control and Prevention. 1993. Prevalence of mobility and self-care disability—United States, 1990. *Morbidity and Mortality Weekly Report* 42: 760-768.

Centers for Disease Control and Prevention. 2001. Prevalence of disabilities and associated health conditions—United States, 1999. *Morbidity and Mortality Weekly Report* 50: 120-125.

Centers for Disease Control and Prevention. 2008. Prevalence of self-reported physically active adults—United States, 2007. *Morbidity and Mortality Weekly Report* 57 (48, December 5): 1297-1300.

Centers for Disease Control and Prevention. 2009. Prevalence and most common causes of disability among adults—United States, 2005. *Morbidity and Mortality Weekly Report* 58: 421-426.

Chad, K.E., D.A. Bailey, H.A. McKay, G.A. Zello, and R.E. Snyder. 1999. The effect of a weight-bearing physical activity program on bone mineral content and estimated volumetric density in children with spastic cerebral palsy. *Journal of Pediatrics* 135 (1, July): 115-117.

Chapman, E.A., H.A. de Vries, and R. Swezey. 1972. Joint stiffness: Effects of exercise on young and old men. *Journal of Gerontology* 27: 218-221.

Chin, A., M.J. Paw, J.G. van Uffelen, I. Riphagen, and W. van Mechelen. 2008. The functional effects of physical exercise training in frail older people: A systematic review. *Sports Medicine* 38 (9): 781-793.

Chow, R.K., J.E. Harrison, C.F. Brown, and V. Hajek. 1986. Physical fitness effect on bone mass in postmenopausal women. *Archives of Physical Medicine and Rehabilitation* 67: 231-234.

Compton, D.M., P.A. Eisenman, and H.L. Henderson. 1989. Exercise and fitness for persons with disabilities. *Sports Medicine* 7: 150-162.

Cowell, L.L., W.G. Squires, and P.B. Raven. 1986. Benefits of aerobic exercise for the paraplegic: A brief review. *Medicine and Science in Sports and Exercise* 18: 501-508.

Coyle, C.P., and M.C. Santiago. 1995. Aerobic exercise training and depressive symptomatology in adults with physical disabilities. *Archives of Physical Medicine and Rehabilitation* 76 (7): 647-652.

Coyle, E.F., W.H. Martin, S.A. Bloomfield, O.H. Lowry, and J.O. Holloszy. 1985. Effects of detraining on responses to submaximal exercise. *Journal of Applied Physiology* 59: 853-859.

Crane, P.B., and D.C. Wallace. 2007. Cardiovascular risks and physical activity in middle-aged and elderly African American women. *Journal of Cardiovascular Nursing* 22 (4, July): 297-303.

Crespo, C.J., S.J. Keteyian, G.W. Heath, and C.T. Sempos. 1996. Leisure-time physical activity among U.S. adults: Results from the Third National Health and Nutrition Examination Survey. *Archives of Internal Medicine* 156: 93-98.

Crespo, C.J., M.R. Palmieri, R.P. Perdomo, D.L. Mcgee, E. Smit, C.T. Sempos, I.M. Lee, and P.D. Sorlie. 2002. The relationship of physical activity and body weight with all-cause mortality: Results from the Puerto Rico Heart Health Program. *Annals of Epidemiology* 12 (8, November): 543-552.

Daniels, R., E. van Rossum, L. de Witte, G.I. Kempen, and W. van den Heuvel. 2008. Interventions to prevent disability in frail community-dwelling elderly: A systematic review. *BMC Health Services Research* 8 (December 30): 278.

Davies, C.T.M., D.O. Thomas, and M.J. White. 1986. Mechanical properties of young and elderly human muscle. *Acta Medica Scandinavica* 220 (Suppl. 711): 219-226.

Davis, G.M. 1993. Exercise capacity of individuals with paraplegia. *Medicine and Science in Sports and Exercise* 25: 423-432.

Day, K. 2006. Active living and social justice: Planning for physical activity in low-income, black, and Latino communities. *Journal of the American Planning Association* 71 (1): 88-99.

Dearwater, S.R., R.E. LaPorte, R.J. Robertson, G. Brenes, L.L. Adams, and D. Becker. 1986. Activity in the spinal cord-injured patient: An epidemiologic analysis of metabolic parameters. *Medicine and Science in Sports* 18: 541-544.

de Groot, P.C., N. Hjeltnes, A.C. Heijboer, W. Stal, and K. Birkeland. 2003. Effect of training intensity on physical capacity, lipid profile and insulin sensitivity in early rehabilitation of spinal cord injured individuals. *Spinal Cord* 41 (12): 673-679.

De Mello, M.T., A.M. Esteves, and S. Tufik. 2004. Comparison between dopaminergic agents and physical exercise as treatment for periodic limb movements in patients with spinal cord injury. *Spinal Cord* 42 (4): 218-221.

de Vries, H.A. 1979. Physiological effects of an exercise training regimen upon men aged 52-88. *Journal of Gerontology* 4: 325-336.

Diabetes Prevention Program Research Group. 1999. Design and methods for a clinical trial in the prevention of type 2 diabetes. *Diabetes Care* 22: 623-634.

Diabetes Prevention Program Research Group. 2009. 10-year follow-up of diabetes incidence and weight loss in the Diabetes Prevention Program Outcomes Study. *Lancet* 374: 1677-1686.

Dodd, K.J., N.F. Taylor, and H.K. Graham. 2003. A randomized clinical trial of strength training in young people with cerebral palsy. *Dev Med Child Neurol* 45 (10): 652-7.

Douglas, P.S., and M. O'Toole. 1992. Aging and physical activity determine cardiac structure and function in the older athlete. *Journal of Applied Physiology* 72: 1969-1973.

Dowler, J.M., and D.A. Jordan-Simpson. 1990. Participation of people with disabilities in selected activities. *Health Reports* 2: 269-277.

Driver, S., J. O'Connor, C. Lox, and K. Rees. 2004. Evaluation of an aquatics programme on fitness parameters of individuals with a brain injury. *Brain Inj* 18 (9): 847-59.

Driver, S. 2005. Social support and the physical activity behaviours of people with a brain injury. *Brain Inj* 19 (13): 1067-75.

Driver, S., K. Rees, J. O'Connor, and C. Lox. 2006. Aquatics, health-promoting self-care behaviours and adults with brain injuries. *Brain Injury* 20 (2): 133-141.

Einarsson, G. 1991. Muscle adaptation and disability in late poliomyelitis. *Scandinavian Journal of Rehabilitation Medicine* 25 (Suppl.): 1-76.

Expert Panel on Detection, Evaluation, and Treatment of High Blood Cholesterol in Adults. 2001. Executive summary of the third report of the National Cholesterol Education Program (NCEP) expert panel on detection, evaluation, and treatment of high blood cholesterol in adults (Adult Treatment Panel III). *Journal of the American Medical Association* 285: 2486-2497.

Eyler, A.E., S. Wilcox, D. Matson-Koffman, K.R. Evenson, B. Sanderson, J. Thompson, J. Wilbur, and D. Rohm-Young. 2002. Correlates of physical activity among women from diverse racial/ethnic groups. *Journal of Women's Health and Gender-Based Medicine* 11 (3, April): 239-253.

Fentem, P.H. 1992. Exercise in the prevention of disease. *British Medical Bulletin* 48: 630-650.

Fentem, P.H. 1994. Benefits of exercise in health and disease. *British Medical Journal* 308: 1291-1295.

Fentem, P.H., and E.J. Bassey. 1985. *50+ All to play for: A guide for those in charge of activity groups.* London: Sports Council.

Fiatarone, M.A., E.F. O'Neill, N.D. Ryan, et al. 1994. Exercise training and nutritional supplementation for physical frailty in very elderly people. *New England Journal of Medicine* 330: 1769-1775.

Findlay, I.N., R.S. Taylor, H.J. Dargie, S. Grant, A.R. Pettigrew, J.T. Wilson, T. Aitchison, J.G. Cleland, A.T. Elliott, B.M. Fisher, G. Gillen, A. Manzie, A.G. Rumley, and J.V.G.A. Durnin. 1987. Cardiovascular effects of training for a marathon run in unfit middle aged men. *British Medical Journal* 295: 521-524.

Fitzgerald, S.J., A.M. Kriska, M.A. Pereira, and M.P. De Courten. 1997. Associations among physical activity, television watching, and obesity in adult Pima Indians. *Medicine and Science in Sports and Exercise* 29 (7): 910-915.

Folsom, A.R., D.K. Arnett, R.G. Hutchinson, F. Liao, L.X. Clegg, and L.S. Cooper. 1997. Physical activity and incidence of coronary heart disease in middle-aged women and men. *Medicine and Science in Sports and Exercise* 29 (7): 901-909.

Ford, E.S., H.W. Kohl III, A.H. Mokdad, and U.A. Ajani. 2005. Sedentary behavior, physical activity, and the metabolic syndrome among U.S. adults. *Obesity Research* 13 (3): 608-614.

Ford, E.S., R.K. Merritt, G.W. Heath, K.E. Powell, R.A. Washburn, A. Kriska, and G. Haile. 1991. Physical activity behaviors in low and high socioeconomic populations. *American Journal of Epidemiology* 133: 1246-1256.

Forrest, K.Y., C.H. Bunker, A.M. Kriska, F.A. Ukoli, S.L. Huston, and N. Markovic. 2001. Physical activity and cardiovascular risk factors in a developing population. *Medicine and Science in Sports and Exercise* 33 (9): 1598-1604.

Frontera, W.R., C.N. Meredith, K.P. O'Reilly, H.G. Knuttgen, and W.J. Evans. 1988. Strength conditioning in older men: Skeletal muscle hypertrophy and improved function. *Journal of Applied Physiology* 64: 1038-1044.

Gaffney, F.A., G. Grimby, B. Danneskiold-Samsøe, and O. Halskov. 1981. Adaptation to peripheral muscle training. *Scandinavian Journal of Rehabilitation Medicine* 13: 11-16.

Gehlsen, G.M., S.A. Grigsby, and D.M. Winant. 1984. Effects of an aquatic fitness program on the muscular strength and endurance of patients with multiple sclerosis. *Physical Therapy* 64: 653-657.

Gilliland, F.D., Y.F. Li, K. Baumgartner, D. Crumley, and J.M. Samet. 2001. Physical activity and breast cancer risk in hispanic and non-hispanic white women. *American Journal of Epidemiology* 154 (5, September 1): 442-450.

Ginis, K.A.M., A.E. Latimer, K. McKechnie, D.S. Ditor, N. McCartney, A.L. Hicks, J. Bugaresti, and B.C. Craven. 2003. Using exercise to enhance subjective well-being among people with spinal cord injury: The mediating influences of stress and pain. *Rehabilitation Psychology* 48 (3): 157-164.

Ginis, K.A., and A.L. Hicks. 2007. Considerations for the development of a physical activity guide for Canadians with physical disabilities. *Can J Public Health* 98 Suppl 2: S135-47.

Gloag, D. 1985. Rehabilitation in rheumatic diseases. *British Medical Journal* 290: 132-136.

Godin, G., A. Colantonio, G.M. Davis, R.J. Shephard, and C. Simard. 1986. Prediction of leisure time exercise behavior among a group of lower-limb disabled adults. *Journal of Clinical Psychology* 42: 272-279.

Gregg, E.W., R.B. Gerzoff, C.J. Caspersen, D.F. Williamson, and K.M. Narayan. 2003. Relationship of walking to mortality among US adults with diabetes. *Archives of Internal Medicine* 163 (12, June 23): 1440-1447.

Grimby, G., A. Aniansson, M. Hedberg, G.B. Henning, U. Grangard, and H. Kvist. 1992. Training can improve muscle strength and endurance in 78- to 84-yr-old men. *Journal of Applied Physiology* 73 (6): 2517-2523.

Grimby, G., G. Einarsson, M. Hedberg, and A. Aniansson. 1989. Muscle adaptive changes in post-polio subjects. *Scandinavian Journal of Rehabilitation Medicine* 21: 19-26.

Hagberg, J.M. 1987. Effect of training on the decline of VO2 max with aging. *Federal Proceedings* 46: 1830-1833.

Hagberg, J.M., D. Goldring, A.A. Ehsani, G.W. Heath, A. Hernandez, K. Schechtman, and J.O. Holloszy. 1983. Effect of exercise training on the blood pressure and hemodynamic features of hypertensive adolescents. *American Journal of Cardiology* 52: 763-768.

Hakim, A.A., H. Petrovitch, C.M. Burchfiel, G.W. Ross, B.L. Rodriguez, L.R. White, K. Yano, J.D. Curb, and R.D. Abbott. 1998. Effects of walking on mortality among nonsmoking retired men. *New England Journal of Medicine* 338 (2, January 8): 94-99.

Ham, S.A., M.M. Yore, J. Kruger, G.W. Heath, and R. Moeti. 2007. Physical activity patterns among Latinos in the United States: Putting the pieces together. *Preventing Chronic Disease* 4 (4): A92.

Hamilton, M.K. 1989. The health and activity limitation survey. *Health Reports* 1: 175-187.

Hardy, L., and D. Jones. 1986. Dynamic flexibility and proprioceptive neuromuscular facilitation. *Research Quarterly for Exercise and Sport* 57: 150-153.

Harkcom, T.M., R.M. Lampman, B.F. Banwell, and C.W. Castor. 1985. Therapeutic value of graded aerobic exercise training in rheumatoid arthritis. *Arthritis Rheum* 28 (1): 32-9.

He, X.Z., and D.W. Baker. 2005. Differences in leisure-time, household, and work-related physical activity by race, ethnicity, and education. *Journal of General Internal Medicine* 20 (3): 259-266.

Heath, G.W. 1994. Physical fitness and aging: Effects of deconditioning. *Science and Sports* 9: 197-200.

Heath, G.W. 2000. Epidemiologic research: A primer for the clinical exercise physiologist. *Clinical Exercise Physiology* 2: 60-67.

Heath, G.W., and P.H. Fentem. 1997. Physical activity among persons with disabilities: A public health perspective. *Exercise and Sport Sciences Reviews* 25: 195-234.

Heath, G.W., J.M. Hagberg, A.A. Ehsani, and J.O. Holloszy. 1981. A physiological comparison of young and older endurance athletes. *Journal of Applied Physiology* 51: 634-640.

Heller, T., K. Hsieh, and J.H. Rimmer. 2004. Attitudinal and psychosocial outcomes of a fitness and health education program on adults with down syndrome. *American Journal of Mental Retardation* 109 (2, March): 175-185.

Herman, T., N. Giladi, L. Gruendlinger, and J.M. Hausdorff. 2007. Six weeks of intensive treadmill training improves gait and quality of life in patients with Parkinson's disease: A pilot study. *Archives of Physical Medicine and Rehabilitation* 88 (9): 1154-1158.

Hicks, A.L., K.A. Martin, D.S. Ditor, A.E. Latimer, C. Craven, J. Bugaresti, and N. McCartney. 2003. Long-term exercise training in persons with spinal cord injury: Effects on strength, arm ergometry performance and psychological well-being. *Spinal Cord* 41 (1): 34-43.

Hickson, R.C., C. Kanakis Jr., J.R. Davis, A.M. Moore, and S. Rich. 1982. Reduced training duration effects on aerobic power, endurance, and cardiac growth. *Journal of Applied Physiology* 53: 225-229.

Hirsch, M.A., T. Toole, C.G. Maitland, and R.A. Rider. 2003. The effects of balance training and high-intensity resistance training on persons with idiopathic Parkinson's disease. *Archives of Physical Medicine and Rehabilitation* 84 (8): 1109-1117.

Hjeltnes, N., and H. Wallberg-Henriksson. 1998. Improved work capacity but unchanged peak oxygen uptake during primary rehabilitation in tetraplegic patients. *Spinal Cord* 36 (10): 691-698.

Hornbuckle, L.M., D.R. Bassett Jr., and D.L. Thompson. 2005. Pedometer-determined walking and body composition variables in African-American women. *Medicine and Science in Sports and Exercise* 37 (6): 1069-1074.

Hoskins, T.A. 1975. Physiologic responses to known exercise loads in hemiplegic patients. *Archives of Physical Medicine and Rehabilitation* 56: 544.

Housley, E. 1988. Treating claudication in five words. *British Medical Journal* 296: 1483.

Hsia, J., L. Wu, C. Allen, A. Oberman, W.E. Lawson, J. Torrens, M. Safford, M.C. Limacher, and B.V. Howard. 2005. Physical activity and diabetes risk in postmenopausal women. *American Journal of Preventive Medicine* 28 (1): 19-25.

Hu, F.B., T.Y. Li, G.A. Colditz, W.C. Willett, and J.E. Manson. 2003. Television watching and other sedentary behaviors in relation to risk of obesity and type 2 diabetes mellitus in women. *Journal of the American Medical Association* 289 (14, April 8): 1785-1791.

Hu, F.B., M.J. Stampfer, C. Solomon, S. Liu, G.A. Colditz, F.E. Speizer, W.C. Willett, and J.E. Manson. 2001. Physical activity and risk for cardiovascular events in diabetic women. *Annals of Internal Medicine* 134 (2, January 18): 96-105.

Hubert, H.B., D.A. Bloch, and J.F. Fries. 1993. Risk factors for physical disability in an aging cohort: The NHANES I epidemiologic follow-up study. *Journal of Rheumatology* 20: 480-488.

Iezzoni, L.I., and V.A. Freedman. 2008. Turning the disability tide: The importance of definitions. *Journal of the American Medical Association* 299 (3, January 23): 332-334.

Irwin, M.L., B.E. Ainsworth, E.J. Mayer-Davis, C.L. Addy, R.R. Pate, and J.L. Durstine. 2002. Physical activity and the metabolic syndrome in a tri-ethnic sample of women. *Obesity Research* 10 (10): 1030-1037.

Ivey, F.M., A.S. Ryan, C.E. Hafer-Macko, A.P. Goldberg, and R.F. Macko. 2007. Treadmill aerobic training improves glucose tolerance and indices of insulin sensitivity in disabled stroke survivors: A preliminary report. *Stroke* 38 (10): 2752-2758.

Jacobs, P.L., M.S. Nash, and J.W. Rusinowski. 2001. Circuit training provides cardiorespiratory and strength benefits in persons with paraplegia. *Medicine and Science in Sports and Exercise* 33 (5): 711-717.

Jacobson, P.C., W. Beaver, S.A. Grubb, T.N. Taft, and R.V. Talmage. 1984. Bone density in women: College athletes and older athletic women. *Journal of Orthopedic Research* 2: 328-332.

Jeong, S., and M.T. Kim. 2007. Effects of a theory-driven music and movement program for stroke survivors in a community setting. *Applied Nursing Research* 20 (3, August): 125-131.

Kaplan, P.E., W. Roden, E. Gilbert, L. Richards, and J.W. Goldschmidt. 1981. Reduction of hypercalciuria in tetraplegia after weight-bearing and strengthening exercises. *Paraplegia* 19: 289-293.

Kasch, F.W., J.L. Boyer, P.K. Schmidt, et al. 1999. Ageing of the cardiovascular system during 33 years of aerobic exercise. *Age and Ageing* 28: 531-536.

Kasch, F.W., and J.P. Wallace. 1976. Physiological variables during 10 years of endurance exercise. *Medicine and Science in Sports* 8: 5-8.

Kinne, S., D.L. Patrick, and E.J. Maher. 1999. Correlates of exercise maintenance among people with mobility impairments. *Disability and Rehabilitation* 21: 15-22.

Knowler, W.C., E. Barrett-Connor, S.E. Fowler, R.F. Hamman, J.M. Lachin, E.A. Walker, and D.M. Nathan. 2002. Reduction in the incidence of type 2 diabetes with lifestyle intervention or metformin. *New England Journal of Medicine* 346 (6, February 7): 393-403.

Kovar, P.A., I.P. Allegrante, C.R. MacKenzie, M.G.E. Peterson, B. Gutin, and M.E. Charlson. 1992. Supervised walking in patients with osteoarthritis of the knee: A randomized controlled trial. *Annals of Internal Medicine* 116: 529-534.

Kristensen, J.H., T.I. Hansen, and B. Saltin. 1980. Cross-sectional and fiber size changes in the quadriceps muscle of man with immobilization and physical training. *Muscle and Nerve* 3: 275-276.

Lai, S.M., S. Studenski, L. Richards, S. Perera, D. Reker, S. Rigler, and P.W. Duncan. 2006. Therapeutic exercise and depressive symptoms after stroke. *Journal of the American Geriatrics Society* 54 (2): 240-247.

Lakatta, E.G., and D. Levy. 2003. Arterial and cardiac aging: Major shareholders in cardiovascular disease enterprises: Part I: Aging arteries: A "set up" for vascular disease. *Circulation* 107: 139-146.

LaPlante, M.P. 1991. Medical conditions associated with disability. In *Disability in the United States: A portrait from national data*, edited by S. Thompson-Hoffman and I. Fitzgerald Storck, pp. 34-72. New York: Springer.

LaPlante, M.P., and D. Carlson. 1996. *Disability in the United States: Prevalence and causes, 1992*. Disability Statistics Report No. 7. Washington, DC: U.S. Department of Education, National Institute of Disability and Rehabilitation Research.

LaPlante, M.P., G.W. Heath, N. Barker, and M.H. Chang. 1996. Prevalence of leisure-time physical activity among people with and without disability: United States, 1990-1991. *Proceedings of the Paralympic Scientific Congress*, Atlanta, Georgia.

Larsson, B., P. Renstrom, K. Svardsudd, L. Welin, G. Grimby, H. Eriksson, L.-O. Ohlson, L. Wilhelmson, and P. Bjorntorp. 1984. Health and ageing characteristics of highly physically active 65-year-old men. *European Heart Journal* 5 (Suppl. E): 31-35.

Laukkanen, P., E. Heikkinen, and M. Kauppinen. 1995. Muscle strength and mobility as predictors of survival in 75-84-year-old people. *Age and Ageing* 24: 468-473.

Launer, L.J., T. Harris, C. Rumpel, and J. Madans. 1994. Body mass index, weight change, and risk of mobility disability in middle-aged and older women: The epidemiologic follow-up study of NHANES I. *Journal of the American Medical Association* 271: 1093-1098.

Lee, P., A. Helewa, H.A. Smythe, C. Bombardier, and C.H. Goldsmith. 1985. Epidemiology of musculoskeletal disorders (complaints) and related disability in Canada. *Journal of Rheumatology* 12: 1169-1173.

Leon, A.S., J. Conrad, D.B. Hunninghake, and R. Serfass. 1979. Effect of a vigorous walking program on body composition, and carbohydrate and lipid metabolism of obese young men. *American Journal of Clinical Nutrition* 33: 1776-1787.

Leroux, A. 2005. Exercise training to improve motor performance in chronic stroke: Effects of a community-based exercise program. *International Journal of Rehabilitation Research* 28 (1, March): 17-23.

Lindeman, E., P. Leffers, F. Spaans, J. Drukker, J. Reulen, M. Kerckhoffs, and A. Koke. 1995. Strength training in patients with myotonic dystrophy and hereditary motor and sensory neuropathy: A randomized clinical trial. *Archives of Physical Medicine and Rehabilitation* 76 (7): 612-620.

Lindeman, E., F. Spaans, J. Reulen, P. Leffers, and J. Drukker. 1999. Progressive resistance training in neuromuscular patients. Effects on force and surface EMG. *Journal of Electromyography and Kinesiology* 9 (6, December): 379-384.

Mack, K.A., L. Anderson, D. Galuska, D. Zablotsky, D. Holtzman, and I. Ahluwalia. 2004. Health and sociodemographic factors associated with body weight and weight objectives for women: 2000 behavioral risk factor surveillance system. *Journal of Women's Health* 13 (9, November): 1019-1032.

Madorsky, J.G., and A. Madorsky. 1983. Wheelchair racing: An important modality in acute rehabilitation after paraplegia. *Archives of Physical Medicine and Rehabilitation* 64: 186-187.

Manini, T.M., J.E. Everhart, K.V. Patel, D.A. Schoeller, L.H. Colbert, M. Visser, F. Tylavsky, D.C. Bauer, B.H. Goodpaster, and T.B. Harris. 2006. Daily activity energy expenditure and mortality among older adults. *Journal of the American Medical Association* 296 (2, July 12): 171-179.

Manson, J.E., P. Greenland, A.Z. LaCroix, M.L. Stefanick, C.P. Mouton, A. Oberman, M.G. Perri, D.S. Sheps, M.B. Pettinger, and D.S. Siscovick. 2002. Walking compared with vigorous exercise for the prevention of cardiovascular events in women. *New England Journal of Medicine* 347 (10, September 5): 716-725.

Marshall, S.J., D.A. Jones, B.E. Ainsworth, J.P. Reis, S.S. Levy, and C.A. Macera. 2007. Race/ethnicity, social class, and leisure-time physical inactivity. *Medicine and Science in Sports and Exercise* 39 (1): 44-51.

Matthews, C.E., K.Y. Chen, P.S. Freedson, M.S. Buchowski, B.M. Beech, R.R. Pate, and R.P. Troiano. 2008. Amount of time spent in sedentary behaviors in the United States, 2003-2004. *American Journal of Epidemiology* 167 (7, April 1): 875-881.

McCurry, S.M., L.E. Gibbons, R.G. Logsdon, M.V. Vitiello, and L. Teri. 2005. Nighttime insomnia treatment and education for Alzheimer's disease: A randomized, controlled trial. *Journal of the American Geriatrics Society* 53 (5): 793-802.

McGruder, H.F., A.M. Malarcher, T.L. Antoine, K.J. Greenlund, and J.B. Croft. 2004. Racial and ethnic disparities in cardiovascular risk factors among stroke survivors: United States 1999 to 2001. *Stroke* 35: 1557-1561.

McTiernan, A., C. Kooperberg, E. White, S. Wilcox, R. Coates, L.L. Adams-Campbell, N. Woods, and J. Ockene. 2003. Recreational physical activity and the risk of breast cancer in postmenopausal

women: The Women's Health Initiative Cohort Study. *Journal of the American Medical Association* 290 (10, September 10): 1331-1336.

Meyer, C.M.H. 1981. Sport and recreation for the severely disabled. *South African Medical Journal* 60: 868-871.

Minor, M.A., and J.E. Hewett. 1995. Physical fitness and work capacity in women with rheumatoid arthritis. *Arthritis Care and Research* 8: 146-154.

Moore, S.C., T.M. Peters, J. Ahn, Y. Park, A. Schatzkin, D. Albanes, A. Hollenbeck, and M.F. Leitzmann. 2009. Age-specific physical activity and prostate cancer risk among white men and black men. *Cancer* 115: 5060-5070.

Morey, M.C., P.A. Cowper, J.R. Feussner, R.C. DiPasquale, G.M. Crowley, D.W. Kitzman, and R.J. Sullivan. 1989. Evaluation of a supervised exercise program in a geriatric population. *Journal of the American Geriatrics Society* 37: 348-354.

Nash, M.S., I. van de Ven, and N. van Elk, and B.M. Johnson. 2007. Effects of circuit resistance training on fitness attributes and upper-extremity pain in middle-aged men with paraplegia. *Archives of Physical Medicine and Rehabilitation* 88 (1): 70-75.

National Council on Disability. 2002. Supreme Court decisions interpreting the Americans With Disabilities Act. Publications and Policy Briefs, National Council on Disability.

National Center for Health Statistics. 2000. *Health, United States, 2000 with adolescent health chartbook*, pp. 229-231. Hyattsville, MD: National Center for Health Statistics.

National Center for Health Statistics. 2007. *Health, United States, 2007 with chartbook on trends in the health of Americans*. Hyattsville, MD: U.S. Department of Health and Human Services, Centers for Disease Control and Prevention.

Newman, M.A., H. Dawes, M. van den Berg, D.T. Wade, J. Burridge, and H. Izadi. 2007. Can aerobic treadmill training reduce the effort of walking and fatigue in people with multiple sclerosis: A pilot study. *Multiple Sclerosis* 13 (1): 113-119.

Nilsson, S., P.H. Staff, and E.D.R. Pruett. 1975. Physical work capacity and the effect of training on subjects with long-standing paraplegia. *Scandinavian Journal of Rehabilitation Medicine* 7: 51-56.

Nordemar, R., U. Berg, B. Ekblom, and L. Edstrom. 1976. Changes in muscle fibre size and physical performance in patients with rheumatoid arthritis after 7 months' physical training. *Scandinavian Journal of Rheumatology* 5: 233-238.

Nordemar, R., B. Ekblom, L. Zachrisson, and K. Lundqvist. 1981. Physical training in rheumatoid arthritis: A controlled long-term study. *Scandinavian Journal of Rheumatology* 10: 17-23.

Noreau, L., R.J. Shephard, C. Simard, G. Pare, and P. Pomerleau. 1993. Relationship of impairment and functional ability to habitual activity and fitness following spinal cord injury. *International Journal of Rehabilitation Research* 16: 265-275.

Ogden, C.L., M.D. Carroll, L.R. Curtin, M.A. McDowell, C.J. Tabak, and K.M. Flegal. 2006. Prevalence of overweight and obesity in the United States, 1999-2004. *Journal of the American Medical Association* 295 (13, April 5): 1549-1555.

Orchard, T.J., M. Temprosa, R. Goldberg, S. Haffner, R. Ratner, S. Marcovina, and S. Fowler. 2005. The effect of metformin and intensive lifestyle intervention on the metabolic syndrome: The Diabetes Prevention Program randomized trial. *Annals of Internal Medicine* 142 (8, April 19): 611-619.

Orsini, N., R. Bellocco, M. Bottai, M. Pagano, S-O. Andersson, J-E. Johansson, J. Giovannucci, and A. Wolk. 2009. A prospective study of lifetime physical activity and prostate cancer incidence and mortality. *British Journal of Cancer* 101: 1932-1938.

Ostbye, T., D.H. Taylor Jr, K.M. Krause, and L. van Scoyoc. 2002. The role of smoking and other modifiable lifestyle risk factors in maintaining and restoring lower body mobility in middle-aged and older Americans: results from the HRS and AHEAD. Health and Retirement Study. Asset and Health Dynamics Among the Oldest Old. *J Am Geriatr Soc* Apr 50 (4): 691-9.

Ouellette, M.M., N.K. LeBrasseur, J.F. Bean, E. Phillips, J. Stein, W.R. Frontera, and R.A. Fielding. 2004. High-intensity resistance training improves muscle strength, self-reported function, and disability in long-term stroke survivors. *Stroke* 35 (6): 1404-1409.

Painter, P., and G. Blackburn. 1988. Exercise for patients with chronic disease. *Postgraduate Medicine* 83: 185-196.

Pang, M.Y., J.J. Eng, A.S. Dawson, H.A. McKay, and J.E. Harris. 2005. A community-based fitness and mobility exercise program for older adults with chronic stroke: A randomized, controlled trial. *Journal of the American Geriatrics Society* 53 (10): 1667-1674.

Pang, M.Y., J.E. Harris, and J.J. Eng. 2006. A community-based upper-extremity group exercise program improves motor function and performance of functional activities in chronic stroke: A randomized controlled trial. *Archives of Physical Medicine and Rehabilitation* 87 (1): 1-9.

Patikas, D., S.I. Wolf, P. Armbrust, K. Mund, W. Schuster, T. Dreher, and L. Doderlein. 2006. Effects of a postoperative resistive exercise program on the knee extension and flexion torque in children with cerebral palsy: A randomized clinical trial. *Archives of Physical Medicine and Rehabilitation* 87 (9): 1161-1169.

Patikas, D., S.I. Wolf, K. Mund, P. Armbrust, W. Schuster, and L. Doderlein. 2005. Effects of a postoperative strength-training program on the walking ability of children with cerebral palsy: A randomized controlled trial. *Archives of Physical Medicine and Rehabilitation* 87 (5): 619-626.

Petajan, J.H., E. Gappmaier, A.T. White, M.K. Spencer, L. Mino, and R.W. Hicks. 1996. Impact of aerobic training on fitness and quality of life in multiple sclerosis. *Annals of Neurology* 39 (4): 432-441.

Phillips, W.T., and W.L. Haskell. 1995. "Muscular fitness" — easing the burden of disability for elderly adults. *Journal of Aging and Physical Activity* 3: 261-289.

Physical Activity Guidelines Advisory Committee. 2008. *Physical Activity Guidelines Advisory Committee report.* Washington, DC: U.S. Department of Health and Human Services.

Pleis, J.R., J.W. Lucas, and B.W. Ward. 2009. Summary health statistics for U.S. adults: National Health Interview Survey, 2008. National Center for Health Statistics. *Vital Health Statistics* 10 (242): 30-42.

Podgorski, C.A., K. Kessler, B. Cacia, D.R. Peterson, and C.M. Henderson. 2004. Physical activity intervention for older adults with intellectual disability: Report on a pilot project. *Mental Retardation* 42 (4, August): 272-283.

Pollock, M.L., C. Foster, D. Knapp, J.L. Rod, and D.H. Schmidt. 1987. Effect of age and training on aerobic capacity and body composition of master athletes. *Journal of Applied Physiology* 62: 725-731.

Ponichtera-Mulcare, J.A. 1993. Exercise and multiple sclerosis. *Medicine and Science in Sports and Exercise* 25: 451-465.

Powell, K.E., P.D. Thompson, C.J. Casperson, and J.S. Kendrick. 1987. Physical activity and the incidence of coronary heart disease. *Annual Review of Public Health* 8: 253-287.

Raab, D.M., J.C. Agre, M. McAdam, and E.L. Smith. 1988. Light resistance and stretching exercise in elderly women: effect upon flexibility. *Arch Phys Med Rehabil* 69 (4): 268-272.

Rampello, A., M. Franceschini, M. Piepoli, R. Antenucci, G. Lenti, D. Olivieri, and A. Chetta. 2007. Effect of aerobic training on walking capacity and maximal exercise tolerance in patients with multiple sclerosis: A randomized crossover controlled study. *Physical Therapy* 87 (5): 545-555.

Rasova, K., E. Havrdova, P. Brandejsky, M. Zalisova, B. Foubikova, and P. Martinkova. 2006. Comparison of the influence of different rehabilitation programmes on clinical, spirometric and spiroergometric parameters in patients with multiple sclerosis. *Multiple Sclerosis* 12 (2): 227-234.

Richardson, C.R., A.M. Kriska, P.M. Lantz, and R.A. Hayward. 2004. Physical activity and mortality across cardiovascular disease risk groups. *Medicine and Science in Sports and Exercise* 36 (11): 1923-1929.

Rimmer, J.H. 2005. Exercise and physical activity in persons aging with a physical disability. *Physical Medicine and Rehabilitation Clinics of North America* 16 (1, February): 41-56.

Rimmer, J.H., D. Braddock, and K.H. Pitetti. 1996. Research on physical activity and disability: An emerging national priority. *Medicine and Science in Sports and Exercise* 28: 1366-1372.

Rimmer, J.H., T. Heller, E. Wang, and I. Valerio. 2004. Improvements in physical fitness in adults with Down syndrome. *American Journal of Mental Retardation* 109 (2, March): 165-174.

Rimmer, J.H., B. Riley, T. Creviston, and T. Nicola. 2000. Exercise training in a predominantly African-American group of stroke survivors. *Medicine and Science in Sports and Exercise* 32 (12): 1990-1996.

Rimmer, J.H., S.S. Rubin, and D. Braddock. 2000. Barriers to exercise in African-American women with physical disabilities. *Archives of Physical Medicine and Rehabilitation* 81: 182-188.

Rimmer, J.H., S.S. Rubin, D. Braddock, and G. Hedman. 1999. Physical activity patterns of African-American women with physical disabilities. *Medicine and Science in Sports and Exercise* 31: 613-618.

Rodgers, M.M., R.E. Keyser, E.K. Rasch, P.H. Gorman, and P.J. Russell. 2001. Influence of training on biomechanics of wheelchair propulsion. *Journal of Rehabilitation Research and Development* 38 (5, September): 505-511.

Santiago, M.C., C.P. Coyle, and W.B. Kinney. 1993. Aerobic exercise effect on individuals with physical disabilities. *Archives of Physical Medicine and Rehabilitation* 74: 1192-1198.

Schenkman, M., T.M. Cutson, M. Kuchibhatla, J. Chandler, C.F. Pieper, L. Ray, and K.C. Laub. 1998. Exercise to improve spinal flexibility and function for people with Parkinson's disease: A randomized, controlled trial. *Journal of the American Geriatrics Society* 46 (10): 1207-1216.

Schneider, V.S., and J. McDonald. 1984. Skeletal calcium homeostasis and countermeasures to prevent disuse osteoporosis. *Calcified Tissue International* 36 (Suppl.): S151-S154.

Schulz, K.H., S.M. Gold, J. Witte, K. Bartsch, U.E. Lang, R. Hellweg, R. Reer, K.M. Braumann, and C. Heesen. 2004. Impact of aerobic training on immune-endocrine parameters, neurotrophic factors, quality of life and coordinative function in multiple sclerosis. *Journal of the Neurological Sciences* 225 (1-2, October 15): 11-18.

Seals, D.R., J.M. Hagberg, B.F. Hurley, A.A. Ehsani, and J.O. Holloszy. 1984. Endurance training in older men and women I. Cardiovascular responses to exercise. *Journal of Applied Physiology* 57: 1024-1029.

Shephard, R.J. 1991. Benefits of sport and physical activity for the disabled: Implications for the individual and for society. *Scandinavian Journal of Rehabilitation Medicine* 23: 51-59.

Shindo, M., S. Komagai, and H. Tanaka. 1987. Physical work capacity and effect of endurance training in visually handicapped boys and young male adults. *European Journal of Applied Physiology* 56: 501-507.

Siegel, W., G. Blomqvist, and J.H. Mitchell. 1970. Effects of a quantitated physical training program on middle-aged sedentary men. *Circulation* 41: 19-29.

Sisson, S.B., S.M. Camhi, T.S. Church, C.K. Martin, C. Tudor-Locke, C. Bouchard, C.P. Earnest, S.R. Smith, R.L. Newton Jr, T. Rankinen, and P.T. Katzmarzyk. 2009. Leisure time sedentary behavior, occupational/domestic physical activity, and metabolic syndrome in U.S. men and women. *Metab Syndr Relat Disord* 7 (6): 529-36

Skinner, J.S., A. Jaskolski, A. Jaskolska, J. Krasnoff, J. Gagnon, A.S. Leon, D.C. Rao, J.H. Wilmore, and C. Bouchard. 2001. Age, sex, race, initial fitness, and response to training: The HERITAGE Family Study. *Journal of Applied Physiology* 90 (5): 1770-1776.

Skrinar, G.S., N.A. Huxley, D.S. Hutchinson, E. Menninger, and P. Glew. 2005. The role of a fitness intervention on people with serious psychiatric disabilities. *Psychiatric Rehabilitation Journal* 29 (2): 122-127.

Slattery, M.L., S. Edwards, M.A. Murtaugh, C. Sweeney, J. Herrick, T. Byers, A.R. Giuliano, and K.B. Baumgartner. 2007. Physical activity and breast cancer risk among women in the southwestern United States. *Annals of Epidemiology* 17 (5): 342-353.

Slattery, M.L., C. Sweeney, S. Edwards, J. Herrick, M. Murtaugh, K. Baumgartner, A. Guiliano, and T. Byers. 2006. Physical activity patterns and obesity in Hispanic and non-Hispanic white women. *Medicine and Science in Sports and Exercise* 38 (1): 33-41.

Smith, E.L. 1981. Bone changes in the exercising older adult. In *Exercise and aging: The scientific basis* (Smith, E.L., and R.C. Serfass, Eds.). Enslow Publishers, Hillsdale, NJ: 179-186.

Sorock, G.S., T.L. Bush, A.L. Golden, L.P. Fried, B. Breuer, and W.E. Hale. 1988. Physical activity and fracture risk in a free-living elderly cohort. *Journal of Gerontology* 43: M134-139.

Sternfeld, B., J. Cauley, S. Harlow, G. Liu, and M. Lee. 2000. Assessment of physical activity with a single global question in a large, multiethnic sample of midlife women. *American Journal of Epidemiology* 152 (7, October 1): 678-687.

Sternfeld, B., H. Wang, C.P. Quesenberry Jr., B. Abrams, S.A. Everson-Rose, G.A. Greendale, K.A. Matthews, J.I. Torrens, and M. Sowers. 2004. Physical activity and changes in weight and waist circumference in midlife women: Findings from the Study of Women's Health Across the Nation. *American Journal of Epidemiology* 160 (9, November 1): 912-922.

Strom, S.S., Y. Yamamura, F.N. Flores-Sandoval, C.A. Pettaway, and D.S. Lopez. 2008. Prostate cancer in Mexican-Americans: identification of risk factors. *Prostate* 1;68 (5): 563-70.

Suominen, H., E. Heikkinen, and T. Parkatti. 1977. Effect of eight weeks' physical training on muscle and connective tissue of the M. vastus lateralis in 69-year-old men and women. *Journal of Gerontology* 32: 33-37.

Surakka, J., A. Romberg, J. Ruutiainen, S. Aunola, A. Virtanen, S.L. Karppi, and K. Maentaka. 2004. Effects of aerobic and strength exercise on motor fatigue in men and women with multiple sclerosis: A randomized controlled trial. *Clinical Rehabilitation* 18 (7, November): 737-746.

Taylor, W.C., T. Baranowski, and D.R. Young. 1998. Physical activity interventions in low-income, ethnic minority, and populations with disability. *American Journal of Preventive Medicine* 15: 334-343.

Teri, L., L.E. Gibbons, S.M. McCurry, R.G. Logsdon, D.M. Buchner, W.E. Barlow, W.A. Kukull, A.Z. LaCroix, W. McCormick, and E.B. Larson. 2003. Exercise plus behavioral management in patients with Alzheimer disease: A randomized controlled trial. *Journal of the American Medical Association* 290 (15, October 15): 2015-2022.

Thompson, R.F., D.M. Crist, M. Marsh, and M. Rosenthal. 1988. Effects of physical exercise for elderly patients with physical impairments. *Journal of the American Geriatrics Society* 36: 130-135.

Troiano, R.P., D. Berrigan, K.W. Dodd, L.C. Masse, T. Tilert, and M. McDowell. 2008. Physical activity in the United States measured by accelerometer. *Medicine and Science in Sports and Exercise* 40 (1): 181-188.

Tseng, B.S., D.R. Marsh, M.T. Hamilton, and F.W. Booth. 1995. Strength and aerobic training attenuate muscle wasting and improve resistance to the development of disability with aging. *J Gerontol A Biol Sci Med Sci* 50 Spec No: 113-9.

U.S. Department of Health and Human Services. 2010. *Healthy people 2020:* www.healthypeople.gov/2020/topicsobjectives2020/pdfs/HP2020objectives.pdf

van der Kooi, E.L., J.S. Kalkman, E. Lindeman, J.C. Hendriks, B.G. van Engelen, G. Bleijenberg, and G.W. Padberg. 2007. Effects of training and albuterol on pain and fatigue in facioscapulohumeral muscular dystrophy. *Journal of Neurology* 254 (7): 931-940.

van der Kooi, E.L., O.J. Vogels, R.J. van Asseldonk, E. Lindeman, J.C. Hendriks, M. Wohlgemuth, S.M. van der Maarel, and G.W. Padberg. 2004. Strength training and albuterol in facioscapulohumeral muscular dystrophy. *Neurology* 63 (4, August 24): 702-708.

Van Deusen, J. 1987. The efficacy of the ROM dance program for adults with rheumatoid arthritis. *American Journal of Occupational Therapy* 41: 90-95.

Wang, B.W., D.R. Ramey, J.D. Schettler, H.B. Hubert, and J.F. Fries. 2002. Postponed development of disability in elderly runners: A 13-year longitudinal study. *Archives of Internal Medicine* 162: 2285-2294.

Wang, Y., and M.A. Beydoun. 2007. The obesity epidemic in the United States—gender, age, socioeconomic, racial/ethnic, and geographic characteristics: A systematic review and meta-regression analysis. *Epidemiologic Reviews* 29: 6-28.

Weinstein, A.R., H.D. Sesso, I.M. Lee, N.R. Cook, J.E. Manson, J.E. Buring, and J.M. Gaziano. 2004. Relationship of physical activity vs body mass index with type 2 diabetes in women. *Journal of the American Medical Association* 292 (10, September 8): 1188-1194.

Wenneberg, S., L.G. Gunnarsson, and G. Ahlstrom. 2004. Using a novel exercise programme for patients with muscular dystrophy. Part II: A quantitative study. *Disability and Rehabilitation* 26 (10, May 20): 595-602.

Whitt-Glover, M.C., W.C. Taylor, G.W. Heath, and C.A. Macera. 2007. Self-reported physical activity among blacks: Estimates from national surveys. *American Journal of Preventive Medicine* 33 (5, November): 412-417.

Williams, R.S., E.E. Logue, J.G. Lewis, T. Barton, N.W. Stead, A.G. Wallace, and S.V. Pizzo. 1980. Physical conditioning augments the fibrinolytic response to venous occlusion in healthy adults. *N Engl J Med* 302 (18): 987-991.

Wilmore, J.H., J.P. Despres, P.R. Stanforth, S. Mandel, T. Rice, J. Gagnon, A.S. Leon, D. Rao, J.S. Skinner, and C. Bouchard. 1999. Alterations in body weight and composition consequent to 20 wk of endurance training: The HERITAGE Family Study. *American Journal of Clinical Nutrition* 70 (3, September): 346-352.

Witmer, J.M., M.R. Hensel, P.S. Holck, A.S. Ammerman, and J.C. Will. 2004. Heart disease prevention for Alaska Native women: A review of pilot study findings. *Journal of Women's Health* 13 (5): 569-578.

Wolin, K.Y., Y. Yan, G.A. Colditz, and I-M. Lee. 2009. Physical activity and colon cancer prevention: A meta-analysis. *British Journal of Cancer* 100: 611-616.

Wood, P.D., W.L. Haskell, S.N. Blair, P.T. Williams, R.N. Krauss, F.T. Lindgren, J.J. Albers, P.H. Ho, and J.W. Farquhar. 1983. Increased exercise level and plasma lipoprotein concentrations: A one-year, randomized, controlled study in sedentary, middle-aged men. *Metabolism* 32: 31-39.

World Health Organization. 2001. *International classification of functioning, disability, and health, ICF.* Geneva: World Health Organization.

Wu, M.K., C.K. Wang, Y.M. Bai, C.Y. Huang, and S.D. Lee. 2007. Outcomes of obese, clozapine-treated inpatients with schizophrenia placed on a six-month diet and physical activity program. *Psychiatr Serv* 58 (4): 544-50.

Yang, D., L. Bernstein, and A.H. Wu. 2003. Physical activity and breast cancer risk among Asian-American women in Los Angeles: A case-control study. *Cancer* 97 (10, May 15): 2565-2575.

Yeh, C-K., and G.A. Rodan. 1984. Tensile forces enhance prostaglandin E synthesis in osteoblastic cells grown on collagen ribbons. *Calcified Tissue International* 36 (Suppl.): S67-S71.

Young, A. 1986. Exercise physiology in geriatric practice. *Acta Medica Scandinavica* 711 (Suppl.): 227-232.

Zahran, H.S., R. Kobau, D.G. Moriarty, M.M. Zack, J. Holt, and R. Donehoo. 2005. Health-related quality of life surveillance—United States, 1993-2002. *MMWR Surveill Summ* 54 (4): 1-35.

CHAPTER 16

Adverse Events and Hazards of Physical Activity

Both excessive and defective exercise destroys the strength.

· Aristotle 384-322 BC ·
Eudemian Ethics

*The secret of my abundant health is that whenever the urge to exercise comes upon me,
I lie down for a while and it passes.*

· R.M. Hutchins ·
President, University of Chicago, 1929-1951

CHAPTER OBJECTIVES

‣ Describe the prevalence rates of common injuries from sports and other physical activities according to population groups

‣ Identify common risk factors for adverse events during physical activity

‣ Discuss the methods used to study hazards and adverse events of physical activity

‣ Discuss the challenges of defining exposure and injury severity in population studies

‣ Describe precautions that might reduce rates and severity of traumatic brain injury, heat injury, and musculoskeletal injury during sport participation

‣ Evaluate whether the strength of evidence allows the conclusion that physical activity causes injury and cardiovascular mortality

‣ Describe potential psychological hazards of abusive exercise in some people

Contrary to the satirical wit of R.M. Hutchins, this book has confirmed that leisure-time physical activity, rather than sedentariness, is associated with lower risk of premature death and several chronic diseases. Nonetheless, there is an ironic grain of truth in the opening quote by Aristotle; vigorous physical activity is not without increased risk of **injury,** and even sudden death, in some circumstances. Just as the precise dose–response relationship between physical activity and lowered health risk is not yet known for most chronic diseases, neither are the types, amounts, and settings of physical activity that increase its hazards and adverse events (i.e., harms of exercise intervention in medical treatment) fully known. Nonetheless, it is likely that the golden mean of Aristotle, "All things in moderation," holds for many of the health benefits of exercise. More is not always better. Knowledge about the association between injury and exposure to different types of physical activity in different settings and environmental conditions is necessary to identify activities that optimize long-term health benefits while minimizing injury and sudden death.

The epidemiologic study of the hazards of occupational physical activity can be traced to the observations of Bernardino Ramazzini in the late 1600s. In his 1713 book *De Morbis Artificum Diatriba (The Diseases of Workers),* Ramazzini recommended moderation to prevent illness in jobs that required severe muscular exertion such as that performed by bricklayers, woodworkers, and printers: "Therefore in work so taxing moderation would be the best safeguard against these maladies, for men and women alike; for the common maxim 'nothing in excess' is one of which I excessively approve" (Ramazzini 1983). However, the modern study of the hazards of leisure-time physical activity did not get organized until about 250 years later, as described by Dr. Jeffrey Koplan, former director of the Centers for Disease Control and Prevention:

> If we are to continue advocating exercise as a health-promoting activity, it is our responsibility as advocates and health professionals to provide the public with information that presents a full and balanced view of exercise, namely, its benefits and risks.

—Koplan, Siscovick, and Goldbaum, 1985

▷ **IN 1713,** Bernardino Ramazzini, possibly the first injury epidemiologist, recommended moderation to prevent illness in jobs that required severe muscular exertion.

Magnitude of the Problem

The spectrum of potentially adverse events and hazards of physical activity participation is broad. It includes, for example, musculoskeletal injuries (the most common), traumatic head injury, heat and cold injuries, infectious diseases, and even cardiac death. However, few precise estimates of the incidence of injuries during leisure-time physical activity among adults of different ages and exposure are available,

either worldwide or in the United States. The 1994 Injury Control and Risk Survey (ICARIS) interviewed over 5000 English-speaking adults by telephone after random-digit dialing of U.S. residential households (Powell et al. 1998). The 30-day injury rates reported among participants in five activities were then estimated for the period of late spring and early summer of 1994 and extrapolated to the U.S. adult population ages 18 years and older. Prevalence rates and numbers were 0.9% (330,000 people) for outdoor bicycling, 1.4% (1,877,000) for walking, 1.4% (2,131,000) for gardening and yard work, 1.6% (394,000) for aerobics, and 2.4% (964,000) for weightlifting.

According to estimates from the National Hospital Ambulatory Medical Care Survey (NHAMCS) conducted between 1997 and 1998, about 1.1 million adults over 24 years of age and 2.6 million children and young adults who played sports or otherwise exercised visited an emergency room as the result of an activity-related injury (Burt and Overpeck 2001). According to that study, 25% of all emergency room injuries among people ages 5 to 24 years resulted from sport participation. The most common emergency room injuries seen in that age range were from basketball (447,000 visits), cycling (421,000 visits), football (271,000 visits), and baseball or softball (245,000). Other risky sports were ice and roller skating, skateboarding, gymnastics, and water and snow sports. Playground injuries led to 137,000 emergency room visits (Burt and Overpeck 2001).

An updated analysis of the NHAMCS between 1997 and 2001 estimated that each year there were 2.5 million visits to emergency rooms for sport injuries by patients younger than 19 years, 23% of all injury-related visits (Simon, Bublitz, and Hambidge 2006). Higher rates were seen among males, whites, and ages over 5 years. The most common injuries (fractures and dislocations, sprains and strains, open wounds, and bruises) occurred during cycling, basketball, playground activity, and football (figure 16.1).

Subsequent analyses by the Centers for Disease Control and Prevention (CDC) of data from the National Electronic Injury Surveillance System-All Injury Program (NEISS-AIP) indicate higher rates of sport- and recreation-related injuries in the U.S. population than estimated by the earlier NHAMCS. In 2001, an estimated 29.7 million people were treated for nonfatal injuries of any kind at U.S. hospital emergency departments (age-adjusted rate, 10.4% of the population) (Vyrostek, Annest, and Ryan 2004). During that approximate period, the rate of sport- and recreation-related injuries treated in U.S. hospital emergency rooms was estimated to be 4.3 million cases (1.54% of the population), accounting for about 15% of all **unintentional injury**–related visits (Gotsch, Annest, and Holmgreen 2002).

▷ **IN THE** United States, nearly 1.5 million adults over 20 years of age and 3 million children and youths visit an emergency room each year as a result of an injury from sports or other leisure-time physical activities.

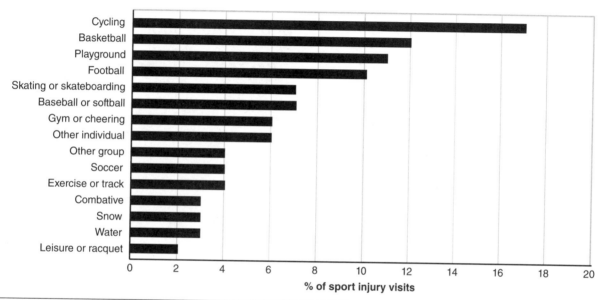

Figure 16.1   Sport-related injuries in youths seen at U.S. emergency rooms.

Data from Simon, Bublitz, and Hambidge 2006.

Eleven Riskiest Activities in the United States

The number (percentage of total) of injury cases from the eight riskiest activities for males and females who received emergency room treatment in the United States from July 2000 to June 2001.

Data from Gotsch, Annest, and Holmgreen 2002.

Males (2,978,423 total cases)	Females (1,272,299 total cases)
Basketball 520,032 (17.5%)	Bicycling 163,012 (12.8%)
Bicycling 434,371 (14.6%)	Basketball 114,644 (9%)
Football 374,072 (12.6%)	Playground 108,023 (8.5%)
Exercise 140,661 (4.7%)	Exercise 98,475 (7.7%)
Baseball 136,632 (4.6%)	Gymnastics 73,405 (5.8%)
Playground 127,028 (4.3%)	Soccer 60,987 (4.8%)
Soccer 104,775 (3.5%)	Softball 56,759 (4.5%)
Skateboarding 84,457 (2.8%)	Horseback riding 45,336 (3.6%)

The percentage of all unintentional injury–related visits associated with sport and recreation was highest for people aged 10 to 14 years (51.5% for boys, 38.0% for girls) and lowest for persons aged >45 years (6.4% for men, 3.1% for women). Types of sport- and recreation-related activities in which the injuries occurred varied by age and sex. Among people aged up to 9 years, the leading types were playground- and bicycle-related injuries. Scooter- and trampoline-related injuries ranked among the top seven types of injuries for both boys and girls aged up to 9 years. For males aged 10 to 19 years, football-, basketball-, and bicycle-related injuries were most common. For females aged 10 to 19 years, basketball-related injuries ranked highest. Among people aged 20 to 24 years, basketball- and bicycle-related injuries were among the three leading types of injuries. Basketball-related injuries ranked highest for men aged 25 to 44 years. Exercise (e.g., weightlifting, aerobics, stretching, walking, jogging, and running) was the leading injury-related activity for women aged >20 years and ranked among the top four types of injuries for men aged >20 years.

Another study described the types and frequencies of musculoskeletal injuries among a cohort of 5028 men and 1285 women, 20 to 85 years of age, who were participants in the Aerobics Center Longitudinal Study (ACLS) and had above-average levels of physical activity (Hootman et al. 2002a). The participants reported detailed information about their physical activity levels and injuries between 1970 and 1982, when their initial clinical examinations occurred, and 1986, when they responded to a mailed survey about their physical activity habits and history of orthopedic injuries. An injury was defined as any self-reported soft tissue or bone injury that occurred during the 12 months preceding the survey. Injuries that participants said occurred as a result of their participation in a formal exercise program were classified as activity-related injuries. Twenty-five percent of the cohort reported that they had experienced musculoskeletal injury during the past year, and 83% of those injuries were activity related, mainly from sport participation. More than two-thirds of the activity-related injuries occurred in the lower extremities, especially the knee. Men and women had similar rates of injuries, which are depicted in figure 16.2.

According to the scientific advisory committee of the 2008 Physical Activity Guidelines for Americans, walking for exercise, gardening or yard work, bicycling or exercise cycling, dancing, swimming, and golf have the lowest injury rates in the United States (Physical Activity Guidelines Advisory Committee 2008).

> ▶ **WALKING FOR** exercise, gardening or yard work, bicycling or exercise cycling, dancing, swimming, and golf have the lowest injury rates in the United States.

High School, Collegiate, and Olympic Sport

According to the High School Sports-Related Injury Surveillance Study, an estimated 1.44 million injuries occurred during practice or competition in the 2005-2006 school year, an average of 2.44 injuries for every 1000 athletes exposed (CDC 2006). Rates were highest in boys' football and wrestling and lowest in boys' baseball and girls' softball (see table 16.1). About half the injuries were sprains or strains, with contusions, fractures, and concussions each accounting for 10% to 15% of the cases.

During 16 years of National Collegiate Athletic Association (NCAA) Injury Surveillance System reports, there were 182,000 injuries and more than 1 million exposure records from 1988-1989 through 2003-2004 (Hootman, Dick, and Agel 2007). Game and practice injuries that required medical attention and resulted in at least one day of time loss were included. Injury rates per 1000 athlete exposures (AE; an athlete exposure = one athlete participating in one practice or game) were higher in games (13.8/1000AE) than in practices (4.0/1000AE), and preseason practice injury rates (6.6) were significantly higher than both in-season (2.3/1000AE) and postseason (1.4/1000AE) practice rates. More than half of injuries were to the lower extremity, with

Most Frequent Types and Sites of Injury in the United States

The most frequent types and body parts of injuries diagnosed during emergency room treatment in the United States from July 2000 to June 2001 (percentage of total cases).

Data from Gotsch, Annest, and Holmgreen 2002.

Type of injury	Site of injury
Strain/sprain (29.1%)	Ankle (12.1%)
Fracture (20.5%)	Finger (9.5%)
Contusion/abrasion (20.1%)	Face (9.2%)
Laceration (13.8%)	Head (8.2%)
	Knee (8.1%)

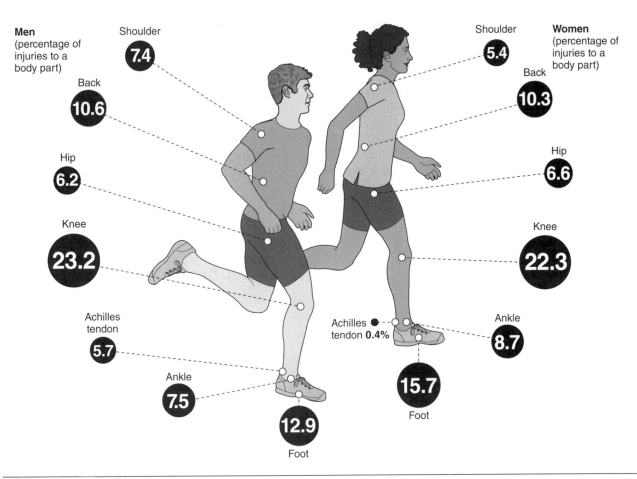

Figure 16.2 Distribution and percentage of activity-related musculoskeletal injuries by body part and gender.

Data from Hootman et al. 2002, "Epidemiology of musculoskeletal injuries among sedentary and physically active adults."

Table 16.1 Sport-Specific Injury Rates in Practice, Competition, and Overall

Sport	Practice	Competition	Overall
Boys' football	2.45	12.09	4.36
Boys' wrestling	2.04	3.93	2.50
Boys' soccer	1.58	4.22	2.43
Girls' soccer	1.10	5.21	2.36
Girls' basketball	1.37	3.60	2.01
Boys' basketball	1.46	2.98	1.89
Girls' volleyball	1.48	1.92	1.64
Boys' baseball	0.87	1.77	1.19
Girls' softball	0.79	1.78	1.13
All sports	**1.69**	**4.63**	**2.44**

Rate per 1000 athletes exposed as investigated by the High School Sports-Related Injury Surveillance Study in the United States for the 2005-2006 school year.

Data from Centers for Disease Control 2006.

ankle ligament sprains most common (15% of all injuries). Rates of concussions and anterior cruciate ligament injuries increased 7% and 1.3%, respectively, each year. Football had the highest injury rates for both practices (9.6/1000AE) and games (35.9/1000AE). Men's baseball had the lowest rate in practice (1.9/1000AE), and women's softball had the lowest rate in games (4.3/1000AE). In football, the rate ratio for games compared to fall practices was greatest for upper leg contusions (18.1), acromioclavicular joint sprains (14.0), knee internal derangements (13.4), ankle ligament sprains (12.0), and concussions (11.1) (Dick et al. 2007).

Although their public health impact is low because of low participation rates, top-level sports confer similar injury rates. At the 2008 Summer Olympic Games, 1055 injuries were reported by 92 national teams (9.6 injuries per 100 registered athletes) (Junge et al. 2009). Nearly three-fourths of the injuries occurred during competition. Half were severe enough to keep the athlete from participating in competition or training. The most prevalent injuries were ankle sprains and thigh strains. The majority (72.5%) of injuries were incurred in competition. The risk of incurring an injury was highest in soccer, taekwondo, hockey, handball, weightlifting, and boxing (all 15% or more of the participating athletes) and lowest for sailing, canoeing/kayaking, rowing, synchronized swimming, diving, fencing, and swimming.

Among athletes with disability who participate in Summer Paralympic events, abrasions, strains, sprains, and contusions are more common than fractures and dislocations but depend on type of disability and sport (Ferrara and Peterson 2000). Lower extremity injuries are more common in ambulatory athletes (those who are visually impaired, amputees, those with cerebral palsy), and upper extremity injuries are more frequent in athletes who use a wheelchair. When injuries were expressed as time lost in participation, 52% resulted in seven days lost or less, 29% in eight to 21 days lost, and 19% in 22 or more days lost. A prospective study showed an injury rate of 9.3 injuries per 1000 athlete exposures, which is similar to the rates among able-bodied participants in American football and soccer (Ferrara et al. 2000). During the 20-day period of the 2002 Winter Paralympics, medical personnel recorded 39 injuries involving 9% of the Paralympic athletes (Webborn, Willick, and Reeser 2006). Most were acute, traumatic injuries in Alpine skiing and sledge hockey. Sprains (32%), fractures (21%), and strains and lacerations (14% each) represented the most common diagnoses. Of the recorded injuries, eight (21%) resulted in time lost from training or competition.

There is a lack of uniformity or standards in methods of reporting injury, particularly injury severity (Alexandrescu, O'Brien, and Lecky 2009). Two ways to judge severity of a sport injury are the number of lost days of participation and whether the injury requires hospitalization. Figure 16.3

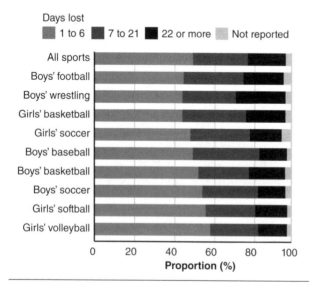

Figure 16.3 Proportion of injuries by number of days lost for various high school sports—High School Sports-Related Injury Surveillance Study, United States, 2005-2006 school year.

*Includes athletes who returned to their teams after >22 days and athletes who were out for the remainder of the season as a result of their injuries.

Data from Centers for Disease Control 2006.

shows, for example, that injuries in boys' football and wrestling and girls' basketball were more likely to keep athletes out of participation for a week or more, whereas injuries in girls' volleyball and softball were more likely to be short-term, keeping athletes out less than a week.

Nationally, high school athletes had an estimated 446,715 injuries from 2005 to 2007 that kept them from participating for more than 21 days (Darrow et al. 2009). The severe injury rate (incidence per 1000 athlete exposures) was greater in competition (0.79/1000AE) than in practice (0.24/1000AE). The most commonly injured body sites were the knee (29%), ankle (12%), and shoulder (11%). The most common injuries were fractures (36%), complete ligament sprains (15%), and incomplete ligament sprains (14%).

Traumatic Brain Injury

The CDC estimates that more than 1 million people with a traumatic brain injury (TBI) are treated and released from U.S. hospital emergency rooms each year, and an additional 235,000 are hospitalized for these injuries (Langlois, Rutland-Brown, and Wald 2006). TBIs can result in long-term memory loss and behavioral changes, including increased risks of depression and dementia.

Head injury during recreational and competitive sport participation reached epidemic status during the past decade (Daneshvar et al. 2011), with an estimated 3.8 million cases annually in the United States; loss of consciousness occurs in about 300,000 cases (CDC 1997; Langlois, Rutland-Brown, and Wald 2006). Among competitive sports, American football has the highest rate of head injuries in the United States; an estimated 4% to 20% of all participants suffer a mild TBI (a concussion) each season (Bailes and Cantu 2001), representing an estimated 8.9% of athletic injuries in high school (Gessell et al. 2007).

In the Nationwide Inpatient Sample, 755 U.S. youths 5 to 18 years of age were hospitalized for a nonfatal sport-related concussion (half the cases lost consciousness) between 2000 and 2004 (Yang et al. 2008). Extrapolated to the population, this represented 3712 hospitalizations and nearly $6 million each year in hospital charges for a day of observation, on average.

Based on reports from 100 high schools and 180 colleges to the High School Reporting Information Online (RIO) and the National Collegiate Athletic Association Injury Surveillance System, concussions were 9% (n = 396) of all high school athletic injuries and 6% (n = 482) of all collegiate athletic injuries during the 2005-2006 school year. Rates were highest in football and soccer and were higher among high school girls in sports played by both boys and girls (i.e., soccer, basketball) (Gessel et al. 2007). The annual rates (%) of concussion in other sports include 7% for hockey, 6% for rugby, 2% for basketball, and 1% for baseball (Bailes and Cantu 2001).

Using the NEISS-AIP database, the CDC estimated that nearly 208,000 patients with nonfatal sport-related

Signs and Symptoms of a Concussion

Physical

Headache

Fuzzy or blurry vision

Cognitive

Difficulty thinking clearly

Feeling slowed down

Difficulty concentrating

Difficulty remembering new information

Emotional

Irritability

Sadness

More emotional

Nervousness or anxiety

Sleep

Sleeping more than usual

Sleeping less than usual

Trouble falling asleep

Reprinted from Centers for Disease Control. Available: http://www.cdc.gov/concussion/signs_symptoms.html.

TBIs were treated in U.S. emergency departments each year during 2001 through 2005. This represented 5% of all emergency department visits related to sport injuries (CDC 2007). See table 16.2. Overall, males accounted for approximately 70.5% of sport-related TBI emergency department visits. The highest rates for both males and females occurred among those aged 10 to 14 years, followed by those aged 15 to 19 years. Activities contributing the greatest number of TBI-related visits to emergency departments included bicycling, football, playground activities, basketball, and riding all-terrain vehicles (ATVs). TBIs accounted for greater than 7.5% of emergency department visits in certain activities, including horseback riding (11.7%), ice skating (10.4%), riding ATVs (8.4%), tobogganing/sledding (8.3%), and bicycling (7.7%).

According to the National Center for Catastrophic Sports Injury Research (NCCSIR), between 1982 and 1996, high school fall sports resulted in 387 direct deaths (caused by performance of the sport) and catastrophic injuries, with 374 (97%) related to football. Indirect deaths (secondary to overexertion while playing a sport) totaled 115, of which 89 (77%) were related to football. Though football had the highest death rates, the incidence rate was less than 1 player per 100,000 participants. High school winter sports during the same period resulted in 70 direct deaths and catastrophic injuries. Direct death rates were highest in wrestling (33 deaths) and basketball (seven deaths) but were less than 1 per 100,000 participants.

From 1945 through 1999, an estimated 497 brain injury–related deaths (86% were subdural hematoma) occurred among American football players. The greatest risks were from 1965 through 1969. There was a dramatic reduction in fatalities from 1975 through 1994 after the 1976 rule change that prohibits initial contact with the head and face during blocking and tackling and the enactment of the National Operating Committee on Standards for Athletic Equipment helmet standard, which occurred in colleges in 1978 and in high schools in 1980 (Cantu and Mueller 2003).

Prospective Cohort Studies

The population-based, observational studies discussed so far used cross-sectional or retrospective designs. Other studies have examined incidence rates over time in a population cohort. For example, Koplan, Rothenberg, and Jones (1995) conducted a 10-year follow-up of a cohort of participants in Atlanta's Peachtree Road Race, the world's largest 10 km race, with over 50,000 runners and walkers each year. During the year following the 1980 race, 37% of about 1400 runners reported that they had suffered an injury that required a reduction in their running distance for at least a week; 14% needed medical treatment (Koplan et al. 1982). About 500 of 1400 runners surveyed initially were surveyed 10 years later by mail regarding physical characteristics, smoking status, education, running and other exercise, body mass index (BMI), injuries, and treatment. Injury was defined as a musculoskeletal ailment that caused respondents to limit or eliminate exercise or that disrupted school or work attendance. Results

Table 16.2   Estimated Hospitalizations for Nonfatal Injuries and Nonfatal TBIs Related to Sports and Recreation in the United States, All Ages, 2001-2005

Activity	All injuries	TBIs	% of TBIs that resulted in hospitalization	% of all injury hospitalizations that resulted from TBI
Bicycling	25,060	6300	16	25
All-terrain vehicle	16,500	3400	30	21
Mini bike/dirt bike	6100	1050	22	17
Football	6800	890	4	13
Baseball/softball	3760	810	6	22
Playground	9670	530	3	6
Basketball	4800	465	3	10
Skateboard	3070	430	8	14
Swimming/diving	3900	350	6	9
Skating	2950	260	5	9
Soccer	2650	200	2	8

Data from Centers for Disease Control 2007.

indicated that 56% of the respondents were still running and 81% continued to exercise in some form. Among men, 31% who no longer ran reported injury as the main reason for stopping. More than 50% of those surveyed reported at least one injury, most of which (32% for men, 28% for women) were to the knee. An inverted-U relationship existed between injuries and weekly distance (those who ran median distances had the most injuries). Overall, injury incidence was 1.02 per 10 person-years for all injuries and 0.58 for those requiring medical attention.

Evaluating Risk

Consistent with the concept of the epidemiologic triangle of host, agent, and environment introduced in chapter 2, before determining whether physical activity represents an independent hazard, it is necessary to consider people's prior risk of injury or death, the type of physical activity, and the environment where activity takes place. Factors that might affect the risk of injury during swimming, for example, are age; sex; whether the ear is predisposed to infection; and such attributes of the activity itself as type of stroke, frequency, speed, distance, and warm-up. For example, someone who swims freestyle often and has a flawed stroke might have increased risk for shoulder problems. A person with a vulnerable ear canal who swims in a warm lake might be at risk for an inner ear infection. The risk of injury during swimming depends not just on time of exposure but also on features of the swimmer and where and how the swimming occurs. About one-fourth of nonfatal heart attacks occur during some form of physical activity. However, the risk of serious cardiovascular complications during exercise is higher in people who have had a prior heart attack than in apparently healthy people.

Contributing factors include uncontrolled hypertension, a recent heavy meal, emotional excitement, and prolonged activity without adequate preparation. Given that exposure is a fundamental risk factor for disease and accidents, it is logical that the most prevalent physical activities should be associated with the highest rates of injury and sudden death. The National Health Interview Survey published in 1991 estimated that, based on percentage of participation, the most popular activities reported by adults 18 years of age or older in the United States were walking (44%), gardening or yard work (29%), stretching exercises (26%), riding a bicycle or stationary exercise cycle (15%), resistance exercise (e.g., weightlifting; 14%), stair climbing (11%), jogging or running (9%), aerobics and aerobic dance (7%), and swimming (6%) (National Center for Health Statistics 1991). Among those activities, evidence about rates and risk factors of injury or death is available only for jogging or running and aerobic dance.

Host Factors

As in previous chapters that dealt with positive health outcomes of physical activity, here it is equally important to judge risk for hazards and adverse events associated with

physical activity according to characteristics of the individual (host). Here we consider age, sex, physical activity experience, injury history, and body mass.

Age

The NEISS-AIP study of U.S. emergency room visits found that unintentional injury–related visits associated with sport and recreation were highest for people aged 10 to 14 years (51.5% for boys, 38.0% for girls) and lowest for persons aged >45 years (Gotsch, Annest, and Holmgreen 2002). However, those rates were not adjusted for time of exposure during participation in risky sports among younger people. Hence, injury rates were likely confounded by sport participation rates. In an early review of running injury studies, van Mechelen (1992) concluded that age was not independently associated with injury. That conclusion was supported by Koplan, Rothenberg, and Jones (1995), who found only a minor increase in the rate of injury among male runners over the age of 50. No other age-related differences were found. Population-based studies examining multiple sports found that sport participants ages 20 to 24 (Kujala et al. 1995; Sandelin et al. 1988; Sandelin and Santavirta 1991) or 16 to 25 (Nicholl, Coleman, and Williams 1995) had a higher incidence of injury than other age groups. However, it may be that people of this age group are more likely to be involved in sports in which injury incidence is high.

▷ **INJURY DURING** vigorous physical activity appears to be independent of age from youth through middle age; it is an equal-opportunity hazard. However, aging becomes a key risk factor among the elderly. Even so, regularly active seniors report fewer injuries from all causes than do physically inactive seniors.

Some studies have looked at injury incidence in particular age groups, namely, school-aged youths and the elderly. Many children's primary exposure to physical activity is in organized sport and physical education classes.

The incidence of injuries from all causes differs according to people's age and their level of physical activity. Among younger people, those who are physically active report more injuries that require medical attention than those who are inactive. In contrast, older people who are inactive report more injuries (see table 16.3) (Carlson et al. 2006).

Sex

The scientific advisory committee of the 2008 Physical Activity Guidelines for Americans concluded that, aside from stress fractures and injuries to the anterior cruciate ligament of the knee, which are more common in females, risks of activity-related injuries appear similar in males and females, especially when rates are adjusted for the commonly lower level of initial physical fitness among females (Physical Activity Guidelines Advisory Committee 2008).

Table 16.3   Annual Incidence* of Self-Reported Injury Requiring Medical Advice by Age Group and Leisure-Time Physical Activity Level

Age group (years)	Overall	Active[H]	Insufficiently active	Inactive[I]
18-24	116.6	126.4	132.5	96.5
25-34	97.3	112.7	85.1	91.8
35-44	87.0	93.0	75.5	91.2
45-64	76.4	72.6	76.5	81.6
65+	68.1	60.6	56.1	74.4

* Incidence per 1000 population.

[H] Meet current physical activity recommendations.

[I] Report no leisure-time light-moderate or vigorous physical activity.

Data from Carlson et al. 2006.

Data from the National Collegiate Athletic Association Injury Surveillance System were used to compare the five-year rate (1989-1993) of knee injuries among 300,000 male and female collegiate athletes participating in soccer and basketball (Arendt and Dick 1995). The incidence of knee injuries among soccer players was higher in females (1.6 cases per 1000 athletes) than males (1.3 cases per 1000 athletes).

The rate of injury (expressed as a percentage of athletes) to the anterior cruciate ligament (ACL) of the knee in women's soccer (0.31%) was double the rate in men's soccer (0.13%), or one ACL injury per 161 activity sessions in women compared to one ACL injury per 385 activity sessions in men. Likewise, in basketball the ACL injury rate of 0.29% (one injury per 247 activity sessions) in women was four times higher than the rate of 0.07% (one injury per 952 activity sessions) in men. Rates of other types of knee injuries did not differ between men and women (Kirkendall and Garrett 2000).

Finnish Youth

The incidence and risk factors for a major knee ligament injury were studied in a population-based cohort of 46,472 Finnish adolescents, ages 14 to 18 years (Parkkari et al. 2008). During an average follow-up of nine years, 0.6% of the cohort (194 males and 71 females) were hospitalized and treated for an anterior or posterior cruciate ligament injury. The injury incidence was 61 cases (95% CI: 54-68) per 100,000 person-years of exposure. After adjustment for socioeconomic, health, and lifestyle factors, the risk among those who participated in organized sport clubs four or more times each week, compared to those who never participated, was twice as high for females (8.5; 95% CI: 4.3-16.4) as for males (4.0; 95% CI: 2.7-6.1).

New Zealand Adults

Data from New Zealand's national no-fault Accident Compensation Corporation for knee ligament injuries between 1 July 2000 and 30 June 2005 were used to estimate incident risks of ACL surgeries in the population of New Zealand (Gianotti et al. 2009). The incidence rate was 36.9 per 100,000 person-years. Sixty-five percent of those injuries occurred during recreation or sport participation. Between ages 20 and 35, males had about twice the incidence rate that females did. However, no attempt was made to equate the sexes on sport participation exposure, and it seems likely that males were more exposed. Rugby, netball, and soccer, which are popular sports for males of those ages, accounted for 70% of the ACL injuries.

United States Military Academy, West Point

In a four-year study of ACL injury incidence among participants in mandatory physical activities at West Point (i.e., intramural, club, or intercollegiate sports; military training; and physical education classes), the injury rate, excluding male-only sports, was about 50% greater in women (rate ratio, 1.51; 95% CI: 1.03-2.21). Rate ratios were higher for women than men in a gymnastics course (5.67; 95% CI: 1.99-16.16), an indoor obstacle course test (3.72; 95% CI: 1.25-11.10), and basketball (2.42; 95% CI: 1.05-5.59) (Mountcastle et al. 2007).

Meta-Analysis

Meta-analytic principles were applied to generate ACL incidences as a function of gender, sport, and prior injury-reduction training (Prodromos et al. 2007). The ratio of female to male ACL tear incidence ratios were as follows: basketball, 3.5; soccer, 2.67; lacrosse, 1.18; and Alpine skiing, 1.0. The collegiate soccer tear rate was 0.32 for female subjects and 0.12 for male subjects. For basketball, the rates were 0.29 and 0.08, respectively. The rate for recreational Alpine skiers was 0.63, and that for experts was 0.03, with no gender variance. Recreational Alpine skiers had the highest incidences of ACL tear, whereas expert Alpine skiers had the lowest incidences. Alpine skiers and lacrosse players showed no gender difference in ACL tear rate. The two volleyball studies showed no ACL tears. Volleyball may in fact be a low-risk sport rather than a high-risk sport. Year-round female athletes who play soccer and basketball have an ACL tear rate of approximately 5%.

Sex Differences and General Injury Risk

Other information on sex differences in exercise-related injury rates is inconclusive. Some studies that investigated sex differences showed that males are at higher risk for injury (Garrick, Gillien, and Whiteside 1986; Nicholl, Coleman, and Williams 1995; Sandelin et al. 1988); others reported higher injury incidence in females (Koplan, Rothenberg, and Jones 1995); and still others showed no differences between the sexes (Backx et al. 1991; de Loes, Jacobsen, and Goldie 1990; Kujala et al. 1995; Zebas et al. 1995). For runners, there appear to be no sex differences in injury risk, though few studies included enough women to allow accurate comparisons (van Mechelen 1992). More injury risk studies are needed that have equivalent participation rates for men and women.

▷ **OTHER THAN** higher rates of tears of the ACL at the knee among females, information available on sex differences in injury rates during vigorous physical activity is sparse or inconclusive.

A prospective, cohort analysis of data from the Aerobics Center Longitudinal Study examined whether sex-specific predictors of lower extremity injury could be identified among 5028 men and 1285 women who participated in running, walking, or jogging for exercise (Hootman et al. 2002b). Possible predictor variables included height, weight, and cardiorespiratory fitness measured at an initial physical examination conducted between 1970 and 1981. Other predictors, along with self-reports of lower extremity (i.e., legs and feet) musculoskeletal injuries and physical activity levels, were obtained from a follow-up mail survey in which participants were asked for their recall over two preceding time periods, five years and 12 months. An injury was defined as any lower extremity injury that required a consultation with a physician. Among men, previous lower extremity injury was the strongest predictor of lower extremity injury (relative risk [RR] = 1.93 to 2.09), regardless of recall period. Among women, mileage exceeding 20 miles/week was the strongest predictor for the five-year period (RR = 2.08), and previous lower extremity injury was the strongest predictor for the 12-month period (RR = 2.81).

Several studies found that the risk of injury during standard U.S. Army basic combat training was about twice as high in women as in men (Bell et al. 2000; Canham et al. 1998; Knapik et al. 2001). For example, in a comparison of 756 men and 474 women, a subsample of 182 men and 168 women completed fitness tests and questionnaires about physical activity and smoking before combat training began (Knapik et al. 2001). All soldiers were then administered the Army Physical Fitness Test consisting of push-ups, sit-ups, and a 3.2 km run. Injuries were registered from medical records. Women had over twice the injury rate of men. For men and women, fewer push-ups, slower 3.2 km run times, lower peak $\dot{V}O_2$, and cigarette smoking were risk factors for time-loss injury. Among the men only, lower levels of physical activity before combat training commenced and both high and low levels of flexibility were also time-loss injury risk factors. Lower peak $\dot{V}O_2$ and cigarette smoking were independent risk factors for time-loss injury for both men and women.

The sex difference in injury rates among soldiers during basic combat training appears to be confounded with differences in fitness among men and women (Bell et al. 2000). Among 861 trainees observed during their eight-week basic combat training course, women experienced twice as many

injuries as men and had 2.5 times higher risk of time-loss injuries than men. However, when the lower fitness and higher fatness of women at the beginning of training were adjusted for, sex was no longer an independent predictor of injury risk. In both men and women, the least-fit 25% of soldiers had about 50% higher risk of time-loss injuries (Knapik 1998). See figure 16.4.

In a study of 251 soldiers at Fort Leonard Wood, Missouri, the risks of injury during combat training were virtually the same and not statistically different between women and men when they were compared within each quartile of sex-specific fitness levels based on 2-mile run performance (table 16.4) (Canham et al. 1998).

Though the explanation is not yet known, males appear to be at higher risk of nontraumatic sport-related death among competitive athletes. In an analysis of data from the National Center for Catastrophic Sports Injury Research over

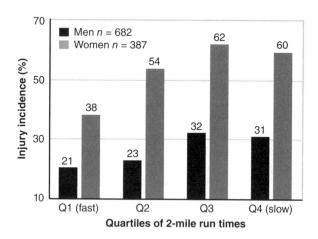

Figure 16.4 Time-loss injuries during basic combat training according to sex and fitness level.

Data from Knapik 1998.

Table 16.4   Risk of Injury Is the Same for Men and Women When Compared on Sex-Specific Fitness Level

Quartile (time in minutes)	Risk (women)	Risk (men)	RR
Q1 + Q2 (<18.00)	33%	29%	1.1
Q3 (18.01-23.00)	47%	41%	1.1
Q4 (20.36-23.00)	58%	43%	1.4
Q5 (23.01+)	60%	80%	0.8

Data from Canham et al. 1998

a 10-year period from July 1983 to June 1993, nontraumatic sport deaths were reported in 126 high school athletes (115 males and 11 females) and 34 college athletes (31 males and three females) (Van Camp et al. 1995). Estimated annual death rates in male athletes (7.5 per million athletes) were five times higher than in female athletes (1.33 per million athletes). Cardiovascular conditions (especially hypertrophic cardiomyopathy and congenital coronary artery anomalies) were the most common causes of death.

Although epidemiologic evidence about risks is scant, current medical opinion is that healthy women with uncomplicated pregnancies can safely participate in most aerobic and recreational activities of moderate intensity (American College of Obstetricians and Gynecologists 2002).

Physical Activity Experience

The SAID (specific adaptations to imposed demands) principle is basic to the effectiveness and safety of physical conditioning. Fitness (i.e., tolerance for physical exertion) is increased when tissues (such as skeletal muscles, ligaments, and bones), organs (such as the heart and liver), joints, and the nervous system adapt after graduated exposure to new demands that are challenging but tolerable without causing damage or injury. Increases in fitness are specific to the type and timing of physical activities. New demands that exceed fitness, that are unusual, or that allow too little time for recovery and adaptation increase the odds of injury.

Van Mechelen (1992) reported that men with less running experience may be more likely to suffer an acute injury when running, but results have been inconclusive. Macera and colleagues (1989) found that runners with less than three years' running experience had an injury odds ratio of 2.2 compared with runners who had more than three years' experience. Among students 14 to 19 years of age, those who were more physically active outside of school (2 or more hours per week) were less likely to be injured than their sedentary peers (de Loes, Jacobsen, and Goldie 1990). Risk factors for exercise injuries during 12 weeks of army infantry training were evaluated among 303 young men (Jones et al. 1993). Physical training was documented on a daily basis, and injuries were registered by medical records. One or more lower extremity injuries (mainly muscle strains, ankle and knee sprains, and overuse syndrome of the knee) accounted for 80% of the injuries. Risk factors were older age, smoking, previous injury (sprained ankles), low levels of previous occupational and physical activity, low frequency of running before entry into the army, flexibility (both high and low), low physical fitness at entry, and high running mileage during training.

Although the risk of musculoskeletal injury during running is related to the amount of running, the risk per mile of exposure diminishes as mileage increases. The rate of injury per mile is about 10 times higher at 5 miles per week (~500 MET-minutes per week) than at 40 miles per week (~4000 MET-minutes per week) (Jones, Cowan, and Knapik 1994; Marti 1988). See figures 16.5 and 16.6.

Similar risks were observed for participants in the Aerobics Center Longitudinal Study (Hootman and Powell 2009). The annual risk of injury for people who spent about 2000 kcal per week (2470 MET-minutes per week) in exercise (mainly walking, jogging, or running) was 22%. The comparable risk was 65% (about 6.5% per 1000 kcal) in people who spent 10,000 kcal per week. On balance, the evidence indicates that adults who meet the current public health recommendation of adding about 500 MET-minutes of moderate to vigorous physical activity each week will be at higher risk of injury if they are currently less active than if they are already active.

▶ **THOUGH EXPOSURE** is a risk factor for hazards during physical activity, previous experience in physical activity or sport seems to reduce the risk of injury.

Injury History

Several epidemiological studies have found a greater risk for injury during physical activity among people who previously suffered an exercise-related injury, especially runners (Jacobs and Berson 1986; Koplan et al. 1982; Macera et al. 1989; Marti et al. 1988; Walter et al. 1989). Van Mechelen (1992) concluded that previous running injuries were an independent risk factor for future running injuries, and Marti and colleagues (1988) found a 65% increase in risk of injury for previously injured runners. In studies of marathon running, those who needed treatment during and immediately after the marathon were more likely to have had an injury before the race (Kretsch et al. 1984). In earlier studies, this effect was not adjusted for other running characteristics such as running distance, and it was not clear whether a previous injury represented additional risk for future injuries after adjustment for distance. However, several studies found a previous injury to be a significant predictor of injury during follow-up, even after controlling for distance (Macera et al. 1989; Marti et al. 1988; Walter et al. 1989). It is not clear whether this finding suggests incomplete healing of the original injury, incomplete rehabilitation of supporting structures, a susceptibility to injury recurrence because of body structure, an uncorrected flaw in running gait, or faulty training practices.

Garrick, Gillien, and Whiteside (1986) reported that participants in group aerobics who had previously experienced a knee, leg, or ankle injury were twice as likely to have a subsequent similar injury as were their peers without a history of orthopedic injury during physical activity. Among male and female participants in the Aerobics Center Longitudinal Study, previous lower extremity injury was one of the strongest predictors of lower extremity injury during the past year (Hootman et al. 2002b).

▶ **A HISTORY OF** previous injury is a risk factor for future injury.

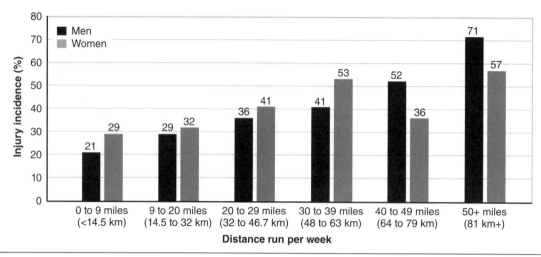

Figure 16.5 Running injury risks according to weekly running distance.

Data from Koplan et al. 1982.

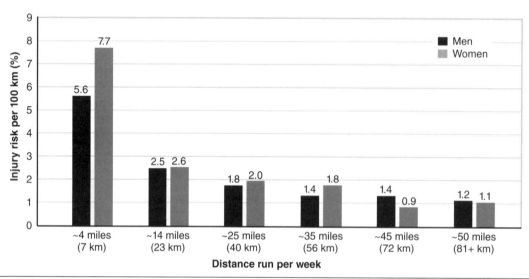

Figure 16.6 Running injury risks according to weekly running distance normalized to total running distance.

Data from Jones, Cowan, and Knapik 1994.

Body Mass

The effects of high or low weight or percent body fat on injury rates have been examined in several ways. Pollock and colleagues (1977) found that among those beginning a running program, those with a high percentage of body fat had more injuries. However, in this study, as in all studies of regular runners, there were very few obese individuals.

Some studies found no convincing evidence that body composition moderated injury rates (Koplan et al. 1982; Macera et al. 1989), whereas other studies reported a U-shaped relationship whereby both the lightest and heaviest groups were at increased risk for injuries compared to groups having average weight (Marti et al. 1988). However, population studies of the effects of body mass or fatness have

not yet adequately controlled for the confounding of body mass and running experience or the sampling bias related to the fact that most long-term runners have low body mass.

Features of the Agent: Physical Activity

Paradoxically, the same features of physical activity that are believed to reduce health risks for mortality and chronic diseases (namely the frequency, duration, intensity, and type of physical activity) also may increase the risk of injury. To date, however, the feature of physical activity most consistently reported as an injury risk factor is total exposure to physical activity (Jones, Cowan, and Knapik 1994). Less is known about the risks that specific features of physical activity,

Reducing Musculoskeletal Sport Injuries

Although stretching is often recommended as a safety measure for preventing injuries (James, Bates, and Osternig 1978), there is a paucity of evidence from population-based studies about its protective effects. Several studies of runners found no difference in injury rates between participants who stretch before running and those who don't stretch (Koplan et al. 1982; Macera et al. 1989), especially after controlling for weekly running distance and previous injury (Walter et al. 1989).

A systematic review of 32 randomized controlled trials including nearly 25,000 participants found evidence of the preventive effect of three types of injury prevention interventions: the use of insoles, use of external joint supports, and multi-intervention training programs (e.g., balance training, ankle discs, functional strengthening) (Aaltonen et al. 2007). In five trials including six different comparisons (2446 participants), custom-made or prefabricated insoles reduced lower limb injuries compared with no insoles in military recruits (risk reduction ≥50% in four comparisons). All seven studies investigating external joint supports

(10,300 participants) showed a tendency to prevent ankle, wrist, or knee injuries (risk reduction ≥50% in five studies). All six multi-intervention training programs (2809 participants) were effective in preventing sport injuries (risk reduction ≥50% in five studies).

Proposed Methods of Injury Prevention

- Stretching: Stretching is not protective against injuries associated with weight-bearing training, including delayed-onset muscle soreness (Thacker et al. 2004; Hart 2005; Herbert and de Noronha 2007).
- Warm-ups: Most studies show some benefit, but the quality of trials is weak (Fradkin, Gabbe, and Cameron 2006; Fradkin, Zazryn, and Smoliga 2010).
- Shock-absorbent insoles and orthotics: Evidence is mixed but leans toward nonprotective (D'hondt et al. 2002; Hume et al. 2008) except for military personnel (Rome, Handoll, and Ashford 2005).

namely frequency, duration, and intensity, each contribute to total physical activity exposure.

Total Exposure

Studies in different populations with different definitions of injury have consistently reported an increase in injuries with an increase in distance run, with risk increasing after about 33 km (20 miles) per week. This factor remained a strong predictor of injury even after adjustment for other running-related practices. Lysholm and Wiklander (1987) also found a positive association in marathon runners between the injury rate during any given month and the training distance covered during the previous month. Cumulative distance is more associated with injury than is the lack of rest between runs (James, Bates, and Osternig 1978). For example, Marti (1988) found no differences in injury rates among runners who ran similar overall weekly distances but ran the distance in two, three, or four training sessions per week.

▶ **WEEKLY MILEAGE** is the main risk factor for running injuries, more than running surface, time of day, or warm-up stretching.

Epidemiologic investigations consistently find that total exposure to physical activity is more strongly associated with increased injury incidence than the specific features of

intensity, frequency, or duration of physical activity (Backx et al. 1991; Jones, Cowan, and Knapik 1994; Koplan, Rothenberg, and Jones 1995; Marti et al. 1988; van Mechelen 1992). However, total exposure is easier to estimate than specific features, so more studies have used total exposure, rather than features, as the dose measure. Hence, the evidence about the dose–response relationships between physical activity and injury risk may be biased by the methods used to define physical activity exposure.

Frequency

The number of exercise sessions per week has been weakly related to physical activity injury incidence; but its influence has been poorly defined in population-based studies. Marti and colleagues (1988) found that injury rates during running were similar for weekly frequencies of two, three, and four sessions after adjusting for total running distance. Conversely, Garrick, Gillien, and Whiteside (1986) reported that aerobics participants who attended only one class per week had twice the injury incidence of those attending four classes per week when injury rates were expressed relative to time of total exposure. In a randomized controlled trial, Pollock and coworkers (1977) found that when distance, duration, and relative intensity were controlled, running injuries occurred twice as often among those who ran five days per week compared with those running one or three days per week.

Duration

The epidemiologic data on exercise duration and musculoskeletal injury are sparse. In the articles examined for this chapter, no data regarding duration of exercise sessions were given. Total exposure (e.g., person-hours or person-years of participation) was provided; and in studies of walking or running, a relative index of miles per week was commonly used (Backx et al. 1991; Koplan, Rothenberg, and Jones 1995; Kujala et al. 1995). Pollock and colleagues (1977) examined the influence of exercise duration on injury incidence while running frequency was held constant at three days per week. Participants who ran for a longer duration (45 min vs. 15 or 30 min) had a greater injury incidence rate.

Intensity

The only sport for which data on exercise intensity (in this case, speed) have been consistently recorded is running. For example, Marti and colleagues (1988) reported that a runner's best time on a 16 km (10 mile) run was associated with increased risk for running injury. However, running pace was not an important risk factor after adjustment for total distance. The paucity of data on the intensity of other types of physical activity prevents clear conclusions about the influence of the intensity of physical activity on injury risk (van Mechelen 1992).

Type of Physical Activity

Regardless of method used to define and measure types of physical activity, it is clear that injury rates differ according to types of physical activity (Backx et al. 1991; de Loes, Jacobsen, and Goldie 1990; Kujala et al. 1995; Nicholl, Coleman, and Williams 1995; Sandelin and Santavirta 1991). Individual and team sports that have high occurrences of physical collisions or contact between participants (e.g., American football, soccer, rugby, ice hockey, wrestling, basketball, karate, judo) have higher injury rates than physical activities that involve less contact or forces directed at other people or objects. Furthermore, more injuries occur during competition than during practice (Kujala et al. 1995). Organized sports have been shown to be responsible for a greater percentage (62%) of the total injuries incurred than physical education and nonorganized sports (Backx et al. 1991).

Unfortunately, several popular types of physical activity, such as golf, swimming, walking, cycling, and calisthenics, remain understudied (Koplan, Siscovick, and Goldbaum 1985). Population studies that compared injury rates among many types of physical activity (e.g., Burt and Overpeck 2001; Gotsch, Annest, and Holmgreen 2002) did not control for time of exposure and features of the participants, activities, and environments sufficiently to permit direct comparisons of independent risks among activities.

Finland

A year-long random survey of the general population in Finland (ages 15 to 74 years) normalized physical activity exposure according to time and time by intensity (i.e., MET-minutes) and found widely differing risk of injury across types of physical activities (table 16.5) (Parkkari et al. 2004).

Latrobe Valley, Australia

A random household telephone survey was conducted quarterly over a 12-month period in a well-defined geographic region, the Latrobe Valley, Australia (Finch and Cassell 2006). Information was collected on participation in sport and active recreation and associated injuries over the previous two weeks for all household members aged over 4 years. Injury rates were calculated per 10,000 population and per 1000 sport participants. Data were collected on 1084 persons from 417 households. Overall, 648 people reported participating in at least one sport or active recreation, and 34 (5.2%; 95% CI: 4.8-5.6%) of these sustained an injury during this activity. Overall, 51.4% of injured cases had a significant impact: 26.5% of the people sought treatment, 34.4% had their activities of daily living adversely affected, and 36.0% had their performance/participation limited. Cricket (51 injuries/10,000 population), horse riding (29/10,000 population), and basketball (25/10,000 population) had the highest injury rates. After adjustment for participation, cricket (242 injuries/1000 participants), horse riding (122/1000 participants), and soccer (107/1000 participants) had the highest injury rates. Cricket and soccer were the sports most associated with "significant" injuries.

Environmental Factors

Even when host factors and features of physical activity are controlled, aspects of the environment where physical activity occurs can affect the risk of injury. Little is yet known about the influence of the myriad potential environmental influences on injury (e.g., street and bike lane design in urban areas).

Exercise Surface

Although clinical studies suggest that a hard running surface or running in the morning is associated with an increased risk of injuries (James, Bates, and Osternig 1978), population studies have not found such differences, especially after controlling for weekly running distance (Macera et al. 1989; Marti et al. 1988; Walter et al. 1989). In a review of running injury studies, van Mechelen (1992) found no differences, at least for men, in injury incidence among running surfaces. Sixty-five percent of injuries

Table 16.5   Injuries per 1000 h of Participation and per 1000 Participants by Activity, Finland

Activity	Injuries per 1000 hours of participation	Estimated injuries per 106 MET-min of participation value (METs)	Injuries per 1000 persons reporting the activity
Commuting activities			
Walking	0.2	0.8 (4)	23.2
Cycling	0.5	1.4 (6)	21.2
Lifestyle activities			
Hunting, fishing, berry picking	0.3	1.3 (4)	20.6
Home repair	0.5	2.1 (4)	78.2
Gardening	1.0	4.2 (4)	92.0
Sports, noncontact			
Golf	0.3	1.1 (4.5)	35.1
Dancing	0.7	2.3 (5)	23.5
Swimming	1.0	2.4 (7)	23.6
Walking	1.2	5.0 (4)	89.7
Rowing	1.5	3.6 (7)	51.9
Pole walking	1.7	5.7 (5)	54.9
Cross-country skiing	1.7	3.5 (8)	67.2
Running	3.6	6.0 (10)	123.2
Track and field sports	3.8	7.9 (8)	318.2
Tennis	4.7	13.1 (6)	188.2
Sports, limited contact			
Cycling	2.0	4.2 (8)	62.4
Aerobics, gymnastics	3.1	7.9 (6.5)	120.6
Horse riding	3.7	15.4 (4)	546.9
Downhill skiing	4.1	11.4 (6)	192.5
In-line skating	5.0	6.7 (12.5)	190.8
Volleyball	7.0	29.2 (4)	447.2
Squash	18.3	25.4 (12)	629.6
Sports, collision and contact			
Karate	6.7	11.2 (10)	611.1
Ice hockey	7.5	15.6 (8)	670.7
Soccer	7.8	18.6 (7)	445.0
Basketball	9.1	25.3 (6)	508.5
Wrestling	9.1	25.3 (6)	625.0
Judo	16.3	27.2 (10)	1363.6

MET values adapted by Advisory Committee Physical Activity Guidelines for Americans, 2008.

Data by Parkkari et al. 2004.

sustained by adolescents during skateboarding occur on public roads, footpaths, and parking lots (Fountain and Meyers 1996). Studies have presented conflicting results about the influence of type of floor surface on injury risk during aerobic dance (Garrick, Gillien, and Whiteside 1986; Richie, Kelso, and Bellucci 1985).

Temperature

The scientific advisory committee of the 2008 Physical Activity Guidelines for Americans concluded that it is safe for healthy people to be physically active in a wide range of typical environmental temperatures and humidity, with proper clothing that insulates in very cold weather and that promotes body heat loss by convection and sweat evaporation during very hot weather (Physical Activity Guidelines Advisory Committee 2008). Physiological acclimatization (e.g., quicker and more sweating) to exertion in warm weather occurs over a few weeks of graduated exposure and increases the safety of warm weather activity (e.g., less risk of heat exhaustion or heatstroke). A similarly protective acclimatization against injury in very cold weather (e.g., frostbite) does not occur.

The American College of Sports Medicine (ACSM) has published detailed safety guidelines for physical activity in extremely cold (ACSM 2006) and hot (ACSM 2007a) temperatures and for proper hydration (avoiding dehydration, which can lead to heat exhaustion and rhabdomyolysis [kidney failure from excessive muscle damage]), especially in American football players, marathon runners, and people with sickle cell trait (Wirthwein et al. 2001), as well as overhydration, which can lead to rare but deadly hyponatremia (excessive sodium loss) (ACSM 2007b).

The influence of environmental temperature on injury risk was indirectly tested in an examination of seasonal differences in injury incidence during U.S. Army basic combat training, which is similar at all times of the year (Knapik et al. 2002). Injury data were retrieved retrospectively from medical records of 1543 men and 1025 women who trained for eight weeks in two separate groups in the summer and two groups in the fall. Among men, the relative risk of a time-loss injury (one that required time away from activity) was 2.5 times higher in the summer than in the fall. Among women, the relative risk of suffering a time-loss injury was 1.7 times higher in the summer than the fall. The injury rates were unchanged after adjustment for age, BMI, and

physical fitness (push-ups, sit-ups, and 2-mile run). Daily temperature was strongly correlated with injury rates ($r = 0.92$ to 0.97), suggesting that environmental temperature is a strong, independent risk factor for injury during strenuous exercise training.

The National High School Sports-Related Injury Surveillance Study for the 2005 through 2009 school years reported 118 cases of environmental heat illness (EHI) among high school athletes from 100 schools that resulted in one or more lost days of participation (1.6 per 100,000 athlete exposures) (CDC 2010). The rate in football (4.5/1000AE) was 10 times higher than the average rate for eight other sports that were studied. Two-thirds of the time-loss heat illnesses occurred during August or during football practice or games. No deaths were reported.

The NCAA reported the EHI rate for football for an 18-year period, comparing the preseason period (from the first practice to the first game) to the entire season (Dick et al. 2007). Overall, the preseason injury rate was 12.73 times higher than that for the entire season. The average injury rate for the preseason period was 5.66/1000AE (range from 2.81/1000AE to 12.49/1000AE), while the season rate was 0.44/1000AE (range from 0.18/1000AE to 0.98/1000AE). Thus, the greatest risk for EHI was during August when football begins. Cooper, Ferrara, and Broglio (2006) analyzed the EHI injury rate in five southeastern schools and found that August accounted for 88% of the EHI events (incident rate = 8.95/1000AE) while September accounted for the remaining 12% of EHI cases (incident rate = 1.70/1000AE). To reduce the risk of EHI in football, the NCAA instituted the five-day acclimatization period for preseason football that went into effect in the 2002-2003 season.

NCAA Football Heat Acclimatization Rules

- During the first 5 days of practice, student-athletes shall not engage in more than 1 on-field practice per day, not to exceed 3 hours in length.

- During the first 2 days of the acclimatization period, helmets are the only piece of protective equipment participants may wear.

- During the third and fourth days of the acclimatization period, helmets and shoulder pads are the only pieces of protective equipment student-athletes may wear.

- During the final day of the 5-day period and on any days thereafter, student-athletes may practice in full pads.
  - After the 5-day acclimatization period: an institution may not conduct multiple on-field practice sessions on consecutive days.

- Student-athletes cannot engage in more than 3 hours of on-field practice activities on those days during which 1 practice is permitted.

- Student-athletes shall not engage in more than 5 hours of on-field activities on those days during which more than 1 practice is permitted.

- On those days when institutions conduct multiple practice sessions, student-athletes must be provided with at least 3 hours of continuous recovery time between the end of the first practice and the start of the last practice that day.

Urban Environment Features

A descriptive epidemiological study of pedestrian injuries among children and adolescents examined environmental and pedestrian factors associated with all motor vehicle crashes occurring in New York City between 1991 and 1997 (DiMaggio and Durkin 2002). Among 693,283 crashes, 97,245 resulted in injuries to 32,578 youth under the age of 20. The rate of pedestrian injuries was 246 per 100,000 people in the population per year, and the fatality rate was 6 per 1000. Younger children (6-14 years) were more likely to be struck midblock, during daylight hours, and during the summer. Adolescents were more likely to be struck at intersections and at night. Road and weather conditions did not influence injury risk.

Air pollution (e.g., organic compounds, chemical particulates, and gases such as ozone) varies among and within cities, depending on roadways and industrial sites. Exposure to air pollution can increase all-cause, cardiovascular, and pulmonary mortality; hospital admissions; emergency room visits; and symptoms. The Environmental Protection Agency has developed the Air Quality Index and, depending upon the value of the index, individuals may be advised to reduce or avoid "prolonged or heavy exertion" out of doors (Environmental Protection Agency 2010).

Methods of Research

Knowledge about the incidence rates and causes of injury during exercise is limited by the methods used by researchers. A mail survey or personal interview has the potential to provide more detailed and accurate information about injuries that do not require medical attention and about the circumstances in which injuries occur than is retrospective examination of hospital or doctor records. However, medical records provide more objective information about injury diagnosis, severity, and treatment than self-reports by participants about their injuries.

A popular method of epidemiologic investigation of injuries has been a mail survey of a selected population (Koplan, Siscovick, and Goldbaum 1985; Nicholl, Coleman, and Williams 1991, 1995; Sandelin et al. 1988). Rates of injuries or illnesses related to physical activity in the United Kingdom were estimated from 17,654 people who responded to a survey mailed to a sample of 28,857 adult inhabitants of England and Wales between the ages of 16 and 45 years during 1989 and 1990 (Nicholl, Coleman, and Williams 1995). The survey asked questions about sport participation, injuries, and general background and habits (e.g., age, weight, smoking, education) during the preceding month. Participation was defined as participation in "sports or other recreational activities involving physical exercise." Injury was defined as any "injury or illness, however minor, through taking part in any of the activities [you] listed." Injuries were further classified as "trivial" or "substantive"; the latter were defined as those that restricted the participant from taking part in usual activities, including work, for a minimum of one day and those for which treatment had been sought. Information was also obtained on whether the injury was new or recurring. Respondents reported 1803 new or recurring injuries. Soccer accounted for more than 25% of all injuries, but the risk of a substantive injury in rugby (96.7 injuries per 1000 occasions of participation and an attributable risk of 29%) for all new injuries was three times higher than in soccer. Over a third of injuries occurred in men aged 16 to 25 years. The most frequently reported injuries were sprains and strains of the lower limbs. Treatment was sought in approximately 25% of the injury cases, and 7% of all new injuries were followed by a visit to a hospital emergency room. After soccer, three fitness activities—running, weight training, and "keeping fit" (i.e., swimming, aerobics, or using an exercise bike)—accounted for most of the injuries. Running accounted for 15.3 injuries per 1000 occasions of participation.

The interview is another frequently used method of inquiry about injuries (Garrick, Gillien, and Whiteside 1986; Sandelin et al. 1988). In 1980, the Central Statistical Office of Finland interviewed 10,405 persons in the Greater Helsinki area (a total population of about 600,000) between the ages of 15 and 75 years about injury occurrence during sports, regardless of severity or treatment, in the preceding year (Sandelin et al. 1988). Injuries were classified into three categories: minor, absence from sport for less than one week; moderate, absence for one to three weeks; and severe, absence for more than three weeks. Results indicated that 75% of those interviewed participated in physical activity for health reasons; and of those participants, 40% said they practiced sports involving large muscle groups and leading to sweating and breathlessness, requiring approximately 50% of cardiorespiratory capacity. The most popular forms of exercise were walking, cycling, and jogging. About 40,000 sport-related injuries were reported, an annual incidence rate of about 670 per 10,000 people. About 70% of the injuries were classified as minor sprains. However, 9% (an estimated 4000 cases) were severe enough to require a visit to a hospital emergency room.

Another method used to assess injury incidence is to retrospectively examine archives of hospital or insurance company records (de Loes, Jacobsen, and Goldie 1990; Kujala et al. 1995; Scheiber and Branche-Dorsey 1995; Zebas et al. 1995). For example, national sport injury insurance registry data in Finland during the period 1987 to 1991 were retrieved to determine incident rates for 62,169 person-years of exposure among participants in soccer, ice hockey, volleyball, basketball, judo, or karate—sports that required insurance enrollment prior to participation. Acute sport injuries that required medical treatment and were reported to the insurance company were analyzed. The age and sex of the person injured and the type of injury, anatomical location, and injury circumstances were described. A total of 54,186 sport injuries were recorded. Injury rates were low in athletes aged under 15, while 20- to 24-year-olds had the highest rates. Results indicated that, even though more time was spent in training than in competition, 46% to 59% of injuries occurred during competition. Also, injury rates were highest in sports that involved body contact. For example, ice hockey had the highest injury incidence. Most injuries occurred to the lower limbs and mainly involved sprains, strains, and contusions.

The Injury Definition Problem

A problem common to the various methods used to measure injury incidence is the general absence of standardization of the definitions of injury (de Loes 1997) and the measures of physical activity or exercise. Definition of injury by a visit to a health care professional is likely not equivalent to injury defined as disruption in regular physical activity. Likewise, the challenge of measuring physical activity in population-based studies as described in chapter 2 has impeded standardization of features of physical activity that may alter injury risks. Thus, decisions made about definitions differ among investigators and undoubtedly influence conclusions about rates of injury and their risk factors.

▶ **STANDARDIZED DEFINITIONS** of injury and physical activity are needed to accurately compare estimates of risk among groups of people and types of physical activity.

The method of reporting injury incidence varies among studies. Incidence rates have been reported as absolute numbers and as rates expressed per person and per time of exposure. As is the case for evaluating the protective effects of physical activity against chronic diseases, the most informative expression of injury rates is injury incidence per time of exposure because using the common denominator of exposure permits a direct comparison of injury rates between different types of physical activity and different participants. It is also important, however, to include properly matched, nonactive controls in order to determine whether injury risk factors are independent influences on injury rates (Koplan, Siscovick, and Goldbaum 1985). These issues are illustrated in the following section about the denominator problem in studies of physical activity injury risks.

▶ **THE MOST** accurate method of expressing injury rates is injury incidence per time of exposure. This allows direct comparisons among different types of physical activity and different people.

The Denominator Problem

Clinical studies have reported high numbers of patients seeking treatment of injuries associated with exercise. However, clinical studies cannot provide information on the prevalence or incidence of exercise-related injuries in a population.

Hence, clinical studies suffer from a "nondenominator" problem (Castelli and Adams 1990; de Loes 1997; Garrick, Gillien, and Whiteside 1986). Conclusions cannot be reached about the public health impact of a series of cases seen by physicians without knowledge of the size of the population from which the clinical cases were drawn. Without such a denominator, the rate of occurrence cannot be computed. Also, it is critical that the appropriate denominator be chosen for comparison; otherwise, a distorted picture of risk can result. For example, an estimated 300,000 cases of traumatic brain injuries occur during sport participation each year in the United States (Sosin, Sniezek, and Thurman 1996). Though about a third of all deaths from injury each year in the United States are attributable to traumatic brain injuries (Sosin, Sniezek, and Waxweiler 1995), most brain injuries during vigorous physical activity are mild to moderate concussions. Mild concussions are seldom fatal, though when repeated over months or years, they can lead to neurological and cognitive **impairment.** Thus, relating sport brain injuries to fatal brain injuries would misleadingly inflate the negative health impact of traumatic brain injury during sport participation.

▶ **ABOUT A** third of all deaths from injury each year in the United States are attributable to traumatic brain injuries, but most brain injuries during vigorous physical activity are mild to moderate concussions, which are seldom fatal. Thus, equating sport brain injuries to fatal brain injuries would yield an overly alarming incidence rate of the negative health impact of traumatic brain injury during sport participation.

The incidence of death during physical activity has been estimated in various population subgroups, including Finnish cross-country skiers; British, American, Finnish, and Israeli military personnel; participants in fitness facilities; and the general young and adult population bases in several countries. Unfortunately, studies have used such varying definitions of injury and such different methods to determine rates that it is difficult to compare their results and reach general conclusions. For example, the definition of a physical activity–related injury varied, and some studies included cases that occurred up to 24 h after participation. The choice of the denominator for computing **death rates** also differed widely among studies.

Coronary heart disease is the main contributing **cause of death** attributable to physical activity, but incidence figures have varied widely, depending on the prevalence of coronary heart disease in the population being studied. For example, the comparatively low rates of sudden death during physical activity among military personnel might be explained by their young ages, their low prevalence of coronary heart disease, and the fact that screening exams exclude from military service or training people who are at cardiac risk because they have potentially fatal malformations of the heart such as aortic stenosis, hypertrophic cardiomyopathy, or Marfan syndrome. Even in military personnel, however, the incidence

Consensus Guidelines for the Measurement of Injury Incidence

1. Provide carefully developed and precisely presented definitions of *injury*.
2. Include denominator data so that injury cases can be related to an at-risk population.
3. Make every effort to minimize selection bias (e.g., samples not representative of population or special subpopulation).
4. Monitor injury experience, activity behavior, and other potential behavioral risk factors concurrently.
5. Employ prospective research designs.

of exercise deaths varies among the groups that are studied. During six weeks of basic training among air force recruits, for example, 17 of 19 sudden cardiac deaths occurred during physical activity (Phillips et al. 1986). Autopsy revealed myocarditis in four of the deaths. That rate of myocarditis (20%) was higher than reported in other studies of military personnel. It might have resulted from viral infections spread by barracks living or recent vaccinations, which are common in recruits but not in older military personnel.

When comparing injury rates among sports, it is necessary to have accurate descriptions of exposure and injuries, including total injury numbers, injury diagnoses, time of injury occurrence, and follow-up treatment. An early review of sport injury studies found that just 11 of 88 studies had used a measure of incidence (Kennedy, Vanderfield, and Kennedy 1977). A few studies of communities have provided better estimates of the incidence or prevalence of activity-related injury. For example, about 670 sport injuries per 10,000 people, 14% of all injuries, were reported in Helsinki, Finland, in 1980 (Sandelin et al. 1988). In a rural city of about 31,000 residents in Sweden, the sport injury rate observed during a year was 150 per 10,000 people, 17% of all injuries, and accounted for 3% of all visits to hospital emergency rooms (de Loes 1990; de Loes and Goldie 1988).

In Rochester, Minnesota, an overall incidence rate of 187 ankle fractures was reported per 100,000 person-years of exposure (Daly et al. 1987); 36% of the fractures occurred during sport participation. About 38% of knee surgeries to repair a torn meniscus were attributed to sport injury in another study (Hede et al. 1990).

Myocardial Infarction and Sudden Death

The cardiovascular complications of vigorous physical activity include cerebrovascular accidents, symptomatic cardiac arrhythmias, aortic dissection, myocardial infarction, and sudden cardiac death (Thompson 1996). The main causes of exercise-related cardiovascular complications are congenital abnormalities in young subjects and atherosclerotic coronary disease in adults. The incidence of exercise deaths is low; about 7.5 and 1.3 per million young male and female athletes and 60 per million middle-aged men die during exertion per year (Thompson 1996). Thus, though the risk of cardiac events is transiently increased during exercise, the absolute risk is low, especially, as will be shown later in this chapter, when compared to the overall risk of cardiac events among people who are sedentary.

In Helsinki, Finland, 3.7% of sudden cardiac deaths (within 1 h of onset of symptoms), 6.3% of delayed cardiac deaths, and 6.8% of nonfatal cardiac events were associated with physical activity (Romo 1972). Furthermore, an additional 9% of sudden cardiac deaths occurred immediately after snow shoveling, sport, or other exceptional physical activity so that physical activity contributed to approximately 14% of all sudden cardiac deaths. Nonetheless, these figures probably underestimate the percentage of exercise events, because unwitnessed deaths, such as those during sleep, were not included in the numerator.

A study of patients in cardiac exercise rehabilitation programs estimated that the risks during exercise were 1 in 112,000 h of participation for cardiac arrest, 1 in 294,000 h of participation for heart attack, and 1 in 784,000 h of participation for cardiac death (Van Camp and Peterson 1986).

Dr. William Castelli, former medical director of the Framingham Heart Study, used two early epidemiologic studies of jogging deaths to illustrate how important it is to use the correct denominator when computing the hazards of physical activity (Castelli and Adams 1990). The first study was conducted in Rhode Island by cardiologist Paul D. Thompson and colleagues. The second study was conducted by Doctor David Siscovick and colleagues in Washington state.

Rhode Island

Twelve men ages 30 to 64 years died while jogging in Rhode Island during a five-year period from 1975 to 1980. To express the number of jogging deaths as an incidence rate, the investigators surveyed the state using a random telephone sample to determine that, among men aged 30 through 64 years, about 7.4% reported jogging at least twice a week (Thompson et al. 1982). Using that group as the denominator, the incidence of death during jogging for men of that age group was one death per year for every 7620 joggers, or about one death per 400,000 person-hours of jogging. Though very low, this mortality rate during jogging was about seven times the estimated death rate during sedentary activities. However, that increased risk was not fully independent of other factors. Resting electrocardiograms were on file for five of the 12 runners, and most were abnormal, so the risk of sudden death during jogging was not completely independent of existing heart disease. A more accurate odds ratio would have used the total number of joggers in Rhode Island who had heart disease in the denominator.

King County, Washington

A subsequent study conducted in King County, Washington, illustrates this point about the importance of choosing the proper denominator (figure 16.7; Siscovick et al. 1984). The physical activity history prior to and during a fatal heart attack was obtained by interview with the wives of 133 men ages 25 to 75 years. Wives of a group of apparently healthy men were similarly questioned about their husbands' exercise habits, which provided the denominator. Among sedentary men, the odds of dying were increased six times during exercise (from a rate of 5 to a rate of 30 cases per 100 million person-hours of exposure).

However, the overall 24-h rate of death from any cause among the regular exercisers (about seven cases) was half that of the sedentary men (about 15 cases). Thus, even though exercise carried a short-term risk, its long-term benefits still outweighed the risks of being sedentary. Similar findings were later reported for women in the Nurses' Health Study.

▶ **THOUGH THE** odds that men with coronary disease will die suddenly of a heart attack are increased about six times during exercise, the overall 24-h rate of death from any cause among regular exercisers is half that of sedentary men. So, even though exercise carries a short-term risk, its long-term benefits still outweigh the risks of being sedentary.

Nurses' Health Study

The risk of sudden cardiac death associated with moderate to vigorous exertion among women was studied using a prospective, nested case-crossover study of 288 cases of sudden cardiac death from the Nurses' Health Study (1980-2004) and a prospective cohort analysis of 69,693 participants without prior cardiovascular disease followed up from 1986 to 2004 (Whang et al. 2006). Absolute risk was very low (one sudden cardiac death per 36.5 million hours of exertion). In case-crossover analyses, the risk of sudden cardiac death was transiently elevated during moderate to vigorous exertion (RR = 2.38; 95% CI: 1.23-4.60) compared with the risk during lesser or no exertion. Habitual moderate to vigorous exertion modified this transient risk, and the risk was no longer significantly elevated among women who exercised 2 or more hours per week. In the cohort analyses, an increasing amount of moderate to vigorous exercise was associated with a lower long-term risk of sudden cardiac death when results were adjusted for age and biomarkers that are risk factors for sudden cardiac death and might explain the influence of habitual physical activity. Regardless of adjustment for confounders or mediators, risk reduction was strong among women who exercised 4 or more hours per week compared with women who did not exercise (adjusted RR = 0.41; 95% CI: 0.20-0.83).

Physical Activity and Existing Heart Disease

An important question is whether someone who has had an exercise-related coronary event would have encountered a similar fate in the near future if he or she had not exercised. Vuori, Makarainen, and Jaaskelainen (1978) were among the first to notice that sudden deaths were more frequent during physical activity. Their observation raised the possibility that the increased metabolic demand placed on the heart during exercise is responsible for the increased fatality rate of any coronary events that happen during exertion. Another view is that physical exertion only hastens the inevitable, as

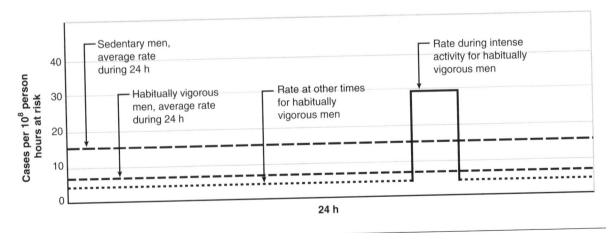

Figure 16.7 A study conducted in King County, Washington, shows the odds of dying from a heart attack in sedentary and physically active men.

Data from Siscovick et al. 1984.

illustrated by a study of the February 1978 Rhode Island blizzard (Faich and Rose 1979). On the day of this storm, the death rate from ischemic heart disease nearly doubled compared with the February average for the previous five years. The death rate remained elevated for several days but then decreased below the usual February average so that the overall death rate in February 1978 was similar to that for the preceding five years. This suggests that the physical and emotional stress of the storm only hastened deaths that would have occurred anyway. However, such a conclusion is tenuous because it is based on the same type of logic described in chapter 2 for the problem of the ecological fallacy, whereby causes of death are inferred from trends of co-occurring events.

Most reported sudden deaths during jogging are due to cardiac arrhythmias secondary to underlying coronary artery disease. People at elevated risk include experienced runners, often those who undertake considerable weekly running distance, who have one or more major coronary risk factors, who started jogging later in life (probably after the development of significant underlying coronary artery disease), and who often ignore prodromal symptoms (i.e., advance warning signs such as chest pain). Other reported causes of death during exercise include myocarditis, idiopathic hypertrophic cardiomyopathy, congenital anomalies of the heart or blood vessels, rupture of the heart or a major blood vessel, heart failure, and heatstroke.

▷ **SEVEN EPIDEMIOLOGIC** studies published between 1984 and 2006 showed that the average risk of sudden adverse cardiac events (i.e., cardiac arrest, sudden death, myocardial infarction) during or soon after vigorous physical activity was five times higher in people who were habitually less active (Physical Activity Guidelines Advisory Committee 2008).

Haskell (1978) surveyed 30 cardiac rehabilitation programs in North America about cardiovascular problems among a cumulative 14,000 patients and 1.6 million patient-hours of exercise exposure. There was one cardiac arrest, one myocardial infarction, and one death for each 33,000, 233,000, and 116,000 patient-hours of participation, respectively. The rehabilitation programs also reported a 4% annual mortality rate, which was the expected rate for postinfarction patients regardless of whether they exercised.

Because of potential cardiac problems during physical exertion, many experts and groups that promote exercise, including the ACSM, recommend a multistage exercise ECG test as part of the medical screening program prior to beginning a strenuous exercise program for sedentary people 45 (men) to 55 (women) years of age or older and for younger people estimated to be at high coronary risk because of family history, premature coronary heart disease, cigarette smoking, obesity, high blood pressure, or elevated levels of serum cholesterol.

Joint and Muscle Injury

Orthopedic and musculoskeletal injuries are much more common than cardiovascular accidents during exercise, especially during running or jogging, yet little is known about the rates and risk factors for activities such as resistance exercise training and stretching for flexibility.

Running and Jogging

Population-based studies of runners have consistently reported annual rates of musculoskeletal injuries that range from 35% (Koplan et al. 1982) to 65% (Lysholm and Wiklander 1987). This variation in injury rates may be due to the diversity of populations studied and the different definitions of injury applied among the studies. Most injuries occur to the lower extremities, especially the knee, foot, and ankle. The most frequently reported types of musculoskeletal injuries are sprains, strains, stress fractures, and various overuse injuries (e.g., patellar or Achilles tendinitis).

Despite poor standardization of methods used to document injury rates and severity, van Mechelen (1992) concluded that the annual incidence rate of running injuries varied from 37% to 56% for the average recreational runner who trains regularly. Expressed as incidence relative to exposure time, those rates approximated a range of 2.5 to 12.1 injuries per 1000 h of running exposure. Most running injuries (70-80%

Potential Risk Factors for Running Injury

Increased Risk	Weak or Mixed Evidence
Previous injury	Warming up
Lack of running experience	Stretching exercises
Running to compete	Body height
Excessive weekly running distances	Malalignment
	Restricted range of motion
No Effect	Running frequency
Age	Intensity of performance
Gender	Stability of running pattern
BMI	Shoes and orthotics
Hill running	Running on one side of the road
Running on hard surfaces	
Participation in other sports	
Time of the year	
Time of the day	

van Mechelen 1992.

of the total) involved the lower extremities, and the most common injuries among different subgroups of runners were tendinitis (competitive runners), stress fractures (boys and girls), and strains and tendinitis (general population). The studies found that injuries led to a reduction or temporary curtailment of running in about 30% to 90% of all injuries; about 20% to 70% of all injuries required medical attention, and less than 5% resulted in lost time from work.

Walking

Walking is the most prevalent form of exercise among adults in North America. The 1994 Injury Control and Risk Survey (ICARIS) of U.S. residential households estimated that 1.4% of adults 18 years or older (about 1,877,000 people) had sustained a walking injury during the preceding month in early summer (Powell et al. 1998). Though walking would seem to have few hazards, injury rates during walking have not been studied much. In a study of injuries associated with physical activity in Helsinki, Finland (Sandelin et al. 1988), walking was the most popular activity, practiced by 75% of the sample surveyed, but it was not listed as having a noteworthy percentage of the observed injuries. Among 698 men and 169 women participants in the Aerobics Center Longitudinal Study who reported a physical activity–related injury requiring physician visits in the previous year, walkers had 25% lower risk of injury than runners among men younger than 45 years and a 33% lower risk among men 45 years or older. Regardless of age, women who walked had about a 25% reduction in risk compared to women who ran, but the reduction wasn't statistically significant because of the small number of women studied. Injury rates were adjusted for age, BMI, previous injury, and strength training, and they were unrelated to the amount of walking (Colbert, Hootman, and Macera 2000).

> ▶ **ADDING A** small and comfortable amount of walking, such as 5 to 15 min two or three times per week, to one's usual daily activities carries a low risk of musculoskeletal injury and no known risk of sudden severe cardiac events (Physical Activity Guidelines Advisory Committee 2008).

Bicycling

The 1994 ICARIS study found that less than 1% of adults aged 18 years or older in the United States (an estimated 330,000 people) reported a bicycling accident during the preceding month of early summer (Powell et al. 1998). Other injury rate estimates have come from clinical studies of cumulative visits to physicians for treatment of injuries from bicycling (though not from stationary cycling). Most of these reports have been of head trauma (Guichon and Myles 1975; Sacks et al. 1991; Thompson, Rivara, and Thompson 1989). Injury rates ranged from 4.6% (Kiburz et al. 1986) to 13% (Kruse and McBeath 1980), but injuries were minor and required no treatment or only self-treatment. A study of urban cyclists found that increased cycling distance and length of cycling time were associated with increased accidents (Sgaglione, Suljaga-Petchell, and Frankel 1982). The difficulty in comparing injury rates and risk factors among the various studies is that the study population varies by type of cycling (recreation, transportation, and sport), and the equipment and riding environment associated with each type of cycling can vary a great deal.

The most common type of cycling injury requiring hospitalization is head trauma (Guichon and Myles 1975). It was estimated that not wearing a helmet led to 107,000 unnecessary bicycle-related head injuries in the United States in 1997 that cost $81 million in direct medical costs and $2.3 billion in indirect health costs (Schulman et al. 2002). A case–control study of head trauma among bicyclists demonstrated the effectiveness of safety helmets in reducing the severity of head trauma (Thompson, Rivara, and Thompson 1989). Other studies have similarly concluded that safety helmets are effective in preventing severe injury and even death (Sacks et al. 1991). A meta-analysis estimated that the use of bicycle helmets reduced the risk of death by nearly 75%, the risk of head injury and brain injury by about 60%, and the risk of facial injury by half (Attewell et al. 2001).

Aerobics or Group Dance Exercise

Aerobics includes a variety of group exercise programs that vary in intensity. The most common feature involves rhythmic movements set to music. The ICARIS study found that less than 1.6% of adults aged 18 years or older in the United States (an estimated 394,000 people) reported an accident associated with aerobics participation during the preceding month (Powell et al. 1998).

Cross-sectional and prospective clinical studies of injuries among aerobic dance participants have yielded consistent results. Overall, about 45% of students and 75% of instructors report injuries (Garrick, Gillien, and Whiteside 1986; Richie, Kelso, and Bellucci 1985; Rothenberger, Chang, and Cable 1988). In one study, the annual injury incidence rate was 2.33 injuries per individual (233 per 100 person-years) (Requa, DeAvilla, and Garrick 1993), similar to the rate of 2.1 injuries per person per year among competitive Irish dancers (Watson 1993). In another study, almost half of the women currently in a program reported having had a previous injury; 23% of these injuries required a visit to a physician (Rothenberger, Chang, and Cable 1988). Although the absolute injury rate for aerobic dance seems high, the rate of long-term limitations on activity appears low. Garrick, Gillien, and Whiteside (1986) reported that 80% of the injuries affected the participant only during the aerobics class. The most common site of injury is the shin, consistently accounting for over 20% of the injuries for both instructors and students.

The only risk factor that has been consistently identified among studies on aerobic dance is frequency of dance class participation. Those participating more than four times per week had a higher injury rate than those participating fewer than four times per week. However, the rate of injury per hour of aerobics decreased as the number of hours of participation increased, similar to results for running discussed earlier for the Peachtree Road Race follow-up study. Higher injury rates also were found in people who had a history of leg and joint problems and who were inexperienced in other types of fitness activities.

Resistance Exercise Training

Injury associated with resistance exercise, like the other activities we have discussed, has been understudied by epidemiological methods. The ICARIS study estimated that 2.4% of U.S. adults 18 years or older (an estimated 964,000 people) had suffered a weightlifting injury during the past month (Powell et al. 1998). Other clinical studies have more recently described the types and impact of such injuries in select subgroups of the population.

Among 45 women who participated in a 24-week training program of weightlifting, running, sprint running, backpacking, and lift and carry drills, 22 (49%) had at least one injury, an injury rate of 2.8 cases per 1000 h of exposure. Total visits to a physician and days lost from training were 89 and 69, respectively. Most injuries were overuse injuries of the lower back, knees, and feet (Reynolds et al. 2001). A clinical case–control study examined the long-term effects of power weightlifting on spinal disc degeneration in 12 pairs of monozygotic (i.e., identical) male twins aged 35 to 69 years who differed according to lifetime histories of participation (on average, 2300 h vs. 200 h of weightlifting). Though twins who differed in endurance exercise participation did not differ in spinal disc degeneration, the men with more participation in power weightlifting had greater disc degeneration in thoracic vertebrae T6-T12 but not in the lumbar spine. Adjustment of the injury rate comparisons for previous back injuries, loading of the spine during occupational work, smoking, and time spent driving did not change the results (Videman et al. 1997). Guidelines for promoting safe increments in progressive resistance training are available from the ACSM (2002).

Injury Features

In assessing the impact of injuries on the health of an individual as well as society as a whole, it is important to characterize injuries by type, location, severity, and consequences.

Type and Location

The most common type of activity-related injury is sprains and strains of the lower limbs, particularly the knee and ankle (Kallinen and Markku 1995; Nicholl, Coleman, and Williams 1995; Zebas et al. 1995). Runners are prone to tendinitis as well (Koplan, Rothenberg, and Jones 1995; van Mechelen 1992). Contact sports have a higher incidence of fractures, contusions, and upper body injuries (Backx et al. 1991; Sandelin et al. 1988).

Severity and Consequences

The majority of physical activity injuries are classified as minor and require little or no medical treatment. Sandelin and colleagues (1988) reported that out of 40,380 total sport injuries, 53% required an adhesive bandage and only 25% necessitated medical treatment involving painkillers. Backx and colleagues (1991) reported that 175 of 399 recorded sport injuries among schoolchildren ages 8 to 17 were not serious enough to report to physicians. In contrast, Marti and coworkers (1988) investigated lifestyle disruption resulting from running injuries and found that 44% of 1994 running injuries resulted in cessation of training for an average of 4.8 weeks, 31% required medical treatment, and 5% led to absence from work. Van Mechelen (1992) concluded that 20% to 70% of all running injuries need medical attention and 30% to 90% result in cessation of training.

When severity in college athletics is defined as missing at least one day of participation and is expressed as incidence per 100,000 athlete exposures, rates range from a high in football for both practices (9.6) and games (35.9) to a low of 1.9 for men's baseball practice. In high school, the rate (incidence per 1000 athlete exposures) of severe injury that keeps athletes from participation for more than 21 days is greater in competition (0.79) than in practice (0.24). Although sport-related concussions account for about 9% of all high school athletic injuries and 6% of all collegiate athletic injuries, less than 1% of sport concussions result in loss of consciousness. Heart patients have a transient fivefold increase in their risk of death while they exercise, but those who regularly exercise still cut their overall risk of cardiac death by half. The estimated risk of exercise-related death during cardiac rehabilitation exercise programs is about 1 death for every 116,000 patient-hours of participation.

Risk of Physical Activity Injuries: The Evidence

To judge the health risks of exercise, it is necessary to use Mill's canons of causality to evaluate the strength of evidence for a cause-and-effect relationship between exercise and the incidence of musculoskeletal injury. Most studies have not used an appropriate control group to provide base rates of injury among people who are sedentary, so the magnitude of the risk ratios reported in many studies is not an accurate indicator of the strength of association between physical activity and injury rates. Dose dependency has been demonstrated in that greater total exposure (frequency × duration × intensity) is associated with increased risk for injury, but the independent effects of specific features of physical activity on injury risk are as yet unestablished.

A few longitudinal and prospective cohort studies have demonstrated a temporal sequence appropriate for a causal relationship between exercise and injury. Consistency has been established in studies examining a large, representative, random sample of people from population bases, although there are relatively few such studies. The moderating effect of age as a risk factor for injury during exercise has been established in several studies; findings for sex are conflicting, and few other factors (e.g., fitness level, sport skill, race, socioeconomic status) have been shown to have moderating effects on injury risk. The independence of features of physical activity and its settings from other confounders of injury risk has been incompletely tested in observational studies. Clinical studies have provided some experimental confirmation of biologically plausible mechanisms of injury, but specific features of people, the environment, and physical activity that influence the rates and severity of injuries have been poorly defined and understudied for most types of physical activity injuries in population-based studies.

▷ **THE SCIENTIFIC** advisory committee of the 2008 Physical Activity Guidelines for Americans concluded that the recommended minimum level of regular physical activity for public health, about 500 MET-minutes per week, has a low (but not precisely measured) risk of musculoskeletal injury.

The clearest evidence of the direct relationship between dose of activity and risk of musculoskeletal injury comes from a handful of studies of running injuries. People who ran 40 miles per week or more (4000 or more MET-minutes per week) were two to three times more likely to have had a running injury in the past 12 months than individuals who ran 5 to 10 miles per week (500-1000 MET-minutes per week) (Physical Activity Guidelines Advisory Committee 2008).

Other Medical Hazards

Various other adverse events and hazards have been associated with participation in medical trials of exercise training or physical activity in the population (table 16.6). They represent a clinical problem that often requires medical treatment. Their preva-

lence and incidence rates during exercise training or in the general population have not been determined, though, so at this point it is not clear how large or widespread a problem they are.

Despite its importance for judging the benefits (i.e., improved health) compared to the harms of medical intervention (Ioannidis et al. 2004), information on adverse events is commonly inadequate in reports of randomized trials. An evaluation of 133 randomized controlled trials published during 2006 in six high-impact medical journals *(New England Journal of Medicine, Lancet, Journal of the American Medical Association, British Medical Journal, Annals of Internal Medicine,* and *PLoS Medicine)* showed that nearly one in five trials reported no information on adverse events (Pitrou et al. 2009). Severity was undefined or vaguely defined in a fourth of the trials, and almost half the trials reported no information on withdrawal of patients because of adverse events; just 13% reported the reasons why the adverse events led to dropout. Furthermore, many trials concluded that adverse events were not significantly higher in the intervention compared to control, even though the trial was too small to yield a statistically powerful test of a difference (Ioannidis 2009).

Table 16.6   Medical Injuries or Illnesses in Vigorous Physical Activity

Type	Hazard
Cardiovascular	Cardiac arrest in heart patients Ruptured aorta
Musculoskeletal	Muscle injury (including delayed-onset muscle soreness) Tendon strains Ligament tears (sprains) Exertional rhabdomyolysis (myoglobin in urine) Joint inflammation
Pulmonary	Exercise-induced bronchospasm
Gastrointestinal	Irritable bowel Gastrointestinal blood loss in runners
Allergic	Exercise-induced anaphylaxis Skin welts
Gynecologic	Delayed menarche Amenorrhea Oligomenorrhea
Endocrinologic	Hypoglycemia in diabetics
Renal	Hematuria (blood in urine) Proteinuria (protein in urine)
Hematologic	Anemia (usually false anemia due to plasma volume expansion, but normal red blood cell count) Gastrointestinal blood loss in runners
Thermal	Heat cramps Heat exhaustion Heatstroke Frostbite Hypothermia

Adapted from Gotsch, Annest, and Holmgreen 2002.

Table 16.7   Adverse Events During Medical Trials of Exercise Training

Study	Medical condition	Type of exercise	Number of trials	Adverse events
Speck et al. 2010	Cancer survivors	Mainly aerobic, resistance, or both	60 randomized controlled trials (RCT) and six nonrandomized	Only half (36 trials) tracked adverse events; 29 reported no adverse events.
Cheema et al. 2008	Breast cancer survivors	Progressive resistance	10 randomized or uncontrolled	No incidence or worsening of lymphedema in eight trials; other events not tracked in four trials. No adverse events in five trials. One yearlong trial reported 13 musculoskeletal events among 85 participants.
Shaw et al. 2006	Obesity	Mainly aerobic, resistance, or both	43 trials	No data on adverse events in any trial.
Liu and Latham 2009	Disability in seniors	Progressive resistance	121 RCT	Adverse events poorly recorded; musculoskeletal complaints, such as joint pain and muscle soreness, were reported in many studies that tracked them. No serious events directly from exercise.
Chien et al. 2008	Chronic heart failure	Home-based exercise	10 trials; only two tracked adverse events	Exercise did not increase the odds of hospitalization for cardiac events (OR = 0.75; 95% CI: 0.19-2.92) more than usual activity. Low power to detect a difference ($n = 143$).
Saunders et al. 2009	Stroke patients	Treadmill exercise training	24 trials involving 1147 participants	One death
de Morton, Keating, and Jeffs 2007	Acute inpatients	Physical therapy	Seven RCT and two controlled trials	No adverse events reported; seven RCT and two pseudo-randomized controlled trials.
Hassett et al. 2008	Traumatic brain injury	Cardiorespiratory fitness training	Six trials involving 303 participants	No adverse events.
Mehrholz et al. 2010	Parkinson's disease	Treadmill training	Eight trials	Adverse events not tracked.
Sigal et al. 2007	Type 2 diabetes	Aerobic, resistance, or both	One RCT	Adverse events (mainly musculoskeletal injury or discomfort) in 71 of 188 (38%) exercisers and 10 of 63 (14%) control participants. Ten participants reported mild hypoglycemia that did not require treatment.

Likewise, reporting of adverse events in trials of exercise intervention in medical patients has been sparse and nonuniform, so the prevalence and severity of harms during exercise training that is otherwise effective for most people are incompletely known. To date, most adverse events reported have been musculoskeletal complaints, not worsening of signs or symptoms of existing medical conditions. See table 16.7.

A study by Bouchard and colleagues (2012) suggests that exercise increases risk factors for cardiovascular disease and diabetes in some people. In six controlled exercise trials including 1,687 adults, two or more outcomes worsened in 7% of participants. Adverse rates for systolic blood pressure (12%), HDL cholesterol (13%), triglycerides (10%), and insulin (8%) exceeded natural variation and measurement error. More research is needed to understand the health impact

of these findings and whether exercise prescriptions can be better based on people's adaptability to exercise.

Psychological Hazards

There is some concern among mental health professionals that the disciplined training and social climate in some sports and leisure-time fitness activities that emphasize lean body composition and dietary restriction can increase the risk of eating problems or add to existing eating problems among participants. Attention has also been recently drawn to the problem of potential steroid and substance abuse among some weightlifters who have a distorted body image. Despite the recognition over 20 years ago that exercise, like food or drugs, can be abused (Dishman 1985; Morgan 1979), it is still not known whether excessive exercise and disordered eating share a common course that is motivated by common goals and followed by common medical outcomes (Davis 2000).

Disordered Eating

Clinical parallels, including elevated anxiety and depression, have been drawn between highly committed runners and patients diagnosed as suffering from anorexia nervosa (i.e., self-starvation). Although some studies of small samples of elite ballet dancers, gymnasts, and wrestlers show higher than expected rates of eating problems, how long they persist and whether they represent goal-appropriate behaviors for the sport rather than medical or psychological pathology have not been established (Dishman 1985). It has been proposed that anorexia athletica (defined as increased risk factors for eating disorders common among some sport groups) is a subclinical syndrome of anorexia nervosa (Sundgot-Borgen 1994). Though 22% of a sample of over 500 elite Norwegian female athletes were judged to be at risk for an eating disorder (Sundgot-Borgen 1994), the prevalence of disordered eating and the independent risk caused by sport and exercise have not yet been established by controlled epidemiologic and clinical studies. In most cases, the eating behaviors of athletes do not appear to signal anorexia nervosa or bulimia (i.e., bingeing and purging; O'Connor and Smith 1999), which have prevalence rates in the United States of about 1% and 4%, respectively.

Nonetheless, disordered eating remains a clinical health concern among top female athletes in some sports. A Norwegian study of female athletes representing the national teams at the junior or senior level, aged 13 to 39 years ($n = 938$), and an age group–matched sample of nonathletes randomly selected from the population ($n = 900$) was designed to determine whether risk factors for eating disorders were uniform between elite athletes and the general population (Torstveit, Rosenvinge, and Sundgot-Borgen 2008). Randomly sampled athletes ($n = 186$) and controls ($n = 145$) were subjects for a clinical interview. More athletes in sports that require leanness (46.7%) were judged to have clinical eating disorders than athletes in other sports (19.8%) and controls (21.4%). Risk factors for eating disorders were menstrual dysfunction in athletes from sports that require leanness, self-reported eating disorder symptoms in other athletes, and self-reported use of pathogenic weight control methods in nonathletes from the population. The results indicated that risk factors for disordered eating are not uniform but rather are unique among elite female athletes depending on participation in sports that require leanness for success at the elite level of competition. The co-occurrence of disordered eating with menstrual dysfunction is a strong health risk among female athletes as well as nonathletes, especially for bone health (ACSM 2007c). Notwithstanding that clinical health concern, among Norwegian adolescents, self-reported disordered eating is more prevalent in nonathletes than in elite athletes, who nonetheless say that losing weight to enhance sport performance is an important reason for their dieting (Martinsen et al. 2010).

Results from more than 50 studies on the topic, including nonelite athletes and recreational exercisers, were inconclusive because the studies merely described symptoms among different groups of active or inactive people without fully considering attributes other than activity history that might account for eating problems (Davis 2000). The studies often lacked standard definitions or valid measures of physical activity or disordered eating. For example, many runners cover 50 miles (80 km) or more each week with no problems at all, whereas other people might not tolerate 20 miles (32 km) a week. Though anorexics often augment food restriction by hyperactivity, because of muscle wasting and anemia their aerobic fitness ($\dot{V}O_2max$) is well below average, in contrast to the above-average aerobic fitness of habitual runners and overtrained athletes. In addition, cross-sectional studies have not revealed a common psychopathology between obligatory (i.e., excessively committed) runners and anorexic patients.

Anorexic Versus Athletic Female

SHARED FEATURES

Dietary faddism

Controlled calorie consumption

Specific carbohydrate avoidance

Low body weight

Resting bradycardia and low blood pressure

Increased physical activity

Amenorrhea or oligomenorrhea

Anemia (may or may not be present)

DISTINGUISHING FEATURES

Athlete	*Anorexic*
Purposeful training	Aimless physical activity
Increased exercise tolerance	Poor or decreasing exercise performance
Good muscular development	Poor muscular development
Accurate body image	Flawed body image (patient believes herself to be overweight)
Body fat level within defined normal range	Body fat level below normal range
	Biochemical abnormalities if abusing laxatives, diuretics, or both

Reprinted, by permission, from J.A. McSherry, 1984, "The diagnostic challenge of anorexia nervosa," *American Family Physician* 29 (2): 144.

Researchers who believe that sport participation increases risk for disordered eating have typically studied small groups of athletes without fully considering the ways in which different sports, levels of competition, behaviors of coaches or teammates, eating or activity histories, and socioeconomic backgrounds affect eating problems. Comparisons of the rates of disordered eating or its risk factors among sports or athletes are not meaningful when other influences on eating behaviors, such as age, personal and family history, personality, or socioeconomic status, are not controlled for. Athletes' risk profiles have not been evaluated against those of nonathletes from the same academic, socioeconomic, or psychological backgrounds. These scientific limitations prevent conclusions that differences or similarities in eating behaviors or attitudes between athletes and patients diagnosed with eating disorders result from involvement in sport or exercise rather than from attributes that existed prior to people's becoming anorexic, bulimic, athletic, or physically active.

Muscle Dysmorphia

Harvard-affiliated researchers Phillips, O'Sullivan, and Pope (1997) proposed a form of body dysmorphic disorder that they have termed **muscle dysmorphia,** in which a person develops a pathological preoccupation with his or her muscularity. They presented case studies in which they concluded that muscle dysmorphia was associated with severe subjective distress, impaired social and occupational functioning, and abuse of anabolic steroids and other substances (Gruber and Pope 2000; Pope et al. 1997).

The investigators next tested the hypothesis that men in Western societies would desire to have a leaner and more muscular body than they had or perceived that they had (Pope et al. 2000). The height, weight, and body fat of college-aged men in Austria ($n = 54$), France ($n = 65$), and the United States ($n = 81$) were measured. Each man chose pictures that he believed represented (1) his own body, (2) the body he ideally would like to have, (3) the body of an average man of his age, and (4) the male body he believed women would prefer. The men's actual body fatness and muscularity were

---

Diagnostic Criteria for Body Dysmorphic Disorder

- The person has a preoccupation with an imagined defect in appearance. If a slight physical anomaly is present, the concern is excessive.
- The preoccupation causes clinically significant distress or impairment in social, occupational, or other important areas of functioning.
- The preoccupation is not better accounted for by another mental disorder (e.g., dissatisfaction with body shape and size as in anorexia nervosa).

Adapted from American Psychiatric Association 2000.

---

compared with those of the four images chosen. Despite modest differences between measured fat and the fatness of the images chosen, men from all three countries chose an ideal body that was an average of 28 lb (12.7 kg) more muscular than their own bodies. The men also believed that women preferred a male body about 30 lb (13.6 kg) more muscular than theirs, even though women in fact said they preferred an average-looking male body. The investigators speculated that the wide discrepancy between men's ideal body image and actual muscularity might help explain muscle dysmorphia and some anabolic steroid abuse.

In another study, 24 men classified as having muscle dysmorphia reportedly had higher body dissatisfaction, riskier eating attitudes, higher prevalence of anabolic steroid use, and greater lifetime prevalence of mood, anxiety, and eating disorders when compared with 30 normal comparison weightlifters recruited from gymnasiums in Boston (Olivardia, Pope, and Hudson 2000). The men with muscle dysmorphia said they frequently experienced shame, embarrassment, and impaired function at work and in social situations. A later study showed that compared to 28 male weightlifters with no symptoms, 15 lifters with current muscle dysmorphia reported more negative thoughts about their bodies, including their muscularity; dissatisfaction with their appearance; checking their appearance; and depending on bodybuilding.

Several cases of body dysmorphia were also reported among 75 female bodybuilders recruited from Boston area gymnasiums (Gruber and Pope 2000). Those with a past or current history of muscle dysmorphia were also likely to have mood or anxiety disorders (Cafri, Olivardia, and Thompson 2008).

It is not yet clear whether either body dysmorphia or muscle dysmorphia is characterized by the symptoms that are common to obsessive–compulsive anxiety disorder or eating disorders (Chosak et al. 2008). A cross-sectional study of a nonrandom sample of 237 male weightlifters aged 18 to 72 years (mean of 33 years), recruited from eight university and community gyms and two nutritional supplement stores in the U.S. South and Midwest, identified five classes of scores on eight measures of body image—dysmorphic, muscle concerned, fat concerned, normal behavioral, and normal (Hildebrandt et al. 2006). Men in the dysmorphic group ($n = 40$, i.e., 17% of the sample) reported overall body image disturbance, drive for muscle size, anxiety about physique, steroid use, and obsessive commitment to diet (including bulimic-type behaviors) and their workout routines (Hildebrandt et al. 2006). The muscle-concerned group ($n = 63$) believed they were not muscular enough and had high drive for muscle size, whereas the fat-concerned group ($n = 66$) had high body dissatisfaction and physique anxiety but not a drive for muscle size. The normal behavioral group ($n = 38$) reported high use of nutritional supplements and exercised often to reduce both muscle and fat weight, in contrast to the so-called normal group ($n = 30$), who desired to increase muscle and decrease body fat but didn't report symptoms of body dissatisfaction or anxiety. Aside from the small, nonrandom sample, a weakness of the study was the absence of any measures of body fatness or muscularity (other than BMI, which is not suitable for measuring body composition in weightlifters) to gauge whether the men's perceptions were realistic or distorted. That would be necessary to determine the extent to which the men's perceptions and motivation were disordered rather than appropriately goal directed. Nonetheless, there is some evidence that anabolic–androgenic steroid use and dependence is an emerging public health problem (Kanayama et al. 2009).

Though these small cross-sectional studies suggest that a clinically meaningful hazard of distorted body image exists, there have not been any controlled population-based studies to determine its prevalence or any prospective cohort studies or randomized clinical studies to determine whether either muscle dysmorphia or body dysmorphia results from participation in resistance exercise training—or whether people who have existing vulnerability to a distorted body image and self-concept are drawn to weightlifting.

Exercise Abuse

There have been case reports of excessive involvement with or dependence on leisure exercise training. William P. Morgan (1979) of the University of Wisconsin first described eight cases of "running addiction," in which commitment to running exceeded prior commitments to work, family, social relations, and medical advice. Similar cases have been labeled *positive addiction, runner's gluttony, fitness fanaticism, athlete's neurosis, obligatory running,* and *exercise abuse.* However, little is understood about the origins, valid diagnosis, or mental health impact of exercise abuse (Davis 2000; Dishman 1985; Bamber et al. 2003; Lejoyeux et al. 2008). Though exercise abuse or addiction is a problem requiring medical treatment for some people, its prevalence is probably not high enough to warrant population interventions. The problem in the United States is too little, not too much, physical activity!

▶ **THOUGH ABUSIVE** or addictive exercise exists as a problem requiring medical treatment for some people, its prevalence is probably not high enough to warrant population interventions. The problem in the United States is too little, not too much, physical activity.

Summary

The descriptive epidemiology of injury during physical activity and adverse events during medical treatment using exercise is less mature than the epidemiology of physical activity and chronic diseases. Knowledge about the risks of injury and the factors that modify those risks during prevalent types of physical activity, such as walking and gardening, is very sparse. The common perception is that walking and gardening involve minimal risks of musculoskeletal injury aside from muscle soreness and joint pain. Whether that is true remains to be determined by proper epidemiologic studies. Likewise, weightlifting or other resistance exercise, aerobic dance or group exercise, and bicycling have become increasingly popular in recent years, yet relatively little is known about the risk factors for injury among participants in these activities. Finally, it is also important to consider that risks to mental health or social adjustment can be associated with extreme dedication to exercise or preoccupation with fitness or physique.

Conditions such as anorexia athletica, muscle dysmorphia, and exercise abuse are not recognized as psychiatric diagnoses, and no controlled prospective studies have yet been conducted to show that they directly result from participation in leisure-time exercise by healthy people. Nonetheless, their appearance in clinical and scientific literature illustrates that their measurement, prevalence, and health consequences require epidemiologic study.

· BIBLIOGRAPHY ·

Aaltonen, S., H. Karjalainen, A. Heinonen, J. Parkkari, and U.M. Kujala. 2007. Prevention of sports injuries: Systematic review of randomized controlled trials. *Archives of Internal Medicine* 167 (15): 1585-1592.

Alexandrescu, R., S.J. O'Brien, and F.E. Lecky. 2009. A review of injury epidemiology in the UK and Europe: Some methodological considerations in constructing rates. *BMC Public Health* 9 (July 10): 226.

American College of Obstetricians and Gynecologists. Committee on Obstetric Practice. 2002. ACOG Committee opinion. Exercise during pregnancy and the postpartum period. *Obstetricsand Gynecology* 99: 171-173.

American College of Sports Medicine. 2002. American College of Sports Medicine position stand: Progression models in resistance training for healthy adults. *Medicine and Science in Sports and Exercise* 34: 364-380.

American College of Sports Medicine. 2006. American College of Sports Medicine position stand: Prevention of cold injuries during exercise. *Medicine and Science in Sports and Exercise* 38: 2012-2029.

American College of Sports Medicine. 2007a. American College of Sports Medicine position stand: Exertional heat illness during training and competition. *Medicine and Science in Sports and Exercise* 39: 556-572.

American College of Sports Medicine. 2007b. American College of Sports Medicine position stand: Exercise and fluid replacement. *Medicine and Science in Sports and Exercise* 39: 377-390.

American College of Sports Medicine. 2007c. American College of Sports Medicine position stand: The Female Athlete Triad. *Medicine and Science in Sports and Exercise* 39 (10): 1867-1882.

American Psychiatric Association. 2000. *Diagnostic and statistical manual of mental disorders.* 4th edition, text revision. Washington, DC: American Psychiatric Association.

Arendt, E., and R. Dick. 1995. Knee injury patterns among men and women in collegiate basketball and soccer. *American Journal of Sports Medicine* 23: 694-701.

Attewell, R.G., K. Glase, and M. McFadden. 2001. Bicycle helmet efficacy: A meta-analysis. *Accident Analysis and Prevention* 33: 345-352.

Backx, F.J., H.J. Beijer, E. Bol, and W. Erich. 1991. Injuries in high-risk persons and high-risk sports. A longitudinal study of 1818 school children. *American Journal of Sports Medicine* 19: 124-130.

Backx, F.J., W.B. Erich, A.B. Kemper, and A.L. Verbeek. 1989. Sports injuries in school-aged children. An epidemiologic study. *American Journal of Sports Medicine* 17: 234-240.

Bailes, J.E., and R.C. Cantu. 2001. Head injuries in athletes. *Neurosurgery* 48: 26-46.

Bamber, D.J., I.M. Cockerill, S. Rodgers, and D. Carroll. 2003. Diagnostic criteria for exercise dependence in women. *British Journal of Sports Medicine* 37 (5): 393-400.

Bell, N.S., T.W. Mangione, D. Hemenway, P.J. Amoroso, and B.H. Jones. 2000. High injury rates among female army trainees: A function of gender? *American Journal of Preventive Medicine* 18 (3 Suppl.): 141-146.

Blair, S.N., H.W. Kohl, and N.N. Goodyear. 1987. Rates and risks for running and exercise injuries: Studies in three populations. *Research Quarterly in Exercise and Sports* 58 (3): 221-228.

Blumenthal, J.A., S. Rose, and J.L. Chang. 1985. Anorexia nervosa and exercise. *Sports Medicine* 2: 237-247.

Bovens, A.M., G.M.E. Janssen, H.G.W. Vermeer, J.H. Hoeberigs, M.P.E. Janssen, and F.T.J. Verstappen. 1989. Occurrence of running injuries in adults following a supervised training program. *International Journal of Sports Medicine* 10: S186-S190.

Burt, C.W., and M.D. Overpeck. 2001. Emergency visits for sports-related injuries. *Annals of Emergency Medicine* 37: 301-308.

Cafri, G., R. Olivardia, and J.K. Thompson. 2008. Symptom characteristics and psychiatric comorbidity among males with muscle dysmorphia. *Comprehensive Psychiatry* 49 (4): 374-379.

Canham, M.L., J.J. Knapik, M.A. Smutok, and B.H. Jones. 1998. Training, physical performance, and injuries among men and women preparing for occupations in the Army. In *Advances in occupational ergonomics and safety: Proceedings of the XIIIth Annual International Occupational Ergonomics and Safety Conference,* edited by S. Kumar, pp. 711-714. Amsterdam, The Netherlands: IOS Press.

Cantu, R.C., and F.O. Mueller. 2003. Brain injury-related fatalities in American football, 1945-1999. *Neurosurgery* 52 (4): 846-852.

Carlson, S.A., J.M. Hootman, K.E. Powell, C.A. Macera, G.W. Heath, J. Gilchrist, C.D. Kimsey, and H.W. Kohl. 2006. Self-reported injury and physical activity levels: United States 2000 to 2002. *Annals of Epidemiology* 16: 712-719.

Castelli, W.P., and D.G. Adams. 1990. Running doesn't kill people with healthy hearts. *Your Patient and Fitness* 2 (2): 12-17.

Centers for Disease Control and Prevention. 1997. Sports-related recurrent brain injuries, United States. *Morbidity and Mortality Weekly Report* 46: 224-227.

Centers for Disease Control and Prevention. 2006. Sports-related injuries among high school athletes—United States, 2005-2006 school year. *Morbidity and Mortality Weekly Report* 55: 1037-1040.

Centers for Disease Control and Prevention. 2007. Nonfatal traumatic brain injuries from sports and recreation activities—United States, 2001–2005 school year. *Morbidity and Mortality Weekly Report* 56 (29): 733-736.

Centers for Disease Control and Prevention. 2010. Heat illness among high school athletes—United States, 2005-2009. *Morbidity and Mortality Weekly Report* 59 (32): 1009-1013.

Cheema, B., C.A. Gaul, K. Lane, and M.A. Fiatarone Singh. 2008. Progressive resistance training in breast cancer: A systematic review of clinical trials. *Breast Cancer Research and Treatment* 109 (1): 9-26.

Chien, C.L., C.M. Lee, Y.W. Wu, T.A. Chen, and Y.T. Wu. 2008. Home-based exercise increases exercise capacity but not quality of life in people with chronic heart failure: A systematic review. *Australian Journal of Physiotherapy* 54 (2): 87-93.

Chosak, A., L. Marques, J.L. Greenberg, E. Jenike, D.D. Dougherty, and S. Wilhelm. 2008. Body dysmorphic disorder and obsessive-compulsive disorder: Similarities, differences and the classification debate. *Expert Review of Neurotherapeutics* 8 (8): 1209-1218.

Colbert, L.H., J.M. Hootman, and C.A. Macera. 2000. Physical activity-related injuries in walkers and runners in the Aerobics Center Longitudinal Study. *Clinical Journal of Sports Medicine* 10: 259-263.

Cooper, E.R., M.S. Ferrara, and S.P. Broglio. 2006. Exertional heat illness and environmental conditions during a single football season in the southeast. *Journal of Athletic Training* 41 (3): 332-326.

Daly, P.J., R.H. Fitzgerald, L.J. Melton, and D.M. Ilstrip. 1987. Epidemiology of ankle fractures in Rochester, Minnesota. *Acta Orthopaedica Scandinavica* 58: 539-544.

Daneshvar, D.H., C.J. Nowinski, A.C. McKee, and R.C. Cantu. 2011. The epidemiology of sport-related concussion. *Clinics in Sports Medicine* 30 (1): 1-17.

Darrow, C.J., C.L. Collins, E.E. Yard, and R.D. Comstock. 2009. Epidemiology of severe injuries among United States high school athletes: 2005-2007. *American Journal of Sports Medicine* 37 (9): 1798-1805.

Davis, C. 2000. Exercise abuse. *International Journal of Sport Psychology* 31: 278-304.

de Loes, M. 1990. Medical treatment and costs of sports-related injuries in a total population. *International Journal of Sports Medicine* 11: 66-72.

de Loes, M. 1997. Exposure data. Why are they needed? *Sports Medicine* 24: 172-175.

de Loes, M., and I. Goldie. 1988. Incidence rate of injuries during sport activity and physical exercise in a rural Swedish municipality: Incidence rates in 17 sports. *International Journal of Sports Medicine* 9 (6): 461-467.

de Loes, M., B. Jacobsen, and I. Goldie. 1990. Risk exposure and incidence of injuries in school physical education at different activity levels. *Canadian Journal of Sport Science* 15 (2): 131-136.

de Morton, N.A., J.L. Keating, and K. Jeffs. 2007. The effect of exercise on outcomes for older acute medical inpatients compared with control or alternative treatments: A systematic review of randomized controlled trials. *Clinical Rehabilitation* 21 (1): 3-16.

D'hondt, N.E., P.A. Struijs, G.M. Kerkhoffs, C. Verheul, R. Lysens, G. Aufdemkampe, and C.N. Van Dijk. 2002. Orthotic devices for treating patellofemoral pain syndrome. *Cochrane Database of Systematic Reviews* (2): CD002267.

Dick, R., M.S. Ferrara, J. Agel, R. Courson, S.W. Marshall, M.J. Hanley, and F. Reifsteck. 2007. Descriptive epidemiology of collegiate men's football injuries: National Collegiate Athletic Association Injury Surveillance System, 1988-1989 through 2003-2004. *Journal of Athletic Training* 42 (2): 221-233.

DiMaggio, C., and M. Durkin. 2002. Child pedestrian injury in an urban setting: Descriptive epidemiology. *Academy of Emergency Medicine* 9: 54-62.

Dishman, R.K. 1985. Medical psychology in exercise and sport. *Medical Clinics of North America* 69: 123-143.

Einerson, J., A. Ward, and P. Hanson. 1988. Exercise responses in females with anorexia nervosa. *International Journal of Eating Disorders* 7: 253-260.

Environmental Protection Agency (EPA). Air Quality Index (AQI) – A guide to air quality and your health. www.airnow.gov/index.cfm?action=aqibasics.aqi.

Faich, G., and R. Rose. 1979. Blizzard morbidity and mortality: Rhode Island, 1978. *American Journal of Public Health* 69: 1050-1052.

Ferrara, M.S., G.R. Palutsis, S. Snouse, and R.W. Davis. 2000. A longitudinal study of injuries to athletes with disabilities. *International Journal of Sports Medicine* 21 (3): 221-224.

Ferrara, M.S., and C.L. Peterson. 2000. Injuries to athletes with disabilities: Identifying injury patterns. *Sports Medicine* 30 (2): 137-143.

Finch, C., and E. Cassell. 2006. The public health impact of injury during sport and active recreation. *Journal of Science and Medicine in Sport* 9: 490-497.

Fountain, J.L., and M.C. Meyers. 1996. Skateboarding injuries. *Sports Medicine* 22: 360-366.

Fradkin, A.J., B.J. Gabbe, and P.A. Cameron. 2006. Does warming up prevent injury in sport? The evidence from randomised controlled trials? *Journal of Science and Medicine in Sport* 9 (3): 214-220.

Fradkin, A.J., T.R. Zazryn, and J.M. Smoliga. 2010. Effects of warming-up on physical performance: A systematic review with meta-analysis. *Journal of Strength and Conditioning Research* 24 (1): 140-148.

Garrick, J.G., D.M. Gillien, and P. Whiteside. 1986. The epidemiology of aerobic dance injuries. *American Journal of Sports Medicine* 14 (1): 67-72.

Gessel, L.M., S.K. Fields, C.L. Collins, R.W. Dick, and R.D. Comstock. 2007. Concussions among United States high school and collegiate athletes. *Journal of Athletic Training* 42 (4): 495-503.

Gianotti, S.M., S.W. Marshall, P.A. Hume, and L. Bunt. 2009. Incidence of anterior cruciate ligament injury and other knee ligament injuries: A national population-based study. *Journal of Science and Medicine in Sport* 12 (6): 622-627.

Gotsch, K., J.L. Annest, and P. Holmgreen. 2002. Nonfatal sports- and recreation-related injuries treated in emergency departments—United States, July 2000–June 2001. *Morbidity and Mortality Weekly Report* 51 (33): 736-740.

Gruber, A.J., and H.G. Pope. 2000. Psychiatric and medical effects of anabolic-androgenic steroid use in women. *Psychotherapy and Psychosomatics* 69: 19-26.

Guichon, D.M.P., and S.T. Myles. 1975. Bicycle injuries: One year sample in Calgary. *Journal of Trauma* 15 (6): 504-506.

Halstead, M.E., and K.D. Walter; Council on Sports Medicine and Fitness. 2010. American Academy of Pediatrics. Clinical report—sport-related concussion in children and adolescents. *Pediatrics* 126 (3): 597-615.

Hart, L. 2005. Effect of stretching on sport injury risk: A review. *Clinical Journal of Sport Medicine* 15 (2): 113.

Haskell, W.L. 1978. Cardiovascular complications during exercise training of cardiac patients. *Circulation* 57: 920-924.

Hassett, L.M., A.M. Moseley, R. Tate, and A.R. Harmer. 2008. Fitness training for cardiorespiratory conditioning after traumatic brain injury. *Cochrane Database of Systematic Reviews,* April 16 (2): CD006123.

Heath, G.W., and J.S. Kendrick. 1989. Outrunning the risks: A behavioral risk profile of runners. *American Journal of Preventive Medicine* 5 (6): 347-352.

Hede, A., D.B. Jensen, P. Blyme, and S. Sonne-Holm. 1990. Epidemiology of meniscal lesions in the knee. *Acta Orthopaedica Scandinavica* 61 (5): 435-437.

Herbert, R.D., and M. de Noronha. 2007. Stretching to prevent or reduce muscle soreness after exercise. *Cochrane Database of Systematic Reviews,* October 17 (4): CD004577.

Herbert, R.D., and M. Gabriel. 2002. Effects of stretching before and after exercising on muscle soreness and risk of injury: Systematic review. *British Medical Journal* 325 (7362): 468-472.

Hildebrandt, T., D. Schlundt, J. Langenbucher, and T. Chung. 2006. Presence of muscle dysmorphia symptomology among male weightlifters. *Comprehensive Psychiatry* 47 (2): 127-135.

Holmich, P., S.W. Christensen, E. Darre, F. Jahnsen, and T. Hartvig. 1989. Non-elite marathon runners: Health, training and injuries. *British Journal of Sports Medicine* 23 (3): 177-178.

Hootman, J.M., R. Dick, and J. Agel. 2007. Epidemiology of collegiate injuries for 15 sports: Summary and recommendations for injury prevention initiatives. *Journal of Athletic Training* 42 (2): 311-319.

Hootman, J.M., C.A. Macera, B.E. Ainsworth, C.L. Addy, M. Martin, and S.N. Blair. 2002a. Epidemiology of musculoskeletal injuries among sedentary and physically active adults. *Medicine and Science in Sports and Exercise* 34: 838-844.

Hootman, J.M., C.A. Macera, B.E. Ainsworth, M. Martin, C.L. Addy, and S.N. Blair. 2002b. Predictors of lower extremity injury among recreationally active adults. *Clinical Journal of Sport Medicine* 12: 99-106.

Hootman, J.M., and K.E. Powell. 2009. Physical activity, fitness, and musculoskeletal injury. In *Epidemiologic methods in physical activity studies,* edited by I-M. Lee, pp. 263-282. New York: Oxford University Press.

Hume, P., W. Hopkins, K. Rome, P. Maulder, G. Coyle, and B. Nigg. 2008. Effectiveness of foot orthoses for treatment and prevention of lower limb injuries: A review. *Sports Medicine* 38 (9): 759-779.

Ioannidis, J.P. 2009. Adverse events in randomized trials: Neglected, restricted, distorted, and silenced. *Archives of Internal Medicine* 169 (19): 1737-1739.

Ioannidis, J.P., S.J. Evans, P.C. Gotzsche, et al.; CONSORT Group. 2004. Better reporting of harms in randomized trials: An extension of the CONSORT statement. *Annals of Internal Medicine* 141 (10): 781-788.

Jacobs, S.J., and B.L. Berson. 1986. Injuries to runners: A study of entrants to a 10,000 meter race. *American Journal of Sports Medicine* 14: 151-155.

James, S.L., B.T. Bates, and L.R. Osternig. 1978. Injuries to runners. *American Journal of Sports Medicine* 6 (2): 40-50.

Jones, B.H., D.N. Cowan, and J.J. Knapik. 1994. Exercise training and injuries. *Sports Medicine* 18 (3): 202-214.

Jones, B.H., D.N. Cowan, J.P. Tomlison, J.R. Robinson, D.W. Polly, and P.N. Frykman. 1993. Epidemiology of injuries associated with physical training among young men in the army. *Medicine and Science in Sports and Exercise* 25 (2): 197-203.

Junge, A., L. Engebretsen, M.L. Mountjoy, J.M. Alonso, P.A. Renström, M.J. Aubry, and J. Dvorak. 2009. Sports injuries during the Summer Olympic Games 2008. *American Journal of Sports Medicine* 37 (11): 2165-2172.

Kallinen, M., and A. Markku. 1995. Aging, physical activity and sports injuries: An overview of common sports injuries in the elderly. *Sports Medicine* 20 (1): 41-52.

Kanayama, G., K.J. Brower, R.I. Wood, J.I. Hudson, and H.G. Pope Jr. 2009. Anabolic-androgenic steroid dependence: An emerging disorder. *Addiction* 104 (12): 1966-1978.

Kennedy, M.C., G.K. Vanderfield, and J.R. Kennedy. 1977. Sport: Assessing the risk. *Medical Journal of Australia* 2: 253-254.

Kiburz, D., R. Jacobs, F. Reckling, and J. Mason. 1986. Bicycle accidents and injuries among adult cyclists. *American Journal of Sports Medicine* 14 (5): 416-419.

Kirkendall, D.T., and W.E. Garrett Jr. 2000. The anterior cruciate ligament enigma: Injury mechanisms and prevention. *Clinical Orthopaedics and Related Research* 372: 64-68.

Knapik, J.J. 1998. U.S. Army Center for Health Promotion and Preventive Medicine (USACHPPM) Technical Report No. 29-HE-8370-98.

Knapik, J.J., M. Canham-Chervak, K. Hauret, M.J. Laurin, E. Hoedebecke, S. Craig, and S.J. Montain. 2002. Seasonal variations in injury rates during US Army basic combat training. *Annals of Occupational Hygiene* 46: 15-23.

Knapik, J.J., K.G. Hauret, S. Arnold, M. Canham-Chervak, A.J. Mansfield, E.L. Hoedebecke, and D. McMillian. 2003. Injury and fitness outcomes during implementation of physical readiness training. *International Journal of Sports Medicine* 24 (5): 372-381.

Knapik, J.J., M.A. Sharp, M. Canham-Chervak, K. Hauret, J.F. Patton, and B.H. Jones. 2001. Risk factors for training-related injuries among men and women in basic combat training. *Medicine and Science in Sports and Exercise* 33: 946-954.

Koplan, J.P., K.E. Powell, R.K. Sikes, R.W. Shirley, and C.C. Campbell. 1982. An epidemiologic study of the benefits and risks of running. *Journal of the American Medical Association* 248 (23): 3118-3121.

Koplan, J.P., R.B. Rothenberg, and E.L. Jones. 1995. The natural history of exercise: A 10-year follow up of a cohort of runners. *Medicine and Science in Sports and Exercise* 27 (8): 1180-1184.

Koplan, J.P., D.S. Siscovick, and G.M. Goldbaum. 1985. The risks of exercise: A public health view of injuries and hazards. *Public Health Reports* 100 (2): 189-195.

Kretsch, A., R. Gragan, P. Duras, F. Allen, J. Sumner, and I. Gillam. 1984. 1980 Melbourne marathon study. *Medical Journal of Australia* 141: 809-814.

Kruse, D.L., and A.A. McBeath. 1980. Bicycle accidents and injuries. *American Journal of Sports Medicine* 8 (5): 342-344.

Kujala, U.I., S. Taimela, I. Antti-Poika, S. Orava, R. Tuominen, and P. Myllynen. 1995. Acute injuries in soccer, ice hockey, volleyball, basketball, judo, and karate: Analysis of national registry data. *British Medical Journal* 311: 1465-1468.

Langlois, J.A., W. Rutland-Brown, and M.M. Wald. 2006. The epidemiology and impact of traumatic brain injury. *Journal of Head Trauma and Rehabilitation* 21: 375-378.

Lejoyeux, M., M. Avril, C. Richoux, H. Embouazza, and F. Nivoli. 2008. Prevalence of exercise dependence and other behavioral addictions among clients of a Parisian fitness room. *Comprehensive Psychiatry* 49 (4): 353-358.

Liu, C.J., and N.K. Latham. 2009. Progressive resistance strength training for improving physical function in older adults. *Cochrane Database of Systematic Reviews,* July 8 (3): CD002759.

Lysholm, J., and J. Wiklander. 1987. Injuries in runners. *American Journal of Sports Medicine* 15 (2): 168-171.

Macera, C.A., R.R. Pate, K.E. Powell, K.L. Jackson, J.S. Kendrick, and T.E. Craven. 1989. Predicting lower-extremity injuries among habitual runners. *Archives of Internal Medicine* 149: 2565-2568.

Marti, B. 1988. Benefits and risks of running among women: An epidemiologic study. *International Journal of Sports Medicine* 9 (2): 92-98.

Marti, B., J.P. Vader, C.E. Minder, and T. Abelin. 1988. On the epidemiology of running injuries: The 1984 Bern Grand-Prix study. *American Journal of Sports Medicine* 16 (3): 285-294.

Martinsen, M., S. Bratland-Sanda, A.K. Eriksson, and J. Sundgot-Borgen. 2010. Dieting to win or to be thin? A study of dieting and disordered eating among adolescent elite athletes and non-athlete controls. *British Journal of Sports Medicine* 44 (1): 70-76.

McSherry, J.A. 1984. The diagnostic challenge of anorexia nervosa. *American Family Physician* 29: 141-145.

Mehrholz, J., R. Friis, J. Kugler, S. Twork, A. Storch, and M. Pohl. 2010. Treadmill training for patients with Parkinson's disease. *Cochrane Database of Systematic Reviews,* January 20 (1): CD007830.

Morgan, W.P. 1979. Negative addiction in runners. *Physician and Sportsmedicine* 7 (2): 57-70.

Morgan, W.P., D.R. Brown, J.S. Raglin, P.J. O'Connor, and K.A. Ellickson. 1987. Psychological monitoring of overtraining and staleness. *British Journal of Sports Medicine* 21: 107-114.

Mountcastle, S.B., M. Posner, J.F. Kragh Jr., and D.C. Taylor. 2007. Gender differences in anterior cruciate ligament injury vary with activity: Epidemiology of anterior cruciate ligament injuries in a young, athletic population. *American Journal of Sports Medicine* 35 (10): 1635-1642.

National Center for Health Statistics, P.F. Adams, and V. Benson. 1991. *Current estimates for the National Health Interview Survey, 1990. Vital and Health Statistics, Series 10,* No. 181. DHHS Publication No. (PHS) 92-1509. Hyattsville, MD: U.S. Department of Health and Human Services, Centers for Disease Control, National Center for Health Statistics.

Nicholl, J.P., P. Coleman, and B.T. Williams. 1991. Pilot study of the epidemiology of sports injuries and exercise-related morbidity. *British Journal of Sports Medicine* 25: 61-66.

Nicholl, J.P., P. Coleman, and B.T. Williams. 1995. The epidemiology of sports and exercise related injury in the United Kingdom. *British Journal of Sports Medicine* 4: 232-238.

O'Connor, P.J., and J.C. Smith. 1999. Physical activity and eating disorders. In *Lifestyle medicine,* edited by J.M. Rippe, pp. 1005-1015. Cambridge, MA: Blackwell Science.

Olivardia, R., H.G. Pope, and J.I. Hudson. 2000. Muscle dysmorphia in male weightlifters: A case–control study. *American Journal of Psychiatry* 157: 1291-1296.

Parkkari, J., P. Kannus, A. Natri, I. Lapinieimu, M. Palvanen, M. Helskanen, I. Vuori, and M. Järvinen. 2004. Active living and injury risk. *International Journal of Sports Medicine* 25: 209-216.

Parkkari, J., K. Pasanen, V.M. Mattila, P. Kannus, and A. Rimpelä. 2008. The risk for a cruciate ligament injury of the knee in adolescents and young adults: A population-based cohort study of 46 500 people with a 9 year follow-up. *British Journal of Sports Medicine* 42 (6): 422-426.

Phillips, K.A., R.L. O'Sullivan, and H.G. Pope. 1997. Muscle dysmorphia. *Journal of Clinical Psychiatry* 58: 361.

Phillips, M., M. Robinowitz, J.R. Higgins, K.J. Boran, T. Reed, and R. Virmani. 1986. Sudden cardiac death in Air Force recruits. *Journal of the American Medical Association* 256: 2696-2699.

Physical Activity Guidelines Advisory Committee. 2008. *Physical Activity Guidelines Advisory Committee report.* Washington, DC: U.S. Department of Health and Human Services.

Pitrou, I., I. Boutron, N. Ahmad, and P. Ravaud. 2009. Reporting of safety results in published reports of randomized controlled trials. *Archives of Internal Medicine* 169 (19): 1756-1761.

Pollock, M.L., L.R. Gettman, C.A. Milesis, M.D. Bah, L. Durstine, and R.B. Johnson. 1977. Effects of frequency and duration of training on attrition and incidence of injury. *Medicine and Science in Sports* 9 (1): 31-36.

Pope, H.G., A.J. Gruber, P. Choi, R. Olivardia, and K.A. Phillips. 1997. Muscle dysmorphia: An underrecognized form of body dysmorphic disorder. *Psychosomatics* 38: 548-557.

Pope, H.G., A.J. Gruber, B. Mangweth, B. Bureau, C. deCol, R. Jouvent, and J.I. Hudson. 2000. Body image perception among men in three countries. *American Journal of Psychiatry* 157: 1297-1301.

Powell, K.E., G.W. Heath, M.J. Kresnow, J.J. Sacks, and C.M. Branche. 1998. Injury rates from walking, gardening, weightlifting, outdoor bicycling, and aerobics. *Medicine and Science in Sports and Exercise* 30 (8): 1246-1249.

Powell, K.E., H.W. Kohl, C.J. Casperson, and S.N. Blair. 1986. An epidemiological perspective on the causes of running injuries. *Physician and Sportsmedicine* 14 (6): 100-114.

Prodromos, C.C., Y. Han, J. Rogowski, B. Joyce, and K. Shi. 2007. A meta-analysis of the incidence of anterior cruciate ligament tears as a function of gender, sport, and a knee injury-reduction regimen. *Arthroscopy* 23 (12): 1320-1325.

Ramazzini, B. 1983. *Diseases of workers: Latin text of 1713 revised with translation and notes by Wilmer Cave Wright.* New York: Classics of Medicine Library, Division of Gryphon Editions.

Requa, R.K., L.N. DeAvilla, and J.G. Garrick. 1993. Injuries in recreational adult fitness activities. *American Journal of Sports Medicine* 21: 461-467.

Reynolds, K.L., E.A. Harman, R.E. Worsham, M.B. Sykes, P.N. Frykman, and V.L. Backus. 2001. Injuries in women associated with a periodized strength training and running program. *Journal of Strength and Conditioning Research* 5 (1): 136-143.

Richie, D.H., S.F. Kelso, and P.A. Bellucci. 1985. Aerobic dance injuries: A retrospective study of instructors and participants. *Physician and Sportsmedicine* 13 (2): 130-140.

Rome, K., H.H. Handoll, and R. Ashford. 2005. Interventions for preventing and treating stress fractures and stress reactions of bone of the lower limbs in young adults. *Cochrane Database of Systematic Reviews,* April 18 (2): CD000450.

Romo, M. 1972. Factors related to sudden death in acute ischaemic heart disease. *Acta Medica Scandinavica* 547 (Suppl. I): 1-92.

Rothenberger, L.A., J.I. Chang, and T.A. Cable. 1988. Prevalence and types of injuries in aerobic dancers. *American Journal of Sports Medicine* 16: 403-407.

Sacks, J.J., P. Holmgreen, S.M. Smith, and D.M. Sosin. 1991. Bicycle-associated head injuries and deaths in the United States from 1984 through 1988. *Journal of the American Medical Association* 266: 3016-3018.

Samet, J.M., T.W. Chick, and C.A. Howard. 1982. Running-related morbidity: A community survey. *Annals of Sports Medicine* 1 (1): 30-34.

Sandelin, J., and S. Santavirta. 1991. Occurrence and epidemiology of sports injuries in Finland. *Annales Chirurgiae et Gynaecologiae* 80: 95-99.

Sandelin, J., S. Santavirta, R. Lattila, P. Vuolle, and S. Sarna. 1988. Sports injuries in a large urban population: Occurrence and epidemiological aspects. *International Journal of Sports Medicine* 9 (1): 61-66.

Saunders, D.H., C.A. Greig, G.E. Mead, and A. Young. 2009. Physical fitness training for stroke patients. *Cochrane Database of Systematic Reviews,* October 7 (4): CD003316.

Scheiber, R.A., and C.M. Branche-Dorsey. 1995. In-line skating injuries: Epidemiology and recommendations for prevention. *Sports Medicine* 19 (2): 427-432.

Schulman, J., J. Sacks, and G. Provensano. 2002. State level estimates of the incidence and economic burden of head injuries stemming from non-universal use of bicycle helmets. *Injury Prevention* 8: 47-52.

Sgaglione, N.A., K. Suljaga-Petchell, and V.H. Frankel. 1982. Bicycle-related accidents and injuries in a population of urban cyclists. *Bulletin of the Hospital for Joint Diseases Orthopaedic Institute* 42 (1): 80-91.

Shaw, K., H. Gennat, P. O'Rourke, and C. Del Mar. 2006. Exercise for overweight or obesity. *Cochrane Database of Systematic Reviews*, October 18 (4): CD003817.

Sigal, R.J., G.P. Kenny, N.G. Boulé, G.A. Wells, D. Prud'homme, M. Fortier, R.D. Reid, H. Tulloch, D. Coyle, P. Phillips, A. Jennings, and J. Jaffey. 2007. Effects of aerobic training, resistance training, or both on glycemic control in type 2 diabetes: A randomized trial. *Annals of Internal Medicine* 147 (6): 357-369.

Simon, T.D., C. Bublitz, and S.J. Hambidge. 2006. Emergency department visits among pediatric patients for sports-related injury: Basic epidemiology and impact of race/ethnicity and insurance status. *Pediatric Emergency Care* 22 (5): 309-315.

Siscovick, D.S., N.S. Weiss, R.H. Fletcher, and T. Lasky. 1984. The incidence of cardiac arrest during vigorous exercise. *New England Journal of Medicine* 311: 874-877.

Sosin, D.M., J.E. Sniezek, and D.J. Thurman. 1996. Incidence of mild and moderate brain injury in the United States, 1991. *Brain Injury* 10: 47-54.

Sosin, D.M., J.E. Sniezek, and R.J. Waxweiler. 1995. Trends in death associated with traumatic brain injury, 1979 through 1992: Success and failure. *Journal of the American Medical Association* 273: 1778-1780.

Speck, R.M., K.S. Courneya, L.C. Mâsse, S. Duval, and K.H. Schmitz. 2010. An update of controlled physical activity trials in cancer survivors: A systematic review and meta-analysis. *Journal of Cancer Survivorship: Research and Practice* 4 (2): 87-100.

Sundgot-Borgen, J. 1994. Risk and trigger factors for the development of eating disorders in female elite athletes. *Medicine and Science in Sports and Exercise* 26: 414-419.

Thacker, S.B., J. Gilchrist, D.F. Stroup, and C.D. Kimsey Jr. 2004. The impact of stretching on sports injury risk: A systematic review of the literature. *Medicine and Science in Sports and Exercise* 36 (3): 371-378.

Thompson, P.D. 1996. The cardiovascular complications of vigorous physical activity. *Archives of Internal Medicine* 156: 2297-2302.

Thompson, P.D., E.J. Funk, R.A. Carleton, and W.Q. Sterner. 1982. Incidence of death during jogging in Rhode Island from 1975 through 1980. *Journal of the American Medical Association* 247: 2535-2538.

Thompson, P.D., M.P. Stern, P. Williams, K. Duncan, W.L. Haskell, and P.D. Wood. 1979. Death during jogging or running: A study of 18 cases. *Journal of the American Medical Association* 242: 1265-1267.

Thompson, R.S., F.P. Rivara, and D.C. Thompson. 1989. A case–control study of the effectiveness of bicycle safety helmets. *New England Journal of Medicine* 320 (21): 1361-1367.

Torstveit, M.K., J.H. Rosenvinge, and J. Sundgot-Borgen. 2008. Prevalence of eating disorders and the predictive power of risk models in female elite athletes: A controlled study. *Scandinavian Journal of Medicine and Science in Sports* 18 (1): 108-118.

U.S. Department of Health and Human Services. 1991. *Healthy people 2000: National health promotion and disease prevention objectives.* Washington, DC: U.S. Department of Health and Human Services.

Van Camp, S.P. 1987a. The hazards of exercise. *Your Patient and Fitness* 1 (4): 18-21.

Van Camp, S.P. 1987b. The hazards of exercise (conclusion). *Your Patient and Fitness* 1 (5): 15-17.

Van Camp, S.P., C.M. Bloor, F.O. Mueller, R.C. Cantu, and H.G. Olson. 1995. Nontraumatic sports death in high school and college athletes. *Medicine and Science in Sports and Exercise* 27: 641-647.

Van Camp, S.P., and R.A. Peterson. 1986. Cardiovascular complications of outpatient cardiac rehabilitation programs. *Journal of the American Medical Association* 256: 1160-1163.

van Mechelen, W. 1992. Running injuries: A review of the epidemiological literature. *Sports Medicine* 14: 320-335.

Videman, T., M.C. Battie, L.E. Gibbons, H. Manninen, K. Gill, L.D. Fisher, and M. Koskenvuo. 1997. Lifetime exercise and disk degeneration: An MRI study of monozygotic twins. *Medicine and Science in Sports and Exercise* 29: 1350-1356.

Vuori, I., M. Makarainen, and A. Jaaskelainen. 1978. Sudden death and physical activity. *Cardiology* 63: 287-304.

Vyrostek, S.B., J.L. Annest, and G.W. Ryan. 2004. Surveillance for fatal and nonfatal injuries—United States, 2001. *Morbidity and Mortality Weekly Report: Surveillance Summaries* 53 (7): 1-57.

Walter, S.D., L.E. Hart, J.M. McIntosh, and J.R. Sutton. 1989. The Ontario cohort study of running-related injuries. *Archives of Internal Medicine* 149: 2561-2564.

Watson, A.W. 1993. Incidence and nature of sports injuries in Ireland: An analysis of four types of sport. *American Journal of Sports Medicine* 21: 137-143.

Webborn, N., S. Willick, and J.C. Reeser. 2006. Injuries among disabled athletes during the 2002 Winter Paralympic Games. *Medicine and Science in Sports and Exercise* 38 (5): 811-815.

Whang, W., J.E. Manson, F.B. Hu, C.U. Chae, L. Rexrode, W.C. Willett, M.J. Stampfer, and C.M. Albert. 2006. Physical exertion, exercise, and sudden cardiac death in women. *Journal of the American Medical Association* 295: 1399-1403.

Wirthwein, D.P., S.D. Spotswood, J.J. Barnard, and J.A. Prahlow. 2001. Death due to microvascular occlusion in sickle-cell trait following physical exertion. *Journal of Forensic Science* 46: 399-401.

Yang, J., G. Phillips, H. Xiang, V. Allareddy, E. Heiden, and C. Peek-Asa. 2008. Hospitalisations for sport-related concussions in US children aged 5 to 18 years during 2000-2004. *British Journal of Sports Medicine* 42 (8): 664-669.

Yates, A., K. Leehey, and C. Shisslak. 1983. Running—an analogue of anorexia? *New England Journal of Medicine* 308: 251-255.

Zebas, C.J., K. Louden, M. Chapman, L. Magee, and S. Bowman. 1995. Musculoskeletal injuries in a college-age population during a 1-semester term. *Journal of American College Health* 44 (1): 32-34.

CHAPTER 17

Adopting and Maintaining a Physically Active Lifestyle

I noticed when I taught slow, heavy, fancy . . . gymnastics, athletics, etc.,
that I would have a very large membership at the first of the year,
but that they would soon drop out.

• Robert Jeffries Roberts •

Director of Physical Education, YMCA, Springfield, Massachusetts, 1887-1889
(quoted in Leonard and Affleck 1947, pp. 315-319)

Train up a child in the way he should go; and when he is old, he will not depart from it.

• The Holy Bible •

King James Version, Book of Proverbs, chapter 22, verse 6

CHAPTER OBJECTIVES

▸ Describe the problems of insufficient physical activity participation in populations and poor adherence to clinical exercise programs

▸ Identify the major determinants (i.e., risk factors) of insufficient physical activity and dropping out of exercise programs

▸ Discuss aspects of the social and built environments associated with physical activity participation

▸ Describe evidence for the genetic basis of physical activity

▸ Contrast putative mediators and moderators of change in physical activity

▸ Discuss prominent theories of behavior change applied to physical activity

▸ Describe the efficacy and effectiveness of interventions used to promote increases in physical activity

Despite the cumulative evidence presented in this book that physical activity promotes health, most Americans are not sufficiently active. The full magnitude of the physical inactivity problem in the United States and other developed nations is clearly illustrated in chapter 3. Getting people to adopt and then getting them to maintain a regular physical activity program are two of the biggest challenges facing public health in developed and developing nations, including the United States. The worldwide prevalence of physical inactivity is estimated to be 17.4%. It is greater in economically advanced nations (28%) and among women and elderly people (Dumith et al. 2011b).

National estimates indicate that 57% of American adults do not meet minimal recommendations for sufficient physical activity, and 36% say they get no leisure-time physical activity (U.S. Department of Health and Human Services 2010). Depending on the strictness of the definitions of sedentariness and regular, moderate-to-vigorous activity, 25% to 40% are not active at all, and only 10% to 25% are active at levels known to increase or maintain cardiorespiratory and muscular fitness. Nearly 30% of adults say they engage in aerobic physical activity of at least moderate intensity for more than 300 min/week, or of vigorous intensity more than 150 min/week, or an equivalent combination (U.S. Department of Health ar n Services 2010); but these are probably exaggera he truth.

▷ **TWENTY-TWO T** of American adults said they did muscle strength tivities on two or more days of the week in 2008. E rcent met that objective and the minimal objecti bic physical activity.

A dramatic decreas n physical activity occurs during adolescence. Among 12,812 U.S. boys and girls 10 to 18 years of age who were participating in the longitudinal Growing Up Today Study, physical activity increased until early adolescence and then declined after age 13 in both boys and girls (Kahn et al. 2008). Averaged across 26 studies (mostly done in the United States), the decline per year in physical activity (mostly self-reported) was −7.0% (95% confidence interval [CI]: −8.8% to −5.2%); the decline among girls was greater in younger ages (9-12 years) but among boys was greater in older ages (13-16 years) (Dumith et al. 2011a). Figure 17.1 shows that by the 12th grade, just 9% of girls and 22% of boys in the United States meet the current guideline of an hour or more of moderate-to-vigorous physical activity each day of the week; these numbers represent declines from 14% for girls and 28% for boys in the 9th grade. Twenty-two percent of girls and 40% of boys say they are active for an hour at least five days a week, down from 31% and 48%, respectively, in the 9th grade.

In 2009, just 18% of U.S. adolescents said they were active enough to meet the current physical activity guideline of an hour or more of aerobic physical activity each day (U.S. Department of Health and Human Services 2010). That rate

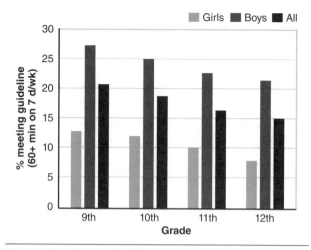

Figure 17.1 Rates of sufficient physical activity during high school in U.S. youths.

Data from Centers for Disease Control, 2010, "Youth risk behavior surveillance - United States, 2009, Surveillance summaries."

had not changed since 2005, when the new guideline was formulated. However, the rate is much lower when an objective measure of physical activity, such as accelerometry, is used. In the United States, 6th-grade girls averaged about 24 min a day in moderate-to-vigorous physical activity (Pate et al. 2006), about the same as for boys and girls in England (Ness et al. 2007); but only 5% of boys and 0.4% of girls in England met the current public health recommendation of at least 1 h of moderate-to-vigorous physical activity each day (Riddoch et al. 2007).

Physical inactivity represents a public health burden that is virtually worldwide in scope; it was the centerpiece for World Health Day in 2002. The most recent estimates of the prevalence of leisure-time physical inactivity and the objectives for changing those rates by the year 2020 are discussed in chapter 1. Selected goals are shown here in table 17.1. Most current goals for people's physical levels by 2020 are 10% increases above the best current estimates. Those goals are more modest increases than were set in 2000 for 2010, but they will still be hard to meet without an organized national campaign that synergizes physical activity interventions in communities.

Change may be harder given emerging evidence for genetic influences on people's physical activity. For example, research on twins in Europe and Australia suggests that 20% to 70% or more of the variation in young to middle-aged adults' physical activity is explainable by genetic traits, with most of the rest explained by **environmental factors** (Stubbe et al. 2006). The genetic influence was less in the older people in that age range (Vink et al. 2011). In Dutch adolescent twins, generation-specific environmental influences shared by twins explained family effects more in girls (52%) than in boys (41%). Family effects explainable by genetics were 42% in boys and 36% in girls (De Moor et al. 2011).

Families can transmit a home culture that promotes or hinders physical activity. Social cultures outside the home

Table 17.1 Selected Objectives for Increasing Physical Activity—Healthy People 2020

Objective	Population	Percentage of total U.S. population	
		Baseline	2020 objective
No leisure-time physical activity	Adults	36.2% (2008)	Reduce to 32.6%
Moderate-intensity aerobic physical activity for at least 150 min per week, or 75 min per week at a vigorous intensity, or an equivalent combination	Adults	43.5% (2008)	Increase to 47.9%
300 min per week of moderate-intensity aerobic physical activity, or 150 min per week at a vigorous intensity, or an equivalent combination	Adults	28.4% (2008)	Increase to 31.3%
Muscle strengthening activities on two or more days of the week	Adults	21.9% (2008)	Increase to 24.1%
Meet objective for aerobic physical activity and for muscle strengthening activity	Adults	18.2% (2008)	Increase to 20.1%
Meet objective for aerobic physical activity and for muscle strengthening activity	Adolescents	18.4% met aerobic guideline (2009)	Increase to 20.2%
Participate in school physical education daily	Adolescents	33.3% (2009)	Increase to 36.6%
Schools requiring daily school physical education	Elementary	3.8% (2006)	Increase to 4.2%
	Middle and junior high	7.9% (2006)	Increase to 8.6%
	Senior high	2.1% (2006)	Increase to 2.3%
Require physical activity programs, equipment, or both for developmental motor activity in child care programs	States	25 states (2006)	Increase to 35 states
Objectives still in development	Adults		Increase trips of 1 mile or less made by walking
	Adults		Increase trips of 5 miles or less by bicycling
	Youth ages 5 to 15 years		Increase trips of 1 mile or less to school
	Youth ages 5 to 15 years		Increase trips of 2 miles or less to school

Based on U.S. Department of Health and Human Services, 2010, *Healthy people 2020.*

also can reinforce physical activity or create learned and built physical barriers to physical activity, which can offset the effectiveness of interventions that focus on a person's individual motivation. Therefore, it is important to understand the physical and social environmental influences that might be changed to increase physical activity, as well as the way in which genetic factors modify the influence of environmental factors and interventions designed to change people's physical activity behavior.

> **STUDIES SUGGEST** that about 50%, on average, of the variation in people's physical activity is explainable by genetic traits, so it is important to identify and change the key environmental factors that influence people's decision to be physically active during their leisure time.

The problem of leisure-time physical inactivity is not just about motivating people to try. In the absence of successful behavioral intervention, the average dropout rate from exercise programs has remained near 50% across the first six to 12 months of participation (shown in figure 17.2) since the first studies on exercise **adherence** were published over 40 years ago (Dishman 1982; Oldridge et al. 1983; Sanne et al. 1973).

Understanding the knowledge, **attitudes,** and behavioral and social skills associated with adopting and maintaining a regular exercise program was a priority identified in *Healthy People 2000,* the U.S. national health goals (U.S. Department of Health and Human Services 1991); and the promotion of physical activity was a key aspect of the next national health goals, *Healthy People 2010* (U.S. Department of Health and Human Services 2000a). The recently released *Healthy People 2020* (U.S. Department of Health and Human Services 2010) emphasizes goals to change policies and practice so that access to physical activity is increased in child care settings, schools (more recess and physical education classes), and workplaces. Specific national goals are set to change policy, and even legislation, about the built environment. The goals assume that national physical activity levels will

rise if people have more access to and availability of physical activity opportunities (such as more parks and trails), if neighborhood designs facilitate transportation by walking or cycling, and if all people have open access to physical activity spaces and facilities at schools outside of normal school hours.

This chapter describes the features of people, environments, and physical activity itself that are potential causes of, or barriers to, physical activity participation. We also discuss theories and interventions that have been used to advance understanding of physical inactivity and to increase moderate to vigorous physical activity and exercise.

Physical activity is not a single behavior, and it requires more effort, and usually more time, than any other lifestyle behavior related to health. Figure 17.3 illustrates that it is a complex set of distinct acts that include, for example, planning for participation, initial **adoption of physical activity,** continued participation or **maintenance,** and overall periodicity of participation (e.g., relapse, resumption of activity, and seasonal variation). Such a complex behavior has many influences, and successful change requires multiple interventions directed at specific features of people and their environments.

Studies have identified about 50 different potential reasons for leisure-time physical inactivity in both adults and youths (Dishman and Sallis 1994; Sallis, Prochaska, and Taylor 2000) (see tables 17.2 through 17.5 later in this chapter); each can influence the decision to increase moderate lifestyle physical activity or to begin or stay with a vigorous exercise program under certain circumstances. Although it is not yet clear which factors are most critical, it appears that for many people, **beliefs** about physical activity (e.g., false expectations of a quick and easy impact on body weight and shape) combine with poor self-control skills to make sustaining an exercise program difficult. Those factors—coupled with social and physical environments that impede physical activity or reinforce other, sedentary behaviors that compete with physical activity when people make choices about how to spend their leisure time—make it easy to understand why so many people in the United States and other economically developed and developing nations are too inactive.

No single variable can predict or fully explain participation in physical activity and exercise. The significance of each potential **determinant** of physical activity has to be viewed in the context of other personal and environmental characteristics and other behavioral choices, as well as features of physical activity. As illustrated in figure 17.3, the determinants of physical activity interact dynamically to influence behavior, and the pattern of this interaction among variables changes over time and age or stage in life. For example, a person's attitudes and physical activity history can interact with environmental variables, such as social support and the weather. After physical activity becomes an established habit, though, the negative influence of bad weather, and the positive influence of social support, on physical activity might become less important.

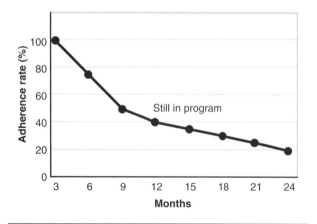

Figure 17.2   Average dropout rate from exercise programs.

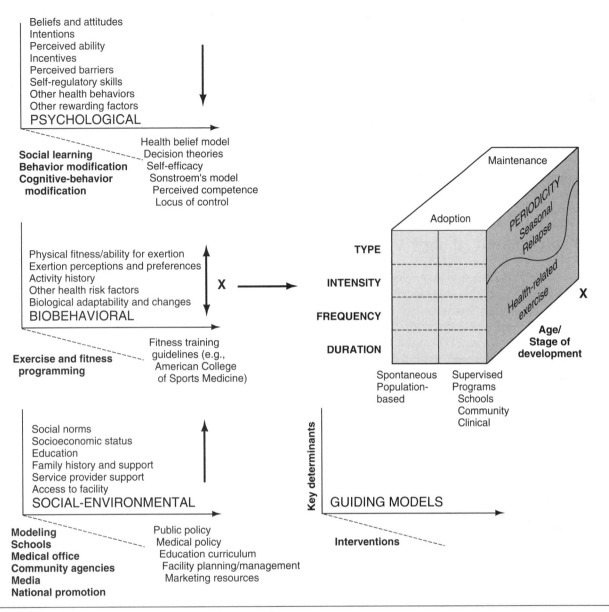

Figure 17.3 A life span interactional model for exercise adherence.

Reprinted, by permission, from R.K. Dishman and A.L. Dunn, 1988, Exercise adherence in children and youth. In *Exercise adherence: Its impact on public health*, edited by R.K. Dishman (Champaign, IL: Human Kinetics), 185

Most research aimed at understanding the personal determinants of physical activity has been cross-sectional or prospective rather than experimental (Dishman 1994b). These determinants can thus be viewed as risk factors for inactivity, even though most studies haven't calculated odds or risk ratios for inactivity or levels of activity. Relatively few randomized controlled trials have been conducted to experimentally manipulate variables presumed to operate as causal determinants. Therefore, throughout this chapter we use the term *determinant* to refer to variables that have established reproducible associations or predictive relationships, rather than proven cause-and-effect connections. Later, however, we introduce the concepts of **mediators** and **moderators** of physical activity and discuss some new studies confirming that changes in such mediators by interventions indeed result in increased physical activity

▷ **DETERMINANTS DENOTE** established, reproducible associations that are potentially causal rather than proven cause-and-effect relationships. Mediators denote variables that explain the effect of an intervention to increase physical activity or variables that explain the effect of another variable in the causal chain of influence on physical activity change. Moderators denote variables that modify the effect of an intervention or another variable on physical activity change.

Motivation is typically synonymous with needs, drives, incentives, or an impetus to action. Many approaches toward understanding and increasing physical activity have focused on motivation without proper attention toward understanding how barriers, both real and perceived, detract from and interact with motivation to determine the direction, intensity, and persistence of human physical activity. Given the high prevalence of sedentariness in developed and developing nations despite widespread attempts to promote physical activity, an alternative focus on barriers can help sharpen thinking about the best ways to intervene in the future.

Individual Barriers to Physical Activity

Costs and barriers associated with a behavior have been recognized as important influences on that behavior since theories about how people make decisions began to proliferate in the 1950s (Janis and Mann 1977). Some barriers to physical activity differ among children and youths, middle-aged people, and older adults and between women and men (Godin et al. 1994). For example, pregnancy and early child rearing can present unique barriers to physical activity for mothers. Also, health conditions that limit mobility increase with age. Nonetheless, not enough is known about the roles of costs and barriers in determining physical activity. Most barriers that are known can be categorized as personal factors, environmental factors, social factors, or features of physical activity (Dishman and Sallis 1994).

Personal Barriers

The descriptive epidemiology of physical activity in the United States presented in chapter 3 illustrates that racial and ethnic minorities, people who have less formal education or low-income jobs, and people who live in rural areas are least physically active during their leisure time. The highest prevalence of physical inactivity is found in the southeastern region of the United States, which is heavily rural. Generally, participation in moderate-intensity activity is similar for males and females, but the rate of participation in vigorous physical activity is lower among females (U.S. Department of Health and Human Services 2000b; Centers for Disease Control and Prevention [CDC] 2010a).

Several personal factors are targets of interventions to increase physical activity because they are potential mediators of people's behavioral choices regarding physical activity. Key personal factors are listed in table 17.2. These include people's beliefs about the outcomes of being physically active or inactive (Steinhardt and Dishman 1989), the **values** they place on those outcomes (Godin and Shephard 1990) compared with other behaviors, satisfaction with their current status and physical activity goals (Dzewaltowski 1994), self-efficacy (i.e., confidence) about being physically active (McAuley and Blissmer 2000) or their ability

Table 17.2 Personal Factors Influencing Physical Activity

Factor	Influence
Demographics	
Increasing age	Negative
Blue-collar occupation	Negative
Higher level of education	Positive
Gender (male)	Positive
High risk for heart disease	Negative
Higher socioeconomic status	Positive
Injury history	Unclear
Overweight/obesity	Negative
Race (nonwhite)	Negative
Pregnancy and early child rearing	Negative
Cognitive variables	
Positive attitude	Positive
Perceived barriers to exercise	Negative
Self-efficacy	Positive
Enjoyment of exercise	Positive
Expected benefits	Positive
Value of expected outcomes	Positive
Self-motivation	Positive
Intention to exercise	Positive
Knowledge of health and exercise	Neutral

to change their current level of physical activity (Sallis et al. 1988), **behavioral intentions** about being active (Godin 1994), and enjoyment of physical activity (Kendzierski and DeCarlo 1991; Motl et al. 2001), among many other factors.

Other personal attributes may be related to levels of physical activity but are not changeable (e.g., age and sex). Nonetheless, such attributes are important to identify and consider when designing physical activity programs or behavioral interventions because they may moderate the effects of interventions to increase physical activity. They can serve as sentinel markers of people who have high risk for being sedentary or who may need special interventions. The personal characteristics that have been considered in determinants research have been organized into demographic factors and social cognitive factors.

Demographic Barriers

Occupation, ethnicity, smoking, education, income, age, and obesity are examples of personal attributes that can present barriers to physical activity or are signals of underlying habits or circumstances that reinforce sedentary living. However, their associations with physical activity can be complex and are still poorly understood.

Occupation

Hourly workers in low-exertion blue-collar occupations are among the least-active Americans in their leisure time and have high risk of dropping out of a rehabilitative exercise program (Oldridge et al. 1983). In one study, eight years after graduation from high school, people who held blue-collar jobs or were unemployed had lower cardiorespiratory fitness than classmates who became civil servants, white-collar workers, or students, even though the two groups had similar fitness levels at the end of high school (Andersen 1996). Many blue-collar or hourly workers may have the attitude that their job requires enough physical activity for health and fitness, but with the use of technology in today's industry, most workers do not expend much energy compared with workers 50 years ago. Nonetheless, physical activity on the job still contributes to overall physical activity. For example, nearly half of 1400 girls in 12th grade from 22 high schools in South Carolina said they had a job and worked nearly 5 h per day outside of school (Dowda et al. 2007b). Nearly one-third of the employed girls' total physical activity occurred while they were at work. Otherwise, the girls with jobs were 20% less active during their leisure time than girls without jobs.

A recent review of 62 studies from 16 nations concluded that people in blue-collar occupations reported higher overall physical activity but lower leisure-time physical activity than white-collar professionals. People in occupations requiring long work hours (more than 45-50 h) and low physical activity on the job appeared to be at high risk for overall inactivity (Kirk and Rhodes 2011). However, more than 80% of the studies used a cross-sectional design (which fails to account for changing work demands), often failed to consider that many blue-collar occupations no longer require physical activity on the job, or didn't adjust for aspects of socioeconomic status (SES) other than job status that can be more influential on leisure-time physical activity (e.g., social networks or dependence on public transport). Thus, the direct and indirect influences of occupation and occupational physical activity remain unclear (Hillsdon 2011).

A longitudinal analysis of the population-based Health and Retirement Study (1996-2002) in the United States found that participation in either work-related or leisure-time physical activity decreased with retirement from a physically demanding job but increased with retirement from a sedentary job (Chung et al. 2009). Lack of wealth made the negative impact of retirement on physical activity worse, whereas wealthy people were more likely to increase their physical activity after retirement.

Age

Physical activity tends to decline with advancing age (Caspersen, Pereira, and Curran 2000), especially when people have age-related disabilities, but age does not necessarily predispose an individual to lower activity. As we just saw, factors associated with a person's job (e.g., conflicts with leisure time or a false perception of adequate physical activity at work) or disposable income (e.g., leisure physical activity may be a low-priority expense) that created barriers to exercise during middle age may diminish during retirement.

Studies have also examined personal determinants of physical activity in younger age groups. A review of 108 studies published between 1970 and 1999 examined determinants of physical activity in children (ages 3-12) and adolescents (ages 13-18; Sallis, Prochaska, and Taylor 2000). Among children, negative associations with physical activity were found for female sex, previous physical inactivity, lack of access to programs or facilities, and time spent indoors. Some of the variables negatively associated with physical activity in adolescents were female sex, ethnicities other than white European, nonparticipation in community sports, being sedentary after school and on weekends, sibling's nonparticipation in physical activity, previous physical inactivity, lack of parents' support or support from significant others, and lack of opportunities to exercise or access to facilities or programs.

Obesity

Excessive body mass can make activities that require weight bearing physically harder than for people of normal weight (Wilfley and Brownell 1994) and contributes to disabilities that can limit physical activity. Also, a history of bad experiences with physical activity, including embarrassment, can contribute to bad attitudes toward physical activity, especially exercise classes with participants of normal weight. An obese person may be less confident about exercising successfully. Indeed, the high failure rate of maintaining weight loss after a diet among people who are obese may lead to lower confidence about staying with an exercise program too. The typical obese person regains one-third of an average 22-lb (10 kg) weight loss within the year after a diet, with all the weight regained within three to five years (Foreyt and Goodrick 1993, 1994).

Psychological Barriers

Personality is weakly associated with physical activity (Rhodes and Smith 2006), but it plausibly could influence spontaneous physical activity or moderate and help explain gene–environment influences on exercise behavior. Psychological factors other than personality can help explain why physical activity varies even among people whose age, education, income, social circumstance, and other demographic factors are very similar. In other words, psychological attributes are important for explaining why some people are active despite circumstances that predict they would be sedentary and why others are sedentary even though they have many opportunities and resources available to them that support physical activity. To put this another way, there are senior citizens who are active despite their age, high school dropouts who are active despite their lack of education, and smokers who exercise. Social and physical environments operating at the levels of families, schools, places of employment, and neighborhoods, all located within communities, can modify how psychological influences on physical activity are formed.

Social Cognitive Determinants of Physical Activity

Social cognitive factors are psychological variables that are transmitted to people from society by learning and **reinforcement** history. Attitudes toward exercising and to a lesser extent social norms about exercise influence intention to exercise, but intentions are often fleeting, influenced by changing priorities and personality factors such as willpower or self-motivation. The intention to exercise can also be influenced by actual (e.g., available leisure time or access to facilities) and perceived personal control over the ability to exercise, especially **self-efficacy.**

How Do People Decide to Be Active?

Theories about how people make decisions to be physically active include theories about forming goals and intentions as well as perceived barriers to behavior. In the following sections we discuss the theories and evaluate their usefulness

for explaining physical activity. Figure 17.4 illustrates relations and interactions among key components of the theories.

A lack of knowledge about appropriate physical activity, as well as negative or indifferent beliefs and attitudes about the benefits of being physically active, certainly can hinder physical activity for many people; but knowledge and positive attitudes about healthy outcomes of being physically active alone are not enough to guarantee that a person will start or stay with a regular exercise program (Sallis et al. 1986). Though education about physical activity and personal fitness is important in helping form attitudes and plans for increasing physical activity, knowing does not directly lead to doing. In a random telephone survey of 2002 American households in the 48 contiguous states and the District of Columbia, 94% of respondents were aware of traditional physical activities that provide a health benefit; but only 68% to 71% were aware of specific exercise guidelines and lifestyle physical activities that benefit health, no matter their age, race or ethnicity, and education (Morrow et al. 2004). In any case, knowledge was unrelated to whether people were physically active at a level sufficient for a health benefit.

McGuire's hierarchy of effects model, used in planning mass-reach communication campaigns (see figure 17.5), illustrates the steps of turning knowledge into intentions and then actions. McGuire's model was tested in Canada's 30-year ParticipACTION campaign to promote physical activity (Craig, Bauman, and Reger-Nash 2010). A cohort

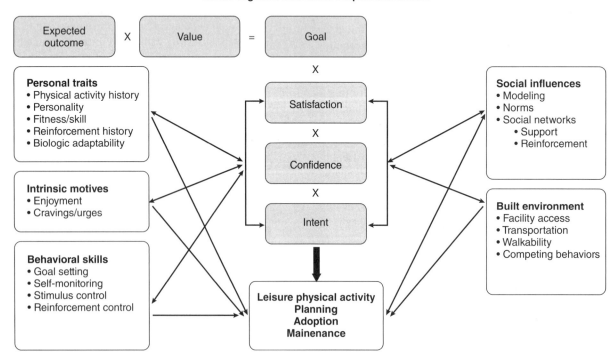

Figure 17.4 Key components of the decision to be physically active and factors that may moderate the effects of those components.
From Dishman 2010.

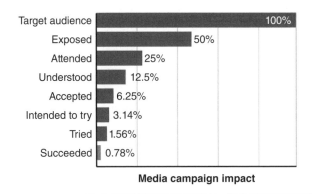

Figure 17.5 McGuire's hierarchy of effects model for mass communication campaigns.

Reprinted, by permission, from R.J. Donovan and N. Owen, 1994, Social marketing and population interventions. In *Advances in exercise adherence,* edited by R.K. Dishman (Champaign, IL: Human Kinetics), 249-290.

of 1106 males and 1356 females from the 1981 Canada Fitness Survey was followed up in 1988, and 1126 people were tested again in 2002 to 2004. Among those inactive at baseline, campaign awareness predicted outcome expectancy, which in turn predicted positive attitude toward physical activity. Positive attitudes predicted high decision balance (i.e., pros > cons), which predicted future intention. Future intention mediated the relationship between decision balance and sufficient activity. Among those sufficiently active at baseline, awareness was unrelated to outcome expectancy and inversely related to positive attitude.

Self-Efficacy Theory

Social cognitive variables (i.e., beliefs that are formed by social learning and reinforcement history) are influences on self-initiated change in health behaviors such as physical activity (Bandura 2004). Self-efficacy is a belief in personal capabilities to organize and execute the courses of action required to attain a behavioral goal. Self-efficacy develops through (1) actual success, (2) watching others like oneself succeed, (3) being persuaded by someone, and (4) emotional or perceived signs of coping ability (e.g., lowered **perceived exertion** after increasing fitness; Bandura 1997b).

Theory of Planned Behavior

According to the theory of planned behavior, attitudes toward physical activity and social norms about physical activity influence the intention to be physically active (Ajzen 1985), which is the main factor leading to physical activity (Hausenblaus, Carron, and Mack 1997). Like self-efficacy, **perceived behavioral control** includes efficacy beliefs about internal factors (e.g., skills, abilities, and self-motivation or willpower) and external factors (e.g., time, opportunity, obstacles, and dependence on other people) that are imposed on behavior.

Although people are more likely to form an intention to behave when they value an expected outcome of the behavior (i.e., they have a positive attitude), that likelihood is increased when a goal is set. People who set goals about being more active and who are dissatisfied with their current activity level are more likely to adopt physical activity, especially if they have high self-efficacy about their ability to be physically active (Dishman et al. 2006). Figure 17.6 shows that like perceived behavioral control, self-efficacy affects behavior directly and also indirectly by influencing intentions. Efficacy beliefs can affect physical activity both directly, by fostering self-management, and indirectly, by influencing perceptions about sociocultural environments that provide assistance for physical activity, which in turn directly influence physical activity. Once formed, self-efficacy, especially beliefs about overcoming barriers to physical activity, can also moderate the relation between perceptions of social facilitators and physical activity change. Thus, beliefs in personal ability to overcome barriers to physical activity can sustain physical activity in the face of increasing barriers or declining opportunities to be active.

Intentions can be transient, though, and are also influenced by personality factors such as willpower or self-motivation and by actual or perceived personal control over physical activity and over the barriers that reduce or prevent it. Intentions seem largely necessary but not sufficient to predict physical activity (Hagger, Chatzisarantis, and Biddle 2002), at best predicting about 25% of people's physical activity. It seems that many people who are physically active are past the point of actively planning for exercise; their past habits and their perceived control over being active are the best predictors of their future physical activity (Godin 1994).

Self-Determination Theory

Self-determination theory is complementary to self-efficacy theory and the theory of planned behavior for understanding physical activity (Hagger and Chatzisarantis 2009). The theory proposes that the social context shapes people's motives by reinforcing or impeding their natural drive toward developing a coherent sense of self (i.e., self-identity) and personally directed behaviors (Ryan and Deci 2000; Ryan et al. 1997). The theory offers yet another way to think about how people develop intrinsic motives to be physically active. It assumes that people strive for autonomy (i.e., behavior is a personal choice), competence (i.e., a sense of mastery or efficacy), and relatedness (i.e., supportive and satisfying social relations). People who are intrinsically motivated choose to be physically active because they enjoy it and find it personally meaningful and valuable. In contrast, people who are extrinsically motivated choose to be physically active more out of a sense of obligation or duty to avoid feelings of guilt. A substantial number of cross-sectional studies, and a few

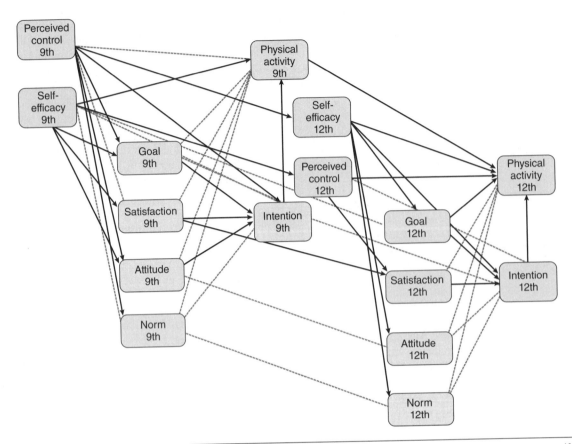

Figure 17.6 Changes in goals and intentions between the 9th and 12th grades helped explain the relation between self-efficacy and change in physical activity in high school girls.

interventions, support the usefulness of self-determination ideas (Hagger and Chatzisarantis 2008; Silva et al. 2011). But how self-determined motives to be a physically active person develop within social contexts of leisure time has not been studied using prospective cohorts, especially during the transition into early adolescence (e.g., Tappe, Duda, and Menges-Ehrnwald 1990) when self-identities are especially malleable.

Psychological factors such as beliefs, values, and intentions influence people's behavior and are especially important for motivating people to take the first steps toward being physically active (e.g., thinking about and planning physical activity or starting a new exercise program). These factors can be changed by personal experience and social norms. Other factors such as **self-motivation** (Dishman and Ickes 1981) are related to skills for regulating personal behavior once the decision to try to be more active has been made. Skills involved with **self-regulation** of behavior include effective **goal setting, self-monitoring** of progress, and self-reward and self-punishment. These skills are important for maintaining physical activity when goals are not easily reached and barriers arise that make physical activity difficult.

Environmental Barriers to Physical Activity

Environmental barriers to physical activity can be divided into physical barriers and social barriers, although the two types interact. In early studies of supervised exercise programs, dropouts reported that program inconvenience was a barrier (e.g., facilities were not easily accessible; the exercise schedule conflicted with other commitments such as work) (see Dishman 1994b for an early a review). Though about 20% to 30% of heart patients dropped out from exercise programs for medical reasons, nonmedical barriers such as work conflicts, relocation, and inaccessibility of exercise facilities accounted for 10% to 40% of dropouts (Andrew and Parker 1979; Oldridge et al. 1983). Today, estimates indicate that people tend to be more physically active if recreational facilities are near their homes; and nearly twice as many people choose to walk or cycle in neighborhoods that are designed for self-powered transportation compared with those designed mainly for automobile transportation (Cervero and Gorham 1995).

Perceived Benefits of and Barriers to Physical Activity

While the aforementioned theoretical models differ according to their pivotal, causal variable, they all include **outcome-expectancy values** as a cornerstone component. An outcome expectancy is the perceived likelihood that performing a behavior will result in a specific outcome. In common language, outcome-expectancy values are similar to attitudes; they refer to the importance people place on their beliefs about the benefits and barriers they hold regarding physical activity. They provide a basis for people's intentions

to behave and for people's goals. These can vary in specific ways according to age, sex, or other personal circumstances (e.g., pregnancy, illness, change in work schedule); but the general categories of perceived benefits of—and perceived barriers to—physical activity are remarkably similar for men and women from college age through middle age (Steinhardt and Dishman 1989) and old age (Stephens and Craig 1990), and they haven't changed much in the past 20 years (e.g., Cerin et al. 2010; Mathews et al. 2010; Petter et al. 2009).

Perceived benefits

1. Stay in shape
2. Feel better in general
3. Maintain good health
4. Maintain proper body weight
5. Improve appearance
6. Enhance self-image and confidence
7. Achieve a positive psychological effect
8. Reduce stress and relax
9. Fun and enjoyment
10. Help cope with life's pressures
11. Lose weight
12. Companionship (friends and family)

Perceived barriers

1. Lack of motivation
2. Too lazy
3. Too busy
4. Not enough time
5. Interference with school
6. Too tired
7. Interference with work
8. Too inconvenient
9. Bad weather
10. Lack of facilities
11. Bored by exercise
12. Fatigued by exercise
13. Family obligations
14. Limiting health
15. Embarrassing

Adapted from Steinhardt and Dishman 1989.

Although the impact of the social environment on physical activity is still incompletely understood, one of the earliest studies of **compliance** with a cardiac rehabilitation exercise program found that one of the best predictors of compliance by the men was the attitude that their wives had toward the men's participation, which was a better predictor than the attitudes held by the men themselves (Heinzelmann and Bagley 1970).

Physical Environment

Access to exercise facilities was the first feature of the physical environment shown to be related to adherence to exercise programs and people's overall physical activity

levels (Sallis et al. 1990b; Teraslinna et al. 1969), although the relationship is complicated. In a study of a community in Southern California, adults who had more commercial exercise facilities located within 1 km (0.6 miles) of their home were more likely to report that they exercised at least three times a week, regardless of age, education, and income (Sallis et al. 1990b). Another study found that access and perceived access to hiking and biking trails were positively related to their use (Troped et al. 2001).

Access can be considered in terms of geography, economics, and safety. For example, running in some urban neighborhoods is risky because of air pollution and high crime rates. Access can also be considered in terms of people's perceptions. Early studies showed that when access to facilities was measured by objective methods (e.g., distance), it was typically related to both the adoption and maintenance of supervised and overall physical activity. However, perceived access was associated mainly with participation in supervised programs (Dishman 1994b). Since those early observations, studies of the association between features of the built environment and participation in physical activity within communities have become widespread. However, because most studies have used cross-sectional designs that are vulnerable to confounding and used self-reports of physical activity and people's self-assessments of the environment, rather than objective measures, the true importance of the environment for promoting physical activity is not yet clear (Brownson et al. 2009). It makes sense that some environments can make it very difficult, or virtually impossible, for people to be physically active for transportation or leisure. However, it seems less likely that merely living in an environment where it is easy and pleasant to be active will directly translate into more activity unless people are otherwise motivated to be active. So, regardless of people's opportunities, their choice to be physically active must be a high priority among all their other options for using their discretionary time.

A review of 150 studies on environmental correlates of physical activity among youths found that most studies used cross-sectional designs and self-ratings of environmental features and physical activity without adjusting for confounders (Ferreira et al. 2006). Overall, however, just 176 of 497 comparisons among children (35%) and 215 of 620 comparisons among adolescents (35%) were statistically significant. A systematic review of 47 studies of social and physical environmental factors and physical activity among adults concluded that availability of physical activity equipment was associated with vigorous physical activity or sports, whereas connectivity of trails was associated with active commuting (Wendel-Vos et al. 2007). Other possible but less consistent correlates of physical activity were availability, accessibility, and convenience of recreational facilities. Among studies that used an objective measure of the environment, only 33 of 129 comparisons (26%) showed a positive association with a feature of the environment (usually access or convenience of a physical activity opportunity). Also, only three of the 47 publications were longitudinal, and just one used an objective measure, showing no association.

Features of the built environment have been measured in three main ways:

1. People's perceptions obtained by telephone interview or by questionnaires
2. Observations by raters (e.g., neighborhood audits) (Colabianchi et al. 2007)
3. Archival data sets (e.g., census records) linked with a **geographic information system (GIS)** (Brownson et al. 2009)

A GIS blends cartography with database technology and statistical analysis to measure, manage, analyze, and model data about geographic locations. A GIS includes **geocoding**, which is finding geographic coordinates (latitude and longitude) from other geographic data, such as a place of residence and neighborhood (e.g., census street addresses linked with street segments and postal zip codes). This type of data provides information that can be used to measure things such as street connectivity (i.e., number and directness of travel route options) and distances to schools, physical activity facilities, and places (e.g., parks and trails). Satellite global positioning system (GPS) measurements can improve the spatial precision of traditional GIS geocoding.

With use of 1994-1995 data from the U.S. National Longitudinal Study of Adolescent Health (wave I; 1994-1995), associations between moderate-to-vigorous physical activity and GIS-coded physical activity facility counts and street connectivity measures within 1, 3, 5, and 8.05 km of each residence were examined in 17,659 boys and girls 11 to 22 years of age (Boone-Heinonen et al. 2010b). Facilities within 3 km buffers and intersection density within 1 km buffers showed the most consistent associations with physical activity. Regardless of sex, race, or ethnicity, household income and education, or region of the country, physical activity was associated with intersection density and the number of facilities or opportunities for physical activity. The authors suggested that the neighborhood area may be larger for physical activity facilities (because of higher incentives to travel) than for intersection density (which may encourage street-based activities such as skateboarding or jogging closer to home).

One of the first clinical studies of the use of exercise to rehabilitate a group of Swedish heart patients found that allowing the men to exercise at home increased their amount of exercise (Sanne et al. 1973), a finding later replicated by researchers at Stanford University (King et al. 1991). In a study of a community in Southern California, half the adults reported exercising at home (Sallis et al. 1986).

Having home exercise equipment does not ensure that it will be used, even though it adds convenience. In 2007, just prior to the 2008 recession, total manufacturers' sales (in wholesale dollars) for the sporting goods and fitness industry in the United States grew at an annual rate of 3.3%. That was down from higher growth rates in 2005 (6.8%) and 2006 (5.8%), but even so, the sporting goods industry outperformed the 2.2% gross domestic product for nondurable goods. In 2009, the two fitness machine categories that generated the most sales were treadmills ($1.027 billion) and elliptical machines ($913 million). Table 17.3 shows estimated home gym use. However, the estimated growth in the number of Americans who said they used a home gym lagged below the growth in overall exercise machine use.

According to figures from the NPD Group, an international sales and marketing research firm, by May 2010 more than 22.6 million Wii users worldwide had purchased Nintendo's exercise game Wii Fit since its launch in April

Table 17.3   Estimated Home Gym Use by Americans

Activity	2009	Change from 2008
Treadmill exercise	51,418	4.1%
Weight or resistance machines	39,752	3.5%
Free weights (dumbbells)	35,744	3.9%
Free weights (barbells)	27,048	3.5%
Elliptical motion trainer	26,521	4.9%
Home gym exercise	24,762	1.0%
Stationary cycling (upright)	24,528	−3.1%

Data from Sporting Goods Manufacturers Association 2010.

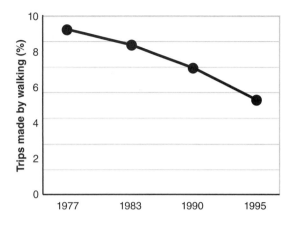

Figure 17.7 Between 1977 and 1995, trips in the United States made by walking declined. This trend poses an important public health problem when the effects of physical inactivity and excess weight are considered.

Data from U.S. Department of Transportation 1997.

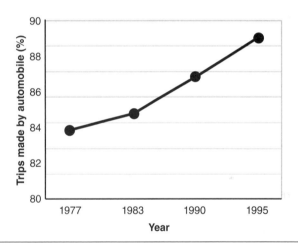

Figure 17.8 Between 1977 and 1995, trips in the United States made by automobile increased. Studies show that one-fourth of all trips people make are 1 mile or less, but three-fourths of these short trips are made by car.

Data from U.S. Department of Transportation 1997.

2008, putting it among the top 20 all-time best-sellers among video games in the United States, alongside *Grand Theft Auto IV*, *Halo 3*, *Call of Duty 4: Modern Warfare*, and *Madden NFL '09*. However, Wii Fit sales dropped by 30% in 2010. A systematic review of 18 studies of energy expenditure during active video game play (12 studies) and physical activity after exposure to active video games (six studies) in youths found a threefold increase in energy expenditure on average, especially for games played mainly using upper body movements (Biddiss and Irwin 2010). However, there was limited evidence on whether youths played the games regularly enough to increase their customary physical activity level. Other evidence indicates that sales of home exercise equipment outpace its actual use. There is a dearth of experimental evidence that availability of exercise equipment or exercise opportunities will result in more physical activity, so access to physical activity settings remains an important area of research and public policy.

The long-term decline of self-powered transportation shown in figure 17.7 and the steady increase in transportation by automobile shown in figure 17.8 signal a key problem for planning urban communities that accommodate physical activity. The U.S. Department of Transportation (1997) estimates that one-fourth of the trips people make today are a mile (1.6 km) or less in distance, but three-fourths of those trips are made by car. Children ages 5 to 15 walk and ride bicycles 40% less today than they did 25 years ago. Fewer than a third of trips to school that are less than a mile (1.6 km) are walked by children; just 2% of trips to school of 2 miles (3.2 km) or less are made by bicycle.

Most modern communities in the United States were designed to accommodate automotive travel and neglected the building of sidewalks and bicycle trails or lanes. Recognition of these trends led to the creation of Active Community Environments (ACEs), a CDC-sponsored initiative to promote walking, bicycling, and the development of accessible recreation facilities. ACEs was developed in response to data from a variety of disciplines, including public health, urban

design, and transportation planning, that implicated several features of the physical community environment in promoting or impeding physical activity: proximity of facilities, street design, density of housing, availability of public transit, and availability of pedestrian and bicycle facilities.

Notwithstanding the transportation barriers to physical activity, other data indicate that the degree of urbanization is associated in a complex way with the level of leisure-time physical activity in the United States. Data from the 1996 Behavioral Risk Factor Surveillance Survey indicated that the overall prevalence of physical inactivity was lowest in central metropolitan areas (27.4%) and in the western United

States (21.1%) (CDC 1998). Physical inactivity was highest (36.6%) in rural areas, particularly in the southeastern United States (43.7%). The inverse relationship between degree of urbanization and physical inactivity is relatively consistent when data are stratified by age, sex, level of education, and household income. A decade later, estimates confirm that states in the south and southeastern United States with large proportions of rural residents (e.g., Alabama, Arkansas, Kentucky, Louisiana, Mississippi, Oklahoma, Tennessee, Texas, West Virginia) also have above-average rates (i.e., near or above 30%) of adults who say they get no physical activity in their leisure time (CDC 2010a). It's still not clear whether effects of the built environment and travel patterns on physical activity differ across regions of the country or how much they differ according to people's sex, age, or race or ethnicity; but evidence is accumulating at a rapid pace.

A review of 50 cross-sectional studies of association between perceived and measured features of the built environment, specifically parks and other recreation settings, concluded that most of the studies showed some positive associations between features of parks and recreation settings with physical activity, more so for leisure activities such as walking than for moderate or vigorous exercise (Kaczynski and Henderson 2008). However, only 19 of the 50 studies (38%) used an objective measure of the environment (e.g., distance of parks or trails from the residence or the number of parks or trails within easy access), and only 21 of the 54 (39%) comparisons made in those 19 studies showed a positive association with physical activity (Kaczinski and Henderson 2007).

More recently, the association between self-reports of physical activity and features of the neighborhood environment (neighborhood was the area within a 10- to 15-min walk from home) was examined in an aggregated sample of 11,541 adults living in cities located in 11 nations: Belgium, Brazil, Canada, Colombia, China (Hong Kong), Japan, Lithuania, New Zealand, Norway, Sweden, and the United States (Sallis et al. 2009). After adjustment for age, gender, and nation, five of seven environmental variables were associated with whether people said they were active enough to meet recommended levels of physical activity: many shops nearby (odds ratio [OR] = 1.29; 95% CI: 1.15-1.44), transit stop in neighborhood (OR = 1.32; 95% CI: 1.16-1.54), sidewalks on most streets (OR: 1.47; 95% CI: 1.32-1.65), bicycle facilities (OR: 1.21; 95% CI: 1.10-1.33), and low-cost recreational facilities (OR = 1.16; 95% CI: 1.05-1.27). See figure 17.9. Single-family homes and perceived crime were not significant. Seventy-seven percent of the participants said they were active enough to meet physical activity guidelines. That seems unusually high and is probably explained by the inclusion of walking for any purpose (but at least 10 min at a time).

In a study of Belgian youths, more than 1400 students 17 years old were recruited in 20 randomly selected schools (Deforche et al. 2010). Physical activity and environmental factors were assessed by self-report questionnaires. Higher land-use-mix diversity, higher street connectivity, more attractive environments, better access to recreational facilities, and higher emotional satisfaction with the neighborhood were associated with more active transportation. Higher

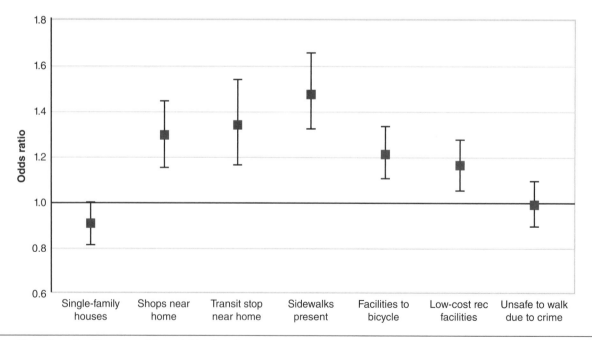

Figure 17.9 Perceived features of the neighborhood environment associated with self-reported physical activity in 11 nations.

Reprinted from *American Journal of Preventive Medicine*, Vol. 36(6), Sallis et al., "Neighborhood environments and physical activity among adults in 11 countries," pgs. 484-490, copyright 2009, with permission of Elsevier.

perceived safety from traffic, better access to recreational facilities, more physical activity equipment at home, and fewer electronic devices in the bedroom were associated with more leisure-time sports. A review of seven cross-sectional studies and interventions on the influence of child care policy and environment on physical activity in preschool-aged children concluded that staff education and training, as well as staff behavior on the playground, were associated with participation in moderate-to-vigorous physical activity in pre-schoolers (Trost, Ward, and Senso 2010). The availability and quality of portable, but not fixed, play equipment also were associated with higher levels of moderate to vigorous physical activity. Lower playground density (fewer children per square meter) and the presence of vegetation and open play areas were positive influences in some studies, but not all.

Fifteen schools located in economically depressed areas in a large city in England each received 20,000 pounds (about $33,000 U.S. in 2003) from the national Sporting Playgrounds Initiative to redesign the playground environment (multicolor playground markings and physical structures) (Ridgers et al. 2007). Eleven schools served as matched socioeconomic controls. Positive intervention effects were observed six weeks and six months later for physical activity measured by heart rate monitors and accelerometers.

Studies in the United States

In a study of nearly 11,000 adults in Atlanta, Georgia, those who lived in walkable neighborhoods were more likely to walk than to drive for transportation and were less obese. The researchers found a 6% elevation in risk of obesity for each hour spent in a car each day and a 5% reduction in risk for each kilometer walked each day (Frank, Andresen, and Schmid 2004). Among Atlantans over age 65, the walkability of neighborhood design (density of residences; connectedness of streets; density of retail stores; and land-use mix of residences, stores, offices, and recreational space) was associated with more walking (OR = 2.02), less time spent traveling in a car (OR = 0.53), and lower odds of being overweight (OR = 0.68) (Frank et al. 2010).

▷ **IN AN** Atlanta study of 11,000 adults, the risk of obesity was elevated by 6% for every hour of driving and reduced by 5% for each kilometer walked per day.

Nearly 2200 adults (20-65 years of age) from 32 neighborhoods in Seattle–King County, Washington, and Baltimore, Maryland–Washington, D.C., rated their neighborhood according to walkability (i.e., residential density, diverse land-use mix, access to mixed land use, street connectivity, walking and cycling facilities, aesthetics, pedestrian/traffic safety, and safety from crime). People who rated their neighborhoods high on walkability spent as much as 13 min each day in moderate-to-vigorous physical activity measured by an accelerometer. They also reported an extra hour each

week of walking for transportation and 75 min more each week in leisure-time activity compared with people living in other neighborhoods (Adams et al. 2011). However, people who are active may be more aware than less active people of physical activity opportunities, falsely inflating the association seen between physical activity and features of the built environment (Adams et al. 2009).

In another study, observers watched people in eight public parks in Los Angeles, California, for 1 h, four times each day, all week, for nearly six months and interviewed 713 park users and 605 area residents who lived within 2 miles of each park. On average, over 2000 individuals were counted in each park (Cohen et al. 2007). Both park use and exercise levels of individuals were predicted by proximity of their residence to the park. Even though the people interviewed said the park was the place where they most commonly exercised, about two-thirds of them were actually engaged in sedentary activities (e.g., sitting and reading, sunbathing) when they were observed. Another survey, of 51 park directors, 4257 park users, and local residents, and observations of 30 parks in the metropolitan area of Los Angeles showed that the strongest correlates of the number of people using the park were the park size and the number of organized activities observed (e.g., sport competitions and other attractions). Neighborhood population density, neighborhood poverty levels, perceptions of park safety, and the presence of a park advisory board were not associated with park use (Cohen et al. 2010).

In a study of 6th-grade girls living in six regions of the United States nearly 1400 reported on whether nine different types of recreational facilities (basketball courts, golf courses, martial arts studios, playing fields, tracks, skating rinks, swimming pools, tennis courts, and dance/gymnastic clubs) were easily accessible (Scott et al. 2007). Next, GIS geocoded (see figure 17.10) all the parks, schools, and commercial sites for physical activity located within a mile of each girl's home. Girls wore accelerometers for measurement of their weekly minutes of moderate-to-vigorous physical activity outside of school. Physical activity was 3% higher for each facility perceived by the girls to be within a mile of their home. However, physical activity was unrelated to objective GIS measures of facility density or access.

A review of 19 cross-sectional studies of rural settings (most adjusted for confounders) and one intervention that examined the association between people's self-reported physical activity and their ratings of features of the built environment (e.g., sidewalks, street lighting, private and public recreational facilities, parks, malls, aesthetics, crime/safety, traffic, walking destinations, and trails) concluded that associations were positive for pleasant aesthetics, trails, safety/crime, parks, and walkable destinations (Frost et al. 2010). However, just 39 of 100 positive comparisons were statistically significant (another five were in the opposite direction), despite the fact that 12 studies had more than 750 participants, which increased the probability of finding an association.

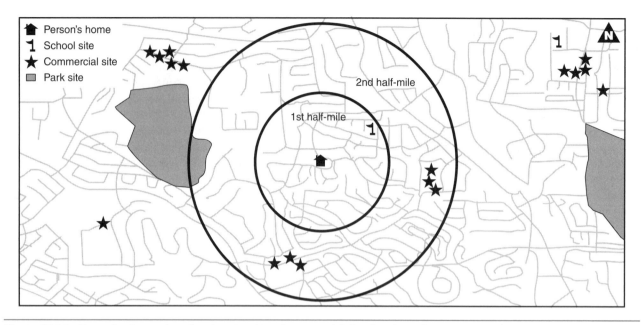

Figure 17.10   Example of mapping of parks, schools, and commercial sites for physical activity research.

If You Build It, Will They Come?

Cross-sectional studies have found that self-reports and objective measures from geographic information systems of the social and built environments (e.g., neighborhood safety and facility accessibility) are inconsistent correlates of physical activity among population-based samples.

When people say that time and inconvenience are barriers to their activity, they may actually be giving excuses for the fact that physical activity is a low-priority choice for using their leisure time. Lack of time can represent a true barrier, merely a perceived barrier, a lack of skills (e.g., self-monitoring or time management) for controlling one's own behavior, or merely an excuse for a lack of motivation to be active. A good way to tell the difference is to ask people which of their current leisure activities they are willing to give up to be replaced by exercise. Adding exercise to an already busy schedule merely invites a schedule conflict or makes lack of time an easy excuse. Unwillingness to replace a current activity with exercise probably signals that exercise is not a priority among all the choices people have for using their discretionary leisure time.

Raynor, Coleman, and Epstein (1998) considered the interaction between accessibility and the reinforcing value of physical activity and sedentary alternatives in a study of 34 sedentary men living in Buffalo, New York. Amount of time that participants spent exercising out of a possible 20 min was compared among four conditions that differed in accessibility to active and sedentary alternatives. The most time (20 min) was spent exercising when the active alternatives were near (in the same room) and the sedentary alternatives were far (a 5-min walk away). Regardless of the accessibility

of the active alternatives, if the sedentary alternatives were near, less than 1 min on average was spent exercising. Participants were active 42% of the time when both alternatives were less accessible. Thus, sedentary men were physically active only when physical activities were more convenient than sedentary activities.

It has not been determined whether perceived access and actual proximity to physical activity settings have direct relations with physical activity, or indirect relations moderated or mediated by social cognitive factors such as social support and efficacy beliefs about overcoming barriers to physical activity, or both. In other words, it is important for studies to show that environmental factors account for variation in physical activity not already explained by personal motivation to be physically active. In one such study, GIS technology was used to map commercial physical activity facilities located within 0.75- and 2.0-mile street network buffers around the homes of 1126 black and white girls in the 12th grade at 22 high schools in South Carolina (Dowda et al. 2009). About 25% of girls had at least one physical activity facility within the 0.75-mile buffer, and 65% of girls had at least one facility within the 2.0-mile buffer. Proximity to multipurpose commercial physical activity facilities was associated with self-reported vigorous physical activity, independently of girls' race, BMI, household income, participation in sport, their self-efficacy for overcoming barriers to physical activity, their perceptions of social support for physical activity, and their perceived access to facilities.

The association between neighborhood active living potential and walking was studied among 2614 middle-aged and older adults living in one of 112 census tracts in Montreal, Canada. Data were linked to observational data on neighborhood active living potential in the 112 census tracts (Gauvin et al. 2008). Greater density of destinations in the census tract was associated with greater likelihoods of walking for any reason at least five days per week for at least 30 min (OR = 1.53; 95% CI: 1.21-1.94). No associations were found between dimensions of neighborhood active living potential and walking for leisure, so the results mainly apply to walking for transportation.

Another study suggests that creating walkable environments may result in higher levels of physical activity and less driving and in slightly lower obesity prevalence, but only for people who prefer to live in a walkable neighborhood. A study of 3500 Atlantans compared travel patterns and obesity after controlling for whether people lived in a type of neighborhood they preferred (Frank et al. 2007). People who preferred and lived in a walkable neighborhood walked the most (33.9% walked), drove the least (25.8 miles per day), and had a lower rate of obesity when compared to people who preferred and lived in a car-dependent neighborhood; they drove 43 miles per day, seldom walked (3.3%), and had twice the rate of obesity (21.6%).

Research on the built environment and physical activity has used mostly cross-sectional designs that can be confounded by residential self-selection bias. That is, people who are otherwise more likely to be physically active may choose and be able to afford to live in neighborhoods that make it easy to be physically active (Boone-Heinonen et al. 2011b). For example, people who are more likely to select a safe, walkable neighborhood with high-quality schools in high-SES areas may also be more likely to choose a physically active lifestyle. Nonetheless, at least one experimental study suggests that interventions can overcome perceived environmental barriers to walking. Among previously inactive middle-aged adults who perceived their walking environment to be unpleasant, those who received a mail-out of a self-help walking program and a pedometer were more likely than controls to increase total walking time and to undertake regular walking (OR = 5.85; 95% CI: 2.60-12.2) (Merom et al. 2009).

Prospective Cohort Studies

Most of the research studies of the built environment and physical activity have used cross-sectional designs that cannot determine cause. Because it has not yet been feasible to conduct population trials, the best evidence about the environment and physical activity participation comes from population-based longitudinal, observational studies of youths and young adults.

National Longitudinal Study of Adolescent Health

A cohort of 12,701 U.S. adolescents was followed from 1994-1995 through 2001-2002 using a time-varying GIS. Longitudinal relations between sessions of moderate-to-vigorous physical activity and built and socioeconomic environment measures (land-cover diversity, pay and public physical activity facilities per 10,000 population, street connectivity, median household income, and crime rate) from adolescence to young adulthood were estimated after adjustment for unmeasured confounders. Moderate-to-vigorous physical activity was positively associated with access to pay facilities in males and inversely associated with higher crime rates in both males and females (Boone-Heinonen et al. 2010b).

CARDIA Study

Four longitudinal surveys from 1985-1986 through 2000-2001 asked 5115 young black and white adults about their frequency of self-reported walking, bicycling, and jogging during the past year. United States census data and GIS geocoding were used to compare time-varying residential locations to neighborhood street network data within a 1 km buffer of each person's place of residence (Hou et al. 2010). After adjustment for time-varying confounders, neighborhood street density was positively associated with walking, bicycling, and jogging in areas of low urbanization; but in middle and high urbanization areas, there were inverse associations in women and no associations in men. After controlling for sociodemographics (age, sex, race) and individual SES, associations of physical activity were lower among blacks living in economically deprived neighborhoods (e.g., proportions of people with an income 150% below the federal poverty level and people 25 years and older without a high school education) but less so in whites (Boone-Heinonen et al. 2011a).

Social Environment

Relationships and interactions with others can have a strong impact on behavior. They can create or resolve barriers to physical activity, as shown in table 17.4. Through words and deeds, family and friends can help or hinder efforts to be physically active. For example, in a large Canadian study, lack of wives' support for exercise involvement was associated

Table 17.4   Social Factors Influencing Physical Activity

Factor	Influence
Class size	Unknown*
Exercise role models	Unknown*
Good group cohesion	Positive*
Physician influence	Positive
Past family influences	Positive
Social support (friends, peers)	Positive
Social support (spouse, family)	Positive
Social support (staff, instructor)	Positive

* Experts predict the influence of these factors, but not enough research has been done to allow firm conclusions.

Reprinted, by permission, from A. Jackson, J. Morrow Jr., D. Hill, and R.K. Dishman, 1999, *Physical activity for health and fitness* (Champaign, IL: Human Kinetics), 325.

with a threefold increase in the dropout rate by men who were recovering from a heart attack (Andrew and Parker 1979; Andrew et al. 1981; Oldridge et al. 1983). Encouragement, praise, sharing chores to free time for exercise, or being an exercise companion can help encourage physical activity. Family and friends can also sabotage efforts by excessive nagging or by distracting a person from personal goals or tempting the person with other activities that are appealing but sedentary. Family and friends also can influence another's behavior less directly; a person learns attitudes and habits from watching and listening to other people.

In an early meta-analysis of studies that examined social influences on exercise, Carron, Hausenblas, and Mack (1996) examined the separate effects of social variables on exercise behavior, beliefs, satisfaction, and attitude. Overall effects were small to medium in size, but moderately large **effect sizes** of 0.62 to 0.69 SD were found for the influence of support by family and important others on attitudes about exercise and for the influence of family support and of task cohesion on exercise behavior. Social support from family and friends has consistently been related to physical activity in cross-sectional and prospective studies. Support from a spouse also appears to be reliably correlated with exercise participation. Individuals who join a fitness center with their spouses demonstrate better exercise adherence than married individuals whose spouses do not join (Wallace, Raglin, and Jastremski 1995). Social interactions and social influences appear to be more important for exercise behavior in women. For example, adherence to a structured exercise program was predicted by women's perception that they received adequate guidance and reassurance of worth, but social provisions did not predict adherence in men (Duncan, Duncan, and McAuley 1993). In contrast, participation in supervised exercise programs is weakly associated with class size, group cohesion, and social support from staff or instructor. No consistent association has been found between exercise models or past family influence and exercise or physical activity. A more recent systematic review of 47 observational studies of social and physical environmental factors and physical activity among adults concluded that only social support and having a companion for physical activity were convincingly associated with different types of physical activity (neighborhood walking, bicycling, vigorous physical activity/sports, active commuting, leisure-time physical activity in general, sedentary lifestyle, moderately intense physical activity, and a combination of moderately intense and vigorous activity) (Wendel-Vos et al. 2007).

A meta-analysis of 30 cross-sectional studies found positive but small associations ($r \sim 0.10$-0.20) of parental encouragement ($r = 0.21$), modeling (i.e., parents being physically active) ($r = 0.10$), and instrumental behaviors (e.g., providing transportation or buying sport equipment) ($r = 0.17$) with child and adolescent physical activity levels (75% used self-reports by parents or children) (Pugliese and Tinsley 2007). Those associations approximate elevations in physical activity of 5% to 10% above chance odds, but they weren't

adjusted for the size of the studies or confounders such as gender, race-ethnicity, and household income or education.

Several cross-sectional studies have shown higher levels of physical activity among youths whose families rate themselves as close or connected, whose parents model and encourage physical activity, or whose parents have an authoritative parenting style (Berge 2009). However, parenting style wasn't predictive of change in physical activity in a large, five-year longitudinal study of 2500 middle school students from 31 schools in Minnesota (Berge et al. 2010).

A systematic review of 35 studies, including 14 randomized controlled trials, of physical activity in healthy youth that included a parental component identified five general procedures for involving parents: (1) face-to-face educational programs or parent training, (2) family participatory exercise programs, (3) telephone communication, (4) organized activities, and (5) educational materials sent home. Two-thirds of the randomized trials were poorly designed or had weak measures, but interventions with educational or training programs during family visits or via telephone communication with parents had the best results. Three of the six studies that included parent training, family counseling, or preventive messages during family visits, as well as two of three studies that reached parents via telephone, had some positive effects. However, most of these studies were pilot studies or trials with control groups that were not randomly assigned. Overall, the authors concluded that there was little evidence for effectiveness of family involvement methods in programs for promoting physical activity in children (O'Connor, Jago, and Baranowski 2009).

Other longitudinal research shows that support from family members may reduce girls' natural decline in physical activity during high school, regardless of their self-efficacy and perceived behavioral control. Among a cohort of 421 girls, those who reported lower family support in the 8th grade had more rapid declines in physical activity through the 9th and 12th grades (Dowda et al. 2007a). A unit change in family support was related to approximately 1/3 of a standard deviation change in total metabolic equivalents (METs).

The decline in physical activity between ages 12 to 17 years in a multiethnic cohort of 371 boys and girls was less in those who had higher self-efficacy to overcome barriers to physical activity or had friends who were active and supportive of physical activity (Duncan et al. 2007). Early-maturing boys were initially the most physically active, but they had a greater decline in physical activity compared to later-maturing boys.

Multilevel Models of Physical Activity Change

Physical activity is no doubt determined by individual decisions and motivation, but also by the interaction of those personal determinants with influences exerted on people by their physical and social environments, including home and family, neighborhoods, places of worship, workplaces, and schools (Duncan et al. 2004; King et al. 2008). For example, preliminary evidence indicates that 3% to 5% of the differences in self-reported walking among people 65 years or older is explainable by the neighborhood they live in (Fisher et al. 2004), and 5% to 10% of the differences in physical activity levels among 10- to 12-year-old boys and girls is explainable by which school they attend. People can be similarly influenced by shared features of their communities, so it likely is the case that people will choose to be physically active if their family or friends are active, if their schools or workplaces provide for and promote physical activity, and if their homes and neighborhoods provide places and opportunities for safe and pleasant physical activities.

▶ **THE DIFFERENT** types of physical activity and places where they can be performed increase the odds that people will find something they enjoy. However, habits are easier to form when a single behavior is reinforced at a specific place and time.

There is wide state-to-state variation in physical activity levels across the United States even after adjustment for age differences in the states. In 2008, 25% of U.S. adults said they got no leisure-time physical activity during the past month, but the rate ranged from 17.9% in Minnesota to 32.4% in Mississippi (CDC 2010a). In 2009, just 18.4% of students in grades 9 through 12 met the current physical activity guideline of an hour or more of moderate-to-vigorous physical activity every day, but the rate ranged from 17% in Massachusetts and South Carolina to nearly 28% in Idaho and Pennsylvania (CDC 2010b). The 2003 National Survey of Children's Health, including nearly 38,000 adolescents aged 10 to 17 years from all U.S. states and the District of Columbia, found, paradoxically, that youths residing in states with higher levels of perceived social trust ("If my child were outside playing and got hurt or scared, there are adults nearby who I trust to help my child") had elevated odds (OR: 9.3; 95% CI: 1.7-49.4) of not meeting current physical activity recommendations (moderate or vigorous activity 20 min or more most days of the week) regardless of poverty level, age, sex, and race-ethnicity (McKay et al. 2007).

In a multilevel, cross-sectional analysis of the Early Childhood Longitudinal Study-Kindergarten Cohort that included 10,694 kindergartners living in 1053 neighborhoods, father's reports of time spent with his child and parent's estimates of family time doing sports accounted for about 19% of children's physical activity, as rated by parents (Beets and Foley 2008). Parental perceptions of a neighborhood's safety for children to play outside was the key feature of neighborhood quality positively associated with children's physical activity. After adjustment for children's weight, motor skills, ethnicity, and television watching, differences between neighborhoods accounted for about 8% of the differences in physical activity among the children.

Unique Features of Physical Activity as a Target for Change

- The goal is to increase a positive health behavior rather than to decrease a negative behavior.
- Physical activity is a biologically based behavior; no other health behavior requires exertion several times greater than rest.
- Physical activity is complex, preceded by chains of psychological, behavioral, and environmental events that require multiple decisions and actions.
- The type and quantity of physical activity vary according to its purpose. This variety can make it harder to form a habit early on.

However, there is as yet very little longitudinal multilevel evidence to confirm how much of physical activity is a personal choice and how much is determined by social and physical environments (Duncan et al. 2004). Figure 17.11 shows that complex models are needed to describe the independent and interactive contributions of key determinants of physical activity at each level to change in physical activity across multiple points in time (Dishman 2008).

A longitudinal study in South Carolina, Transition and Activity in Kids (TRACK), is following a cohort of 1000 black and white boys and girls as they transition from the 5th grade through middle school to observe the influence of the physical and social environments in their family, neighborhoods, and schools on their personal motivation to be physically active.

Genetics of Physical Activity

Not all physical activity results from thought-out plans. Studying twins is an approach commonly used to estimate how much of the difference in physical activity among people is accounted for by genetic inheritability. Comparing the correlation between monozygotic (MZ; identical) twins and dizygotic (DZ; fraternal) twins parses out influences of twin resemblance on physical activity. If physical activity levels are more similar between MZ twins, who share all the same genes, than between DZ twins, who share only half their genes, then there is a genetic component to physical activity. If the correlation of physical activity levels within twin pairs is similar for MZ and DZ twins, common environmental factors shared by each twin seem to explain variation in physical activity, regardless of genes. Because MZ twins share the same environment and the same genes, a correlation within pairs of MZ twins that is less than perfect (i.e., less than 1.0) indicates that the variation in physical activity is likely explainable by unique environmental experiences not shared

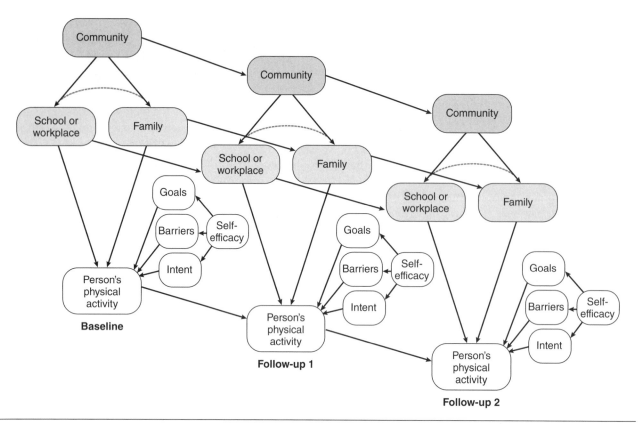

Figure 17.11 Conceptual multilevel model of influences on physical activity measured at the level of the person and features of the environment where people live, work, or go to school at different times.

by the twins (plus unknown errors in the measure of physical activity). Finally, if the correlation of physical activity levels within fraternal, DZ, twins (i.e., twins of the opposite sex) is lower than within same-sex DZ twins, then males and females would appear to have different environmental or genetic influences on physical activity. A better test, of course, would be to compare adult identical twins separated at birth, because they would have experienced different environments.

Perhaps the biggest study to use this approach evaluated physical activity surveys in 13,676 pairs of MZ twins and 23,375 pairs of DZ twins aged 19 to 40 years from seven countries participating in the GenomEUtwin project: Denmark, Finland, the Netherlands, Norway, Sweden, the United Kingdom, and Australia). Figure 17.12 shows that genetic heritability of physical activity level was similar for the most part across nations (mean of 51%).

▷ **TWIN AND** family studies have estimated that the heritability of physical activity ranges from 20% to 70%.

Candidate Genes for Physical Activity

Little is known about how genes, the environment, and their interactions influence people's spontaneous physical activity or their conscious decisions to regularly exercise. Physical

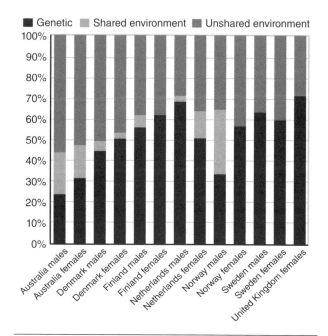

Figure 17.12 Genetic and environmental influence on physical activity in adults in the GenomEUtwin study. The genetic and shared environment bars represent the portion of the variation in physical activity that could be explained by each of those factors. The unshared environment sections represent variation not explained by either factor.

Data from Stubbe et al. 2006.

activity is a complex, multifactorial trait likely influenced mainly by polygenes that each explain small portions (~1%) of the variance in physical activity. However, in contrast to the literature on obesity, in which at least 22 genes have been supported by at least five studies, less than 10 association studies and two linkage studies have examined candidate genes for physical activity, without much replication of results (Dishman 2008). Most candidate genes for physical activity suggested by linkage or association studies have been selected for study based on understanding of energy intake pathways that influence energy balance, more so than models of otherwise motivated behavior. However, some genes that have been studied might be involved in regulation of motivation systems for both feeding and physical activity. Evidence has been mixed on whether alleles of dopamine receptor and serotonin genes (see the discussion of brain neurotransmitters in chapter 14 on mental health) explain variations in personality (e.g., novelty seeking and extraversion), which plausibly could explain a portion of leisure or spontaneous physical activity (Dishman 2008).

Biology of Motivation for Physical Activity

In contrast to the factors that limit skeletal muscle control of locomotion under conditions of impairment, the neurobiological regulation of voluntary, nonstrenuous physical activity by healthy animals has received little study (Dishman et al. 2006). Reduced dopamine (DA) release or loss of DA receptors in the brain appears related to the age-associated decline in physical activity observed among many species. The mesolimbic (i.e., ventral tegmentum–nucleus accumbens) DA system is a critical component of the forebrain circuitry that regulates activational aspects of motivation. Activation of brain cells in reward regions of the hypothalamus during spontaneous running by rats was established 40 years ago, and electrical self-stimulation of the ventral tegmental area has been used to artificially motivate treadmill running and weightlifting in rats. However, little is known about the role of the mesolimbic DA system in the motivation of voluntary physical activity (Werme et al. 2002).

Environmental Intervention and Self-Regulation

The preceding theories and models of how people reach a decision to be physically active view behavior as influenced by expectations that valued outcomes outweigh anticipated costs of or barriers to a given behavior. However, those theoretical models do not necessarily do a good job of explaining why such choices often do not result in sustainable behavior change. The models do not adequately address how features of the environment impede or foster physical activity; nor do they consider how people can use behavioral skills such as decision making, self-monitoring, goal setting, stimulus control, and reinforcement control to prompt and reinforce their own behavior.

The following sections describe how behavior modification and cognitive–behavior modification address the ways in which the environment and self-regulation can influence physical activity. People often must make several attempts at behavior change before they experience success. For these reasons, successful behavior change must be viewed as an ongoing endeavor. Increasing the physical activity of Americans requires interventions at the community level (including physicians' offices, schools, churches, families, and local government) with approaches that span multiple levels of change (personal, interpersonal, organizational, environmental, institutional, and legislative) and aim to reach diverse segments of the population otherwise missed by traditional health care.

Behavior Modification

Behavior modification is the planned, systematic application of principles of learning to the modification of behavior. According to behavior modification theory, changes in behavior result from associations between external stimuli and the consequences of a specific behavior. The role of people's thoughts, motives, and perceptions is minimized. What precedes and what follows a behavior influence the frequency of that behavior; that is, behavior is cued and reinforced. According to behavior modification theory, the key to behavior change lies in the identification of the target behavior (e.g., walking at lunch or stationary cycling while studying) and effective cues and reinforcers for it. Behavioral approaches, such as written agreements, behavioral contracts, lotteries, and stimulus and reinforcement control have been successful in exercise intervention studies.

Cognitive–Behavior Modification

Many people seem to lack the behavioral skills needed to pursue their commitments to long-range physical activity goals. These may be valued goals, but they are remote and require diligence for many weeks or months before rewarding changes are seen. Also, later gains occur more slowly than initial ones. This is very frustrating when constant improvements are expected. The daily pleasures of sedentary behaviors can erode the good intentions of pursuing physical activity goals.

Cognitive–behavior modification is based on the assumption that people can learn behavioral skills that help them self-regulate their behavior. Hence, psychological variables are viewed as key links between the environment and behavior. A wide range of maladaptive behaviors result from an individual's irrational, unproductive thoughts. Learning or insight can serve to restructure, augment, or replace faulty thoughts with behaviorally effective beliefs and skills. Simply put, thoughts and feelings moderate behavior, and they can be changed. People are educated about the relationship of cognitions, feelings, and behaviors and are taught skills to identify and control antecedents and **consequences** that prompt and reinforce behavior. Cognitive–behavioral approaches, including self-monitoring, goal setting, feedback, and decision making, have been effective in increasing exercise adherence when used alone or in combination.

Self-monitoring is keeping and displaying an objective record of behavior (e.g., frequency, time, and place). This objective measure of actual behavior can be compared with goals and gains. It also reduces people's rationalizations that they are already sufficiently physically active when they are not.

Stimulus control involves manipulating antecedent conditions, or cues, that can prompt a behavior. Prompts can be verbal, physical, or symbolic. The goal is to increase cues for the desired behavior and decrease cues for competing behaviors. Examples of cues to increase exercise behavior are posters, slogans, notes, placement of exercise equipment in visible locations, recruiting social support, and exercising at the same time and place every day. Before going home after work and first thing in the morning are times when distracting cues are lessened.

Reinforcement control entails understanding and modifying the consequences of a target behavior to increase or decrease its occurrence. Reinforcement is commonly thought of as rewarding a behavior to increase its frequency. Positive reinforcement is the addition of a stimulus that leads to increased frequency of behavior. Negative reinforcement increases behavior by the removal of a stimulus from the environment. In contrast, **punishment** is the addition or removal of a stimulus after which the frequency of behavior is reduced.

Goal setting is used to accomplish a specific task in a specific period of time. Goals can be simple and time limited or complex and long-term. Goals serve as immediate regulators of human behavior, providing direction, mobilizing effort, and fostering persistence in the search for task strategies. Goal setting provides a plan of action that focuses and directs activity and emphasizes a clear link between behavior and outcome. Specific, measurable goals make it easier to monitor progress, make adjustments, and know when the goal has been attained. Goals must be reasonable and realistic. A goal might be achievable, but personal and situational constraints can make it unrealistic. For example, losing 2 lb (0.9 kg) a week through diet and exercise is reasonable for many people but almost impossible for a working mother of three who has minimal time for exercise and cooking. Unrealistic goals set the participant up to fail, which can damage self-efficacy and adherence to the program of behavior change.

Stage Theory

Exercise behavior theorists began to recognize the need for dynamic models of exercise that include the idea of stages nearly 30 years ago (Dishman 1982; Godin, Valois, and Desharnais 1995; Sallis and Hovell 1990; Sonstroem 1988).

However, those ideas didn't have much impact on interventions designed to increase physical activity. In the early 1990s, Marcus and others (e.g., Marcus et al. 1992; Marcus and Simkin 1993) began applying the **transtheoretical model (TTM) of stages of change** to the study of physical activity. The TTM is a general model of intentional behavior change that includes the use of different cognitive and behavioral processes at different stages of change. Prochaska and DiClemente (1983) developed the TTM in the late 1970s and early 1980s based on an analysis of 18 leading systems of psychotherapy. They observed smokers trying to quit without professional intervention and found that these self-changers passed through specific stages as they tried to stop smoking. Although the TTM was developed to describe changes in addictive behavior, it has expanded to include the adoption of preventive health behaviors and the use of medical services, including physical activity (Prochaska et al. 1994).

The model describes health behavior adoption and maintenance as a process that occurs through a series of five behaviorally and motivationally defined stages (figure 17.13).

Three key factors are hypothesized to influence behavior change. They include self-efficacy, incorporated from the **social cognitive theory**; **decisional balance,** which is the

---

Exercise Stages of Change

Precontemplation stage: Individuals are inactive and have no intention to start exercising. They are not seriously thinking about changing their level of exercise within the next six months, or they deny the need to change.

Contemplation stage: Individuals are also inactive, but they intend to start regular exercise within the next six months.

Preparation stage: Individuals are active below a criterion level (typically defined as at least three times per week for 20 min or longer) but intend to become more active in the near future (within the next 30 days).

Action stage: Individuals have engaged in regular exercise at the criterion level for less than six months. Motivation and investment in behavior change are sufficient at this stage, and the perceived benefits are greater than the perceived cost. However, this is the least-stable stage. Individuals in the action stage are at greatest risk of a relapse.

Maintenance stage: Individuals have been exercising regularly for more than six months. Exercise behavior is more established than in the other stages, and the risk of a relapse is low.

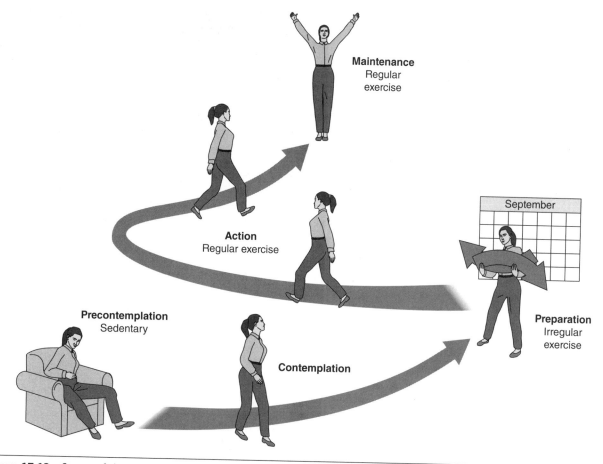

Figure 17.13   Stages of change model.

Reprinted, by permission, from J. Buckworth and R.K. Dishman, 2001, *Exercise psychology* (Champaign, IL: Human Kinetics), 220.

evaluation of the benefits and costs of the target behavior; and **processes of change,** which are the tactics used to change behavior.

There are presumably 10 processes or tactics to change behavior; five are cognitive-experiential and five are behavioral. Cognitive–experiential processes are the processes whereby an individual's own actions or experiences generate relevant information. Examples are consciousness raising, when people become more aware of opportunities to be active, and self-reevaluation, in which values regarding inactivity are reappraised. Behavioral processes are the processes whereby environmental events and behaviors, such as **stimulus control** and **reinforcement control,** generate information.

The level-of-change dimension is the context in which the target behavior occurs. Stages of change and processes of change are the components of the transtheoretical model that have been used to develop and implement interventions to enhance the adoption and maintenance of regular exercise. Different strategies are applied based on an individual's stage of change. For example, cognitive strategies, such as increasing knowledge about personal benefits of physical activity,

can be directed toward someone in the precontemplation or contemplation stages. Someone in the preparation or action stages might benefit more from behavioral strategies such as reinforcement management and stimulus control.

The key tactic for moving people from precontemplation to contemplation is to get their attention using messages that show relevance. Beliefs about the benefits of exercise should be strengthened and perceived costs reduced. Health risk appraisals and fitness testing are examples of interventions that can prompt contemplation, even though they don't directly lead to long-term behavior change.

The goal with contemplators and people in the preparation stage is to help them take action. Marketing and media campaigns promoting exercise, as well as accurate, easy-to-understand information about how to start an exercise program geared toward people's goals, can help move people into the action stage by increasing knowledge, improving attitudes, and increasing intentions to adopt physical activity. Initial goals should thus be challenging but realistic in order to foster exercise self-efficacy. Environmental and social supports and barriers should also be evaluated and modified to promote the new behaviors.

Individuals in the action phase are still at high risk of dropping out of an exercise program. Social support is critical in this stage. Instruction in self-regulatory skills, such as stimulus control, reinforcement management, and self-monitoring of progress are also useful strategies.

The usefulness of the transtheoretical model for exercise interventions has been mixed, and the instruments used to measure stages of change and processes of change have been poorly validated for exercise (Marshall and Biddle 2001) until recently (Dishman, Jackson, and Bray 2010). Also, a recent longitudinal study (Dishman et al. 2010b) supports earlier cross-sectional findings (Rosen 2000) indicating that, contrary to theory, people appear to use both cognitive–experiential and behavioral processes while they attempt to increase or maintain their physical activity. In a multiethnic cohort of 500 adults living in Hawaii who were observed at six-month intervals three or more times for two years, people who maintained or attained the Healthy People 2010 guidelines for regular participation in moderate or vigorous physical activity were more likely to retain higher scores on self-efficacy and both experiential and behavioral processes of change across the two years of observation (Dishman et al. 2010b). However, the stages were not useful for predicting change in physical activity (Dishman et al. 2009c). They were more likely to falsely classify people as meeting the guideline than to falsely classify them as not meeting it. Probabilities of predicting six-month transitions were about 50% for the stable class of meeting the guideline each time and just 25% for transitions between meeting and not meeting the guideline.

Readiness for change does not explain why people have difficulty maintaining a change. Even among people who are habitually active, unexpected changes in activity routines or settings can interrupt or end a previously continuous exercise program. Relocation, medical events, and travel can disrupt the continuity of activity and create new activity barriers. Interventions may be needed until physical activity becomes intrinsically rewarding (e.g., fun) to the person.

Relapse Prevention

Most of the theories described so far can be applied to the adoption and maintenance of behavior change. The **relapse prevention** model focuses exclusively on the maintenance of voluntary self-control efforts. The goal of the model is to help people who are attempting to modify their behavior cope effectively with situations that could tempt them to return to the old, undesired behavior pattern. Marlatt and Gordon (1985) originally designed the model to enhance abstinence from high-frequency, undesired, addictive behaviors such as smoking, substance abuse, and overeating; but the model has also been used to change physical activity (King and Frederiksen 1984; Knapp 1988). In this model, maintenance of behavioral change is focused on a person's ability to cope with relapses cognitively and behaviorally.

Components of Relapse Prevention

- Identifying situations that put a person at high risk for relapse
- Revising plans to avoid or cope with high-risk situations (e.g., time management, relaxation training, confidence building, reducing barriers to activity)
- Correcting positive outcome expectancies for inactivity so that consequences of not exercising are placed in proper perspective
- Expecting and planning for lapses, such as scheduling alternative activities while on vacation or after injury
- Minimizing the abstinence violation effect, whereby a temporary lapse is catastrophized into feelings of total failure, which lead to loss of confidence and complete cessation
- Correcting a lifestyle imbalance in which "shoulds" outweigh "wants"
- Avoiding urges to relapse by blocking self-dialogues and images of the benefits of not exercising

Relapse begins with a **high-risk situation,** which is a situation that challenges a person's confidence in his or her ability to adhere to a desired behavioral change. An adequate coping response leads to increased self-efficacy and decreased probability of relapse. Inadequate coping or no coping leads to decreased self-efficacy and possibly positive expectations of what will happen if the behavioral change is skipped. For example, people tired at the end of the workday may expect to feel refreshed if they rest rather than exercise. They actually may feel guilty, however, while the activity would likely have been invigorating. The more rigid the "rule" is, the more obvious the slip. For example, if the rule is to exercise three days per week at 6:15 a.m. for 35 min, starting 10 min late can be perceived as a slip. Perception of slipping may lead to the **abstinence violation effect,** which has both cognitive and emotional components. This effect includes cognitive dissonance, in which there is an incongruity between thoughts or feelings and behavior. For example, the slip behavior does not match the self-concept of being in control of exercise behavior. Another cognitive component of the abstinence violation effect is all-or-nothing thinking, such as defining oneself as either a success or a failure, which also can increase emotional stress. The emotional components of abstinence violation include catastrophic thinking when a temporary slip is exaggerated into a sense of failure, self-blame, lowered self-esteem, guilt, and perceived loss of control, setting the stage for relapse.

▶ **HIGH-RISK SITUATIONS** and rigid rules increase the risk of relapse.

A lifestyle imbalance in which "shoulds" exceed "wants" also predisposes a person to relapse. People who spend more time doing what should be done at the expense of doing what they want to do feel deprived, and the desire for indulgence or self-gratification increases. Exercise might be viewed not as pleasurable but as another obligation. Thus, positive expectations of not adhering to the behavioral change make relapse more attractive.

Conceptually, the relapse prevention model seems useful for exercise adherence, given that 50% of those who begin a regular exercise program drop out within the first six months, most within the first three months. However, the model was developed for maintaining cessation of high-frequency, undesired behaviors, and exercise is a low-frequency, desired behavior. It is clear when someone relapses from smoking cessation, but it is hard to operationally define a slip from regular exercise and identify when a slip becomes relapse. An exercise lapse may be hard to recognize or deal with in time to forestall relapse.

Effectiveness of Physical Activity Interventions

Behavior modification techniques can increase participation rates by about 15% to 35% above the common dropout level of 50% that occurs without behavioral intervention. Nonetheless, long-term maintenance of increased physical activity after the interventions has not been established. An early quantitative meta-analysis was conducted of 127 studies that examined the efficacy of interventions for increasing physical activity among 131,000 subjects in community, worksite, school, home, and health care settings in the United States and a few other countries (Dishman and Buckworth 1996). The researchers reported 445 effects as Pearson correlation coefficients (r) as they varied according to moderating variables important for community and clinical intervention. The mean effect was moderately large, $r = 0.34$, approximately 3/4 of a standard deviation, or an increase in binomial success rate from 50% to 67%. The estimated population effect weighted by sample size was larger, $r = 0.75$, approximately 2 standard deviations, or increased success to 88%. Figures 17.14 through 17.16 illustrate the contrasts between levels of independent moderating variables. Effects were larger when the interventions employed the principles of behavior modification, targeted community groups, and measured active leisure of low intensity.

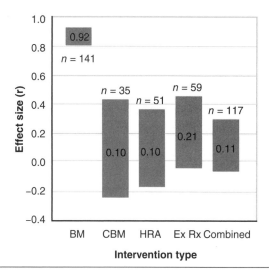

Figure 17.14   Effect of intervention to increase physical activity was largest for behavior modification (BM). CBM = cognitive–behavior modification; HRA = health risk appraisal; Ex Rx = traditional exercise prescription; Combined = multiple intervention.

Adapted, by permission, from R.K. Dishman and J. Buckworth, 1996, "Increasing physical activity: A quantitative synthesis," *Medicine and Science in Sports and Exercise* 28: 706-719.

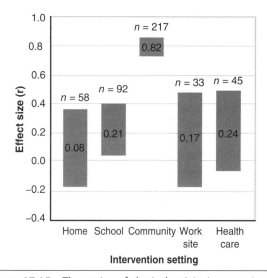

Figure 17.15   The setting of physical activity intervention had an effect size r that was largest for community-based interventions; 95% CI excluded zero.

Adapted, by permission, from R.K. Dishman and J. Buckworth, 1996, "Increasing physical activity: A quantitative synthesis," *Medicine and Science in Sports and Exercise* 28: 706-719.

Only about 25% of intervention studies included long-term follow-up to determine whether the interventions had lasting effects once they ended. Therefore, the positive effects of interventions must presently be viewed as short-term. The results showed that physical activity *can* be increased by intervention. That is to say, selected interventions have been shown to have efficacy (i.e., they increased

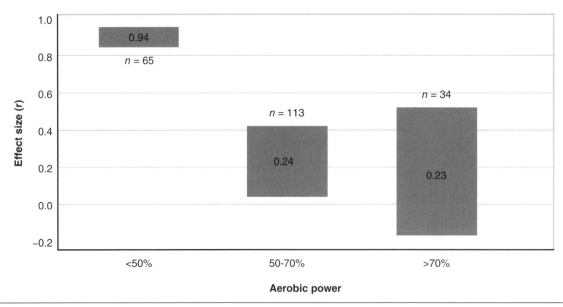

Figure 17.16 Physical activity intervention had an effect size *r* that was largest for low-intensity interventions; 95% CI excluded zero.

Adapted, by permission, from R.K. Dishman and J. Buckworth, 1996, "Increasing physical activity: A quantitative synthesis," *Medicine and Science in Sports and Exercise* 28: 706-719.

The RE-AIM Framework
for Evaluating Population-Based Behavioral Interventions

Reach: The absolute number, proportion, and population representativeness of people who are willing to participate in an intervention

Efficacy: The impact of an intervention on the primary outcome targeted by the intervention, which can also include desirable secondary outcomes such as quality of life and economic outcomes, as well as undesirable, adverse events such as injury or death

Adoption: The absolute number, proportion, and representativeness of settings and interventionists who are willing to initiate a program

Implementation: The degree of fidelity to the various elements of an intervention's administrative protocol, including consistency of intended delivery and time and cost of the intervention

Maintenance: The extent to which a program or policy becomes institutionalized or part of routine organizational practices and policies or, at the individual level, the long-term effects of a program on outcomes six or more months after the most recent intervention contact

Modified from Glasgow, Vogt, and Boles 1999.

---

physical activity within the context of the experimental intervention and the people who were measured). However, the optimal ways for selecting intervention components, settings, and population segments to maintain increases in physical activity require experimental confirmation through randomized controlled trials. Moreover, the public health significance of an efficacious intervention also depends on whether the intervention reaches a high proportion of the target population, whether it is adopted and implemented fully and well within the target population by the responsible organizations, and whether the effects of the intervention are maintained after it ends (Glasgow, Vogt, and Boles 1999; Glasgow et al. 2002).

Interventions to Increase Physical Activity

The key sets of actions required globally to increase physical activity, especially in developing nations, include (1) efforts to disseminate individual-level behavior change programs to reach much larger populations rather than volunteers; (2)

social marketing and mass communication campaigns to change social norms in the community and among professionals and policy makers; (3) efforts to influence the social and physical environments to make them more conducive to physical activity; and (4) the development and implementation of national physical activity plans and strategies, with sufficient time lines and resources to achieve measurable change (Bauman, Finegood, and Matsudo 2009).

National Physical Activity Plans

In preparation for developing the National Physical Activity Plan for the United States (Pate 2009), an evaluation of national physical activity plans from six countries (Australia, United Kingdom, Scotland, Sweden, Northern Ireland, and Norway) concluded that most plans had the essential elements recommended by the CDC/WHO Collaborating Center for Physical Activity and Health Promotion (Pratt et al. 2009). These included consultation with key stakeholders; development of coalitions across government, nongovernment, and private sectors; use of individual and environmental strategies for intervention; implementation at different levels (community, state, and national); integration of physical activity with other related agenda (nutrition, environment, public health); special consideration for subpopulation groups (children, women, disabled people, indigenous people); time lines for realization of goals and objectives; and plan identity (logos, branding, and slogans). Only Northern Ireland's plan documented details for funding and executing the plan's goals and evaluating the plan's success (Bornstein, Pate, and Pratt 2009).

Consistent with the ideas of the National Physical Activity Plan for the United States (Pate 2009), Active Living by Design was a five-year community grant program of the Robert Wood Johnson Foundation, established to help 25 communities create environments that support active living. Each funded site established a multidisciplinary community partnership and implemented the 5P strategies: preparation, promotions, programs, policy, and physical projects (Bors et al. 2009). The community partnerships worked within neighborhoods, schools, worksites, and various organizations to increase physical and social supports for physical activity. Time will tell whether these types of community interventions are sustainable and effective (Glasgow and King 2009).

Successful physical activity promotion must also synergize with planning and policy in other sectors of government. For example, after more than a decade of strong public communications about evidence-based practices in physical activity and public health in Australia, a national physical activity policy framework for the health sector emerged, but not as a policy vision that was inclusive of the other essential sectors such as education, transport, and urban planning as well as sport and recreation (Bellew et al. 2008). In addition, public and political interest in elite sport and, later, childhood obesity and type 2 diabetes tended to overwhelm the physical activity and public health initiative.

Recommendations for Community Interventions

The Task Force on Community Preventive Services is an independent, nonfederal panel consisting of 15 members, including a chair, appointed by the director of the CDC. It oversees preparation of the *Guide to Community Preventive Services* (popularly called the Community Guide), a periodic report that provides public health decision makers with recommendations about population-based interventions for the promotion of health and the prevention of disease, injury, disability, and premature death for use by communities and health care systems. The task force reviewed and assessed evidence on the quality and effectiveness of 94 community-based interventions for increasing physical activity or aerobic capacity (Kahn et al. 2002).

As summarized in table 17.5, the task force recommended six interventions: two informational approaches (i.e., community-wide campaigns and point-of-decision prompts to encourage use of stairs); three behavioral and social approaches (i.e., school-based physical education, social support interventions in community settings, and individually adapted health behavior change programs); and one intervention to increase physical activity by using environmental and policy approaches (i.e., creation of or enhanced access to places for physical activity, combined with informational outreach activities).

The task force found an insufficient number of studies of mass media campaigns, college physical education, and **health education**. The group could not yet recommend classroom-based health education focusing on reducing television viewing and video game playing because no link was demonstrated between reduced television watching or video game playing and increased physical activity.

Examples of Successful Community Interventions

The interventions described in this section were carried out in several countries and in a variety of community settings. Consistent with the Task Force on Community Preventive Services recommendations for successful community interventions to increase physical activity, the successful interventions used informational approaches (community-wide campaigns and point-of-decision prompts to encourage use of stairs), behavioral and social approaches (school-based physical education, social support interventions in community settings, and individually adapted health behavior change programs), and one intervention to increase physical activity by using environmental and policy approaches (creation of or enhanced access to places

Table 17.5   Recommendations From the Task Force on Community Preventive Services Regarding Use of Selected Interventions to Increase Physical Activity Behaviors and Improve Physical Fitness

Interventions (number of qualifying studies)	Intervention description	Task force recommendation for use
Informational approaches to increasing physical activity		
Community-wide campaigns	These large-scale, highly visible, multicomponent campaigns direct their messages to large audiences using a variety of approaches, including television, radio, newspapers, movie theaters, billboards, and mailings.	Recommended with strong evidence
Behavioral and social approaches to increasing physical activity		
Individually adapted health behavior change programs	These programs are tailored to a person's specific interests or readiness to make a change in physical activity habits. Teaching behavioral skills such as goal setting, building social support, self-rewards, problem solving, and relapse prevention, the programs help people learn to incorporate physical activity into their daily routines.	Recommended with strong evidence
School-based physical education (PE)	This approach seeks to modify school curricula and policies to increase the amount of time students spend in moderate to vigorous activity while in PE class. Schools can accomplish this either by increasing the amount of time spent in PE class or by increasing students' activity levels during PE classes.	Recommended with strong evidence
Social support interventions in community contexts	The goal of this approach is to increase physical activity by creating or strengthening social networks. Examples include exercise buddies, exercise contracts, and walking groups.	Recommended with strong evidence
Environmental and policy approaches to increasing physical activity		
Creating or improving access to places for physical activity combined with informational outreach	Examples include building walking or biking trails or making it possible for people to use exercise facilities in community centers or in the workplace. Informational outreach includes activities such as providing training on equipment, seminars, counseling, risk screening, and health forums and workshops.	Recommended with strong evidence
Point-of-decision prompts to encourage stair use	These signs are placed by elevators and escalators and encourage people to use nearby stairs instead.	Recommended with sufficient evidence
Community-scale urban design land-use policies and practices	Examples involve the efforts of urban planners, architects, engineers, developers, and public health professionals to change the physical environment of urban areas of several square miles or more in ways that support physical activity.	Recommended with sufficient evidence
Street-scale urban design and land-use policies	Examples involve the efforts of urban planners, architects, engineers, developers, and public health professionals to change the physical environment of small geographic areas, generally limited to a few blocks, in ways that support physical activity.	Recommended with sufficient evidence

Adapted from Task Force on Community Preventive Services 2001.

for physical activity, combined with informational outreach activities).

Informational Approaches

Community-wide campaigns represent an intervention approach classified as an informational approach to promoting physical activity. These campaigns represent large-scale, high-intensity, high-visibility programming and often use TV, radio, newspapers, and other media to raise program awareness, disseminate targeted and segmented health messages, and reinforce behavior change. This strategy often employs multicomponent, multisector, and multisite interventions. The Stanford Heart Disease Prevention Program (Young et al. 1996) and the Wheeling Walks intervention (Reger et al. 2002) are examples of effective community-wide campaigns in regions of the United States. A highly visible, multilevel community intervention in São Paulo, Brazil, *Agita São Paulo* (Move São Paulo), has targeted the entire state of São Paulo, about 34 million people, since 1995 and served as the main model and venue for the WHO's World Health Day in 2002, *Agita Mundo* (Move the World). Sponsored by the São Paulo Ministry of Health and spearheaded by physician Victor Matsudo, the *Agita São Paulo* campaign has successfully penetrated the São Paulo culture with brand recognition of its icon, the 30-Minute Man, who appears in all kinds of communications, from billboards to monthly utility bills mailed to individual citizens (Matsudo et al. 2002, 2003). The *Agita São Paulo* and *Agita Mundo* experiences taught that local, national, and global programs, coalitions, partnerships, and networks at all levels are essential to guarantee the success of physical activity promotion as a public health strategy (Matsudo and Matsudo 2006).

Another extensive public policy initiative for sports and health occurred in Finland during the early 1990s and resulted in two national programs. The initial Finland on the Move program was designed to stimulate new local projects through national financial support, training and consultation services, and media promotion. The ongoing Fit for Life program is based on the experience gained from the initial intervention but focuses mainly on an intensive mass media approach that targets people ages 40 to 60 years. The Finnish experience has demonstrated that deliberate efforts to communicate scientific knowledge can lead to a better acceptance of physical activity on the national level and that well-planned and sensitive state-level support of grassroots activities can succeed (Vuori, Paronen, and Oja 1998). An example of a nationally based health initiative that included the promotion of physical activity is the ParticipACTION mass campaign, which ran in Canada from 1979 to 2001 and was launched again in 2007 (Tremblay and Craig 2009).

Another informational approach developed in Brazil and implemented mainly in Latin America (Hoehner et al. 2008) uses regular, short physical activity–related educational and motivational messages often delivered by a health-educator communicator and focused on key community sites, including worksites, senior centers, and community centers rather than broad mass media campaigns.

In the United States, the VERB campaign targeted a cohort of 2729 "tweens," young people ages 9 to 13, in communities across the United States with mass media efforts, Internet links, and community events and programs designed to increase and maintain physical activity (Berkowitz et al. 2008). After one year, 74% of children surveyed were aware of the VERB campaign. The average 9- to 10-year-old aware of the campaign engaged in 34% more free-time physical activity sessions per week than did 9- to 10-year-old youths who were unaware of the campaign (Huhman et al. 2005). Of course, it is also possible that already active children were more likely to notice information about physical activity.

Behavioral and Social Approaches

An exemplary intervention that represents this strategy, as reported by Kriska and colleagues (1986), was one in which women living in and around Pittsburgh, Pennsylvania were organized into walking clubs within their neighborhoods and received communications (e.g., newsletters, phone prompts) designed to reinforce and sustain their walking network. Another example comes from the work of Lombard and colleagues (1995), who organized walking partners and small groups in communities. They conducted initial training on walking and behavioral principles and provided neighborhood maps and other supports. Phone networks and regular prompts and updates were used to reinforce behaviors and provide opportunities for participants to ask questions.

Individual-focused interventions usually consist of an assessment of a participant's physical activity level and readiness to change, a tailored activity plan, and navigation to community interventions by a centralized health provider or promoter (Dunn et al. 1999). This approach, which focuses on lifestyle physical activity, has been shown to be cost-effective when compared to supervised physical activity programs (Sevick et al. 2000). Providing physical activity classes in community settings (e.g., public parks and plazas, worksites, and community centers) also has been identified as a promising practice (Hoehner et al. 2008; Martins and Duarte 2000; Pain et al. 2001).

Schools

School physical education and health education curricula provide methods of promoting youth physical activity, and many of these strategies have been shown to be effective (Stone et al. 1998). A systematic review of 26 controlled trials implemented in a school setting, and aimed at increasing physical activity in children and adolescents 6 to 18 years of age, concluded that there is good evidence that school-based physical activity interventions (requiring at least a combination of printed educational materials and changes to the school curriculum) have a positive impact on duration of physical activity and $\dot{V}O_2$max, but generally no effect on leisure-time physical activity rates outside of school (Dobbins et al. 2009). Another systematic review that gauged 19 interventions to increase physical activity in Latin America according to the standards of the U.S. Community Guide concluded that only for school-based physical education classes was the strength of the evidence from Latin America sufficient to support a practice recommendation (Hoehner et al. 2008). Five studies (three were randomized) from Brazil, Chile, and the U.S.–Mexico border showed increases in physical activity during physical education classes and walking or biking to school.

Overall, interventions have had a moderately large effect (more than half a standard deviation) on physical activity observed during school, but small effects on self-reported physical activity outside of school and no effects on physical activity outside of school measured objectively by accelerometers (see figure 17.17).

Most early studies of interventions in schools targeted upper elementary students. However, daily participation in a physical education class by high school students decreased from 42% in 1991 to 27% in 1997 (CDC 1998). It was just 23% in 2009, dropping from 47% in the 9th grade to 22% in the 12th grade (CDC 2010). As figure 17.18 illustrates, the percentage of high school students in the United States who attended daily physical education classes in 2009 varied

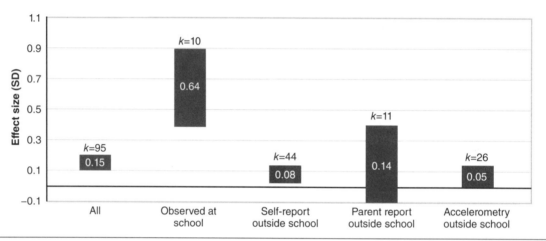

Figure 17.17 Effects of school-based interventions on physical activity in children and adolescents 1996 through 2007 (k = number of effects).

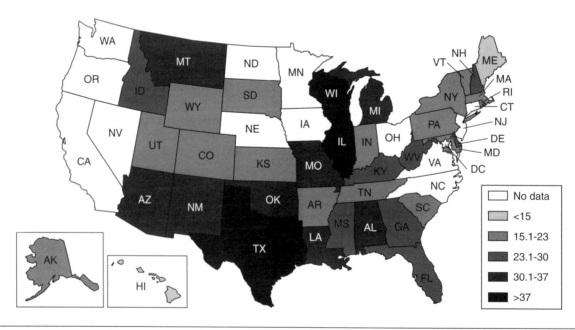

Figure 17.18 Percentage of U.S. high school students enrolled in daily physical education class in 2009.

Data from Centers for Disease Control, 2010, "Youth risk behavior surveillance - United States, 2009."

> ### Five Components of a Comprehensive School Physical Activity Program
>
> - Physical education
> - Physical activity during school
> - Physical activity before and after school
> - Staff involvement
> - Family and community involvement

widely, from 5% in Maine to 68% in Illinois, and was lower among girls in most states and overall (19% in girls vs. 27% in boys). About 51% of girls and 62% of boys said they participated on at least one sport team (CDC 2010).

Because physical activity declines during adolescence (Kahn et al. 2008), more community opportunities for recreational activities and sports should be considered. Other directions for interventions through the schools could include curricula that target behavioral skills necessary for lifelong physical activity, the integration of physical activity in other academic classes (e.g., computing target heart rate zone in math class or writing essays on making exercise fun in English class), noncompetitive and inclusive after-school recreation programs, and programs that involve parents.

The National Association for Sport and Physical Education (NASPE), an association of the American Alliance of Health, Physical Education, Recreation and Dance, recently launched Let's Move in School (LMIS), a national initiative to increase physical activity before, during, and after school. Let's Move in School invites all U.S. schools to help kids achieve 60 min of movement a day and improve health and academic performance. To date, close to 780 schools totaling 675,000 students have registered for a Let's Move in School event.

The goal of Let's Move in School is "to ensure that every school provides a comprehensive school physical activity program with quality physical education as the foundation so that youth will develop the knowledge, skills, and confidence to be physically active for a lifetime." Let's Move in School urges physical educators, parents, school administrators, and policy makers to get involved in bringing quality physical education and physical activity to schools through a comprehensive school physical activity program (Allensworth and Kolbe 1987).

The Child and Adolescent Trial for Cardiovascular Health (CATCH)

This was a randomized trial carried out in California, Louisiana, Minnesota, and Texas that targeted children in grades 3, 4, and 5. The intervention, which was based on social cognitive theory and organizational change, was implemented in class, with the family, and through policy changes in schools

randomly assigned to an experimental (56 schools) or control group (40 schools). Participants in the CATCH program increased moderate to vigorous physical activity in class and vigorous activity outside of class.

Middle-School Physical Activity and Nutrition (M-SPAN)

This was a trial for students at 24 middle schools in San Diego, California and its surrounding area that targeted physical activity change across the school environment both in physical education class and during other periods throughout the school day, although the trial also had a nutrition component (Sallis et al. 2003). School staff and students were engaged in policy change efforts, but there was no classroom health education. Based on structured observations of physical education class and other school physical activity environments, at two years there was an increase in physical activity at school in the intervention schools relative to control schools for boys (about 1 SD), but not girls.

Trial of Activity in Adolescent Girls (TAAG)

TAAG was a multicenter, two-year, group-randomized trial designed to reduce the usual decline in moderate-to-vigorous physical activity between the 6th and 8th grades among girls randomly selected from middle schools in six regions of the United States: Baltimore, Maryland; Columbia, South Carolina; Minneapolis, Minnesota; New Orleans, Louisiana; San Diego, California; and Tucson, Arizona (Webber et al. 2008). The goals were to increase opportunities, support, and incentives for increased physical activity. Components included programs linking schools and community agencies, physical education, health education, and social marketing. A third-year intervention used school and community personnel to direct intervention activities. There was no effect of the intervention on girls' physical activity, measured by accelerometers, in the 8th grade. However, after the third year, girls in intervention schools were more physically active than girls in control schools. The difference was small, though, about 1.6 min of daily physical activity or 80 kcal per week.

Lifestyle Education for Activity Project (LEAP)

The LEAP intervention, carried out in 24 high schools in South Carolina, included nearly 3000 girls during their 8th- and 9th-grade years (Pate et al. 2005). It was organized according to the Coordinated School Health Program (CSHP) model (Allensworth and Kolbe 1987). With help from the intervention staff, teachers at each school developed behavioral skills in instructional units that emphasized the acquisition and practice of self-regulatory behaviors (e.g., goal setting, time management, identifying and overcoming barriers, and self-reinforcement); the units were implemented in health education, biology, family and consumer science, or physical education, depending upon how each school provided health education. The LEAP physical education component, known as LEAP PE, included a one-year curriculum designed by the teachers at each school to develop motor skills in a variety of physical activities that were popular with high school girls, including aerobics, weight training, dance, and self-defense, using approaches that favored small groups and cooperative and successful learning experiences. In addition to facilitating noncompetitive mastery of skills, instruction used modeling of success, encouragement, and moderately intense exercise directed toward enhancing self-efficacy and enjoyment. The intervention led to a significant increase in overall physical activity, not just physical activity during school, that was maintained at the 12th grade in the schools that most fully implemented and then retained core features of the intervention three years after LEAP ended (Pate et al. 2007).

Other School Programs

Active transport by walking and cycling to and from school can provide substantial physical activity for children and youth. Communities can leverage federal dollars set aside to promote cycling and pedestrian activities with assistance from state departments of transportation.

An example is the California Department of Transportation, which provided $66 million in funding over three years for "Safe Routes to Schools" grants to 270 schools (Boarnet et al. 2005). In Marin County, walking to school increased 64% and biking increased 114% after a combined intervention (Staunton, Hubsmith, and Kallins 2003). A statewide evaluation of 10 schools found that students who passed by the improvements on their way to school increased walking and biking by 15% compared to 4% for those who did not pass by the improvements (Boarnet et al. 2005).

Worksites

An early meta-analysis of 26 workplace interventions in the United States between 1972 and 1997, yielding 45 effects on 9000 people, reported a small overall effect (0.22 SD) of increased physical activity (Dishman et al. 1998) that was confirmed (0.21 SD; 95% CI: 0.11-0.31) in a later analysis of 41 effects (Conn et al. 2009). Workplace programs may provide information and encouragement to get employees to begin exercising, but additional studies using valid research designs and measures are needed to confirm this. Two worksite-based studies demonstrating the role of policy and environmental approaches to promoting physical activity are the Los Angeles Lift-Off (Yancey et al. 2004) and Move to Improve (Dishman et al. 2009a).

Los Angeles Lift-Off

Yancey and colleagues (2004) conducted a randomized controlled posttest-only trial to evaluate the level of participation in a physical activity promotion program designed to integrate a single 10-min exercise break into regularly occurring meetings or events during work time at Los Angeles County Department of Health Services worksites. The unique focus of this intervention was a "minimal" environmental change specifically targeting underserved populations. Results indicated

that more than 90% of meeting attendees participated in the exercises. The investigators concluded that captive audiences, such as those attending mandatory meetings and events, may be engaged in brief bouts of exercise as a part of the workday, regardless of physical activity level or stage of change.

Move to Improve

A multisite group randomized controlled trial consisting of a 12-week intervention increased moderate-to-vigorous physical activity among employees at 16 worksites in the United States and Canada of a large retail company by targeting features of the workplace environment as well as employee motivation using personal and team goal setting (Dishman et al. 2009a). Participants in the intervention had greater increases in moderate-to-vigorous physical activity and walking compared to participants in a health education control condition. The proportion of participants that met the Healthy People 2010 recommendation for regular participation in either moderate or vigorous physical activity remained near 25% at control sites during the study but increased to 50% at intervention sites. During the last six weeks of the study, intervention participants exceeded 300 min weekly of self-reported moderate-to-vigorous physical activity and 9000 daily pedometer steps, which each were positively related to the goals set by the participants (Dishman et al. 2010c).

Policy and Environmental Approaches

Interventions designed to create or provide access to places where people can be physically active often involve the combined efforts of worksites, schools, coalitions, government agencies, and community members (Kahn et al. 2002). These interventions provide improved access to exercise facilities, such as fitness centers (both proprietary and nonprofit), community centers, and walking–bicycle trails, as well as providing access to school grounds (Kahn et. al. 2002; Heath et al. 2006). An exemplary intervention of this type, described by Linenger and colleagues (1991), included new infrastructure (i.e., bike paths), access to facilities (e.g., expanded hours of operation, lighted and integrated paths), and improved programming on a residential naval air station in San Diego, California (Linenger, Chesson, and Nice 1991). Recent studies have documented that developing such infrastructure is reasonable from a cost perspective (Wang et al. 2004).

An emerging strategy consists of community-wide policies and planning that place physical activity within the public policy agendas of communities, emphasize promotion of physical activity guidelines, provide organizational incentives, address institutional and environmental barriers, and use media effectively (Hoehner et al. 2008).

Community Organizations

Many U.S. community organizations provide physical activity facilities or programs, or they could do so. In the private sector, health clubs, dance studios, martial arts organizations, swimming clubs, and sport leagues are familiar examples.

Nonprofit organizations include YMCAs and YWCAs and Boys and Girls Clubs as well as sport leagues. Faith-based organizations often have physical activity facilities and programs for their members, which could be made available to others in the community. Private and public housing developments have recreational and fitness facilities. Thus, many resources throughout the nation can be used for recreational physical activity, and with improved promotion they can become better utilized. However, there do not appear to be any systematic studies of how the facilities and programs of community organizations contribute to physical activity in the surrounding communities.

Public Recreation Facilities

Public parks and recreation facilities are widely used, with about 80% of people in many regions of the United States making some use of municipal facilities and a smaller but substantial percentage using park programs and services (Godbey et al. 2005). Various studies have shown that 30% to 65% of park users were engaged in physical activities or sports (Godbey et al. 2005). The contribution of public recreation facilities and programs to physical activity could be enhanced through optimization of the design of the facilities to support physical activity of various population groups and promotion of use of the facilities.

The National Recreation and Park Association partnered with the National Heart, Lung, and Blood Institute on the three-year Hearts N' Parks Program, whose goal was to promote physical activity in parks to reduce health disparities among high-risk, underserved population groups. Youth efforts emphasized after-school and summer camp programs. Adult target populations were senior center attendees, city employees, and the general population of adult park users. A recent evaluation of magnet centers that developed multiple physical activity promotion programs found that 50 Hearts N' Parks magnet centers were operating in 11 states. Participants in programs were shown to improve knowledge, attitudes, and physical activity behavior using standardized survey procedures (National Recreation and Park Association 2004).

Promoting the Use of Facilities

The Missouri state health department, with the assistance of a community heart health coalition, helped to fund construction of walking trails in two communities through the Department of Transportation (DOT). To promote use of the existing trails, the state funded the health department to conduct an awareness campaign and trail enhancement activities in one of the communities with a year-old trail. The health department and a heart health coalition conducted the resulting Take Our Trail Campaign for three months (Brownson et al. 1996). The campaign kicked off with a 3-mile Family Fun-Walk, with T-shirts and refreshments donated by local businesses.

For the length of the campaign, signs were placed throughout the community to raise awareness of the trail. A simple brochure on the importance of physical activity, tips to increase walking, and information about safe use of the trail and joining a walking club was sent to all programs in the local health department, as well as to clinics, church leaders, and the heart health coalition. The local television station created a public service announcement during the evening news to promote the trail and the importance of regular physical activity. The public transportation system placed signs inside buses. The heart health coalition helped develop walking clubs at worksites, churches, and social organizations. Local law enforcement officials agreed to patrol the walking trail periodically. The coalition worked with local businesses, city government, and churches to raise money to enhance the trail, adding amenities such as lights, benches, mile markers, painted lanes, and a water fountain. The Take Our Trail community had a 35% increase in trail use between one month before and one month after the springtime campaign compared with a 10% increase in the community without the campaign. More than 60% of trail users in both communities indicated an increase in walking since development of the trail. When asked about how they became aware of the trail, most respondents indicated that they lived or worked near the trail or that they heard about it at church or at work, from their physicians, or from friends or family; they usually were unaware of the promotional campaign.

Costs/Benefits and Funding

Wang and colleagues (2004) examined the cost of trail development and the number of users of four trails in Lincoln, Nebraska. The first year of trail development cost $289,035, of which 73% was construction cost. Of the 3986 trail users, 88% were active at least three days a week. The average annual per capita cost for people who became more physically active was $98; for people who became active for general health improvement, it was $142; and for those who became active for weight loss, $884. The study provides a set of basic cost-effectiveness measures by compiling actual cost items of trail development, estimating the number and type of trail users, and identifying several physical activity–related outcomes and items. Roux and colleagues (2008), using econometric modeling of data from a list of exemplary community-based interventions, including interventions shaped by policy and environmental supports, concluded that such programs provide a good return on investment through their effectiveness in bringing about improvements in physical activity among persons exposed to such programs.

Mediators and Moderators of Physical Activity Change and Interventions

It is disappointing that cognitive–behavior modification and health education interventions designed to increase physical activity have usually been ineffective, but this may partly be explained by poor methods used to implement or evaluate those types of interventions (Dishman and Buckworth 1996; Dishman et al. 1998). Also, nearly all of these types of interventions did not clearly target or actually measure changes in the cognitive variables that were presumably targeted by the intervention to mediate change in physical activity (Baranowski, Anderson, and Carmack 1998; Dishman 1991; Lewis et al. 2002; Luban et al. 2008). That is, the studies didn't identify or confirm mediators of change.

Mediators of Physical Activity Change

Mediators are variables in a causal sequence that transmit the relation or effect of an independent variable on a dependent variable (MacKinnon, Fairchild, and Fritz 2007). Analyses shown in figures 17.19 and 17.20 indicate that increases in self-efficacy (Dishman et al. 2004) and enjoyment (Dishman

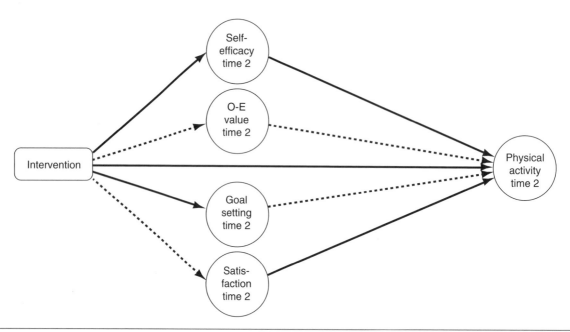

Figure 17.19 Increases in self-efficacy partly explained the effectiveness of a school-based intervention to increase physical activity among adolescent girls. Solid lines denote significant relationships. Broken lines denote nonsignificant relationships. Time 2 = scores in 9th grade.

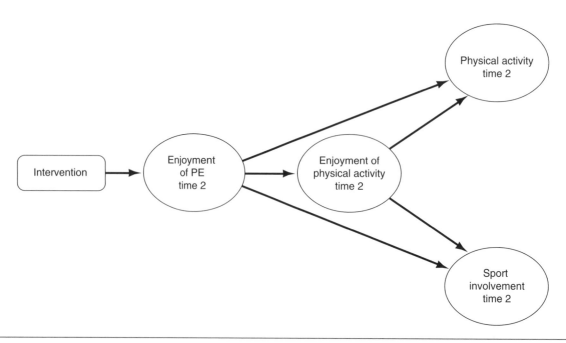

Figure 17.20 Increases in enjoyment of physical education and physical activity partly explained the effectiveness of a school-based intervention to increase physical activity among adolescent girls. Time 2 = scores in 9th grade.

et al. 2005) partly mediated the effectiveness of a school-based intervention designed to increase girls' leisure-time physical activity during the 8th and 9th grades, a period when physical activity begins to decline among adolescent girls.

Moderators of Physical Activity Change

Moderators (i.e., effect modifiers) are variables that are not in a causal sequence but that alter the relation or effect between an independent variable and a dependent variable (MacKinnon, Fairchild, and Fritz 2007). Those constructs help explain how people set and strive to attain specific behavioral goals. Little is known about the role of personality (Rhodes and Smith 2006) or of general motivational traits that may act as moderators of the influence of social cognitive variables on exercise adherence. For example, concepts related to willpower or self-motivation are acknowledged in social cognitive theory as possible influences on persistence during behavior change (Azjen 2002; Bandura 1997a), but they have been understudied as moderators of exercise adherence (Dishman 2010). In one example, a three-year longitudinal study of South Carolina girls during high school, self-efficacy was stable and moderated the relation between changes in physical activity and perceived social support. Figure 17.21 shows that girls who maintained a perception of strong social support had less of a decline in physical activity if they also had high self-efficacy. However, girls having high self-efficacy had a greater decline in physical activity if they perceived declines in social support (Dishman et al. 2009b).

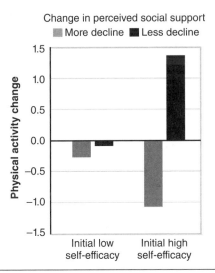

Figure 17.21 Results of moderator analysis. The effect of the interaction of initial status of self-efficacy with the longitudinal change in perceived social support on declines in physical activity.

Reprinted from R.K. Dishman et al., *Journal of Pediatric Psychology* "Self-efficacy moderates the relation between declines in physical activity and perceived social support in high school girls," 2009, 34(4): 441-451, by permission of Oxford University Press.

Features of Physical Activity That Promote Adoption and Maintenance

In addition to establishing national or international standards for physical activity participation based on epidemiologic evidence for the dose–response relationship between physical activity and health (Physical Activity Guidelines Advisory Committee 2008) or guidelines for increasing or maintaining fitness (e.g., Pollock et al. 1998), it is important to determine whether activity characteristics encourage or impede participation by some people. Regardless of exercise intensity, injuries from weight-bearing exercise, including running, can lead directly to dropouts. However, injuries typically do not occur often until durations of 45 min or frequencies of five days per week are approached by previously untrained individuals (Pollock 1988). Dropouts resulting from injuries are not more prevalent in elderly people when walking is the physical activity (Pollock et al. 1991). However, the impact of injury on subsequent physical activity has not been established in population-based studies.

The typical exercise program based on standard guidelines in sports medicine (e.g., Pollock et al. 1998) has been ineffective in promoting sustained participation without adding a behavior modification component, and behavior modification has been most successful when the physical activities targeted were leisure-time activities at intensities of less than 50% of aerobic capacity (Dishman and Buckworth 1996). Only 10% to 25% of U.S. adults follow the typical **exercise prescription,** the exercise intensity, duration, and frequency optimal for fitness. For example, in a study of California adults, more men (11%) than women (5%) adopted vigorous exercise such as running during a year, but a comparatively higher proportion of women (33%) than men (26%) took up moderate activities such as routine walking, stair climbing, and gardening (Sallis et al. 1986). Both sexes were more likely to adopt regular activities of a moderate intensity than high-intensity fitness activities. Moderate activities showed a dropout rate of 25% to 35%, roughly half that seen for vigorous exercise (50%). Hence, if large numbers of people are unwilling or unable to participate with the frequency or at the duration or intensity recommended by professional consensus for fitness, it is possible that other guidelines for participation could complement fitness standards to increase the activity of a population by reducing total sedentariness.

With this in mind, in 1993 the American College of Sports Medicine (ACSM) and the CDC began promoting an active lifestyle program as a complement to exercise prescription. The recommendation to accumulate 30 min or more of moderate-intensity physical activity most days of the week was designed to encourage sedentary people to pursue activities such as walking, gardening, and household chores (Pate et al. 1995), possibly in multiple (three to five) bouts of short duration (e.g., 5-10 min) daily. This approach could reduce some currently perceived barriers to participation, such as time, effort, and injury. However, experimental evidence is lacking to demonstrate that this approach actually increases physical activity participation. Two randomized controlled trials compared the effects of multiple short bouts of exercise (i.e., intermittent 10-min sessions totaling about 40 min each day) with traditional long sessions (i.e., 40 min each session) on physical activity, weight loss, and fitness during 20-week (Jakicic et al. 1995) and 18-month (Jakicic et al. 1999) weight loss interventions among overweight and obese middle-aged women. In general, the multiple short bouts led to similar, but not greater, long-term increases in physical activity, cardiorespiratory fitness, and weight loss compared to traditional long sessions. Regardless of approach, weight loss at 18 months was directly related to the average amount of time spent exercising each week. Women who exercised more than 200 min each week lost an average of 13 kg, compared with an 8.5 kg loss in women who exercised 150 to 200 min and a 3.5 kg loss in those who exercised less than 150 min each week.

Consistent with those findings, the Food and Nutrition Board of the Institute of Medicine recommended that adults and children spend at least 1 h each day participating in moderately intense physical activity in order to maintain optimal cardiovascular health regardless of body weight (Couzin 2002). Though that recommendation is similar to the upper end of the amounts of weekly physical activity recommended by the ACSM for weight loss and maintenance among adults (i.e., 300 min each week) (Jakicic et al. 2001), it is more than double the ACSM position that significant health benefits occur with a minimum of 150 min of moderate physical activity each week (Jakicic et al. 2001; Pate et al. 1995; U.S. Department of Health and Human Services 2008). The ACSM subsequently expressed concerns that the focus on 60 min per day might confuse people, causing them to doubt whether 30 min a day, or shorter bursts of activity such as three 10-min walks, provides any health benefit, perhaps discouraging many sedentary people from adopting any program of moderate activity because they view 60 min each day as an insurmountable goal.

The actual impact of these different recommendations requires experimental comparison in randomized clinical trials. Currently, assumptions about the superiority of one approach over the others for increasing and maintaining physical activity in the population are based on expert opinion, not fact. For example, though some health outcomes of physical activity do not require much time and effort among previously sedentary people, other outcomes of exercise valued by many people, such as weight loss or maintenance and improved body image, require more time and effort. Thus, there may be a time–effort paradox with regard to sustaining an exercise program for some people. People who are sedentary may be more apt to adopt an exercise recommendation that requires little time and effort. However, if they expect high fitness or large improvements in physique, they may drop out after becoming frustrated by

little or no gain, which is likely if they have invested little time or effort in the exercise program.

A meta-analysis of adherence in 27 randomized exercise trials concluded that the effects of prescribed frequency (SD = 0.08), intensity (SD = 0.02), duration (SD = 0.05), and mode of activity (SD ranged from 0.03 to 0.10) were small or trivial (Rhodes, Warburton, and Murray 2009). However, most of the trials manipulated only a single feature of exercise exposure and used very different definitions of adherence (e.g., attendance at supervised sessions, maintenance of heart rate [HR] within a prescribed intensity range, exercising for the prescribed duration and weekly frequency according to personal diaries). Only a few of the trials defined adherence according to whether people dropped out, which has been the hallmark definition of exercise adherence for the past 35 years. One trial reported 85% attendance, but 42% of the participants had dropped out! In fact, studies that reported only dropout rates were excluded from the review. Half the trials lasted less than six months, which has been the standard time frame used to define maintenance of an exercise program. The dropout rate averaged 18% (522 of 2829 participants), ranging from 0% in a home-based program that relied on people's diaries to verify adherence to 30% to 40% in some six-month and two-year trials. Only 25% of the trials adjusted their adherence measure for the number of people who dropped out. Finally, a number of the trials actively used behavior modification approaches to improve overall adherence, thus confounding a true test of whether features of physical activity modify adherence rates.

Another recent review of studies that targeted short bouts of physical activity (i.e., ≤10-15 min) integrated into the daily routine of organizations (particularly schools and workplaces) concluded that the results had been modest but consistently favorable for promoting feasible and sustainable increases in physical activity that are more appealing to segments of the sedentary population (Barr-Anderson et al. 2011). However, of the 40 studies evaluated, just five studies in schools and two studies at workplaces were randomized controlled trials that used a measure of physical activity as an outcome. Just one three-year trial of the five school-based trials (the others lasted 5 to 20 months) and two of two workplace trials lasting 10 to 12 weeks reported a significant increase in physical activity.

Perceived Exertion

When the goal of an exercise program is to promote regular participation, traditional exercise prescriptions and programming should be modified by considerations such as perceived exertion and preferred activities (Dishman 1994c). The limitations of using HR as the only index of appropriate exercise intensity among people without heart disease have been recognized for many years. The ACSM recommends using rating of perceived exertion (RPE) among healthy adults to complement the monitoring of HR for deciding on the appropriate intensity of aerobic exercise for each person (see table 17.6).

Table 17.6　Classification of Physical Activity Intensity Based on Physical Activity Lasting Up to 60 min

Intensity	Endurance-type activity							Resistance-type activity
	Relative intensity			Absolute intensity (METs) in healthy adults (age in years)				Relative intensity*
	$\dot{V}O_2R$ (%) heart rate reserve (%)	Maximal heart rate (%)	RPE†	Young (20-39 years)	Middle-aged (40-64 years)	Old (65-79 years)	Very old 80+ years)	Maximal voluntary contraction (%)
Very light	<20	<35	<10	<2.4	<2.0	<1.6	1.0	<30
Light	20-39	35-54	10-11	2.4-4.7	2.0-3.9	1.6-3.1	1.1-1.9	30-49
Moderate	40-59	55-69	12-13	4.8-7.1	4.0-5.9	3.2-4.7	2.0-2.9	50-69
Hard	60-84	70-89	14-16	7.2-10.1	6.0-8.4	4.8-6.7	3.0-4.25	70-84
Very hard	85	90	17-19	10.2	8.5	6.8	4.25	85
Maximal**	100	100	20	12.0	10.0	8.0	5.0	100

* Based on eight to 12 repetitions for persons under age 50 years and 10 to 15 repetitions for persons aged 50 years and older.

† Borg Rating of Perceived Exertion 6-20 scale (Borg 1962).

** Maximal values are mean values achieved during maximal exercise by healthy adults. Absolute intensity (MET) values are approximate mean values for men. Mean values for women are approximately 1 to 2 METs lower than those for men. $\dot{V}O_2R$ = oxygen uptake reserve.

Reprinted, by permission, from M.L. Pollock et al., 1998, "The recommended quantity and quality of exercise for developing and maintaining cardiorespiratory and muscular fitness, and flexibility in healthy adults," *Medicine and Science in Sports and Exercise* 30: 978.

Swedish psychologist Gunnar Borg conceived of RPE as a subjective integration of many sensory and physiological responses to exercise (including sensations of muscular force, strain, pain, heavy breathing, body and skin temperature, and sweat). He developed rating scales for practical measurement of perceived exertion (Borg 1962, 1998). Ratings of perceived exertion between 11 and 16 on Borg's 6-to-20 category rating scale usually correspond with exercise intensities between 50% and 75% of maximum METs or 50% to 85% of HR reserve. After people learn to use their whole perceptual range, from no exertion to the highest level they can imagine, the use of RPE permits the exercise intensity to be self-adjusted to the level corresponding to the target HR.

Because perceived exertion is more closely linked in most circumstances with relative oxygen consumption than with relative HR (Robertson and Noble 1997), the subjective strain associated with a typical target HR can vary widely. Hence, it is not surprising that some participants given age-predicted HR ranges frequently complain that the exercise intensity is either too easy or too hard. Studies show that when most people exercise at a pace that feels "somewhat hard," their breathing is not too labored and their pulse rates are likely to be in a range of 120 to 150 beats/min. At this level, most healthy people can safely increase fitness and health while avoiding discomfort.

The Accuracy of RPE for Relative Exercise Intensity

The errors with use of RPE to reproduce a level of oxygen consumption of between 50% and 70% $\dot{V}O_2$max during exercise are not greater than the errors that occur using target

HR (Dunbar et al. 1992). Many studies have used percent HR reserve as the standard for judging the accuracy of RPE production in prescribed exercise, based on the assumption that relative HR best yields the rate of energy expenditure that is optimal for increasing aerobic capacity (i.e., $\dot{V}O_2$max). But the only evidence that percent HR reserve and percent $\dot{V}O_2$max are equivalent across exercise intensities came from studies of small groups of highly trained men. Research on a large group of men and women of various ages showed that a target HR based on percent HR reserve underestimates percent $\dot{V}O_2$max by about 5% to 10% at intensities between 50% and 60% HR reserve but overestimates percent $\dot{V}O_2$max by about 4% to 8% at intensities between 80% and 85% HR reserve (figure 17.22) (Wier and Jackson 1992).

Hence, for many people, percent HR reserve is an inaccurate index of low and high relative exercise intensities and thus the wrong standard for prescribing exercise intensity. Rating of perceived exertion during low-intensity aerobic exercise depends mainly on the perception of force; but as the exercise intensity increases, sensations associated with increasing blood lactate and hyperventilation play a more significant role (Robertson and Noble 1997). Ventilatory and lactate thresholds have been associated with ratings of 13 to 15, which correspond with subjective categories of "somewhat hard" to "hard" on Borg's 6-to-20 RPE scale. These intensities may be uncomfortable for many beginning exercisers, even healthy college students, and may discourage them from resuming or starting an exercise program.

As fitness level improves after regular exercise, a standard intensity of exercise is perceived as less effortful because it represents a lower percentage of the person's capacity. However, studies show that perceived exertion after exercise

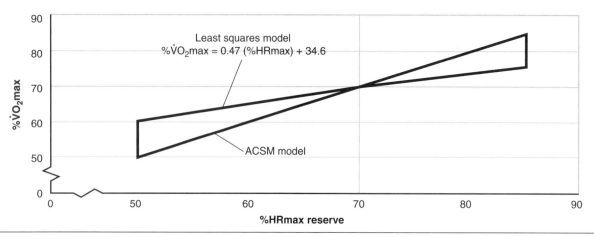

Figure 17.22   Errors of percent heart rate reserve as an estimate of percent aerobic capacity.
Data from Wier and Jackson 1992.

training is more closely linked with blood lactate than percent $\dot{V}O_2$max (Boutcher et al. 1989; Demello et al. 1987; Seip et al. 1991). One hallmark of endurance exercise training is that extra lactic acid does not appear in the blood until a higher relative $\dot{V}O_2$max is reached. The extra lactic acid lowers the pH of muscle and stimulates hyperventilation; each change contributes to pain and perceived exertion. All this means that a person can more comfortably exercise at a higher percentage of aerobic capacity after training because blood lactate levels are lower.

Preferred Exertion

Borg also introduced the idea of **preferred exertion** or "preference level" as the intensity of exercise perceived as being just about right or comfortable (Borg 1962). High physiological strain relative to perceived exertion may increase risks for musculoskeletal and orthopedic injuries that can lead to inactivity. If inactive people select, or are prescribed, an exercise intensity that is perceived as very effortful relative to their physiological responses, they may be less likely to continue participation. Conversely, some individuals prefer to exceed conventional prescriptions. In a one-year randomized exercise trial of middle-aged, sedentary adults, similar adherence was observed for groups assigned to comparatively low (60-73% HRmax) or high (73-88% HRmax) intensities (King et al. 1991). However, the authors reported that each group selected intensities during the year that regressed toward a common level corresponding to mean daily exercise RPEs of about 12 to 13. Farrell and colleagues (1982) instructed trained male runners to run for 30 min at a freely chosen pace and compared responses with 30-min runs at fixed intensities of 60% and 80% $\dot{V}O_2$max. The preferred intensity was approximately 75% $\dot{V}O_2$max and ranged from 65% to 90%. Ratings of perceived exertion during the preferred run initially averaged 9.2 and increased to 11.5. These ratings were between the mean RPE values of 8.8 and 12.3 for the 60% and 80% $\dot{V}O_2$max runs. When we asked young and middle-

aged men to select either a power output while cycling or a treadmill speed at zero grade that was comfortable, they chose intensities that were about 60% $\dot{V}O_2$max, with an RPE of 11 to 14, which is moderately hard (Dishman, Farquhar, and Cureton 1994). Trained runners appear to prefer intensities ranging from 65% to 90% $\dot{V}O_2$max.

Summary

Though the numbers are far from settled, the best estimates today are that people's physical activity during leisure time is determined about 20% to 70% by genetic traits. Another 25% to 40% is explainable by beliefs and motivations shaped by learning, and an additional 10% to 50% may be explainable by physical and social environments. These estimates don't add up in part because studies haven't simultaneously measured the independent effects of each type of influence. More importantly, perhaps, it is not yet known how those three domains of influence interact to ultimately determine a person's decision to be physically active on a regular basis. For example, people's genes partly determine how they adapt to exercise training, which could make it easier for some people to reach their exercise goals (figure 17.23). Genetic traits don't guarantee that someone will be active or doom

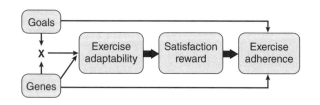

Figure 17.23   People's genes may partly determine whether they reach their exercise goals.

Reprinted, by permission, from R.K. Dishman, 2008, "Gene-physical activity interactions in the etiology of obesity: behavioral considerations," *Obesity* 16(Suppl 3): S60-65.

someone to inactivity. Likewise, creating an environment that makes physical activity easy doesn't ensure that a person living in that environment will be motivated to use it. Successful interventions can lead to 15% to 35% increases in physical activity in the short term, but most of those increases are lost in the long term.

It is not easy to alter personal preferences or longstanding habits. For those who are fortunate, regular, moderate physical activity or vigorous exercise is a natural part of the day. For most people, though, changing from a sedentary lifestyle to one that includes regular physical activity is plain hard work and requires planning before a new physical activity habit is formed. Changing physical activity is not like changing most other health behaviors.

On the plus side, the variety of forms of physical activity increases the odds that people can find types that they will enjoy. However, this variety also makes physical activity complex for beginners and can make it harder to establish a habit early on. Habits are easier to form when a single behavior is reinforced at a specific place and time. Though replacing sedentary behaviors with physical activity is important, the goal for physical activity is to adopt and maintain a positive health behavior rather than to give up or stop a negative health behavior, such as drinking too much alcohol or smoking cigarettes. The exertional nature of physical activity also makes it unique among health behaviors. No other health behavior requires that metabolism be raised several times higher than rest. The sensations of physical exertion can yield complex interactions with psychological aspects of physical activity for some people. For example, discomfort, fatigue, and soreness are common early outcomes of a new exercise program and can discourage a beginning exerciser.

Recognizing personal and social environmental barriers to physical activity is a first step toward increasing physical activity. This chapter outlines those that have been identified. Until physical activity becomes habitual or enjoyable, sustained participation requires active behavior modification. Most behavior modification techniques for changing physical activity center on (1) goal setting based on initial fitness and desired outcomes; (2) identification of personal costs and expected barriers to adoption and maintenance of an activity routine; (3) strategies for preventing or minimizing the impact of barriers to participation and for increasing support and reinforcement from friends and family; (4) planning a gradual progression of difficulty to optimize success so that the participant has growing confidence in both physical abilities and the ability to maintain the new pattern of activity; (5) feedback from fitness testing and self-monitoring of activity and progress by the participant; and (6) personal strategies for returning to activity after a period of relapse to inactivity due to flagging motivation, injury, vacation, and so on.

An ecological model for understanding and changing physical activity can be added to the traditional approaches to expand our ability to identify and overcome barriers to physical activity, which are also defined on different levels. Personal barriers can be psychological, such as low exercise self-efficacy or perceived lack of time, or physical, such as past injuries. Barriers can also be interpersonal, as when peers support and encourage sedentary behaviors. Environmental barriers can be natural (e.g., inclement weather) or constructed (lack of transportation to an exercise facility or unsafe neighborhoods). Life transitions, such as graduation, marriage, childbirth, or divorce, can interrupt an established physical activity habit, and seasonal variations in opportunities for physical activity require study.

Increasing the physical activity of Americans and people in other nations requires interventions at the community level (including physicians' offices, schools, churches, families, and local government) with approaches that span multiple levels of change (personal, interpersonal, organizational, environmental, institutional, and policy or legislative) and aim to reach diverse segments of the population otherwise missed by the traditional health care system (King 1994). To guide these efforts, more multilevel studies of personal and environmental mediators and moderators of change in objectively measured physical activity will be needed (Dishman 2010).

· BIBLIOGRAPHY ·

Adams, M.A., S. Ryan, J. Kerr, J.F. Sallis, K. Patrick, L.C. Frank, and G.I. Norman. 2009. Validation of the Neighborhood Environment Walkability Scale (NEWS) items using geographic information systems. *Journal of Physical Activity and Health* 6 (Suppl. 1): S113-123.

Adams, M.A., J.F. Sallis, J. Kerr, T.L. Conway, B.E. Saelens, L.D. Frank, G.J. Norman, and K.L. Cain. 2011. Neighborhood environment profiles related to physical activity and weight status: A latent profile analysis. *Preventive Medicine,* March 4. [Epub ahead of print]

Ajzen, I. 1985. From intentions to actions: A theory of planned behavior. In *Action-control: From cognition to behavior,* edited by J. Kuhl and J. Beckman, pp. 11-39. Heidelberg: Springer.

Ajzen, I. 1988. *Attitudes, personality and behavior.* Chicago: Dorsey Press.

Ajzen, I. 2002. Perceived behavioral control, self-efficacy, locus of control, and the theory of planned behavior. *Journal of Applied Social Psychology* 32: 1-20.

Allensworth, D.D., and L.J. Kolbe. 1987. The comprehensive school health program: Exploring an expanded concept. *Journal of School Health* 57: 409-412.

Alves, R.V., J. Mota, M.C. Costa, and J.G.B. Alves. 2004. Aptidão física relacionada a saúde de idosos: Influência da hidroginástica. *Revista Brasileira de Medicina do Esporte* 10: 31-37.

Andersen, L.B. 1996. Tracking of risk factors for coronary heart disease from adolescence to young adulthood with special emphasis on physical activity and fitness: A longitudinal study. *Danish Medical Bulletin* 43 (December): 407-418.

Andrew, G.M., N.B. Oldridge, J.O. Parker, D.A. Cunningham, P.A. Rechnitzer, N.L. Jones, C. Buck, T. Kavanagh, R.J. Shephard, and J.R. Sutton. 1981. Reasons for dropout from exercise programs in post-coronary patients. *Medicine and Science in Sports and Exercise* 13: 164-168.

Andrew, G.M., and J.O. Parker. 1979. Factors related to dropout of post myocardial infarction patients from exercise programs. *Medicine and Science in Sports and Exercise* 11: 376-378.

Auweele, Y.A., R. Rzewnicki, and V. Van Mele. 1997. Reasons for not exercising and exercise intentions: A study of middle-aged sedentary adults. *Journal of Sports Sciences* 15: 151-165.

Bandura, A. 1994. Health promotion by social cognitive means. *Health Education & Behavior* 31: 143-164.

Bandura, A. 1986. *Social foundations of thought and action.* Englewood Cliffs, NJ: Prentice Hall.

Bandura, A. 1997a. Editorial: The anatomy of stages of change. *American Journal of Health Promotion* 12 (1): 8-10.

Bandura, A. 1997b. *Self-efficacy: The exercise of control.* New York: Freeman.

Baranowski, T., C. Anderson, and C. Carmack. 1998. Mediating variable framework in physical activity interventions: How are we doing? How might we do better? *American Journal of Preventive Medicine* 15: 266-297.

Baron, R.M., and D.A. Kenny. 1986. The moderator–mediator variable distinction in social psychological research: Conceptual, strategic, and statistical considerations. *Journal of Personality and Social Psychology* 51: 1173-1182.

Barr-Anderson, D.J., M. AuYoung, M.C. Whitt-Glover, B.A. Glenn, and A.K. Yancey. 2011. Integration of short bouts of physical activity into organizational routine a systematic review of the literature. *American Journal of Preventive Medicine* 40 (1): 76-93.

Bauman, A., D.T. Finegood, and V. Matsudo. 2009. International perspectives on the physical inactivity crisis—structural solutions over evidence generation? *Preventive Medicine* 49 (4): 309-312.

Beets, M.W., and J.T. Foley. 2008. Association of father involvement and neighborhood quality with kindergartners' physical activity: A multilevel structural equation model. *American Journal of Health Promotion* 22 (3): 195-203.

Bellew, B., S. Schöeppe, F.C. Bull, and A. Bauman. 2008. The rise and fall of Australian physical activity policy 1996-2006: A national review framed in an international context. *Australia and New Zealand Health Policy* 5: 18.

Berge, J.M. 2009. A review of familial correlates of child and adolescent obesity: What has the 21st century taught us so far? *International Journal of Adolescent Medicine and Health* 21 (4): 457-483.

Berge, J.M., M. Wall, K. Loth, and D. Neumark-Sztainer. 2010. Parenting style as a predictor of adolescent weight and weight-related behaviors. *Journal of Adolescent Health* 46 (4): 331-338.

Berkowitz, J.M., M. Huhman, and M.J. Nolin. 2008. Did augmenting the VERB™ Campaign advertising in select communities have an effect on awareness, attitudes, and physical activity? *American Journal of Preventive Medicine* 34 (6S): S257-S266.

Beunen, G., and M. Thomis. 1999. Genetic determinants of sports participation and daily physical activity. *International Journal of Obesity and Related Metabolic Disorders* 23 (Suppl. 3): S55-S63.

Biddiss, E., and J. Irwin. 2010. Active video games to promote physical activity in children and youth: A systematic review. *Archives of Pediatric and Adolescent Medicine* 164 (7): 664-672.

Biddle, S.J.H., and C.R. Nigg. 2000. Theories of exercise behavior. *International Journal of Sport Psychology* 31 (2): 290-304.

Blair, S.N., M. Booth, I. Gyarfas, H. Iwane, B. Marti, V. Matsudo, M.S. Morrow, T. Noakes, and R. Shephard. 1996. Development of public policy and physical activity initiatives internationally. *Sports Medicine* 21 (3): 157-163.

Blair, S.N., D.R. Jacobs, and K.E. Powell. 1985. Relationships between exercise or physical activity and other health behaviors. *Public Health Reports* 100: 172-180.

Blamey, A., N. Mutrie, and T. Aitchison. 1995. Health promotion by encouraged use of stairs. *British Medical Journal* 311: 289-290.

Boarnet, M.G., C.L. Anderson, K. Day, T. McMillan, and M. Alfonzo. 2005. Evaluation of the California Safe Routes to School legislation: Urban form changes and children's active transportation to school. *American Journal of Preventive Medicine* 28 (2S2): 134-140.

Bookchin, M. 1982. *The ecology of freedom: The emergence and dissolution of hierarchy.* Palo Alto, CA: Cheshire Books.

Bookchin, M. 1995. *The philosophy of social ecology: Essays on dialectical naturalism.* 2nd edition, revised. Montreal: Black Rose Books.

Boone-Heinonen, J., A.V. Diez Roux, C.I. Kiefe, C.E. Lewis, D.K. Guilkey, and P. Gordon-Larsen. 2011a. Neighborhood socioeconomic status predictors of physical activity through young to middle adulthood: The CARDIA study. *Social Science and Medicine* 72 (5): 641-649.

Boone-Heinonen, J., P. Gordon-Larsen, D.K. Guilkey, D.R. Jacobs Jr., and B.M. Popkin. 2011b. Environment and physical activity dynamics: The role of residential self-selection. *Psychology of Sport and Exercise* 12: 54-60.

Boone-Heinonen, J., D.K. Guilkey, K.R. Evenson, and P. Gordon-Larsen. 2010a. Residential self-selection bias in the estimation of built environment effects on physical activity between adolescence and young adulthood. *International Journal of Behavioral Nutrition and Physical Activity* 7 (October 4): 70.

Boone-Heinonen, J., B.M. Popkin, Y. Song, and P. Gordon-Larsen. 2010b. What neighborhood area captures built environment features related to adolescent physical activity? *Health and Place* 16 (6): 1280-1286.

Booth, M.L., N. Owen, A. Bauman, O. Clavisi, and E. Leslie. 2000. Social-cognitive and perceived environmental influences associated with physical activity in older Australians. *Preventive Medicine* 31: 15-22.

Borg, G.A.V. 1962. *Physical performance and perceived exertion. Studia psychologica et paedagogica,* Vol. 11. *Series Altera.* Lund, Sweden: Gleerup.

Borg, G.A.V. 1998. *Borg's perceived exertion and pain scales.* Champaign, IL: Human Kinetics.

Bornstein, D.B., R.R. Pate, and M. Pratt. 2009. A review of the national physical activity plans of six countries. *Journal of Physical Activity and Health* 6 (Suppl. 2): S245-264.

Bors, P., M. Dessauer, R. Bell, R. Wilkerson, J. Lee, and S.L. Strunk. 2009. The Active Living by Design National Program Community Initiatives and lessons learned. *American Journal of Preventive Medicine* 37 (6S2): S313-S321.

Boutcher, S.H., R.L. Seip, R.K. Hetzler, E.F. Pierce, D. Snead, and A. Weltman. 1989. The effects of specificity of training on rating of perceived exertion at the lactate threshold. *European Journal of Applied Physiology and Occupational Physiology* 59: 365-369.

Brassington, G.S., A.A. Atienza, R.E. Perczek, T.M. DiLorenzo, and A.C. King. 2002. Intervention-related cognitive versus social mediators of exercise adherence in the elderly. *American Journal of Preventive Medicine* 23 (2 Suppl.): 80-86.

Brownell, K., A.J. Stunkard, and J. Albaum. 1980. Evaluation and modification of exercise patterns in the natural environment. *American Journal of Psychiatry* 136: 1540-1545.

Brownson, R.C., C.M. Hoehner, K. Day, A. Forsyth, and J.F. Sallis. 2009. Measuring the built environment for physical activity: State of the science. *American Journal of Preventive Medicine* 36 (4 Suppl.): S99-123.e12.

Brownson, R.C., C.A. Smith, M. Pratt, et al. 1996. Preventing cardiovascular disease through community-based risk reduction: The Bootheel Heart Health Project. *American Journal of Public Health* 86 (2): 206-213.

Bruce, E., R. Frederick, R.A. Bruce, and L.D. Fisher. 1976. Comparison of active participants and dropouts in CAPRI cardiopulmonary rehabilitation programs. *American Journal of Cardiology* 37: 53-60.

Bruce, R.A., T.A. DeRouen, and K.F. Hossack. 1980. Pilot study examining the motivational effects of maximal exercise testing to modify risk factors and health habits. *Cardiology* 66 (2): 111-119.

Brynteson, P., and T.M.I. Adams. 1993. The effects of conceptually based physical education programs on attitudes and exercise habits of college alumni after 2 to 11 years of follow-up. *Research Quarterly for Exercise and Sport* 64: 208-212.

Buckworth, J., and R.K. Dishman. 2001. *Exercise psychology.* Champaign, IL: Human Kinetics.

Bull, F.C., K. Jamrozik, and B.A. Blanksby. 1998. Tailoring advice on exercise: Does it make a difference? *American Journal of Preventive Medicine* 16 (3): 230-239.

Burke, E.J., and M.L. Collins. 1984. Using perceived exertion for the prescription of exercise in healthy adults. In *Clinical sports medicine.* Lexington, MA: Callamore Press.

Calfas, K.J., B.J. Long, J.F. Sallis, W. Wooten, M. Pratt, and K. Patrick. 1996. A controlled trial of physician counseling to promote the adoption of physical activity. *Preventive Medicine* 25 (3): 225-233.

Calfas, K.J., J.F. Sallis, B. Oldenburg, and M. French. 1997. Mediators of change in physical activity following an intervention in primary care: PACE. *Preventive Medicine* 26: 297-304.

Carande-Kulis, V.G., M.V. Maciosek, P.A. Briss, et al. 2000. Methods for systematic reviews of economic evaluations for the Guide to Community Preventive Services. *American Journal of Preventive Medicine* 18 (1S): 75-91.

Cardinal, B.J. 1999. Extended stage model of physical activity behavior. *Journal of Human Movement Studies* 37: 37-54.

Carron, A.V., H.A. Hausenblas, and D. Mack. 1996. Social influence and exercise: A meta-analysis. *Journal of Sport and Exercise Psychology* 18: 1-16.

Caspersen, C.J., G.M. Christenson, and R.A. Pollard. 1985. Status of the 1990 physical fitness and exercise objectives: Evidence from HNIS 1985. *Public Health Reports* 101: 587-592.

Caspersen, C.J., M.A. Pereira, and K.M. Curran. 2000. Changes in physical activity patterns in the United States, by sex and cross-sectional age. *Medicine and Science in Sports and Exercise* 32 (9): 1601-1609.

Castro, C., J.F. Sallis, S.A. Hickmann, R.E. Lee, and A.H. Chen. 1999. A prospective study of psychosocial correlates of physical activity for ethnic minority women. *Psychology and Health* 14 (2): 277-293.

Centers for Disease Control and Prevention. 1998. Self-reported physical inactivity by degree of urbanization—United States, 1996. *Morbidity and Mortality Weekly Report* 47 (50): 1097-1100.

Centers for Disease Control and Prevention. 2000. *Fact sheet: Youth risk behavior trends from CDC's 1991, 1993, 1995, 1997, and 1999 Youth Risk Behavior Surveys.* Atlanta: U.S. Department of Health and Human Services, Centers for Disease Control and Prevention, National Center for Chronic Disease Prevention and Health Promotion.

Centers for Disease Control and Prevention. 2001a. Increasing physical activity: A report on recommendations of the Task Force on Community Preventive Services. *Morbidity and Mortality Weekly Report* 50 (RR-18): 1-16.

Centers for Disease Control and Prevention. 2001b. Physical activity trends—United States, 1990–1998. *Morbidity and Mortality Weekly Report* 50 (9): 166-169.

Centers for Disease Control and Prevention. 2007. Prevalence of regular physical activity among adults—U.S., 2001 and 2005. *Morbidity and Mortality Weekly Report* 56 (46): 1209-1212.

Centers for Disease Control and Prevention. 2008. Prevalence of self-reported physically active adults—U.S., 2007. *Morbidity and Mortality Weekly Report* 57 (48): 1297-1300.

Centers for Disease Control and Prevention. 2010a. *State indicator report on physical activity, 2010.* Atlanta: U.S. Department of Health and Human Services.

Centers for Disease Control and Prevention. 2010b. Youth Risk Behavior Surveillance—United States, 2009. Surveillance Summaries. *Morbidity and Mortality Weekly Report* 59 (SS-5): 117-126.

Cerin, E., E. Leslie, T. Sugiyama, and N. Owen. 2010. Perceived barriers to leisure-time physical activity in adults: An ecological perspective. *Journal of Physical Activity and Health* 7 (4): 451-459.

Cervero, R., and R. Gorham. 1995. Commuting in transit versus automobile neighborhoods. *Journal of the American Planning Association* 61: 210-225.

Chung, S., M.E. Domino, S.C. Stearns, and B.M. Popkin. 2009. Retirement and physical activity: Analyses by occupation and wealth. *American Journal of Preventive Medicine* 36 (5): 422-428.

Cohen, D.A., T. Marsh, S. Williamson, K.P. Derose, H. Martinez, C. Setodji, and T.L. McKenzie. 2010. Parks and physical activity: Why are some parks used more than others? *Preventive Medicine* 50 (Suppl. 1, January): S9-12.

Cohen, D.A., T.L. McKenzie, A. Sehgal, S. Williamson, D. Golinelli, and N. Lurie. 2007. Contribution of public parks to physical activity. *American Journal of Public Health* 97 (3): 509-514.

Colabianchi, N., M. Dowda, K.A. Pfeiffer, D.E. Porter, M.J. Almeida, and R.R. Pate. 2007. Towards an understanding of salient neighborhood boundaries: Adolescent reports of an easy walking distance and convenient driving distance. *International Journal of Behavioral Nutrition and Physical Activity* 4: 66.

Conn, V.S., A.R. Hafdahl, P.S. Cooper, L.M. Brown, and S.L. Lusk. 2009. Meta-analysis of workplace physical activity interventions. *American Journal of Preventive Medicine* 37 (4): 330-339.

Cooper, K.M., D. Bilbrew, P.M. Dubbert, K. Kerr, and K. Kirchner. 2001. Health barriers to walking for exercise in elderly primary care. *Geriatric Nursing* 22: 258-262.

Courneya, K.S., and T.M. Bobick. 2000. Integrating the theory of planned behavior with the processes and stages of change in the exercise domain. *Psychology of Sport and Exercise* 1: 41-56.

Courneya, K.S., and L.M. Hellsten. 1998. Personality correlates of exercise behavior, motives, barriers, and preferences: An application of the five-factor model. *Personality and Individual Differences* 24 (5): 625-633.

Courneya, K.S., and E. McAuley. 1994. Are there different determinants of the frequency, intensity, and duration of physical activity? *Behavioral Medicine* 20 (2): 84-90.

Courneya, K.S., and E. McAuley. 1995. Cognitive mediators of the social influence-exercise adherence relationship: A test of the Theory of Planned Behavior. *Journal of Behavioral Medicine* 18 (5): 499-515.

Couzin, J. 2002. Nutrition research. IOM panel weighs in on diet and health. *Science* 297 (5588): 1788-1789.

Craig, C.L., A. Bauman, and B. Reger-Nash. 2010. Testing the hierarchy of effects model: ParticipACTION's serial mass communication campaigns on physical activity in Canada. *Health Promotion International* 25 (1): 14-23.

Crespo, C.J., E. Smit, R.E. Andersen, O. Carter-Pokras, and B.E. Ainsworth. 2000. Race/ethnicity, social class and their relation to physical inactivity during leisure time: Results from the third National Health and Nutrition Examination Survey, 1988–1994. *American Journal of Preventive Medicine* 18 (1): 46-53.

Davis, T.M., and D.D. Allensworth. 1994. Program management: A necessary component for the comprehensive school health program. *Journal of School Health* 64: 400-404.

Deforche, B., D. Van Dyck, M. Verloigne, and I. De Bourdeaudhuij. 2010. Perceived social and physical environmental correlates of physical activity in older adolescents and the moderating effect of self-efficacy. *Preventive Medicine* 50 (Suppl. 1): S24-29.

DeJoy, D.M., and D.J. Southern. 1993. An integrative perspective on worksite health promotion. *Journal of Occupational Medicine* 35: 1221-1230.

Demello, J.J., K.J. Cureton, R.E. Boineau, and M.M. Singh. 1987. Ratings of perceived exertion at the lactate threshold in trained and untrained men and women. *Medicine and Science in Sports and Exercise* 19: 354-362.

De Moor, M.H., G. Willemsen, I. Rebollo-Mesa, J.H. Stubbe, E.J. De Geus, and D.I. Boomsma. 2011. Exercise participation in adolescents and their parents: Evidence for genetic and generation specific environmental effects. *Behavior Genetics* 41 (2): 211-222.

Dennison, B.A., J.H. Straus, E.D. Mellits, and E. Charney. 1988. Childhood physical fitness tests: Predictor of adult physical activity levels? *Pediatrics* 82: 324-330.

Dietz, W.H. 1996. The role of lifestyle in health: The epidemiology and consequences of inactivity. *Proceedings of the Nutrition Society* 55: 829-840.

Dishman, R.K. 1982. Compliance/adherence in health-related exercise. *Health Psychology* 1 (3): 237-267.

Dishman, R.K. 1988. Supervised and free-living physical activity: No differences in former athletes and nonathletes. *American Journal of Preventive Medicine* 4: 153-160.

Dishman, R.K. 1990. Determinants of participation in physical activity. In *Exercise, fitness, and health: A consensus of current knowledge,* edited by C. Bouchard, R.J. Shephard, T. Stephens, J.R. Sutton, and B.D. McPherson, pp. 78-101. Champaign, IL: Human Kinetics.

Dishman, R.K. 1991. Increasing and maintaining exercise and physical activity. *Behavior Therapy* 22: 345-378.

Dishman, R.K. 1993. Exercise adherence. In *Handbook of research on sport psychology,* edited by R.N. Singer, M. Murphey, and L.K. Tennant, pp. 779-798. New York: Macmillan.

Dishman, R.K., ed. 1994a. *Advances in exercise adherence.* Champaign, IL: Human Kinetics.

Dishman, R.K. 1994b. The measurement conundrum in exercise adherence research. *Medicine and Science in Sports and Exercise* 26: 1382-1390.

Dishman, R.K. 1994c. Prescribing exercise intensity for healthy adults using perceived exertion. *Medicine and Science in Sports and Exercise* 26: 1087-1094.

Dishman, R.K. 2008. Gene-physical activity interactions in the etiology of obesity: Behavioral considerations. *Obesity (Silver Spring)* 16 (Suppl. 3): S60-65.

Dishman, R.K. 2010. Psychological factors and physical activity level. In *Physical activity and obesity,* 2nd edition, edited by C. Bouchard and P.T. Katzmarzyk. Champaign, IL: Human Kinetics.

Dishman, R.K., and J. Buckworth. 1996. Increasing physical activity: A quantitative synthesis. *Medicine and Science in Sports and Exercise* 28: 706-719.

Dishman, R.K., D.M. DeJoy, M.G. Wilson, and R.J. Vandenberg. 2009a. Move to Improve: A randomized workplace trial to increase physical activity. *American Journal of Preventive Medicine* 36 (2): 133-141.

Dishman, R.K., and A.L. Dunn. 1988. Exercise adherence in children and youth: Implications for adulthood. In *Exercise adherence: Its impact on public health,* edited by R.K. Dishman, pp. 155-200. Champaign, IL: Human Kinetics.

Dishman, R.K., A.L. Dunn, J.F. Sallis, R.J. Vandenberg, and C.A. Pratt. 2010a. Social-cognitive correlates of physical activity in a multi-ethnic cohort of middle-school girls: Two-year prospective study. *Journal of Pediatric Psychology* 35 (2): 188-198.

Dishman, R.K., R.P. Farquhar, and K.J. Cureton. 1994. Responses to preferred intensities of exertion in men differing in activity levels. *Medicine and Science in Sports and Exercise* 26: 783-790.

Dishman, R.K., and W.J. Ickes. 1981. Self-motivation and adherence to therapeutic exercise. *Journal of Behavioral Medicine* 4: 421-438.

Dishman, R.K., W.J. Ickes, and W.P. Morgan. 1980. Self-motivation and adherence to habitual physical activity. *Journal of Applied Social Psychology* 10: 115-131.

Dishman, R.K., A.S. Jackson, and M.S. Bray. 2010. Validity of processes of change in physical activity among college students in the TIGER study. *Annals of Behavioral Medicine* 40 (2): 164-175.

Dishman, R.K., R.W. Motl, R. Saunders, G. Felton, D.S. Ward, M. Dowda, and R.R. Pate. 2005. Enjoyment mediates effects of a school-based physical-activity intervention. *Medicine and Science in Sports and Exercise* 37: 478-487.

Dishman, R.K., R.W. Motl, R. Saunders, G. Felton, D.S. Ward, M. Dowda, and R.R. Pate. 2004. Self-efficacy partially mediates the effect of a school-based physical-activity intervention among adolescent girls. *Preventive Medicine* 38: 628-636.

Dishman, R.K., B. Oldenburg, H.A. O'Neal, and R.J. Shephard. 1998. Worksite physical activity interventions. *American Journal of Preventive Medicine* 15 (4): 344-361.

Dishman, R.K., and J.F. Sallis. 1994. Determinants and interventions for physical activity and exercise. In *Physical activity, fitness and health: International proceedings and consensus statement*, edited by C. Bouchard, T. Stephens, and R.J. Shephard, pp. 214-238. Champaign, IL: Human Kinetics.

Dishman, R.K., R.P. Saunders, G. Felton, D.S. Ward, M. Dowda, and R.R. Pate. 2006. Goals and intentions mediate efficacy beliefs and declining physical activity in high school girls. *American Journal of Preventive Medicine* 31: 475-483.

Dishman, R.K., R.P. Saunders, R.W. Motl, M. Dowda, and R.R. Pate. 2009b. Self-efficacy moderates the relation between declines in physical activity and perceived social support in high school girls. *Journal of Pediatric Psychology* 34 (4): 441-451.

Dishman, R.K., N.J. Thom, C.R. Rooks, R.W. Motl, C. Horwath, and C.R. Nigg. 2009c. Failure of post-action stages of the transtheoretical model to predict change in regular physical activity: A multiethnic cohort study. *Annals of Behavioral Medicine* 37 (3): 280-293.

Dishman, R.K., R.J. Vandenberg, R.W. Motl, and C.R. Nigg. 2010b. Using constructs of the transtheoretical model to predict classes of change in regular physical activity: A multi-ethnic longitudinal cohort study. *Annals of Behavioral Medicine* 40 (2): 150-163.

Dishman, R.K., R.J. Vandenberg, R.W. Motl, M.G. Wilson, and D.M. DeJoy. 2010c. Dose relations between goal setting, theory-based correlates of goal setting and increases in physical activity during a workplace trial. *Health Education Research* 25 (4): 620-631.

Dobbins, M., K. De Corby, P. Robeson, H. Husson, and D. Tirilis. 2009. School-based physical activity programs for promoting physical activity and fitness in children and adolescents aged 6-18. *Cochrane Database of Systematic Reviews*, January 21 (1): CD007651.

Donovan, R.J., and N. Owen. 1994. Social marketing and population interventions. In *Advances in exercise adherence*, edited by R.K. Dishman, pp. 249-290. Champaign, IL: Human Kinetics.

Douglas, K.A., J.L. Collins, C.W. Warren, L. Kann, R. Gold, S. Clayton, J.G. Ross, and L.J. Kolbe. 1997. Results from the 1995 National College Health Risk Behavior Survey. *Journal of American College Health* 46: 55-66.

Dowda, M., R.K. Dishman, K.A. Pfeiffer, and R.R. Pate. 2007a. Family support for physical activity in girls from 8th to 12th grade in South Carolina. *Preventive Medicine* 44 (2): 153-159.

Dowda, M., R.K. Dishman, D. Porter, R.P. Saunders, and R.R. Pate. 2009. Commercial facilities, social cognitive variables, and physical activity of 12th grade girls. *Annals of Behavioral Medicine* 37 (1): 77-87.

Dowda, M., K.A. Pfeiffer, R.K. Dishman, and R.R. Pate. 2007b. Associations among physical activity, health indicators, and employment in 12th grade girls. *Journal of Women's Health (Larchmt)* 16 (9): 1331-1339.

Dumith, S.C., D.P. Gigante, M.R. Domingues, and H.W. Kohl 3rd. 2011a. Physical activity change during adolescence: A systematic review and a pooled analysis. *International Journal of Epidemiology*, January 18. [Epub ahead of print]

Dumith, S.C., P.C. Hallal, R.S. Reis, and H.W. Kohl 3rd. 2011b. Worldwide prevalence of physical inactivity and its association with human development index in 76 countries. *Preventive Medicine*, February 28. [Epub ahead of print]

Dunbar, C.C., R.J. Robertson, R. Baun, M.F. Blandin, K. Metz, R. Burdett, and F.L. Goss. 1992. The validity of regulating exercise intensity by ratings of perceived exertion. *Medicine and Science in Sports and Exercise* 24: 94-99.

Duncan, T.E., S.C. Duncan, and E. McAuley. 1993. The role of domain and gender-specific provisions of social relations in adherence to a prescribed exercise regimen. *Journal of Sport and Exercise Psychology* 15: 220-231.

Duncan, S.C., T.E. Duncan, L.A. Strycker, and N.R. Chaumeton. 2004. A multilevel approach to youth physical activity research. *Exercise and Sport Sciences Reviews* 32 (3): 95-99.

Duncan, S.C., T.E. Duncan, L.A. Strycker, and N.R. Chaumeton. 2007. A cohort-sequential latent growth model of physical activity from ages 12 to 17 years. *Annals of Behavioral Medicine* 33 (1): 80-89.

Duncan, T.E., and E. McAuley. 1993. Social support and efficacy cognitions in exercise adherence: A latent growth curve analysis. *Journal of Behavioral Medicine* 16: 199-218.

Dunn, A.L., R.E. Andersen, and J.M. Jakicic. 1998. Lifestyle physical activity interventions: History, short- and long-term effects, and recommendations. *American Journal of Preventive Medicine* 15: 398-412.

Dunn, A.L., B.H. Marcus, J.B. Kampert, M.E. Garcia, H.W. Kohl III, and S.N. Blair. 1999. Comparison of lifestyle and structured interventions to increase physical activity and cardiorespiratory fitness: A randomized trial. *Journal of the American Medical Association* 281 (4): 327-334.

Dunton, G.F., J. Kaplan, J. Wolch, M. Jerrett, and K.D. Reynolds. 2009. Physical environmental correlates of childhood obesity: A systematic review. *Obesity Reviews* 10 (4): 393-402.

Dwyer, J., and R. Bybee. 1983. Heart rate indices of the anaerobic threshold. *Medicine and Science in Sports and Exercise* 15: 72-76.

Dzewaltowski, D.A. 1994. Physical activity determinants: A social cognitive approach. *Medicine and Science in Sports and Exercise* 26: 1395-1399.

Dzewaltowski, D.A., J.M. Noble, and J.M. Shaw. 1990. Physical activity participation: Social cognitive theory versus the theories of reasoned action and planned behavior. *Journal of Sport and Exercise Psychology* 12: 388-405.

Eden, K.B., C.T. Orleans, C.D. Mulrow, N.J. Pender, and S.M. Teutsch. 2002. Does counseling by clinicians improve physical activity? A summary of the evidence for the U.S. Preventive Services Task Force. *Annals of Internal Medicine* 137: 208-215.

Edmundson, E., G.S. Parcel, H.A. Feldman, J. Elder, C.L. Perry, C.C. Johnson, B.J. Williston, E.J. Stone, M. Yang, L. Lytle, and L. Webber. 1996. The effects of the Child and Adolescent Trial for Cardiovascular Health upon psychosocial determinants of diet and physical activity. *Preventive Medicine* 25: 442-454.

Epstein, L.H. 1998. Integrating theoretical approaches to promote physical activity. *American Journal of Preventive Medicine* 15: 257-265.

Epstein, L.H., and J.N. Roemmich. 2001. Reducing sedentary behavior: Role in modifying physical activity. *Exercise and Sport Sciences Reviews* 29 (3): 103-108.

Epstein, L.H., B.E. Saelens, M.D. Myers, and D. Vito. 1997. Effects of decreasing sedentary behaviors on activity choice in obese children. *Health Psychology* 16: 107-113.

Estabrooks, P.A. 2000. Sustaining exercise participation through group cohesion. *Exercise and Sport Sciences Reviews* 28: 63-67.

Ewart, C.K., K.J. Stewart, and R.E. Gillilan. 1986. Usefulness of self-efficacy in predicting overexertion during programmed exercise in coronary artery disease. *American Journal of Cardiology* 57: 557-561.

Ewart, C.K., C.B. Taylor, C.B. Reese, and R.F. DeBusk. 1983. Effects of early postmyocardial infarction exercise testing on self-perception and subsequent physical activity. *American Journal of Cardiology* 51: 1076-1080.

Farrell, P.A., W.K. Gates, M.G. Maksud, and W.P. Morgan. 1982. Increases in plasma b-endorphin/b-lipotropin immunoreactivity after treadmill running in humans. *Journal of Applied Physiology* 52: 1245-1249.

Ferreira, I., K. van der Horst, W. Wendel-Vos, S. Kremers, F.J. van Lenthe, and J. Brug. 2006. Environmental correlates of physical activity in youth - a review and update. *Obesity Reviews* 8 (2): 129-154.

Fisher, K.J., F. Li, Y. Michael, and M. Cleveland. 2004. Neighborhood-level influences on physical activity among older adults: A multilevel analysis. *Journal of Aging and Physical Activity* 12 (1): 45-63.

Fletcher, G.F., S.N. Blair, J. Blumenthal, C. Casperson, B. Chaitman, and S. Epstein. 1992. Statement on exercise: Benefits and recommendations for physical activity programs for all Americans. *Circulation* 86: 340-344.

Foreyt, J.P., and G.K. Goodrick. 1993. Evidence for success of behavior modification in weight loss and control. *Annals of Internal Medicine* 119: 698-701.

Foreyt, J.P., and G.K. Goodrick. 1994. Impact of behavior therapy on weight loss. *American Journal of Health Promotion* 8: 466-468.

Frank, L.D., M.A. Andresen, and T.L. Schmid. 2004. Obesity relationships with community design, physical activity, and time spent in cars. *American Journal of Preventive Medicine* 27 (2): 87-96.

Frank, L., J. Kerr, D. Rosenberg, and A. King. 2010. Healthy aging and where you live: Community design relationships with physical activity and body weight in older Americans. *Journal of Physical Activity and Health* 7 (Suppl. 1): S82-90.

Frank, L.D., B.E. Saelens, K.E. Powell, and J.E. Chapman. 2007. Stepping towards causation: Do built environments or neighborhood and travel preferences explain physical activity, driving, and obesity? *Social Science in Medicine* 65 (9): 1898-1914.

Frisch, R.E., G. Wyshak, N.L. Albright, I. Schiff, K.P. Jones, J. Witschi, E. Shiang, E. Koff, and M. Marguglio. 1985. Lower prevalence of breast cancer and cancers of the reproductive system among former college athletes compared to non-athletes. *British Journal of Cancer* 52: 885-891.

Frost, S.S., R.T. Goins, R.H. Hunter, S.P. Hooker, L.L. Bryant, J. Kruger, and D. Pluto. 2010. Effects of the built environment on physical activity of adults living in rural settings. *American Journal of Health Promotion* 24 (4, March-April): 267-283.

Garcia, A.W., and A.C. King. 1991. Predicting long-term adherence to aerobic exercise: A comparison of two models. *Journal of Sport and Exercise Psychology* 13: 394-410.

Gauvin, L., M. Riva, T. Barnett, L. Richard, C.L. Craig, M. Spivock, S. Laforest, S. Laberge, M.C. Fournel, H. Gagnon, and S. Gagné. 2008. Association between neighborhood active living potential and walking. *American Journal of Epidemiology* 167 (8): 944-953.

Gettman, L.R., M.L. Pollock, and A. Ward. 1983. Adherence to unsupervised exercise. *Physician and Sportsmedicine* 11: 56-66.

Giles-Corti, B., M.H. Broomhall, M. Knuiman, C. Collins, K. Douglas, K. Ng, A. Lange, and R.J. Donovan. 2005. Increasing walking: How important is distance to, attractiveness, and size of public open space? *American Journal of Preventive Medicine* 28 (2S2): 169-176.

Glasgow, R.E., S.S. Bull, C. Gillette, L.M. Klesges, and D.H. Dzewaltowski. 2002. Behavior change intervention research in health care settings: A review of recent reports, with emphasis on external validity. *American Journal of Preventive Medicine* 23: 62-69.

Glasgow, R.E., and D.K. King. 2009. Implications of Active Living by Design for broad adoption, successful implementation, and long-term sustainability. *American Journal of Preventive Medicine* 37 (6 Suppl. 2): S450-S452.

Glasgow, R.E., T.M. Vogt, and S.M. Boles. 1999. Evaluating the public health impact of health promotion interventions: The RE-AIM framework. *American Journal of Public Health* 89: 1323-1327.

Godbey, G.C., L.L. Caldwell, M. Floyd, and L.L. Payne. 2005. Contributions of leisure studies and recreation and park management research to the active living agenda. *American Journal of Preventive Medicine* 28 (2S2): 150-158.

Godin, G. 1994. Theories of reasoned action and planned behavior: Usefulness for exercise promotion. *Medicine and Science in Sports and Exercise* 26: 1391-1394.

Godin, G., R. Desharnais, P. Valois, L. Lepage, J. Jobin, and R. Bradet. 1994. Differences in perceived barriers to exercise between high and low intenders: Observations among different populations. *American Journal of Health Promotion* 8: 279-285.

Godin, G., and G. Kok. 1996. The theory of planned behavior: A review of its applications to health-related behaviors. *American Journal of Health Promotion* 11: 87-98.

Godin, G., and R.J. Shephard. 1990. Use of attitude–behavior models in exercise promotion. *Sports Medicine* 10 (2): 103-121.

Godin, G., P. Valois, and R. Desharnais. 1995. Combining behavioral and motivational dimensions to identify and characterize the stages in the process of adherence to exercise. *Psychology and Health* 10: 333-344.

Godin, G., P. Valois, and R. Desharnais. 2001. A typology of stages of adherence to exercise behavior: A cluster analysis. *Journal of Applied Social Psychology* 31: 1979-1994.

Gómez, L.F., J.C. Mateus, and G. Cabrera. 2004. Leisure-time physical activity among women in a neighbourhood in Bogotá, Colombia: Prevalence and sociodemographic correlates. *Cadernos de Saúde Pública* 20: 1103-1109.

Gordon-Larsen, P., R.G. McMurray, and B.M. Popkin. 1999. Adolescent physical activity and inactivity vary by ethnicity: The National Longitudinal Study of Adolescent Health. *Journal of Pediatrics* 135: 301-306.

Graves, L.E., N.D. Ridgers, K. Williams, G. Stratton, G. Atkinson, and N.T. Cable. 2010. The physiological cost and enjoyment of Wii Fit in adolescents, young adults, and older adults. *Journal of Physical Activity and Health* 7 (3): 393-401.

Hagger, M.S., and N.L. Chatzisarantis. 2008. Self-determination theory and the psychology of exercise. *International Review of Sport and Exercise Psychology* 1: 79-103.

Hagger, M.S., and N.L. Chatzisarantis. 2009. Integrating the theory of planned behaviour and self-determination theory in health behaviour: A meta-analysis. *British Journal of Health Psychology* 14 (2): 275-302.

Hagger, M.S., N. Chatzisarantis, and S.J. Biddle. 2002. A meta-analytic review of the theories of reasoned action and planned behaviour in physical activity: Predictive validity and the contribution of additional variables. *Journal of Sport and Exercise Psychology* 24: 3-32.

Hausenblaus, H.A., A.V. Carron, and D.E. Mack. 1997. Application of the theories of reasoned action and planned behavior to exercise behavior: A meta-analysis. *Journal of Sport and Exercise Psychology* 19: 36-51.

Heath, G.W., R.C. Brownson, J. Kruger, R. Miles, K.E. Powell, and L.T. Ramsey. 2006. The effectiveness of urban design and land use and transport policies and practices to increase physical activity: A systematic review. *Journal of Physical Activity and Health* 1: S55-S71.

Heinzelmann, F., and R.W. Bagley. 1970. Response to physical activity programs and their effects on health behavior. *Public Health Reports* 86: 905-911.

Heirich, M.A., A. Foote, J.C. Erfurt, and B. Konopka. 1993. Work-site physical fitness programs: Comparing the impact of different program designs on cardiovascular risks. *Journal of Occupational Medicine* 35: 510-517.

Hensley, L.D. 2000. State of required physical education in colleges and universities. *Research Quarterly for Exercise and Sport* 71: A71-A72.

Hillsdon, M. 2011. Occupational social class, occupational physical activity, and leisure-time physical activity. *American Journal of Preventive Medicine* 40 (4): 494-495.

Hoehner, C.M., J. Soares, D. Parra Perez, I.C. Ribeiro, C.E. Joshu, M. Pratt, B.D. Legetic, D.C. Malta, V.R. Matsudo, L.R. Ramos, E.J. Simões, and R.C. Brownson. 2008. Physical activity interventions in Latin America: A systematic review. *American Journal of Preventive Medicine* 34 (3): 224-233.

Hofstetter, C.R., M.F. Hovell, C. Macera, J.F. Sallis, V. Spry, E. Barrington, and C. Callender. 1991. Illness, injury, and correlates of aerobic exercise and walking: A community study. *Research Quarterly for Exercise and Sport* 62: 1-9.

Hou, N., B.M. Popkin, D.R. Jacobs Jr., Y. Song, D. Guilkey, C.E. Lewis, and P. Gordon-Larsen. 2010. Longitudinal associations between neighborhood-level street network with walking, bicycling, and jogging: The CARDIA study. *Health and Place* 16 (6): 1206-1215.

Hovell, M.F., J.F. Sallis, C.R. Hofstetter, V.M. Spry, J.P. Elder, P. Faucher, and C.J. Caspersen. 1989. Identifying correlates of walking for exercise: An epidemiologic prerequisite for physical activity promotion. *Preventive Medicine* 18: 856-866.

Hoyt, M.F., and I.L. Janis. 1975. Increasing adherence to a stressful decision via a motivational balance-sheet procedure: A field experiment. *Journal of Personality and Social Psychology* 31: 833-839.

Huhman, M., L.D. Potter, F.L. Wong, S.W. Banspach, J.C. Duke, and C.D. Heitzler. 2005. Effects of a mass media campaign to increase physical activity among children: Year-1 results of the VERB campaign. *Pediatrics* 116 (2, August): e277-284.

Jakicic, J.M., K. Clark, E. Coleman, J.E. Donnelly, J. Foreyt, E. Melanson, J. Volek, and S.L. Volpe. 2001. American College of Sports Medicine position stand: Appropriate intervention strategies for weight loss and prevention of weight regain for adults. *Medicine and Science in Sports and Exercise* 33: 2145-2156.

Jakicic, J.M., R.R. Wing, B.A. Butler, and R.J. Robertson. 1995. Prescribing exercise in multiple short bouts versus one continuous bout: Effects on adherence, cardiorespiratory fitness, and weight loss in overweight women. *International Journal of Obesity and Related Metabolic Disorders* 19: 893-901.

Jakicic, J.M., C. Winters, W. Lang, and R.R. Wing. 1999. Effects of intermittent exercise and use of home exercise equipment on adherence, weight loss, and fitness in overweight women. *Journal of the American Medical Association* 282: 1554-1560.

Janis, I.L., and L. Mann. 1977. *Decision making: A psychological analysis of conflict, choice, and commitment.* New York: Free Press.

Jeffery, R.W., R.R. Wing, C. Thorson, and L.R. Burton. 1998. Use of personal trainers and financial incentives to increase exercise in a behavioral weight-loss program. *Journal of Consulting and Clinical Psychology* 66: 777-783.

Kaczynski, A.T., and K.A. Henderson. 2007. Environmental correlates of physical activity: A review of evidence about parks and recreation. *Leisure Sciences* 29: 315-354.

Kaczynski, A.T., and K.A. Henderson. 2008. Parks and recreation settings and active living: A review of associations with physical activity function and intensity. *Journal of Physical Activity and Health* 5 (4): 619-632.

Kahn, E.B., L.T. Ramsey, R.C. Brownson, G.W. Heath, E.H. Howze, K.E. Powell, and E.J. Stone. 2005. Physical activity. In *The guide to community preventive services: What works to promote health,* edited by S. Zaza, P.A. Briss, and K.W. Harris. New York: Oxford University Press.

Kahn, E.B., L.T. Ramsey, R.C. Brownson, G.W. Heath, E.H. Howze, K.E. Powell, E.J. Stone, M.W. Rajab, and P. Corso. 2002. The effectiveness of interventions to increase physical activity. A systematic review. *American Journal of Preventive Medicine* 22 (4 Suppl.): 73-107.

Kahn, J.A., B. Huang, M.W. Gillman, A.E. Field, S.B. Austin, G.A. Colditz, and A.L. Frazier. 2008. Patterns and determinants of physical activity in U.S. adolescents. *Journal of Adolescent Health* 42 (4): 369-377.

Kann, L., S.A. Kinchen, B.I. Williams, J.G. Ross, R. Lowry, J.A. Grunbaum, and L.J. Kolbe. 2000. Youth risk behavior surveillance—United States, 1999. *Morbidity and Mortality Weekly Report* 49 (SS-5): 1-96.

Kann, L., S.A. Kinchen, B.I. Williams, J.G. Ross, R. Lowry, C.V. Hill, J.A. Grunbaum, P.S. Blumson, J.L. Collins, and L.J. Kolbe. 1998. CDC surveillance summaries: Youth risk behavior survey—United States, 1997. *Morbidity and Mortality Weekly Report* 47 (SS-3): 1-89.

Kann, L., C.W. Warren, W.A. Harris, J.L. Collins, B.I. Williams, J.G. Ross, and L.J. Kolbe. 1996. Youth risk behavior surveillance—United States, 1995. *Morbidity and Mortality Weekly Report* 45 (SS-4): 1-83.

Kaplan, R.M., C.J. Atkins, and S. Reinsch. 1984. Specific efficacy expectations mediate exercise compliance in patients with COPD. *Health Psychology* 3: 223-242.

Kendzierski, D., and K.J. DeCarlo. 1991. Physical activity enjoyment scale: Two validation studies. *Journal of Sport and Exercise Psychology* 13 (1): 50-64.

Kirk, M.A., and R.E. Rhodes. 2011. Occupation correlates of adults' participation in leisure-time physical activity: A systematic review. *American Journal of Preventive Medicine* 40 (4): 476-485.

King, A.C. 1994. Community and public health approaches to the promotion of physical activity. *Medicine and Science in Sports and Exercise* 26: 1405-1412.

King, A.C., C. Castro, S. Wilcox, A.A. Eyler, J.F. Sallis, and R.S. Brownson. 2000. Personal and environmental factors associated with physical inactivity among different racial-ethnic groups of U.S. middle-aged and older-aged women. *Health Psychology* 19: 354-364.

King, A.C., W.L. Haskell, H.C. Taylor, and R.F. DeBusk. 1991. Group- vs. home-based exercise training in healthy older men and women. *Journal of the American Medical Association* 266: 1535-1542.

King, A.C., W.A. Satariano, J. Marti, and W. Zhu. 2008. Multilevel modeling of walking behavior: Advances in understanding the interactions of people, place, and time. *Medicine and Science in Sports and Exercise* 40 (7 Suppl.): S584-S593.

King, A.C., C.B. Taylor, W.L. Haskell, and R.F. DeBusk. 1988. Strategies for increasing early adherence to and long-term maintenance of home-based exercise training in healthy middle-aged men and women. *American Journal of Cardiology* 61: 628-632.

King, A.L., and L.W. Frederiksen. 1984. Low-cost strategies for increasing exercise behavior: Relapse preparation training and support. *Behavior Modification* 3: 3-21.

Knapp, D.N. 1988. Behavioral management techniques and exercise promotion. In *Exercise adherence: Its impact on public health,* edited by R.K. Dishman, pp. 203-236. Champaign, IL: Human Kinetics.

Kohl, H.W., and W. Hobbs. 1998. Development of physical activity behavior among children and adolescents. *Pediatrics* 101 (Suppl. 5): 549-554.

Kriska, A.M., C. Bayles, J.A. Cauley, R.E. LaPorte, R.B. Sandler, and G. Pambianco. 1986. A randomized exercise trial in older women: Increased activity over two years and the factors associated with compliance. *Medicine and Science in Sports and Exercise* 18: 557-562.

Kronsberg, S.S., S.R. Daniels, P.B. Crawford, Z.I. Sabry, and K. Liu. 2002. Decline in physical activity in black girls and white girls during adolescence. *New England Journal of Medicine* 347: 709-715.

Leonard, F.E., and G.B. Affleck. 1947. *A guide to the history of physical education.* Philadelphia: Lea & Febiger.

Leslie, E., P.B. Sparling, and N. Owen. 2001. University campus settings and the promotion of physical activity in young adults: Lessons from research in Australia and the USA. *Health Education* 3: 116-125.

Lewis, B.A., B.H. Marcus, R.R. Pate, and A.L. Dunn. 2002. Psychosocial mediators of physical activity behavior among adults and children. *American Journal of Preventive Medicine* 23 (2 Suppl.): 26-35.

Linenger, J.M., C.V. Chesson, and D.S. Nice. 1991. Physical fitness gains following simple environmental change. *American Journal of Preventive Medicine* 7 (5): 298-310.

Lombard, D.N., T.N. Lombard, and R.A. Winett. 1995. Walking to meet health guidelines: The effects of prompting frequency and prompt structure. *Health Psychology* 14 (2): 164-170.

Luepker, R.V., D.M. Murray, D.R. Jacobs, M.B. Mittelmark, N. Bracht, R. Carlaw, R. Crow, P. Elmer, J.R. Finnegan, A.R. Folsom, et al. 1994. Community education for cardiovascular disease prevention: Risk factor changes in the Minnesota Heart Health Program. *American Journal of Public Health* 84: 1383-1393.

Luepker, R.V., C.L. Perry, S.M. McKinlay, P.R. Nader, G.S. Parcel, E.J. Stone, L.S. Webber, J.P. Elder, H.A. Feldman, and C.C. Johnson. 1996. Outcomes of a field trial to improve children's dietary patterns and physical activity: The Child and Adolescent Trial for Cardiovascular Health. *Journal of the American Medical Association* 275: 768-776.

Lyons, E.J., D.F. Tate, D.S. Ward, J.M. Bowling, K.M. Ribisl, and S. Kalyararaman. 2011. Energy expenditure and enjoyment during video game play: Differences by game type. *Medicine and Science in Sports and Exercise,* February 28. [Epub ahead of print]

MacKinnon, D.P., A.J. Fairchild, and M.S. Fritz. 2007. Mediation analysis. *Annual Review of Psychology* 58: 593-614.

Marcus, B.H., C.A. Eaton, J.S. Rossi, and L.L. Harlow. 1994. Self-efficacy, decision-making and the stages of change: An integrative model of physical exercise. *Journal of Applied Social Psychology* 24: 489-508.

Marcus, B.H., N. Owen, L.H. Forsyth, N.A. Cavill, and F. Fridinger. 1998. Physical activity interventions using mass media, print media, and information technology. *American Journal of Preventive Medicine* 15: 362-378.

Marcus, B.H., V.C. Selby, R.S. Niaura, and J.S. Rossi. 1992. Self-efficacy and the stages of exercise behavior change. *Research Quarterly for Exercise and Sport* 63 (1): 60-66.

Marcus, B.H., and L.R. Simkin. 1993. The stages of exercise behavior. *Journal of Sports Medicine and Physical Fitness* 33: 83-88.

Marcus, B.H., and A.L. Stanton. 1993. Evaluation of relapse prevention and reinforcement interventions to promote exercise adherence in sedentary females. *Research Quarterly for Exercise and Sport* 64: 447-452.

Marlatt, G.A., and J. Gordon. 1985. *Relapse prevention.* New York: Guilford Press.

Marshall, S.J., and S.J. Biddle. 2001. The transtheoretical model of behavior change: a meta-analysis of applications to physical activity and exercise. *Annals of Behavioral Medicine* 23: 229-246.

Martin, J.E., P.M. Dubbert, A.D. Katell, J.K. Thompson, J.R. Raczynski, M. Lake, P.O. Smith, J.S. Webster, T. Sikova, and R.E. Cohen. 1984. The behavioral control of exercise in sedentary adults: Studies 1 through 6. *Journal of Consulting Clinical Psychology* 52: 795-811.

Martins, C., and M.F. Duarte. 2000. Efeitos da ginastica laboral em servidores da reitoria da UFSC. *Revista Brasileira de Ciencia e Movimento* 12: 14-18.

Mathews, A.E., S.B. Laditka, N. Laditka, S. Wilcox, S.J. Corwin, R. Liu, D.B. Friedman, R. Hunter, W. Tseng, and R.G. Logsdon. 2010. Older adults' perceived physical activity enablers and barriers: A multicultural perspective. *Journal of Aging and Physical Activity* 18 (2): 119-140.

Matsudo, S.M., and V.R. Matsudo. 2006. Coalitions and networks: Facilitating global physical activity promotion. *Promotion and Education* 13 (2): 133-138, 158-163.

Matsudo, S.M., V.R. Matsudo, T.L. Araujo, D.R. Andrade, E.L. Andrade, L.C. de Oliveira, and G.F. Braggion. 2003. The Agita São Paulo Program as a model for using physical activity to promote health. *Revista Panamerica de Salud Pública* 14 (4): 265-272.

Matsudo, V.R., S.M. Matsudo, D. Andrade, T. Araujo, E. Andrade, L.C. de Oliveira, and G. Braggion. 2002. Promotion of physical activity in a developing country: The Agita São Paulo experience. *Public Health Nutrition* 5 (1A): 253-261.

McAuley, E., and B. Blissmer. 2000. Self-efficacy determinants and consequences of physical activity. *Exercise and Sport Sciences Reviews* 28: 85-88.

McKay, C.M., B.A. Bell-Ellison, K. Wallace, and J.M. Ferron. 2007. A multilevel study of the associations between economic and social context, stage of adolescence, and physical activity and body mass index. *Pediatrics* 119 (Suppl. 1): S84-91.

Melillo, K.D., E. Williamson, S.C. Houde, M. Futrell, C.Y. Read, and M. Campasano. 2001. Perceptions of older Latino adults regarding physical fitness, physical activity, and exercise. *Journal of Gerontology Nursing* 27: 38-46.

Merom, D., A. Bauman, P. Phongsavan, E. Cerin, M. Kassis, W. Brown, B.J. Smith, and C. Rissel. 2009. Can a motivational intervention overcome an unsupportive environment for walking—findings from the Step-by-Step Study. *Annals of Behavioral Medicine* 38 (2): 137-146.

Meyer, A., J. Nash, A. McAlister, N. Maccoby, and J.W. Farquhar. 1980. Skills training in a cardiovascular health education campaign. *Journal of Consulting and Clinical Psychology* 48: 129-142.

Miyachi, M., K. Yamamoto, K. Ohkawara, and S. Tanaka. 2010. METs in adults while playing active video games: A metabolic chamber study. *Medicine and Science in Sports and Exercise* 42 (6): 1149-1153.

Moody, J.S., J.J. Prochaska, J.F. Sallis, T.L. McKenzie, M. Brown, and T.L. Conway. 2004. Viability for parks and recreation centers as sites for youth physical activity promotion. *Health Promotion and Practice* 5: 438-443.

Morrow, J.R. Jr., J.A. Krzewinski-Malone, A.W. Jackson, T.J. Bungum, and S.J. FitzGerald. 2004. American adults' knowledge of exercise recommendations. *Research Quarterly for Exercise and Sport* 75 (3): 231-237.

Motl, R.W., R.K. Dishman, G. Felton, and R.R. Pate. 2003. Self-motivation and physical activity among black and white adolescent girls. *Medicine and Science in Sports and Exercise* 35: 128-136.

Motl, R.W., R.K. Dishman, R. Saunders, M. Dowda, G. Felton, and R.R. Pate. 2001. Measuring enjoyment of physical activity in adolescent girls. *American Journal of Preventive Medicine* 21: 110-117. Erratum in *American Journal of Preventive Medicine,* 2001, 21: 332.

Motl, R.W., R.K. Dishman, D.S. Ward, R. Saunders, M. Dowda, G. Felton, and R.R. Pate. 2002. Examining social-cognitive determinants of intention and physical activity in adolescent girls using structural equation modeling. *Health Psychology* 21: 459-467.

National Institute of Child Health and Human Development Study of Early Child Care and Youth Development Network. 2003. Frequency and intensity of activity of third-grade children in physical education. *Archives of Pediatrics and Adolescent Medicine* 157: 185-190.

National Recreation and Park Association. 2004. Hearts N' Parks—Report of 2004. Magnet Center Performance Data. www.nhlbi.nih.gov/health/prof/heart/obesity/hrt_n_pk/2004_report.pdf

Ness, A.R., S.D. Leary, C. Maddocks, et al. 2007. Objectively measured physical activity and fat mass in a large cohort of children. *PLoS Medicine* 4: e97.

Norman, R.M.G. 1986. The nature and correlates of health behavior. In *Health promotion studies series,* No. 2, pp. 1-163. Ottawa: Health and Welfare, Canada.

O'Connor, T.M., R. Jago, and T. Baranowski. 2009. Engaging parents to increase youth physical activity: A systematic review. *American Journal of Preventive Medicine* 37 (2): 141-149.

Oldridge, N.B. 1979. Compliance of past myocardial infarction patients from exercise programs. *Medicine and Science in Sports* 11: 373-375.

Oldridge, N.G., A. Donner, C.W. Buck, N.L. Jones, G.A. Anderson, J.O. Parker, D.A. Cunningham, T. Kavanagh, P.A. Rechnitzer, and J.R. Sutton. 1983. Predictive indices for dropout: The Ontario Exercise Heart Collaborative Study Experience. *American Journal of Cardiology* 51: 70-74.

Owen, N., E. Leslie, J. Salmon, and M.J. Fotheringham. 2000. Environmental determinants of physical activity and sedentary behavior. *Exercise and Sport Sciences Reviews* 28: 153-158.

Pain, B.M., S.M.M. Matsudo, E.L. Andrade, G.F. Graggion, and V.K. Matsudo. 2001. Effect of a physical activity program on physical fitness and self-perception of physical fitness of women over 50 years-old. *Revista de Atividade Fisica e Saude* 6: 50-64.

Parcel, G.S., B. Simons-Morton, N.M. O'Hara, T. Baranowski, and B. Wilson. 1989. School promotion of healthful diet and physical activity: Impact on learning outcomes and self-reported behavior. *Health Education Quarterly* 16 (2): 181-199.

Pate, R.R. 2009. A national physical activity plan for the United States. *Journal of Physical Activity and Health* 6 (Suppl. 2): S157-158.

Pate, R.R., G.W. Heath, M. Dowda, and S.G. Trost. 1996. Associations between physical activity and other health behaviors in a representative sample of US adolescents. *American Journal of Public Health* 86 (11): 1577-1581.

Pate, R.R., M. Pratt, S.N. Blair, W.L. Haskell, C.A. Macera, C. Bouchard, D. Buchner, W. Ettinger, G.W. Heath, A.C. King, et al. 1995. Physical activity and public health. A recommendation from the Centers for Disease Control and Prevention and the American College of Sports Medicine. *Journal of the American Medical Association* 273: 402-407.

Pate, R.R., R. Saunders, R.K. Dishman, C. Addy, M. Dowda, and D.S. Ward. 2007. Long-term effects of a physical activity intervention in high school girls. *American Journal of Preventive Medicine* 33 (4): 276-280.

Pate, R.R., J. Stevens, C. Pratt, et al. 2006. Objectively measured physical activity in sixth-grade girls. *Archives of Pediatric and Adolescent Medicine* 160: 1262-1268.

Pate, R.R., D.S. Ward, R.P. Saunders, G. Felton, R.K. Dishman, and M. Dowda. 2005. Promotion of physical activity among high-school girls: A randomized controlled trial. *American Journal of Public Health* 95 (9): 1582-1587.

Pearman, S.N., R.F. Valois, R.G. Sargent, R.P. Saunders, J.W. Drane, and C.A. Macera. 1997. The impact of a required college health and physical education course on the health status of alumni. *Journal of American College Health* 4: 77-85.

Perusse, L., A. Tremblay, C. Leblanc, and C. Bouchard. 1989. Genetic and familial environmental influences on level of habitual physical activity. *American Journal of Epidemiology* 129: 1012-1022.

Petter, M., C. Blanchard, K.A. Kemp, A.S. Mazoff, and S.N. Ferrier. 2009. Correlates of exercise among coronary heart disease patients: Review, implications and future directions. *European Journal of Cardiovascular Prevention and Rehabilitation* 16 (5): 515-526.

Physical Activity Guidelines Advisory Committee. 2008. *Physical Activity Guidelines Advisory Committee report.* Washington, DC: U.S. Department of Health and Human Services.

Pinto, B.M., H. Lynn, B.H. Marcus, J. DePue, and M.G. Goldstein. 2001. Physician-based activity counseling: Intervention effects on mediators of motivational readiness for physical activity. *Annals of Behavioral Medicine* 23: 2-10.

Pollock, M.L. 1988. Prescribing exercise for fitness and adherence. In *Exercise adherence: Its impact on public health,* edited by R.K. Dishman, pp. 259-277. Champaign, IL: Human Kinetics.

Pollock, M.L., J.F. Carroll, J.E. Graves, S.H. Leggett, R.W. Braith, M. Limacher, and J.M. Hagberg. 1991. Injuries and adherence to walk/jog and resistance programs in the elderly. *Medicine and Science in Sports and Exercise* 23: 1194-1200.

Pollock, M.L., G.A. Gaesser, J.D. Butcher, J. Despres, R.K. Dishman, B.A. Franklin, and C.E. Garber. 1998. American College of Sports Medicine position stand: Recommended quantity and quality of exercise for developing and maintaining cardiorespiratory and muscular fitness, and flexibility in healthy adults. *Medicine and Science in Sports and Exercise* 30: 975-991.

Pratt, M., J.N. Epping, and W.H. Dietz. 2009. Putting physical activity into public health: A historical perspective from the CDC. *Preventive Medicine* 49: 301–302

Prochaska, J.O., and C.C. DiClemente. 1983. The stages and processes of self-change in smoking: Towards an integrative model of change. *Journal of Consulting and Clinical Psychology* 51: 390-395.

Prochaska, J.O., and B.H. Marcus. 1994. The transtheoretical model: Applications to exercise. In *Advances in exercise adherence,* edited by R.K. Dishman, pp. 161-180. Champaign, IL: Human Kinetics.

Prochaska, J.O., W.F. Velicer, J.S. Rossi, M.G. Goldstein, B.H. Marcus, W. Rakowski, C. Fiore, L.L. Harlow, C.A. Redding, D. Rosenblum, and S.R. Rossi. 1994. Stages of change and decisional balance for 12 problem behaviors. *Health Psychology* 13 (1): 39-46.

Pugliese, J., and B. Tinsley. 2007. Parental socialization of child and adolescent physical activity: A meta-analysis. *Journal of Family Psychology* 21 (3): 331-343.

Raynor, D.A., K.J. Coleman, and L.H. Epstein. 1998. Effects of proximity on the choice to be physically active or sedentary. *Research Quarterly for Exercise and Sport* 69: 99-103.

Reed, G.R. 1999. Adherence to exercise and the transtheoretical model of behavior change. In *Adherence issues in sport and exercise,* edited by S. Bull, pp. 19-45. New York: Wiley.

Reger, B., S. Booth-Butterfield, H. Smith, A. Bauman, M. Wootan, S. Middlestadt, B. Marcus, and F. Greer. 2002. Wheeling Walks: A community campaign using paid media to encourage walking among sedentary older adults. *Preventive Medicine* 35 (3): 285-292.

Rhodes, R.E., and N.E. Smith. 2006. Personality correlates of physical activity: A review and meta-analysis. *British Journal of Sports Medicine* 40: 958-965.

Rhodes, R.E., D.E. Warburton, and H. Murray. 2009. Characteristics of physical activity guidelines and their effect on adherence: A review of randomized trials. *Sports Medicine* 39 (5): 355-375.

Riddoch, C.J., C. Mattocks, K. Deere, J. Saunders, J. Kirby, K. Tilling, S.D. Leary, S.N. Blair, and A.R. Ness. 2007. Objective measurement of levels and patterns of physical activity. *Archives of Disease in Childhood* 92: 963-969.

Ridgers, N.D., G. Stratton, S.J. Fairclough, and J.W. Twisk. 2007. Long-term effects of a playground markings and physical structures on children's recess physical activity levels. *Preventive Medicine* 44 (5): 393-397.

Robertson, R.J., and B.J. Noble. 1997. Perception of physical exertion: Methods, mediators, and applications. *Exercise and Sport Sciences Reviews* 25: 407-452.

Rosen, C.S. 2000. Is the sequencing of change processes by stage consistent across health problems? A meta-analysis. *Health Psychology* 19 (6): 593-604.

Rosenstock, I.M. 1974. Historical origins of the health belief model. *Health Education Monographs* 2: 1-9.

Roux, L., M. Pratt, T.O. Tengs, M.M. Yore, T.L. Yanagawa, J. Van Den Bos, C. Rutt, R.C. Brownson, K.E. Powell, G. Heath, H.W. Kohl 3rd, S. Teutsch, J. Cawley, I.M. Lee, L. West, and D.M. Buchner. 2008. Cost effectiveness of community-based physical activity interventions. *American Journal of Preventive Medicine* 35 (6): 578-588.

Rowland, T.W. 1998. The biological basis of physical activity. *Medicine and Science in Sports and Exercise* 30 (3): 392-399.

Ryan, R.M., and E.L. Deci. 2000. Self-determination theory and the facilitation of intrinsic motivation, social development, and well-being. *American Psychologist* 55 (1): 68-78.

Ryan, R.M., C.M. Frederick, D. Lepes, N. Rubio, and K.M. Sheldon. 1997. Intrinsic motivation and exercise adherence. *International Journal of Sport Psychology* 28 (4): 335-354.

Sallis, J.F. 1993. Epidemiology of physical activity and fitness in children and adolescents. *Critical Reviews in Food Science and Nutrition* 33: 405-408.

Sallis, J.F., H.R. Bowles, A. Bauman, B.E. Ainsworth, F.C. Bull, C.L. Craig, M. Sjöström, I. De Bourdeaudhuij, J. Lefevre, V. Matsudo, S. Matsudo, D.J. Macfarlane, L.F. Gomez, S. Inoue, N. Murase, V. Volbekiene, G. McLean, H. Carr, L.K. Heggebo, H. Tomten, and P. Bergman. 2009. Neighborhood environments and physical activity among adults in 11 countries. *American Journal of Preventive Medicine* 36 (6): 484-490.

Sallis, J.F., K.J. Calfas, J.F. Nichols, J.A. Sarkin, M.F. Johnson, S. Caparosa, S. Thompson, and J.E. Alcaraz. 1999. Evaluation of a university course to promote physical activity: Project GRAD. *Research Quarterly for Exercise and Sport* 70 (1): 1-10.

Sallis, J.F., T.L. Conway, J.J. Prochaska, T.L. McKenzie, S.P. Marshall, and M. Brown. 2001. The association of school environments with youth physical activity. *American Journal of Public Health* 91: 618-620.

Sallis, J.F., R.M. Grossman, R.B. Pinski, T.L. Patterson, and P.R. Nader. 1987. The development of scales to measure social support for diet and exercise behaviors. *Preventive Medicine* 16: 825-836.

Sallis, J.F., W.L. Haskell, S.P. Fortmann, K.M. Vranizan, C.B. Taylor, and D.S. Solomon. 1986. Predictors of adoption and maintenance of physical activity in a community sample. *Preventive Medicine* 15: 331-346.

Sallis, J.F., and M.F. Hovell. 1990. Determinants of exercise behavior. *Exercise and Sport Sciences Reviews* 11: 307-330.

Sallis, J.F., M.F. Hovell, and C.R. Hofstetter. 1992. Predictors of adoption and maintenance of vigorous physical activity in men and women. *Preventive Medicine* 21: 237-251.

Sallis, J.F., M.F. Hovell, C.R. Hofstetter, J.P. Elder, P. Faucher, V.M. Spry, E. Barrington, and M. Hackley. 1990a. Lifetime history of relapse from exercise. *Addictive Behaviors* 15: 573-579.

Sallis, J.F., M.F. Hovell, C.R. Hofstetter, J.P. Elder, M. Hackley, C.J. Caspersen, and K.E. Powell. 1990b. Distance between homes and exercise facilities related to frequency of exercise among San Diego residents. *Public Health Reports* 105: 179-185.

Sallis, J.F., T.L. McKenzie, T.L. Conway, J.P. Elder, J.J. Prochaska, M. Brown, M.M. Zive, S.J. Marshall, and J.E. Alcaraz. 2003. Environmental interventions for eating and physical activity: A randomized controlled trial in middle schools. *American Journal of Preventive Medicine* 24 (3): 209-217.

Sallis, J.F., R.B. Pinski, R.M. Grossman, T.L. Patterson, and P.R. Nader. 1988. The development of self-efficacy scales for health-related diet and exercise behaviors. *Health Education Research* 3: 283-292.

Sallis, J.F., J.J. Prochaska, and W.C. Taylor. 2000. A review of correlates of physical activity of children and adolescents. *Medicine and Science in Sports and Exercise* 32: 963-975.

Sallis, J.F., B.G. Simons-Morton, E.J. Stone, C.B. Corbin, L.H. Epstein, N. Faucette, R.J. Iannotti, J.D. Killen, R.C. Klesges, C.K. Petray, et al. 1992. Determinants of physical activity and interventions in youth. *Medicine and Science in Sports and Exercise* 24 (6): S248-S257.

Sanne, H.M., D. Elmfeldt, G. Grimby, C. Rydin, and L. Wilhelmsen. 1973. Exercise tolerance and physical training of non-selected patients after myocardial infarction. *Acta Medica Scandinavica* 551 (Suppl.): 1-124.

Schmitz, K., S.A. French, and R.W. Jeffery. 1997. Correlates of changes in leisure time physical activity over 2 years: The Healthy Worker Project. *Preventive Medicine* 26: 570-579.

Scott, M.M., K.R. Evenson, D.A. Cohen, and C.E. Cox. 2007. Comparing perceived and objectively measured access to recreational facilities as predictors of physical activity in adolescent girls. *Journal of Urban Health* 84 (3): 346-359.

Seip, R.L., D. Snead, E.F. Pierce, P. Stein, and A. Weltman. 1991. Perceptual responses and blood lactate concentration: Effect of training state. *Medicine and Science in Sports and Exercise* 23: 80-87.

Sevick, M.A., A.L. Dunn, M.S. Morrow, B.H. Marcus, G.J. Chen, and S.N. Blair. 2000. Cost-effectiveness of lifestyle and structured exercise interventions in sedentary adults. Results of project ACTIVE. *American Journal of Preventive Medicine* 19: 1-8.

Silva, M.N., D. Markland, E.V. Carraça, P.N. Vieira, S.R. Coutinho, C.S. Minderico, M.G. Matos, L.B. Sardinha, and P.J. Teixeira. 2011. Exercise autonomous motivation predicts 3-yr weight loss in women. *Medicine and Science in Sports and Exercise* 43:728-737.

Simkin, L.R., and A.M. Gross. 1994. Assessment of coping with high-risk situations for exercise relapse among healthy women. *Health Psychology* 13 (3): 274-277.

Sonstroem, R.J. 1988. Psychological models. In *Exercise adherence: Its impact on public health,* edited by R.K. Dishman. Champaign, IL: Human Kinetics.

Ståhl, T., A. Rutten, D. Nutbeam, A. Bauman, L. Kannas, T. Abel, G. Luschen, D.J. Rodriquez, J. Vinck, and J. van der Zee. 2001. The importance of the social environment for physically active lifestyle: Results from an international study. *Social Science and Medicine* 52: 1-10.

Staunton, C.E., D. Hubsmith, and W. Kallins. 2003. Promoting safe walking and biking to school: The Marin County success story. *American Journal of Public Health* 93: 1431-1434.

Steinhardt, M.A., and R.K. Dishman. 1989. Reliability and validity of expected outcomes and barriers for habitual physical activity. *Journal of Occupational Medicine* 31: 536-546.

Stephens, T., and C.L. Craig. 1990. *The well-being of Canadians: Highlights of the 1988 Campbell's Survey.* Ottawa: Canadian Fitness and Lifestyle Research Institute.

Steptoe, A., J. Wardle, R. Fuller, A. Holte, J. Justo, R. Sanderman, and L. Wichstrom. 1997. Leisure-time physical exercise: Prevalence, attitudinal correlates, and behavioral correlates among young Europeans from 21 countries. *Preventive Medicine* 26 (6): 845-854.

Stokols, D. 1992. Establishing and maintaining health environments: Toward a social ecology of health promotion. *American Psychologist* 47: 6-22.

Stone, E.J., T.L. McKenzie, G.J. Welk, and M. Booth. 1998. Effects of physical activity interventions in youth: Review and synthesis. *American Journal of Preventive Medicine* 15 (4): 298-315.

Stubbe, J.H., D.I. Boomsma, J.M. Vink, B.K. Cornes, N.G. Martin, A. Skytthe, K.O. Kyvik, R.J. Rose, U.M. Kujala, J. Kaprio, J.R. Harris, N.L. Pedersen, J. Hunkin, T.D. Spector, and E.J. de Geus. 2006. Genetic influences on exercise participation in 37,051 twin pairs from seven countries. *PLoS One* 1 (December 20): e22.

Tappe, M.K., J.L. Duda, and P. Menges-Ehrnwald. 1990. Personal investment predictors of adolescent motivational orientation toward exercise. *Canadian Journal of Sport Sciences* 15 (3): 185-192.

Taylor, S.E. 1999. Health behaviors. In *Health psychology,* 4th edition, pp. 50-93. Boston: McGraw-Hill.

Teraslinna, P., T. Partanen, A. Koskela, K. Partanen, and P. Oja. 1969. Characteristics affecting willingness of executives to participate in an activity program aimed at coronary heart disease prevention. *Journal of Sports Medicine and Physical Fitness* 9: 224-229.

Tremblay, M.S., and C.L. Craig. 2009. ParticipACTION: Overview and introduction of baseline research on the "new" ParticipACTION. *International Journal of Behavioral Nutrition and Physical Activity* 6: 84.

Troped, P.J., and R.P. Saunders. 1998. Gender differences in social influence on physical activity at different stages of exercise adoption. *American Journal of Health Promotion* 13: 112-115.

Troped, P.J., R.P. Saunders, R.R. Pate, B. Reininger, J.R. Ureda, and S.J. Thompson. 2001. Associations between self-reported and objective physical environmental factors and use of a community rail-trail. *Preventive Medicine* 32 (2): 191-200.

Trost, S.G., D.S. Ward, and M. Senso. 2010. Effects of child care policy and environment on physical activity. *Medicine and Science in Sports and Exercise* 42 (3): 520-525.

Turk, D.C., T.E. Rudy, and P. Salovey. 1984. Health protection: Attitudes and behaviors of LPNs, teachers, and college students. *Health Psychology* 3: 189-210.

U.S. Department of Health and Human Services. 1991. *Healthy people 2000: National health promotion and disease prevention objectives.* DHHS Publication No. (PHS) 91-50212. Washington, DC: Government Printing Office.

U.S. Department of Health and Human Services. 1996. *Physical activity and health: A report of the Surgeon General.* Atlanta: U.S. Department of Health and Human Services, Centers for Disease Control, National Center for Chronic Disease Prevention and Health Promotion.

U.S. Department of Health and Human Services. 1999. *Chronic diseases and their risk factors: The nation's leading causes of death.* Atlanta: Centers for Disease Control and Prevention.

U.S. Department of Health and Human Services. 2000a. *Healthy people 2010: National health promotion and disease prevention objectives.* DHHS (PHS) 91-50212. Washington, DC: Government Printing Office.

U.S. Department of Health and Human Services. 2000b. *Healthy people 2010: Understanding and improving health.* 2nd edition. Washington, DC: Government Printing Office.

U.S. Department of Health and Human Services. 2008. *2008 Physical activity guidelines for Americans.* www.health.gov/paguidelines/.

U.S. Department of Health and Human Services. 2010. *Healthy people 2020: National health promotion and disease prevention objectives.* Office of Disease Prevention and Health Promotion. Publication No. B0132. Washington, DC: Government Printing Office.

U.S. Department of Transportation. 1997. *Nationwide personal transportation survey.* Lanham, MD: Federal Highway Commission.

Vink, J.M., D.I. Boomsma, S.E. Medland, M.H. de Moor, J.H. Stubbe, B.K. Cornes, N.G. Martin, A. Skytthea, K.O. Kyvik, R.J. Rose, U.M. Kujala, J. Kaprio, J.R. Harris, N.L. Pedersen, L. Cherkas, T.D. Spector, and E.J. de Geus. 2011. Variance components models for physical activity with age as modifier: A comparative twin study in seven countries. *Twin Research and Human Genetics* 14 (1): 25-34.

Vuori, I.M., P. Oja, and O. Paronen. 1994. Physically active commuting to work—testing its potential for exercise promotion. *Medicine and Science in Sports and Exercise* 26 (7): 844-850.

Vuori, I., O. Paronen, and P. Oja. 1998. How to develop local physical activity promotion programmes with national support: The Finnish experience. *Patient Education and Counseling* 33 (Suppl. 1): S111-S119.

Wallace, J.P., J.S. Raglin, and C. Jastremski. 1995. Twelve month adherence of adults who joined a fitness program with a spouse vs. without a spouse. *Journal of Sports Medicine and Physical Fitness* 35: 206-213.

Wallace, L.S., J. Buckworth, T.E. Kirby, and W.M. Sherman. 2000. Characteristics of exercise behavior among college students: Application of social cognitive theory to predicting stage of change. *Preventive Medicine* 31: 494-505.

Wang, G., C.A. Macera, B. Scudder-Soucie, T. Schmid, M. Pratt, D. Buchner, and G. Heath. 2004. Cost analysis of the built environment: The case of bike and pedestrian trails in Lincoln, Neb. *American Journal of Public Health* 94 (4): 549-553.

Wankel, L.M., and C. Thompson. 1977. Motivating people to be physically active: Self-persuasion vs. balanced decision-making. *Journal of Applied Social Psychology* 7: 332-340.

Wankel, L.M., J.K. Yardley, and J. Graham. 1985. The effects of motivational interventions upon the exercise adherence of high and low self-motivated adults. *Canadian Journal of Applied Sport Sciences* 10: 147-156.

Ward, A., and W.P. Morgan. 1984. Adherence patterns of healthy men and women enrolled in an adult exercise program. *Journal of Cardiac Rehabilitation* 4: 143-152.

Webber, L.S., D.J. Catellier, L.A. Lytle, D.M. Murray, C.A. Pratt, D.R. Young, J.P. Elder, T.G. Lohman, J. Stevens, J.B. Jobe, R.R. Pate; TAAG Collaborative Research Group. 2008. Promoting physical activity in middle school girls: Trial of Activity for Adolescent Girls. *American Journal of Preventive Medicine* 34 (3): 173-184.

Weinstein, N.D., A.J. Rothman, and S.R. Sutton. 1998. Stage theories of health behavior: Conceptual and methodological issues. *Health Psychology* 17 (3): 290-299.

Wendel-Vos, W., M. Droomers, S. Kremers, J. Brug, and F. van Lenthe. 2007. Potential environmental determinants of physical activity in adults: A systematic review. *Obesity Reviews* 8 (5): 425-440.

Werme, M, C. Messer, L. Olson, L. Gilden, P. Thorén, E.J. Nestler, and S. Brené. 2002. Delta FosB regulates wheel running. *Journal of Neuroscience* 22: 8133-8138.

Whaley, M.H., P.H. Brubaker, L.A. Kaminsky, and C.R. Miller. 1997. Validity of rating of perceived exertion during graded exercise testing in apparently healthy adults and cardiac patients. *Journal of Cardiopulmonary Research* 17 (July-August): 261-267.

Wier, L.T., and A.S. Jackson. 1992. Percent VO2max and percent HRmax reserve are not equal methods of assessing exercise intensity. *Medicine and Science in Sports and Exercise* 24 (Suppl. 5): 1057.

Wilfley, D., and K.D. Brownell. 1994. Exercise and weight maintenance. In *Advances in exercise adherence,* edited by R.K. Dishman. Champaign, IL: Human Kinetics.

Yancey, A.K., W.J. McCarthy, W.C. Taylor, A. Merlo, C. Gewa, et al. 2004. The Los Angeles Lift Off: A sociocultural environmental change intervention to integrate physical activity into the workplace. *Preventive Medicine* 38: 848-856.

Young, D.R., W.L. Haskell, C.B. Taylor, and S.P. Fortmann. 1996. Effect of community health education on physical activity knowledge, attitudes, and behavior. *American Journal of Epidemiology* 144: 264-274.

GLOSSARY

absolute intensity—Work rate expressed as an absolute value that is the same for all people, for example, running at 6 mi/h (9.7 km/h).

absolute risk—The incidence rate of disease, injury, or death in a group.

abstinence violation effect—When a temporary slip or lapse during an attempt to change a habit is catastrophized by the person into feelings of total failure, lost confidence, and a subsequent relapse to the past habit.

accelerometer—Mechanical device that measures the acceleration and thus movement of the body in one or more planes through use of transducers.

acetylcholine—Neurotransmitter at cholinergic synapses that causes cardiac inhibition, vasodilation, gastrointestinal peristalsis, and other parasympathetic effects; also acts in an excitatory manner between motor neurons and skeletal muscles.

activity limitations—Problems in performance of everyday functions such as communication, self-care, mobility, learning, and behavior.

acute exercise—A single session of exercise; is typically short but can last for 4 h or more (e.g., a marathon).

acute-phase response—Early immune response to an infection, signaled by pro-inflammatory cytokines secreted by monocytes and inflammatory proteins produced by the liver and commonly followed by transient leukocytosis.

adaptive immunity—Acquired memory of the immune system that enhances specific recognition of and defense against an antigen, permitting a quicker and larger immune response upon a subsequent exposure.

adherence—In medicine, faithfully following an agreed-upon plan of treatment, such as a person's continuation in an exercise program. Otherwise, maintenance of a self-initiated change in behavior.

adhesion molecule—A homing receptor on a lymphocyte that regulates transient adhesion to the blood vascular endothelium. Some examples are L-selectin, LFA-1, VLA-4, and CD44.

adipose—Composed of fat cells.

adoption of physical activity—Behavioral and cognitive components, including some degree of psychological commitment, of beginning regular, purposeful, structured physical activity.

adrenal cortex—The outer covering of the adrenal gland, which is adjacent to the kidney and secretes glucocorticoid, mineralocorticosteroid, and sex hormones.

adrenaline—See *epinephrine.*

adrenal medulla—The inner core of the adrenal gland; secretes epinephrine, norepinephrine, and enkephalins.

adrenergic receptors—Cells or fibers of the autonomic or central nervous system that use epinephrine as their neurotransmitter.

adrenocorticotropic hormone (ACTH)—A hormone released by the anterior lobe of the hypophysis (anterior pituitary) that controls the production and release of hormones of the adrenal cortex.

afferent nerve—A neural axon that carries nerve impulses away from a sensory organ to the central nervous system.

α_1-receptors—A subclass of α-adrenergic receptors that are widespread, with clinically important concentrations in the liver, heart, vascular, intestinal, and genitourinary smooth muscle and in the central and peripheral nervous systems.

α_2-receptors—A subclass of α-adrenergic receptors found on pancreatic beta cells, platelets, and vascular smooth muscle, as well as both pre- and postsynaptically in the central and peripheral nervous systems.

alpha wave activity—Brain wave activity in the range of 8 to 12 Hz, commonly described as relaxed wakefulness.

amygdala—A group of nuclei located in the limbic system that is involved in the control of appropriate behavior for social situations, emotional memory, and the generation of fear and anger.

angina pectoris—A paroxysmal thoracic pain with a feeling of suffocation and impending death, most often due to anoxia of the myocardium, that is precipitated by effort or excitement.

angiography—Radiographic visualization of blood vessels.

angiotensin I—A physiologically inactive peptide formed from angiotensinogen by the enzyme renin.

angiotensin II—Formed by angiotensin-converting enzyme (ACE) from biologically inactive angiotensin I. Angiotensin II causes contraction of vascular smooth muscle and thus increases blood pressure and stimulates the release of aldosterone from the adrenal gland.

angiotensin-converting enzyme (ACE)—The enzyme that converts angiotensin I to angiotensin II in the lungs by removing two amino acid residues.

angiotensinogen—A peptide produced by the liver that is converted to angiotensin I by renin.

antibody—A protein secreted by plasma cells of the immune system that protects against a specific antigen.

antigen-presenting cell—A cell, such as a macrophage or a dendritic cell, that engulfs antigens and presents them to B or T lymphocytes in a recognizable form (e.g., in an MHC class II molecule).

antioxidant—An enzyme or other organic substance, such as vitamin E or beta-carotene, that is capable of counteracting the damaging effects of oxidation in animal tissue.

anxiety—A response to a perceived threat that consists of feelings of tension, apprehension, and nervousness; unpleasant thoughts or worries; and physiological changes.

anxiety disorder—A mental illness characterized by apprehension or worry that is accompanied by restlessness, muscular tension, elevated heart rate, and breathlessness. Anxiety disorders include phobias, panic disorders, obsessive–compulsive disorders, and generalized anxiety disorder.

anxiolytic—Having the effect of decreasing anxiety.

apoprotein—One of a class of regulatory proteins that combine with enzymes and lipoproteins to regulate their actions.

arteriosclerosis—Induration, or hardening, of arteries.

assistive technology—Under the Assistive Technology Act of 1998 (Public Law 105-394), technology to be utilized in "any item, piece of equipment, or product system, whether acquired commercially, modified, or customized, that is used to increase, maintain, or improve the functional capabilities of individuals with disabilities."

atheroma—A fatty deposit in the inner lining of an artery.

atherosclerosis—Arteriosclerotic disease characterized by deposits of fatty plaques on the inner linings of medium and large arteries.

attitude—An evaluation of and reaction to an object, person, event, or idea, which includes cognitive, affective, and behavioral components.

attributable risk—See *risk difference*.

autonomic nervous system (ANS)—Part of the peripheral nervous system that innervates smooth muscle, cardiac muscle, and glands; composed of the sympathetic, parasympathetic, and enteric divisions.

Ayurveda—Sanskrit for "knowledge of living." The ancient Indian system of medicine.

basophil—Granulocyte containing heparin and histamine that is involved in hypersensitivity responses to an antigen (e.g., allergies). Other than having a segmented nucleus, a basophil has a shape and function similar to a those of a mast cell.

Bayes' theorem—When applied to diagnostic tests, the odds of event A (e.g., disease) being dependent upon event B (e.g., positive test result) are an inverse function of the prior probability of A and B before the test is administered.

behavioral epidemiology—The observation and study of behaviors, including physical inactivity, that lead to disease, injury, or premature death and the distribution of these behaviors.

behavioral intention—What a person aims to do or accomplish; intention is incremental (e.g., It is somewhat likely that I will do something) rather than dichotomous (e.g., I will or won't do something).

behaviorism—A field of psychology, which developed out of learning theory, that describes behavior through the associations among observable stimulus, response, and outcome, with no role for personality or mental states in predicting and describing behavior.

beliefs—Expectations, convictions, or opinions.

β_1-receptors—A subclass of β-adrenergic receptors equally sensitive to epinephrine and norepinephrine. They are found in the heart, in juxtoglomerular cells in the kidney, and in the central and peripheral nervous systems.

bias—Any deviation of results or inferences from the truth, or a process leading to such deviations. Bias can result from several sources: systematic variation in measurement from the true value (systematic error), flaws in study design, flawed data, and so on.

biological plausibility—One of Mill's canons, which states that the observed association between a risk factor and a disease outcome must be explainable by existing knowledge about possible biological mechanisms of the disease in order to establish causality.

B lymphocyte—A short-lived lymphocyte not derived in the thymus gland that is a key cell of humoral immunity and a precursor of the plasma cell that secretes immunoglobulins.

body composition—Proportions of fat, water, protein, and mineral that constitute body mass.

body mass index (BMI)—The ratio of body weight (in kilograms) to height (in meters) squared. Individuals with a BMI of 25 to 29.9 are considered overweight, whereas individuals with a BMI of 30 or more are considered obese.

bone involution—The loss of endosteal bone at a faster rate than exosteal bone is deposited, which results in osteopenia, a major risk factor of osteoporosis, and usually begins around age 30 or 40.

breast carcinoma in situ—A cancer that is confined to lobules (milk glands) or ducts (milk passages) and has not spread to surrounding fat cells in the breast or to other organs.

calcitonin—A polypeptide hormone produced by C cells of the thyroid gland that causes a reduction of calcium ions in the blood, inhibits bone resorption, and increases vitamin D receptors in osteoblasts.

calorimetry—A method of measuring energy expenditure by recording increases in temperature in a controlled environment.

cancer—A family of related diseases that result from uncontrolled growth and spread of abnormal cells, which usually become a malignant tumor.

carcinogen—A substance or agent that causes cancer.

carcinoma—A malignant tumor of epithelial cells.

cardiac arrhythmia—Any variation from the normal rhythm of the heartbeat, including, for example, sinus arrhythmia, premature beats, heart block, and ventricular fibrillation.

cardiorespiratory fitness—The capacity of the cardiorespiratory system to take up and use oxygen; the capability to carry out activities that use large muscle groups at moderate intensities, that use oxygen for the production of energy, and that can be sustained for more than a few minutes.

case–control study—A research design in which people with a disease or injury or people who have died from that condition (i.e., cases) are compared with healthy people (i.e., controls) on the prevalence of a suspected causal risk factor after the cases have been matched with controls on exposure to other key risk factors that might be confounders.

catecholamines—Class of synaptic neurotransmitters, including dopamine, norepinephrine, and epinephrine, that also act as hormones and that contain a single amine group (monoamines).

cause of death—A single underlying condition to which a death is attributed, based on information reported on a death certificate and the international rules for selecting the underlying cause of death from reported conditions.

cerebrovascular disease—Any of a variety of diseases affecting the arteries that supply the brain via the obstructive effects of atherosclerosis.

chemokines—A class of pro-inflammatory cytokines released by phagocytes, endothelial cells, fibroblasts, and smooth muscle cells in response to bacteria, viruses, and cell damage at the site of infection; they chemically attract and activate leukocytes in infected tissue.

chemotactic—Facilitating the attraction or repulsion of a cell along a chemical concentration gradient.

cholesterol—The most abundant steroid found in animal tissue. A waxy constituent of cell membranes, hormones, and atheroma.

cholesterol ester transfer protein (CETP)—A protein that regulates the transfer of cholesterol ester from HDL-C to LDL-C, VLDL-C, and chylomicrons in exchange for triglycerides.

chronic exercise—Bouts of exercise that are repeated on a fairly regular basis over a period of time; exercise training or regular exercise that is defined by the type, intensity, duration, weekly frequency, and time period (e.g., weeks, months) of activity.

chylomicron—A very low density lipoprotein, composed of about 95% triglycerides, produced by the small intestine.

cingulate cortex—A band of limbic cortex lying above the corpus collosum and along the lateral walls of the longitudinal fissure that separates the hemispheres of the cerebrum.

clinical trial—A research study conducted with patients, usually to evaluate a new treatment.

clonal expansion—The proliferation of activated, genetically identical B lymphocytes and T lymphocytes; enables the body to have sufficient numbers of antigen-specific lymphocytes to mount an effective immune response.

coagulability—The tendency of a liquid to thicken or to be transformed to a solid, as in the clotting of blood.

cognition—Mental process of knowing, including aspects such as awareness, perception, reasoning, and judgment.

cognitive–behavior modification—A technique of behavioral change, based on principles from learning theory, that focuses on modifying the cognitions and behaviors related to the target behavior and on cues and reinforcers of the target behavior.

cohort—A large group of individuals identified by a common characteristic that are studied over a period of time as part of a scientific or medical investigation. The term *cohort* is derived from one of the 10 divisions of a Roman legion, consisting of 300 to 600 soldiers.

collagen—The fibrous protein that makes up connective tissue, including bone.

colony-stimulating factors—Protein–carbohydrate compounds found in the blood that stimulate the proliferation of bone marrow cells and the formation of colonies of granulocytes and/or macrophages.

complement system—About 20 proteins that augment the action of phagocytic cells by opsonization.

compliance—Following a prescribed standard of behavior, usually related to immediate and short-term health advice to alleviate symptoms, such as taking a specific regimen of medications; a sense of coerced obedience.

confidence interval—A range of values for a variable of interest constructed to have a specified probability of including the true value of the variable.

confounder—An extraneous factor that is not a consequence of exposure to the risk factor under study or an experimental manipulation but that affects the outcome and thus distorts the study's findings. Confounders are determinants or correlates of the outcome under study that are unequally distributed among the exposed and unexposed individuals, making it difficult or impossible to interpret the relationships among the other variables.

confounding—A situation in which the effects of two or more processes are not separate; the distortion of the apparent effect of an exposure or risk brought about by association with other factors that can influence the outcome.

consequence—Abstract or concrete event that follows a target behavior, either immediately or after some time, and can either reinforce and thus increase the frequency of the target behavior or punish and thus decrease the frequency of the target behavior.

consistency—One of Mill's canons, which states that, to establish causality, the observed association between a risk factor and a disease outcome must always be observed when the risk factor is present.

construct—An abstract idea developed to describe the relationship among phenomena or for other research purposes that exists theoretically but is not directly observable.

control—In experimental research, a group or condition that does not experience the treatment that the researcher is studying, for the sake of comparison with the treatment groups or conditions.

coronary heart disease (CHD)—Atherosclerosis of the medium-sized and large arteries that supply the myocardium (heart muscle).

cortical bone—The superficial thin layer of compact bone found in the shafts of adult long bones; the nontrabecular portion of bone that consists largely of small canals through which blood vessels pass, called osteons, surrounded by concentric layers, or lamellae, of bone.

corticotropin-releasing hormone (CRH)—Hormone released by the paraventricular nucleus (cells separating the lateral ventricles of the brain) of the anterior hypothalamus that controls the diurnal rhythms of adrenocorticotropic hormone release.

cortisol—A steroid hormone; the major glucocorticoid secreted by the adrenal cortex, which plays a primary role in the stress response and in central nervous dysregulation associated with mood disorders and is also involved in stimulating the formation and storage of glycogen and maintenance of blood glucose.

C-reactive protein—An acute-phase protein that binds to some bacteria and fungi, serving as both an opsonin and a complement catalyst during inflammation.

cross-sectional study—Research plan in which data are collected at a single point in time and participants are classified by predictor (independent) and outcome (dependent) variables.

cytokine—Any of a class of antibody proteins released by cells that mediate cellular actions of other cells. Lymphokines and interleukins are specific types found in the immune system.

cytolytic—Pertaining to dissolution of a cell.

cytotoxic—Relating to or producing injury or death of a cell.

death rate—The number of deaths in a population in a given period divided by the total population at the middle of that period.

decisional balance—One of the three components of the transtheoretical model of stages of change; the balance between the perceived benefits of the target behavior and the perceived costs.

dependent variable—A measurable outcome that is influenced by an independent variable.

descriptive epidemiology—The assessment of variation in a behavior or disease prevalence by age, sex, race or ethnicity, health status, geographic location, and so on.

desirable weight—Body weight judged by normative (i.e., averaged among people) weights and associated with socially defined attractiveness, physical performance, or risks for disease and mortality.

determinant—In exercise behavior research, a variable that has an established, reproducible association or predictive relationship with an outcome variable; a correlate, but not necessarily a confirmed cause.

diabetes mellitus—A group of diseases characterized by high levels of blood glucose resulting from defects in insulin production, insulin action, or both.

diacylglycerol O-acyltransferase (DGAT)—Enzyme that influences esterification of diacylglycerol to yield triglycerides.

diapedesis—Transmigration of the leukocyte through the vascular wall into the infected tissue; the last step of extravasation.

disability—The interactions between individuals with health conditions and barriers in their environment.

disease—An interruption, cessation, or disorder of body organs, systems, or functions, usually having a known cause, distinct signs and symptoms, or altered morphology.

distraction hypothesis—Explanation for the beneficial psychological effects of exercise as time out from worrisome thoughts and daily stressors.

dopamine—Neurotransmitter that is the precursor for norepinephrine and epinephrine.

dose response—One of Mill's canons, which states that to establish causality, the risk of disease associated with a risk factor must be greater with stronger exposure to the risk factor.

doubly labeled water (DLW)—A method of estimating free-living energy expenditure by having subjects ingest a measured amount of water labeled with stable isotopes ($^2H^1H^{18}O$). CO_2 production, and hence energy use, is estimated from the difference in the elimination rates from the body of ^{18}O (which is eliminated as both water and carbon dioxide) and ^2H (which is eliminated only as water) from urine samples obtained over a seven- to 14-day period.

downregulation—Tolerance developed after repeated administration of a pharmacologically or physiologically active substance or in response to excessively high levels of a substance, which is often characterized by an initial decrease in the affinity of receptors for the substance and a subsequent decrease in the number of receptors.

dual X-ray absorptiometry (DXA)—A radiographic method of determining bone mineral and fat mass by measuring the uptake of radiation energy during a body scan.

dysregulation—Disruption in self-regulation.

dysthymia—Mild, chronic form of major depression.

ecological fallacy—False conclusion that the co-occurrence of a risk factor with a health marker observed in an ecological study indicates cause and effect.

ecological study—Specific type of cross-sectional investigation in which the incidence of a risk factor is observed concurrently with the incidence of a health outcome in a given geographic region.

effectiveness—The ability of an intervention or method to work in other settings, to be practically applied outside of a laboratory setting to yield a successful outcome.

effect modifier—A variable that changes the association between a risk factor and morbidity or mortality. For example, overweight people who are physically fit have less CHD risk than similarly overweight people who are unfit. Thus, physical fitness modifies or moderates the effect of overweight on CHD.

effect size—Measure of the strength of an association or a relationship, often considered an indication of practical significance; the difference in the outcome for the average subject who received a treatment from the outcome for the average subject who did not.

efferent nerve—A neural axon that carries nerve impulses away from the central nervous system to an organ.

efficacy—The ability of an intervention or method to do what it was intended to do.

elastin—The main structural protein that makes up elastic fibers.

electroencephalogram (EEG)—A recording of gross electrical activity of the brain using large electrodes placed on the scalp in a standardized pattern.

electromyogram (EMG)—A recording of the gross electrical activity of muscle contraction.

electrophysiological measure—Measure of neural activity in the brain using electrodes positioned in the brain cortex or in specific regions of brain neurons to record electrical potentials during behavior or in response to stress.

embolism—The sudden blocking of an artery by a clot or foreign material that has been brought to the site by blood flow.

emotion—An intense mental state that arises subjectively rather than through conscious effort and is accompanied by physiological changes related to autonomic activation; brief responses of negative or positive feelings.

endocannabinoids—Endogenous physiological ligands that bind to the same cannabinoid receptors that mediate the psychoactive effects of Cannabis (i.e., marijuana).

endogenous—Produced within the body.

endorphin—Endogenous opioid peptide that can act as a neurotransmitter, neuromodulator, and hormone.

endorphin hypothesis—Unsubstantiated proposition that the mood enhancement associated with exercise is due to actions of endorphins secreted during exercise.

endosteum—The layer of vascular connective tissue lining the medullary cavity of bone.

endothelium—The layer of flat cells that line the cavities of the heart and blood vessels and the serous cavities of the body.

enkephalin—An endogenous opioid, a class of compounds that exert effects like those of opium, such as reduced pain sensitivity.

enteric nervous system—The branch of the autonomic nervous system that regulates the intestines.

environmental factors—The policies, systems, social contexts, and physical barriers or facilitators that affect a person's participation in activities, including work, school, leisure, and community events.

eosinophil—Antiparasitic leukocyte.

epidemic—Occurrence of a disease that has a greater than expected frequency in a population during a specific period of time.

epidemiology—The study of the distribution and determinants of health-related states and events in the population.

epinephrine—A compound secreted by the adrenal medulla and by postganglionic sympathetic nerves that acts as a hormone and as a neurotransmitter and plays an important role in preparing to respond to stress. Also known as *adrenaline*.

esterification (of cholesterol)—Removal of water from cholesterol via removal of the OH from its acid and alcohol groups. Esterified cholesterol is hydrophobic (i.e., repels water molecules) and moves to the core of the HDL-C molecule, creating a concentration gradient that augments transfer of cholesterol from cell membranes (e.g., endothelial cells) or other lipoproteins to the surface of the HDL-C molecule.

etiology—The causes, development, and pathophysiology of a disease.

exercise—A subset of physical activity consisting of planned, structured, repetitive bodily movements with the purpose of improving or maintaining one or more components of physical fitness or health.

exercise prescription—Recommendation for a specific exercise mode, intensity, duration, and frequency per week to meet specific goals.

exosteum—Bone cells outside the central medullary cavity.

extravasation—Margination and emigration of leukocytes from the blood across vessel walls into infected tissues.

fibrillation—Rapid, asynchronous twitching of individual muscle fibers, commonly in the atria or ventricles of the heart, which causes irregular pulse and can lead to sudden cardiac death.

fibrin—The insoluble protein formed from fibrinogen by the proteolytic action of thrombin during the normal clotting of blood. Fibrin forms the essential portion of the blood clot.

fibrinogenesis—Conversion of the blood protein fibrinogen to fibrin in the presence of ionized calcium by the hydrolytic protease enzyme thrombin.

fibrinolysis—Solubilization of fibrin in blood clots, chiefly by the proteolytic action of plasmin.

fibroblast—A cell that produces connective tissue such as fibrin.

fibrosis—Formation of excessive fibrous tissue.

5-hydroxyindoleacetic acid (5-HIAA)—A major metabolite of serotonin.

flexibility—The range of motion at a specific joint or linked joints during both passive and dynamic movements.

free radical—A chemically active atom or molecular fragment containing a chemical charge due to an excess or deficiency of electrons. Free radicals seek to receive or release electrons to achieve a more stable configuration, a process that can damage the large molecules within cells.

functional magnetic resonance imaging (FMRI)—Method of determining brain activity that applies magnetic resonance to find out which parts of the brain are activated by various types of physical sensations or motor activity.

galanin—Amino acid peptide neurotransmitter that hyperpolarizes noradrenergic neurons and inhibits locus coeruleus firing in vitro.

gamma-aminobutyric acid (GABA)—Major inhibitory transmitter in the nervous system.

generalized anxiety disorder (GAD)—Disorder characterized by excessive or pathologic worry about multiple concerns, exaggerated vigilance, and somatic symptoms of stress and anxiety such as muscular tension.

genotype—The sum of all of the genetic information in an organism.

geocoding—The process of finding geographic coordinates from geographic data such as street addresses, postal codes, or the satellite global positioning system.

geographic information systems—A method that blends cartography with database technology and statistical analysis to measure, manage, analyze, and model data about geographic locations.

gestational diabetes—A form of glucose intolerance that occurs in some women during pregnancy. Gestational diabetes occurs more frequently among African Americans, Hispanic Americans, and Native Americans than among non-Hispanic white Americans. It is also more common among obese women and women with a family history of diabetes.

glucocorticoid—Class of hormones that affect carbohydrate metabolism and are released by the adrenal cortex, for example in response to stress.

goal setting—Process by which specific plans are established in order to achieve a desired outcome.

granulocyte—Any of a class of mature leukocytes having a lobed nucleus, including neutrophils, eosinophils, and basophils.

gymnastics—Subdiscipline of ancient Greek medicine based on therapeutic exercise. It persisted through the European Renaissance.

health—Optimal functioning of an organism without signs of disease or abnormality.

health disparities—Inequalities or inequities in environment, access to, use, or quality of health care, health outcomes, and health status that deserve scrutiny.

health education—Programs and strategies designed to promote health behavior through educational programs and mass media campaigns.

health-related physical fitness—Components of physical fitness that have been empirically associated with overall health and ability to perform daily tasks and activities, including cardiorespiratory fitness, body composition, flexibility, muscular strength and endurance, and metabolic variables such as glucose tolerance.

hematocrit—Relative volume of blood cells occupied by erythrocytes. An average figure for humans is 45%.

hemispheric asymmetry—Differences in neural circuits between the left and right hemispheres of the brain.

hemostasis—The stoppage of blood flow through a vessel or body part, such as clotting to stop hemorrhage.

hepatic lipoprotein lipase (HPL)—Enzyme that catalyzes the hydrolysis of HDL-C in the liver by the hydrolysis of its triglyceride and phospholipid content. Its net effect is the conversion of HDL2 back to HDL-C in the liver.

high-density lipoprotein cholesterol (HDL-C)—A fraction, about one-fourth to one-third, of the total blood cholesterol. HDL-C is known as the "good" cholesterol because a high level of it seems to protect against heart attack. Basic studies suggest that HDL-C tends to carry cholesterol away from the arteries and back to the liver to be disposed from the body.

high-risk situation—Any situation that challenges confidence in one's ability to maintain a healthy behavior or to abstain from an unhealthy behavior.

Hill's criteria—Named for English epidemiologist Sir Austin Bradford Hill (1897–1991). Key criteria (strength of association, temporal sequence, dose response, consistency, and biological plausibility) that, if satisfied, indicate the likelihood that a statistical association between a risk factor and a disease outcome is causal.

hippocampus—Portion of the limbic system thought to be important in learning and memory.

Hoffmann reflex—A neuromuscular reflex that provides a measure of the efficacy of synaptic transmission between type Ia afferent sensory nerve fibers and alpha motor neurons in the spinal cord. Also termed the H-reflex.

homocysteine—A natural intermediate amino acid formed during the metabolism of an essential amino acid, methionine. A risk factor for atherosclerosis.

homocystinuria—Abnormally high levels of homocysteine because of deficiencies in metabolic enzymes.

hydrolysis—Splitting of a compound into two or more simpler compounds by water.

hygiene—Science or practice of health and its maintenance.

hypercholesterolemia—High levels of blood cholesterol; a risk factor for cardiovascular disease.

hyperglycemia—An abnormally high level of sugar in the blood.

hyperlipidemia—An elevated concentration of any or all of the lipids in the plasma, such as cholesterol, triglycerides, and lipoproteins.

hypertension—Persistently high arterial blood pressure, which may have no known cause (essential or idiopathic hypertension) or may be associated with other primary diseases (secondary hypertension). This condition is considered a risk factor for the development of heart disease, peripheral vascular disease, stroke, and kidney disease.

hypothalamic-pituitary-adrenocortical axis (HPA axis)—The hypothalamus, pituitary gland, and adrenal cortex.

hypothalamus—Part of the diencephalon that controls vegetative functions, regulates hormone balance, and plays a role in emotional behavior.

immune system—An integrated network of molecules, cells, tissues, and organs that defends an organism against infection by foreign substances (e.g., bacteria and viruses) and against mutated native cells (i.e., tumors); also helps to repair damaged tissues and to clean up the debris of dead cells.

immunoglobulin (Ig)—Any of a class of antibody proteins secreted by plasma cells formed from B lymphocytes. Immunoglobulins are classified by their relative basal levels in human blood: IgG, 80%; IgA, 10% to 15%; IgM, 5% to 10%; IgD, less than 0.1%; IgE, less than 0.01%.

immunology—The study of the immune system.

impaired fasting glucose—A prediabetic condition, possibly reversible, in which the fasting blood sugar level is elevated to between 110 and 125 mg/dl after an overnight fast but is not high enough to be classified as diabetes.

impaired glucose tolerance (IGT)—A prediabetic condition, possibly reversible, in which the blood sugar level is elevated to between 140 and 199 mg/dl after a 2-h oral glucose tolerance test but is not high enough to be classified as diabetes.

impairment—A chronic physiological, psychological, or anatomical abnormality of bodily structure or function caused by disease or injury.

incident cases—New cases of a disease or condition that occur in a given population during a time frame of interest.

independence—Dissociation from confounders.

independent variable—A measurable factor that is experimentally manipulated, or fluctuates naturally, to influence an outcome (i.e., the dependent variable).

indirect calorimetry—A method of estimating energy expenditure based on the known relationship of oxygen consumption with the caloric output of burning fat, carbohydrate, and protein.

inflammation—A localized response of increased blood flow and capillary permeability in response to injury or to an abnormal physical, chemical, or biological stimulus, associated with an influx of neutrophils and macrophages and secretion of cytokines to remove the source of infection and repair the injury. Signs and symptoms include redness, heat, swelling, pain, and impaired function.

injury—Damage to tissue caused by the exchange of kinetic, thermal, chemical, electrical, or radiation energy at levels intolerable to tissue, or the deprivation of oxygen due to suffocation.

innate immunity—Natural, nonspecific recognition and defense against an antigen by the immune system without prior exposure.

insular cortex—An island of involuted cerebral cortex contained beneath the sylvian fissure near the temporal lobe; believed important in regulating emotional responses, especially cardiovascular responses.

integrin molecules—Adhesion receptors expressed on leukocytes that bind with adhesion molecules on the endothelial surface; assists homing of lymphocytes to specific lymphoid sites so that leukocytes stop rolling and become loosely attached to the endothelium, forming the marginal pool.

intensity—The degree of exertion during physical activity, expressed as force (e.g., Newton-meters), as the rate of power output (e.g., watts), as a value relative to maximal capacity (e.g., 70% of maximal aerobic capacity), or as perceived exertion.

interferon-gamma (IFN-γ)—A cytokine produced by activated lymphocytes that plays a major role in antimicrobial, antitumor, and antiviral responses.

interleukins—Generic name for a category of cytokines that are produced by leukocytes and other cell types. Particularly important in cytokine networks that regulate inflammatory and immune responses.

interleukin-1 (IL-1)—A lymphokine and polypeptide hormone produced mainly by macrophages that activates acute-phase responses during the first few hours of infection or tissue damage. Such responses include fever, redistribution of amino acids (including muscle protein catabolism), and increased liver production of antimicrobial plasma proteins. IL-1 also activates the cascade of humoral and cellular immune responses against infection.

interleukin-2 (IL-2)—A lymphokine and polypeptide hormone produced mainly by activated lymphocytes whose main functions are activating other humoral immune cells, clonal expansion of T lymphocytes, increased expression of its receptors, and stimulating the release of other cytokines such as IFN.

interleukin-6 (IL-6)—A lymphokine and polypeptide hormone produced mainly by activated lymphocytes and blood monocytes. Its main functions are to stimulate B and T cells and to induce acute-phase protein synthesis during acute-phase responses, thus regulating the antiinflammatory response.

interleukin-8 (IL-8)—A chemokine secreted by macrophages and epithelial cells in damaged tissue; attracts neutrophils and fibroblasts involved with healing wounds.

interleukin-10 (IL-10)—An anti-inflammatory cytokine produced by T_{H-2} lymphocytes.

interleukin-12 (IL-12)—A cytokine secreted by macrophages and B cells. Activates T_{H-1} and cytotoxic lymphocytes and natural killer cells.

interleukin-15 (IL-15)—Structurally and functionally similar to IL-2. Secreted by monocytes and macrophages after viral infection. It modulates T and B lymphocytes and induces proliferation of NK cells.

International Classification of Diseases (ICD-10)—A classification of the nature of illness and injuries developed by the World Health Organization.

International Classification of Functioning, Disability and Health (ICF)—The World Health Organization's conceptual and coding framework for describing the functioning and disability associated with a person's health condition.

intima—Innermost lining, usually referring to the endothelium of arteries.

invasive breast carcinoma—Cancer cells that spread in the breast and to other parts of the body.

in vitro—Referring to a biological test or procedure done outside the body, as in a laboratory dish.

in vivo—Within a living body, usually with reference to a test or procedure done with intact, live subjects.

ischemia—A low oxygen state, or hypoxia, in the tissue, usually due to obstruction of the arterial blood supply or inadequate blood flow.

isomorphic—Referring to an animal model of disease that evokes the same features as the human disease, which abate after administration of drugs that are clinically useful in humans; the features generated may not have the same etiology or course of development as in the human disease.

ketosis—A toxic, acidotic state resulting from abnormal glucose metabolism, common in uncontrolled diabetes, that leads to cell damage, especially in small blood vessels and nerves.

kyphosis—Exaggeration of the normal posterior curve of the thoracic spine, often caused by compression fractures of the vertebrae.

latency—Length of time between the application of a stimulus and the response.

lecithin—Yellowish or brownish waxy phospholipid that is an essential component of cells and that yields two fatty acids when hydrolyzed.

lecithin:cholesterol acyltransferase (LCAT)—Enzyme that catalyzes the esterification of free cholesterol and the transfer of a free fatty acid from a phospholipid (lecithin) located on the shell of an HDL-C molecule to another cholesterol molecule.

leukocyte—A white blood cell differentiated from stem cells in bone marrow and lymphoid tissue.

leukocytosis—An abnormally high level of leukocytes, most commonly neutrophils, circulating in the blood in response to infection or stress.

lipoprotein—Compound containing lipid (e.g., triglyceride and cholesterol) and protein that is soluble in blood.

lipoprotein lipase (LPL)—Enzyme that catalyzes the hydrolysis of lipoproteins and regulates the concentration of HDL2 in plasma. Increased LPL activity increases the hydrolysis of VLDL and chylomicrons, increasing the formation of lower-density lipoprotein remnants that can be cleared by the liver and can yield cholesterol more easily to HDL-C.

locus coeruleus—Located in the pons, the major brain nucleus for the production of norepinephrine; it has a major role in inhibition of spontaneous firing in areas of the brain that it innervates.

low-density lipoprotein cholesterol (LDL-C)—A fraction of total blood cholesterol that normally circulates in the blood. However, when too much LDL-C is present, it can slowly build up in the walls of the arteries that feed the heart and brain. Together with other substances, it can form a thick, hard deposit called a plaque that can block those arteries.

lymph—A clear, sometimes yellowish fluid containing leukocytes (mainly lymphocytes) collected from bodily tissues and carried through lymphatic vessels and lymph nodes to the venous blood circulation via the thoracic duct.

lymphocyte—A type of leukocyte differentiated from stem cells in lymphatic tissue such as lymph nodes, spleen, thymus gland, tonsils, Peyer's patches, and bone marrow. Lymphocytes make up 20% to 30% of leukocytes in the blood.

lymphoid—Pertaining to the lymph, lymphatic tissue, or the lymphatic system.

lymphokine—Any of a class of cytokines secreted by lymphocytes that augment cellular immunity by activating monocytes, macrophages, lymphocytes, and natural killer cells.

lymph system—Coordinated system composed mainly of lymph, lymphatic tissues (e.g., lymph nodes, spleen, thymus gland, tonsils, Peyer's patches, and bone marrow), lymphocytes, and lymphokines.

lysis—Destruction of a cell.

macrophage—A relatively long-lived phagocytic cell of mammalian tissues derived from blood monocytes.

maintenance—Sustaining a regular exercise program for a specific period of time, usually at least six months.

major depression—One of two major categories of mood disorders (the other being manic–depressive disorder) characterized by depressed mood or loss of interest or pleasure and other behavioral and psychological symptoms.

manic–depressive disorder—One of two major categories of mood disorders (the other being major depression) characterized by periods of depression alternating with periods of elevated mood and associated behavior.

marginal pool—Sequestration of leukocytes in blood vessels by transient adhesion to endothelial cells.

margination—Movement of circulating leukocytes to the edge of the bloodstream, thereby increasing their contact with endothelial cells that line the vessels; facilitates extravasation.

mast cell—Granular, basophilic, connective tissue cell that contains heparin and histamine and is involved in inflammatory responses, especially in the upper respiratory system.

maximal aerobic power—The maximal amount of oxygen that the body can take up and use.

mediator—Intervening causal variable necessary to complete a cause–effect pathway between an intervention and physical activity, or a variable that transmits the effects of another variable on physical activity.

melancholia—A severe form of major depressive episode. Key features are a pervasive loss of pleasure or interest in pleasurable activities, dark mood that is worse in the morning, early morning awakening, psychomotor retardation or agitation, weight loss, and extreme feelings of guilt.

menarche—The onset of pubertal menstruation.

menopause—Permanent cessation of menses.

messenger RNA—RNA produced by transcription that reflects the exact nucleotide sequence of the genetically active DNA; it carries the code for a particular protein from the nuclear DNA to a ribosome in the cytoplasm, where protein is made in the amino acid sequences specified by the messenger RNA.

MET—Metabolic equivalent, the energy expended in kilocalories divided by resting energy expenditure in kilocalories, either measured or estimated from body size. 1 MET is approximately $1 \text{ kcal} \cdot \text{kg}^{-1} \cdot \text{h}^{-1}$ on average.

meta-analysis—Quantitative procedure for summarizing the effects of a number of research studies on a common topic.

metabolic syndrome—Co-occurrence of obesity (especially visceral adiposity) with diabetes, hypertension, and hyperlipidemia, a constellation of risk factors of coronary heart disease.

metastasize—To spread by metastasis, the process whereby tumors spread to parts of the body other than the originating part.

microsomal triglyceride transfer protein (MTP)—Needed for the assembly and secretion of apolipoprotein B–containing lipoproteins.

Mill's canons—Named for British philosopher John Stuart Mill (1806–1873). Principles of logical, inductive reasoning that provided origins of key criteria (dose response, consistency, and independence from confounding factors) that, if satisfied, indicate the likelihood that a statistical association between a risk factor and a disease outcome is causal.

mineralocorticosteroids—A group of hormones (the most important being aldosterone) that regulate the balance of water and electrolytes (ions such as sodium and potassium) in the body. The hormones act on the kidneys, specifically on the kidney tubules.

moderator—A variable that influences the relationship between two other variables or that influences how an intervention or mediator affects the outcome.

monocyte—A large white blood cell (i.e., leukocyte) differentiated from stem cells in bone marrow that has a single nucleus. Monocytes constitute about 5% of the leukocytes circulating in the blood.

mood—An affective state that is accompanied by anticipation, even unconscious, of pleasure or pain; moods can last less than a minute or as long as days, even weeks or months when disordered.

morbidity—The state of being diseased.

motivation—Synonymous with needs, drives, incentives, or an impetus to action. Concept that explains the direction, intensity, and persistence of behavior.

muscle dysmorphia—Pathological preoccupation with muscularity that can occur in both men and women.

muscular endurance—The capacity to exert force repeatedly.

muscular strength—The capacity to exert force against resistance.

myocardial infarction—Irreversible injury or death of heart muscle cells resulting from sudden insufficiency of blood flow; commonly called a heart attack.

natural history—Observed fluctuation in people's attributes, behavior, or health that is not the result of controlled experimental manipulation.

natural killer (NK) cell—One of a class of distinct lymphocytes that have innate immune properties and are key cells in natural surveillance and destruction of viruses, tumor cells, bacteria, protozoa, and other foreign microorganisms.

negative likelihood ratio—The odds that a negative test result will give an accurate prediction of the absence of disease. It is calculated as the prior odds multiplied by a (NLR) = ([1 − sensitivity]/specificity).

neuroimaging—Methods to measure brain activity using techniques such as functional magnetic resonance imaging.

neuropeptide Y—Amino acid peptide that inhibits the locus coeruleus from firing in vitro, providing feedback inhibition to locus coeruleus neurons.

neurotransmitter—Any specific chemical agent that is released by a presynaptic nerve cell upon excitation and that crosses the synapse to stimulate, inhibit, or modify the postsynaptic cell, serving as the basis of communication between neurons.

neutrophil—The most active phagocytic granulocyte. Neutrophils constitute about 80% of granulocytes and 50% to 65% of all leukocytes in the blood.

noradrenaline—See *norepinephrine.*

noradrenergic—Relating to cells or fibers of the autonomic or central nervous system that use norepinephrine as their neurotransmitter.

norepinephrine—The main neurotransmitter of peripheral sympathetic nerves and a key neuromodulator in the brain. Also acts as a hormone released by the adrenal medulla; its principal effects are excitatory. Also known as *noradrenaline.*

nucleus accumbens—A collection of neural cell bodies located in the basal forebrain near the ventral striatum. Helps regulate reward-motivated behavior.

nulliparity—Condition of not having given birth.

number needed to treat (NNT)—The number of patients that must be treated by a certain intervention in order to prevent one additional bad outcome (death, heart attack, depression episode, etc.). It is calculated as the inverse of the absolute risk reduction (i.e., 1/[control group event rate − treatment group event rate]) and is expressed as the nearest whole number.

obesity—An excessively high amount of body fat or adipose tissue in relation to lean body mass. The amount of body fat includes both the distribution of fat throughout the body and the size of the adipose tissue deposits. Body fat distribution can be estimated by skinfold measurements, waist-to-hip ratio, ultrasound, dual X-ray absorptiometry, computed tomography, or magnetic resonance imaging.

obsessive–compulsive disorder (OCD)—A disorder characterized by a recurrent, persistent, and unwanted idea, thought, or impulse to carry out an unwanted act that the individual cannot voluntarily suppress, typified by repetitive acts or rituals to relieve anxiety.

odds ratio (OR)—The ratio of the odds of exposure to a risk factor (i.e., chance of having vs. not having the risk factor) in the diseased group, *a/b,* to the odds of exposure to the risk factor in the nondiseased group, *c/d.* Used in cross-sectional or case–control studies where exposure to risk cannot be observed.

oncogenes—Genes that promote abnormal cell division, usually by transforming the DNA of a host cell.

opsonization—Coating by antibodies or complement of the cell walls of bacteria or viruses, making it easier for immune cells to inject cytotoxic enzymes into foreign cells.

osteoblasts—Cells that arise from fibroblasts and, as they mature, are associated with the production of bone.

osteoclasts—Large, multinucleate cells formed from differentiated macrophages, responsible for the breakdown of bone.

osteocytes—Osteoblasts that have become embedded within the bone matrix, occupying a flat oval cavity and sending slender cytoplasmic processes through the canaliculi (tiny channels), which make contact with other osteocytes.

osteoid matrix—A framework composed of newly formed osteocytes prior to calcification that provides the infrastructure for the mineralization of bone (e.g., by calcium and phosphorus) and, along with trabecular bone, gives bone its mechanical, elastic, and tensile strength.

osteopenia—Reduced bone mass due to inadequate osteoid synthesis. May lead to osteoporosis.

osteoporosis—A disease characterized by abnormally low bone mass and microstructural deterioration of bone tissue that leads to brittle bones and increased risk of fractures after minimal trauma. Osteoporosis is commonly defined as a bone mineral density more than 2.5 standard deviations below the average in young adults.

osteosarcoma—Cancer of bone.

outcome-expectancy value—The value or valence placed on an outcome expectation.

overweight—Excessive body weight. Usually expressed in relation to height compared with some standard of acceptable or desirable weights.

oxidation—A chemical reaction whereby the atoms in a compound lose electrons during combination with oxygen.

pandemic—An epidemic that spreads widely across a region or the world.

parasympathetic nervous system—One of three divisions of the autonomic nervous system. The parasympathetic nervous system arises from the cranial nerves and the sacral portions of the spinal cord and is involved primarily in energy conservation.

parathyroid hormone—A peptide hormone that stimulates osteoclasts to increase blood calcium, the effect opposite to that of calcitonin.

parity—Condition of having given birth.

pathogen—A microorganism that causes a disease.

perceived behavioral control—The degree to which an individual believes that he or she is able to have an effect on a specific outcome, which ranges along a continuum from no control to total control.

perceived exertion—The subjective judgment of strain or effort during physical activity, involving quantity rather than quality of sensations.

performance-related fitness—The ability to perform physical tasks. Components of performance-related fitness include psychomotor skills, maximal and submaximal cardiorespiratory power, muscular strength, power and endurance in the limbs and trunk for propulsion, body size, and body composition.

periaqueductal gray area—Gray matter that surrounds the duct between the third and fourth ventricles of the brain; processes neural signals associated with pain and aversive behavior.

person with a disability—A person who has been identified as having an activity limitation or who uses assistance or perceives him- or herself as having a disability.

person-year—A commonly used denominator in the computation of rates that equalizes risk exposure among groups. One person observed for one year equals one person-year.

Peyer's patches—Glandular, mucosal masses of lymphatic tissue located in the small intestine and tonsils.

phagocytic cell—A cell that can ingest and digest other cells. Neutrophils ingest mainly bacteria. Macrophages and monocytes scavenge mainly degenerated cells and dead tissue.

phagocytosis—The process of ingestion and digestion by cells of other cells, bacteria, dead tissue, and other organic and inorganic matter.

phobia—An obsessive, persistent, and unrealistic fear of an external situation or object that is out of proportion to the actual threat or danger.

phospholipase—Enzyme that catalyzes the hydrolysis of phosphate from a phospholipid.

phospholipid—A lipid compound, such as lecithin, that contains phosphorus and is found in lipoproteins.

physical activity—Bodily movement produced by skeletal muscle contraction that requires energy expenditure. Characterized by features including frequency, intensity, timing, and type.

physical activity survey—A self-report questionnaire used to assess physical activity, usually administered by mail, telephone, fax, or Internet.

physical fitness—The capacity to meet the present and potential physical challenges of life successfully; a set of personal attributes, such as muscular strength, cardiorespiratory capacity, and agility, that relate to the ability to perform physical activity.

plasmin—A proteolytic enzyme that hydrolyzes (i.e., dissolves) fibrin. Formed in the blood from plasminogen by tissue-type plasminogen activator (tPA) and trypsin or by drugs such as streptokinase.

plasminogen—The biologically inactive precursor of plasmin.

polyp—A mass (a tumor, inflammation, lesion, or malformation) that projects outward from a tissue surface.

polysomnography—Simultaneous measurement of multiple physiological indicators of sleep stages, such as brain waves, respiration, and muscle and chin movements to detect rapid eye movement.

population attributable risk—Theoretical percentage reduction in morbidity or mortality rate that might occur if all individuals with a specific risk factor eliminated that factor.

positive likelihood ratio—The odds that a positive test result will give an accurate prediction of the presence of a disease. It is calculated as sensitivity/(1 − specificity) multiplied by the prior odds of the disease (prevalence/[1 − prevalence]).

positron emission tomography (PET)—Method of measuring the dynamic activity of a living brain by detecting positrons emitted by radioactive glucose, or analog chemicals, administered orally or by injection.

posttraumatic stress disorder—Anxiety and behavioral disturbances that develop within the first month after exposure to an extreme trauma.

preferred exertion—The level of exertion that someone finds comfortable and is motivated to endure.

prefrontal cortex—The inferior part of the frontal cerebral cortex; believed to store memories of the consequences of behaviors or experiences that were aversive or pleasurable, permitting an emotion to be sustained long enough to direct behavior toward the goal that is appropriate for that emotion.

prevalent cases—The number of persons in a population who have a particular disease or condition at some specific point in time.

primary osteoporosis—Age-related (type I or senile) bone loss and postmenopausal (type II) bone loss.

primary prevention—Preventing the development of disease in a susceptible population.

processes of change—One of the three components of the transtheoretical model of stages of change; 10 covert and overt activities that are used to change thinking or affect behavior or relationships.

prodromal symptom—An early or premonitory symptom of a disease.

prospective cohort study—A research design in which baseline information on potential risk factors is collected from members of a large group of people having a common characteristic (i.e., a cohort) and the people are followed over time to track the incidence of disease.

prostaglandins—A class of hormone-like amino acid derivatives that regulate the dilation and constriction of smooth muscle and play a key role in inflammation. Prostaglandins are found in blood vessels, the intestines, the lungs, and the uterus and in hormones that have an antagonistic influence on lipid metabolism.

protease—An enzyme that catalyzes the splitting of the interior peptide bonds in a protein.

punishment—Consequences of a specific behavior that decrease the frequency of the behavior.

randomized controlled trial—A research design in which participants are selected for study and are randomly assigned to receive an experimental manipulation or a control condition. Measurements are made before and after the intervention period in both groups to assess the degree of change in the outcomes of interest between the intervention and control conditions.

raphe nucleus—One of the major nuclei for the production of serotonin, located in the center line of the brain stem.

reasonable weight—A realistically attainable body weight that is influenced by the impact of weight gain on a person, the person's individual history, and the circumstances that contribute to his or her "settling point" and likelihood of successfully maintaining weight loss.

receptor—A structural protein molecule, usually on the cell surface or within the cytoplasm, that combines with a specific factor, such as a hormone or neurotransmitter; the interaction of the factor and the receptor results in a change in cell function.

reciprocal determinism—The central concept of causation for social cognitive theory, which describes the bidirec-

tional, interacting influence of determinants of behavior; a mutually influencing relationship among two or more variables.

reinforcement—Consequences of a target behavior that increase the frequency of the behavior.

reinforcement control—Behavior change strategy that manipulates the consequences of the target behavior to increase the frequency of the behavior.

relapse prevention—Set of strategies designed to help keep people from returning to undesired behavior after successful behavior modification.

relative intensity—Work rate expressed in relation to maximal intensity, maximal aerobic capacity, or maximal workload.

relative risk (RR)—The ratio of the risk of disease in an exposed group, $a/(a + b)$, to the risk in an unexposed group, $c/(c + d)$, where a and c are incident cases and b and d are nonincident cases. Used in prospective studies where exposure to risk can be observed. Also known as the *risk ratio*.

reliability—Characteristic of a measure that includes precision, accuracy, and stability over time; freedom from measurement error or random error.

research design—Manner in which study participants are grouped or classified according to levels of the independent variable, modifiers, and confounders to determine influences on the dependent variable.

residual confounding—Occurs when all potential confounders are not measured or analyzed or when adjustments are not made for confounders that change across time.

reverse cholesterol transport—Return of excess cholesterol from extrahepatic tissue to the liver for metabolism. Reverse cholesterol transport involves esterification and storage of cholesterol in the core of the HDL molecule by the enzyme lecithin:cholesterol acyltransferase, which is regulated by apolipoprotein A1.

risk difference—An estimate of the amount of risk attributed to a risk factor, calculated as the risk (i.e., incidence rate) of disease in the group exposed to the risk factor minus the risk of disease in the unexposed group. Also called the *attributable risk*.

risk factor—A clearly defined characteristic that has been associated with the increased rate of a subsequently occurring disease.

risk ratio (RR)—See *relative risk*.

sarcoma—A tumor of connective tissue cells, usually malignant.

saturated fat—A fatty acid with all potential hydrogen-binding sites filled (totally hydrogenated), which is associated with high risk of atherosclerosis.

secondary osteoporosis—Osteoporosis that is caused by another disease but may not be independent of age or menopause.

secondary prevention—Early diagnosis and prompt treatment to shorten the duration of an illness, reduce its severity, and limit sequelae (subsequent effects).

secular trend—A naturally occurring change in the population.

selectin molecules—A type of adhesion molecule expressed by the endothelium of venules, which bind with leukocytes and cause them to roll along a "sticky" endothelial surface of the blood vessel; mediate the first step of extravasation.

self-concept—Organized configuration of perceptions about one's attributes and qualities that are within conscious awareness.

self-efficacy—Perception of one's capability to carry out a behavior with a known outcome; expectations of personal mastery regarding initiation and persistence of a behavior.

self-esteem—A person's evaluation of his or her self-concept and feelings associated with that evaluation.

self-monitoring—An individual's assessment of the antecedents, consequences, and characteristics of attempts to engage in or avoid a target behavior.

self-motivation—Internal factor that arouses, directs, and integrates a person's behavior; sustains a person to evaluate his or her own performance and then to seek to meet personal standards of achievement in the absence of external reinforcement.

self-regulation—Ways in which a person modifies his or her own behavior based on the assumption that behavior is under the person's direct control and is guided by internalized standards whose achievement will elicit positive self-evaluation.

sensitivity—A diagnostic test that is sensitive doesn't fail to detect a disease if it is present. It will yield a high proportion of true positives and few false negatives.

serotonergic—Denoting or relating to activity of neurons that produce or respond to serotonin.

serotonin—A synaptic transmitter produced and secreted by the raphe nuclei; general suppressor of neural gain. Also known as 5-hydroxytryptamine (5-HT).

set point theory—The idea that the body has an internal control mechanism—that is, a set point—located in the lateral hypothalamus of the brain that regulates metabolism to maintain a certain level of body fat.

settling point theory—The idea that weight loss and gain in most humans are determined mainly by the patterns of diet and physical activity that they "settle" into as habits based on the interaction of their genetic dispositions, learning, and environmental cues to behavior.

sinoatrial node—A small mass of specialized cardiac muscle cells located in the right atrium of the heart; emits the electrical signal that determines the intrinsic rate of the heartbeat.

social cognitive theory—A theory of human behavior, which evolved from social learning theory, that views behavior as a function of social cognitions; its key concept is that the characteristics of a person, environment, and behavior mutually influence one another.

social ecology—The study of human and natural ecosystems, the interrelations of culture and nature, and especially how people function in natural systems during change. Applied to physical activity, it suggests that interventions should blend personal and environmental resources to focus on developing social support networks and community partnerships to promote physical activity.

specificity—A diagnostic test that is specific doesn't falsely detect a disease that isn't present. A specific test has a high proportion of true negatives and few false positives.

state anxiety—The immediate response to a conscious or unconscious threat that has somatic and cognitive symptoms, including elevated heart rate, muscle tension, visceral motility, transient feelings of lack of control, low confidence, and uncertainty.

statin—One of a family of drugs (e.g., lovastatin, pravastatin, and simvastatin) that lower LDL levels by inhibiting the enzyme HMG-CoA reductase.

stenosis—Narrowing or stricture of a duct (e.g., a blood vessel) or a canal.

stimulus control—Strategies to change the frequency of a target behavior by modifying the antecedents of the behavior.

strength of association—One of Mill's canons, which states that there must be a large and clinically meaningful difference in disease risk between those exposed and those not exposed to a risk factor in order to establish causality.

stressor—A force that acts on a biological system to cause stress; an imbalance or disruption in homeostasis.

stroke—The loss or impairment of bodily function resulting from injury or death of brain cells after insufficient blood supply.

surveillance—The tracking of population trends in a behavior, such as physical activity, over time.

sympathetic nervous system (SNS)—One of three divisions of the autonomic nervous system. The sympathetic nervous system arises from the thoracic and lumbar portions of the spinal cord and is involved primarily in activities that require energy expenditure.

telomerase—An enzyme that blocks the shrinking of telomeres, thus resulting in uncontrolled division of a cell into a tumor.

telomeres—Structures located at the end of chromosomes that shrink each time a cell divides until they reach a critical length, usually at maturation, that inhibits the cell from dividing further, after which the cell dies.

temperament—Mainly stable, core component of personality that affects an individual's emotional responsiveness and predisposition to changing moods.

temporal sequence—One of Mill's canons, which states that exposure to a risk factor must precede development of the disease in order to establish causality.

thalamus—A brain region in the diencephalon composed of sensory relay nuclei with bidirectional connections to many areas in the cerebral cortex.

theory—Formulation of underlying principles of certain observed phenomena that have been verified to some degree and are used to explain and predict; a symbolic model used to guide the design, execution, and interpretation of research.

3-methoxy-4-hydroxyphenylglycol (MHPG)—The major metabolite of norepinephrine, secreted in the urine.

thrombin—A proteolytic enzyme in blood that converts fibrinogen to fibrin by hydrolysis.

thrombosis—Formation, development, or presence of a blood clot within a vessel.

tissue-type plasminogen activator (tPA)—Activates conversion of plasminogen from plasmin in the blood. Released from endothelial cells in blood vessels.

T lymphocyte—A long-lived (months to years) lymphocyte derived in the thymus gland. A key cell of cell-mediated, adaptive immunity possessing cytotoxic or memory abilities.

total peripheral resistance (TPR)—The total resistance to blood flow in the systemic circulation; the quotient produced when the mean arterial pressure is divided by the cardiac output.

trabecular bone—Adult bone consisting of mineralized, regularly ordered parallel collagen fibers that are more loosely organized than those of cortical bone; found in adult flat bones, vertebrae, and ends of long bones.

trait—The tendency to respond to an internal or external event in a particular manner. Traits are relatively consistent over time, but changes in traits are also possible.

trait anxiety—Chronic generalized anxiety that predisposes a person to appraise events as threatening.

transforming growth factor-beta (TGF-β)—A cytokine secreted by platelets, macrophages, and lymphocytes that increases IL-1 production by macrophages, increases IgA formation, attracts monocytes and macrophages, and aids wound healing by inhibiting inflammation after cell injury.

transient ischemic attack (TIA)—A temporary paralysis, numbness, speech difficulty, or other neurological symptoms that start suddenly but disappear within 24 h (typically within several hours).

transtheoretical model (TTM) of stages of change—A dynamic model of intentional behavior change that is based on the stages and processes individuals go through to bring about long-term behavior change.

triglyceride—The main constituent of fats and oils; an ester composed of three fatty acid molecules and one glycerol molecule.

trypsin—Proteolytic enzyme formed in the small intestine that activates conversion of plasmin to plasminogen in the blood.

tumor necrosis factor-alpha (TNF-α)—A cytokine produced primarily by monocytes and lymphocytes that activates the killing of tumor cells by macrophages, plays a role in antiviral activity, and is a major mediator of the inflammatory acute-phase response. High levels of TNF-α have harmful effects, including inflammation and muscle wasting.

tumor necrosis factor-beta (TNF-β)—A cytokine secreted by T lymphocytes that activates tumor lysis, enhances phagocytosis by macrophages, and mediates inflammation.

tumor suppressor gene—A gene that slows down or terminates cell division before progression to a tumor.

type 1 diabetes—A form of diabetes that develops when the body's immune system destroys pancreatic beta cells, the only cells in the body that make the hormone insulin, which regulates blood glucose. This form of diabetes usually strikes children and young adults, who need supplemental insulin daily to survive. Also called *insulin-dependent diabetes mellitus (IDDM)* or *juvenile-onset diabetes*.

type 2 diabetes—A form of diabetes that usually begins as insulin resistance, a disorder in which the cells do not use insulin properly. As the need for insulin rises, the pancreas gradually loses its ability to produce insulin. Type 2 diabetes is increasingly being diagnosed in children and adolescents. Also called *non-insulin-dependent diabetes mellitus (NIDDM)* or *adult-onset diabetes*.

unintentional injury—An injury that is judged to have occurred without anyone intending that harm be done.

upregulation—Increased sensitivity developed after repeated administration of a pharmacologically or physiologically active substance or in response to abnormally low levels of a substance, which is often characterized by an initial increase in the affinity of receptors for the substance or an increase in the number of receptors.

vagal tone—Basal level of parasympathetic activation of the vagus nerve.

value (of an outcome)—The reinforcement or incentive value of an expected outcome, which can be something an individual wants to obtain or to avoid.

ventral striatum—Area of the brain around the lateral ventricle that includes the caudate nucleus and putamen; the ventral striatum and the globus pallidus (or pallidum) form the corpus striatum.

ventral tegmental area (VTA)—A group of neural cell bodies in the underside of an area at the top of the brain stem, between the pons and the fourth ventricle of the brain, containing neurons that secrete dopamine and project to the frontal cortex and the nucleus accumbens; believed to regulate arousal, reinforcement, and pleasure.

very low density lipoprotein cholesterol (VLDL-C)—A subfraction of the total blood cholesterol, composed mainly of triglycerides and cholesterol, that is a precursor to the formation of LDL-C in the blood.

viscosity—A physical property of fluids that determines the internal resistance to shear forces; thickness.

vitamin D—A vitamin produced by the body in response to sunlight exposure that plays an important role in calcium and phosphorus metabolism.

waist circumference—A common measure used to assess abdominal fat content. The presence of excess body fat in the abdomen, disproportionate to total body fat, is considered an independent predictor of ailments associated with obesity.

waist-to-hip ratio—The ratio of waist circumference to hip circumference. For men, a ratio of 0.90 or less is considered safe. For women, a ratio of 0.80 or less is considered safe.

INDEX

Note: The italicized *f* and *t* following page numbers refer to figures and tables, respectively.

A

absolute intensity 68
absolute risk 23
accelerometers, portable 41*t*, 43-46, 45*f*
acetylcholine 151, 151*f*
ACL (anterior cruciate ligament) injuries 477-478
Active Community Environments (ACE) 515
Active Commuting in CARDIA 153
Active Commuting in Finland 153
activities of daily living (ADL) 448, 454, 455, 459
actual incidence rates 19-20
acute exercise
    cognitive function and 423-424
    fibrinolysis and 114
    immune system and 359-360, 360*t*, 362*t*, 367
adaptive immunity 348, 349
addictive exercise 496
adenocarcinoma 335
adherence, exercise 506, 506*f*, 507*f. See also*
    lifestyle changes for physical activity
adhesion molecules 356-358, 356*f*, 367
adipokines 353, 354
adiponectin 230, 251, 321, 353
adjusted rates 20, 20*t*
adolescents and youths. *See also* children
    anxiety disorders in 417
    body fatness and physical activity in 208-209
    depression in 402
    dyslipidemia in 169, 183
    health-related fitness of 51*f*
    hypertension in 153, 156
    inflammation and exercise in 363
    injuries in 472-474, 473*f*, 476
    obesity in 199, 201
    physical activity decreases in 504, 504*f*
    physical activity interventions for 225-226,
        531-533, 532*f*
    physical activity levels of 66-68, 66*f*, 67*f*, 444*t*
    suicide risk in 381, 382
adrenergic receptors 151
adrenocorticotropic hormone (ACTH) 358,
    405-406
aerobic exercise training
    cognitive function and 422
    depression and 399, 400-401
    dyslipidemia and 182-186, 184*f*, 185*f*
    injuries in 490-491
Aerobics Center Longitudinal Study (ACLS)
    on all-cause mortality 85-86, 88
    on cancer 312, 312*f*
    on cardiovascular disease 108, 109
    on depression 398, 398*f*
    on diabetes 257-258, 258*f*
    on dyslipidemia 180-181
    features of 8, 24
    on hypertension 153-154, 154*f*
    on inflammation and physical activity 113
    on injuries 472, 478, 479
    on obesity 212-213, 213*f*, 217-218, 219-220
    strength of association in 90
    on stroke 135

on weight cycling 219-220
afferent nerves 410
African Americans. *See also* race and ethnicity
    breast cancer in 322, 325, 446
    cancer prevalence in 311
    cardiovascular health of 445, 445*f*
    depression in 396
    diabetes in 245, 247, 247*f*
    with disabilities 451, 451*f*
    dyslipidemia in 169, 170*f*
    endometrial cancer in 336
    fitness and all-cause mortality in 87
    hypertension in 148, 148*f*, 149, 152-153,
        157, 159, 185
    inflammation and physical activity and 113
    mental health disorders in 381-382, 383*f*
    metabolic syndrome in 207, 447
    obesity in 202-203, 202*f*, 203*f*, 447
    osteoporosis in 275, 275*f*
    percent body fat in 206
    physical activity levels of 65*f*, 66*f*, 442, 442*f*,
        444*t*, 445
    prostate cancer in 446
    stroke in 126
    type 2 diabetes in 448
age
    of adults with disabilities 450*f*, 451
    bone loss and 279
    breast cancer risk and 325
    cardiorespiratory fitness and 51
    cholesterol levels and 173*t*
    as confounder and effect modifier 32-33,
        32*f*, 33*f*
    energy expenditure measures and 68
    fat-free body mass and 50-51
    hypertension and 145*f*, 148, 148*t*, 159
    injuries and 476, 477*t*
    leading causes of death and 79, 79*t*
    MEV values and 68, 69*t*
    physical activity levels and 62, 65*f*, 66, 66*f*,
        444*t*, 509
    stroke risk and 127
aging. *See* older adults
Agita São Paulo (Move São Paulo) 531
agoraphobia 416, 416*f*
AIDS. *See* HIV/AIDS
air pollution, exercise in 485
Alameda County Study 394-395
Alaska Natives 202-203. *See also* American
    Indians and Alaska Natives
alcohol use
    breast cancer and 326
    death rates and xviii
    hypertension and 150, 155, 158*t*
    lipoproteins and 173*t*, 174
    stroke and 128
all-cause mortality 77-92
    causation from observational studies 89-90
    leisure-time physical activity and 80-84
    life expectancy at birth 78-79, 78*t*
    major causes of 79, 79*t*

occupational physical activity and 80
physical activity and relative risk 79-80
physical activity recommendations 91-92
physical fitness and 85-88, 86*f*
race/ethnicity and physical activity 443, 445
sedentary behavior and 84-85
strength of evidence 90-91
alpha wave activity 419
Alzheimer's dementia 420-421, 425. *See also*
    dementia and cognitive function
American College of Sports Medicine (ACSM)
    active lifestyle recommendations by 537-538
    F.I.T.T. principles of 52-54, 53*t*
    on hot and cold weather exercise 484
    on physical activity for weight loss 209
    on physical inactivity 9
American Heart Association 9
American Indians and Alaska Natives. *See also*
    race and ethnicity
    breast cancer in 325
    diabetes in 247, 255, 259
    hypertension in 148, 148*f*
    inflammation and physical activity in 113
    metabolic syndrome in 447
    obesity in 202-203, 202*f*, 203*f*, 218
    physical activity levels of 65*f*, 66*f*, 444*t*
    stroke in 126, 126*f*
    suicide in 382
    type 2 diabetes in 38
American Indian Schoolchildren–PATHWAYS
    218
Americans with Disabilities Act (ADA) 448
AMP-activated protein kinase (AMPK) 253-
    254, 253*f*, 264
Amsterdam Growth and Health Longitudinal
    Study 286
amygdala 386*f*, 387, 411
angina pectoris 96
angiotensin-converting enzyme (ACE) inhibitors
    149-150
anorexia nervosa 494-495
anterior cingulate cortex 386*f*, 387
anterior cruciate ligament (ACL) injuries 477-478
antidepressants 387-388, 388*f*, 389-391
antigen-presenting cells (APC) 350, 350*f*
anxiety disorders 408-420
    biological plausibility of findings on 418-
        420, 419*f*
    body dysmorphia and 495
    body warming and 419
    brain EEG asymmetry and 419, 419*f*
    cognitive and social factors in 418
    costs of 381
    distraction hypothesis and 415
    dose–response in studies of 417, 418
    endorphins and 405, 419
    etiology of 410
    exercise treatment studies 415-417, 416*f*
    generalized anxiety disorder 409, 410, 412,
        416-417
    Hoffmann reflex and 419

insulin
adipose tissue and 251
colon cancer and 321
diabetes and 247
glucose transport and 249-250, 250f
hypertension and 160
increased sensitivity after exercise 263-264
insulin resistance 251, 251f, 264, 321
tumor growth factor 321
insulin-dependent diabetes mellitus (IDDM).
See diabetes mellitus; type 1 diabetes
insulin resistance 251, 251f, 264, 321
integrins 356f, 357
intima 97
intensity of exercise. *See also* acute exercise
absolute *vs.* relative 68
all-cause mortality and 81, 91
in coronary heart disease 56, 56f, 115-116
corrected for age, gender, and weight 68, 69t
injury rate and 482
preferred exertion and 540
rating of perceived exertion and 538-540,
539t, 549f
recommendations for 53-54, 53t
from total volume of exercise 116
interferons (IFNs)
exercise and 367, 367t, 369
in innate immune reaction 351, 353, 354
multiple sclerosis and 344
interleukins
characteristics of specific 354
exercise and 360, 367-368, 367t
in immune response 349, 350f, 351f, 352-
358, 353f, 355f, 356f
insulin sensitivity and 252, 253
International Classification of Diseases (ICD-
10) 384-385
International Classification of Functioning, Disability and Health (ICF) xix, 448
International Congress on Physical Activity and
Public Health 10
International Society for Physical Activity and
Health 10
INTERSTROKE study 127
interventions, physical activity 528-535. *See
also* lifestyle changes for physical activity
interview data 485
invasive breast carcinoma (IBC) 323
ion channels 151, 152f
Iowa Women's Health Study 81-82, 155
ischemia 97
ischemic heart disease 104f
ischemic stroke. *See also* stroke
characteristics of 124, 124f
physical activity and 131f, 133f
prevalence of 126
risk factors in 127, 128t
transient 124, 135
Israel studies 101

J

Japanese studies 133-134, 155
Jenner, Edward 345-346, 346f
jogging. *See* running
joints 457-458, 489-491
Justification for the Use of Statins in Prevention
(JUPITER) study 176
juvenile diabetes. *See* diabetes mellitus; type 1
diabetes

K

Kandel, Eric 386
ketosis 247
King County study 102, 102f, 488, 488f
Kiribati diabetes study 255
knee injuries 477-478
Kuopio and North Karelia, Finland study 211,
211f
kyphosis 277

L

lacunar infarcts 129
large granular lymphocytes (LGL) 350-351
LDL-C. *See* low-density lipoprotein cholesterol
lecithin 171
lecithin:cholesterol acyltransferase (LCAT)
171, 172, 178, 188, 189t
leptin 223-224, 251, 353
Let's Move in School (LMIS) 533
leukocytes 349, 356-357, 356f, 358f
leukocytosis 353, 355, 357-358, 358f, 367
Levin, Morton 28
life expectancy
at birth 78-79, 78t
by country 78t
health care spending and xvi
obesity and 199
physical activity increases and 88
in the United States xix-xx, 75, 78t
life span interactional model 507f
lifestyle changes for physical activity 503-541
activity goals 504, 505t
adolescent physical activity levels 504, 504f
behavioral and social approaches 531
behavior modification 523
cognitive–behavior modification 523-524
costs/benefits and funding 535
decision to be physically active 510-512,
511f, 512f
dopamine and 523
dropout rate from exercise programs 506,
506f
effectiveness of interventions 527-528, 527f,
528f
genetic factors and 506, 521-523, 522f, 540-
541, 540f
Healthy People 2020 objectives 505t
individual barriers to physical activity 508-
509, 508t
informational approaches 531
life span interactional model for adherence
507f
mediators and moderators of 535-537, 536f
multilevel models of physical activity change
520-521, 522f
National Physical Activity Plan 10-11, 529
perceived benefits and barriers in 513
perceived exertion and 538-540, 539t, 540f
physical activity interventions 528-535
physical environmental barriers in 512-519,
515f, 516f, 518f
policy and environmental approaches 534-535
preferred exertion and 540
prevalence of physical inactivity 504, 504f
psychological barriers 509-510
recommendations (exercise prescription)
537-538
relapse prevention 526-527

school interventions 531-534, 532f
social environment and 519-520, 519t
stage theory 524-526, 525f
web resources on 505
worksite interventions 534
Lifestyle Education for Activity Project (LEAP)
533-534
Lifestyle Interventions and Independence for
Elders (LIFE) Trial 363
likelihood ratios 29t, 30
Lipid Research Clinics Mortality Study 212
Lipid Research Clinics Prevalence Study 108,
108f
lipodystrophy syndrome 364
lipoprotein lipase (LPL) 171, 178t, 188, 189t
lipoproteins. *See also* cholesterol; dyslipidemia;
high-density lipoprotein cholesterol; low-
density lipoprotein cholesterol
characteristics of 170-171, 170f, 170t
in coronary heart disease 97-98
physical activity and 179-189
very low density lipoproteins 170t, 171,
173f, 186, 187
lithium 390, 391
lobular carcinoma in situ (LCIS) 323
London Bus Conductors Study 100
longitudinal research design 21. *See also* prospective cohort studies
Look AHEAD trial 261, 265
Los Angeles Atherosclerosis Study 181
Los Angeles Lift-Off 534
Los Angeles Public Safety Employees study 108
Losartan Intervention for Endpoint Reduction in
Hypertension (LIFE) Study 134, 259
loss to follow-up 89, 110-111
low-density lipoprotein cholesterol (LDL-C).
See also dyslipidemia
characteristics of 170f, 170t, 171
in coronary heart disease 97-99, 98f, 168-
169, 168t, 169f
drug treatment for 174t, 175-177
physical activity and 168, 179-188, 180f
plant sterols and 187
risk factors 177
treatment goals for 169, 176, 176t
lung cancer 335
lymphedema 337
lymphocytes. *See also* B lymphocytes; T lymphocytes
dendritic cells 349f, 352
exercise and 359-360, 360t
in immune response 349f, 350-351, 351f, 352f
lymphokines 279

M

macrophages
in atherogenesis 97-98
exercise and 359, 362t
in immune response 348, 349, 349f, 352, 353f
Male Health Professionals study 216
Malmo, Sweden study 258, 259
manic–depressive disorders 384, 391
MAPK proteins 254
Marathon study 180
mass-to-height ratio, breast cancer and 333
mast cells 352
Mauritius study 255
maximal aerobic power 51, 68, 135, 137
Mayer, Jean 198

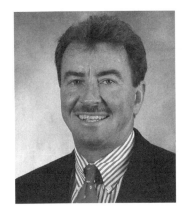

Rod K. Dishman, PhD, is a professor of exercise science, adjunct professor of psychology, and the director of the Exercise Psychology Laboratory at the University of Georgia at Athens. He is also adjunct professor in the Arnold School of Public Health at the University of South Carolina at Columbia. Dr. Dishman is a reviewer for more than 50 journals, including *Journal of the American Medical Association (JAMA)* and *American Journal of Public Health*. He has served on editorial boards of numerous journals in preventive medicine and public health, such as *Exercise and Sport Science Reviews, Medicine & Science in Sports & Exercise,* and *Health Psychology* and as an exercise consultant to public health agencies in the United States, Canada, and Europe. He has published approximately 150 peer-reviewed articles and written or edited several books related to physical activity and health.

Dr. Dishman is an American College of Sports Medicine fellow, where he has served as a member of the Research Advisory Committee and the Board of Trustees. He was a member of the jury for selection of the Olympic Prize in Sport Sciences awarded by the International Olympic Committee's Medical Commission and served on the scientific advisory committee for the 2008 Physical Activity Guidelines for Americans. He resides in Athens, Georgia.

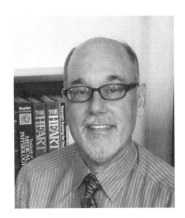

Gregory Heath, DHSc, MPH, has been contributing to the field of exercise science and health promotion for over 25 years. Dr. Heath is Guerry professor and head of the department of health and human performance at the University of Tennessee at Chattanooga. Previously, he worked at the Centers for Disease Control and Prevention as lead health scientist in the Physical Activity and Health Branch. He has extensive experience in conducting studies and data analyses in the areas of physical activity epidemiology and public health practice.

Dr. Heath is a fellow in the Council on Epidemiology and Prevention, the American Heart Association, and the American College of Sports Medicine. He earned his doctor of health science degree in applied physiology and nutrition and his master's of public health in epidemiology from Loma Linda University.

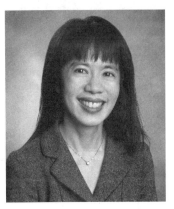

I-Min Lee, MBBS, MPH, ScD, is an associate professor of medicine at Harvard Medical School, an associate professor of epidemiology at Harvard School of Public Health, and associate epidemiologist at Brigham and Women's Hospital in Boston. Her main research interest is in the role of physical activity in promoting health and preventing chronic disease. This extends to characteristics associated with a physically active way of life, such as maintenance of ideal body weight. She also is concerned with issues relating to women's health. Lee has published more than 190 peer-reviewed articles and is a frequent invited presenter, teacher, and speaker at local, national, and international levels.

A reviewer for 30 journals, including *Lancet* and *New England Journal of Medicine*, Lee also serves on the editorial board for *Harvard Women's Health Watch, Medicine & Science in Sports & Exercise,* and the *Brazilian Journal of Physical Activity and Health.*

Lee is an elected member of the American Epidemiological Society and a member of the Society for Epidemiologic Research, the American Heart Association, and the International Society for Physical Activity and Health. She is a member and fellow of the American College of Sports Medicine (ACSM) and has served on the ACSM's Research Advisory Committee and Board of Trustees. Dr. Lee also served on the scientific advisory committee for the *2008 Physical Activity Guidelines for Americans.*

Lee is the recipient of numerous awards and recognitions, in particular the Young Epidemiologist Award from the Royal Society of Medicine in the United Kingdom (1999); the William G. Anderson Award from the American Alliance for Health, Physical Education, Recreation and Dance (2007); the Charles C. Shepard Award from the Centers for Disease Control and Prevention (2009); and the ACSM's Citation Award (2011).

Lee resides in Brookline, Massachusetts.

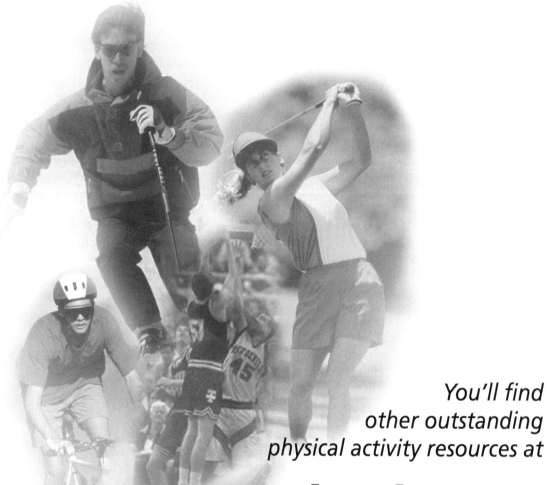

You'll find
other outstanding
physical activity resources at

www.HumanKinetics.com

In the U.S. call

1-800-747-4457

Australia..08 8372 0999
Canada 1-800-465-7301
Europe.......................................+44 (0) 113 255 5665
New Zealand..0800 222 062

HUMAN KINETICS
The Information Leader in Physical Activity & Health
P.O. Box 5076 • Champaign, IL 61825-5076 USA